DENTAL PRACTITIONERS' FORMULARY
1992–94

DENTAL PRACTITIONERS' FORMULARY

1992–94

together with
BRITISH NATIONAL FORMULARY
Number 24 (September 1992)

for use in the
NATIONAL HEALTH SERVICE

British Dental Association
British Medical Association
Royal Pharmaceutical Society of Great Britain

Copyright 1992 © by the British Medical Association and the Royal Pharmaceutical Society of Great Britain

Copies may be obtained through any bookseller or, in any case of difficulty, direct from the publishers:

British Medical Association
Tavistock Square
London WC1H 9JP, England

The Pharmaceutical Press
Royal Pharmaceutical Society of Great Britain
1 Lambeth High Street
London SE1 7JN, England

ISBN: 0 85369 280 7   ISSN: 0263-6417

All rights reserved. No part of this publication may be reproduced, stored in a retrieval system, or transmitted in any form or by any means—electronic, mechanical, photocopying, recording or otherwise—without the prior written permission of the joint copyright holders.

Typeset in Great Britain by Page Bros, Norwich, Norfolk NR6 6SA and printed and bound by The Bath Press, Bath, Avon BA2 3BL.

Joint Formulary Committee 1992–93

Chairman
C. F. George, BSc, MD, FRCP, FFPM

Deputy Chairman
C. R. Hitchings, BPharm, MSc, FRPharmS, MCPP

Committee Members

Alison Blenkinsopp, PhD, BPharm, MRPharmS
P. E. Green, BSc, MSc, LLM, MRPharmS
P. A. Leech, MRCS, LRCP, DMJ(clin)
F. P. Marsh, MA, MB, BChir, FRCP
G. M. Mitchell, KStJ, MB, ChB, FRPharmS
Jane Richards, MB BS, MRCS, LRCP, FRCGP, D(Obst)RCOG, DCH
P. C. Waller, MD, MRCP
N. L. Wood, BPharm, MRPharmS

Dental Formulary Subcommittee 1991–92

Chairman
H. D. Edmondson, MB, ChB, DDS, FDSRCS, MRCS, LRCP, DA

Committee Members

B. Caplan, LDS, RFPS(Glas)
C. F. George, BSc, MD, FRCP, FFPM
C. Howard, BDS, LDS, DDPH, RCS Eng
J. S. Robson, BDS
D. K. Stables, BDS, DDPH, RCS Eng

Joint Secretaries
Natalie-Jane Macdonald, MB, ChB, MRCP

Sara Morris, BSc

A. Wade, BPharm, MPhil, FRPharmS

Executive Editor
Anne B. Prasad, FRPharmS

Senior Assistant Editor
Sheenagh M. Townsend-Smith, BSc, DipLib

Editorial Assistant
Sunayana A. Shah, BPharm, MRPharmS

Executive Secretary
Susan M. Thomas, BSc(Econ), MA

Contents

	Page
Preface	ix
Arrangement of Information	x
Drug Information Services	x
GUIDANCE ON PRESCRIBING	1
Medical Emergencies in Dental Practice	2
Antibiotic Prophylaxis	4
Endocarditis prophylaxis	4
Cardiovascular Disease	6
Oral Side-effects of Drugs	7
Adverse Reactions to Drugs	8
CLASSIFIED NOTES ON DRUGS AND PREPARATIONS	
Antiseptics and Cleansers	10
Antibacterial Drugs	11
Penicillins	11
Cephalosporins	13
Tetracyclines	14
Erythromycin	14
Clindamycin	15
Metronidazole	15
Sodium Fusidate	16
Co-trimoxazole	16
Antifungal Drugs	17
Antiviral Drugs	18
Corticosteroids and other Drugs for Oral Ulceration and Inflammation	19
Analgesics	21
Hypnotics and Anxiolytics	24
Vitamins	25
Fluorides	26
Antihistamines	27
Nasal Decongestants	27
APPENDIXES	
Appendix 1: Interactions	28
Appendix 2: Liver Disease	30
Appendix 3: Renal Impairment	31
Appendix 4: Pregnancy	32
Appendix 5: Breast-feeding	33
LIST OF DENTAL PREPARATIONS	34
Additions	35
Deletions	35
Changes of Title	35
INDEX	36

Preface

This edition of the DPF is a revision of the 1990 edition. It is designed for use in dental treatment given under Part II of the National Health Service Acts. It contains only preparations which dental surgeons can prescribe for patients receiving NHS treatment, for which Form FP14 (GP14 in Scotland) should be used. The Act and Regulations do not set any limitations upon the number and variety of substances which the dental surgeon may administer to patients in the surgery or may order by private prescription. Providing the relevant legal requirements are observed the dental surgeon may use or order whatever is required for the clinical situation.

The Subcommittee has agreed that if the prescriber has decided that a drug in the DPF is suitable for the patient's condition then when possible a full range of appropriate dosage forms and strengths should be available for prescribing. In most cases the BP no longer specifies the strength of tablets and capsules, therefore, unless otherwise specified, any strength complying with the BP standard may be prescribed. Strengths known to be available have been included.

Basic net prices continue to be included in the DPF; these prices are not suitable for quoting to patients seeking private prescriptions or contemplating over-the-counter purchases, for further details see BNF p. 1.

There is no statutory requirement for the dental surgeon to communicate with a patient's general medical practitioner when prescribing for dental use. There are, however, occasions when this would be in the patient's interest and such communication is to be encouraged.

To save undue repetition, extensive cross-reference has been made to sections of the BNF of relevance to users of the DPF. The BNF will also be found useful for information about drugs being prescribed medically or being purchased by patients for their own use, and for assessing the possibility of interactions with materials used or prescribed in dental practice.

This edition of the DPF has been prepared as a supplement to the BNF, with which it is bound. In preparing this edition the text on analgesics has also been extensively revised and the guidelines on antibiotic prophylaxis have been adjusted to reflect the latest recommendations of the British Society for Antimicrobial Chemotherapy.

The Dental Formulary Subcommittee wishes to acknowledge the expert assistance of A. J. Duxbury, BDS, MSc, PhD, DDS, FDSRCPS. The advice and comments of H. Cannell, MD, MSc, FDSRCS, LRCP, MRCS, DPMSA are also gratefully acknowledged.

> Comments and constructive criticism will be welcome, and should be sent to:
> Executive Editor,
>   DPF/BNF,
>   c/o Royal Pharmaceutical Society of Great Britain,
>   1 Lambeth High Street,
>   London SE1 7JN.

Arrangement of Information

The arrangement of information in this edition generally follows that of the BNF (see p. ix) with the following exceptions:

1. The range of preparations available for prescribing has been divided into sections instead of the more extensive division into chapters used in the BNF.
2. In each section, notes for prescribers on particular groups of drugs are followed by entries on the drugs and any of their preparations that are included in the list approved by the appropriate Secretaries of State.
   The titles used in the list should be used for prescribing in the NHS; whenever possible they are identical with titles of official preparations in the BP or BPC. Details of equivalent proprietary preparations may be found on the appropriate pages of the BNF. All preparations in the DPF should be prescribed by approved name therefore proprietary names are not included.

> **Sugar**
> Although liquid preparations are particularly suitable for children, many contain sugar which encourages dental decay. Sugar-free preparations should be used whenever possible; products in both the DPF and BNF which do not contain glucose, fructose, or sucrose are marked 'sugar-free'.
> In order to avoid the need for diluents (which often contained sugar) when fractional doses are prescribed oral liquid medicines are no longer diluted to a 5-mL dose. Instead, an oral syringe is supplied, see BNF p. 2

Drug Information Services

Information on any aspect of drug therapy relating to dental treatment can be obtained, free of charge, by telephoning the following number:

Manchester   061-225 2063 Direct Line
or   061-276 6270

Note. For information on general aspects of drug therapy see Drug Information Services in BNF.

Prices
See BNF p. 1 for explanation.

Guidance on Prescribing

For general guidance see BNF, pp. 2–5

In reading the BNF, information for doctors should be taken to apply to dental surgeons. In addition, particular attention is drawn to the following.

DOSES. The doses stated in the DPF are intended for general guidance and represent, unless otherwise stated, the usual range of doses that are generally regarded as being suitable for adults; unless otherwise indicated the quantities are those generally suitable for administration on one occasion.

USE OF THE FORMULARY. The DPF is intended for the guidance of dental surgeons and other workers who have the necessary training and experience to interpret the information it provides. It is intended as a pocket reference book, and should be supplemented as necessary from specialised publications. Manufacturers' data sheets prepared in accordance with the Medicines (Data Sheet) Regulations 1972 are available for most proprietary medicines and these should also be consulted.

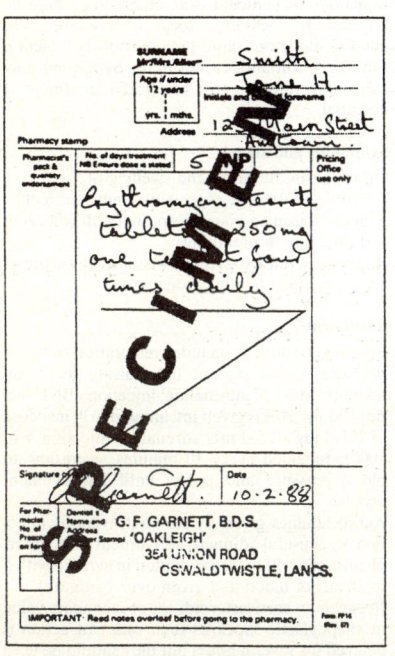

HEALTH AND SAFETY. When handling chemical or biological materials particular attention should be given to the possibility of allergy, fire, explosion, radiation, or poisoning. Some substances, including corticosteroids, antibiotics, phenothiazines, and many cytotoxics, are irritant or very potent and should be handled with caution. Contact with the skin and inhalation of dust should be avoided.

LABELLING OF DISPENSED MEDICINES. The Representative Board of the British Dental Association has made an agreement on 'NP' labelling with the Council of the Royal Pharmaceutical Society similar to that stated in the BNF (p. 3).

PRESCRIBING FOR THE ELDERLY. Old people, especially the very old, require special care and consideration. Dosage should generally be substantially lower than for younger patients and it is common to start with about 50% of the adult dose.

For further guidance see BNF, p. 14.

CONTROLLED DRUGS AND DRUG DEPENDENCE. The use of controlled drugs in dental practice is very limited but the dental surgeon should be aware of the regulations governing their use, in particular the requirements for Controlled Drug prescriptions. *Details are given in the BNF*, pp. 7–9, but in addition dental prescriptions must incorporate the words 'for dental treatment only'.

Dental surgeons should take care that they do not unwittingly become a source of supply for addicts. The methods of addicts include visiting more than one surgery, fabricating stories to substantiate demands, and forging prescriptions. A dental surgeon should therefore be very wary of prescribing for strangers and in particular of requests for prescriptions for opioid analgesics or benzodiazepines.

PATIENTS WITH SYSTEMIC DISEASE. Patients may attend the dental surgeon for treatment of an oral disorder but at the same time have another disease or be under treatment that might modify their management. If the dental surgeon notes or suspects that the patient has systemic disease or is taking other medication, the matter may need to be discussed with the patient's general medical practitioner or hospital consultant.

Medical Emergencies in Dental Practice

This section provides guidelines on the management of the more common medical emergencies which may arise in dental practice. Dental surgeons and their staffs should be familiar with standard resuscitation procedures, but in all circumstances it is advisable to summon medical assistance as soon as possible. For an **algorithm** of the procedure for **cardiopulmonary resuscitation**, see BNF p. 99.

Syncope

Insufficient blood supply to the brain results in loss of consciousness. The commonest cause is a vasovagal attack or simple faint (syncope) due to emotional stress.

Symptoms and signs
Patient feels faint.
Pallor and sweating.
Yawning and slow pulse.
Nausea and vomiting.
Dilated pupils.
Muscular twitching.

Treatment
Lay the patient flat and raise the legs to improve cerebral circulation.
Loosen any tight clothing around the neck.
Once consciousness is regained, give sugar in water or a cup of sweet tea.

Other possible causes
POSTURAL HYPOTENSION can be a consequence of rising abruptly or of standing upright for too long; antihypertensive drugs predispose to this. When rising, susceptible patients should take their time. Management is as for a vasovagal attack.

ADRENAL INSUFFICIENCY may be caused by administration of corticosteroids and can persist for years after stopping long-term therapy. A patient with adrenal insufficiency may become hypotensive under the stress of a dental visit (see also BNF section 6.3.4).
Treatment is as follows:
  lay patient flat and inject *at least* 200 mg of hydrocortisone (preferably as sodium succinate) intravenously. Give oxygen and call for medical assistance.

ARRHYTHMIAS may lead to a sudden fall in cardiac output with loss of consciousness. Medical assistance should be summoned.

HYPERVENTILATION. Under stressful circumstances, some patients hyperventilate. This gives rise to feelings of faintness but does not usually result in syncope. In most cases reassurance is all that is necessary; rebreathing from cupped hands or the reservoir bag of an anaesthetic machine may be helpful but calls for careful supervision.

The drugs referred to in this section are:
Adrenaline Injection, adrenaline 1 in 1000, (adrenaline 1 mg/mL as acid tartrate), 1-mL amps
Chlorpheniramine Injection, chlorpheniramine maleate 10 mg/mL, 1-mL amps
Diazepam Injection, diazepam 5 mg/mL, 2-mL amps
Glucagon Injection, glucagon (as hydrochloride), 1-unit and 10-unit vials (with solvent)
Glucose—50 g for one drink
Glucose Intravenous Infusion, glucose 50% (500 mg/mL), 50-mL amps
Glyceryl Trinitrate Tablets and Sprays
Hydrocortisone Injection, hydrocortisone 100 mg (preferably as sodium succinate vials with 2-mL solvent)
Oxygen
Salbutamol Injection, salbutamol (as sulphate) 500 micrograms/mL, 1-mL amps

---

Anaphylaxis

A severe allergic reaction may follow oral or parenteral administration of a drug. Allergic reactions in dentistry most commonly follow injections of penicillin but other drugs may be implicated, including local anaesthetics. In general, the more rapid the onset of the reaction the more profound it tends to be. Symptoms may develop within minutes and rapid treatment is essential.

Symptoms and signs
Paraesthesia, flushing, and swelling of face.
Generalised itching, especially hands and feet.
Bronchospasm and laryngospasm (with wheezing and difficulty in breathing).
Rapid weak pulse together with fall in blood pressure and pallor; finally cardiac arrest.

Treatment
First-line treatment includes restoration of blood pressure, laying patient flat, raising feet, and administration of **adrenaline**[1] injection (BNF section 3.4.3). This is given **intramuscularly** in a dose of 0.5–1 mg (0.5–1 mL adrenaline injection 1 in 1000), repeated every 10 minutes, according to blood pressure and pulse, until improvement occurs.
Antihistamines given by slow intravenous injection are a useful adjunctive treatment (e.g. chlorpheniramine 10 to 20 mg diluted in syringe with 5 to 10 mL of blood and given over 1 minute).
Intravenous **corticosteroids** are of secondary value in anaphylactic shock as their onset of action is delayed for several hours but they should be used to prevent further deterioration in severely affected patients. Usually hydrocortisone (preferably as sodium succinate) is given by intravenous injection in a dose of 100 to 300 mg.

---

1. In patients on non-cardioselective beta-blockers severe anaphylaxis may not respond to adrenaline injection, calling for addition of salbutamol by intravenous injection.

Cardiac emergencies

ANGINA. If there is a history of angina the patient will probably carry glyceryl trinitrate tablets or spray (or isosorbide dinitrate tablets) and should be allowed to use them.

MYOCARDIAL INFARCTION. The pain of myocardial infarction is similar to that of angina but generally more severe and more prolonged.

Symptoms and signs

Sudden onset of severe, crushing pain across front of chest; pain may radiate towards the shoulder and down arm, or into neck and jaw.
Skin becomes pale and clammy.
Nausea and vomiting are common.
Breathing is shallow.
Pulse is weak and blood pressure falls.

Treatment

Call for medical assistance or an ambulance immediately.
Allow patient to rest in the position that feels most comfortable; in presence of breathlessness this is likely to be sitting position, whereas syncopal patient will want to lie flat; often an intermediate position (dictated by patient) will be most appropriate.
Intramuscular injection of drugs does not provide useful relief of pain because absorption is too slow (particularly when cardiac output is reduced) but a mixture of nitrous oxide 50% and oxygen 50% (Entonox®) can be effective if given continuously; it is safe in this situation.
Reassure patient as much as possible to relieve further anxiety.
If patient collapses and loses consciousness attempt standard resuscitation measures. For an **algorithm** of the procedure for **cardiopulmonary resuscitation**, see BNF p. 99.

Hypoglycaemia

Diabetic patients occasionally administer their standard dose of insulin before dental treatment but omit the usual meal (although they should not). This can lead to the blood glucose falling to an abnormally low level (hypoglycaemia). Patients can often recognise the symptoms themselves and this state responds to sugar in water or a few lumps of sugar. Children may not have such prominent changes but may appear unduly lethargic.

Symptoms and signs

Shaking and trembling.
Sweating.
'Pins and needles' in lips and tongue.
Hunger.
Palpitations.
Headache (occasionally).
Double vision.
Difficulty in concentration.
Slurring of speech.
Confusion.
Change of behaviour.
Truculence.
Unconsciousness.

Treatment

In early stages, glucose or 3–4 lumps of sugar with a little water. If necessary this may be repeated in 10–15 minutes.
If patient unconscious, up to 50 mL of 50% glucose given intravenously, *or* glucagon 1 mg (1 unit) injected by any route (subcutaneous, intramuscular, or intravenous) (useful when intravenous injection of glucose difficult or impossible to administer).

Epileptic seizure

Patients with epilepsy must continue with their normal dosage of anticonvulsant drugs when attending for dental treatment. It is not uncommon for epileptic patients not to volunteer the information but there should be little difficulty in recognising a tonic-clonic (grand mal) seizure.

Symptoms and signs

There may be a brief warning (but variable).
Sudden loss of consciousness, patient becomes rigid, falls, may give a cry, and becomes cyanotic (tonic phase).
After 30 seconds, there are jerking movements of limbs; tongue may be bitten (clonic phase).
There may be frothing from mouth and urinary incontinence.
Seizure typically lasts a few minutes; patient may then become flaccid but remain unconscious.
After a variable time patient regains consciousness but may remain confused for a while.

Treatment

During a convulsion try to ensure that patient is not at risk from injury but make no attempt to put anything in mouth or between teeth (in mistaken belief that this will protect tongue).
Do not attempt to restrain convulsive movements.
After convulsive movements have subsided place patient in coma position and check airway.
After convulsion patient may be confused ('post-ictal confusion') and may need reassurance and sympathy. Patient should not be sent home until fully recovered but it is not necessary to seek medical attention or transfer to hospital unless convulsion was atypical, prolonged (or repeated), or if injury occurred.
Medication should only be given if convulsive seizures are prolonged (convulsive movements lasting 15 minutes or longer) or repeated rapidly. Intravenous administration of diazepam 10 mg is often effective but should be used with caution because of risk of respiratory depression (for further details see BNF section 4.8.2).
Partial seizures similarly need very little active management (in an automatism only minimum amount of restraint should be applied to prevent injury). Again patient should be observed until post-ictal confusion has completely resolved.

Antibiotic Prophylaxis

Joint prostheses

Advice of a Working Party of the British Society for Antimicrobial Chemotherapy (*Lancet*, 1992, *339*, 301) is that patients with **prosthetic joint implants** (including total hip replacements) do not require antibiotic prophylaxis for dental treatment. The Working Party considers that it is unacceptable to expose patients to the adverse effects of antibiotics when there is no evidence that such prophylaxis is of any benefit, but that those who develop any intercurrent infection require prompt treatment with antibiotics to which the infecting organisms are sensitive.

The Working Party has commented that joint infections have rarely been shown to follow dental procedures and are even more rarely caused by oral streptococci.

Immunosuppressed patients and those with indwelling intraperitoneal catheters

Advice of a Working Party of the British Society for Antimicrobial Chemotherapy is that patients who are immunosuppressed (including transplant patients) and patients with indwelling intraperitoneal catheters do not require antibiotic prophylaxis for dental treatment provided there is no other indication for prophylaxis.

The Working Party has commented that there is little evidence that dental treatment is followed by infection in immunosuppressed and immunodeficient patients nor is there evidence that dental treatment is followed by infection in patients with indwelling intraperitoneal catheters.

Infective Endocarditis

Patients with *cardiac defects* (congenital, rheumatic, etc) or who have had a *prosthetic replacement* of a damaged valve are at risk from infective endocarditis following dental procedures.

Those who have had one or more episodes of infective endocarditis in the past appear to be particularly susceptible.

There is no evidence that patients with prosthetic heart valves are any more susceptible to infective endocarditis after dental operations than those with damaged natural valves, but if it develops treatment may be more difficult.

Although almost any dental procedure is capable of causing bacteraemia, infective endocarditis is a rare and unpredictable complication even in susceptible patients. It is virtually impossible therefore to assess the relative effectiveness of different prophylactic regimens; nevertheless there is now some consensus among cardiologists and microbiologists. The recommendations which follow are those of a Working Party of the British Society for Antimicrobial Chemotherapy, *Lancet*, 1982, *2*, 1323–26; *idem*, 1986, *1*, 1267; *idem*, 1990, *335*, 88–9; *idem*, 1992, *339*, 1292.

Although there are theoretical advantages in giving antibiotics by injection (to ensure rapid absorption and high plasma concentrations), this presents difficulties in general dental practice. It is agreed therefore that wherever possible it is more practical to give antibiotics by mouth for prophylaxis in dental out-patients.

IDENTIFICATION OF PATIENTS AT RISK. All patients must be questioned about a history of rheumatic fever or heart defects and especially whether they have previously had infective endocarditis. The value of such a history is limited in that the patient may be unaware of a vulnerable heart lesion, but this is the best that can be done. Turbulence around the valves has been identified as a risk factor. Heart murmurs in children are often of no significance but whenever there is any doubt a cardiologist should be consulted.

The peak incidence of infective endocarditis is now in the sixth and seventh decades, so that the elderly are at greater risk than young persons.

PROCEDURES THAT NEED COVER. Dental procedures that require antibiotic prophylaxis are:

extractions
scaling
surgery involving gingival tissues

REDUCTION OF ORAL SEPSIS. A history of a dental procedure preceding an attack of infective endocarditis is obtained in only a minority of patients but oral bacteria enter the blood stream on many other occasions. The frequency and severity of bacteraemia is also related to the severity of the gingival sepsis. Maintenance of the highest possible standards of oral hygiene in patients at risk reduces:

need for dental extractions or other surgery;
chances of severe bacteraemia if dental surgery has to be carried out;
chance or frequency of 'spontaneous' bacteraemia.

Application of an antiseptic such as chlorhexidine gel (1%) to the dry gingival margin or the use of a chlorhexidine mouthwash (0.2%) 5 minutes before the dental procedure should reduce the severity of bacteraemia and may be used to supplement antibiotic prophylaxis in those at risk.

Intraligamentary injection of local anaesthetic solutions may carry a risk of severe bacteraemia and is best **avoided** in patients susceptible to endocarditis.

POSTOPERATIVE CARE. It is imperative to warn every patient at risk to report to the doctor or dentist *if any minor illness develops after dental treatment*, whether or not antibiotics have been given, as infective endocarditis has an insidious onset and many failures of treatment are the result of late diagnosis. If endocarditis develops it is likely to be within a month of dental treatment.

Infective endocarditis 5

RECOMMENDATIONS FOR ENDOCARDITIS PROPHYLAXIS

Under local or no anaesthesia (taken in presence of dentist or dental nurse):
Patients not allergic to pencillin and who have not received a penicillin more than once in the previous month including those with a prosthetic valve (but not those who have had endocarditis, see special risk patients below)
ADULT single dose of amoxycillin[1] 3 g by mouth 1 hour before procedure
CHILD under 5 years, quarter adult dose; 5–10 years, half adult dose

Patients allergic to penicillin or who have received a penicillin more than once in the previous month including those with a prosthetic valve (but not those who have had endocarditis, see special risk patients below)
ADULT single dose of clindamycin 600 mg by mouth[2] 1 hour before procedure
CHILD under 5 years quarter adult dose; 5–10 years, half adult dose

Under general anaesthesia:
Patients not allergic to penicillin and who have not received a penicillin more than once in the previous month (but not those with a prosthetic valve or who have had endocarditis, see special risk patients below)
ADULT amoxycillin 1 g by intramuscular or intravenous injection[3] at induction then 500 mg by mouth 6 hours later
CHILD under 5 years quarter adult dose; 5–10 years, half adult dose[4]

or

ADULT amoxycillin 3 g by mouth 4 hours before induction then a further 3 g as soon as possible after procedure
CHILD under 5 years, quarter adult dose; 5–10 years, half adult dose

or

ADULT amoxycillin 3 g by mouth and probenecid 1 g by mouth 4 hours before procedure

Special risk patients who should be referred to hospital:
Patients with prosthetic valves who are to have a general anaesthetic
Patients who are allergic to penicillin who are to have a general anaesthetic
Patients who have had a penicillin more than once in the previous month who are to have a general anaesthetic
All patients who have had a previous attack of endocarditis
For recommendations for these patients see BNF section 5.1, table 2

---

1. Amoxycillin is liable to cause irritating rashes, especially in people with infectious mononucleosis (glandular fever) in whom it should be avoided.
2. Oral clindamycin now replaces oral erythromycin (which caused nausea and vomiting). If clindamycin is given, periodontal or other multistage procedures should not be repeated at intervals of less than 2 weeks.
3. If the intramuscular or intravenous route is considered necessary it may be preferable for the procedure to be carried out in hospital. To reduce the pain, intramuscular injection is given in 2.5 mL of lignocaine hydrochloride 1% injection.
4. Whenever possible painful intramuscular injections should be avoided in children.

Cardiovascular Disease

Arrhythmias

Patients, especially those who have suffered a myocardial infarction, may have unstable cardiac rhythm or a degree of heart failure. Current medication should be carefully checked. Premedication (e.g. with temazepam) may be useful in some instances for very anxious patients.

See below for reference to vasoconstrictors and unstable cardiac rhythm.

Hypertension

Patients with hypertension may be under treatment with antihypertensive drugs such as those described in section 2.5 of the BNF. Their blood pressure may fall to dangerously low levels when they are given general anaesthesia and this should only be administered in hospital when appropriate precautions can be taken.

See also under Vasoconstrictors (below).

Thrombo-embolic disease

Patients receiving **heparin** or oral anticoagulants such as **warfarin**, **nicoumalone**, or **phenindione** may be liable to excessive bleeding after extraction of teeth. Often dental surgery can be delayed until the anticoagulant therapy is discontinued.

Occasionally, an extraction during anticoagulant treatment may be unavoidable. The patient's physician should be consulted and the anticoagulant level adjusted (with laboratory control) so that the prothrombin time is not more than twice the control figure. If possible, a single simple extraction should be done first. If this goes well further teeth may be extracted, two or three at a time. Some dental surgeons suture the gum lightly over the socket to hold in place a haemostatic such as oxidised cellulose.

Aspirin is contra-indicated in patients on anticoagulant therapy, and in those with any disorder of haemostasis, see **interactions**, p. 28.

Vasoconstrictors in local anaesthetic solutions

Lignocaine 2 per cent with **adrenaline** 1 in 80 000 is probably the most widely used local anaesthetic agent. For the vast majority of patients, experience over many years indicates that it is a safe and effective preparation.

There is no indication for the use of **noradrenaline** as a vasoconstrictor for local anaesthetics since it presents no advantages. Administration of local anaesthetics containing noradrenaline 1 in 25 000 has been followed by a small number of severe hypertensive episodes. These few episodes emphasise the possible danger of using local anaesthetics containing noradrenaline, especially in high concentrations.

In patients with severe hypertension or unstable cardiac rhythm, the use of adrenaline in a local anaesthetic may be hazardous if inadvertently given intravenously. For these patients **prilocaine** with or without felypressin can be used but there is no clinical evidence that it is any safer.

There is no clinical evidence of dangerous interactions between **adrenaline**-containing local anaesthetics and monoamine-oxidase inhibitors (MAOIs) or tricyclic antidepressants.

Oral Side-effects of Drugs

Drug-induced disorders of the mouth may be due to a local action on the mouth or to a systemic effect manifested by oral changes.

Oral mucosa

Medicaments applied directly to the oral mucosa can lead to inflammation and ulceration.

Elderly patients may have difficulty swallowing tablets; if left in the mouth, ulceration may develop. They should always take their tablets or capsules with fluid, and in some cases it may be wise to prescribe capsules if available.

Aspirin tablets allowed to dissolve in the sulcus for the treatment of toothache can lead to a white patch followed by painful ulceration. **Choline salicylate** gels are also irritant and are particularly troublesome if placed under dentures.

Potassium chloride modified-release tablets are irritant to the mucosa.

Crystal violet, another irritant, is no longer used on mucous membranes (for explanation see BNF, p. 434).

Flavouring agents, particularly **essential oils**, may cause contact hypersensitivity of the skin, but mucosal swelling is not usually prominent.

The oral mucosa is particularly vulnerable to ulceration in patients treated with cytotoxic drugs, especially **methotrexate**.

An occasional complication of long-term **phenytoin** treatment is macrocytic anaemia, leading to oral manifestations such as sore tongue or severe aphthous stomatitis.

Systemic administration of some NSAIDs, e.g. indomethacin, may cause ulceration of the mucosa; this is not a topical effect but the precise mechanism is not clear. Other drugs capable of causing severe oral ulceration include **methyldopa**, **allopurinol**, **gold** (auranofin and aurothiomalate), and **penicillamine**. **Captopril** can cause stomatosis.

Erythema multiforme may follow the use of certain drugs, especially **sulphonamides, co-trimoxazole, antiepileptics, penicillin**, and **chlorpropamide**. The oral mucosa may be extensively ulcerated, with characteristic target lesions on the skin. Oral lesions of toxic epidermal necrolysis have been reported for a similar range of drugs.

Lichenoid eruptions can be clinically indistinguishable from lichen planus. Drugs associated with the appearance of white striae and plaques, atrophic changes and ulceration include **NSAIDs, methyldopa, chloroquine, oral antidiabetics, diuretics, phenothiazines**, and **gold** (auranofin and aurothiomalate).

Thrush and other types of candidiasis complicate treatment with **antibiotics** and **immunosuppressants**. Oropharyngeal thrush is an occasional side-effect of **corticosteroid** inhalers.

Teeth

Brown staining of the teeth frequently follows the use of **chlorhexidine** mouthwash or gel; this can readily be removed by polishing at the end of the course of treatment. **Ferric** salts in liquid form can stain the enamel black.

Intrinsic staining of the teeth is most commonly due to **tetracyclines**. They will affect the teeth if given at any time from about the fourth month *in utero* until the age of twelve years. All tetracyclines cause this; the colour varies from yellow to grey.

Excessive ingestion of **fluoride** leads to dental fluorosis with mottling of the enamel and areas of hypoplasia or pitting; fluoride tablets or drops may cause mild mottling (white patches) if the dose is too large for the child's age or for the fluoride content of the local drinking water.

Periodontium

Gingivitis and ulceration are common in patients receiving **cytotoxics** or **immunosuppressants**.

Hyperplasia of the gingivae is a side-effect of **phenytoin** and sometimes of **cyclosporin** or **nifedipine**. The degree of hyperplasia varies but can reach the extent that the crowns of the teeth are virtually covered.

Thrombocytopenia may be drug related, and cause bleeding of the gingival margins, which may follow mild trauma, such as toothbrushing, or eventually be spontaneous.

Salivary glands

The main effect of drugs on the salivary glands is a reduction in flow (xerostomia). Patients with a persistently dry mouth may develop a burning or scalded sensation, and have poor oral hygiene, increased dental caries, periodontal disease, intolerance of dentures, and oral infections (particularly candidiasis).

Many drugs have been implicated in xerostomia, particularly **antimuscarinics** (anticholinergics) and tricyclic **antidepressants**. Excessive use of **diuretics** can also result in xerostomia.

Increased production of saliva is not a problem unless the patient has difficulty in swallowing.

Pain in the salivary glands has been reported following the use of some **antihypertensives** (e.g. bethanidine, clonidine, methyldopa) and of the **vinca alkaloids**.

Swelling of the salivary glands may be idiopathic but it has been described rarely in association with **iodides, antithyroid drugs, phenothiazines**, and **sulphonamides**.

Taste

Taste acuity may be decreased or there can be an alteration in taste sensation. Drugs implicated include penicillamine, griseofulvin, captopril and enalapril, lincomycin, carbimazole, clofibrate, phenindione, lithium salts, gold (auranofin and aurothiomalate), and metronidazole.

Adverse Reactions to Drugs

Any drug may produce unwanted or unexpected adverse reactions. Detection and recording of these is of vital importance.

Dental surgeons are urged to help by reporting adverse reactions to:

CSM
Freepost
London SW8 5BR
(071-627 3291)

Yellow prepaid lettercards for reporting are available from the above address or by dialling 100 and asking for 'CSM Freefone'; also, forms are bound in this book (inside back cover).

A 24-hour Freefone service is now available to all parts of the United Kingdom, for dentists seeking advice and information on adverse reactions; it may be obtained by dialling 100 and asking for 'CSM Freefone'. Outside office hours a telephone-answering machine will take messages.

The following regional centres also collect data:

CSM Mersey
Freepost
Liverpool L3 3AB
(051-236 4620 Extn 2126)

CSM West Midlands
Freepost
Birmingham B15 1BR
(021-627 2179 Direct Line)

CSM Northern
Freepost 1085
Newcastle upon Tyne NE1 1BR
(091-232 1525 Direct Line)

CSM Wales
Freepost
Cardiff CF4 1ZZ
(0222 759541 Direct Line)

Suspected adverse reactions to *any* therapeutic agent should be reported, including drugs, blood products, vaccines, X-ray contrast media, dental or surgical materials, intra-uterine devices, and contact lens fluids.

ADROIT

Adverse Drug Reactions On-line Information Tracking (ADROIT) has now been introduced to facilitate the monitoring of adverse drug reactions.

NEWER DRUGS. These are indicated by the sign ▼. Dentists are asked to report *all* suspected reactions (i.e. any adverse or any unexpected event, however minor, which could conceivably be attributed to the drug). Reports should be made despite uncertainty about a causal relationship, irrespective of whether the reaction is well recognized, and even if other drugs have been given concurrently.

ESTABLISHED DRUGS. Dentists are asked to report *all* serious suspected reactions, including those that are fatal, life-threatening, disabling, incapacitating, or which result in or prolong hospitalisation; they should be reported even if the effect is well recognised.

Examples include anaphylaxis, blood disorders, endocrine disturbances, effects on fertility, haemorrhage from any site, renal impairment, jaundice, ophthalmic disorders, severe CNS effects, severe skin reactions, reactions in pregnant women, and any drug interactions. Reports of serious adverse reactions are required to enable risk/benefit ratios to be compared with other drugs of a similar class. For established drugs dentists are asked not to report well-known, relatively minor side-effects, such as dry mouth with tricyclic antidepressants, constipation with opioids, or nausea with digoxin.

Special problems

See BNF p. 10.

Prevention of adverse reactions

Adverse reactions may be prevented as follows:

1. Never use any drug unless there is a good indication. If the patient is pregnant do not use a drug unless the need for it is imperative.
2. It is very important to recognise allergy and idiosyncrasy as causes of adverse drug reactions. Ask if the patient had previous reactions.
3. Ask if the patient is already taking other drugs *including self-medication*; remember that interactions may occur.
4. Age and hepatic or renal disease may alter the metabolism or excretion of drugs, so that much smaller doses may need to be prescribed. Pharmacogenetic factors may also be responsible for variations in the rate of metabolism, notably of isoniazid and the tricyclic antidepressants.
5. Prescribe as few drugs as possible and give very clear instructions to the elderly or any patient likely to misunderstand complicated instructions.
6. When possible use a familiar drug. With a new drug be particularly alert for adverse reactions or unexpected events.
7. If serious adverse reactions are liable to occur warn the patient.

Defective Medicines

During the manufacture or distribution of a medicine an error or accident may occur whereby the finished product does not conform to its specification. While such a defect may impair the therapeutic effect of the product and could adversely affect the health of a patient, it should **not** be confused with an Adverse Drug Reaction where the product conforms to its specification. The Defect Medicines Report Centre operates a 24-hour service to assist with the investigation of problems arising from licensed medicinal products thought to be defective, and to co-ordinate any necessary protective action. Reports on suspect defective medicinal products should include the brand or the non-proprietary name, the name of the manufacturer or supplier, the strength and dosage form of the product, the product licence number, the batch number or number of the product, the nature of the defect, and an account of any action already taken in consequence. The Centre can be contacted at:

The Defect Medicines Report Centre
Medicines Control Agency
Room 1801, Market Towers
1 Nine Elms Lane
London SW8 5NQ
071-273 0574 (weekdays 8.30 am–5.30 pm)
or 071-210 5368 or 5371 (any other time)

Classified Notes on Drugs and Preparations

Antiseptics and Cleansers

Superficial infections of the mouth are often helped by warm mouthwashes; they have a mechanical cleansing effect and cause some local hyperaemia. However, they must be used both frequently and vigorously to have any effect, and some can lead to irritation of the oral mucosa. A warm saline mouthwash is ideal and can be prepared either by dissolving half a teaspoonful of salt in a tumblerful of warm water or by diluting **sodium chloride compound mouthwash** with an equal volume of warm water.

Mouthwashes containing an oxidising agent, such as **hydrogen peroxide**, may be useful in the treatment of acute ulcerative gingivitis (Vincent's infection) as the organisms responsible are anaerobes. Hydrogen peroxide also has a mechanical cleansing action since it froths on contact with oral debris. **Sodium perborate** has a similar effect, but should not be used for periods longer than 7 days because of possible absorption of borate.

Chlorhexidine is an effective antiseptic which has the advantage of inhibiting plaque formation on the teeth. It does not, however, completely control plaque deposition and is not a substitute for effective toothbrushing. Moreover it does not penetrate significantly into stagnation areas and is therefore of little value in the control of dental caries or of periodontal disease once pocketing has developed.

Chlorhexidine can be used as a mouthwash for secondary infection in mucosal ulceration. The mouthwash or the gel may be used for controlling gingivitis, as an adjunct to other oral hygiene measures. The mouthwash or the gel may also be used as an alternative to toothbrushing where there is a painful periodontal condition (e.g. primary herpetic stomatitis) or if the patient has a haemorrhagic disorder, or is handicapped.

Povidone-iodine is another effective antiseptic. The mouthwash is a useful preparation in dealing with mucosal infections but does not inhibit plaque accumulation. It should not be used for periods longer than 14 days as a significant amount of iodine is absorbed.

Neither chlorhexidine nor povidone-iodine mouthwashes have any beneficial effect in the control of acute ulcerative gingivitis.

Thymol is a weak antiseptic of negligible value for treating oral infections. Mouthwash solution-tablets are used to rinse out the mouth to remove unpleasant tastes. Compound thymol glycerin may be used as a mechanical rinse instead of a saline mouthwash.

For further information see BNF section 12.3.

CHLORHEXIDINE GLUCONATE

Indications: oral hygiene (including endocarditis prophylaxis, p. 5); plaque inhibition
Side-effects: idiosyncratic mucosal irritation; reversible brown staining of teeth

Chlorhexidine Dental Gel DPF, chlorhexidine gluconate 1%. Net price 50 g = 83p
Brush on teeth once or twice daily

Chlorhexidine Mouthwash DPF, chlorhexidine gluconate 0.2% (aniseed- or mint-flavoured). Net price 300 mL = £1.25
Rinse mouth with 10 mL for about 1 minute twice daily
Note. A spray presentation (chlorhexidine gluconate 0.2%) can also be prescribed, net price 60 mL = £2.80 (mint-flavoured). The spray presentation should be applied as required to the tooth and gingival surfaces using up to max. of 12 actuations (approx. 0.14 mL per actuation) twice daily.

OXIDISING AGENTS

Indications: oral hygiene

Hydrogen Peroxide Mouthwash DPF, consists of Hydrogen Peroxide Solution (6% ≡ approx. 20-volume) BP
Rinse mouth for 2–3 minutes with 15 mL in half a tumblerful of warm water 2–3 times daily

Sodium Perborate Mouthwash, DPF, sodium perborate 68.6% (buffered). Net price 20 × 1.7-g sachet-pack = £1.40
Use 1 sachet in 30 mL of water 3 times daily after meals
Cautions: Do not use for longer than 7 days because of possible absorption of borate; not recommended in renal impairment or for children under 5 years

POVIDONE-IODINE

Indications: oral hygiene
Cautions: pregnancy; breast-feeding
Side-effects: idiosyncratic mucosal irritation and hypersensitivity reactions

Povidone-iodine Mouthwash DPF, povidone-iodine 1%. Net price 250 mL = 82p
Adults and children over 6 years, up to 10 mL undiluted or diluted with an equal quantity of warm water up to 4 times daily for up to 14 days

SODIUM CHLORIDE

Indications: oral hygiene

Sodium Chloride Mouthwash, Compound, BP, sodium chloride 1.5% (see BNF p. 398).
Use diluted with equal volume of warm water

THYMOL

Indications: oral hygiene

Compound Thymol Glycerin BP, glycerol 10%, thymol 0.05%, with colouring and flavouring
Use undiluted or diluted with 3 volumes of warm water

Mouthwash Solution-tablets DPF, consist of tablets which may contain antimicrobial, colouring, and flavouring agents in a suitable soluble effervescent basis to make a mouthwash suitable for dental purposes. Net price 20 = 32p
Dissolve 1 tablet in a tumblerful of warm water
Note. Mouthwash solution-tablets may contain ingredients such as thymol.

Antibacterial Drugs

Additional information on antibacterial drugs may be found in BNF section 5.1

Bacterial sialadenitis requires treatment with antibiotics, as do severe infections such as osteomyelitis, cellulitis, and actinomycosis. Fortunately, these infections are rare.

Antibiotics may be helpful in the temporary treatment of an acute alveolar abscess but only if drainage or extraction has to be delayed. They should never be used as an alternative to either extraction of the tooth or drainage through the root canals. In some cases of spreading infection, however, it may be useful to give antibiotics following surgical intervention.

Another use of antibiotics is in the protection of patients with cardiac valvular disease against infective endocarditis following dental operations (see p. 4).

CHOICE OF A SUITABLE DRUG. Before selecting an antibiotic the clinician must first consider two factors—the patient and the known or likely causative organism. Factors related to the patient which must be considered include history of allergy, renal and hepatic function, resistance to infection (i.e. whether immunocompromised), ability to tolerate drugs by mouth, severity of illness, ethnic origin, age, and, if female, whether pregnant, breast-feeding, or taking an oral contraceptive.

The known or likely organism and its antibiotic sensitivity, in association with the above factors, will suggest one or more antibiotics, the final choice depending on the microbiological, pharmacological, and toxicological properties. Antibiotics should never be given haphazardly for some painful swelling of a doubtful nature. Were this to be a malignant neoplasm the delay in diagnosis could reduce the patient's chance of survival.

BEFORE STARTING THERAPY. The following precepts should be considered before starting antibiotic therapy:

Viral infections should not be treated with antibiotics. Examples are primary herpetic stomatitis, herpangina, herpes labialis, herpes zoster (shingles), and mumps.

The **'blind'** prescribing of an antibiotic for a patient with pyrexia, cervical lymphadenopathy, or facial swelling can lead to further difficulty in establishing the diagnosis. There must be no doubt that the lesion under consideration is due to a bacterial infection.

An up-to-date knowledge of **prevalent organisms** and their current sensitivity is of great help in choosing an antibiotic before bacteriological confirmation is available.

Bacteriological sampling should always be carried out in severe infections, using a specimen of exudate or pus, to determine the causative organism and its antibiotic sensitivities.

The **dose** of an antibiotic will vary according to a number of factors including age, weight, renal function, and severity of infection. Small doses may be ineffective and are likely to encourage resistant strains of bacteria to multiply.

The **route** of administration of an antibiotic will often depend on the severity of the infection. In dentistry the oral route and intramuscular injection usually suffice although rarely intravenous administration may be necessary.

Duration of therapy depends on the nature of the infection and the response to treatment. Courses should not be unduly prolonged as they are wasteful and may lead to side-effects. Many acute infections of dental origin respond to a course of antibiotics lasting from 4 to 7 days. Longer treatment is needed for chronic infections, especially actinomycosis where it may have to be continued for several weeks. Otherwise an antibiotic should not be continued if the infection does not respond within a few days. In such cases bacteriological examination should be carried out or the antibiotic changed.

Combined antibiotic therapy has little justification in dentistry: if bactericidal antibiotics (e.g. penicillin) are used along with bacteriostatic antibiotics (especially tetracycline) the action of one can antagonise that of the other. Regimens of combined antibiotic therapy proposed for the prevention of infective endocarditis are the exception.

Penicillins

The penicillins are bactericidal and act by interfering with bacterial cell wall synthesis. They diffuse well into body tissues and fluids, but penetration into the cerebrospinal fluid is poor except when the meninges are inflamed. They are excreted in the urine in therapeutic concentrations. Probenecid blocks the renal tubular excretion of the penicillins, producing higher and more prolonged plasma concentrations.

The most important side-effect of penicillins is hypersensitivity, which causes rashes and, occasionally, anaphylaxis, which can be fatal. Patients who are allergic to one penicillin will be allergic to all as the hypersensitivity is related to the basic penicillin structure. A rare but serious toxic effect of penicillins is encephalopathy due to cerebral irritation. This may result from excessively high doses but can also develop with normal doses given to patients with renal impairment.

Before prescribing a penicillin it is essential to ask whether the patient has ever had any ill-effect, however slight, from penicillin in the past. If there has been any such reaction, penicillin should not be given in any form; if a reaction develops during treatment, the drug should be stopped immediately. Patients with a history of atopic allergy (asthma, eczema, hay fever, etc.) are more likely to be allergic to penicillin. The management of anaphylactic reactions is outlined on p. 2. Penicillin or other antibiotics should not be given for trivial infections or where the diagnosis is doubtful.

Diarrhoea is common during oral penicillin therapy, particularly with ampicillin and its derivatives which can also cause pseudomembranous colitis.

BENZYLPENICILLIN AND PHENOXYMETHYLPENICILLIN

Benzylpenicillin (penicillin G), the first of the penicillins, remains a useful antibiotic for most dental infections. In some cases of osteomyelitis and cellulitis as well as actinomycosis, benzylpenicillin may be started intramuscularly and followed by phenoxymethylpenicillin orally. Benzylpenicillin is destroyed by gastric acid and is therefore only suitable for parenteral administration.

Procaine penicillin is a sparingly soluble salt of benzylpenicillin. It is used in combination with benzylpenicillin and benethamine penicillin.

Benethamine penicillin is a benzylpenicillin salt with a very low solubility giving a prolonged action after intramuscular injection, though producing low plasma concentrations. It is only used in combination with benzylpenicillin and procaine penicillin.

Phenoxymethylpenicillin (penicillin V) has a similar antibacterial spectrum to benzylpenicillin, but is less active. It is gastric acid-stable, so is suitable for oral administration.

BENZYLPENICILLIN SALTS

Indications: osteomyelitis, cellulitis, actinomycosis, prophylaxis in fractures of the jaw
Cautions: history of allergy; renal impairment
Contra-indications: penicillin hypersensitivity
Side-effects: sensitivity reactions including urticaria, fever, joint pains; angioedema; anaphylactic shock in hypersensitive patients

PoM **Benzylpenicillin Injection BP,** powder for reconstitution, benzylpenicillin sodium (unbuffered). Net price 600-mg vial = 35p
Dose: by intramuscular injection, 1.2 g daily in 4 divided doses, increased if necessary to 2.4 g daily; CHILD see BNF section 5.1.1.1

PoM **Penicillin Triple Injection BPC,** powder for reconstitution, benethamine penicillin 475 mg, procaine penicillin 250 mg, benzylpenicillin sodium 300 mg. Net price per vial = 40p
Dose: by deep intramuscular injection, 1 vial every 2–3 days

PHENOXYMETHYLPENICILLIN
(Penicillin V)

Indications: osteomyelitis, cellulitis, actinomycosis, prophylaxis in fractures of the jaw
Cautions; Contra-indications; Side-effects: see under Benzylpenicillin; diarrhoea; **interactions:** see p. 29
Dose: 250–500 mg every 6 hours, at least 30 minutes before food; CHILD, every 6 hours, 1–5 years 125 mg, 6–12 years 250 mg

PoM **Phenoxymethylpenicillin Tablets BP,** phenoxymethylpenicillin (as potassium salt) 250 mg, net price 20 = 33p. Label: 9, 23

PoM **Phenoxymethylpenicillin Oral Solution BP,** (Phenoxymethylpenicillin Elixir), phenoxymethylpenicillin (as potassium salt) for reconstitution with water, 125 mg/5 mL, net price 100 mL = 47p; 250 mg/5 mL, 100 mL = 71p. Label: 9, 23

BROAD-SPECTRUM PENICILLINS

Ampicillin is active against certain Gram-positive and Gram-negative organisms but is inactivated by penicillinases including those produced by *Staphylococcus aureus* and by common Gram-negative bacilli such as *Escherichia coli*. Almost all staphylococci, 50% of *E. coli* strains, and 15% of *Haemophilus influenzae* strains are now resistant.

Amoxycillin is a derivative of ampicillin which differs by only one hydroxyl group and has a similar antibacterial spectrum. It is, however, better absorbed when given by mouth, producing higher plasma and tissue concentrations; unlike ampicillin, absorption is not affected by the presence of food in the stomach.

Both may be given by mouth (ampicillin before food) and by injection, and are well excreted in the bile and urine. They are indicated for the treatment of soft-tissue infections, sinusitis, and bacterial sialadenitis.

Maculopapular rashes commonly occur with amoxycillin and ampicillin but are not usually related to true penicillin allergy. They are almost invariable in patients with glandular fever; they are also common in patients with chronic lymphatic leukaemia and in patients infected with the human immunodeficiency virus (HIV).

AMOXYCILLIN

Indications: soft-tissue infections, sialadenitis, sinusitis, prophylaxis of endocarditis
Cautions; Contra-indications; Side-effects: see under Benzylpenicillin; diarrhoea; rashes (see notes above); **interactions:** see p. 28
Dose: by mouth, 250 mg every 8 hours *or* 375 mg every 12 hours, doubled in severe infections; CHILD under 10 years 125 mg every 8 hours, doubled in severe infections
Short-course oral therapy, dental abscess, 3 g repeated after 8 hours
Prophylaxis of endocarditis, see p. 5
By intramuscular or intravenous injection—see BNF section 5.1.1.3

PoM **Amoxycillin Capsules BP,** amoxycillin (as trihydrate) 250 mg, net price 20 = £2.82; 500 mg, 20 = £5.67. Label: 9

PoM **Amoxycillin Tablets, Dispersible, DPF,** amoxycillin (as trihydrate), sugar-free, 375 mg, net price 10-tab pack = £2.62; 500 mg, 21-tab pack = £8.48; 750 mg, 10-tab pack = £5.25. Label: 9, 13

Antibacterial drugs

PoM **Amoxycillin Oral Powder DPF,** amoxycillin (as trihydrate) (sugar-free), 750 mg/sachet, net price 4-sachet pack = £2.86; 3 g/sachet, 2-sachet pack = £4.73. Label: 9, 13

PoM **Amoxycillin Oral Suspension BP,** (Amoxycillin Mixture) amoxycillin (as trihydrate) for reconstitution with water, 125 mg/5 mL, net price 100 mL = £1.98; 250 mg/5 mL, 100 mL = £3.24. Label: 9

Note. A sugar-free formulation can be requested.

PoM **Amoxycillin Injection DPF,** powder for reconstitution, amoxycillin (as sodium salt). Net price 250-mg vial = 36p; 500-mg vial = 66p; 1-g vial = £1.31

AMPICILLIN

Indications; Cautions; Contra-indications; Side-effects: see under Amoxycillin; **interactions:** see p. 28

Dose: 0.25–1 g every 6 hours, at least 30 minutes before food; CHILD under 10 years, half adult dose

PoM **Ampicillin Capsules BP,** ampicillin 250 mg, net price 20 = 67p; 500 mg, 20 = £1.44. Label: 9, 23

PoM **Ampicillin Oral Suspension BP,** (Ampicillin Mixture), ampicillin for reconstitution with water, 125 mg/5 mL, net price 100 mL = 76p; 250 mg/5 mL, 100 mL = £1.23. Label: 9, 23

Cephalosporins

The cephalosporins are broad-spectrum antibiotics but in spite of the number of cephalosporins currently available there are few absolute indications for their use. All have a similar antibacterial spectrum although individual agents have differing activity against certain organisms. The pharmacology of the cephalosporins is similar to that of the penicillins, excretion being principally renal and blocked by probenecid. Cephalexin and cephradine are active when given by mouth.

The principal side-effect of the cephalosporins is hypersensitivity and about 10% of penicillin-sensitive patients will also be allergic to the cephalosporins.

It has been shown that infections due to oral streptococci (often termed *Streptococcus viridans*) which become resistant to penicillin are usually also resistant to cephalosporins. This is of importance in the case of patients who have had rheumatic fever and are on long-term penicillin therapy.

CEPHALEXIN

Indications: soft-tissue infections, osteomyelitis
Cautions: penicillin sensitivity; renal impairment; false positive urinary glucose (if tested for reducing substances) and false positive Coombs' test; **interactions:** p. 28

Contra-indications: cephalosporin hypersensitivity; porphyria (see BNF section 9.8.2)

Side-effects: diarrhoea and rarely pseudo-membranous colitis (CSM has warned both more likely with higher doses), nausea and vomiting; allergic reactions including rashes, pruritus, urticaria, serum sickness-like reactions with rashes, fever and arthralgia, and anaphylaxis; erythema multiforme, toxic epidermal necrolysis reported; eosinophilia and rarely thrombocytopenia or neutropenia; disturbances in liver enzymes, transient hepatitis and cholestatic jaundice; other side-effects reported include reversible interstitial nephritis, hyperactivity, nervousness, sleep disturbances, confusion, hypertonia, and dizziness

Dose: 250 mg every 6 hours *or* 500 mg every 8–12 hours, increased to 1–1.5 g every 6–8 hours for severe infections; CHILD 1–5 years, 125 mg every 8 hours; 6–12 years, 250 mg every 8 hours

PoM **Cephalexin Capsules BP,** cephalexin 250 mg, net price 20 = £2.44; 500 mg, 20 = £4.80. Label: 9

PoM **Cephalexin Tablets BP,** cephalexin 250 mg, net price 20 = £2.44; 500 mg, 20 = £4.80; 1 g (scored), 14-tab pack = £8.72. Label: 9

PoM **Cephalexin Oral Suspension DPF,** (Cephalexin Mixture), cephalexin for reconstitution with water, 125 mg/5 mL, net price 100 mL = £1.27; 250 mg/5 mL, 100 mL = £2.55; 500 mg/5 mL, 100 mL = £6.19. Label: 9 *or* cephalexin ready-prepared suspension 125 mg/5 mL, net price 100 mL = £1.59, 250 mg/5 mL, 100 mL = £3.19. Label: 9

CEPHRADINE

Indications: soft-tissue infections, osteomyelitis

Cautions; Contra-indications; Side-effects: see under Cephalexin

Dose: by mouth, 250–500 mg every 6 hours *or* 0.5–1 g every 12 hours; CHILD 25–50 mg/kg daily in divided doses

By intramuscular injection or intravenous injection or infusion, 0.5–1 g every 6 hours, increased to 8 g daily in severe infections; CHILD see BNF section 5.1.2

PoM **Cephradine Capsules BP,** cephradine 250 mg, net price 20-cap pack = £3.55; 500 mg, 20-cap pack = £7.00. Label: 9

PoM **Cephradine Oral Solution DPF,** (Cephradine Mixture), cephradine 250 mg/5 mL when reconstituted with water. Net price 100 mL = £4.22. Label: 9

PoM **Cephradine Injection DPF,** powder for reconstitution, cephradine. Net price 500-mg vial = 99p; 1-g vial = £1.95

Tetracyclines

The tetracyclines are broad-spectrum antibiotics whose value has decreased owing to increasing bacterial resistance.

Tetracycline rinsed in the mouth has been advocated mainly for recurrent oral aphthae and there is some evidence that it is effective; it may also be effective in herpes infections in the mouth.

Tetracyclines are particularly likely to promote superinfection such as oral thrush when used topically in the mouth.

The tetracyclines are deposited in growing bone and teeth (being bound to calcium) causing staining and occasionally dental hypoplasia, and should **not** be given to children under 12 years or to pregnant women. With the exception of doxycycline and minocycline the tetracyclines may exacerbate renal failure and should not be given to patients with kidney disease. Absorption of tetracyclines is decreased by milk (except doxycycline and minocycline), antacids, and calcium, iron and magnesium salts.

TETRACYCLINE

Indications: systemic, destructive (refractory) forms of periodontal disease; topical, severe recurrent aphthous ulceration; oral herpes (p. 18)

Cautions: breast-feeding; hepatic impairment; renal impairment (avoid if severe); rarely causes photosensitivity; **interactions:** see p. 29

Contra-indications: severe renal impairment, pregnancy, children under 12 years of age; systemic lupus erythematosus

Side-effects: nausea, vomiting, diarrhoea; erythema (discontinue treatment); headache and visual disturbances may indicate benign intracranial hypertension; pseudomembranous colitis reported

Dose: 250 mg every 6 hours, increased in severe infections to 500 mg every 6–8 hours; as oral rinse, see below

COUNSELLING. Tablets or capsules should be swallowed whole with plenty of fluid while sitting or standing

PoM **Tetracycline Capsules BP,** tetracycline hydrochloride 250 mg. Net price 20 = 30p. Label: 7, 9, 23, counselling, posture, see above
ORAL RINSE. For an oral rinse the contents of a 250-mg capsule can be stirred in a small amount of water and held in the mouth for 2–3 minutes 3 times daily for not longer than 3 days followed by a break of at least 3 days before treatment is recommenced (to avoid oral thrush); the rinse should preferably not be swallowed

PoM **Tetracycline Tablets BP,** coated, tetracycline hydrochloride 250 mg. Net price 20 = 30p. Label: 7, 9, 23, counselling, posture, see above

DOXYCYCLINE

Indications: sinusitis (see BNF section 5.1, table 1)

Cautions; Contra-indications; Side-effects: see under Tetracycline, but may be used in renal impairment; avoid in porphyria (see BNF section 9.8.2)

Dose: 200 mg on first day, then 100 mg daily
COUNSELLING. Capsules should be swallowed whole with plenty of fluid during meals while sitting or standing

PoM **Doxycycline Capsules 100 mg BP,** doxycycline 100 mg (as hydrochloride). Net price 20 = £9.32. Label: 6, 9, 27, counselling, posture, see above

OXYTETRACYCLINE

Indications; Cautions; Contra-indications; Side-effects: see under Tetracycline; avoid in porphyria (see BNF section 9.8.2)

Dose: 250–500 mg every 6 hours

PoM **Oxytetracycline Capsules BP,** oxytetracycline (as hydrochloride) 250 mg. Net price 28-cap pack = 96p. Label: 7, 9, 23
PoM **Oxytetracycline Tablets BP,** coated, oxytetracycline dihydrate 250 mg. Net price 20 = 24p. Label: 7, 9, 23

Erythromycin

Erythromycin has a similar, although not identical, antibacterial spectrum to that of penicillin; it is thus an alternative in penicillin-allergic patients. Indications include treatment of some acute dental infections (e.g. acute dento-alveolar abscess, lateral periodontal abscess) in penicillin-allergic patients.

For prophylaxis of infective endocarditis in patients allergic to penicillin, single-dose oral clindamycin now replaces oral erythromycin (which caused nausea and vomiting).

ERYTHROMYCIN

Indications: see notes

Cautions: hepatic and renal impairment; avoid in porphyria (see BNF section 9.8.2); **interactions:** see p. 28

Side-effects: nausea, vomiting, abdominal discomfort, diarrhoea after large doses; reversible hearing loss also reported after large doses; if given for more than 14 days may occasionally cause cholestatic jaundice

Dose: by mouth, ADULT and CHILD over 8 years, 250–500 mg every 6 hours *or* 0.5–1 g every 12 hours; up to 4 g daily in severe infections; CHILD 2–8 years, 250 mg every 6 hours; doses doubled in severe infections

By intravenous route, see BNF section 5.1.5

PoM **Erythromycin Tablets BP,** e/c, erythromycin 250 mg, net price 20 = 86p; 500 mg, 20 = £2.03. Label: 5, 9, 25
PoM **Erythromycin Stearate Tablets BP,** erythromycin (as stearate) 250 mg, net price 20 = £2.13; 500 mg, 20 = £4.48. Label: 9

Antibacterial drugs 15

PoM **Erythromycin Ethyl Succinate Tablets DPF**, f/c, erythromycin 500 mg (as ethyl succinate). Net price 28-tab pack = £6.47. Label: 9

PoM **Erythromycin Ethyl Succinate Oral Suspension DPF**, erythromycin (as ethyl succinate) for reconstitution with water, 250 mg/5 mL, net price 100 mL = £2.17; 500 mg/5 mL, 100 mL = £3.59. Label: 9

Note. A sugar-free formulation can be requested, net price 140 mL (250 mg/5 mL) = £4.28

PoM **Erythromycin Ethyl Succinate Oral Suspension, Paediatric, DPF**, erythromycin 125 mg (as ethyl succinate)/5 mL when reconstituted with water. Net price 100 mL = £1.47. Label: 9

Note. A sugar-free formulation can be requested, net price 140 mL = £2.20

PoM **Erythromycin Lactobionate Intravenous Infusion BP**, powder for reconstitution, erythromycin (as lactobionate). Net price 1-g vial = £8.63

Clindamycin

Clindamycin has very limited use because of its **serious side-effects**. It is active against Gram-positive cocci, including penicillin-resistant staphylococci and also against many anaerobes, especially *Bacteroides fragilis*. It is well concentrated in bone and excreted in bile and urine.

The most serious toxic effect of clindamycin is **pseudomembranous colitis** which may be fatal and is most common in middle-aged and elderly females, especially following operation. This complication may occur with most antibiotics but is more frequently seen with clindamycin and is due to a toxin produced by *Clostridium difficile*, an anaerobic organism resistant to many antibiotics including clindamycin. It is sensitive to vancomycin or metronidazole administered by mouth (BNF section 1.5).

Clindamycin is the treatment of choice for some staphylococcal bone and joint infections resistant to other antimicrobials, but should only be prescribed on **specialist advice**. Hypersensitivity to penicillin is not shared by clindamycin and there is no cross-resistance between it and penicillin.

For **single-dose** clindamycin prophylaxis of infective endocarditis in patients allergic to penicillin, see p. 5.

CLINDAMYCIN

Indications: see notes above
Cautions: discontinue immediately if diarrhoea or colitis develops; hepatic or renal impairment; **interactions:** see p. 28
Contra-indications: diarrhoeal states
Side-effects: diarrhoea (discontinue treatment), abdominal discomfort, nausea, vomiting, pseudomembranous colitis; rash; jaundice and altered liver function tests; neutropenia, eosinophilia, agranulocytosis and thrombocytopenia reported; pain, induration, and abscess after intramuscular injection; thrombophlebitis after intravenous injection

Dose: by mouth, 150–300 mg every 6 hours; up to 450 mg every 6 hours in severe infections; CHILD, 3–6 mg/kg every 6 hours
Prophylaxis of endocarditis, see p. 5 (**important:** single-dose only)
COUNSELLING. Patients should discontinue immediately and contact doctor if diarrhoea develops; capsules should be swallowed with a glass of water
By intramuscular injection or slow intravenous infusion, see BNF section 5.1.6

PoM **Clindamycin Capsules BP**, clindamycin (as hydrochloride) 75 mg, net price 20 = £4.92; 150 mg, 20 = £9.07. Label: 9, 27, counselling, see above (diarrhoea)

PoM **Clindamycin Oral Suspension, Paediatric, DPF**, (Clindamycin Mixture, Paediatric), clindamycin 75 mg (as palmitate hydrochloride)/5 mL when reconstituted with purified water (freshly boiled and cooled). Net price 100 mL = £6.62. Label: 9, 27, counselling, see above (diarrhoea)

PoM **Clindamycin Injection DPF**, clindamycin 150 mg (as phosphate)/mL. Net price 2-mL amp = £5.17; 4-mL amp = £10.29

Metronidazole

Metronidazole is an antimicrobial drug with high activity against anaerobic bacteria and protozoa. It is most effective in the treatment of acute ulcerative gingivitis (Vincent's infection) and pericoronitis where it is used in conjunction with local hygiene measures. For these purposes it is usually sufficient to prescribe 200 mg 3 times daily for 3 days although the duration of treatment may be longer in pericoronitis.

METRONIDAZOLE

Indications: see notes above
Cautions: disulfiram-like reaction with alcohol; hepatic impairment, pregnancy and breast-feeding (manufacturer advises avoidance of high-dose regimens); **interactions:** see p. 29
Side-effects: nausea, vomiting, unpleasant taste, and gastro-intestinal disturbances; rashes, urticaria and angioedema; rarely drowsiness, headache, dizziness, ataxia, and darkening of urine; on prolonged or intensive therapy peripheral neuropathy, transient epileptiform seizures, and leucopenia
Dose: 200 mg every 8 hours for 3–7 days (see notes above); CHILD 1–3 years 50 mg every 8 hours; 3–7 years 100 mg every 12 hours; 7–10 years 100 mg every 8 hours

PoM **Metronidazole Tablets BP**, metronidazole 200 mg, net price 20 = 70p; 400 mg, 20 = £1.45. Label: 4, 9, 21, 25, 27

PoM **Metronidazole Oral Suspension DPF**, (Metronidazole Mixture), metronidazole 200 mg (as benzoate)/5 mL. Net price 100 mL = £4.53. Label: 4, 9, 23

Sodium fusidate

An ointment containing sodium fusidate is indicated in the fissures of angular cheilitis where *Staphylococcus aureus* has been isolated.

For further information see BNF section 13.10.1.2

SODIUM FUSIDATE
Indications: see notes above
Cautions: avoid contact with eyes
Side-effects: rarely local hypersensitivity reactions

PoM **Sodium Fusidate Ointment BP,** (former title: Fusidic Acid Ointment DPF), sodium fusidate 2%, in an anhydrous greasy basis. Net price 15 g = £2.40; 30 g = £4.07
Apply 3–4 times daily

Co-trimoxazole

The importance of the sulphonamides as chemotherapeutic agents has decreased as a result of increasing bacterial resistance and their replacement by antibiotics which are generally more active and less toxic.

Sulphonamide preparations other than **co-trimoxazole** are not included as there are no indications for prescribing them alone in general dental practice.

Sulphamethoxazole and trimethoprim have been used in combination (as co-trimoxazole) because of their synergistic activity. Increasing bacterial resistance to sulphonamides and the high incidence of sulphonamide-related side-effects have, however, diminished the value of co-trimoxazole.

Indications for co-trimoxazole include soft-tissue infections and sialadenitis.

Sulphonamides are potentially capable of causing a wide variety of side-effects but only rashes are relatively common. Very occasionally Stevens-Johnson syndrome (erythema multiforme exudativum) appears to have resulted from treatment with sulphonamides and causes severe labial, oral and other mucosal ulceration, rashes, and sometimes ocular damage.

> Side-effects of co-trimoxazole are similar to those of the sulphonamides, but a particular watch should be kept for haematological effects and special care should be taken in patients who may be folate deficient such as the elderly and chronic sick. There have been recent reports of deaths in patients over the age of 65 years being treated with co-trimoxazole and almost certainly associated with the sulphonamide component. For this reason co-trimoxazole should be used with care in the elderly and preferably only if there is no acceptable alternative. The effect on the fetus is unknown and co-trimoxazole should not be used in pregnancy.

CO-TRIMOXAZOLE

A mixture of trimethoprim and sulphamethoxazole in the proportions of 1 part to 5 parts
Indications: soft-tissue infections, sialadenitis
Cautions: blood counts in prolonged treatment, maintain adequate fluid intake, renal impairment, breast-feeding; photosensitivity; elderly patients (**important:** see notes above); **interactions:** see BNF p. 484
Contra-indications: pregnancy, infants under 6 weeks (risk of kernicterus), renal or hepatic failure, jaundice, blood disorders; porphyria (see BNF section 9.8.2)
Side-effects: nausea, vomiting, glossitis, rashes, erythema multiforme (includes Stevens-Johnson syndrome), epidermal necrolysis, eosinophilia, agranulocytosis, granulocytopenia, purpura, leucopenia; megaloblastic anaemia due to trimethoprim
Dose: 960 mg every 12 hours, increased to 1.44 g in severe infections; 480 mg every 12 hours if treated for more than 14 days; CHILD, every 12 hours, 6 months to 5 years, 240 mg; 6–12 years, 480 mg
Note. 480 mg of co-trimoxazole consists of sulphamethoxazole 400 mg and trimethoprim 80 mg.

PoM **Co-trimoxazole Tablets BP,** co-trimoxazole 480 mg, net price 20 = £1.00; 960 mg, 20 = £3.23. Label: 9

PoM **Co-trimoxazole Tablets, Dispersible, BP,** co-trimoxazole 480 mg. Net price 20 = 97p. Label: 9, 13

PoM **Co-trimoxazole Tablets, Paediatric, BP,** co-trimoxazole 120 mg. Net price 20 = 64p. Label: 9
Note. Some brands of co-trimoxazole paediatric tablets have been discontinued, therefore supplies may be difficult to obtain

PoM **Co-trimoxazole Oral Suspension BP,** (Co-trimoxazole Mixture), co-trimoxazole 480 mg/5 mL. Net price 100 mL = £3.00. Label: 9

PoM **Co-trimoxazole Oral Suspension, Paediatric, BP,** (Co-trimoxazole Mixture, Paediatric), co-trimoxazole 240 mg/5 mL. Net price 100 mL = £2.09. Label: 9

Antifungal Drugs

Fungal infections of the mouth are usually due to *Candida* spp. and may take the form of thrush, denture stomatitis, or chronic hyperplastic candidiasis. Thrush, apart from that seen in infants or in debilitating disease, may develop for a variety of reasons but often appears following the use of broad-spectrum antibiotics or corticosteroids. It is a common feature of the early stages of AIDS.

Thrush and denture stomatitis should be treated with **nystatin** or **amphotericin** which are used topically and are not absorbed from the gut. Thrush should respond within a few days.

Patients with denture stomatitis should be instructed to cleanse their dentures thoroughly and, ideally, to leave them out during treatment but this has a low rate of compliance. As a compromise miconazole oral gel can be placed in the fitting surface of the denture before insertion (for a short period only).

Miconazole may be more effective for some types of candidiasis, particularly chronic mucocutaneous candidiasis or candidal leukoplakia, the diagnosis of which depends on laboratory examinations. Candidal leukoplakia is not clinically distinguishable from other types of leukoplakia and the possibility of future malignant change must be assessed by biopsy. If in spite of such considerations these agents are used and there is no obvious response within one or two weeks of use, then the patient should be sent for investigation to confirm the diagnosis and, if candidiasis is present, to eliminate the possibility of any underlying disease, such as the prodromal stage of AIDS. Persistent infections may be due to re-infection from the genitourinary tract or alimentary canal and a course of tablets (amphotericin, nystatin) may be prescribed.

Folds at the angles of the mouth may be an age change or due to faulty dentures, or very occasionally, to a nutritional deficiency. They may become infected with *Candida* spp. While the underlying cause is being established it is often helpful to apply an antifungal ointment to the fissures. These lesions may also be infected with *Staphylococcus aureus* or β-haemolytic streptococci (see fusidic acid).

For further information see BNF sections 5.2; 12.3.2; and 13.10.2.

AMPHOTERICIN

Indications: oral and perioral fungal infections

PoM Amphotericin Tablets DPF, amphotericin 100 mg. Net price 20-tab pack = £2.97. Label: 9
Dose: intestinal candidiasis (see notes above), 100–200 mg every 6 hours

PoM Amphotericin Lozenges BP, amphotericin 10 mg. Net price 6 × 10-lozenge pack = £3.95. Label: 9, 24, counselling, after food
Dose: Dissolve 1 lozenge slowly in the mouth 4 times daily, may require 10–15 days' treatment (continued for 48 hours after lesions have resolved); increased to 8 daily if infection severe

PoM Amphotericin Oral Suspension DPF, (Amphotericin Mixture), amphotericin 100 mg/mL (sugar-free). Net price 12 mL with pipette = £2.31. Label: 9, counselling, use of pipette, hold in mouth, after food
Dose: Place 1 mL in the mouth after food and retain near lesions 4 times daily for 14 days (continued for 48 hours after lesions have resolved)

MICONAZOLE

Indications: oral fungal infections
Cautions: pregnancy; avoid in porphyria (see BNF section 9.8.2)

PoM ¹Miconazole Oral Gel DPF, miconazole 25 mg/mL (sugar-free). Net price 80 g = £5.00. Label: 9, counselling, hold in mouth, after food
Dose: Place 5–10 mL in the mouth after food and retain near lesions, 4 times daily; CHILD under 2 years 2.5 mL twice daily; 2–6 years 5 mL twice daily; over 6 years 5 mL 4 times daily
Localised lesions, smear affected area with clean finger; a 15-g tube (net price £1.70) also available
1. A 15-g tube can be sold to the public

With hydrocortisone (cream and ointment), see p. 20

NYSTATIN

Indications: oral and perioral fungal infections

PoM Nystatin Tablets BP, coated, nystatin 500 000 units. Net price 56-tab pack = £4.70. Label: 9
Dose: intestinal candidiasis (see notes above), 500 000 units every 6 hours, doubled in severe infections

PoM Nystatin Oral Suspension BP, (Nystatin Mixture), nystatin 100 000 units/mL. Net price 30 mL = £2.50. Label: 9, counselling, use of pipette, hold in mouth, after food
Dose: Place 1 mL in the mouth after food and retain near the lesions 4 times daily, usually for 7 days (continued for 48 hours after lesions have resolved)
Note. A sugar-free formulation can be requested, net price 24 mL = £1.67

PoM Nystatin Pastilles DPF, nystatin 100 000 units. Net price 28-pastille pack = £3.95. Label: 9, 24, counselling, after food
Dose: suck 1 pastille slowly 4 times daily after food

PoM Nystatin Ointment BP, nystatin 100 000 units/g. Net price 30 g = £2.14
Apply 2–4 times daily, continuing for 7 days after lesions have healed

Antiviral Drugs

The specific therapy of virus infections is generally unsatisfactory and treatment is, therefore, primarily symptomatic. Fortunately, the majority of infections resolve spontaneously.

Acyclovir is active against herpes viruses but does not eradicate them. It is effective only if started at the onset of infection.

Idoxuridine is also only effective if started at the onset of infection; it is too toxic for systemic use.

HERPETIC GINGIVO-STOMATITIS. The management of primary herpetic gingivo-stomatitis is a soft diet, adequate fluid intake, analgesics as required, and the use of **chlorhexidine** mouthwash to control plaque accumulation if toothbrushing is painful. In the case of severe herpetic stomatitis, systemic acyclovir is required.

Herpes infections of the mouth may also respond to tetracycline rinsed in the mouth (see p. 14).

Idoxuridine 0.1% paint has been superseded by more effective preparations.

HERPES LABIALIS. Acyclovir cream can be used for the treatment of initial and recurrent herpes labialis; it must be applied at the earliest possible stage, namely when prodromal changes of sensation are felt in the lip and before vesicles appear.

Idoxuridine solution (5% in dimethyl sulphoxide) is used less frequently for herpes labialis since acyclovir is more effective; it too must be applied at the earliest possible stage; it should not be used in the mouth.

See also BNF sections 5.3; 12.3.2; and 13.10.3.

ACYCLOVIR

Indications: herpes simplex; varicella-zoster, see BNF section 5.3

Cautions: maintain adequate hydration; reduce dose in renal impairment; pregnancy; **interactions:** see BNF p. 477 (systemic only)

Side-effects: rashes; gastro-intestinal disturbances; rises in bilirubin and liver-related enzymes, increases in blood urea and creatinine, decreases in haematological indices, headache, neurological reactions, fatigue; topical application: transient stinging or burning on topical application; occasionally erythema or drying of the skin

Dose: by mouth

Herpes simplex, treatment, 200 mg (400 mg in the immunocompromised) 5 times daily, usually for 5 days; CHILD under 2 years, half adult dose; over 2 years, adult dose

Herpes zoster, see BNF section 5.3

Note. Prophylactic doses not included here—see BNF section 5.3.

PoM **Acyclovir Tablets 200 mg DPF,** acyclovir 200 mg, net price 25-tab pack = £28.89. Label: 9

PoM **Acyclovir Oral Suspension DPF,** acyclovir 200 mg/5 mL, sugar-free. Net price 125 mL = £28.89. Label: 9

Note. Acyclovir oral suspension is intended to be swallowed for a systemic effect as an alternative to tablets in patients who cannot swallow the tablets; it is **not** merely intended for local use in the mouth

PoM **Acyclovir Cream DPF,** acyclovir 5% in an aqueous cream basis. Net price 2 g = £8.37; 10 g = £25.22

Apply to lesions every 4 hours (5 times daily) for 5 days, started at first sign of attack. Not to be used in the mouth

IDOXURIDINE IN DIMETHYL SULPHOXIDE

Indications: see notes above

Cautions: avoid contact with eyes, mucous membranes, and textiles; breast-feeding

Contra-indications: pregnancy (toxicity in *animal* studies)

Side-effects: stinging on application, changes in taste; excessive use may lead to maceration

PoM **Idoxuridine 5% in Dimethyl Sulphoxide DPF,** idoxuridine 5% in dimethyl sulphoxide. Net price 5 mL (with applicator) = £7.04

Apply to lesions 4 times daily for 3–4 days. Not to be used in the mouth

Corticosteroids and other Drugs for Oral Ulceration and Inflammation

Ulceration of the oral mucosa may be caused by trauma (physical or chemical), recurrent aphthae, infections, carcinoma, dermatological disorders, nutritional deficiencies, gastro-intestinal disease, haematopoietic disorders, and drug therapy. It is important to establish the diagnosis in each case as the majority of these lesions require specific management in addition to local treatment. Local treatment aims at protecting the ulcerated area, or at relieving pain or reducing inflammation.

SIMPLE MOUTHWASHES. A **saline** or **compound thymol glycerin** mouthwash may relieve the pain of traumatic ulceration. The mouthwash is made up with warm water and used at frequent intervals until the discomfort and swelling subsides. *For preparations see p.* 10.

ANTISEPTIC MOUTHWASHES. Secondary bacterial infection may be a feature of any mucosal ulceration; it can increase discomfort and delay healing. Use of a **chlorhexidine** or **povidone-iodine** mouthwash is often beneficial and may accelerate healing of recurrent aphthae. *For preparations see p.* 10.

CORTICOSTEROIDS. Topical corticosteroid therapy may be used for different forms of oral ulceration. In the case of aphthous ulcers it is most effective if applied in the prodromal phase.

Thrush or other types of candidiasis are recognised complications of corticosteroid treatment.

Hydrocortisone lozenges are allowed to dissolve next to an ulcer and are useful in recurrent aphthae, erosive lichen planus, discoid lupus erythematosus, and benign mucous membrane pemphigoid.

Triamcinolone dental paste is designed to keep the corticosteroid in contact with the mucosa for long enough to permit penetration of the lesion, but is difficult for patients to apply properly.

Hydrocortisone cream is used in treating uninfected inflammatory lesions on the lips and perioral skin. **Hydrocortisone and miconazole cream** or ointment is useful where infection by susceptible organisms and inflammation co-exist, particularly for initial treatment (up to about 7 days). Organisms susceptible to miconazole include candida spp. and many Gram-positive bacteria including streptococcus and staphylococcus.

Systemic corticosteroid therapy for severe conditions such as pemphigus vulgaris is best reserved for the physician because of potential side-effects.

LOCAL ANALGESICS. Local analgesics have a limited role in the management of oral ulceration. When applied topically their action is of a relatively short duration so that analgesia cannot be maintained continuously throughout the day. The main indication for a topical local analgesic is to relieve the pain of otherwise intractable oral ulceration particularly when it is due to major aphthae. For this purpose **lignocaine 5% ointment** is applied to the ulcer. Care must be taken not to produce anaesthesia of the pharynx before meals as this might lead to choking.

Benzydamine mouthwash may be useful in palliating the discomfort associated with a variety of ulcerative conditions. It reduces the discomfort of post-irradiation mucositis. If the full-strength preparation causes some stinging it can be diluted with an equal volume of water. The spray may also be useful.

Choline salicylate dental gel has some analgesic action and may provide relief for recurrent aphthae, but excessive application or confinement under a denture irritates the mucosa and can itself cause ulceration. Benefit in teething may merely be due to pressure of application (comparable with biting a teething ring); excessive use can lead to salicylate poisoning.

See also BNF section 12.3.

MECHANICAL PROTECTION. **Carmellose gelatin paste** may relieve some discomfort arising from ulceration, by protecting the ulcer site. The paste adheres to the mucosa, but is difficult to apply effectively to some parts of the mouth.

DRY MOUTH. This condition may be caused by irradiation of the head and neck region, damage to or disease of the salivary glands, or by the administration of drugs with antimuscarinic (anticholinergic) side-effects, for example antispasmodics, tricyclic antidepressants, and some antipsychotic drugs. It may be relieved in many patients by simple measures such as frequent sips of cool drinks, sucking pieces of ice or sugar-free fruit pastilles, or by the use of an artificial saliva (see next page).

BENZYDAMINE HYDROCHLORIDE
Indications: painful inflammatory conditions of oropharynx
Side-effects: occasional numbness or stinging

Benzydamine Mouthwash DPF, benzydamine hydrochloride 0.15%. Net price 300 mL = £4.25
Rinse or gargle, using 15 mL (diluted if stinging occurs), every 1½–3 hours as required, usually for not more than 7 days; not suitable for childen under 12 years

Benzydamine Oral Spray DPF, benzydamine hydrochloride 0.15%. Net price 30-mL unit = £3.39
4–8 puffs onto affected area every 1½–3 hours; CHILD under 6 years 1 puff per 4 kg to max. 4 puffs every 1½–3 hours; 6–12 years 4 puffs every 1½–3 hours

CARMELLOSE SODIUM
Indications: mechanical protection of oral and perioral lesions

Carmellose Gelatin Paste DPF, carmellose sodium 16.58%, pectin 16.58%, gelatin 16.58% in Plastibase®. Net price 30 g = £1.50; 100 g = £3.32
Apply a thin layer when necessary after meals

CORTICOSTEROIDS
Indications: oral and perioral lesions
Contra-indications: untreated oral infection
Side-effects: occasional exacerbation of local infection

PoM **Hydrocortisone Lozenges BPC,** hydrocortisone 2.5 mg (as sodium succinate). Net price 20 = £1.40
One lozenge 4 times daily, allowed to dissolve slowly in the mouth in contact with the ulcer; if ulcers recur rapidly treatment may be continued for a period at reduced dosage

PoM **Hydrocortisone Cream BP,** hydrocortisone 1%[1]. Net price 15 g = 47p. Label: 28
Apply thinly 2–3 times daily reducing frequency as condition responds
1. The BP does not specify one particular strength but when hydrocortisone cream is prescribed by a dental practitioner on form FP14 (GP14 in Scotland) a cream containing 1% will be dispensed.

PoM **Triamcinolone Dental Paste BP,** triamcinolone acetonide 0.1% in an adhesive basis. Net price 10 g = £1.27
Apply a thin layer 2–4 times daily; do not rub in

With antifungal
PoM **Hydrocortisone and Miconazole Cream DPF,** hydrocortisone 1% and miconazole nitrate 2%, net price 30 g = £2.24. Label: 28
PoM **Hydrocortisone and Miconazole Ointment DPF,** hydrocortisone 1% and miconazole nitrate 2%, net price 30 g = £3.10. Label: 28
For angular cheilitis apply sparingly 2–3 times daily; do not use for longer than 7 days

LIGNOCAINE HYDROCHLORIDE
Indications: relief of pain in oral lesions
Cautions: avoid prolonged use; hypersensitivity may occur

Lignocaine 5% Ointment DPF, lignocaine 5% in a suitable basis. Net price 15 g = 83p
Rub gently into affected areas. Max. dose for 70 kg man 200 mg lignocaine (= ¼ tube)

SALICYLATES
Indications: mild oral and perioral lesions
Cautions: frequent application, especially in children, may give rise to salicylate poisoning
Note. CSM warning on aspirin and Reye's syndrome does not apply to non-aspirin salicylates or to topical preparations such as teething gels, but for comment on these see BNF section 12.3.1

Choline Salicylate Dental Gel BP (former title: Choline Salicylate Dental Paste DPF), choline salicylate 8.7% in a flavoured gel basis. Net price 10 g = 72p; 15 g (sugar-free) = £1.11
Apply ½-inch of gel with gentle massage not more often than every 3 hours; CHILD over 4 months ¼-inch of gel not more often than every 3 hours; max. 6 applications daily

ARTIFICIAL SALIVA
Indications: dry mouth

Artificial Saliva DPF, *Oral spray,* sorbitol 1.8 g, carmellose sodium (sodium carboxymethylcellulose) 390 mg, dibasic potassium phosphate 48.23 mg, potassium chloride 37.5 mg, monobasic potassium phosphate 21.97 mg, calcium chloride 9.972 mg, magnesium chloride 3.528 mg, sodium fluoride 258 micrograms/60 mL, with preservatives and colouring agents. Net price 60-mL unit = £3.96
Saliva deficiency, 2–3 sprays onto oral mucosa up to 4 times daily, or as directed
See BNF p. 557 for the brand of artificial saliva corresponding to this definition

Analgesics

Analgesics should be used **judiciously** in dental care as a **temporary** measure until causative factors have been brought under control. A general dental practitioner will usually find **paracetamol, aspirin, ibuprofen** or **diflunisal** adequate for most purposes and need rarely prescribe opioids.

Dental pain of inflammatory origin, such as that associated with *pulpitis, apical infection, localised osteitis (dry socket)* or *pericoronitis* is usually best treated by the control of infection, together with the provision of drainage, restorative procedures and other local measures. The role of analgesics is to provide temporary relief of pain (usually for about one to seven days) until the causative factors have been brought under control. In the case of *pulpitis, intraosseous infection* or *abscess*, reliance on analgesics alone is usually inappropriate.

Similar principles apply to the management of *acute problems affecting the oral mucosa* (e.g. acute herpetic gingivostomatitis, erythema multiforme). The pain and discomfort associated with such problems may be relieved with benzydamine, used as a mouthwash or spray. Where a patient is *febrile*, however, the antipyretic action of aspirin or paracetamol is often helpful. A chlorhexidine mouthwash may also be useful, both for *oral hygiene and to control secondary infection*.

Postoperative dental pain can usually be controlled with an appropriate analgesic given in a suitable dose for about 24 to 72 hours. Any analgesic given pre-operatively should be one (e.g. paracetamol) that is not likely to increase the risk of postoperative bleeding.

All analgesics have limitations in respect of their overall pain-relieving ability and their propensity for causing unwanted effects. In general, those most suitable for use in dental pain are **paracetamol, aspirin** and **ibuprofen**. Opioid analgesics (which include **dihydrocodeine** and **pethidine**) are relatively ineffective in dental pain and their side-effects can be unpleasant.

The **choice** of an analgesic for dental purposes should be based on its suitability for the patient. The dose depends on the degree of pain relief needed (or able to be achieved) bearing in mind that with some analgesics little additional benefit can be achieved by increasing the dose. The interval between doses is related to factors such as the duration of action of the drug and the need to avoid side-effects. In the case of postoperative pain, taking an analgesic before the effect of the local anaesthetic has worn off can result in better overall control.

Most dental pain is effectively relieved by non-steroidal anti-inflammatory drugs (NSAIDs) which act by blocking the synthesis of prostaglandins. Paracetamol acts in a related manner but has no anti-inflammatory effect. Opioid analgesics such as dihydrocodeine and pethidine act on the central nervous system and are traditionally used for moderate to severe pain. However, their greater efficacy in the control of dental pain compared with adequate doses of non-opioid analgesics has yet to be demonstrated.

There is some evidence that a combination of a non-opioid and an opioid analgesic can provide greater relief of dental pain than a non-opioid analgesic given alone. This only applies, however, when an appropriate dose combination is used. Most combination analgesic preparations available have not been shown to provide greater relief of pain than the same dose of the non-opioid component given alone. Moreover, they have the disadvantage of an increased number of side-effects.

NSAIDs

> **CSM advice (peptic ulceration).**
> 1. NSAIDs should not be given to patients with active peptic ulceration.
> 2. In patients with a history of peptic ulcer disease and in the elderly they should be given only after other forms of treatment have been carefully considered.
> 3. In all patients it is prudent to start at the bottom end of the dose range.
>
> **CSM Warning (asthma).**
> Any degree of worsening of asthma may be related to the ingestion of NSAIDs, either prescribed or (in the case of ibuprofen and others) purchased over the counter.

Aspirin is effective against mild to moderate dental pain. Dispersible tablets provide a rapidly absorbed form of aspirin adequate for most purposes. The side-effects of aspirin are uncommon relative to the scale on which it is taken. The main side-effect is gastro-intestinal irritation; gastric bleeding can be a serious complication. Aspirin is also associated with bronchospasm and sensitivity reactions (patients should therefore be asked if they are allergic to aspirin). Aspirin should **not** be prescribed for children owing to its association with Reye's syndrome.

> **CSM advice (Reye's syndrome).**
> The CSM has considered available evidence on possible links between Reye's syndrome and aspirin use by feverish children, and recommends that aspirin should no longer be given to children aged under 12 years, unless specifically indicated, e.g. for juvenile rheumatoid arthritis. It is therefore important to advise families that aspirin is not, on the evidence now available, a suitable medicine for children with minor illnesses. Paracetamol (see below) is an effective alternative treatment for fever in children.

Diflunisal is an aspirin derivative but both its clinical effects and its side-effects more closely resemble those of ibuprofen. Like aspirin and ibuprofen, diflunisal is used for mild to moderate dental pain. It has a long duration of action and need only be given twice daily, which can be an advantage for some patients. There is one unconfirmed study which showed an increased incidence of localised osteitis (dry socket) following its use for postoperative analgesia.

Ibuprofen is also effective against mild to moderate dental pain. Like aspirin it causes gastro-intestinal irritation and may cause bronchospasm. Ibuprofen can be used in children and a paediatric preparation is now on the dental list.
For further information see BNF sections 4.7 and 10.1.1.

ASPIRIN
Indications: mild to moderate pain, pyrexia
Cautions: asthma, allergic disease, renal or hepatic impairment (avoid if severe), dehydration, pregnancy; G6PD-deficiency (see BNF section 9.1.5); **interactions:** see p. 28
Contra-indications: children under 12 years and in breast-feeding (Reye's syndrome—see notes above); gastro-intestinal ulceration, haemophilia, avoid in gout
Side-effects: generally mild and infrequent but high incidence of gastro-intestinal irritation with slight asymptomatic blood loss, increased bleeding time, and bronchospasm and skin reactions in hypersensitive patients
Dose: 300–900 mg every 4–6 hours when necessary; max. 4 g daily

Aspirin Tablets, Dispersible, BP, aspirin 300 mg in a suitable dispersible basis. Net price 20 = 9p. Label: 13, 21, 32
Note. When dispersible or soluble aspirin tablets are prescribed and no strength is stated, dispersible aspirin tablets containing 300 mg will be dispensed.

DIFLUNISAL
Indications: mild to moderate pain and inflammation
Cautions: history of gastro-intestinal disease; allergy; elderly; pregnancy; breast-feeding; cardiac, renal and hepatic impairment (**important:** see pp. 30 and 31); increases bleeding time; **interactions:** see p. 28
Contra-indications: gastro-intestinal bleeding or ulceration, history of asthma precipitated by aspirin or other NSAIDs, or sensitivity to salicylates
Side-effects: gastro-intestinal discomfort (occasionally bleeding) and allergy (bronchospasm, rashes, angioedema); other side-effects reported for NSAIDs include headache, dizziness, tinnitus, haematuria, and rarely blood disorders, papillary necrosis or interstitial fibrosis, aseptic meningitis (see BNF p. 359)
Dose: 250–500 mg twice daily preferably after food

PoM **Diflunisal Tablets BP,** coated, diflunisal 250 mg, net price 20 = £1.80; 500 mg, 20 = £3.61. Label: 21, 25, counselling, avoid aluminium hydroxide

IBUPROFEN
Indications: mild to moderate pain and inflammation

Cautions: elderly, history of peptic ulceration, allergic disorders (particularly asthma and hypersensitivity to salicylates), pregnancy, cardiac, renal and hepatic impairment (**important:** see pp. 30 and 31); **interactions:** see p. 29
Contra-indications: gastro-intestinal bleeding or ulceration; history of asthma precipitated by aspirin or other NSAIDs
Side-effects: gastro-intestinal discomfort (occasionally bleeding) and allergy (bronchospasm, rashes, angioedema); other side-effects reported for NSAIDs include headache, dizziness, tinnitus, haematuria and rarely blood disorders, papillary necrosis or interstitial fibrosis, aseptic meningitis (see BNF p. 359)
Dose: 1.2–1.8 g daily in 3–4 divided doses preferably after food; increased if necessary to max. of 2.4 g daily; CHILD see under preparation below

PoM **Ibuprofen Tablets BP,** coated, ibuprofen 200 mg, net price 20 = 26p; 400 mg, 20 = 51p; 600 mg, 20 = £1.36. Label: 21
Note. Proprietary brands of ibuprofen tablets are on sale to the public (see BNF p. 359)

PoM **Ibuprofen Oral Suspension DPF,** ibuprofen 100 mg/5 mL (sugar-free). Net price 150 mL = £2.41. Label: 21
Dose: CHILD 1–2 years 2.5 mL 3–4 times daily, 3–7 years 5 mL, 8–12 years 10 mL

PARACETAMOL
Paracetamol's analgesic efficacy is probably less than that of aspirin, but it has the advantage that it does not affect bleeding time or interact significantly with warfarin. Moreover, it does not cause gastric irritation. Paracetamol is a suitable analgesic for children; sugar-free versions are available and can be requested by specifying "sugar-free" on the prescription. Of special concern with paracetamol is its hepatic toxicity in overdosage—*dosage schedules should be strictly adhered to and **not** exceeded.*
Important. Overdosage with paracetamol, alone or with dextropropoxyphene, is dangerous, see BNF, p. 18.

PARACETAMOL
Indications: mild to moderate pain, pyrexia
Cautions: hepatic and renal impairment, alcohol dependence; **interactions:** see p. 29
Side-effects: side-effects rare, but rashes, blood disorders, and acute pancreatitis reported; **important:** liver damage (and less frequently renal damage) following overdosage, see under Emergency Treatment of Poisoning (BNF p. 18)
Dose: 0.5–1 g every 4–6 hours to a max. of 4 g daily; CHILD 1–5 years 120–250 mg, 6–12 years 250–500 mg; these doses may be repeated every 4–6 hours when necessary (max. 4 doses in 24 hours)

Analgesics

Paracetamol Tablets BP, paracetamol 500 mg. Net price 20 = 9p. Label: 29, 30

Paracetamol Tablets, Dispersible, DPF, paracetamol 500 mg in a suitable dispersible basis. Net price 60-tab pack = £1.43. Label: 13, 29, 30

Paracetamol Oral Suspension, Paediatric, BP, paracetamol 120 mg/5 mL. Net price 100 mL = 50p. Label: 30

Note. BP directs that when Paediatric Paracetamol Oral Suspension or Paediatric Paracetamol Mixture is prescribed and no strength is stated Paracetamol Oral Suspension 120 mg/5 mL should be dispensed. Sugar-free versions are available and can be ordered by specifying 'sugar-free' on the prescription.

OPIOID ANALGESICS

Dihydrocodeine is an opioid analgesic with an efficacy similar to that of codeine. Like other opioids, dihydrocodeine often causes nausea and vomiting which limits its value in dental pain; if taken for more than a few doses it is also liable to cause constipation. Dihydrocodeine is not very effective in postoperative dental pain. The dose of dihydrocodeine by mouth should not usually exceed 30 mg every 4 hours; doubling it to 60 mg may provide some additional pain relief but this may be at the cost of more nausea and vomiting.

Pethidine is a synthetic opioid analgesic which provides prompt but short-lasting analgesia; even in high doses it is less effective than morphine. It can be taken by mouth, but for optimal use needs to be given by injection. Its efficacy in postoperative dental pain is open to question and its overall use in dentistry is likely to be minimal. Pethidine has the same side-effects as dihydrocodeine and, apart from being less constipating, is also more likely to cause them. The severity of its interaction with monoamine-oxidase inhibitors (MAOIs) is a further special hazard. Dependence is unlikely to be a problem if very few tablets are prescribed on very few occasions; nevertheless, dental practitioners need to be aware of the possibility that addicts may seek to acquire supplies.

DIHYDROCODEINE TARTRATE

Indications: moderate to severe pain (but see notes above)

Cautions: history of drug abuse; hypotension, asthma, decreased respiratory reserve, hypothyroidism, hepatic or renal impairment; pregnancy, breast-feeding; reduce dose in elderly and debilitated; **interactions:** see p. 28

Contra-indications: avoid in raised intracranial pressure or head injury

Side-effects: constipation, dizziness, sedation, respiratory depression, cough suppression; urinary retention, nausea, vomiting; tolerance; liable to cause dependence

Dose: 30 mg every 4–6 hours when necessary, preferably after food (see also notes above); CHILD see BNF section 4.7.2

PoM **Dihydrocodeine Tablets BP,** dihydrocodeine tartrate 30 mg. Net price 20 = 62p. Label: 2, 21

Note. A proprietary brand of an analgesic containing dihydrocodeine and paracetamol is on sale to the public, see BNF p. 175

PETHIDINE HYDROCHLORIDE

Indications: severe pain (but see notes above)

Cautions; Side effects: see under Dihydrocodeine Tartrate; in therapeutic doses pethidine is even more liable than dihydrocodeine to produce adverse effects and convulsions have been reported in overdosage; avoid in severe renal impairment; see also notes above; **important:** interaction with MAOIs is special hazard; **interactions:** see p. 29

Dose: 50–150 mg every 4 hours; CHILD see BNF section 4.7.2

CD **Pethidine Tablets BP,** pethidine hydrochloride 50 mg, net price 20 = 39p. Label: 2

ORAL AND FACIAL PAIN

Although **carbamazepine** is not an analgesic it is very effective for the treatment of the severe pain associated with trigeminal neuralgia and (less commonly) glossopharyngeal neuralgia. Other causes of facial pain should be excluded and it should only be prescribed in collaboration with the patient's medical practitioner. A dose of 100 mg once or twice daily is given initially and slowly increased according to response; most patients require 200 mg three to four times daily but a few may require up to 1.6 g daily; plasma concentration monitoring is needed when high doses are given. Carbamazepine has numerous side-effects including, rarely, serious blood disorders. Careful patient monitoring is therefore an essential aspect of patient care. Occasionally extreme dizziness is encountered which is a further reason for starting treatment with a small dose and increasing it slowly.

CARBAMAZEPINE

Indications: trigeminal neuralgia, glossopharyngeal neuralgia

Cautions: see notes above; pregnancy—**important** see p. 32, breast-feeding; hepatic impairment; may decrease efficacy of oral contraceptives; **interactions:** see BNF pp. 185 and 482

Contra-indications: atrioventricular conduction abnormalities (unless paced); porphyrias (see BNF section 9.8.2); patients on MAOIs or within 2 weeks of MAOI therapy (theoretical grounds only)

Side-effects: gastro-intestinal disturbances, dizziness, drowsiness, headache, ataxia, confusion and agitation (elderly), visual disturbances (especially double vision and often associated with peak plasma concentrations); constipation, anorexia; generalised erythematous rash may occur in about 3% of patients; leucopenia and other blood disorders have occurred rarely; cholestatic jaundice, acute renal failure. Stevens-Johnson syndrome, toxic epidermal necrolysis, alopecia, thromboembolism, fever, proteinuria, lymph node enlargement, cardiac conduction disturbances, and hepatitis reported; hyponatraemia and oedema also reported (with higher doses)

Dose: during acute stage only, initially, 100–200 mg 1–2 times daily, increased gradually to a usual dose of 200 mg 3–4 times daily, according to the patient's needs; in some cases 1.6 g daily may be needed

Note. Need for plasma concentration monitoring, see BNF, pp. 182 and 186.

PoM **Carbamazepine Tablets BP,** carbamazepine 100 mg, net price 20 = 64p; 200 mg, 20 = £1.14; 400 mg, 20 = £2.29. Label: 3

Tricyclic antidepressants. Chronic oral and facial pain (e.g. atypical facial pain or arthritic pain) may call for more prolonged use of analgesics or for other appropriate drugs. Tricyclic antidepressants may be useful for facial pain, particularly if associated with depression (but are not on the list of drugs that may be prescribed by general dental practitioners within the NHS). Long-term prescribing for disorders of this type should only follow a full investigation of the problem and usually involves other specialists. It should always be remembered that patients on long-term therapy need to be monitored both for progress and for side-effects.

Hypnotics and Anxiolytics

> **CSM advice.**
> 1. Benzodiazepines are indicated for the short-term relief (two to four weeks only) of anxiety that is severe, disabling or subjecting the individual to unacceptable distress, occurring alone or in association with insomnia or short-term psychosomatic, organic or psychotic illness.
> 2. The use of benzodiazepines to treat short-term 'mild' anxiety is inappropriate and unsuitable.
> 3. Benzodiazepines should be used to treat insomnia only when it is severe, disabling, or subjecting the individual to extreme distress.

Hypnotics

A drug which acts as an anxiolytic in low dose will act as a hypnotic in a high dose.

The main use of hypnotics in dentistry is to prevent an anxious patient from losing sleep before undergoing a dental operation. Such patients may benefit from the use of a hypnotic for 1 to 3 nights before the dental appointment. Hypnotics do not relieve pain; if pain interferes with sleep an appropriate analgesic should be given.

Temazepam and **nitrazepam** are benzodiazepines used as hypnotics. Nitrazepam has a prolonged action; it may give rise to residual effects on the following day and with repeated dosage tends to be cumulative. Temazepam acts for a shorter time and has little or no hangover effect; withdrawal phenomena are more common with the short-acting benzodiazepines.

For further information see BNF section 4.1.1.

Anxiolytics

These drugs diminish unpleasant feelings of tension, anxiety, and panic (however, particularly when used for deep sedation they can sometimes induce sexual fantasies).

Anxiolytic treatment should be limited to the lowest possible dose for the shortest possible time (see CSM advice above).

Although anxiolytics may help in the treatment of some patients they are no substitute for sympathy, reassurance, and gentle handling by the dental surgeon.

Diazepam has a long half-life and therefore a sustained action; repeated dosage is cumulative.

Temporomandibular joint pain-dysfunction syndrome can be related to anxiety in some patients who may clench or grind their teeth during the day or night. The muscle spasm (which appears to be the main source of pain) may be treated empirically with an overlay appliance which provides a free sliding occlusion and may also interfere with grinding. In addition, **diazepam**, which has muscle relaxant as well as anxiolytic properties, may be helpful but should only be prescribed on a short-term basis during the acute phase. Analgesics such as **aspirin** or **ibuprofen** may also be required.

Diazepam and **temazepam** are often effective anxiolytics for dental treatment in adults; they are less suitable for children. Diazepam can be given to adults in a dose of 5 mg on the preceding night and followed by 5 mg the next day an hour before surgery. **Temazepam** which has a shorter duration of action can be given in a dose of 10 to 30 mg, one hour before surgery. Patients should be warned **not** to drive a car.

GENERAL ANAESTHESIA, SEDATION AND RESUSCITATION

For details of the framework within which general anaesthesia, sedation, and resuscitation can be carried out in general dental practice, see:

> Report of an Expert Working Party on General Anaesthesia, Sedation and Resuscitation in Dentistry, Standing Dental Advisory Committee, London, Department of Health, 1990 and associated documents.

For general information on drugs used in anaesthesia, see BNF chapter 15.

DIAZEPAM

Indications: short-term use in anxiety or insomnia

Cautions: respiratory disease, muscle weakness, history of drug abuse, marked personality disorder, pregnancy, breast-feeding; reduce dose in elderly and debilitated, and in hepatic and renal impairment; avoid prolonged use (and abrupt withdrawal thereafter); special precautions for intravenous injection; **interactions:** see p. 28.

DRIVING. Drowsiness may affect performance of skilled tasks (e.g. driving); effects of alcohol enhanced

Contra-indications: respiratory depression; acute pulmonary insufficiency; phobic or obsessional states, chronic psychosis; porphyria (see BNF section 9.8.2)

Side-effects: drowsiness and lightheadedness which may persist to the next day; confusion and ataxia (especially in the elderly); amnesia may occur; dependence; *occasionally:* headache, vertigo, hypotension, salivation changes, gastro-intestinal disturbances, rashes, visual disturbances, changes in libido, urinary retention; blood disorders and jaundice reported; on intravenous injection, pain, thrombophlebitis and rarely apnoea or hypotension

Dose: 5 mg on night before dental procedure then 5 mg the following day 1 hour before procedure
See also BNF section 4.1.2

PoM **Diazepam Tablets BP,** diazepam 2 mg, net price 20 = 2p; 5 mg, 20 = 2p; 10 mg, 20 = 5p. Label: 2 *or* 19

PoM **Diazepam Oral Solution BP,** (Diazepam Elixir), diazepam 2 mg/5 mL. Net price 100 mL = £1.54. Label: 2 *or* 19

NITRAZEPAM

Indications: insomnia (short-term use)
Cautions; Contra-indications; Side-effects: see under Diazepam
Dose: 5–10 mg at bedtime; ELDERLY (or debilitated), 2.5–5 mg

PoM **Nitrazepam Tablets BP,** nitrazepam 5 mg, net price 20 = 7p. Label: 19

TEMAZEPAM

Indications: insomnia (short-term use)
Cautions; Contra-indications; Side-effects: see under Diazepam; shorter-acting
Dose: 10–30 mg at bedtime; ELDERLY or debilitated, half adult dose

PoM **Temazepam Capsules DPF,** soft gelatin capsules, gel-filled, temazepam 10 mg, net price 20 = 48p; 15 mg, 20 = 62p; 20 mg, 20 = 84p; 30 mg, 20 = £1.24. Label: 19
Note. The Advisory Council on the Misuse of Drugs has warned that the gel-filled capsules may be subject to abuse.

PoM **Temazepam Tablets DPF,** temazepam 10 mg, net price 20 = 48p; 20 mg, 20 = 84p. Label: 19

PoM **Temazepam Oral Solution BP,** (Temazepam Elixir) temazepam 10 mg/5 mL. Net price 100 mL = £2.65. Label: 19

Vitamins

Vitamin deficiency due to inadequate dietary intake is rare in Britain but can develop in elderly people or alcoholics. Most other patients who develop a nutritional deficiency have malabsorption and if this is suspected the patient should be referred to a physician.

It is unjustifiable to treat stomatitis or glossitis with mixtures of vitamin preparations; this delays diagnosis and correct treatment.

Severe cases of scurvy cause gingival swelling and bleeding margins as well as petechiae on the skin. This is, however, exceedingly rare and a patient with this appearance is more likely to have leukaemia. Investigation should not be delayed by a trial period of vitamin treatment.

For further information on vitamins see BNF section 9.6.

ASCORBIC ACID
(Vitamin C)

Indications: prevention and treatment of scurvy
Dose: prophylactic, 25–75 mg daily; therapeutic, not less than 250 mg daily in divided doses

Ascorbic Acid Tablets BP, ascorbic acid 25 mg, net price 20 = 9p; 50 mg, 20 = 7p; 100 mg, 20 = 24p; 200 mg, 20 = 28p; 500 mg (Label: 24), 20 = 68p

Vitamin B Tablets, Compound, Strong, BPC, brown, f/c or s/c, nicotinamide 20 mg, pyridoxine hydrochloride 2 mg, riboflavine 2 mg, thiamine hydrochloride 5 mg. Net price 20 = 9p

Dose: treatment of vitamin B deficiency, 1–2 tablets 3 times daily

Fluorides

Availability of adequate fluoride confers significant resistance to dental caries. It is now considered that the topical action of fluoride on enamel and plaque is more important than the systemic effect.

Where the natural fluoride content of the drinking water is significantly less than 1 mg per litre (one part per million) artificial fluoridation is the most economical method of supplementing fluoride intake.

Daily administration of tablets or drops is a suitable alternative, but systemic fluoride supplements should not be prescribed without prior reference to the fluoride content of the local water supply; they are not advisable when the water contains more than 700 micrograms per litre (0.7 parts per million). In addition, the British Association for the Study of Community Dentistry now recommends that infants need not receive fluoride supplements until the age of 6 months.

Use of dentifrices which incorporate sodium fluoride and/or monofluorophosphate is also a convenient source of fluoride.

Individuals who are either particularly caries prone or medically compromised may be given additional protection by use of fluoride rinses or by application of fluoride gels. Rinses may be used daily or weekly; daily use of a less concentrated rinse is more effective than weekly use of a more concentrated one. Gels must be applied on a regular basis under professional supervision; extreme caution is necessary to prevent the child from swallowing any excess. Less concentrated gels have recently become available for home use. Varnishes are also available and are particularly valuable for young or handicapped children since they adhere to the teeth and set in the presence of moisture.

SODIUM FLUORIDE

Note. Sodium fluoride 2.2 mg provides approx. 1 mg fluoride ion

Indications: prophylaxis of dental caries—see notes above

Contra-indications: not for areas where drinking water is fluoridated

Side-effects: occasional white flecks on teeth with recommended doses; rarely yellowish-brown discoloration if recommended doses are exceeded

Dose: expressed as fluoride ion (F^-):

Water content less than 300 micrograms F^-/litre,
CHILD up to 6 months, none;
6 months–2 years, 250 micrograms F^- daily;
2–4 years, 500 micrograms F^- daily;
over 4 years, 1 mg F^- daily

Water content between 300 and 700 micrograms F^-/litre,
CHILD up to 2 years, none;
2–4 years, 250 micrograms F^- daily;
over 4 years, 500 micrograms F^- daily

Water content above 700 micrograms F^-/litre, supplements not advised (see notes above)

For details of brands and strengths of **sodium fluoride tablets** and **oral drops** available, see BNF p. 349

Mouthwashes
Mouthwashes are not prescribable on form FP14 (GP14 in Scotland) but for details of those available see BNF p. 349

From 1 January 1993 fluoride tablets and oral drops will be prescribable on form FP14 (GP14 in Scotland).

There are also arrangements for health authorities to supply fluoride tablets in the course of pre-school dental schemes, and they may also be supplied in school dental schemes.

Antihistamines

There is no evidence that any one of the older antihistamines is superior to another in antihistamine activity but they differ in duration of action and incidence of the main side-effects, namely antimuscarinic (anticholinergic) effects and drowsiness.

Most antihistamines are relatively short-acting but some, (e.g. **promethazine**), act for up to 12 hours. All are of potential value in nasal allergy, urticaria, and allergic rashes associated with drug allergy. The majority have the serious disadvantage of causing drowsiness (some of the newer antihistamines less so, see BNF section 3.4.1).

Antihistamines are widely used as anti-emetics; it has been suggested that these drugs may be useful in dental surgery for patients with an over-active vomiting reflex, but diazepam is likely to be more effective.

For further information see BNF sections 3.4.1 and 4.6.

CHLORPHENIRAMINE MALEATE
Indications: symptomatic relief of allergy such as hay fever, urticaria
Cautions; Side-effects: see notes and under Promethazine Hydrochloride
DRIVING. Drowsiness may affect performance of skilled tasks (e.g. driving); effects of alcohol enhanced
Dose: 4 mg every 4–6 hours, max. 24 mg daily; CHILD see BNF section 3.4.1

Chlorpheniramine Tablets BP, chlorpheniramine maleate 4 mg. Net price 20 = 9p. Label: 2

PROMETHAZINE HYDROCHLORIDE
Indications: symptomatic relief of allergy such as hay fever, urticaria; anti-emetic
Cautions: epilepsy, prostatic hypertrophy, glaucoma, hepatic disease; avoid in porphyria (see BNF section 9.8.2); **interactions:** see p. 29
DRIVING. Drowsiness may affect performance of skilled tasks (e.g. driving); effects of alcohol enhanced
Side-effects: drowsiness, (rarely paradoxical stimulation, particularly in high dosage and in children), headache, antimuscarinic effects such as urinary retention, dry mouth, blurred vision, gastro-intestinal disturbances; occasional rashes and photosensitivity
Dose: 25 mg at night increased to 50 mg if necessary *or* 10–20 mg 2–3 times daily; CHILD 5–10 years 10–25 mg daily

Promethazine Hydrochloride Tablets BP, coated, promethazine hydrochloride 10 mg, net price 56-tab pack = £1.03; 25 mg, 56-tab pack = £1.53. Label: 2
Note. A proprietary brand of promethazine hydrochloride tablets 20 mg (Sominex®) is on sale to the public for the treatment of occasional insomnia in adults

Promethazine Oral Solution BP, (Promethazine Hydrochloride Elixir), promethazine hydrochloride 5 mg/5 mL. Net price 100 mL = £1.15. Label: 2

Nasal Decongestants

Sinusitis affecting the maxillary antrum can cause pain in the upper jaw; where this is associated with blockage of the opening from the sinus into the nasal cavity it is helpful to use an inhalation or nasal drops.

For the preparation of an **inhalation**, the compound is added to a bowl of hot, not boiling, water and the warm moist air together with the volatile medicaments inhaled; this is assisted by covering the head with a towel. It is probable that it is the moist air which is useful.

Nasal preparations containing sympathomimetic drugs such as **ephedrine** produce vasoconstriction of mucosal blood vessels and decrease in the thickness of the swollen nasal mucosa, giving relief to the nasal obstruction. Prolonged use, however, leads to rebound secondary vasodilatation with recurrences of nasal congestion; further applications of the sympathomimetic preparations result eventually in the development of tolerance, diminished therapeutic effect, and damage to the nasal cilia.

Ephedrine Nasal Drops is effective within 1 minute, and lasts for several hours; tolerance develops rapidly. Ephedrine can be absorbed through the nasal mucosa, therefore the drops should not be used in patients taking MAOIs; see also Interactions, BNF p. 495 (Sympathomimetics)

For further information see BNF sections 3.8 and 12.2.2.

Ephedrine Nasal Drops BP, ephedrine hydrochloride in a suitable aqueous vehicle (see BNF section 12.2.2)
Instil 1–2 drops into each nostril up to 3 or 4 times daily when required
Note. The BP directs that if no strength is specified 0.5% drops should be supplied; net price 10 mL = 80p.

Menthol and Eucalyptus Inhalation BP 1980 (see BNF section 3.8). Net price 50 mL = 19p
Directions for use: add one teaspoonful to a pint of hot, **not** boiling, water and inhale the vapour

Appendix 1: Interactions

Two or more drugs given at the same time may exert their effects independently or may interact. The interaction may be potentiation or antagonism of one drug by another, or occasionally some other effect.

The following list of interactions is a shortened version of the table in the BNF (see pp. 477–98). Some interactions involve drugs that are not on the dental list. For comment on vasoconstrictor interactions see DPF, p. 4.

HAZARDOUS INTERACTIONS. The symbol • has been placed against interactions that are **potentially hazardous** and where combined administration of the drugs involved should be **avoided** (or only undertaken with caution and appropriate monitoring).

Interactions that have no symbol do not usually have serious consequences.

Interactions relevant to drugs in the DPF

Acyclovir *see* BNF p. 477 (systemic only)
Amoxycillin *see* Penicillins
Amphotericin *see* BNF p. 478 (systemic only)
Ampicillin *see* Penicillins
Antihistamines
  Alcohol: enhanced sedative effect
  • Antibacterials: *erythromycin* inhibits *terfenadine* metabolism (*see* BNF p. 127)
  Antidepressants; *tricyclics* increase antimuscarinic and sedative effects
  • Antifungals: *ketoconazole* inhibits *terfenadine* metabolism (cardiac toxicity reported)
  Antimuscarinics: increased antimuscarinic side-effects
  Anxiolytics and Hypnotics: enhanced sedative effect
  Betahistine: antagonism (theoretical)
Aspirin
  Antacids and Adsorbents: excretion of *aspirin* increased in alkaline urine
  • Anticoagulants: increased risk of bleeding due to antiplatelet effect
  Antiepileptics: enhancement of effect of *phenytoin* and sodium valproate
  • Cytotoxics: reduced excretion of *methotrexate* (increased toxicity)
  Diuretics: antagonism of diuretic effect of *spironolactone*; reduced excretion of *acetazolamide* (risk of toxicity)
  Domperidone and Metoclopramide: *metoclopramide* enhances effect of *aspirin* (increased rate of absorption)
  Mifepristone: manufacturer recommends avoid aspirin until 8–12 days after *mifepristone*
  Uricosurics: effect of *probenecid* and *sulphinpyrazone* reduced
Benzodiazepines and other Anxiolytics and Hypnotics
  Alcohol: enhanced sedative effect
  Anaesthetics: enhanced sedative effect
  Analgesics: *opioid analgesics* enhance sedative effect
  Antibacterials: *erythromycin* inhibits metabolism of *midazolam* (increased plasma concentration, **important:** see also BNF p. 465); *isoniazid* inhibits metabolism of *diazepam*; *rifampicin* increases metabolism of *diazepam*

Benzodiazepines (*continued*)
  Anticoagulants: *choral hydrate* may transiently enhance effect of *nicoumalone and warfarin*
  Antidepressants: enhanced sedative effect
  Antiepileptics: metabolism of *clonazepam* accelerated (reduced effect)
  Antihistamines: enhanced sedative effect
  Antihypertensives: enhanced hypotensive effect; enhanced sedative effect with *alpha-blockers*
  Antipsychotics: enhanced sedative effect
  Disulfiram: metabolism of *diazepam and chlordiazepoxide* inhibited (enhanced sedative effect)
  Dopaminergics: *benzodiazepines* occasionally antagonise effect of *levodopa*
  Muscle Relaxants: *baclofen* enhances sedative effect
  Nabilone: enhanced sedative effect
  Ulcer-healing Drugs: *cimetidine* inhibits metabolism of *benzodiazepines and chlormethiazole* (increased plasma concentrations); *omeprazole* inhibits metabolism of *diazepam* (increased plasma concentrations)
Carbamazepine
  Owing to its enzyme-inducing activity carbamazepine interacts with a very large number of drugs, for details see BNF, p. 482
Cephalosporins
  Alcohol: disulfiram-like reaction with *cephamandole*
  • Anticoagulants: anticoagulant effect of *warfarin and nicoumalone* enhanced by *cephamandole* and possibly others
  Probenecid: reduced excretion of *cephalosporins* (increased plasma concentrations)
Chlorpheniramine *see* Antihistamines
Clindamycin
  Cholinergics: antagonism of effect of *neostigmine and pyridostigmine*
  Muscle relaxants: enhancement of effect of *non-depolarising muscle relaxants such as tubocurarine*
Co-trimoxazole and Sulphonamides *see* BNF p. 484
Diazepam *see* Benzodiazepines
Diflunisal *see* NSAIDs
Dihydrocodeine *see* Opioid Analgesics
Doxycycline *see* Tetracyclines
Ephedrine *see* Sympathomimetics
Erythromycin
  Analgesics: plasma concentration of *alfentanil* increased
  • Anti-arrhythmics: plasma concentration of *disopyramide* increased (risk of toxicity)
  • Anticoagulants: effect of *nicoumalone and warfarin* enhanced
  Antiepileptics: inhibition of metabolism of *carbamazepine* (increased plasma-carbamazepine concentration)
  • Antihistamines: inhibition of metabolism of *terfenadine* (*see* BNF p. 127)
  Anxiolytics and Hypnotics: inhibition of metabolism of *midazolam* (increased plasma concentration, **important:** see also BNF p. 465)
  Cardiac Glycosides: effect of *digoxin* enhanced
  • Cyclosporin: inhibition of metabolism (increased plasma-cyclosporin concentration)
  Dopaminergics: plasma concentration of *bromocriptine* increased
  Ergotamine: ergotism reported
  • Theophylline: inhibition of metabolism (increased plasma-theophylline concentration)

Appendix 1: Interactions   29

Ibuprofen see NSAIDs
Metronidazole
  Alcohol: disulfiram-like reaction
• Anticoagulants: effect of *nicoumalone and warfarin* enhanced
• Antiepileptics: *metronidazole* inhibits metabolism of *phenytoin* (increased plasma-phenytoin concentration); *phenobarbitone* accelerates metabolism of *metronidazole* (reduced plasma-metronidazole concentration)
  Disulfiram: pyschotic reactions reported
  Lithium: increased toxicity reported
  Ulcer-healing Drugs: *cimetidine* inhibits metabolism of *metronidazole* (increased plasma-metronidazole concentration)
Miconazole see BNF p. 490 (systemic only)
Nitrazepam see Benzodiazepines
NSAIDs (see also Aspirin)
  Anion-exchange Resins: *cholestyramine* reduces absorption of *phenylbutazone*
  Antacids and Adsorbents: *antacids* reduce absorption of *diflunisal*
• Antibacterials: *NSAIDs* increase risk of convulsions with *4-quinolones*
  Anticoagulants: see Warfarin, BNF p. 497
• Antidiabetics: effect of *sulphonylureas* enhanced by *azapropazone and phenylbutazone*
• Antiepileptics: effect of *phenytoin* enhanced by *azapropazone and phenylbutazone*
  Antihypertensives: antagonism of hypotensive effect; increased risk of renal failure with *ACE inhibitors* and increased risk of hyperkalaemia on administration of *ACE inhibitors* with *indomethacin and possibly other NSAIDs*
  Cardiac Glycosides: *NSAIDs* may exacerbate heart failure, reduce GFR, and increase plasma-cardiac glycoside concentration
• Cyclosporin: increased risk of nephrotoxicity
• Cytotoxics: excretion of *methotrexate* reduced by *aspirin, azapropazone, diclofenac, indomethacin, ketoprofen, naproxen, phenylbutazone* and probably other NSAIDs (increased risk of toxicity)
  Diuretics: risk of nephrotoxicity of *NSAIDs* increased; *NSAIDs* notably indomethacin antagonise diuretic effect; *indomethacin and possibly other NSAIDs* increase risk of hyperkalaemia with *potassium-sparing diuretics*; occasional reports of decreased renal function when *indomethacin* given with *triamterene*
• Lithium: excretion of *lithium* reduced by *diclofenac, ibuprofen, indomethacin, mefenamic acid, naproxen, phenylbutazone, piroxicam, and probably other NSAIDs* (possibility of toxicity)
  Mifepristone: manufacturer recommends avoid aspirin, and *NSAIDs* until 8–12 days after *mifepristone* administration
  Thyroxine: false low total plasma-thyroxine concentration with *phenylbutazone*
  Uricosurics: *probenecid* delays excretion of *indomethacin, ketoprofen, and naproxen* (raised plasma concentrations)

Opioid Analgesics
  Anti-arrhythmics: delayed absorption of *mexiletine*
  Antibacterials: *rifampicin* accelerates metabolism of *methadone* (reduced effect); *erythromycin* increases plasma concentration of *alfentanil*
• Anticoagulants: *dextropropoxyphene* may enhance effect of *nicoumalone and warfarin*
  Antidepressants: CNS excitation or depression (hypertension or hypotension) if *pethidine and possibly other opioid analgesics* given to patients receiving *MAOIs*
• Antiepileptics: *dextropropoxyphene* enhances effect of *carbamazepine*
  Anxiolytics and Hypnotics: enhanced sedative effect
  Cisapride: possible antagonism of gastro-intestinal effect
  Domperidone and Metoclopramide: antagonism of gastro-intestinal effects
  Dopaminergics: hyperpyrexia and CNS toxicity reported with *selegiline*
  Ulcer-healing Drugs: *cimetidine* inhibits metabolism of opioid analgesics notably *pethidine* (increased plasma concentration)
Oxytetracycline see Tetracyclines
Paracetamol
  Anion-exchange Resins: *cholestyramine* reduces absorption of *paracetamol*
  Anticoagulants: prolonged regular use of *paracetamol* possibly enhances *warfarin*
  Antivirals: regular use of *paracetamol* possibly reduces metabolism of *zidovudine* (increased risk of neutropenia)
  Domperidone and Metoclopramide: *metoclopramide* accelerates absorption of *paracetamol* (enhanced effect)
Penicillins
  Antacids: reduced absorption of *pivampicillin*
  Anticoagulants: see Phenindione (BNF p. 492) and Warfarin (BNF p. 497)
  Guar Gum: reduced absorption of *phenoxymethylpenicillin*
  Probenecid: reduced excretion of *penicillins*
  Sex Hormones: see Contraceptives, Oral, BNF p. 484
Pethidine see Opioid Analgesics
Phenoxymethylpenicillin see Penicillins
Promethazine see Antihistamines
Sympathomimetics see BNF p. 495
Temazepam see Benzodiazepines
Tetracyclines
  Antacids: reduced absorption
  Anticoagulants: see Phenindione (BNF p. 492) and Warfarin (BNF p. 497)
  Antiepileptics: *carbamazepine, phenobarbitone, phenytoin, and primidone* increase metabolism of *doxycycline* (reduced plasma concentration)
  Antihypertensives: *quinapril* reduces absorption (tablets contain magnesium carbonate excipient)
  Barbiturates: see under Antiepileptics, above
  Calcium Salts: reduced absorption of *tetracyclines*
  Dairy products: reduced absorption (except *doxycycline* and *minocycline*)
  Iron: absorption of *oral iron* reduced by *tetracyclines* and vice versa
  Sex Hormones: see Contraceptives, Oral, BNF p. 484
  Ulcer-healing Drugs: *bismuth chelate* and *sucralfate* reduce absorption
  Zinc Salts: reduced absorption (and vice versa)

Appendix 2: Liver disease

Liver disease may alter the response to drugs in several ways, and prescribing should be kept to a minimum in all patients with severe liver disease.

Recommendations on the drugs listed in the DPF that should be avoided or used with caution in liver disease are shown in the following table, which is a shortened version of the table given in the BNF (see pp. 499–502).

Table of drugs in the DPF to be avoided or used with caution in liver disease

Drugs	Comment
Aspirin	Avoid—increased risk of gastro-intestinal bleeding
Chlorpheniramine	Avoid—may precipitate coma
Clindamycin	Reduce dose
Diazepam	Can precipitate coma
Diflunisal	Increased risk of gastro-intestinal bleeding and can cause fluid retention
Dihydrocodeine	Avoid—may precipitate coma
Erythromycin	May cause idiosyncratic hepatotoxicity
Ibuprofen	Increased risk of gastro-intestinal bleeding and can cause fluid retention
Lignocaine	Avoid (or reduce dose) in severe liver disease
Metronidazole	Reduce dose in severe liver disease
Nitrazepam	Can precipitate coma
Paracetamol	Dose-related toxicity—avoid large doses
Pethidine	Avoid—may precipitate coma
Promethazine	Avoid—may precipitate coma
Temazepam	Avoid—may precipitate coma
Tetracycline	Avoid—dose-related toxicity by i/v route

Appendix 3: Renal impairment

The use of drugs in patients with reduced renal function can give rise to problems for several reasons. Failure to excrete a drug or its metabolites may produce toxicity; sensitivity to some drugs is increased even if elimination is unimpaired; many side-effects are tolerated poorly by patients with renal impairment; and some drugs cease to be effective when renal function is reduced. Many of these problems can be avoided by reducing the dose or by using alternative drugs. Discussion with the general medical practitioner is advisable.

Recommendations on the drugs listed in the DPF that should be avoided or used with caution in patients with renal impairment are shown in the following table, which is a shortened version of the table given in the BNF (see pp. 503–9). Dose recommendations are based on the severity of renal impairment.

Dialysis and renal transplants

Heparin is only active for about 6 hours and the optimum time for dental treatment is on the day after dialysis when the dialysis is having its maximum effect and the effect of the heparin has worn off. Precautions regarding the use of drugs in renal impairment should be observed in dialysis patients.

Renal transplant and immunosuppressed patients should be treated on the merits of the individual case, if necessary with specialist referral. See also advice on p. 4.

Table of drugs in the DPF to be avoided or used with caution in renal impairment

Drugs	Dosage recommendations	Comments
Acyclovir	Reduce dose	Possible transient increase in plasma urea
Amoxycillin	Reduce dose	Rashes more common
Amphotericin	Use only if no alternative	Nephrotoxic
Ampicillin	Reduce dose	Rashes more common
Aspirin	Avoid	Fluid retention; deterioration in renal function; increased risk of gastro-intestinal bleeding
Benzylpenicillin	Max. 6 g daily in severe impairment	Neurotoxicity—high doses may cause convulsions
Cephalexin	Max. 500 mg daily in severe impairment	
Cephradine	Reduce dose	
Co-trimoxazole	Reduce dose	Rashes and blood disorders; may cause further deterioration in renal function
Diazepam	Start with small doses	Increased cerebral sensitivity
Diflunisal	Avoid if possible	Excreted by kidney; sodium and water retention and deterioration in renal function (**important:** see BNF p. 359)
Dihydrocodeine	Avoid	Increased and prolonged effect
Erythromycin	Max. 1.5 g daily in severe impairment	Ototoxicity
Ibuprofen	Avoid if possible	Sodium and water retention and deterioration in renal function (**important:** see BNF p. 359)
Nitrazepam	Start with small doses	Increased cerebral sensitivity
Pethidine	Avoid	Increased CNS toxicity
Temazepam	Start with small doses	Increased cerebral sensitivity
Tetracyclines (except doxycycline)	Avoid	Anti-anabolic effect, increased plasma urea, further deterioration in renal function

Appendix 4: Pregnancy

Drugs can have harmful effects on the fetus at any time during pregnancy. Experience with many drugs in pregnancy is limited.

During the *first trimester* they may produce congenital malformations (teratogenesis), and the period of greatest risk is from the third to the eleventh week of pregnancy.

During the *second* and *third trimesters* drugs may affect the growth and functional development of the fetus or have toxic effects on fetal tissues; and drugs given shortly before term or during labour may have adverse effects on the neonate after delivery.

Recommendations on the drugs listed in the DPF that should be avoided or used with caution in pregnancy are shown in the following table which is a shortened version of the table given in the BNF (see pp. 510–16).

Drugs should be prescribed in pregnancy only if the expected benefit to the mother is thought to be greater than the risk to the fetus, and all drugs should be avoided if possible during the first trimester. Drugs which have been extensively used in pregnancy and appear to be usually safe should be prescribed in preference to new or untried drugs; and the smallest effective dose should be used.

Few drugs have been shown conclusively to be teratogenic in man but no drug is safe beyond all doubt in early pregnancy. Screening procedures are available where there is a known risk of certain defects.

It should be noted that the DPF provides independent advice and may not always agree with the data sheets.

Absence of a drug from the list does not imply safety.

Table of drugs in the DPF to be avoided or used with caution in pregnancy

Drugs (trimester of risk)	Comments
Antihistamines *see* BNF p. 511	
Aspirin (3)	Impaired platelet function and risk of haemorrhage; delayed onset and increased duration of labour with increased blood loss; avoid analgesic doses if possible in last week of pregnancy; with high doses, closure of fetal ductus arteriosus *in utero* and possibly persistent pulmonary hypertension of newborn; kernicterus in jaundiced neonates
Benzodiazepines (3)	Depress neonatal respiration; cause neonatal drowsiness, hypotonia, and withdrawal symptoms; avoid large doses and regular use; short-acting benzodiazepines preferable to long-acting
Carbamazepine	Avoid in neuralgia (but for epilepsy see BNF p. 186)
Co-trimoxazole (1)	Possible teratogenic risk (trimethoprim a folate antagonist)
(3)	Neonatal haemolysis and methaemoglobinaemia; fear of increased risk of kernicterus in neonates appears to be unfounded
Diazepam *see* Benzodiazepines	
Diflunisal *see* NSAIDs	
Dihydrocodeine *see* Opioid Analgesics	
Doxycycline *see* Tetracyclines	
Ibuprofen *see* NSAIDs	
Idoxuridine in Dimethyl Sulphoxide	Avoid
Metronidazole	Manufacturer advises avoidance of high-dose regimens
Nitrazepam *see* Benzodiazepines	
NSAIDs (3)	With regular use closure of fetal ductus arteriosus *in utero* and possibly persistent pulmonary hypertension of the newborn
	Delayed onset and increased duration of labour
Opioid Analgesics (3)	Depress neonatal respiration; withdrawal effects in neonates of dependent mothers; gastric stasis and risk of inhalation pneumonia in mother during labour
Oxytetracycline *see* Tetracyclines	
Pethidine *see* Opioid Analgesics	
Povidone-iodine (2, 3)	Sufficient iodine may be absorbed to affect fetal thyroid
Temazepam *see* Benzodiazepines	
Tetracyclines (2, 3)	Dental discoloration; maternal hepatotoxicity with large parenteral doses

Appendix 5: Breast-feeding

The following is a shortened version of the table given in the BNF (for full table, see BNF pp. 517–21).

It lists drugs:
which should be used only with caution or which are contra-indicated in breast-feeding;
which, on present evidence, may be given to the mother during breast-feeding, because they are excreted in milk in amounts which are too small to be harmful to the infant;
which are not known to be harmful to the infant although they are present in milk in significant amounts.

Because of the inadequacy of currently available information on drugs in breast milk the following table should be used only as a guide; absence from the table does not imply safety.

Table of drugs in the DPF excreted in breast milk

Drugs	Comments
Antihistamines	Significant amount of some but not known to be harmful
Aspirin	Avoid—possible risk of Reye's syndrome; regular use of high doses could impair platelet function and produce hypoprothrombinaemia in infant if neonatal vitamin K stores low
Benzodiazepines	Avoid repeated doses; lethargy and weight loss may occur in infant
Carbamazepine	Avoid in neuralgia but for epilepsy, see BNF, p. 186
Chlorpheniramine *see* Antihistamines	
Co-trimoxazole	Small risk of kernicterus in jaundiced infants and of haemolysis in G6PD-deficient infants (due to sulphamethoxazole)
Diazepam *see* Benzodiazepines	
Doxycycline *see* Tetracyclines	
Ephedrine	Irritability and disturbed sleep reported
Ibuprofen	Amount too small to be harmful
Idoxuridine	May possibly make milk taste unpleasant
Metronidazole	Significant amount in milk; avoid for 24 hours after large single doses; may give a bitter taste to the milk
Nitrazepam *see* Benzodiazepines	
Oxytetracycline *see* Tetracyclines	
Paracetamol	Amount too small to be harmful
Povidone-iodine	Avoid—iodine absorbed is concentrated in milk
Promethazine *see* Antihistamines	
Temazepam *see* Benzodiazepines	
Tetracyclines	Some authorities recommend avoidance but absorption and therefore discoloration of teeth in infant probably prevented by chelation with calcium in milk

List of Dental Preparations

The following list has been approved by the appropriate Secretaries of State, and the preparations therein may be prescribed by dental practitioners on form FP14 (GP14 in Scotland).

If requested, **sugar-free** versions will be dispensed where available

Acyclovir Cream, DPF
Acyclovir Oral Suspension, DPF
Acyclovir Tablets 200 mg, DPF
Amoxycillin Capsules, BP
Amoxycillin Injection, DPF
Amoxycillin Oral Powder, DPF
Amoxycillin Oral Suspension, BP
Amoxycillin Tablets, Dispersible, DPF
Amphotericin Lozenges, BP
Amphotericin Oral Suspension, DPF
Amphotericin Tablets, DPF
Ampicillin Capsules, BP
Ampicillin Oral Suspension, BP
Artificial Saliva, DPF
Ascorbic Acid Tablets, BP
Aspirin Tablets, Dispersible, BP[1]
Benzydamine Mouthwash, DPF
Benzydamine Oral Spray, DPF
Benzylpenicillin Injection, BP
Carbamazepine Tablets, BP
Carmellose Gelatin Paste, DPF
Cephalexin Capsules, BP
Cephalexin Oral Suspension, DPF
Cephalexin Tablets, BP
Cephradine Capsules, BP
Cephradine Injection, DPF
Cephradine Oral Solution, DPF
Chlorhexidine Gluconate gels containing at least 1 per cent
Chlorhexidine Mouthwash, DPF[2]
Chlorpheniramine Tablets, BP
Choline Salicylate Dental Gel, BP
Clindamycin Capsules, BP
Clindamycin Injection, DPF
Clindamycin Oral Suspension, Paediatric, DPF
Co-trimoxazole Oral Suspension, BP
Co-trimoxazole Oral Suspension, Paediatric, BP
Co-trimoxazole Tablets, BP
Co-trimoxazole Tablets, Dispersible, BP
Co-trimoxazole Tablets, Paediatric, BP
Diazepam Oral Solution, BP
Diazepam Tablets, BP
Diflunisal Tablets, BP
Dihydrocodeine Tablets, BP
Doxycycline Capsules 100 mg, BP
Ephedrine Nasal Drops, BP
Erythromycin Ethyl Succinate Oral Suspension, DPF
Erythromycin Ethyl Succinate Oral Suspension, Paediatric, DPF
Erythromycin Ethyl Succinate Tablets, DPF
Erythromycin Lactobionate Intravenous Infusion, BP
Erythromycin Stearate Tablets, BP
Erythromycin Tablets, BP
Hydrocortisone Cream, BP
Hydrocortisone Lozenges, BPC
Hydrocortisone and Miconazole Cream, DPF
Hydrocortisone and Miconazole Ointment, DPF
Hydrogen Peroxide Mouthwash, DPF
Ibuprofen Oral Suspension, DPF
Ibuprofen Tablets, BP
Idoxuridine 5% in Dimethyl Sulphoxide, DPF
Lignocaine 5% Ointment, DPF
Menthol and Eucalyptus Inhalation, BP 1980[3]
Metronidazole Oral Suspension, DPF
Metronidazole Tablets, BP
Miconazole Oral Gel, DPF
Mouthwash Solution-tablets, DPF
Nitrazepam Tablets, BP
Nystatin Ointment, BP
Nystatin Oral Suspension, BP
Nystatin Pastilles, DPF
Nystatin Tablets, BP
Oxytetracycline Capsules, BP
Oxytetracycline Tablets, BP
Paracetamol Oral Suspension, Paediatric, BP[4]
Paracetamol Tablets, BP
Paracetamol Tablets, Dispersible, DPF
Penicillin Triple Injection, BPC
Pethidine Tablets, BP
Phenoxymethylpenicillin Capsules, BP
  [not currently available]
Phenoxymethylpenicillin Oral Solution, BP
Phenoxymethylpenicillin Tablets, BP
Povidone-iodine Mouthwash, DPF
Promethazine Hydrochloride Tablets, BP
Promethazine Oral Solution, BP
Sodium Chloride Mouthwash, Compound, BP
Sodium Fluoride Oral Drops, DPF[5]
Sodium Fluoride Tablets, DPF[5]
Sodium Fusidate Ointment, BP
  (former title Fusidic Acid Ointment, DPF)
Sodium Perborate Mouthwash, DPF
Temazepam Capsules, DPF
Temazepam Oral Solution, DPF
Temazepam Tablets, DPF
Tetracycline Capsules, BP
Tetracycline Tablets, BP
Thymol Glycerin, Compound, BP
Triamcinolone Dental Paste, BP
Vitamin B Tablets, Compound, Strong, BPC
Zinc Sulphate Mouthwash, DPF
  [not currently available]

---

1. Addendum 1989 to BP 1988 has directed that when soluble aspirin tablets are prescribed, dispersible aspirin tablets should be dispensed
2. This includes spray presentation
3. This preparation does not appear in BP 1988
4. BP 1988 directs that when Paediatric Paracetamol Oral Suspension or Paediatric Paracetamol Mixture is prescribed and no strength stated Paracetamol Oral Suspension 120 mg/5 mL should be dispensed
5. With effect from 1 January, 1993

Additions

Ibuprofen Oral Suspension, DPF
Sodium Fluoride Oral Drops, DPF (with effect from 1 January 1993)

Sodium Fluoride Tablets, DPF (with effect from 1 January 1993)

Deletions

Amphotericin Ointment, DPF
Diazepam Capsules, BP
Erythromycin Ethyl Succinate Oral Powder, DPF

Procaine Penicillin Injection, BP
Tetracycline Oral Suspension, BP

Changes of Title

The following changes of name are in accordance with new approved names issued by the British Pharmacopoeia Commission:

Old	New
Erythromycin Lactobionate Injection, DPF	Erythromycin Lactobionate Intravenous Infusion, BP
Temazepam Oral Solution, DPF	Temazepam Oral Solution, BP

Index

A

Abbreviations, *inside front cover*
Abscess, 11
Acknowledgements, ix
Actinomycosis, 11, 12
Acyclovir, 18
  interactions, *see* BNF
  preparations, 18
  renal impairment, 31
Additions, 35
Adrenal suppression, 2
Adrenaline
  allergic emergencies, 2
  local anaesthesia, 6
ADROIT, 8
Adverse reactions to drugs, 8
Allergic disorders, 27
Allergic emergencies, 2
Amoxycillin, 12
  endocarditis, 5
  interactions, 28
  preparations, 12–13
  renal impairment, 31
Amphotericin, 17
  interactions, *see* BNF
  preparations, 17
    ointment, 35
  renal impairment, 31
Ampicillin, 12, **13**
  interactions, 28
  preparations, 13
  renal impairment, 31
Analgesics, 21–4
  anti-inflammatory, 21
  local, 19
  non-opioid, 21
  NSAIDs, 21
    interactions, 29
    pregnancy, 32
  opioid, 23
    interactions, 29
    pregnancy, 32
  topical, 19
  see also individual drugs
Anaphylaxis, 2
Angina, 2
Angular cheilitis, 16, 17, 20
Antibacterial drugs, 11–16
  endocarditis prophylaxis, 5
Antibiotics *see* Antibacterial drugs
Anticoagulants, surgery and, 6
Antifungal drugs, 17
Antihistamines, 27
  breast-feeding, 33
  interactions, 28
  pregnancy, *see* BNF
Antihypertensives, anaesthesia and, 6
Antiseptics, mouth, 10
Antiviral drugs, 18
Anxiety, 24
Anxiolytics, 24
  see also Benzodiazepines
Aphthous ulcers, 14, **19**
Arrangement of information, x
Arrhythmias, 2, 6
Artificial saliva, 19, 20
Ascorbic acid, 25
  tablets, 25
Aspirin, 21, **22**
  breast-feeding, 33
  interactions, 28
  liver disease, 30
  pregnancy, 32
  renal impairment, 31
  Reye's syndrome and, 21
  tablets,
    dispersible, 22
    soluble, 22

B

Bacterial endocarditis, 4–5
Benethamine penicillin, 12
Benzodiazepines, 24
  breast-feeding, 33
  interactions, 28
  pregnancy, 32
Benzydamine, 19
  preparations, 20
Benzylpenicillin, 12
  injection, 12
  renal impairment, 31
Bone infections, 15
Breast-feeding, prescribing in, 33

C

Candidiasis, 17
Carbamazepine, 23
  breast-feeding, 33
  interactions, *see* BNF
  pregnancy, 32
  tablets, 24
Cardiovascular disease, prescribing in, 6
Carmellose gelatin paste, 19, **20**
Cellulitis, 11, 12
Cephalexin, 13
  preparations, 13
  renal impairment, 31
Cephalosporins, 13
  interactions, 28
Cephradine, 13
  preparations, 13
  renal impairment, 31
Cheilitis, angular 16, 17, 20

Children, prescribing for, *see* BNF
Chlorhexidine, 10
  endocarditis, 4
  preparations, 10
Chlorpheniramine, 27
  injection, 2
  liver disease, 30
  tablets, 27
  see also Antihistamines
Choline salicylate dental gel, 19, **20**
  oral mucosa and, 7
Cleansers, mouth, 10
Clindamycin, 15
  endocarditis, 5
  interactions, 28
  liver disease, 30
  preparations, 15
Contents, vii
Convulsions, 3
Corticosteroids,
  adrenal suppression, 2
  oral ulceration, 19
Co-trimoxazole, 16
  breast-feeding, 33
  interactions, *see* BNF
  pregnancy, 32
  preparations, 16
  renal impairment, 31

D

Decongestants, nasal, 27
Defective medicines, 8
Deletions, 35
Dental preparations, list of, 34
Denture stomatitis, 17
Dentures, painful, 19
Dextrose, *see* Glucose
Diabetes mellitus, 3
Dialysis patients, 31
Diazepam, 24, **25**
  epileptic seizures, 3
  liver disease, 30
  preparations, 25
    capsules, 35
  renal impairment, 31
  see also Benzodiazepines
Diflunisal, 21, **22**
  liver disease, 30
  renal impairment, 31
  tablets, 22
  see also Analgesics, NSAIDs
Dihydrocodeine, 23
  liver disease, 30
  renal impairment, 31
  tablets, 23
  see also Analgesics, opioid
Doses, 1

Index 37

Doxycycline, 14
  capsules, 14
  see also Tetracycline
Drug information services, x
Dry mouth, 19

E

Elderly, prescribing for, 1
Emergencies, medical, 2
  drugs for use in, 2
Endocarditis, prophylaxis, 4–5
Ephedrine, 27
  breast-feeding, 33
  interactions, see BNF
  nasal drops, 27
Epilepsy, 3
Erythromycin, 14
  endocarditis, 14
  interactions, 28–9
  liver disease, 30
  preparations, 14–15
  renal impairment, 31
Erythromycin ethyl succinate oral powder, 35

F

Facial pain, 23
Fainting, 2
Felypressin, 6
Fluoride, 26
  preparations, see BNF
Fungal infections, 17
Fusidic acid ointment, 16

G

Gas cylinders, identification of, see BNF
Gingival hyperplasia, 7
Gingivitis,
  acute ulcerative, 10, 15
  as side-effect, 7
Glossopharyngeal neuralgia, 23
Glucagon, 3
Glucose, 3
Glyceryl trinitrate, preparations, 3

H

Heparin, 6
Herpes labialis, 18
Herpes zoster, see BNF
Herpetic stomatitis, 18
Hip replacement, prophylaxis, 4

Hydrocortisone, 19
  miconazole and, 19
  preparations, 20
    injection, 2
    miconazole and, 20
Hydrogen peroxide mouth-wash, 10
Hypertension, 6
Hyperventilation, 2
Hypnotics, 24
  see also Benzodiazepines
Hypoglycaemia, 3

I

Ibuprofen, 22
  breast-feeding, 33
  liver disease, 30
  preparations, 22
  renal impairment, 31
  see also Analgesics, NSAIDs
Idoxuridine, 18
  5% in dimethyl sulphoxide, 18
  breast-feeding, 33
  pregnancy, 32
Immunosuppression, prophylaxis, 4
Infections,
  bacterial, 11–16
  fungal, 17
  viral, 18
Infective endocarditis, 4–5
Inflammation, oral, 19
Information services, drugs, x
Inhalations, 27
Insomnia, 24
Interactions, 28–9

J

Joint infections, 15
  see also Osteomyelitis
Joint prostheses, prophylaxis, 4

K

Kidney impairment, 31

L

Labelling of medicines, 1
  cautionary and advisory, see BNF
Leukoplakia, 17
Lichen planus, erosive, 19
Lignocaine, 19
  5% ointment, 20
  liver disease, 30
  vasoconstrictors and, 6

List of dental preparations, 34
Liver disease, prescribing in, 30
Local anaesthetic solutions, vasoconstrictors in, 6
Local analgesics, 19
Lupus erythematosus, discoid, 19

M

MAOIs, opioid analgesics and, 23
Menthol and eucalyptus inhalation, 27
Metronidazole, 15
  breast-feeding, 33
  interactions, 29
  liver disease, 30
  pregnancy, 32
  preparations, 15
Miconazole, 17
  hydrocortisone and, 19, **20**
  interactions, see BNF
  oral gel, 17
Milk, drugs in, 33
Mouthwash solution-tablets, 10
Mouthwashes, 10
Mucosa, oral, side-effects on, 7
Muscle spasm, 24
Myocardial infarction, 3

N

Nasal decongestants, 27
Neuralgia, 23
Nicoumalone, 6
Nitrazepam, 24, **25**
  liver disease, 30
  renal impairment, 31
  tablets, 25
  see also Benzodiazepines
Nitrous oxide-oxygen, myocardial infarction, 3
Noradrenaline, hypertensive episodes, 6
'NP' labelling, 1
NSAIDs (Non-steroidal anti-inflammatory drugs) see Analgesics
Nutritional deficiency, 25
Nystatin, 17
  preparations, 17

O

Opioid analgesics see Analgesics, opioid
Oral infections, local treatment of, 10
Oral inflammation, 19
Oral syringe, x
Oral ulceration, 19

Osteomyelitis, 11, 12
Oxytetracycline, 14
   preparations, 14
   see also Tetracycline

P

Pain, 21
   facial, 23
Panic, 24
Paracetamol, 22
   breast-feeding, 33
   interactions, 29
   liver disease, 30
   preparations, 23
Pemphigoid, benign mucous membrane, 19
Penicillin G *see* Benzylpenicillin
Penicillin V *see* Phenoxymethylpenicillin
Penicillin triple injection, 12
Penicillins, 11
   anaphylactic reactions, 11
   broad-spectrum, 12
Pericoronitis, 15
Pethidine, 23
   liver disease, 30
   MAOIs and, 23
   renal impairment, 31
   tablets, 23
   see also Analgesics, opioid
Phenindione, 6
Phenoxymethylpenicillin, 12
   interactions, 29
   preparations, 12
      capsules, 34
Plaque, inhibition of, 10
Poisons information services, *inside front cover* (see also BNF)
Povidone-iodine, 10
   breast-feeding, 33
   mouthwash, 10
   pregnancy, 32
Preface, ix
Pregnancy, prescribing in, 32
Prescription writing, 1
Prilocaine, 6
Procain penicillin, 12
   injection, 35
Promethazine, 27
   liver disease, 30
   preparations, 27
   see also Antihistamines

Prophylaxis,
   endocarditis, 4–5
   immunosuppression, 4
   joint prostheses, 4
   transplants, 4
Pseudomembranous colitis, 12, **15**

R

Renal impairment, prescribing in, 31
Rheumatic heart disease, 4

S

Salbutamol, medical emergencies, 2
Salicylates, topical, 19, **20**
Saline mouthwash, 10
Saliva, artificial, 19, 20
Salivary glands, side-effects on, 7
Scurvy, 25
Sialadenitis, 11, 12, 16
Sinusitis, 12, 14
Sodium chloride compound mouthwash, 10
Sodium fluoride, 26
   preparations, *see* BNF
Sodium fusidate ointment, 16
Sodium perborate mouthwash, 10
Soft-tissue infection, 12–13, 16
Sport, prescribing and, *see* BNF
Status epilepticus, 3
Stomatitis,
   denture, 17
   herpetic, 18
Sugar, x
Sulphamethoxazole, 16
Sulphonamides, 16
Sympathomimetic nasal decongestants, 27
Syncope, 2
Syringe, oral, x

T

Taste disturbance, 7
Teeth, grinding, 24
Teeth, staining of, 7

Teething, topical salicylates, 19
Temazepam, 24, **25**
   liver disease, 30
   preparations, 25
   renal impairment, 31
   see also Benzodiazepines
Temporomandibular joint pain-dysfunction syndrome, 24
Tetracycline, 14
   breast-feeding, 33
   interactions, 29
   liver disease, 30
   pregnancy, 32
   preparations, 14
      suspension, 35
   renal impairment, 31
   staining of teeth, 7
Tetracyclines *see* Tetracycline
Thrush, 17
Thymol, 10
   glycerin, compound, 10
Triamcinolone dental paste, 19, **20**
Trigeminal neuralgia, 23
Trimethoprim, 16

U

Ulceration, 19
   as side-effect, 7

V

Vasoconstrictors, local anaesthetics and, 6
Vincent's infection, 10, 15
Viral infections, 18
Vitamin B tablets, compound, strong, 25
Vitamin C, 25
Vitamins, 25
Vomiting reflex, over-active, 27

W

Warfarin, 6

Z

Zinc sulphate mouthwash, 34

BRITISH NATIONAL FORMULARY

September 1992

BRITISH NATIONAL FORMULARY

Number 24
(September 1992)

British Medical Association
and
Royal Pharmaceutical Society of Great Britain

Copyright 1992 © by the British Medical Association and the Royal Pharmaceutical Society of Great Britain

Copies may be obtained through any bookseller or, in any case of difficulty, direct from the publishers:

British Medical Association
Tavistock Square
London WC1H 9JP, England

The Pharmaceutical Press
Royal Pharmaceutical Society of Great Britain
1 Lambeth High Street
London SE1 7JN, England

ISBN: 0 85369 254 8. ISSN: 0260–535X

All rights reserved. No part of this publication may be reproduced, stored in a retrieval system, or transmitted in any form or by any means—electronic, mechanical, photocopying, recording or otherwise—without the prior written permission of the joint copyright holders.

Typeset in Great Britain by Page Bros, Norwich, Norfolk NR6 6SA and printed and bound by The Bath Press, Bath, Avon BA2 3BL.

Joint Formulary Committee 1992–93

Chairman
C. F. George, BSc, MD, FRCP, FFPM

Deputy Chairman
C. R. Hitchings, BPharm, MSc, FRPharmS, MCPP

Committee Members

Alison Blenkinsopp, PhD, BPharm, MRPharmS
P. E. Green, BSc, MSc, LLM, MRPharmS
P. A. Leech, MRCS, LRCP, DMJ(clin)
F. P. Marsh, MA, MB, BChir, FRCP
G. M. Mitchell, KStJ, MB, ChB, FRPharmS
Jane Richards, MB BS, MRCS, LRCP, FRCGP, D(Obst)RCOG, DCH
P. C. Waller, MD, MRCP
N. L. Wood, BPharm, MRPharmS

Joint Secretaries
Natalie-Jane Macdonald, MB, ChB, MRCP
A. Wade, BPharm, MPhil, FRPharmS

Executive Editor
Anne B. Prasad, FRPharmS

Senior Assistant Editor
Sheenagh M. Townsend-Smith, BSc, DipLib

Assistant Editors
D. K. Mehta, BPharm, MSc, MRPharmS
Anjana Patel, BPharm, MSc, PhD, MRPharmS

Editorial Assistants
Pamela M. Mason, BSc, MSc, PhD, MRPharmS
Sunayana A. Shah, BPharm, MRPharmS
M. J. Timmis, BPharm, MRPharmS

Executive Secretary
Susan M. Thomas, BSc(Econ), MA

Contents

	Page
Arrangement of Information	ix
Preface	x
Changes	xi
Drug Information Services	xiv

GUIDANCE ON PRESCRIBING — 1

    General Guidance — 2
    Prescription Writing — 4
    Controlled Drugs and Drug Dependence — 7
    Adverse Reactions to Drugs — 10
    Prescribing for Children — 11
    Prescribing in Terminal Care — 12
    Prescribing for the Elderly — 14

EMERGENCY TREATMENT OF POISONING — 15

CLASSIFIED NOTES ON DRUGS AND PREPARATIONS

1: **Gastro-intestinal System** — 24
    1.1 Antacids — 24
    1.2 Antispasmodics and other drugs altering gut motility — 27
    1.3 Ulcer-healing drugs — 31
    1.4 Antidiarrhoeal drugs — 35
    1.5 Treatment of chronic diarrhoeas — 37
    1.6 Laxatives — 40
    1.7 Preparations for haemorrhoids — 45
    1.8 Stoma care — 47
    1.9 Drugs affecting intestinal secretions — 58

2: **Cardiovascular System** — 61
    2.1 Positive inotropic drugs — 61
    2.2 Diuretics — 63
    2.3 Anti-arrhythmic drugs — 69
    2.4 Beta-adrenoceptor blocking drugs — 75
    2.5 Antihypertensive therapy — 81
    2.6 Nitrates and calcium-channel blockers — 90
    2.7 Sympathomimetics — 98
    2.8 Anticoagulants and protamine — 102
    2.9 Antiplatelet drugs — 105
    2.10 Fibrinolytic drugs — 106
    2.11 Antifibrinolytic drugs and haemostatics — 107
    2.12 Lipid-lowering drugs — 109
    2.13 Local sclerosants — 112

3: **Respiratory System** — 113
    3.1 Bronchodilators — 113
    3.2 Corticosteroids — 122
    3.3 Cromoglycate and related therapy — 125
    3.4 Antihistamines, hyposensitisation, and allergic emergencies — 126
    3.5 Respiratory stimulants and surfactants — 131

Drug Information Services

Information on any aspect of drug therapy can be obtained, free of charge, from Regional and District Drug Information Services. Details regarding the *local* services provided within your Region can be obtained by telephoning the following numbers.

England

Birmingham	021-311 1974	Direct Line
	or 021-378 2211	Extn 2296/2297
Bristol	0272 282867	Direct Line
Guildford	0483 504312	Direct Line
Ipswich	0473 704430	Direct Line
	or 0473 704431	Direct Line
Leeds	0532 430715	Direct Line
Leicester	0533 555779	Direct Line
Liverpool	051-236 4620	Extn 2126/2127/2128
London (Guy's Hospital)	071-955 5000	Extn 3594/5892
	or 071-378 0023	Direct Line
London (London Hospital)	071-377 7487	Direct Line
	or 071-377 7488	Direct Line
London (Northwick Park)	081-869 3973	Direct Line
Manchester	061-225 2063	Direct Line
	or 061-276 6270	Direct Line
Newcastle	091-232 1525	Direct Line
Oxford	0865 221808	Direct Line
	or 0865 221836	Direct Line
Southampton	0703 796908	Direct Line
	or 0703 796909	Direct Line

Northern Ireland

Belfast	0232 248095	Direct Line
Londonderry	0504 45171	Extn 3262

Scotland

Aberdeen	0224 681818	Extn 52316
Dundee	0382 60111	Extn 2351
Edinburgh	031-229 2477	Extn 2094/2416/2443
	or 031-229 3901	Direct Line
Glasgow	041-552 4726	Direct Line
Inverness	0463 234151	Extn 288
	or 0463 220157	Direct Line

Wales

Cardiff	0222 742979	Direct Line

Poisons Information Services

Belfast	0232 240503
Birmingham	021-554 3801
Cardiff	0222 709901
Dublin	0001 379964 *or* 0001 379966
Edinburgh	031-229 2477
	or 031-228 2441 (Viewdata)
Leeds	0532 430715 *or* 0532 432799
London	071-635 9191 *or* 071-955 5095
Newcastle	091-232 5131

Note. Some of these centres also advise on laboratory analytical services which may be of help in the diagnosis and management of a small number of cases.

New Preparations (continued)

▼ PoM Lamisil® (Sandoz)
Cream, terbinafine hydrochloride 1%. Net price 15 g = £4.98; 30 g = £8.98. BNF section 13.10.2
Additives: benzyl alcohol, polysorbate 60
Administration: fungal skin infections, apply thinly 1–2 times daily for up to 1 week in tinea pedis, 1–2 weeks in tinea corporis and tinea cruris, 2 weeks in cutaneous candidiasis and pityriasis versicolor; CHILD not yet recommended
Side-effects: redness, itching, or stinging at site of application; rarely allergic reactions (discontinue treatment)

Oramorph® Unit Dose Vials (Boehringer Ingelheim)
PoM *Oral vials*, morphine sulphate 10 mg/5-mL vial, net price 25 vials = £3.31. Label: 2. BNF section 4.7.2
CD *Oral vials*, morphine sulphate 30 mg/5-mL vial, net price 25 vials = £9.30; 100 mg/5-mL vial, 25 vials = £31.00. Label: 2

▼ PoM Recormon® S (Boehringer Mannheim)
Injection (for subcutaneous use), powder for reconstitution, epoetin beta. Net price 1000-unit vial = £9.00; 2000-unit vial = £18.00 (both with syringe and water for injections). BNF section 9.1.3

PoM Timoptol® (MSD)
Preservative-free eye-drops, timolol (as maleate) 0.25%, net price 30 × 0.25 mL = £9.60; 0.5%, 30 × 0.25 mL = £10.97. BNF section 11.6

PoM Zumenon® (Duphar)
Tablets, blue, f/c, oestradiol 2 mg, net price 28-tab pack = £2.55. BNF section 6.4.1.1
Dose: menopausal symptoms (but not osteoporosis prophylaxis), with progestogen for 10–14 days per cycle if uterus intact, starting on the 5th day of menstruation (or any time if cycles have ceased or are infrequent) 1–2 tablets daily

---

Preparations included in appropriate sections of BNF No. 24

Adalat LA, p.95
AeroBec-100, p. 123
Alnide, p. 381
Alomide, p. 380
Becloforte Diskhaler, p. 124
Calcichew D3, p. 352
Clarityn syrup, p. 127
Codafen Continus, p. 360
Creon-25000, p. 60
Cystrin, p. 298
Depixol Low Volume, p. 154

Diamox SR, p. 384
Elantan LA-25, p. 93
Estracombi, p. 270
Havrix, p. 447
Haemophilus influenza vaccine, p. 447
HeplexAmine, p. 343
Histoacryl, p. 430
Ibugel, p. 375
Imigran tablets, p. 183
Lactitol powder, p. 44

Li-Liquid, p. 156
Liquifilm Tears (preservative-free), p. 386
Lithofalk, p. 59
Lyclear dermal cream, p. 430
Metrogel, p. 425
Ocufen, p. 386
One-alpha injection, p. 353
Prepulsid suspension, p. 30
Proleukin, p. 321
Remedeine, p. 175

Salofalk, p. 39
Sevredol suppositories, p. 179
Suprecur, p. 282
Tarivid infusion, p. 233
Triadene, p. 293
Trosyl cream, p. 427
Typhim Vi, p. 454
Unicap preparations, p. 329
Vivotif, p. 454

Note. Neo-Naclex-K remains available

Discontinued Preparations

Preparations discontinued during the compilation of BNF No. 24

Abidec capsules
Alka-Donna-P
Alka-Donna-P
Aludrox SA
Antepar tablets
Antoin
Aradolene
Bactrim paediatric tablets
Barquinol HC
Baypen
BC 500 with Iron
Bronchilator
Cardiacap
Cedilanid
Colgen
Cotazym
Cyclospasmol

Diamox Sustets
Elyzol suppositories
Ergometrine tablets
Glykola
Golytely
Gynatren
Hibidil
Hypercal
Hyperdrol
Lachesine eye-drops
Ledercort ointment
Lincocin
Mynah-200
Naxogin-500
Noratex
Normetic
Orovite syrup

Panmycin
Polybactrin Soluble GU
Polycrol
Polycrol Forte
Propaderm-A
Rabro
Rikospray Silicone
Savloclens
Savlodil
Septrin dispersible paediatric tablets
Sintisone
Synogist
Syraprim
Talpen
Tanderil Chloramphenicol
Teflox

Temazepam capsules (hard gelatin)
Temazepam Planpak
Tercoda
Thovaline
Timoped
Tonocard injection
Torecan suppositories
Travogyn cream
Trimovate ointment
V-Cil-K
Velosulin Cartridge
Zinc sulphate lotion
Zinc sulphate mouthwash

Note. Product licences for triazolam preparations (including Halcion®) have been suspended.

New Preparations

New monographs

ACITRETIN (BNF section 13.5)
Indications; Cautions; Contra-indications; Side-effects: see under Etretinate, p. 415
Dose: administered in accordance with expert advice, 25–30 mg daily (Darier's disease 10 mg daily) for 2–4 weeks, then adjusted according to response, usually within range 25–50 mg daily (in some cases up to max. 75 mg daily) for further 6–8 weeks (in Darier's disease and ichthyosis not more than 50 mg daily for up to 6 months); CHILD see data sheet

▼ **Neotigason**® (Roche)
Capsules, acitretin 10 mg (brown/white), net price 56-cap pack = £26.53; 25 mg (brown/yellow), 56-cap pack = £61.57 (**hosp. only**, specialist dermatological supervision) Label: 10 patient information leaflet, 21

ESMOLOL HYDROCHLORIDE (BNF section 2.4)
Indications: short-term treatment of supraventricular arrhythmias (including atrial fibrillation, atrial flutter, sinus tachycardia); tachycardia and hypertension in peri-operative period
Cautions; Contra-indications; Side-effects: see under Propranolol Hydrochloride, p. 77
Dose: by intravenous infusion, consult data sheet for details of dose titration

▼ PoM **Brevibloc**® (Du Pont)
Injection, esmolol hydrochloride 10 mg/mL, net price 10-mL vial = £5.90; 250 mg/mL (for dilution before infusion), 10-mL amp = £65.90

FINASTERIDE (BNF section 6.4.2)
Indications: benign prostatic hyperplasia
Cautions: obstructive uropathy, prostate cancer; use of condoms recommended if sexual partner is pregnant or is likely to become pregnant (finasteride excreted in semen); women of child-bearing potential should avoid handling crushed or broken tablets
Side-effects: impotence, decreased libido and ejaculate volume
Dose: 5 mg daily, review treatment after 6 months

▼ PoM **Proscar**® (MSD)
Tablets, blue, f/c, finasteride 5 mg. Net price 28-tab pack = £24.90

NICOTINE PRODUCTS (BNF section 4.10)
Indications: adjunct to smoking cessation
Cautions: cardiovascular disease (avoid if severe); hyperthyroidism; diabetes mellitus; renal and hepatic impairment; exacerbation of gastritis and peptic ulcers
Contra-indications: pregnancy, breast-feeding
Side-effects: headache and cold and influenza-like symptoms; dizziness and nausea; insomnia; myalgia
Dose: see under preparations, below

PoM **Nicotinell TTS**® (Geigy)
'10' *patch*, self-adhesive, yellowish-ochre, releasing nicotine approx. 7 mg/24 hours when in contact with skin. Net price 28 = £32.83. Label: 10 patient information leaflet, counselling, see administration below
'20' *patch*, self-adhesive, yellowish-ochre, releasing nicotine approx. 14 mg/24 hours when in contact with skin. Net price 28 = £34.56. Label: 10 patient information leaflet, counselling, see administration below
'30' *patch*, self-adhesive, yellowish-ochre, releasing nicotine approx. 21 mg/24 hours when in contact with skin. Net price 28 = £36.28. Label: 10 patient information leaflet, counselling, see administration below
ADMINISTRATION: apply to dry, non-hairy skin on trunk or upper arm, removing after 24 hours and siting replacement patch on a different area (avoid using the same area for several days); individuals smoking 20 cigarettes daily or fewer, initially '20' patch daily; individuals smoking more than 20 cigarettes daily, initially '30' patch daily; withdraw nicotine replacement gradually over 3–4 weeks; review treatment if abstinence not achieved in 3 months

---

Existing monographs

PoM **Half Securon SR**® (Knoll)
Tablets, m/r, f/c, verapamil hydrochloride 120 mg. Net price 100-tab pack = £25.00. Label: 25. BNF section 2.6.2
Dose: hypertension, 120 mg daily, increased if necessary to max. 480 mg daily (doses above 240 mg daily as 2 divided doses)
Angina, see p. 96 (may be used for dose titration)

▼ PoM **Isotrex**® (Stiefel)
Gel, isotretinoin 0.05%. Net price 30 g = £6.96. Label: 10 patient information leaflet. BNF section 13.6
Additives: butylated hydroxytoluene
Administration: acne vulgaris, apply sparingly to clean skin 1–2 times daily
Cautions; Contra-indication; Side-effects: as for Tretinoin, p. 418

Changes

The BNF is revised twice yearly and numerous changes are made between issues. All copies of BNF No. 23 (March 1992) should therefore be withdrawn and replaced by BNF No. 24 (September 1992).
Significant changes have been made in the following sections for BNF No. 24:

Prescribing and sport, p. 23
Stoma appliances [more detail on associated products] (section 1.8)
Antihypertensive therapy [elderly and systolic hypertension] (section 2.5)
Vasoconstrictor sympathomimetics [ephedrine monograph] (section 2.7.2)
Adrenoceptor stimulants [clarification] (section 3.1.1)
Theophylline [editorial changes] (section 3.1.3)
Peak flow meters [notes added] (section 3.1.5)
Corticosteroids for asthma (section 3.2)
Compound cough preparations (section 3.9.2)
Oral antipsychotics [equivalent doses] (section 4.2.1)
Compound analgesics [reorganisation and inclusion of over-the-counter products] (section 4.7.1)
Epilepsy [classification] (section 4.8.1)
Status epilepticus [guidelines] (section 4.8.2)

Endocarditis prophylaxis [revised recommendations] (section 5.1, table 2)
Breast pain (section 6.7.2)
Vaginal preparations [effect on condoms and diaphragms] (section 7.2)
Oral contraceptives [interactions] (section 7.3.1)
HRT and surgery (section 7.3.1)
Progestogen-only contraceptives [missed pill] (section 7.3.2)
Appliances for urinary disorders [more detail, particularly catheters] (section 7.5)
Rheumatic disease [antimalarials and ocular toxicity] (section 10.1.3)
Sunscreens [preparations with SPF less than 15 no longer prescribable] (section 13.8.1)
Vaccines [revised Department of Health guidelines] (chapter 14)
Appendix 7 [indications amended]
Appendix 8 [rationalisation of notes]

Dose Changes

Preparations affected by changes in dose statements introduced into BNF No. 24:

Amoxycillin [gonorrhoea], p. 206
Ampicillin [gonorrhoea], p. 207
Cephamandole [child], p. 214
Chlormethiazole [more detail], p. 141
Clindamycin [more detail], p. 221
Cyclosporin, p. 320
Desmopressin [more detail], pp. 278–9
Flecainide, p. 72
Halofantrine [child], p. 241
Inhalations, aromatic [age limits], p. 134
Isoprenaline, p. 100

Loratadine [child], p. 127
Lorazepam [anaesthesia], p. 465
Medicoal, p. 17
Mefloquine [duration], p. 244
Metoprolol [hypertension], p. 79
MFV-Ject [child], p. 448
Oxybutynin [elderly], p. 298
Sulphinpyrazone [maintenance], p. 371
Thiopentone [child], p. 460
Trasidrex, p. 80
Zidovudine [child], p. 239

Classification Changes

4.1.2 Hydroxyzine now in 3.4.1
5.1.6 Clindamycin [title change]
6.7.2 Danazol, gestrinone and gonadorelin analogues [title change]
8.2.5 Aldesleukin [new section]
13.10.5 Preparations for minor cuts and abrasions [title change]

Name Changes

Old name	New Name
HA-1A	Nebacumab

New Names

The following approved names have been adopted:

Co-magaldrox, compounded preparations of magnesium hydroxide and aluminium hydroxide; the proportions are expressed in the form x/y where x and y are the strengths in milligrams per unit dose of magnesium hydroxide and aluminium hydroxide respectively (available as Maalox®, Mucogel®).

Co-triamterzide, compounded preparations of triamterene and hydrochlorothiazide in the mass proportions 2 parts to 1 part respectively (available as Dyazide®, Triamco®).

Preface

The present format of the British National Formulary was introduced in February 1981. Information is included on most products available to prescribers in the United Kingdom. The product entries, are preceded by relevant notes to help in the choice of appropriate treatment.

Basic net prices are included to provide better indications of relative cost. Where there is a choice of suitable preparations for a particular disease or condition the relative cost may be used in making a selection. It should be emphasised, however, that cost-effective prescribing must take into account other factors (such as dose frequency and duration of treatment) that affect the total cost. The use of more expensive drugs is justified if it will result in better treatment of the patient or a reduction of the length of an illness or the time spent in hospital.

The BNF is intended to be a pocket book for rapid reference and so cannot contain all the information necessary for prescribing and dispensing. It should be supplemented as necessary from specialised publications. Manufacturers' data sheets prepared in accordance with the Medicines (Data Sheet) Regulations 1972 are available for most proprietary medicines and these should also be consulted. Less detail is given in the chapters on malignant disease and immunosuppression, and anaesthesia, as it is expected that those undertaking treatment will have specialised knowledge and will consult specialist literature. Supplementary information may be available from local drug information services.

The Joint Formulary Committee acknowledges the help of individuals and organisations that provided information or advised on specific matters. The principal contributors for this edition were J. M. Aitken, S. P. Allison, D. G. Arkell, C. G. Barnes, L. Beeley, R. H. Behrens, R. J. Buckley, I. Burgess, C. M. Castleden, D. A. Chamberlain, B. T. Colvin, C. Diamond, R. Dinwiddie, A. J. Duxbury, H. M. Elliston, A. M. Geddes, A. H. Ghodse, E. C. Gordon-Smith, J. Guillebaud, C. H. Hawkes, M. J. S. Langman, T. H. Lee, P. N. Leigh, R. Levinsky, R. Marks, M. W. McNicol, G. M. Mead, M. R. Moore, D. J. Oliver, L. E. Ramsay, P. A. Routledge, R. S. Sawers, M. C. Sheppard, S. D. Shorvon, M. Tarr, A. Tattersfield, R. N. Thin, G. R. Thompson, V. R. Tindall, M. D. Vickers, D. G. Waller, D. A. Warrell, P. Watkins, K. Watson, G. B. Wyatt. The Committee also wishes to express its thanks to correspondents in the pharmaceutical industry who provided information and made numerous comments on points of detail, to colleagues who have advised members of the committee and the editorial staff on specific matters, and to J. Holmes and T. M. Roberts for clerical assistance. Finally, the Committee would like to thank those doctors, pharmacists, nurses, and others who sent comments and suggestions.

> Comments and constructive criticism will be welcome, and should be sent to:
> Executive Editor,
>   British National Formulary,
>   c/o Royal Pharmaceutical Society of Great Britain,
>   1 Lambeth High Street,
>   London SE1 7JN.

Arrangement of Information

Guidance on prescribing
This part includes information on prescription writing, prescribing for children and elderly patients, and prescribing in terminal care. Information is also given on adverse reactions, controlled drugs, and dependence.

Emergency treatment of poisoning
The main intention of this chapter is to provide information on the management of acute poisoning when first seen in the home, although aspects of hospital-based treatment are mentioned.

Classified notes on drugs and preparations
The main text consists of classified notes on drugs and preparations used in the treatment of diseases and conditions. These notes are divided into 15 chapters, each of which is related to a particular system of the human body or to another main subject. Each chapter is then divided into sections which begin with appropriate *notes for prescribers*. These notes are intended to provide information to doctors, pharmacists, nurses etc. to facilitate the selection of suitable treatment. The notes are followed by details of relevant drugs and preparations.

DRUGS appear under pharmacopoeial or other non-proprietary titles. When there is an *appropriate current monograph* (Medicines Act 1968, Section 65) preference is given to a name at the head of that monograph; otherwise a British Approved Name, if available, is used. If there is an acknowledged reference drug, information on it is usually given first; otherwise the drugs are arranged alphabetically.

PREPARATIONS usually follow immediately after the drug which is their main ingredient. They are printed in text-sized type but those considered by the Committee to be less suitable for prescribing are described in smaller type. Small type is also used for the entries describing foods for special diets, stoma and urinary appliances, and wound management products. Preparations are included under a non-proprietary title only if:
   (a) they are marketed under such a title,
   (b) they are not otherwise prescribable under the NHS, or
   (c) they may be prepared extemporaneously.
If proprietary preparations are of a distinctive colour this is stated, but flavour is not usually mentioned.
   In the case of compound preparations the indications, cautions, contra-indications, side-effects, and interactions of all constituents should be taken into account in prescribing; usually the ingredients should be looked up separately.

PREPARATIONS NOT AVAILABLE FOR NHS PRESCRIPTION. The symbol NHS has been placed against those preparations included in the BNF that are not prescribable under the NHS. Those prescribable only for specific disorders have a foot-note specifying the condition(s) for which the preparation remains available. Prescribers are reminded that some preparations which are not *prescribable* by brand name under the NHS may nevertheless be *dispensed* using the brand name in question providing that the prescription has been written in the form of an appropriate non-proprietary name.

PRESCRIPTION-ONLY MEDICINES. The symbol PoM has been placed against those preparations that are available only on medical or dental prescription. For more detailed information see *Medicines, Ethics and Practice*, No. 8, London, Pharmaceutical Press, 1992 (and subsequent editions as available). The symbol **CD** indicates that the preparation is subject to the prescription requirements of the Misuse of Drugs Act. For regulations governing prescriptions for such preparations see pages 7–9.

PRICES (see p. 1) have been calculated whenever possible from the basic cost used in pricing NHS prescriptions dispensed in February 1992, see p. 1 for further details.

Appendixes and indexes
The appendixes include information on interactions, liver disease, renal impairment, pregnancy, breast-feeding, intravenous additives, borderline substances, and cautionary and advisory labels for dispensed medicines. Where relevant they are designed for use in association with the main body of the text.
   The Dental Practitioners' List is also included in this section. The indexes consist of the Index of Manufacturers and the Main Index.

	11.4	Corticosteroids and other anti-inflammatory preparations	379
	11.5	Mydriatics and cycloplegics	381
	11.6	Treatment of glaucoma	382
	11.7	Local anaesthetics	385
	11.8	Miscellaneous ophthalmic preparations	385
	11.9	Contact lenses	387
12:	Ear, Nose, and Oropharynx		388
	12.1	Drugs acting on the ear	388
	12.2	Drugs acting on the nose	391
	12.3	Drugs acting on the oropharynx	394
13:	Skin		399
	13.1	Vehicles	399
	13.2	Emollient and barrier preparations	400
	13.3	Local anaesthetics and antipruritics	403
	13.4	Topical corticosteroids	404
	13.5	Preparations for psoriasis and eczema	411
	13.6	Preparations for acne	415
	13.7	Preparations for warts and calluses	418
	13.8	Sunscreens and camouflagers	420
	13.9	Shampoos and some other scalp preparations	421
	13.10	Anti-infective skin preparations	423
	13.11	Disinfectants and cleansers	431
	13.12	Antiperspirants	434
	13.13	Wound management products	435
	13.14	Topical circulatory preparations	441
14:	Immunological Products and Vaccines		442
	14.1	Active immunity	442
	14.2	Passive immunity	444
	14.3	Storage and use	444
	14.4	Vaccines and antisera	444
	14.5	Immunoglobulins	454
	14.6	International travel	457
15:	Anaesthesia		458
	15.1	General anaesthesia	458
	15.2	Local anaesthesia	472

APPENDIXES AND INDEXES

Appendix 1: Interactions	476
Appendix 2: Liver Disease	499
Appendix 3: Renal Impairment	503
Appendix 4: Pregnancy	510
Appendix 5: Breast-feeding	517
Appendix 6: Intravenous Additives	522
Appendix 7: Borderline Substances	534
Appendix 8: Cautionary and Advisory Labels	546
Dental Practitioners' Formulary (List of Dental Preparations)	556
Index of Manufacturers	558
INDEX	566

Contents vii

	3.6	Oxygen	132
	3.7	Mucolytics	133
	3.8	Aromatic inhalations	134
	3.9	Antitussives	134
	3.10	Systemic nasal decongestants	136
4:	Central Nervous System		138
	4.1	Hypnotics and anxiolytics	138
	4.2	Drugs used in psychoses and related disorders	145
	4.3	Antidepressant drugs	157
	4.4	Central nervous stimulants	165
	4.5	Appetite suppressants	166
	4.6	Drugs used in nausea and vertigo	167
	4.7	Analgesics	172
	4.8	Antiepileptics	185
	4.9	Drugs used in parkinsonism and related disorders	192
	4.10	Drugs used in substance dependence	197
5:	Infections		199
	5.1	Antibacterial drugs	199
	5.2	Antifungal drugs	234
	5.3	Antiviral drugs	237
	5.4	Antiprotozoal drugs	240
	5.5	Anthelmintics	247
6:	Endocrine System		250
	6.1	Drugs used in diabetes	250
	6.2	Thyroid and antithyroid drugs	260
	6.3	Corticosteroids	262
	6.4	Sex hormones	267
	6.5	Hypothalamic and pituitary hormones and anti-oestrogens	275
	6.6	Drugs affecting bone metabolism	279
	6.7	Other endocrine drugs	281
7:	Obstetrics, Gynaecology, and Urinary-tract Disorders		284
	7.1	Drugs used in obstetrics	284
	7.2	Treatment of vaginal and vulval conditions	287
	7.3	Contraceptives	290
	7.4	Drugs for genito-urinary disorders	296
	7.5	Appliances for urinary disorders	300
8:	Malignant Disease and Immunosuppression		310
	8.1	Cytotoxic drugs	310
	8.2	Drugs affecting the immune response	319
	8.3	Sex hormones and antagonists in malignant disease	321
9:	Nutrition and Blood		326
	9.1	Anaemias and some other blood disorders	326
	9.2	Fluids and electrolytes	334
	9.3	Intravenous nutrition	342
	9.4	Oral nutrition	345
	9.5	Minerals	345
	9.6	Vitamins	349
	9.7	Bitters and tonics	355
	9.8	Metabolic disorders	355
10:	Musculoskeletal and Joint Diseases		357
	10.1	Drugs used in rheumatic diseases and gout	357
	10.2	Drugs used in neuromuscular disorders	371
	10.3	Drugs for the relief of soft-tissue inflammation	374
11:	Eye		376
	11.1	Administration of drugs to the eye	376
	11.2	Control of microbial contamination	376
	11.3	Anti-infective eye preparations	376

Guidance on Prescribing

Prices in the BNF

Basic **net prices** have been introduced into the BNF in order to provide better indications of relative cost. Whenever possible they have been calculated from the basic cost used in pricing NHS prescriptions dispensed in February 1992; unless an original pack is available these prices are based on the largest pack size of the preparation in use in community pharmacies. The price for an extemporaneously prepared preparation has been omitted where the net cost of the ingredients used to make it would give a misleadingly low impression of the final price.

The unit of 20 is still sometimes used as a basis for comparison, but where suitable original packs are available these are priced instead.

Gross prices vary as follows:
1. Costs to the NHS are greater than the net prices quoted and include professional fees and overhead allowances;
2. Private prescription charges are calculated on a separate basis;
3. Over-the-counter sales are at retail price, as opposed to basic net price, and include VAT.

BNF prices are NOT, therefore, suitable for quoting to patients seeking private prescriptions or contemplating over-the-counter purchases.
A fuller explanation of costs to the NHS may be obtained from the Drug Tariff.
It should be noted that separate Drug Tariffs are operative in England and Wales, Scotland, and Northern Ireland. Prices in the different tariffs may vary.

PACT and SPA

PACT (Prescribing Analyses and Cost) and SPA (Scottish Prescribing Analysis) automatically provide general practitioners with information about their prescribing. The information is sent on a quarterly basis direct from the Prescription Pricing Authority. It is available at three levels of complexity:
Level 1 reports compare practice prescribing with that of the local Family Health Services Authority (FHSA) or Health Board (in Scotland) and national averages—they are produced once a quarter for each general practitioner;
Level 2 reports are produced for general practitioners with above average costs—they can also be requested;
Level 3 reports are available only on request—they are effectively a list of all items prescribed by the general practitioner, grouped into the BNF therapeutic categories, giving detailed cost information. These reports are termed level 2 in Scotland since the intermediate level is not produced.

General Guidance

Medicines should be prescribed only when they are essential, and in all cases the benefit of administering the medicine should be considered in relation to the risk involved. This is particularly important during pregnancy where the risk to both mother and fetus must be considered (for further details see Prescribing in Pregnancy, Appendix 4).

ABBREVIATION OF TITLES. In general, titles of drugs and preparations should be written *in full*. Unofficial abbreviations should not be used as they may be misinterpreted; obsolete titles, such as Mist. Expect. and Mist. Tussis should not be used.

NON-PROPRIETARY TITLES. Where non-proprietary ('generic') titles are given, they should be used in prescribing. This will enable any suitable product to be dispensed, thereby saving delay to the patient and sometimes expense to the health service. The only exception is where bioavailability problems are so important that the patient should always receive the same brand; in such cases, the brand name or the manufacturer should be stated. Non-proprietary titles should **not** be invented for the purposes of prescribing generically since this can lead to confusion, particularly in the case of compound and modified-release preparations.

Titles used as headings for monographs may be used freely in Great Britain and Northern Ireland but in other countries may be subject to restriction.

Many of the non-proprietary titles used in this book are titles of monographs in the European Pharmacopoeia, British Pharmacopoeia or British Pharmaceutical Codex 1973. In such cases the preparations must comply with the standard (if any) in the appropriate publication, as required by the Medicines Act (section 65).

PROPRIETARY TITLES. Names followed by the symbol® are or have been used as proprietary names in the United Kingdom. These names may in general be applied only to products supplied by the owners of the trade marks.

DOSES. The doses stated in the BNF are intended for general guidance and represent, unless otherwise stated, the usual range of doses that are generally regarded as being suitable for adults; unless otherwise indicated the quantities are those generally suitable for administration on one occasion.

ORAL SYRINGES. Since 1 July 1992, when fractional doses are prescribed, *oral liquid medicines* are **no longer** diluted to a 5-mL dose (or multiple thereof). Instead the pharmacist supplies an **oral syringe**. The oral syringe is marked in 0.5 mL divisions from 1 to 5 mL to measure doses of less than 5 mL. The 5-mL spoon will continue in use for doses of 5 mL (or multiple thereof). The oral syringe is provided with an adaptor and an instruction leaflet.

STRENGTHS AND QUANTITIES. The strength or quantity to be contained in capsules, lozenges, tablets, etc. should be stated by the prescriber.

If a pharmacist receives an incomplete prescription for a systemically administered preparation other than a prescription for a controlled drug and considers it would not be appropriate for the patient to return to the doctor, the following procedures will apply:

(a) an attempt must always be made to contact the prescriber to ascertain the intention;
(b) if the attempt is successful the pharmacist must, where practicable, subsequently arrange for details of quantity, strength where applicable, and dosage to be inserted by the prescriber on the incomplete form;
(c) where, although the prescriber has been contacted, it has not proved possible to obtain the written intention regarding an incomplete prescription, the pharmacist may endorse the form 'p.c.' (prescriber contacted) and add details of the quantity and strength where applicable of the preparation supplied, and of the dose indicated. The endorsement should be initialled and dated by the pharmacist;
(d) where the prescriber cannot be contacted and the pharmacist has sufficient information to make a professional judgment the preparation may be dispensed. If the quantity is missing the pharmacist may supply sufficient to complete up to 5 days' treatment; except that where a combination pack (i.e. a proprietary pack containing more than one medicinal product) or oral contraceptive is prescribed by name only, the smallest pack shall be dispensed. In all cases the prescription must be endorsed 'p.n.c.' (prescriber not contacted) the quantity, the dose, and the strength (where applicable) of the preparation supplied must be indicated, and the endorsement must be initialled and dated;
(e) if the pharmacist has any doubt about exercising discretion, an incomplete prescription must be referred back to the prescriber.

ADDITIVES. Oral liquid preparations in the BNF that do not contain *fructose*, *glucose* or *sucrose* are labelled "sugar-free".

Where the presence of *gluten* or of *tartrazine* is specified on a data sheet this is indicated in the BNF against the preparation in question; not all data sheets provide details of additives therefore if it is essential to know whether a preparation is free of gluten or of tartrazine the manufacturer should be contacted.

Information is provided on *preservatives* in eye-drops.

Information is provided on *selected additives* in skin preparations (for details see section 13.1).

EXTEMPORANEOUS PREPARATION. The BP direction that a preparation must be *freshly prepared* indicates that it must be made not more than 24 hours before it is issued for use. The direction that a preparation should be *recently prepared* indicates that deterioration is likely if the preparation is stored for longer than about 4 weeks at 15° to 25°.

DRUGS AND DRIVING. Prescribers should advise patients if treatment is likely to affect their ability to drive motor vehicles. This applies particularly to drugs with sedative effects and patients should be warned that these effects are increased by alcohol. See also Appendix 8.

DRUGS AND SPORT. For details see p. 23.

NOTICE CONCERNING PATENTS. In the BNF certain drugs have been included notwithstanding the existence of actual or potential patent rights. In so far as such substances are protected by Letters Patent, their inclusion in this Formulary neither conveys, nor implies, licence to manufacture.

HEALTH AND SAFETY. When handling chemical or biological materials particular attention should be given to the possibility of allergy, fire, explosion, radiation, or poisoning. Some substances, including corticosteroids, antibiotics, phenothiazines, and many cytotoxics, are irritant or very potent and should be handled with caution. Contact with the skin and inhalation of dust should be avoided.

SAFETY IN THE HOME. Patients must be warned to keep all medicines out of the reach of children. All solid dose oral medicines should be dispensed either in reclosable *child-resistant containers* complying with the British Standard or in unit packaging of strip or blister type, unless:
 (i) they are in manufacturers' original packs so designed that transfer to a reclosable child-resistant container would be a retrograde or unnecessary procedure;
 (ii) the patient is elderly or handicapped and would have difficulty in opening a child-resistant container;
 (iii) the patient specifically requests otherwise.

In cases (ii) and (iii) the pharmacist should make a particular point of advising that the medicines be kept well out of the reach of children.

All patients should be advised to dispose of *unwanted medicines* by returning them to a supplier for destruction.

NAME OF MEDICINE. The name of the medicine should appear on the label unless the prescriber indicates otherwise.
1. Subject to the conditions of paragraphs 4 and 6 below, the name of the prescribed medicine is stated on the label unless the prescriber deletes the letters 'NP' which appear on NHS prescription forms.
2. The strength is also stated on the label in the case of tablets, capsules, and similar preparations that are available in different strengths.
3. If it is the wish of the prescriber that a description such as 'The Sedative Tablets' should appear on the label, the prescriber should write the desired description on the prescription form.
4. The arrangement will extend to approved names, proprietary names or titles given in the BP, BPC, BNF, or DPF. The arrangement does not apply when a prescription is written so that several ingredients are given.
5. The name written on the label is that used by the prescriber on the prescription.
6. If more than one item is prescribed on one form and the prescriber does not delete the letters 'NP', each dispensed medicine is named on the label, subject to the conditions given above in paragraph 4. If the prescriber wants only selected items on such a prescription to be so labelled this should be indicated by deleting the letters 'NP' on the form and writing 'NP' alongside the medicines to be labelled.
7. When a prescription is written other than on an NHS prescription form the name of the prescribed preparation will be stated on the label of the dispensed medicine unless the prescriber indicates otherwise.
8. The Council of the Royal Pharmaceutical Society advises that the labels of dispensed medicines should indicate the total quantity of the product dispensed in the container to which the label refers. This requirement applies equally to solid, liquid, internal, and external preparations. If a product is dispensed in more than one container, the reference should be to the amount in each container.

Scope of the BNF

The BNF is intended for the guidance of medical practitioners, pharmacists, dentists, nurses, and other workers who have the necessary training and experience to interpret the information it provides. It is intended as a reference book for the pocket, and should be supplemented by a study of more detailed publications when required.

Security and validity of prescriptions

The Councils of the British Medical Association and the Royal Pharmaceutical Society have issued a joint statement on the security and validity of prescriptions.

In particular, prescription forms should:
 (i) not be left unattended at reception desks;
 (ii) not be left in a car where they may be visible; and
 (iii) when not in use, be kept in a locked drawer within the surgery and at home.

Where there is any doubt about the authenticity of a prescription, the pharmacist should contact the prescriber. If this is done by telephone, the number should be obtained from the directory rather than relying on the prescription form information, which may be false.

Prescription Writing

> The following recommendations are acceptable for **prescription-only medicines** (PoM). For items marked **CD** see Controlled Drugs and Drug Dependence p. 7.

Prescriptions should be written legibly in ink or otherwise as to be indelible[1], should be dated, should state the full name and address of the patient, and should be signed in ink by the prescriber[2]. The age of the patient should preferably be stated, and is a legal requirement in the case of prescription-only medicines for children under 12 years of age.

In general practice the following should be noted:

(a) For solids, quantities of 1 gram or more should be written as 1 g etc.

Quantities less than 1 gram should be written in milligrams, e.g. 500 mg, not 0.5 g.

Quantities less than 1 mg should be written in micrograms, e.g. 100 micrograms, not 0.1 mg.

When decimals are unavoidable a zero should be written in front of the decimal point where there is no other figure, e.g. 0.5 mL, not .5 mL.

Use of the decimal point is acceptable to express a range, e.g. 0.5 to 1 g.

(b) 'Micrograms' and 'nanograms' should **not** be abbreviated. Similarly 'units' should **not** be abbreviated.

(c) The term 'millilitre' (ml or mL)[3] is used in medicine and pharmacy, and cubic centimetre, c.c., or cm³ should not be used.

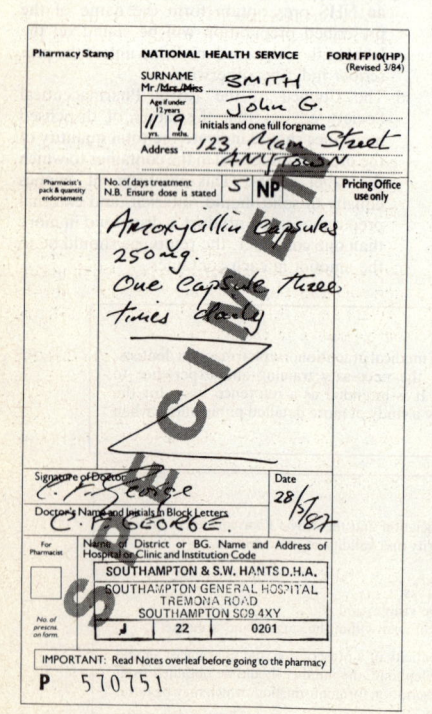

(d) Dose and dose frequency should be stated; in the case of preparations to be taken 'as required' a **minimum dose interval** should be specified.

For oral liquid preparations of the *linctus* or *elixir* type and for *preparations for children*, doses should preferably be stated in terms of 5-mL spoonfuls.

For *mixtures for adults*, doses should preferably be stated in 10-mL quantities; unless the prescription states otherwise, the patient will be directed to take the dose with water.

When doses other than 5 or 10 mL are prescribed the dose-volume will be provided by means of an *oral syringe*, see p. 2 (except for preparations intended to be measured with a pipette).

Suitable quantities:
Elixirs, Linctuses, and Paediatric
  Mixtures (5-mL dose), 50, 100, or 150 mL
Adult Mixtures (10-mL dose), 200 or 300 mL
Ear Drops, Eye-drops, and Nasal Drops,
  10 mL (or the manufacturer's pack)
Eye Lotions, Gargles, and Mouth-washes, 200 mL
Liniments, 100 mL

(e) For suitable quantities of dermatological preparations, see section 13.1.

(f) The names of drugs and preparations should be written clearly and **not** abbreviated, using approved titles **only**.

(g) The symbol 'NP' on NHS forms should be deleted if it is required that the name of the preparation should not appear on the label. For full details see p. 3.

(h) The quantity to be supplied may be stated by indicating the number of days of treatment required in the box provided on NHS forms. In most cases the exact amount will be supplied. This does not apply to items directed to be used as required; if the dose and frequency are not given the quantity to be supplied should be stated.

When several items are ordered on one form the box can be marked with the number of days of treatment providing the quantity is added for any item for which the amount cannot be calculated.

(i) Although directions should preferably be in **English without abbreviation**, it is recognised that some Latin abbreviations are used (for details see Inside Back Cover).

(j) A prescription for a preparation that has been withdrawn or needs to be specially imported for a named patient should be handwritten. The name of the preparation should be endorsed with the prescriber's signature and the letters 'WD' (withdrawn or specially-imported drug); there may be considerable delay in obtaining a withdrawn medicine.

---

1. It is permissible to issue carbon copies of NHS prescriptions as long as they are signed in ink.
2. Computer-generated facsimile signatures do not meet the legal requirement.
3. The use of capital 'L' in mL is a printing convention throughout the BNF; both mL and ml are recognised abbreviations for SI units.

Computer-issued Prescriptions

For computer-issued prescriptions the following recommendations of the Joint Computing Group of the General Medical Services Committee and the Royal College of General Practitioners should also be noted:

1. The computer must print out the date[1], the patient's surname, one forename, other initials, and address, and may also print out the patient's title. The age of children under 12 years must be printed in the box available; a facility may exist to print out the age of older children and adults as well.
2. The doctor's name[2] must be printed at the bottom of the prescription form; this will be the name of the doctor responsible for the prescription (who will normally sign it). The doctor's surgery address, reference number, and Family Health Services Authority (FHSA)[3] are also necessary. In addition, the surgery telephone number should be printed.
3. When prescriptions are to be signed by trainees, assistants, locums, or deputising doctors, the name of the doctor printed at the bottom of the form must still be that of the responsible principal. To avoid difficulties for the pharmacist checking the prescription, the name of the signing doctor may be printed in the signature box, to be signed over on prescribing.
4. Names of medicines must come from a dictionary held in the computer memory, to provide a check on the spelling and ensure that the name is written in full. The computer can be programmed to recognise both the non-proprietary and the proprietary name of a particular drug and to print out the preferred choice, but must not print out both names. For medicines not in the dictionary, separate checking mechanisms are required—the user must be warned that no check was possible and the entire prescription must be entered into the lexicon.
5. The dictionary may contain information on the usual doses, formulations, and (where relevant) pack sizes to produce standard predetermined prescriptions for common preparations, and to provide a check on the validity of an individual prescription on entry.
6. The prescription must be printed in English without abbreviation; information may be entered or stored in abbreviated form. The dose must be in numbers, the frequency in words, and the quantity in numbers in brackets, thus: 40 mg four times daily (112).

It must also be possible to prescribe by indicating the length of treatment required, see (h) above.

7. The BNF recommendations should be followed as in (a), (b), (c), (d), and (e) above.
8. Checks may be incorporated to ensure that all the information required for dispensing a particular drug has been filled in. Instructions such as 'as directed' should be avoided. For the instruction 'when required' the maximum daily dose should normally be specified.
9. Numbers and codes used in the system for organising and retrieving data must never appear on the form.

> Generic names of **compound preparations** which appear in the BNF are those approved by the British Pharmacopoeia Commission; whenever possible they reflect the names of the active ingredients.
>
> Prescribers should avoid creating their own compound names for the purposes of generic prescribing; such names do not have an approved definition and can be misinterpreted.
>
> Special care should be taken to avoid errors when prescribing compound preparations; in particular the hyphen in the prefix 'co-' should be retained.
>
> Special care should also be taken to avoid creating generic names for **modified-release** preparations where the use of these names could lead to confusion between formulations with different lengths of action.

10. Supplementary warnings or advice should be written in full, should not interfere with the clarity of the prescription itself, and should be in line with any warnings or advice in the BNF; numerical codes should not be used.
11. A mechanism (such as printing a series of non-specific characters) may be incorporated to cancel out unused space, or wording such as 'no more items on this prescription' may be added after the last item. Otherwise the doctor should delete the space manually.
12. To avoid forgery the computer may print on the form the number of items to be dispensed (somewhere separate from the box for the pharmacist). The number of items per form need be limited only by the ability of the printer to produce clear and well-demarcated instructions with sufficient space for each item and a spacer line before each fresh item.
13. Handwritten alterations should only be made in exceptional circumstances—it is preferable to print out a new prescription. Any alterations that are made must be written in the doctor's own handwriting and countersigned.
14. Prescriptions for controlled drugs cannot be produced by a printer[4]. If there is a record of such a prescription in the computer, it must not be printed. Instead the computer may print out a blank form with the doctor's name[1] and other details printed at the bottom.
15. The strip of paper on the side of the FP10[5](Comp) may be used for various purposes but care should be taken to avoid including confidential information. It may be advisable for the patient's name to appear at the top, but this should be preceded by 'confidential'.
16. In rural dispensing practices prescription requests (or details of medicines dispensed) will normally be entered in one surgery. The prescriptions (or dispensed medicines) may then need to be delivered to another surgery or location; if possible the computer should hold up to 10 alternatives.

---

1. The exemption for own handwriting regulations for phenobarbitone does not apply to the date; a computer-generated date need not be deleted but the date must also be added by the prescriber.
2. Except in Scotland where it does not appear.
3. Health Board in Scotland.
4. Except in the case of phenobarbitone (but see also footnote 1) or where the prescriber has been exempted from handwriting requirements, for details see Controlled Drugs and Drug Dependence p. 7.
5. GP10 in Scotland.

Emergency Supply of PoM at Patient's Request[1]

The Medicines (Products Other Than Veterinary Drugs) (Prescription Only) Order 1983, as amended, allows exemptions from the Prescription Only requirements for emergency supply to be made by a person lawfully conducting a retail pharmacy business provided:
(a) that the pharmacist has interviewed the person requesting the prescription-only medicine and is satisfied:
  (i) that there is immediate need for the prescription-only medicine and that it is impracticable in the circumstances to obtain a prescription without undue delay;
  (ii) that treatment with the prescription-only medicine has on a previous occasion been prescribed by a doctor[2] for the person requesting it;
  (iii) as to the dose which it would be appropriate for the person to take;
(b) that no greater quantity shall be supplied than will provide five days' treatment except when the prescription-only medicine is:
  (i) an ointment, cream, or preparation for the relief of asthma in an aerosol dispenser when the smallest pack can be supplied;
  (ii) an oral contraceptive when a full cycle may be supplied;
  (iii) an antibiotic in liquid form for oral administration when the smallest quantity that will provide a full course of treatment can be supplied;
(c) that an entry shall be made in the prescription book stating:
  (i) the date of supply;
  (ii) the name, quantity and, where appropriate, the pharmaceutical form and strength;
  (iii) the name and address of the patient;
  (iv) the nature of the emergency;

(d) that the container or package must be labelled to show:
  (i) the date of supply;
  (ii) the name, quantity and, where appropriate, the pharmaceutical form and strength;
  (iii) the name of the patient;
  (iv) the name and address of the pharmacy;
  (v) the words 'Emergency supply'.
(e) that the prescription-only medicine is not a substance specifically excluded from the emergency supply provision, and does not contain a Controlled Drug specified in schedules 1, 2, or 3 to the Misuse of Drugs Regulations 1985 except for phenobarbitone or phenobarbitone sodium for the treatment of epilepsy: for details see *Medicines, Ethics and Practice*, No. 8, London, Pharmaceutical Press, 1992 (and subsequent editions as available).

ROYAL PHARMACEUTICAL SOCIETY'S GUIDELINES
(1) The pharmacist should consider the medical consequences, if any, of **not** supplying.
(2) The pharmacist should identify the patient by means of documentary evidence and/or personal knowledge.
(3) The doctor who prescribed on a previous occasion should be identified and contacted, if possible.
(4) The patient should be asked whether the doctor has stopped the treatment.
(5) The patient should be asked whether any other medicine is being taken at the same time to check drug interactions.
(6) An emergency supply should not be made if the item requested was prescribed previously more than six months prior to the request. Variations may be made in the case of illnesses which occur infrequently, e.g. hay fever, asthma attack, or migraine.
(7) Consideration should be given to providing less than five days' supply if this is justified.
(8) Labelling should be clear and legible and there should be some suitable identification of emergency supply entries in the prescription book.

---

1. For emergency supply at the request of a doctor see *Medicines, Ethics and Practice*, No. 8, London, Pharmaceutical Press, 1992 (and subsequent editions as available).
2. The doctor must be a UK-registered doctor.

> **Plasma concentrations** in the BNF are expressed in mass units per litre (e.g. mg/litre). The approximate equivalent in terms of amount of substance units (e.g. micromol/litre) is given in brackets.

Approximate Conversions and Units

lb	kg
1	0.45
2	0.91
3	1.36
4	1.81
5	2.27
6	2.72
7	3.18
8	3.63
9	4.08
10	4.54
11	4.99
12	5.44
13	5.90
14	6.35

stones	kg
1	6.35
2	12.70
3	19.05
4	25.40
5	31.75
6	38.10
7	44.45
8	50.80
9	57.15
10	63.50
11	69.85
12	76.20
13	82.55
14	88.90
15	95.25

mL	fl. oz
50	1.8
100	3.5
150	5.3
200	7.0
500	17.6
1000	35.2

Mass
1 kilogram (kg) = 1000 grams (g)
1 gram (g) = 1000 milligrams (mg)
1 milligram (mg) = 1000 micrograms
1 microgram = 1000 nanograms
1 nanogram = 1000 picograms

Volume
1 litre = 1000 millilitres (mL)
1 millilitre = 1000 microlitres
1 pint ≈ 568 mL

Other units
1 kilocalorie (kcal) = 4186.8 joules (J)
1000 kilocalories (kcal) = 4.1868 megajoules (MJ)
1 megajoule (MJ) = 238.8 kilocalories (kcal)
1 millimetre of mercury (mmHg) = 133.3 pascals (Pa)
1 kilopascal (kPa) = 7.5 mmHg (pressure)

Controlled Drugs and Drug Dependence

PRESCRIPTIONS. Preparations which are subject to the prescription requirements of the Misuse of Drugs Regulations 1985, i.e. preparations specified in schedules 2 and 3, are distinguished throughout the BNF by the symbol **CD** (Controlled Drugs). The principal legal requirements relating to medical prescriptions are listed below.

Prescriptions ordering Controlled Drugs subject to prescription requirements must be *signed* and *dated*[1] by the prescriber and specify the prescriber's *address*. The prescription must always state *in the prescriber's own handwriting*[2] in ink or otherwise so as to be indelible:

1. The name and address of the patient;
2. In the case of a preparation, the form[3] and where appropriate the strength of the preparation;
3. The total quantity of the preparation, or the number of dose units, *in both words and figures*;
4. The dose.

A prescription may order a Controlled Drug to be dispensed by instalments; the amount of the instalments and the intervals to be observed must be specified.[4] Prescriptions ordering 'repeats' on the same form are **not** permitted.

It is an offence for a doctor to issue an incomplete prescription and a pharmacist is **not** allowed to dispense a Controlled Drug unless all the information required by law is given on the prescription. Failure to comply with the regulations concerning the writing of prescriptions will result in inconvenience to patients and delay in supplying the necessary medicine.

DEPENDENCE AND MISUSE. The prevalence of drug dependence and misuse in Great Britain, particularly amongst young people, continues to give cause for concern to teachers, social workers, and the police, as well as doctors.

The most serious drugs of addiction are **diamorphine** (heroin), **morphine**, and the **synthetic opioids**; illicit **cocaine** is now also a problem.

Despite marked reduction in the prescribing of **amphetamines** there is concern that abuse of illicitly produced amphetamine and related compounds is widespread.

The principal **barbiturates** are now Controlled Drugs, but phenobarbitone and phenobarbitone sodium or a preparation containing either of these are exempt from the handwriting requirement (**important:** the exemption does **not** apply to the date; a computer-generated date need not be deleted but the date must also be added by the prescriber). Moreover, for the treatment of epilepsy phenobarbitone and phenobarbitone sodium are available under the emergency supply regulations (p. 6).

Cannabis (Indian hemp) has no approved medicinal use and cannot be prescribed by doctors (except under licence from the Home Secretary). Its use is illegal but has become widespread in certain sections of society. Cannabis is a mild hallucinogen seldom accompanied by a desire to increase the dose; withdrawal symptoms are unusual. **Lysergide** (lysergic acid diethylamide, LSD) is a much more potent hallucinogen; its use can lead to severe psychotic states in which life may be at risk.

---

1. A prescription is valid for 13 weeks from the date stated thereon.
2. Unless the prescriber has been specifically exempted from this requirement or unless the prescription contains no controlled drug other than phenobarbitone or phenobarbitone sodium or a preparation containing either of these. The exemption does **not** apply to the date; a computer-generated date need not be deleted but the date must also be added by the prescriber.
3. The dosage form (e.g. tablets) must be included on a Controlled Drugs prescription irrespective of whether it is implicit in the proprietary name (e.g. Tenuate Dospan®) or of whether only one form is available.
4. A special form, FP10(HP)(ad), in Scotland HBP(A), is available to doctors in NHS drug treatment centres for prescribing cocaine, dextromoramide, diamorphine, dipipanone, methadone, morphine, or pethidine by instalments for addicts. In Scotland general practitioners can prescribe by instalments on form GP10. In England and Wales forms FP10 and FP10(HP) are not suitable for this purpose but form FP10(MDA) is available. **Important:** in all cases a special licence is necessary to prescribe cocaine, diamorphine, or dipipanone for addicts except for treatment of organic disease or injury, for details see p. 9.

PRESCRIBING DRUGS LIKELY TO CAUSE DEPENDENCE OR MISUSE. The prescriber has three main responsibilities:

1. To avoid creating dependence by introducing drugs to patients without sufficient reason. In this context, the proper use of the morphine-like drugs is well understood. The dangers of other controlled drugs are less clear because recognition of dependence is not easy and its effects, and those of withdrawal, are less obvious. Perhaps the most notable result of uninhibited prescribing is that a very large number of patients in the country take tablets which do them neither much good nor much harm, but are committed to them indefinitely because they cannot readily be stopped.

2. To see that the patient does not gradually increase the dose of a drug, given for good medical reasons, to the point where dependence becomes more likely. This tendency is seen especially with hypnotics and anxiolytics (for CSM advice see section 4.1). The prescriber should keep a close eye on the amount prescribed to prevent patients from accumulating stocks that would enable them to arrange their own dosage or even that of their families and friends. A minimal amount should be prescribed in the first instance, or when seeing a new patient for the first time.

3. To avoid being used as an unwitting source of supply for addicts. Methods include visiting more than one doctor, fabricating stories, and forging prescriptions. A doctor should therefore be wary of prescribing for strangers and may be able to get information about suspected opioid addicts from the Home Office (for details see p. 9).

Patients under temporary care should be given only small supplies of drugs unless they present an unequivocal letter from their own doctors. Doctors should also remember that their own patients may be doing a collecting round with other doctors, especially in hospitals. It is sensible to decrease dosages steadily or to issue weekly or even daily prescriptions for small amounts if it is apparent that dependence is occurring.

The stealing and misuse of prescription forms could be minimised by the following precautions:
(a) do not leave unattended if called away from the consulting room or at reception desks; do not leave in a car where they may be visible; when not in use, keep in a locked drawer within the surgery and at home;
(b) draw a diagonal line across the blank part of the form under the prescription;
(c) write the quantity in words and figures when prescribing drugs prone to abuse; this is obligatory for controlled drugs (see Prescriptions, above);
(d) alterations are best avoided but if any are made they should be clear and unambiguous; add initials against altered items;
(e) if prescriptions are left for collection they should be left in a safe place in a sealed envelope.

TRAVELLING ABROAD. Prescribed drugs listed in schedules 4 and 5 to the Misuse of Drugs Regulations 1985 are not subject to import or export licensing but doctors are advised that patients travelling abroad may only carry 15 days' supply of any schedule 2 or 3 prescribed controlled drug without a licence. If especially high doses are prescribed, however, or if prescriptions are for a longer period, an import or export licence may be required. Licences are issued by the Home Secretary, Home Office, Drugs Branch, Queen Anne's Gate, London SW1H 9AT, telephone 071-273 3806.

There is no standard application form but applications must be supported by a letter from a doctor giving details of:
> the patient's name and current address;
> the quantities of drugs to be carried;
> the strength and form in which the drugs will be dispensed;
> the dates of travel to and from the United Kingdom.

Ten days should be allowed for processing the application.

Individual doctors who wish to take Controlled Drugs abroad while accompanying patients, may similarly be issued with licences. Licences are not normally issued to doctors who wish to take Controlled Drugs abroad solely in case a family emergency should arise.

These import/export licences for named individuals do not have any legal status outside the UK and are only issued to comply with the Misuse of Drugs Act and facilitate passage through UK Customs control. For clearance in the country to be visited it would be necessary to approach that country's embassy or High Commission in the UK.

The Misuse of Drugs Act, 1971

This Act was passed in 1971 to provide more flexible and more comprehensive control over the misuse of drugs of all kinds than was possible under the earlier Dangerous Drugs Act. The Act as amended prohibits certain activities in relation to 'Controlled Drugs', in particular their manufacture, supply, and possession. The penalties applicable to offences involving the different drugs are graded broadly according to the *harmfulness attributable to a drug when it is misused* and for this purpose the drugs are defined in the following three classes:

> **Class A** includes: alfentanil, cocaine, dextromoramide, diamorphine (heroin), dipipanone, lysergide (LSD), methadone, morphine, opium, pethidine, phencyclidine, and class B substances when prepared for injection
> **Class B** includes: oral amphetamines, barbiturates, cannabis, cannabis resin, codeine, ethylmorphine, glutethimide, pentazocine, phenmetrazine, and pholcodine
> **Class C** includes: certain drugs related to the amphetamines such as benzphetamine and chlorphentermine, buprenorphine, diethylpropion, mazindol, meprobamate, pemoline, pipradrol, and most benzodiazepines

The Misuse of Drugs Regulations 1985 define the classes of person who are authorised to supply and possess controlled drugs while acting in their professional capacities and lay down the conditions under which these activities may be carried out. In the regulations drugs are divided into five schedules each specifying the requirements governing such activities as import, export, production, supply, possession, prescribing, and record keeping which apply to them.

> **Schedule 1** includes drugs such as cannabis and lysergide which are not used medicinally. Possession and supply are prohibited except in accordance with Home Office authority.

Schedule 2 includes drugs such as diamorphine (heroin), morphine, pethidine, quinalbarbitone, glutethimide, amphetamine, and cocaine and are subject to the full controlled drug requirements relating to prescriptions, safe custody, the need to keep registers, etc. (unless exempted in schedule 5).

Schedule 3 includes the barbiturates (except quinalbarbitone, now schedule 2), buprenorphine, diethylpropion, mazindol, meprobamate, pentazocine, and phentermine. They are subject to the special prescription requirements (except for phenobarbitone, see p. 7) but not to the safe custody requirements (except for buprenorphine and diethylpropion) nor to the need to keep registers (although there are requirements for the retention of invoices for 2 years).

Schedule 4 includes 34 benzodiazepines and pemoline which are subject to minimal control. In particular, controlled drug prescription requirements do not apply and they are not subject to safe custody.

Schedule 5 includes those preparations which, because of their strength, are exempt from virtually all Controlled Drug requirements other than retention of invoices for two years.

Notification of Addicts

The Misuse of Drugs (Notification of and Supply to Addicts) Regulations 1973 require that any doctor who attends a person who the doctor considers or has reasonable grounds to suspect, is addicted to any drug shall, within seven days of the attendance, furnish in writing particulars of that person to:

Chief Medical Officer,
Home Office, Drugs Branch,
Queen Anne's Gate, London SW1H 9AT.

The drugs commonly in use to which the Regulations apply are:

Cocaine	Methadone
Dextromoramide	Morphine
Diamorphine	Opium
Dipipanone	Oxycodone
Hydrocodone	Pethidine
Hydromorphone	Phenazocine
Levorphanol	Piritramide

Note. Dipipanone is only legally available as Diconal® Tablets. These have been much misused by opiate addicts in recent years; only medical practitioners with a special licence may now prescribe them for addicts to treat addiction. Doctors and others should be suspicious of young people who ask for them, especially as temporary residents.

Particulars[1] to be notified to the Chief Medical Officer are:

Name and address
Sex
Date of birth
National Health Service number
Date of attendance
Name of drugs of addiction
Whether patient injects any drug (whether or not notifiable)

Notification must be confirmed annually in writing if the patient is still being treated by the practitioner. Notified information is incorporated in an Index of Addicts which is maintained in the Home Office and information from this is available on a confidential basis to doctors; in fact, it is good medical practice to check all new cases of addiction or suspected addiction with the Index before prescribing or supplying controlled drugs since this is a safeguard against addicts obtaining supplies simultaneously from two or more doctors. Enquiries can be made either in writing to the Chief Medical Officer or, preferably, by telephoning 071-273 2213. To keep notified information confidential, such enquiries are normally answered by means of a return telephone call. The reply will come from lay staff who are not qualified to give guidance on the clinical handling of cases; a recorded telephone service is available for out-of-office hours.

The preceding paragraph applies only to medical practitioners in England, Scotland, and Wales. In Northern Ireland notification should be sent to:

Chief Medical Officer,
Department of Health and Social Services,
Dundonald House,
Belfast BT4 3SF.
Enquiries should also be made to that Department, telephone 0232 650111 extension 229.

Prescribing of diamorphine (heroin), dipipanone, and cocaine for addicts

The Misuse of Drugs (Notification of and Supply to Addicts) Regulations 1973 also provide that only medical practitioners who hold a special licence issued by the Home Secretary may prescribe diamorphine, dipipanone (Diconal®), or cocaine for addicts; other practitioners must refer any addict who requires these drugs to a treatment centre. Whenever possible the addict will be introduced by a member of staff from the treatment centre to a pharmacist whose agreement has been obtained and whose pharmacy is conveniently sited for the patient. Prescriptions for weekly supplies will be sent to the pharmacy by post and will be dispensed on a daily basis as indicated by the doctor. If any alterations of the arrangements are requested by the addict, the portion of the prescription affected must be represcribed and not merely altered. *General practitioners and other doctors may still prescribe diamorphine, dipipanone, and cocaine for patients (including addicts) for relief of pain due to organic disease or injury without a special licence.*

For prescription-writing guidelines, see p. 7.

---

1. Only the particulars of which the doctor has knowledge need be notified immediately; the remainder may be notified at a later date. General practitioners and hospital doctors may now obtain notification forms from their Regional Health Authority Database Administrator; private doctors, police surgeons, and prison medical officers may obtain form HSA2/1(rev) for notification from their Family Health Services Authority (FHSA).

Adverse Reactions to Drugs

Any drug may produce unwanted or unexpected adverse reactions. Detection and recording of these is of vital importance. Doctors are urged to help by reporting adverse reactions to:

CSM
Freepost
London SW8 5BR
(071-627 3291)

Yellow prepaid lettercards for reporting are available from the above address or by dialling 100 and asking for 'CSM Freefone'; also, forms are bound in this book (inside back cover).

A 24-hour Freefone service is now available to all parts of the United Kingdom, for doctors seeking advice and information on adverse reactions; it may be obtained by dialling 100 and asking for 'CSM Freefone'. Outside office hours a telephone-answering machine will take messages.

The following regional centres also collect data:

CSM Mersey
Freepost
Liverpool L3 3AB
(051-236 4620 Extn 2126)

CSM Northern
Freepost 1085
Newcastle upon Tyne
NE1 1BR
(091-232 1525 Direct Line)

CSM Wales
Freepost
Cardiff CF4 1ZZ
(0222 759541 Direct Line)

CSM West Midlands
Freepost
Birmingham B15 1BR
(021-627 2179 Direct Line)

Suspected adverse reactions to *any* therapeutic agent should be reported, including drugs, blood products, vaccines, X-ray contrast media, dental or surgical materials, intra-uterine devices, and contact lens fluids.

ADROIT

Adverse Drug Reactions On-line Information Tracking (ADROIT) has now been introduced to facilitate the monitoring of adverse drug reactions.

NEWER DRUGS. These are indicated by the sign ▼. Doctors are asked to report *all* suspected reactions (i.e. any adverse or any unexpected event, however minor, which could conceivably be attributed to the drug). Reports should be made despite uncertainty about a causal relationship, irrespective of whether the reaction is well recognized, and even if other drugs have been given concurrently.

ESTABLISHED DRUGS. Doctors are asked to report *all* serious suspected reactions, including those that are fatal, life-threatening, disabling, incapacitating, or which result in or prolong hospitalisation; they should be reported even if the effect is well recognised.

Examples include anaphylaxis, blood disorders, endocrine disturbances, effects on fertility, haemorrhage from any site, renal impairment, jaundice, ophthalmic disorders, severe CNS effects, severe skin reactions, reactions in pregnant women, and any drug interactions. Reports of serious adverse reactions are required to enable risk/benefit ratios to be compared with other drugs of a similar class. For established drugs doctors are asked not to report well-known, relatively minor side-effects, such as dry mouth with tricyclic antidepressants, constipation with opioids, or nausea with digoxin.

Special problems

Delayed drug effects. Some reactions (e.g. cancers, chloroquine retinopathy, and retroperitoneal fibrosis) may become manifest months or years after exposure. Any suspicion of such an association should be reported.

The elderly. Doctors are asked to be particularly alert to adverse reactions in the elderly.

Congenital abnormalities. When an infant is born with a congenital abnormality or there is a malformed aborted fetus doctors are asked to consider whether this might be an adverse reaction to a drug and to report all drugs (including self-medication) taken during pregnancy.

Vaccines. Doctors are asked to report all suspected reactions to both new and established vaccines. The balance between risks and benefits needs to be kept under continuous review.

Prevention of adverse reactions

Adverse reactions may be prevented as follows:

1. Never use any drug unless there is a good indication. If the patient is pregnant do not use a drug unless the need for it is imperative.
2. It is very important to recognise allergy and idiosyncrasy as causes of adverse drug reactions. Ask if the patient had previous reactions.
3. Ask if the patient is already taking other drugs *including self-medication*; remember that interactions may occur.
4. Age and hepatic or renal disease may alter the metabolism or excretion of drugs, so that much smaller doses may need to be prescribed. Pharmacogenetic factors may also be responsible for variations in the rate of metabolism, notably of isoniazid and the tricyclic antidepressants.
5. Prescribe as few drugs as possible and give very clear instructions to the elderly or any patient likely to misunderstand complicated instructions.
6. When possible use a familiar drug. With a new drug be particularly alert for adverse reactions or unexpected events.
7. If serious adverse reactions are liable to occur warn the patient.

Defective Medicines

During the manufacture or distribution of a medicine an error or accident may occur whereby the finished product does not conform to its specification. While such a defect may impair the therapeutic effect of the product and could adversely affect the health of a patient, it should **not** be confused with an Adverse Drug Reaction where the product conforms to its specification.

The Defect Medicines Report Centre operates a 24-hour service to assist with the investigation of problems arising from licensed medicinal products thought to be defective, and to co-ordinate any necessary protective action. Reports on suspect defective medicinal products should include the brand or the non-proprietary name, the name of the manufacturer or supplier, the strength and dosage form of the product, the product licence number, the batch number or numbers of the product, the nature of the defect, and an account of any action already taken in consequence. The Centre can be contacted at:

The Defect Medicines Report Centre
Medicines Control Agency
Room 1801, Market Towers
1 Nine Elms Lane
London SW8 5NQ
071-273 0574 (weekdays 8.30 am–5.30 pm)
or 071-210 5368 or 5371 (any other time)

Prescribing for Children

All children, and particularly neonates, differ from adults in their response to drugs. Special care is needed in the neonatal period (first 30 days of life) and doses should always be calculated according to weight. At this age, the risk of toxicity is increased by inefficient renal filtration, relative enzyme deficiencies, differing target organ sensitivity, and inadequate detoxifying systems causing delayed excretion. In childhood dosage should be adjusted for weight until 50 kg or puberty is reached.

Whenever possible painful intramuscular injections should be **avoided** in children.

PRESCRIPTION WRITING. Prescriptions should be written according to the guidelines in Prescription Writing (p. 4). Inclusion of age is a legal requirement in the case of prescription-only medicines for children under 12 years of age, but it is preferable to state the age for **all** prescriptions for children.

It is particularly important to state the strengths of capsules or tablets. Although liquid preparations are particularly suitable for children, many contain sucrose which encourages dental decay. When taken over a long period, sugar-free tablets and liquid medicines should be used when possible.

When a prescription for a liquid oral preparation is written and the dose ordered is smaller than 5 mL, the preparation will no longer be diluted. Instead an **oral syringe** will be supplied, for full details, see p. 2. Parents should be advised not to add any medicines to the contents of the infant's feeding bottle, since the drug may interact with the milk or other liquid in it; moreover the ingested dosage may be reduced, if the child does not drink all the contents.

Parents must be warned to keep **all** medicines out of the reach of children, see Safety in the Home, p. 3.

Dosage in Children

Children's doses in the BNF are stated in the individual drug entries as far as possible, except where paediatric use is not recommended or there are special hazards.

Doses are generally based on body-weight (in kilograms) or the following age ranges:

first month (neonate)
up to 1 year (infant)
1–5 years
6–12 years

Where a single dose is quoted for a given range, it applies to the middle of the age range and some extrapolation may be necessary to obtain doses for ages at the lower and upper limits of the stated range.

DOSE CALCULATION. Children's doses may be calculated from adult doses by using age, body-weight, or body-surface area, or by a combination of these factors. The most reliable methods are those based on body-surface area.

Body-weight may be used to calculate doses expressed in mg/kg. Young children may require a higher dose per kilogram than adults because of their higher metabolic rates. Other problems need to be considered. For example, calculation by body-weight in the obese child would result in much higher doses being administered than necessary; in such cases, dose should be calculated from an ideal weight, related to height and age.

Body-surface area (BSA) estimates are more accurate for calculation of paediatric doses than body-weight since many physical phenomena are more closely related to body-surface area. The average body-surface area of a 70-kilogram human is about 1.8 m^2. Thus, to calculate the dose for a child the following formula may be used:

Approximate dose for patient =

$$\frac{\text{surface area of patient (m}^2\text{)}}{1.8} \times \text{adult dose}$$

The **percentage method** below may be used to calculate paediatric doses of commonly prescribed drugs that have a wide margin between the therapeutic and the toxic dose.

Age	Ideal body-weight kg	lb	Height cm	in	Body-surface m^2	Percentage of adult dose
Newborn*	3.4	7.5	50	20	0.23	12.5
1 month*	4.2	9	55	22	0.26	14.5
3 months*	5.6	12	59	23	0.32	18
6 months	7.7	17	67	26	0.40	22
1 year	10	22	76	30	0.47	25
3 years	14	31	94	37	0.62	33
5 years	18	40	108	42	0.73	40
7 years	23	51	120	47	0.88	50
12 years	37	81	148	58	1.25	75
Adult						
Male	68	150	173	68	1.8	100
Female	56	123	163	64	1.6	100

* The figures relate to full term and not preterm infants who may need reduced dosage according to their clinical condition.

More precise body-surface values may be calculated from height and weight by means of a table (e.g. *Martindale: The Extra Pharmacopoeia*, 29th Edition, London, Pharmaceutical Press, 1989) or a nomogram (e.g. J. Insley, *A Paediatric Vade-Mecum*, 12th Edition, London, Edward Arnold, 1990).

DOSE FREQUENCY. Doses for antibiotics are usually stated as every 6 hours. Some flexibility should be allowed in children to avoid waking them during the night. For example, the night-time dose may be given at the parent's bedtime.

Where new or potentially toxic drugs are used, the manufacturers' recommended doses should be carefully followed.

Prescribing in Terminal Care

In recent years there has been increased interest in providing better treatment and support for patients with terminal illness. The aim is to keep them as comfortable, alert, and free of pain as possible. If patients are to end their days in serenity it may also be necessary to direct attention to emotional, financial, social, or family problems. The patient's minister or the hospital chaplain may give invaluable help.

DOMICILIARY CARE. If they wish, whenever possible, patients should end their days in their own homes. Although families may at first be afraid of caring for the patient at home, they will usually do so if extra support from district nursing services and social services is provided. Families may be reassured if an assurance is given that the patient will be admitted to a hospital or hospice if they cannot cope.

HOSPITAL OR HOSPICE CARE. The most important lesson to be drawn from the experience of hospices is that both doctors and nurses must give time to listen to the patient. This gives great support and comfort to a patient who may otherwise suffer intolerable loneliness. Often problems come to light that can easily be dealt with—adjusting a blind in the late afternoon, an irritating noise to be avoided, drinks to be placed in easier reach, someone to read the newspaper, or the TV to be replaced by radio. The staff should not exclude the family from contributing to the patient's care; if prevented they may be resentful or subsequently suffer a feeling of guilt.

DRUG TREATMENT. The number of drugs should be as few as possible, for even the taking of medicine may be an effort. Oral medication is usually satisfactory unless there is severe nausea and vomiting, dysphagia, weakness, or coma, in which case parenteral medication may be necessary.

PAIN

Analgesics are always more effective in preventing the development of pain than in the relief of established pain.

The **non-opioid** analgesics **aspirin** or **paracetamol** given regularly will often make the use of opioids unnecessary. Aspirin (or other NSAIDs if preferred) may also control the pain of *bone secondaries*; naproxen, flurbiprofen, and indomethacin (see section 10.1.1) are valuable and if necessary can be given rectally. **Corticosteroids** or **radiotherapy** are also often useful for pain due to bone metastases.

Morphine is the most useful of the **opioid analgesics**. In addition to relief of pain, it confers a state of euphoria and mental detachment.

Nausea and vomiting may occur in the initial stages of morphine therapy but can be prevented by giving an anti-emetic such as haloperidol or prochlorperazine. An anti-emetic is usually only necessary for the first 4 or 5 days therefore fixed-combination opioid preparations containing an anti-emetic are not recommended since they lead to unnecessary anti-emetic therapy (often with undesirable drowsiness). *Constipation* is almost invariable and should be prevented by the regular administration of a laxative.

Morphine is given *by mouth* as an oral solution regularly every 4 hours, the initial dose depending largely on the patient's previous treatment. A dose of 5–10 mg is enough to replace a weaker analgesic (such as paracetamol or co-proxamol), but 10–20 mg or more is required to replace a strong one (comparable to morphine itself). If the first dose of morphine is no more effective than the previous analgesic it should be increased by 50%, the aim being to choose the lowest dose which prevents pain. Although a dose of 5–20 mg is usually adequate there should be no hesitation in increasing it to 30–60 mg or occasionally to 90–150 mg or higher if necessary. If pain occurs between doses the next dose due is increased; in the interim an additional dose is given.

Modified-release tablets of morphine (MST Continus® tablets or SRM-Rhotard® tablets) are an alternative to the oral solution; they have the advantage that they need only be taken every 12 hours. The starting dose of MST Continus® tablets or SRM-Rhotard® tablets is usually 10–20 mg every 12 hours if no other analgesic (or only paracetamol) has previously been taken, but to replace a weaker opioid analgesic (such as co-proxamol) the starting dose is usually 20–30 mg every 12 hours. Increments should be made to the dose, not to the frequency of administration, which should remain at every 12 hours.

The effective dose of MST Continus® tablets or SRM-Rhotard® tablets can alternatively be found by giving the oral solution of morphine every 4 hours in increasing doses until the pain has been controlled, and then transferring the patient to the same total 24-hour dose of morphine given as the modified-release tablet (divided into two portions for 12-hourly administration). The first dose of the modified-release tablet is given 4 hours after the last dose of the oral solution.

If the patient becomes unable to swallow, the equivalent intramuscular dose of morphine is half the oral solution dose; in the case of the modified-release tablets it is half the total 24-hour dose (which is then divided into 6 portions to be given every 4 hours). **Diamorphine** is preferred for injection because being more soluble it can be given in a smaller volume. The equivalent intramuscular (or subcutaneous) dose of diamorphine is only about a quarter to a third of the oral dose of morphine; *subcutaneous infusion via syringe driver* can be useful. The patient's symptoms are preferably stabilised with regular intramuscular (or subcutaneous) injections before commencing the subcutaneous infusion. It is common practice to add haloperidol, methotrimeprazine, or cyclizine as an anti-emetic; hyoscine may be added for excessive respiratory secretions or intestinal colic.

Morphine is also available for *rectal administration* as suppositories; alternatively **oxycodone** suppositories can be obtained on special order.

Nerve blocks may be considered when pain is localised to a specific area.

Prescribing in terminal care

GASTRO-INTESTINAL PAIN. The pain of *intestinal colic* may be reduced by loperamide 2–4 mg 4 times daily. Hyoscine hydrobromide may also be helpful, given sublingually at a dose of 300 micrograms 3 times daily as Kwells® (Nicholas) tablets, or as a continuous subcutaneous infusion of 0.6–2.4 mg over 24 hours using a syringe driver.

Gastric distension pain due to pressure on the stomach may be helped by a preparation incorporating an antacid with an antiflatulent (see section 1.1.1.1) and by domperidone 10 mg 3 times daily before meals.

MUSCLE SPASM. The pain of muscle spasm can be helped by a muscle relaxant such as diazepam 5–10 mg daily or baclofen 5–10 mg 3 times daily.

NERVE PAIN. Pain due to *nerve compression* may be reduced by a corticosteroid such as dexamethasone 8 mg daily, which reduces oedema around the tumour, thus reducing compression.

Dysaesthetic or stabbing pain resulting from *nerve irritation* may be reduced by amitriptyline 25–75 mg at night, or by carbamazepine 200 mg 3 times daily.

MISCELLANEOUS CONDITIONS

RAISED INTRACRANIAL PRESSURE. Headache due to *raised intracranial pressure* often responds to a high dose of a corticosteroid, such as dexamethasone 16 mg daily for 4 to 5 days, subsequently reduced to 4 to 6 mg daily if possible.

INTRACTABLE COUGH. *Intractable cough* may be relieved by moist inhalations or may require regular administration of an oral morphine hydrochloride solution in an initial dose of 5 mg every 4 hours. Methadone linctus should be avoided as it has a long duration of action and tends to accumulate.

DYSPNOEA. *Dyspnoea* may be relieved by regular oral morphine hydrochloride solution in carefully titrated doses, starting at 5 mg every 4 hours. Diazepam 5–10 mg daily may be helpful; a corticosteroid, such as dexamethasone 4 to 8 mg daily, may also be helpful if there is *bronchospasm* or *partial obstruction*.

EXCESSIVE RESPIRATORY SECRETION. *Excessive respiratory secretion* (death rattle) may be reduced by subcutaneous injection of hyoscine hydrobromide 400 to 600 micrograms every 4 to 8 hours.

RESTLESSNESS AND CONFUSION. *Restlessness and confusion* may require treatment with haloperidol 1 to 3 mg by mouth every 8 hours. Chlorpromazine 25–50 mg by mouth every 8 hours is an alternative, but causes more sedation. Methotrimeprazine is also used occasionally for restlessness.

HICCUP. *Hiccup due to gastric distension* may be helped by a preparation incorporating an antacid with an antiflatulent (see section 1.1.1.1). If this fails, metoclopramide 10 mg every 6 to 8 hours by mouth or by intramuscular injection can be added; if this also fails, chlorpromazine 10 to 25 mg every 6 to 8 hours can be tried.

ANOREXIA. *Anorexia* may be helped by prednisolone 15 to 30 mg daily or dexamethasone 2 to 4 mg daily.

CONSTIPATION. *Constipation* is a very common cause of distress and should be prevented if possible by the regular administration of laxatives; a faecal softener with a peristaltic stimulant (e.g. co-danthramer), or lactulose solution with a senna preparation should be used (see sections 1.6.2 and 1.6.3).

FUNGATING GROWTH. *Fungating growth* may be treated by cleansing with a mixture of 1 part of 4% povidone-iodine skin cleanser solution and 4 parts of liquid paraffin. Oral administration of metronidazole (see section 5.1.11) may eradicate the anaerobic bacteria responsible for the odour of fungating tumours; topical application (see section 13.10.1.2) is also used but may increase the likelihood of resistance.

CAPILLARY BLEEDING. *Capillary bleeding* may be reduced by applying gauze soaked in adrenaline solution (1 in 1000).

DRY MOUTH. *Dry mouth* may be due to candidiasis which can be treated by nystatin oral suspension or pastilles, amphotericin lozenges, or miconazole oral gel after food; alternatively, fluconazole can be given by mouth (see section 5.2). Dry mouth can also be a side-effect of morphine.

PRURITUS. *Pruritus*, even when associated with *obstructive jaundice*, often responds to simple measures such as emollients. In the case of obstructive jaundice, further measures include administration of cholestyramine or an anabolic steroid, such as stanozolol 5–10 mg daily; antihistamines can be helpful (see section 3.4.1).

CONVULSIONS. Patients with *cerebral tumours* or *uraemia* may be susceptible to convulsions. Prophylactic treatment with phenytoin or carbamazepine (see section 4.8.1) should be considered. When oral medication is no longer possible, diazepam as suppositories 10–20 mg every 4 to 8 hours, or phenobarbitone by injection 50–200 mg twice daily is continued as prophylaxis.

DYSPHAGIA. A corticosteroid such as dexamethasone 8 mg daily may help, temporarily, if there is an obstruction due to *tumour*. See also under Dry Mouth.

INSOMNIA. Patients with advanced cancer may not sleep because of discomfort, cramps, night sweats, joint stiffness, or fear. There should be appropriate treatment of these problems before hypnotics are used. Benzodiazepines, such as temazepam, may be useful (see section 4.1.1).

NAUSEA AND VOMITING. *Nausea and vomiting* are very common in patients with advanced cancer. The cause should be diagnosed before treatment with anti-emetics (see section 4.6) is started.

HYPERCALCAEMIA. See section 9.5.1.2.

Prescribing for the Elderly

Old people, especially the very old, require special care and consideration from prescribers.

Elderly patients are apt to receive multiple drugs for their multiple diseases. This greatly increases the risk of drug interactions as well as other adverse reactions. Moreover, symptoms such as headache, sleeplessness, and lightheadedness which may be associated with social stress, as in widowhood, loneliness, and family dispersal can lead to further prescribing, especially of psychotropics. The use of drugs in such cases can at best be a poor substitute for effective social measures and at worst pose a serious threat from adverse reactions.

In very old subjects, manifestations of normal ageing may be mistaken for disease and lead to inappropriate prescribing. For example, drugs such as prochlorperazine are commonly misprescribed for giddiness due to age-related loss of postural stability. Not only is such treatment ineffective but the patient may experience serious side-effects such as drug-induced parkinsonism, postural hypotension, and mental confusion.

Self-medication with over-the-counter products or with drugs prescribed for a previous illness (or even for another person) may be an added complication. Discussion with relatives and a home visit may be needed to establish exactly what is being taken.

The ageing nervous system shows increased *susceptibility* to many commonly used drugs, such as opioid analgesics, benzodiazepines, and antiparkinsonian drugs, all of which must be used with caution.

PHARMACOKINETICS. While drug distribution and metabolism may be significantly altered, the most important effect of age is reduction in renal clearance, frequently aggravated by the effects of prostatism, nephrosclerosis, or chronic urinary tract infection. Many aged patients thus possess only limited reserves of renal function, excrete drugs slowly, and are highly susceptible to nephrotoxic drugs. Acute illness may lead to rapid reduction in renal clearance, especially if accompanied by dehydration. Hence, a patient stabilised on a drug with a narrow margin between the therapeutic and the toxic dose (e.g. digoxin) may rapidly develop adverse effects in the aftermath of a myocardial infarction or a respiratory tract infection.

The net result of pharmacokinetic changes is that tissue concentrations are commonly increased by over 50%, and aged and debilitated patients may show even larger changes.

COMMON ADVERSE REACTIONS. Adverse reactions often present in the elderly in a vague and non-specific fashion. *Mental confusion* is often the presenting symptom (caused by almost any of the commonly used drugs). Other common manifestations are *constipation* (with antimuscarinics and many tranquillisers) and postural *hypotension* and *falls* (with diuretics and many psychotropics).

Many hypnotics with long half-lives have serious hangover effects of drowsiness, unsteady gait, and even slurred speech and confusion. Those with short half-lives should be used but they too can present problems (see section 4.1.1). Short courses of hypnotics are occasionally useful for helping a patient through an acute illness or some other crisis but every effort must be made to avoid dependence.

Diuretics are overprescribed in old age and should not be used on a long-term basis to treat simple gravitational oedema which will usually respond to increased movement, raising the legs, and support stockings. A few days of diuretic treatment may speed the clearing of the oedema but it should rarely need continued drug therapy.

Other drugs which commonly cause adverse reactions are antiparkinsonian drugs, antihypertensives, psychotropics, and digoxin; the usual maintenance dose of digoxin in very old patients is 125 micrograms daily (62.5 micrograms is often inadequate, and toxicity is common in those given 250 micrograms).

Drug-induced blood disorders are much more common in the elderly. Therefore drugs with a tendency to cause bone marrow depression (e.g. co-trimoxazole, mianserin) should be avoided unless there is no acceptable alternative.

Bleeding associated with aspirin and other NSAIDs is more common in the elderly, and the outcome tends to be more serious.

The elderly generally require a lower maintenance dose of warfarin than younger adults; once again, the outcome of bleeding tends to be more serious.

GUIDELINES. First one must always pose the question of whether a drug is indicated at all.

It is a sensible policy to prescribe from a limited range of drugs and to be thoroughly familiar with their effects in the elderly.

Dosage should generally be substantially lower than for younger patients and it is common to start with about 50% of the adult dose. Some drugs (e.g. chlorpropamide) should be avoided altogether.

Review repeat prescriptions regularly. It may be possible to stop the drug (e.g. digoxin can often be withdrawn) or it may be necessary to reduce the dose to match diminishing renal function.

Simplify regimens. Elderly patients cannot normally cope with more than three different drugs and, ideally, these should not be given more than twice daily. In particular, regimens which call for a confusing array of dosage intervals should be avoided.

Write full instructions on every prescription (*including* repeat prescriptions) so that containers can be properly labelled with full directions. Avoid imprecisions like 'as directed'. Child-resistant containers may be unsuitable.

Instruct patients what to do when drugs run out, and also how to dispose of any that are no longer necessary.

If these guidelines are followed most elderly people will cope adequately with their own medicines. If not then it is essential to enrol the help of a third party, usually a relative but sometimes a home help, neighbour, or a sheltered-housing warden.

Emergency Treatment of Poisoning

Poisons Information Services

Belfast	0232 240503
Birmingham	021-554 3801
Cardiff	0222 709901
Dublin	0001 379964
	or 0001 379966
Edinburgh	031-229 2477
	031-228 2441
	(Viewdata)
Leeds	0532 430715
	or 0532 432799
London	071-635 9191
	or 071-955 5095
Newcastle	091-232 5131

Note. Some of these centres also advise on laboratory analytical services which may be of help in the diagnosis and management of a small number of cases.

CONSULT POISONS INFORMATION CENTRES DAY AND NIGHT

These notes deal with the initial management of acute poisoning in the home; brief mention only is given of hospital-based treatment. The notes are only guidelines and it is strongly recommended that **poisons information services** (see previous page) be consulted in cases where there is doubt about the degree of risk or about appropriate management.

HOSPITAL ADMISSION. All patients who show features of poisoning should generally be admitted to hospital. Patients who have taken poisons with delayed actions should also be admitted, even if they appear well; delayed-action poisons include aspirin, iron, paracetamol, tricyclic antidepressants, co-phenotrope (diphenoxylate with atropine, *Lomotil*®), and paraquat, also modified-release capsules or tablets. A note should be sent of what is known and what treatment has been given.

It is often impossible to establish with certainty the identity of the poison and the size of the dose. Fortunately this is not usually important because only a few poisons (such as opioids, paracetamol, and iron) have specific antidotes and few patients require active removal of the poison. Most patients must be treated symptomatically. Nevertheless, knowledge of the type of poisoning does help in anticipating the course of events. Patients' reports may be of little help, as they may be confused or may only be able to say that they have taken an undefined amount, possibly of mixed drugs. Parents may think a child has taken something which could be poisonous and may exaggerate or underplay the risks out of anxiety or guilt. Sometimes symptoms are due to an illness such as appendicitis. Accidents can arise from a number of domestic and industrial products (the contents of which are not generally known).

> The **poisons information services** (see p. 15) will provide advice on all aspects of poisoning day and night.

General care

RESPIRATION

Respiration is often impaired in unconscious patients. An obstructed airway requires immediate attention. Pull the tongue forward, remove dentures and oral secretions, hold the jaw forward, insert an oropharyngeal airway if one is available, and turn the patient semiprone. The risk of inhaling vomit is minimised with the patient positioned semiprone and head down.

Most poisons that impair consciousness also depress respiration. Assisted ventilation by mouth-to-mouth or Ambu bag inflation may be needed. Oxygen is not a substitute for adequate ventilation, though it should be given in the highest concentration possible in poisoning with carbon monoxide and irritant gases.

Respiratory stimulants do not help and are **potentially dangerous**.

BLOOD PRESSURE

Hypotension is common in severe poisoning with central nervous system depressants. A systolic blood pressure of less than 70 mmHg may lead to irreversible brain damage or renal tubular necrosis. The patient should be carried head downwards on a stretcher and nursed in this position in the ambulance. Oxygen should be given to correct hypoxia and an intravenous infusion should be set up if at all practicable. Vasopressor drugs should **not** be used.

Fluid depletion without hypotension is common after prolonged coma and after aspirin poisoning due to vomiting, sweating, and hyperpnoea.

HEART

Cardiac conduction defects and arrhythmias may occur in acute poisoning, notably with tricyclic antidepressants. Arrhythmias often respond to correction of underlying hypoxia or acidosis. Ventricular arrhythmias that have been confirmed by emergency ECG and which are causing serious hypotension may require treatment with lignocaine 50–100 mg by slow intravenous injection. Supraventricular arrhythmias are seldom life-threatening and drug treatment is best withheld until the patient reaches hospital.

BODY TEMPERATURE

Hypothermia may develop in patients of any age who have been deeply unconscious for some hours particularly following overdose with barbiturates or phenothiazines. It may be missed unless temperature is measured rectally using a low-reading rectal thermometer. It is best treated by wrapping the patient in blankets to conserve body heat. Hot-water bottles are of little value and may cause burns.

CONVULSIONS

Single short-lived convulsions do not require treatment. Diazepam, up to 10 mg by slow intravenous injection, preferably in emulsion form, should be given if convulsions are protracted or recur frequently; it should not be given intramuscularly.

Removal and elimination

REMOVAL FROM THE STOMACH

The dangers of attempting to empty the stomach have to be balanced against the toxicity of the ingested poison, as assessed by the quantity ingested, the inherent toxicity of the poison, and the time since ingestion. Gastric emptying is clearly unnecessary if the risk of toxicity is small or if the patient presents too late.

Emptying the stomach by **gastric lavage** or **emesis** is of doubtful value if attempted more than 4 hours after ingestion. However, a worthwhile recovery of salicylates can be achieved up to 24 hours after ingestion and of tricyclic antidepressants (which delay gastric emptying) up to 8 hours after ingestion. The chief danger of gastric aspiration and lavage is inhalation of stomach contents, and it should **not** be attempted in drowsy or comatose patients unless there is a good enough cough reflex or the airway can be protected by a cuffed endotracheal tube. Stomach tubes should **not** be passed after corrosive poisoning.

Petroleum products are more dangerous in the lungs than in the stomach and therefore removal from the stomach is **not** advised because of the risk of inhalation.

On balance gastric lavage is seldom practicable or desirable before the patient reaches hospital.

Emesis induced by using **ipecacuanha** (Paediatric Ipecacuanha Emetic Mixture BP) tends to be used in children. It may be given safely in the home providing that the patient is fully conscious and that the poison ingested is neither a corrosive nor a petroleum distillate, and is not liable to cause rapid onset of coma or convulsions.

Salt solutions, copper sulphate, apomorphine, and mustard are dangerous and should **not** be used.

IPECACUANHA

Indications: induction of emesis in selected patients, see notes above

Cautions: avoid in poisoning with corrosive or petroleum products owing to risk of aspiration (see notes above); also avoid if risk of aspiration, in shock, or if risk of convulsions; cardiovascular disease

Side-effects: excessive vomiting and mucosal damage; cardiac effects if absorbed

Dose: see under preparation below

Ipecacuanha Emetic Mixture, Paediatric (BP)
Paediatric Ipecacuanha Emetic
  Note. Paediatric Ipecacuanha Emetic Mixture is equivalent in strength to Ipecac Syrup USP
  Mixture, ipecacuanha liquid extract 0.7 mL, hydrochloric acid 0.025 mL, glycerol 1 mL, syrup to 10 mL
  Dose: ADULT 30 mL; CHILD 6–18 months 10 mL, older children 15 mL; the dose is followed by a tumblerful of water and repeated after 20 minutes if necessary

PREVENTION OF ABSORPTION

Given by mouth, **activated charcoal** can bind many poisons in the stomach, thereby *reducing their absorption*. The **sooner** it is given the **more effective** it is—but it may still be effective up to 4 hours after ingestion (longer in the case of modified-release preparations). It is safe and is particularly useful for the prevention of absorption of poisons which are toxic in small amounts, e.g. antidepressants.

For the use of charcoal in active elimination techniques, see below.

Carbomix® (Penn)
  Powder, activated charcoal. Net price 50-g bottle = £10.93
  Dose: reduction of absorption, 50 g; CHILD, 25 g (50 g in severe poisoning)
  Active elimination, see below

Medicoal® (Torbet)
  Granules, effervescent, activated charcoal 5 g/sachet. Net price 5-sachet pack = £3.28, 30-sachet pack = £16.50
  Dose: reduction of absorption, initially 1–2 sachets repeated every 15–20 minutes until dose of charcoal given is 5–10 times that of poison ingested (if amount known) *or* (if amount not known) until max. 10 sachets have been given; each sachet suspended in approx. 100 mL water (volume of suspension may need to be reduced for children)

ACTIVE ELIMINATION TECHNIQUES

Repeated doses of **activated charcoal** by mouth *enhance the elimination* of some drugs after they have been absorbed; repeated doses are given after overdosage with:

Aspirin
Carbamazepine
Dapsone
Digitoxin
Digoxin
Phenobarbitone
  and other barbiturates
Phenytoin
Quinine
Theophylline

The usual adult dose of activated charcoal is 50 g initially then 25 g every 4 hours.

Other techniques intended to enhance the elimination of poisons after absorption are only practicable in hospital and are only suitable for a small number of severely poisoned patients. Moreover, they only apply to a limited number of poisons. Examples include:
  Forced alkaline diuresis for salicylates and phenobarbitone (but haemodialysis now preferred)
  Haemodialysis for salicylates, phenobarbitone, methyl alcohol (methanol), ethylene glycol, and lithium
  Haemoperfusion for medium- and short-acting barbiturates, chloral hydrate, meprobamate, and theophylline

Specific drugs

ALCOHOL

Acute intoxication with alcohol (ethanol) is common in adults but also occurs in children. The features include ataxia, dysarthria, nystagmus, and drowsiness, which may progress to coma, with hypotension and acidosis. Aspiration of vomit is a special hazard and hypoglycaemia may occur in children and some adults. Patients are managed supportively with particular attention to maintaining a clear airway and measures to reduce the risk of aspiration of gastric contents. The blood glucose is measured and glucose given if indicated.

ANALGESICS (NON-OPIOID)

ASPIRIN. Absorption of aspirin and other salicylates may be delayed, especially if enteric-coated tablets have been taken; blood concentrations taken within the first 6 hours may therefore be misleadingly low.

The chief features of poisoning are hyperventilation, tinnitus, deafness, vasodilatation, and sweating. Coma is uncommon but indicates very severe poisoning. The associated acid-base disturbances are complex.

Gastric emptying is carried out in all cases; a worthwhile recovery of salicylates can be achieved up to 24 hours after ingestion.

Treatment must be in hospital where plasma salicylate, pH, and electrolytes can be measured. Fluid losses are replaced and forced alkaline diuresis is considered when the plasma-salicylate concentration is greater than

500 mg/litre (3.6 mmol/litre) in adults *or*
300 mg/litre (2.2 mmol/litre) in children.

NSAIDs. Mefenamic acid is the most significant member of this group encountered in overdosage. Convulsions are the most important feature of toxicity and are treated with diazepam.

Ibuprofen may cause nausea, vomiting, and tinnitus, but more serious toxicity is very uncommon. Gastric emptying is indicated if more than 100 mg/kg has been ingested within the preceding 4 hours, followed by symptomatic measures.

PARACETAMOL. As little as 10–15 g (20–30 tablets) of paracetamol may cause severe hepatocellular necrosis and, less frequently, renal tubular necrosis. Nausea and vomiting, the only early features of poisoning, usually settle within 24 hours. Persistence beyond this time, often associated with the onset of right subcostal pain and tenderness, usually indicates development of hepatic necrosis. Liver damage is maximal 3–4 days after ingestion and may lead to encephalopathy, haemorrhage, hypoglycaemia, cerebral oedema, and death.

Therefore, despite a lack of significant early symptoms, patients who have taken an overdose of paracetamol should be transferred to hospital urgently.

Gastric emptying is carried out if the overdose was taken within 4 hours of admission.

Antidotes such as **acetylcysteine** and **methionine** protect the liver if given within 10–12 hours of ingestion; acetylcysteine may also be effective up to and possibly beyond 24 hours but expert advice is **essential**.

Patients at risk of liver damage and therefore requiring treatment can be identified from a single measurement of the plasma-paracetamol concentration, related to the time from ingestion, provided this time interval is not less than 4 hours; earlier samples may be misleading. The concentration is compared against a reference line joining plots of 200 mg/litre (1.32 mmol/litre) at 4 hours and 30 mg/litre (0.2 mmol/litre) at 15 hours, on a semi-logarithmic graph. Those whose concentrations are above that line are treated either with acetylcysteine intravenously or with methionine by mouth. Patients on enzyme-inducing drugs (e.g. carbamazepine, phenobarbitone, phenytoin, rifampicin, and alcohol) may develop toxicity at **lower** plasma-paracetamol concentrations; they should receive acetylcysteine if their plasma-paracetamol concentrations are 50% or more of the standard reference line.

In remote areas, emesis should be induced if the patient presents within 4 hours of the overdose. Methionine (2.5 g) should be given by mouth once vomiting has occurred; it is seldom practicable to give acetylcysteine outside hospital. Once the patient reaches hospital the need to continue treatment with the antidote will be assessed from the plasma-paracetamol concentration (related to the time from ingestion).

See also Co-proxamol, under Analgesics (opioid).

ACETYLCYSTEINE

Indications: paracetamol overdosage (see notes above)
Cautions: asthma
Side-effects: rashes, anaphylaxis
Dose: by intravenous infusion, in glucose intravenous infusion 5%, initially 150 mg/kg in 200 mL over 15 minutes, followed by 50 mg/kg in 500 mL over 4 hours, then 100 mg/kg in 1000 mL over 16 hours

PoM **Parvolex**® (Evans)
Injection, acetylcysteine 200 mg/mL. Net price course of 12 amps of 10 mL = £31.75

METHIONINE

Indications: paracetamol overdosage, see notes above
Dose: by mouth, 2.5 g initially, followed by 3 further doses of 2.5 g every 4 hours

Methionine Tablets (Evans), DL-methionine 250 mg. Net price course of 40 tabs = £8.32

ANALGESICS (OPIOID)

Opioids (narcotic analgesics) cause varying degrees of coma, respiratory depression, and pinpoint pupils. The specific antidote **naloxone** is indicated if there is coma or bradypnoea. Since naloxone is short-acting repeated injections are necessary according to the respiratory rate and depth of coma. Alternatively, it may be given by continuous intravenous infusion, the rate of administration being adjusted according to response.

CO-PROXAMOL. Combinations of dextropropoxyphene and paracetamol (co-proxamol) are frequently taken in overdosage. The initial features are those of acute opioid overdosage with coma, respiratory depression, and pinpoint pupils. Patients may die of acute cardiovascular collapse before reaching hospital (particularly if alcohol has also been consumed) unless adequately resuscitated or given **naloxone** as antidote to the dextropropoxyphene. Paracetamol hepatotoxicity may develop later and should be anticipated and treated as indicated above.

NALOXONE HYDROCHLORIDE

Indications: overdosage with opioids; for postoperative respiratory depression, see section 15.1.7
Cautions: physical dependence on opioids; cardiac irritability; naloxone is short-acting, see notes above
Dose: by intravenous injection, 0.8–2 mg repeated at intervals of 2–3 minutes to a max. of 10 mg if respiratory function does not improve (then question diagnosis); CHILD 10 micrograms/kg; subsequent dose of 100 micrograms/kg if no response

By subcutaneous or intramuscular injection, as intravenous injection but only if intravenous route not feasible (onset of action slower)
By continuous intravenous infusion, 2 mg diluted in 500 mL intravenous infusion solution at a rate adjusted according to the response

PoM **Naloxone** (Non-proprietary)
Injection, naloxone hydrochloride 400 micrograms/mL. Net price 1-mL amp = £4.92
PoM **Min-I-Jet®** **Naloxone** (IMS)
Injection, naloxone hydrochloride 400 micrograms/mL. Net price 1-mL disposable syringe = £5.17; 2-mL disposable syringe = £9.66
PoM **Narcan®** (Du Pont)
Injection, naloxone hydrochloride 400 micrograms/mL, net price 1-mL amp = £4.92, 1-mL disposable syringe = £5.44; 1 mg/mL, 2-mL amp = £22.00
Neonatal preparations —see section 15.1.7

ANTIDEPRESSANTS

Tricyclic and related antidepressants cause dry mouth, coma of varying degree, hypotension, hypothermia, hyperreflexia, extensor plantar responses, convulsions, respiratory failure, cardiac conduction defects, and arrhythmias. Dilated pupils and urinary retention also occur. Metabolic acidosis may complicate severe poisoning; delirium with confusion, agitation, and visual and auditory hallucinations, is common during recovery.

Symptomatic treatment and activated charcoal by mouth may reasonably be given in the home before transfer but hospital admission is strongly advised, and supportive measures to ensure a patent airway and adequate ventilation during transfer are mandatory. Intravenous diazepam may be required for control of convulsions (preferably in emulsion form). Although arrhythmias are worrying, some will respond to correction of hypoxia and acidosis; the use of anti-arrhythmic drugs is best avoided. Diazepam given by mouth is usually adequate to sedate delirious patients but large doses may be required.

HYPNOTICS AND ANXIOLYTICS

BARBITURATES. These cause drowsiness, coma, respiratory depression, hypotension, and hypothermia. The duration and depth of cerebral depression vary greatly with the drug, the dose, and the tolerance of the patient. The severity of poisoning is often greater with a large dose of barbiturate hypnotics than with the longer-acting phenobarbitone. The majority of patients survive with supportive measures alone. Forced alkaline diuresis may be considered in severe phenobarbitone poisoning. Charcoal haemoperfusion is the treatment of choice for the small minority of patients with very severe barbiturate poisoning who fail to improve, or who deteriorate despite good supportive care.

BENZODIAZEPINES. Benzodiazepines taken alone cause drowsiness, ataxia, dysarthria, and occasionally minor and short-lived depression of consciousness. They potentiate the effects of other central nervous system depressants taken concomitantly. Flumazenil, a benzodiazepine antagonist, may be used in the *differential diagnosis* of unclear cases of multiple drug overdose but expert advice is **essential**.

IRON SALTS

Iron poisoning is commonest in childhood and is usually accidental. The symptoms are nausea, vomiting, abdominal pain, diarrhoea, haematemesis, and rectal bleeding. Hypotension, coma, and hepatocellular necrosis occur later. Mortality is reduced with intensive and specific therapy with **desferrioxamine**, which chelates iron. The stomach should be emptied at once, preferably by inducing vomiting as this is quickest. Gastric lavage in hospital should follow as soon as possible, leaving a solution of 5–10 g of desferrioxamine mesylate in 50–100 mL water in the stomach. The serum-iron concentration is measured as an emergency and parenteral desferrioxamine given to chelate absorbed iron in excess of the expected iron binding capacity.

DESFERRIOXAMINE MESYLATE
Indications: removal of iron from the body in poisoning; for use in chronic iron overload, see section 9.1.3
Cautions: avoid prochlorperazine
Side-effects: pain at site of intramuscular injection, anaphylactic reactions, and hypotension when given too rapidly by intravenous injection
Dose: by mouth after gastric lavage, see notes above
By intramuscular injection, 1–2 g in 10–20 mL of water for injections every 3–12 hours; max. 6 g in 24 hours
By continuous intravenous infusion, up to 15 mg/kg/hour; max. 80 mg/kg in 24 hours

PoM **Desferal®** (Ciba)
Injection, powder for reconstitution, desferrioxamine mesylate. Net price 500-mg vial = £2.53

LITHIUM

Most cases of lithium intoxication occur as a complication of long-term therapy and are caused by reduced excretion of the drug due to a variety of factors including dehydration, deterioration of renal function, infections, and co-administration of diuretics or NSAIDs (or other drugs that interact). Acute deliberate overdoses may also occur with delayed onset of symptoms (12 hours or more) due to slow entry of lithium into the tissues and continuing absorption from modified-release formulations.

The early clinical features are non-specific and may include apathy and restlessness which could be confused with mental changes due to the patient's depressive illness. Vomiting, diarrhoea, ataxia, weakness, dysarthria, muscle twitching, and tremor may follow. Severe poisoning is associated with convulsions, coma, renal failure, electrolyte imbalance, dehydration, and hypotension.

Therapeutic lithium concentrations are within the range of 0.4–1.0 mmol/litre; concentrations in excess of 2.0 mmol/litre are usually associated with serious toxicity and such cases may need treatment with forced diuresis or dialysis (if there is renal failure). In acute overdosage much higher serum concentrations may be present without features of toxicity and measures to increase urine production are usually all that are necessary. Otherwise treatment is supportive with special regard to electrolyte balance, renal function, and control of convulsions.

PHENOTHIAZINES AND RELATED DRUGS

Phenothiazines cause less depression of consciousness and respiration than other sedatives. Hypotension, hypothermia, sinus tachycardia, and arrhythmias (particularly with thioridazine) may complicate poisoning. Dystonic reactions can occur with therapeutic doses, (particularly with prochlorperazine and trifluoperazine) and convulsions may occur in severe cases. Drugs to control arrhythmias and convulsions may be needed. Dystonic reactions are rapidly abolished by injection of drugs such as benztropine or procyclidine (see section 4.9.2).

STIMULANTS

AMPHETAMINES. These cause wakefulness, excessive activity, paranoia, hallucinations, and hypertension followed by exhaustion, convulsions, hyperthermia, and coma. The early stages can be controlled by chlorpromazine and, if necessary, beta-blockers. Later, tepid sponging, anticonvulsants, and artificial respiration may be needed. Amphetamine excretion can be increased by forced acid diuresis but this is seldom necessary.

COCAINE. Cocaine can be smoked, sniffed, or injected. It stimulates the central nervous system causing agitation, dilated pupils, tachycardia, hypertension, hallucinations, hypertonia, and hyperreflexia. Convulsions, coma and metabolic acidosis may develop in the worst cases. Sedation, with intravenous diazepam, may be all that is necessary but intravenous propranolol may be indicated for severe intoxication.

THEOPHYLLINE

Theophylline and related drugs are often prescribed as modified-release formulations and toxicity may therefore be delayed. They cause vomiting (which may be severe and intractable), agitation, restlessness, dilated pupils, and sinus tachycardia. More serious effects are haematemesis, convulsions, and supraventricular and ventricular arrhythmias. Profound hypokalaemia may develop rapidly.

The stomach should be emptied as early as possible. Elimination of theophylline may be enhanced by repeated doses of activated charcoal by mouth (see also under Active Elimination Techniques). Hypokalaemia is corrected by intravenous infusion of potassium chloride and may be so severe as to require 60 mmol/hour (high doses under ECG monitoring). Convulsions should be controlled by intravenous administration of diazepam (emulsion preferred). Sedation with diazepam may be necessary in agitated patients. Providing the patient is **not** an asthmatic, extreme tachycardia, hypokalaemia, and hyperglycaemia may be reversed by intravenous administration of propranolol (see section 2.4).

Other poisons

> CONSULT POISONS INFORMATION CENTRES DAY AND NIGHT—see p. 15

CYANIDES

Cyanide antidotes include dicobalt edetate, given alone, and sodium nitrite, followed by sodium thiosulphate. These antidotes are held for emergency use in hospitals as well as in centres where cyanide poisoning is a risk such as factories and laboratories.

DICOBALT EDETATE

Indications: acute poisoning with cyanides
Cautions: owing to toxicity to be used only when patient tending to lose, or has lost, consciousness; not to be used as a precautionary measure
Side-effects: transient hypotension, tachycardia, and vomiting
Dose: by intravenous injection, 300 mg (20 mL) over 1 minute, followed by 50 mL of glucose intravenous infusion 50%, both repeated once or twice if necessary

PoM **Kelocyanor**® (Lipha)
Injection, dicobalt edetate 300 mg/20 mL. Net price 20-mL amp = £2.66

SODIUM NITRITE

Indications: poisoning with cyanides (used in conjunction with sodium thiosulphate)
Side-effects: flushing and headache due to vasodilatation

PoM **Sodium Nitrite Injection**
Injection, sodium nitrite 3% (30 mg/mL) in water for injections
Dose: 10 mL by intravenous injection over 3 minutes, followed by 25 mL of sodium thiosulphate injection 50%, by intravenous injection over 10 minutes
Available from Martindale, Penn, etc. (special order)

SODIUM THIOSULPHATE

Indications: poisoning with cyanides (used in conjunction with sodium nitrite)

PoM **Sodium Thiosulphate Injection**
Injection, sodium thiosulphate 50% (500 mg/mL) in water for injections
Dose: see above under Sodium Nitrite Injection
Available from Martindale, Penn, etc. (special order)

HEAVY METALS

Heavy metal antidotes include dimercaprol, penicillamine, and sodium calciumedetate.

Other poisons

DIMERCAPROL
(BAL)

Indications: poisoning by antimony, arsenic, bismuth, gold, mercury, thallium; adjunct (with sodium calciumedetate) in lead poisoning
Cautions: hypertension
Contra-indications: not indicated for iron or cadmium poisoning; severe hepatic impairment
Side-effects: hypertension, tachycardia, malaise, nausea, vomiting, lachrymation, sweating, burning sensation (mouth and eyes), constriction of throat and chest, headache, muscle spasm, abdominal pain, tingling of extremities; pyrexia in children; pain on injection
Dose: by intramuscular injection, 2.5–3 mg/kg every 4 hours for 2 days, 2–4 times on the 3rd day, then 1–2 times daily for 10 days or until recovery

PoM **Dimercaprol Injection** (Boots), dimercaprol 50 mg/mL. Net price 2-mL amp = 70p

PENICILLAMINE

Indications: poisoning by certain toxic metal ions, particularly by copper and lead
Cautions; Contra-indications; Side-effects: see section 10.1.3
Dose: 1–2 g daily in divided doses before food until urinary lead is stabilised at less than 500 micrograms/day; CHILD 20 mg/kg daily

Preparations
See section 10.1.3

SODIUM CALCIUMEDETATE

Indications: poisoning by heavy metals, especially lead
Cautions: renal impairment
Side-effects: nausea, cramp; in overdosage renal damage
Dose: by intravenous infusion, adults and children, up to 40 mg/kg twice daily in sodium chloride intravenous infusion 0.9% or glucose intravenous infusion 5% for up to 5 days, repeated if necessary after 48 hours

PoM **Ledclair®** (Sinclair)
Injection, sodium calciumedetate 200 mg/mL. Net price 5-mL amp = £3.81

NOXIOUS GASES

CARBON MONOXIDE. Carbon monoxide poisoning is now usually due to inhalation of smoke, car exhaust, or fumes caused by blocked flues or incomplete combustion of fuel gases in confined spaces. Its toxic effects are entirely due to hypoxia.

Immediate treatment is essential. The person should be removed into the fresh air, the airway cleared, and **oxygen** 100% administered as soon as available. Artificial respiration should be given as necessary and continued until adequate spontaneous breathing starts, or stopped only after persistent and efficient treatment of cardiac arrest has failed. Admission to hospital is desirable because complications may arise after a delay of hours or days. Cerebral oedema should be anticipated in severe poisoning and is treated with an intravenous infusion of mannitol (see section 2.2.5). Referral for hyperbaric oxygen treatment should be discussed with the poisons information services if the victim is or has been unconscious or has a blood carboxyhaemoglobin concentration of more than 40%.

SULPHUR DIOXIDE, CHLORINE, PHOSGENE, AMMONIA. The immediate effect of all except phosgene is coughing and choking. Pulmonary oedema, with severe breathlessness and cyanosis may develop suddenly up to 36 hours after exposure. Death may occur. Patients are kept under observation and those who develop pulmonary oedema are given corticosteroids and oxygen. Assisted ventilation may be necessary in the most serious cases.

PESTICIDES

PARAQUAT. Concentrated liquid paraquat preparations (e.g. Gramoxone®), available to farmers and horticulturalists, contain 10–20% paraquat and are extremely toxic. Granular preparations, for garden use, contain only 2.5% paraquat and have caused few deaths.

Paraquat has local and systemic effects. Splashes in the eyes irritate and ulcerate the cornea and conjunctiva. Copious washing of the eye and instillation of antibacterial eye-drops, should aid healing but it may be a long process. Skin irritation, blistering, and ulceration can occur from prolonged contact both with the concentrated and dilute forms. Inhalation of spray, mist, or dust containing paraquat may cause nose bleeding and sore throat but not systemic toxicity.

Ingestion of concentrated paraquat solutions is followed by nausea, vomiting, and diarrhoea. Painful ulceration of the tongue, lips, and fauces may appear after 36 to 48 hours together with renal failure. Some days later there may be dyspnoea with pulmonary fibrosis due to proliferative alveolitis and bronchiolitis.

Treatment should be started immediately. The single most useful measure is oral administration of either **Fuller's earth** or **bentonite** to adsorb paraquat and reduce absorption. The stomach is then emptied by careful gastric lavage and 300 mL of a suspension containing 30 g of Fuller's earth and 15 g of magnesium sulphate should be left in the stomach. Further quantities of 300 mL of a 30% Fuller's earth suspension are given after 2 and after 4 hours; magnesium sulphate or mannitol is given as required to produce diarrhoea and empty the gut. Some authorities prefer regimens employing 15% Fuller's earth suspensions. **Activated charcoal** is also effective and is given in a dose of 100 g by mouth if Fuller's earth or bentonite are not available immediately. Intravenous fluids and analgesics are given as necessary. Oxygen therapy should be avoided if possible since this may exacerbate damage to the lungs. Measures to enhance elimination of absorbed paraquat are probably valueless but should be discussed with the poisons information services who will also give guidance on predicting the likely outcome from plasma concentrations. Paraquat absorption can be confirmed by a simple qualitative urine test.

ORGANOPHOSPHORUS INSECTICIDES. Organophosphorus insecticides are usually supplied as powders or dissolved in organic solvents. All are absorbed through the bronchi and intact skin as well as through the gut and inhibit cholinesterase activity thereby prolonging and intensifying the effects of acetylcholine. Toxicity between different compounds varies considerably, and onset may be delayed after skin exposure.

Anxiety, restlessness, dizziness, headache, miosis, nausea, hypersalivation, vomiting, abdominal colic, diarrhoea, bradycardia, and sweating are common. Muscle weakness and fasciculation may develop and progress to generalised flaccid paralysis including the ocular and respiratory muscles. Convulsions, coma, pulmonary oedema with copious bronchial secretions, hypoxia, and arrhythmias occur in severe cases. Hyperglycaemia and glycosuria without ketonuria may also be present.

Further absorption should be prevented by emptying the stomach, removing the patient to fresh air, or removing soiled clothing and washing contaminated skin. In severe poisoning it is vital to ensure a clear airway, frequent removal of bronchial secretions, and adequate ventilation and oxygenation. **Atropine** will reverse the muscarinic effects of acetylcholine and is given in a dose of 2 mg as atropine sulphate injection (intramuscularly or intravenously according to the severity of poisoning) every 20 to 30 minutes until the skin becomes flushed and dry, the pupils dilate, and tachycardia develops.

Pralidoxime mesylate (P2S), a cholinesterase reactivator, is indicated, as an adjunct to atropine, in moderate or severe poisoning but is only effective if given within 24 hours. It may be obtained from designated centres, the names of which are held by the poisons information services (see p. 15). A dose of 1 g by intramuscular injection or, diluted with 10–15 mL water for injections, by slow intravenous injection should produce improvement in muscle power within 30 minutes but repeated doses or, in severe cases, an intravenous infusion of up to 500 mg/hour may be required.

PRALIDOXIME MESYLATE

Indications: adjunct to atropine in the treatment of organophosphorus poisoning
Cautions: renal impairment, myasthenia gravis
Contra-indications: poisoning due to carbamates and to organophosphorus compounds without anticholinesterase activity
Side-effects: drowsiness, dizziness, disturbances of vision, nausea, tachycardia, headache, hyperventilation, and muscular weakness
Dose: by intramuscular injection, 1 g initially followed by 1–2 further doses if necessary; in very severe poisoning the initial dose can be doubled; usual max. 12 g in 24 hours
By slow intravenous injection (diluted to 10–15 mL with water for injections and given over 5–10 minutes), 1 g initially followed by 1–2 further doses if necessary; in very severe poisoning the initial dose can be doubled; usual max. 12 g in 24 hours
CHILD 20–60 mg/kg as required depending on severity of poisoning and response

PoM **Pralidoxime Mesylate Injection,** pralidoxime mesylate 200 mg/mL. Available as 5-mL amps (from designated centres)

SNAKE BITES AND INSECT STINGS

SNAKE BITE. Acute envenoming from snake bite is rare in the United Kingdom and the only indigenous venomous snake is the adder (*Vipera berus*). The bite may cause local and systemic effects. Local effects include pain, swelling, bruising, and tender enlargement of regional lymph nodes. Systemic effects include early transient hypotension with syncope, angioedema, abdominal colic, diarrhoea, and vomiting, with later persistent or recurrent hypotension, ECG abnormalities, spontaneous systemic bleeding, coagulopathy, adult respiratory distress syndrome, and acute renal failure. There is a small risk of fatal envenoming especially in children and the elderly.

Indications for antivenom treatment include systemic envenoming, especially hypotension (see above), polymorphonuclear leucocytosis and local envenoming if, after bites on the hand or foot, swelling extends beyond the wrist or ankle within 4 hours of the bite. Two ampoules of **Zagreb antivenom** (Regent) are diluted with 2–3 volumes of sodium chloride intravenous infusion 0.9% and given by slow intravenous injection (not more than 2 mL of diluted antivenom per minute) or by intravenous infusion. The **same dose** should be used for **adults** and **children**. The dose can be repeated in 1–2 hours if there is no clinical improvement. Adrenaline injection must be immediately to hand for treatment of anaphylactic antivenom reactions (for full details see section 3.4.3).

Antivenom is available for certain foreign snakes and spiders. For information on identification, management, and supply, telephone:

Oxford	(0865) 220968
	or (0865) 741166
Liverpool	051-708 9393
Liverpool (Walton Hospital Pharmacy)	
(supply only)	051-525 3611
London	071-635 9191

INSECT STINGS. Stings from ants, wasps, bees, and hornets cause local pain and swelling but seldom cause severe toxicity. If the sting is in the mouth or on the tongue marked swelling may cause respiratory distress. The stings from these insects are usually treated by cleaning the area, applying a cooling lotion (such as a calamine preparation), and giving an antihistamine by mouth. Bee stings should be removed by scraping them off with a finger nail or knife before cleaning the area. Anaphylactic reactions require treatment with **adrenaline**. Inhalation of adrenaline (Medihaler-epi®, see section 3.4.3) may be sufficient for mild bronchospasm, but self-administered subcutaneous adrenaline is the best first-aid treatment for patients with severe hypersensitivity. For full details of the management of anaphylaxis, see section 3.4.3.

Classified Notes on Drugs and Preparations

DOPING CONTROL IN SPORT
SPORTS COUNCIL
INTERNATIONAL OLYMPIC COMMITTEE
DOPING CLASSES AND METHODS: EXAMPLES

STIMULANTS e.g. amphetamine, cocaine, ephedrine and related compounds
NARCOTIC ANALGESICS e.g. codeine, morphine, pethidine and related compounds
ANABOLIC STEROIDS e.g. nandrolone, stanozolol, testosterone and related compounds
BETA BLOCKERS e.g. acebutolol, atenolol, propranolol and related compounds
DIURETICS e.g. frusemide, hydrochlorothiazide, triamterine & related compounds
PEPTIDE HORMONES & ANALOGUES e.g. growth hormone, HCG, EPO
BLOOD DOPING, INCLUDING ERYTHROPOIETIN (EPO),
PHARMACOLOGICAL, CHEMICAL AND PHYSICAL MANIPULATION
Classes of drugs subject to certain restrictions
ALCOHOL, MARIJUANA (not prohibited but may be restricted)
LOCAL ANAESTHETICS, CORTICOSTEROIDS (except for approved treatments)

TREATMENT GUIDELINES:
EXAMPLES OF PERMITTED AND PROHIBITED SUBSTANCES
(based upon International Olympic Committee Doping Classes)

ASTHMA: ALLOWED - Terbutaline, salbutamol, Ventolin, Intal, Becotide. N.B. Inhalers Only.
COUGH: ALLOWED - steam and menthol inhalations. Benylin Expectorant. All antibiotics.
BANNED - products containing codeine, ephedrines, phenylpropanolamine.
DIARRHOEA: ALLOWED - Dioralyte, Lomotil, Motilium.
BANNED - products containing codeine or morphine.
HAYFEVER: ALLOWED - Antihistamines, Triludan, Piriton, Histryl, Beconase, Otrivine, Opticrom eye drops.
BANNED - products containing ephedrine, pseudoephedrine.
HEADACHE: ALLOWED - Paracetamol, aspirin, Anadin.
BANNED - Products containing codeine, dextropropoxyphene.
SORE THROAT: ALLOWED - Soluble paracetamol gargle.
VOMITING: ALLOWED - Dioralyte, Rehidrat, Maxolon.

WARNING: THE ABOVE ARE ONLY EXAMPLES OF SUBSTANCES CURRENTLY PERMITTED OR PROHIBITED BY THE IOC.
IF IN DOUBT, CHECK WITH YOUR GOVERNING BODY OR WITH THE SPORTS COUNCIL, DOPING CONTROL UNIT 071 383 5667 or 071 383 5411. REMEMBER - YOU ARE RESPONSIBLE. JANUARY 1991

1: Drugs acting on the
GASTRO-INTESTINAL SYSTEM

The drugs and preparations in this chapter are described under the following sections:

1.1 Antacids
1.2 Antispasmodics and other drugs altering gut motility
1.3 Ulcer-healing drugs
1.4 Antidiarrhoeal drugs
1.5 Treatment of chronic diarrhoeas
1.6 Laxatives
1.7 Preparations for haemorrhoids
1.8 Stoma care
1.9 Drugs affecting intestinal secretions

1.1 Antacids

1.1.1 Aluminium- and magnesium-containing
1.1.2 Sodium bicarbonate
1.1.3 Calcium- and bismuth-containing

Antacids are still useful for treating gastro-intestinal disease; they can often relieve symptoms in both *ulcer* and *non-ulcer dyspepsia*, and in *reflux oesophagitis*. They are best given when symptoms occur or are expected, usually between meals and at bedtime, four or more times daily; additional doses may be required up to once an hour. Conventional doses e.g. 10 mL three or four times daily of liquid magnesium–aluminium antacids promote ulcer healing, possibly less well than antisecretory agents (section 1.3); proof of a relationship between healing and neutralising capacity is lacking. Liquid preparations are more effective than solids.

INTERACTIONS. Antacids should not be taken at the same time as other drugs as they may impair their absorption. Antacids may also damage enteric coatings designed to prevent dissolution in the stomach.

1.1.1 Aluminium- and magnesium-containing antacids

Aluminium- and **magnesium-containing** antacids, such as magnesium carbonate, hydroxide and trisilicate, and aluminium glycinate and hydroxide, being relatively insoluble in water, are long-acting if retained in the stomach. They are suitable for most antacid purposes. Magnesium-containing antacids tend to be laxative whereas aluminium-containing antacids may be constipating. Aluminium accumulation does not appear to be a risk if renal function is normal (see also appendix 3).

Compound preparations have no clear advantages over simpler preparations: neutralising capacity may be the same.

Complexes, such as **hydrotalcite** and **magaldrate**, confer no special advantage.

> **Low Na$^+$**
> The words low Na$^+$ added after some preparations indicate a sodium content of less than 1 mmol per tablet or 10-mL dose.

ALUMINIUM HYDROXIDE

Indications: dyspepsia; for use in hyperphosphataemia, see section 9.5.2.2
Cautions: see notes above; porphyria, see section 9.8.2; interactions: Appendix 1 (antacids and adsorbents)
Contra-indications: hypophosphataemia

Aluminium-only preparations
Aluminium Hydroxide (Non-proprietary)
Tablets, dried aluminium hydroxide 500 mg. Net price 20 = 29p
  Dose: 1–2 tablets chewed 4 times daily and at bedtime or as required
Mixture (gel), about 4% w/w Al$_2$O$_3$ in water, with a peppermint flavour. Net price 200 mL = 36p
  Dose: antacid, 5–10 mL 4 times daily between meals and at bedtime or as required; CHILD 6–12 years, up to 5 mL 3 times daily
  Note. The brand name NHS Aludrox® (Charwell) is used for aluminium hydroxide mixture; net price 200 mL = 77p. For NHS Aludrox® tablets see preparations with magnesium, below.

Alu-Cap® (3M)
Capsules, green/red, dried aluminium hydroxide 475 mg (low Na$^+$). Net price 120-cap pack = £3.84
  Dose: antacid, 1 capsule 4 times daily and at bedtime

With magnesium
NHS **Aludrox®** (Charwell)
Tablets, aluminium hydroxide-magnesium carbonate co-dried gel 282 mg, magnesium hydroxide 85 mg. Net price 60 = £1.69
  Dose: 1 or 2 tablets chewed 4 times daily between meals and at bedtime when required

NHS **Dijex®** (Crookes)
Tablets, pink, aluminium hydroxide-magnesium carbonate co-dried gel 400 mg (low Na$^+$). Net price 30 = 63p
  Dose: 1–2 tablets chewed every 2–4 hours when required
Liquid, aluminium hydroxide gel 4.9 g, magnesium hydroxide 85 mg/5 mL. Net price 200 mL = £1.24
  Dose: 5–10 mL every 2–4 hours when required

NHS **Gastrils®** (Jackson)
Pastilles, green (mint-flavoured) or yellow (fruit-flavoured), s/c, aluminium hydroxide-magnesium carbonate co-dried gel 500 mg. Net price 45 g = 62p
  Dose: 2 pastilles sucked when required; CHILD 1 pastille 3 times daily

NHS **Gelusil®** (W-L)
Tablets, dried aluminium hydroxide 250 mg, magnesium trisilicate 500 mg (low Na$^+$). Net price 50 = £1.91
  Dose: 1–2 tablets chewed or sucked after meals or when required; CHILD half adult dose

Abbreviations and symbols, see inside front cover   Prices are **net**, see p. 1

1.1 Antacids

Maalox® (Rhône-Poulenc Rorer)
Tablets, dried aluminium hydroxide 400 mg, magnesium hydroxide 400 mg (low Na⁺). Net price 100 = £1.40
Dose: 1–2 tablets chewed 20 minutes–1 hour after meals and at bedtime or when required
Suspension, sugar-free, dried aluminium hydroxide 220 mg, magnesium hydroxide 195 mg/5 mL (low Na⁺). Net price 500 mL = £1.95; 20 × 10-mL sachets = 78p
Dose: 5–10 mL 20 minutes–1 hour after meals and at bedtime or when required

Maalox TC® (Rhône-Poulenc Rorer)
Tablets, dried aluminium hydroxide 600 mg, magnesium hydroxide 300 mg (low Na⁺). Net price 100 = £3.60
Suspension, sugar-free, dried aluminium hydroxide 600 mg, magnesium hydroxide 300 mg/5 mL (low Na⁺). Net price 500 mL = £3.60
Dose: antacid, 1–2 tablets chewed or 5–10 mL suspension 4 times daily 20 minutes–1 hour after meals and at bedtime or as required; duodenal ulcer, 3 tablets or 15 mL suspension 4 times daily (treatment) *or* twice daily (prevention of recurrence)

Mucogel® (Pharmax)
Suspension, sugar-free, dried aluminium hydroxide 220 mg, magnesium hydroxide 195 mg/5 mL (low Na⁺). Net price 500 mL = £1.96
Dose: 10–20 mL 3 times daily, 20 minutes–1 hour after meals, and at bedtime or when required

MAGNESIUM CARBONATE

Indications: dyspepsia
Cautions: renal impairment; see also notes above; **interactions:** Appendix 1 (antacids and adsorbents)
Contra-indications: hypophosphataemia
Side-effects: diarrhoea; belching due to liberated carbon dioxide

Aromatic Magnesium Carbonate Mixture (BP) (Aromatic Magnesium Carbonate Oral Suspension)
Oral suspension, light magnesium carbonate 3%, sodium bicarbonate 5%, in a suitable vehicle containing aromatic cardamom tincture. Extemporaneous preparations should be recently prepared according to the following formula: light magnesium carbonate 300 mg, sodium bicarbonate 500 mg, aromatic cardamom tincture 0.3 mL, double-strength chloroform water 5 mL, water to 10 mL. Contains about 6 mmol Na⁺/10 mL. Net price 200 mL = 19p
Dose: 10 mL 3 times daily in water

For compound preparations with aluminium, see under Aluminium Hydroxide (previous page)

MAGNESIUM TRISILICATE

Indications: dyspepsia
Cautions; Contra-indications: see under Magnesium Carbonate
Side-effects: diarrhoea

Magnesium Trisilicate Tablets, Compound (BP)
Tablets, magnesium trisilicate 250 mg, dried aluminium hydroxide 120 mg. Net price 20 = 20p
Dose: 1–2 tablets chewed when required

Magnesium Trisilicate Mixture (BP) (Magnesium Trisilicate Oral Suspension)
Oral suspension, 5% each of magnesium trisilicate, light magnesium carbonate, and sodium bicarbonate in a suitable vehicle with a peppermint flavour. Extemporaneous preparations should be recently prepared according to the following formula: magnesium trisilicate 500 mg, light magnesium carbonate 500 mg, sodium bicarbonate 500 mg, concentrated peppermint emulsion 0.25 mL, double-strength chloroform water 5 mL, water to 10 mL. Contains about 6 mmol Na⁺/10 mL. Net price 200 mL = 20p
Dose: 10 mL 3 times daily in water

Magnesium Trisilicate Oral Powder, Compound (BP)
Oral powder, magnesium trisilicate 250 mg, chalk 250 mg, heavy magnesium carbonate 250 mg, sodium bicarbonate 250 mg/g. Contains about 3 mmol Na⁺/g. Net price 20 g = 7p. Label: 13
Dose: 1–5 g in liquid when required

For compound preparations with aluminium, see under Aluminium Hydroxide (previous page)

ALUMINIUM-MAGNESIUM COMPLEXES

HYDROTALCITE

Aluminium magnesium carbonate hydroxide hydrate
Indications: dyspepsia
Cautions: see notes above; **interactions:** Appendix 1 (antacids and adsorbents)

Hydrotalcite (Non-proprietary)
Tablets, hydrotalcite 500 mg. Net price 56-tab pack = 81p
Dose: 2 tablets chewed between meals and at bedtime; CHILD 6–12 years 1 tablet
Suspension, hydrotalcite 500 mg/5 mL. Net price 500-mL pack = £1.96
Dose: 10 mL between meals and at bedtime; CHILD 6–12 years 5 mL
Note. The brand name NHS Altacite® (Roussel) is used for hydrotalcite suspension and tablets; see section 1.1.1.1 for Altacite Plus® preparations.

MAGALDRATE

A synthetic combination of aluminium and magnesium hydroxides and sulphuric acid
Indications: dyspepsia
Cautions: see notes above; **interactions:** Appendix 1 (antacids and adsorbents)

Magaldrate (Non-proprietary)
Suspension, magaldrate 800 mg/5 mL. Net price 100 mL = 38p
Dose: 5–10 mL after meals and at bedtime; CHILD 6–12 years 2.5–5 mL
Note. The brand name NHS Dynese® (Galen) is used for magaldrate suspension; it is sugar-free and low Na⁺.

1.1.1.1 Aluminium- and magnesium-containing antacids with additional ingredients

Activated dimethicone (simethicone), given alone or added to an antacid as an antifoaming agent to relieve flatulence, is of uncertain value. Alginates added as protectants against *reflux oesophagitis* may be useful, but surface anaesthetics (e.g. oxethazaine) added to improve symptom relief are of doubtful efficacy. The amount of additional ingredient or antacid in individual preparations varies widely, as does their sodium content, so that preparations may not be freely interchangeable.

Preparations containing activated dimethicone with an antacid may be useful for the relief of *hiccup in terminal care*.

NHS Actonorm® (Wallace Mfg)
Gel, dried aluminium hydroxide 220 mg, activated dimethicone 25 mg, magnesium hydroxide 200 mg/5 mL (low Na⁺). Net price 200 mL = £1.70
Dose: 5–20 mL when required

Algicon® (Rhône-Poulenc Rorer)
Tablets, aluminium hydroxide-magnesium carbonate co-dried gel 360 mg, magnesium alginate 500 mg, magnesium carbonate 320 mg, potassium bicarbonate 100 mg, sucrose 1.5 g (low Na⁺). Net price 60-tab pack = £2.40
Dose: 1–2 tablets 4 times daily (chewed after meals and at bedtime)
Suspension, yellow, aluminium hydroxide-magnesium carbonate co-dried gel 140 mg, magnesium alginate 250 mg, magnesium carbonate 175 mg, potassium bicarbonate 50 mg/5 mL (low Na⁺). Net price 500 mL = £2.60
Dose: 10–20 mL 4 times daily (chewed after meals and at bedtime)

Altacite Plus® (Roussel)
NHS *Tablets*, co-simalcite 250/500 (activated dimethicone 250 mg, hydrotalcite 500 mg) (low Na⁺). Net price 20-tab pack = £1.05
Dose: 2 tablets chewed between meals and at bedtime when required; CHILD 8–12 years 1 tablet
Suspension, sugar-free, co-simalcite 125/500 (activated dimethicone 125 mg, hydrotalcite 500 mg)/5 mL (low Na⁺). Net price 500 mL = £1.85
Dose: 10 mL between meals and at bedtime when required; CHILD 8–12 years 5 mL

Asilone® (Boots)
NHS *Tablets*, dried aluminium hydroxide 500 mg, activated dimethicone 270 mg (low Na⁺). Net price 24-tab pack = £1.39
Dose: 1–2 tablets chewed or sucked before meals and at bedtime
Suspension, sugar-free, dried aluminium hydroxide 420 mg, activated dimethicone 135 mg, light magnesium oxide 70 mg/5 mL (low Na⁺). Net price 500 mL = £1.95
Dose: 5–10 mL before meals and at bedtime
Note. Asilone® Liquid contains the same active ingredients as Asilone® Suspension but is in a 200-mL pack (net price £1.24)

NHS Carbellon® (Torbet)
Tablets, black, activated charcoal 100 mg, magnesium hydroxide 100 mg, peppermint oil 0.003 mL. Net price 50-tab pack = £1.20
Dose: 2–4 tablets chewed 3 times daily; CHILD 6–12 years 2 tablets 3 times daily

Diovol® (Pharmax)
Suspension, sugar-free, aluminium hydroxide 200 mg, dimethicone 25 mg, magnesium hydroxide 200 mg/5 mL (low Na⁺). Net price 300 mL = £1.16
Dose: 5–10 mL when required

Gastrocote® (Boehringer Mannheim)
Tablets, alginic acid 200 mg, dried aluminium hydroxide 80 mg, magnesium trisilicate 40 mg, sodium bicarbonate 70 mg. Contains about 1 mmol Na⁺/tablet. Net price 100-tab pack = £3.76
Dose: 1–2 tablets chewed 4 times daily (after meals and at bedtime)
Liquid, sugar-free, peach-coloured, dried aluminium hydroxide 80 mg, magnesium trisilicate 40 mg, sodium alginate 220 mg, sodium bicarbonate 70 mg/5 mL. Contains 1.8 mmol Na⁺/5 mL. Net price 500 mL = £2.86
Dose: 5–15 mL 4 times daily (after meals and at bedtime)

Gastron® (Sanofi Winthrop)
Tablets, alginic acid 600 mg, dried aluminium hydroxide 240 mg, magnesium trisilicate 60 mg, sodium bicarbonate 210 mg. Contains about 3 mmol Na⁺/tablet. Net price 100-tab pack = £3.90
Dose: 1–2 tablets chewed 3 times daily after meals and 2 tablets at bedtime

Gaviscon® (R&C)
Tablets, alginic acid 500 mg, dried aluminium hydroxide 100 mg, magnesium trisilicate 25 mg, sodium bicarbonate 170 mg. Contains 2 mmol Na⁺/tablet. Net price 60-tab pack = £2.25
Dose: 1–2 tablets chewed after meals and at bedtime, followed by water; CHILD 1 tablet
Liquid, pink, sugar-free, sodium alginate 250 mg, sodium bicarbonate 133.5 mg, calcium carbonate 80 mg/5 mL. Contains about 3 mmol Na⁺/5 mL. Net price 100 mL = 54p
Dose: 10–20 mL after meals and at bedtime; CHILD 5–10 mL

Infant Gaviscon® (R&C)
Oral powder, sugar-free, sodium alginate 225 mg, magnesium alginate 87.5 mg, dried aluminium hydroxide 112.5 mg with colloidal silica and mannitol/dose (half dual-sachet). Contains 0.92 mmol Na⁺/dose. Net price 15 dual-sachets (30 doses) = £2.46
Dose: INFANT under 4.5 kg 1 dose (half dual-sachet) mixed with feeds (or water in breast-fed infants) when required; over 4.5 kg 2 doses (1 dual-sachet); CHILD 2 doses (1 dual-sachet) in water after each meal
Note. Not to be used in premature infants, or where excessive water loss likely (e.g. fever, diarrhoea, vomiting, high room temperature)
IMPORTANT. This is a new formulation; each half of the dual-sachet is identified as 'one dose'. To avoid errors prescribe as 'dual-sachet' with directions in terms of 'dose'

PoM Mucaine® (Wyeth)
Suspension, sugar-free, aluminium hydroxide mixture 4.75 mL, magnesium hydroxide 100 mg, oxethazaine 10 mg/5 mL. Net price 200-mL pack = 76p
Dose: 5–10 mL (without fluid) 3–4 times daily (15 minutes before meals and at bedtime or when required)

Maalox Plus® (Rhône-Poulenc Rorer)
NHS *Tablets*, white/yellow, dried aluminium hydroxide 200 mg, activated dimethicone 25 mg, magnesium hydroxide 200 mg (low Na$^+$). Net price 50 = £1.67
Dose: 1–2 tablets chewed 4 times daily after meals and at bedtime or when required
Suspension, sugar-free, dried aluminium hydroxide 220 mg, activated dimethicone 25 mg, magnesium hydroxide 195 mg/5 mL (low Na$^+$). Net price 500 mL = £1.95
Dose: 5–10 mL 4 times daily (after meals and at bedtime or when required)

NHS **Simeco®** (Wyeth)
Tablets, pink/white, aluminium hydroxide–magnesium carbonate co-dried gel 282 mg, activated dimethicone 25 mg, magnesium hydroxide 85 mg. Net price 60-tab pack = £3.15
Dose: 2 tablets to be chewed after or between meals and at bedtime
Suspension, aluminium hydroxide 215 mg, activated dimethicone 25 mg, magnesium hydroxide 80 mg/5 mL. Net price 200 mL = £1.35
Dose: 10 mL after or between meals and at bedtime; CHILD 6–12 years, up to 5 mL 3 times daily

Topal® (Innovex)
Tablets, alginic acid 200 mg, dried aluminium hydroxide 30 mg, light magnesium carbonate 40 mg with lactose 220 mg, sucrose 880 mg (low Na$^+$). Net price 42-tab pack = £1.67
Dose: 1–3 tablets chewed 4 times daily (after meals and at bedtime); CHILD half adult dose

NHS **Unigest®** (Unigreg)
Tablets, dried aluminium hydroxide 450 mg, dimethicone 400 mg (low Na$^+$). Net price 12 = 98p
Dose: 1–2 tablets chewed or sucked after meals and at bedtime or when required

DIMETHICONE ALONE

Infacol® (Pharmax)
Liquid, sugar-free, activated dimethicone 40 mg/mL (low Na$^+$). Net price 50 mL = £1.42. Counselling, use of dropper
Dose: gripes, colic or wind pains, INFANT 0.5–1 mL before feeds

1.1.2 Sodium bicarbonate

Sodium bicarbonate, being soluble in water, is rapid-acting, but absorbed bicarbonate can cause alkalosis in excessive doses. Like other carbonate-containing antacids it liberates carbon dioxide which causes belching. Sodium bicarbonate and antacid preparations with a high sodium content, such as magnesium trisilicate mixture, should be avoided in patients on salt-restricted diets (in heart failure and hepatic and renal impairment).

SODIUM BICARBONATE
Indications: rapid relief of dyspepsia
Cautions: renal impairment; patients on a sodium-restricted diet; avoid prolonged use; **interactions:** Appendix 1 (antacids and adsorbents)
Side-effects: belching due to liberated carbon dioxide and, with prolonged use, alkalosis

Sodium Bicarbonate (BP). Contains about 12 mmol Na$^+$/g. Label: 13
Dose: 1–5 g in water when required
Sodium Bicarbonate Tablets, Compound (BP) (Soda Mint Tablets), sodium bicarbonate 300 mg. Contains about 4 mmol Na$^+$/tab
Dose: 2–6 tablets sucked when required

1.1.3 Calcium- and bismuth-containing antacids

Bismuth-containing antacids (unless chelates) are best avoided because absorbed bismuth can be neurotoxic, causing encephalopathy; they tend to be constipating. Calcium-containing antacids can induce rebound acid secretion: with modest doses the clinical significance is doubtful, but prolonged high doses also cause hypercalcaemia and alkalosis, and can precipitate the milk alkali syndrome. **Interactions:** Appendix 1 (antacids and adsorbents).

NHS **Nulacin®** (Bencard)
Tablets, calcium carbonate 130 mg, heavy magnesium carbonate 30 mg, heavy magnesium oxide 130 mg, magnesium trisilicate 230 mg, with milk solids, dextrins and maltose (low Na$^+$). Net price 25 = 82p
Additives: include gluten
Dose: 1 tablet chewed or sucked when required between meals and at bedtime; max. 8 tablets daily

NHS **Roter®** (Roterpharma)
Tablets, pink, bismuth subnitrate 300 mg, frangula 25 mg, magnesium carbonate 400 mg, sodium bicarbonate 200 mg. Net price 20 = 48p
Dose: 1–2 tablets dispersed in warm water 3 times daily after meals

1.2 Antispasmodics and other drugs altering gut motility

The smooth muscle relaxant properties of antimuscarinic and other antispasmodic drugs may be useful as adjunctive treatment in *non-ulcer dyspepsia*, in the *irritable bowel syndrome*, and in *diverticular disease*. The gastric antisecretory effects of conventional antimuscarinic drugs are of little practical significance since dosage is limited by atropine-like side-effects. Moreover, they have been superseded by more powerful and specific antisecretory drugs, including the histamine H$_2$-receptor antagonists and the selective antimuscarinic pirenzepine.

The dopamine-receptor antagonists metoclopramide and domperidone have different properties, tending to stimulate transit in the gut.

Cautionary label wordings, see inside back cover   Prices are **net**, see p. 1

ANTIMUSCARINICS

The antimuscarinics (less correctly termed 'anti-cholinergics') can be divided into atropine and its related alkaloids (including the belladonna alkaloids), and synthetic antimuscarinics. The synthetic antimuscarinics can, in turn, be divided into **tertiary amine** (dicyclomine hydrochloride) and **quaternary ammonium compounds** (mepenzolate bromide, pipenzolate bromide, poldine methylsulphate, and propantheline bromide). The tertiary amine dicyclomine hydrochloride has a much less marked antimuscarinic action than atropine and may also have some direct action on smooth muscle.

Quaternary ammonium compounds are less lipid soluble than atropine and so may be less likely to cross the blood–brain barrier; they are also less well absorbed. Although central atropine-like side-effects, such as confusion, are thereby reduced, peripheral atropine-like side-effects remain common with dry mouth, difficult visual accommodation, hesitant micturition, and constipation at doses which act as gut neuromuscular relaxants or inhibitors of acid secretion. The elderly are particularly susceptible; glaucoma and urinary retention may occur.

Antimuscarinics tend to relax the oesophageal sphincter and should be avoided in patients with symptomatic reflux; all antispasmodics should be avoided in paralytic ileus. Despite these side-effects antimuscarinics are nevertheless useful in some *dyspeptics*, in the *irritable bowel syndrome*, and in *diverticular disease*. Nonselective antimuscarinics (e.g. belladonna alkaloids) are outmoded as ulcer treatments, any clinical virtues being outweighed by atropinic side-effects.

The quaternary ammonium compound, **hyoscine butylbromide** is advocated as a gastro-intestinal antispasmodic, but it is poorly absorbed and its action is brief; the injection is a useful antispasmodic in endoscopy and radiology.

ATROPINE SULPHATE and BELLADONNA ALKALOIDS

Indications: see notes above; atropine sulphate, see also section 15.1.3
Cautions: elderly; urinary retention, prostatic enlargement, tachycardia, cardiac insufficiency, paralytic ileus, ulcerative colitis, and pyloric stenosis; may aggravate gastro-oesophageal reflux; pregnancy and breast-feeding; **interactions:** Appendix 1 (antimuscarinics)
Contra-indications: closed-angle glaucoma
Side-effects: dry mouth with difficulty in swallowing and thirst, dilatation of the pupils with loss of accommodation and sensitivity to light, increased intra-ocular pressure, flushing, dry skin, bradycardia followed by tachycardia, palpitations and arrhythmias, difficulty with micturition, and constipation; rarely fever, confusional states and rashes

Compound preparations
NHS **Actonorm**® (Wallace Mfg)
Powder, atropine sulphate 100 micrograms, aluminium hydroxide gel 50 mg, calcium carbonate 145 mg, magnesium carbonate 381.4 mg, magnesium trisilicate 50 mg, sodium bicarbonate 373 mg, peppermint oil 500 micrograms/g. Net price 85 g = £1.86. Label: 13
Dose: one level 5-mL spoonful (2 g) in liquid 3–4 times daily; elderly, initially 5 mL twice daily

NHS **Aluhyde**® (Sinclair)
Tablets, scored, belladonna liquid extract 7.8 mg, dried aluminium hydroxide 245 mg, magnesium trisilicate 245 mg. Net price 50-tab pack = £3.99
Dose: 2 tablets 3 times daily

NHS **Bellocarb**® (Sinclair)
Tablets, beige, scored, belladonna dry extract 10 mg (equivalent to 100 micrograms of hyoscyamine), magnesium carbonate 300 mg, magnesium trisilicate 300 mg. Net price 50-tab pack = £3.43
Dose: 1–2 tablets 4 times daily

DICYCLOMINE HYDROCHLORIDE

Indications: adjunct in gastro-intestinal disorders characterised by smooth muscle spasm
Cautions; Contra-indications; Side-effects: see under Atropine Sulphate; contra-indicated in infants under 6 months
Dose: 10–20 mg 3 times daily; CHILD 6–24 months 5–10 mg up to 3–4 times daily, 15 minutes before feeds, 2–12 years 10 mg 3 times daily

PoM ¹**Merbentyl**® (Merrell)
Tablets, dicyclomine hydrochloride 10 mg. Net price 20 = 58p
Syrup, dicyclomine hydrochloride 10 mg/5 mL. Net price 100 mL = 88p
1. Dicyclomine hydrochloride can be sold to the public provided that the maximum single dose is 10 mg and the maximum daily dose is 60 mg

PoM **Merbentyl 20**® (Merrell)
Tablets, dicyclomine hydrochloride 20 mg. Net price 84-tab pack = £4.89

Compound preparations
Kolanticon® (Merrell)
Gel, sugar-free, dicyclomine hydrochloride 2.5 mg, dried aluminium hydroxide 200 mg, light magnesium oxide 100 mg, activated dimethicone (simethicone USP) 20 mg/5 mL. Net price 200 mL = £1.33; 500 mL = £1.90
Dose: 10–20 mL every 4 hours when required

HYOSCINE BUTYLBROMIDE

Indications: adjunct in gastro-intestinal disorders characterised by smooth muscle spasm
Cautions; Contra-indications; Side-effects: see under Atropine Sulphate and notes above; avoid in porphyria (see section 9.8.2)
Dose: by mouth, 20 mg 4 times daily; CHILD 6–12 years, 10 mg 3 times daily
By intramuscular or intravenous injection (acute spasm), 20 mg, repeated after 30 minutes if necessary

1.2 Antispasmodics

PoM [1]**Buscopan**® (Boehringer Ingelheim)
Tablets, coated, hyoscine butylbromide 10 mg. Net price 56-tab pack = £2.38 (not recommended, see notes above)
1. Can be sold to the public provided single dose does not exceed 20 mg, daily dose does not exceed 80 mg, and pack does not contain a total of more than 240 mg. Net price 24 × 10 mg-tab pack = £1.70.
Injection, hyoscine butylbromide 20 mg/mL. Net price 1-mL amp = 19p

MEPENZOLATE BROMIDE

Indications: adjunct in gastro-intestinal disorders characterised by smooth muscle spasm
Cautions; Contra-indications; Side-effects: see under Atropine Sulphate and notes above
Dose: 25–50 mg 3–4 times daily

PoM Cantil® (Boehringer Mannheim)
Tablets, yellow, scored, mepenzolate bromide 25 mg. Net price 50-tab pack = £2.75
Additives: include tartrazine

PIPENZOLATE BROMIDE

Indications: adjunct in gastro-intestinal disorders characterised by smooth muscle spasm
Cautions; Contra-indications; Side-effects: see under Atropine Sulphate and notes above
Dose: 5 mg 3 times daily and 5–10 mg at night

PoM Piptal® (Boehringer Mannheim)
Tablets, peach, pipenzolate bromide 5 mg. Net price 50 = £1.14

Compound preparations
PoM Piptalin® (Boehringer Mannheim)
Suspension, orange, sugar-free, pipenzolate bromide 4 mg, activated dimethicone 40 mg/5 mL. Net price 100 mL = £1.11
Dose: 10 mL 3–4 times daily before meals; CHILD up to 10 kg 2.5 mL, 10–20 kg 2.5–5 mL, 20–40 kg 5 mL, 3–4 times daily 15 minutes before meals (or feeds)

POLDINE METHYLSULPHATE

Indications: adjunct in gastro-intestinal disorders characterised by smooth muscle spasm
Cautions; Contra-indications; Side-effects: see under Atropine Sulphate and notes above
Dose: 2–4 mg 4 times daily

PoM Nacton® (Bencard)
Tablets, scored, poldine methylsulphate 2 mg. Net price 112-tab pack = £1.89
Tablets forte, orange, scored, poldine methylsulphate 4 mg. Net price 112-tab pack = £3.61

PROPANTHELINE BROMIDE

Indications: adjunct in gastro-intestinal disorders characterised by smooth muscle spasm; for use in urinary frequency, see section 7.4.2
Cautions; Contra-indications; Side-effects: see under Atropine Sulphate and notes above
Dose: 15 mg 3 times daily at least 1 hour before meals and 30 mg at night, max. 120 mg daily

Cautionary label wordings, see inside back cover

PoM Pro-Banthine® (Baker Norton)
Tablets, pink, s/c, propantheline bromide 15 mg. Net price 100 = £2.34. Label: 23

OTHER ANTISPASMODICS

Alverine citrate, mebeverine hydrochloride, and peppermint oil are believed to be direct relaxants of intestinal smooth muscle and may relieve pain in the *irritable bowel syndrome* and *diverticular disease*. They have no serious adverse effects but, like all antispasmodics, should be avoided in paralytic ileus. Peppermint oil occasionally causes heartburn.

ALVERINE CITRATE

Indications: adjunct in gastro-intestinal disorders characterised by smooth muscle spasm; dysmenorrhoea
Cautions: pregnancy
Contra-indications: paralytic ileus
Dose: 60–120 mg 1–3 times daily; CHILD 8–12 years, 60 mg 3 times daily

Spasmonal® (Norgine)
Capsules, blue/grey, alverine citrate 60 mg. Net price 20 = £2.24

Compound preparations
[1]**Alvercol**® (Norgine)
Granules, beige, coated, sterculia 62%, alverine citrate 0.5%. Net price 500 g = £12.50. Label: 25, 27, counselling, see below
Dose: irritable bowel syndrome, 1–2 heaped 5-mL spoonfuls swallowed without chewing with water once or twice daily after meals; CHILD 6–12 years, half adult dose
COUNSELLING. Preparations that swell in contact with liquid should always be carefully swallowed with water and should not be taken immediately before going to bed
1. Formerly Normacol Antispasmodic

MEBEVERINE HYDROCHLORIDE

Indications: adjunct in gastro-intestinal disorders characterised by smooth muscle spasm
Cautions: paralytic ileus; avoid in porphyria (see section 9.8.2.)

PoM Colofac® (Duphar)
Tablets, s/c, mebeverine hydrochloride 135 mg. Net price 20 = £1.67. Label: 22
Dose: ADULT and CHILD over 10 years, 1 tablet 3 times daily preferably 20 minutes before meals
Note. Tablets containing mebeverine hydrochloride 135 mg also available from APS, Berk (Fomac®), Cox, Generics, Hillcross
Liquid, yellow, sugar-free, mebeverine hydrochloride 50 mg (as embonate)/5 mL. Net price 300 mL = £3.50. Label: 22
Dose: ADULT and CHILD over 10 years, 15 mL 3 times daily, preferably 20 minutes before food

Prices are **net**, see p. 1

Compound preparations

PoM Colven® (R&C)

Granules, yellowish-brown, effervescent, ispaghula husk 3.5 g, mebeverine hydrochloride 135 mg/sachet. Contains 6.1 mmol Na$^+$/sachet; caution in renal impairment. Net price 60 sachets = £15.00. Label: 13, 22, counselling, see below

Dose: irritable bowel syndrome, 1 sachet in water morning and night 30 minutes before food; an additional sachet may also be taken before the midday meal if necessary

COUNSELLING. Preparations that swell in contact with liquid should always be carefully swallowed with water and should not be taken immediately before going to bed

PEPPERMINT OIL

Indications: relief of abdominal colic and distension, particularly in irritable bowel syndrome
Cautions: ulcerative colitis, paralytic ileus, rarely sensitivity to menthol
Side-effects: heartburn, rarely, allergy

LOCAL IRRITATION. Capsules should not be broken or chewed because this would release peppermint oil causing irritation of mouth or oesophagus

Colpermin® (Tillotts)

Capsules, e/c, light blue/dark blue, green band, peppermint oil 0.2 mL. Net price 100-cap pack = £12.76. Label: 5, 22, 25

Dose: 1–2 capsules, swallowed whole with water, 3 times daily before meals for up to 2–3 months if necessary

Mintec® (Innovex)

Capsules, e/c, green/ivory, peppermint oil 0.2 mL. Net price 100-cap pack = £12.80. Label: 5, 22, 25

Dose: 1–2 capsules, swallowed whole with water, 3 times daily before meals for up to 2–3 months if necessary

MOTILITY STIMULANTS

Metoclopramide and **domperidone** are dopamine antagonists which stimulate gastric emptying and small intestinal transit, and enhance the strength of oesophageal sphincter contraction. Metoclopramide is used in some patients with *non-ulcer dyspepsia*, for speeding the transit of barium during intestinal follow-through examination, and as accessory treatment for *oesophageal reflux*. Both metoclopramide and domperidone are useful in nonspecific or cytotoxic-induced *nausea and vomiting* (see section 4.6).

Metoclopramide and, occasionally, domperidone induce extrapyramidal reactions with facial and skeletal muscle spasms and oculogyric crises. These are more common in the young (especially girls and young women) and the very old, usually occur shortly after starting treatment, and subside within 24 hours of stopping the drug. Injection of an antiparkinsonian agent such as procyclidine (see section 4.9.2) will abort attacks. Other side-effects include gynaecomastia and galactorrhoea; diarrhoea can occur. Dosage of both should be reduced in renal impairment and both should be avoided immediately after abdominal surgery.

Cisapride is a newly introduced motility stimulant believed to promote release of acetylcholine in the gut wall; it does not have dopamine-antagonist properties. It is of use in treating *oesophageal reflux and gastric stasis* and in the short-term management of *non-ulcer dyspepsia*.

CISAPRIDE

Indications: see under dose
Cautions: halve dose initially in hepatic and renal impairment; elderly; **interactions:** Appendix 1 (cisapride)
Contra-indications: where gastro-intestinal stimulation dangerous; pregnancy
Side-effects: abdominal cramps and diarrhoea, occasional headaches and lightheadedness; convulsions and extrapyramidal effects reported
Dose: ADULT and CHILD over 12 years
Symptoms and mucosal lesions associated with gastro-oesophageal reflux, 10 mg 3–4 times daily; 12-week course recommended
Symptoms of impaired gastric motility secondary to disturbed and delayed gastric emptying associated with diabetes, systemic sclerosis and autonomic neuropathy, 10 mg 3–4 times daily initially for 6 weeks (but longer treatment may be necessary)
Symptoms of dyspepsia (peptic ulcer or other lesions excluded), 10 mg 3 times daily (usual course 4 weeks)

COUNSELLING. Advise patient to take 15–30 minutes before meals and at bedtime (to control night symptoms)

PoM Alimix® (Cilag)

Tablets, scored, cisapride (as monohydrate) 10 mg, net price 120-tab pack = £38.57.
Counselling, administration, see above

PoM Prepulsid® (Janssen)

Tablets, scored, cisapride (as monohydrate) 10 mg, net price 120-tab pack = £38.57.
Counselling, administration, see above
Suspension, cisapride (as monohydrate) 5 mg/5 mL. Net price 500 mL = £16.00.
Counselling, administration, see above

DOMPERIDONE

See section 4.6

METOCLOPRAMIDE HYDROCHLORIDE

Indications: see notes above; for use in nausea and vomiting, see section 4.6

PATIENTS UNDER 20 YEARS. Use restricted to severe intractable vomiting of known cause, vomiting of radiotherapy and cytotoxics, aid to gastro-intestinal intubation, pre-medication

Cautions; Side-effects; Dose: see notes above and section 4.6

Preparations: see section 4.6

1.2.1 Compound antispasmodic preparations

These preparations should be **avoided**, especially where they contain barbiturates. Sedatives should only be used in gastro-intestinal disease on their own individual merits.

NHS APP Stomach Tablets® (Consolidated)
Tablets, homatropine methylbromide 1.5 mg, dried aluminium hydroxide 15 mg, bismuth subcarbonate 12.5 mg, calcium carbonate 183 mg, heavy magnesium carbonate 180 mg, magnesium trisilicate 108 mg. Net price 50-tab pack = £1.05
Dose: 1 tablet chewed 3–4 times daily after meals

NHS APP Stomach Powder® (Consolidated)
Powder, homatropine methylbromide 1 mg, dried aluminium hydroxide 30 mg, bismuth subcarbonate 20 mg, calcium carbonate 379 mg, heavy magnesium carbonate 370 mg, magnesium trisilicate 200 mg/g. Net price 100 g = 95p. Label: 13
Dose: 5-mL spoonful in liquid 3–4 times daily after meals

1.3 Ulcer-healing drugs

1.3.1 H$_2$-receptor antagonists
1.3.2 Selective antimuscarinics
1.3.3 Chelates and complexes
1.3.4 Prostaglandin analogues
1.3.5 Proton pump inhibitors
1.3.6 Other ulcer-healing drugs

Peptic ulceration commonly involves the stomach, duodenum, and lower oesophagus; after gastric surgery it involves the gastro-enterostomy stoma.

General measures, including stopping smoking and taking **antacids**, promote healing as do the use of a wide variety of antisecretory and other treatments. **H$_2$-receptor antagonists** (cimetidine, famotidine, nizatidine, ranitidine) are all very effective in *gastric and duodenal ulcer* and to a lesser extent in *oesophageal disease*. Relapse is common when treatment ceases, and can be managed by further short courses of treatment or by maintenance H$_2$-receptor antagonist therapy. **Pirenzepine** (a selective antimuscarinic) and **misoprostol** (a prostaglandin analogue) also inhibit acid secretion; **bismuth chelate** and **sucralfate** act by as yet poorly understood means. **Carbenoxolone**, a liquorice derivative, causes fluid retention too commonly for routine use; a **deglycyrrhizinised liquorice** preparation is of doubtful efficacy. The proton pump inhibitor **omeprazole** is an effective treatment for *gastric and duodenal ulcers* and particularly for *erosive oesophagitis*.

Associated infection with *Helicobacter pylori* can be suppressed temporarily by bismuth chelate; it may possibly be suppressed permanently when antibiotics (amoxycillin or tetracycline, with metronidazole) are given at the same time, but antibiotic-associated colitis is an important risk and metronidazole resistance in *H. pylori* is easily acquired.

NSAID-associated peptic ulceration can be treated with the conventional range of drugs. Short-term treatment in patients taking NSAIDs may prevent the development of peptic ulcers but has not been shown to prevent complications of bleeding or perforation.

1.3.1 H$_2$-receptor antagonists

All H$_2$-receptor antagonists heal *gastric and duodenal ulcers* by reducing gastric acid output as a result of H$_2$-receptor blockade; like cimetidine and ranitidine, the newer ones (famotidine and nizatidine) can also be expected to relieve *peptic oesophagitis* and, in high doses, to reduce gastric acid output in the *Zollinger–Ellison syndrome*.

Maintenance treatment with half doses prevents *ulcer relapse*, but does not modify the natural course of the disease when treatment has ceased; it is probably best given in courses of 4–6 weeks with further short courses if symptoms recur. Maintenance treatment is best suited to those with frequent severe recurrences and to the elderly who suffer ulcer complications.

Treatment of *undiagnosed dyspepsia* may be acceptable in younger patients but is undesirable in older people because the diagnosis of gastric cancer may be delayed.

Therapy can promote healing of NSAID-associated ulcers but there is no proof that the ulcer complications are prevented.

Clear proof that treatment is beneficial in *haematemesis* and *melaena* is lacking, but prophylactic use reduces the frequency of bleeding from gastroduodenal erosions in *hepatic coma*, and possibly in other conditions requiring *intensive care*. Treatment also reduces the frequency of *acid aspiration* in obstetric patients at delivery (Mendelson's syndrome).

SIDE-EFFECTS. H$_2$-receptor antagonists are well tolerated and side-effects are uncommon with few significant differences between available drugs. Dizziness, somnolence or fatigue, and rash have occasionally been reported with all of them, and there are rare reports of headache, liver dysfunction, and blood disorders. Other rare reports include bradycardia or AV block, confusion, interstitial nephritis (cimetidine), and urticaria and angioedema. Cimetidine is also associated with occasional gynaecomastia and rare reports of impotence and myalgia. Causal relationships of other reports, such as pancreatitis, are unclear.

INTERACTIONS. Cimetidine retards oxidative hepatic drug metabolism by binding to microsomal cytochrome P450. It should be avoided in patients stabilised on warfarin, phenytoin, and theophylline (or aminophylline), but other interactions (see **Appendix 1**) may be of less clinical relevance. Famotidine, nizatidine, and ranitidine do not share the drug metabolism inhibitory properties of cimetidine.

CIMETIDINE

Indications: benign gastric and duodenal ulceration, stomal ulcer, reflux oesophagitis, Zollinger-Ellison syndrome, other conditions where gastric acid reduction is beneficial (see notes above and section 1.9.4)

Cautions: see notes above; renal and hepatic impairment (reduce dose); pregnancy and breast-feeding; preferably avoid intravenous injection (infusion is preferable) particularly in high dosage (may rarely cause arrhythmias) and in cardiovascular impairment; **interactions:** Appendix 1 (histamine H$_2$-antagonists) and notes above

Side-effects: altered bowel habit, dizziness, rash, tiredness; reversible confusional states, reversible liver damage, headache; rarely, decreased blood counts, muscle or joint pain, bradycardia and AV block; interstitial nephritis and acute pancreatitis reported; gynaecomastia is also an occasional problem with cimetidine but usually only in high dosage (see also notes above)

Dose: by mouth, 400 mg twice daily (with breakfast and at night) *or* 800 mg as a single daily dose at night (benign gastric and duodenal ulceration). Doses should be taken for at least 4 weeks (6 weeks in gastric ulceration, 8 weeks in NSAID-associated ulceration); when necessary the dose may be increased to 400 mg 4 times daily or rarely (e.g. as in stress ulceration) to a max. of 2.4 g daily in divided doses; CHILD 20–30 mg/kg daily in divided doses

Maintenance, 400 mg at night *or* 400 mg morning and night

Reflux oesophagitis, 400 mg 4 times daily for 4–8 weeks, Zollinger-Ellison syndrome, 400 mg 4 times daily or occasionally more

Gastric acid reduction (prophylaxis of acid aspiration; do not use syrup), obstetrics 400 mg at start of labour, then up to 400 mg every 4 hours if required (max. of 2.4 g daily); surgical procedures 400 mg 90–120 minutes before induction of general anaesthesia

Short-bowel syndrome, 400 mg twice daily (with breakfast and at bedtime) adjusted according to response

To reduce degradation of pancreatic enzyme supplements, 0.8–1.6 g daily in 4 divided doses according to response 1–1½ hours before meals

By intramuscular injection, 200 mg every 4–6 hours; max. 2.4 g daily

By slow intravenous injection, 200 mg given over at least 2 minutes; may be repeated every 4–6 hours; if a larger dose is needed or there is cardiovascular impairment, the dose should be diluted and given over at least 10 minutes (infusion is preferable); max. 2.4 g daily

By intravenous infusion, 400 mg in 100 mL of sodium chloride 0.9% intravenous infusion infused over ½–1 hour (may be repeated every 4–6 hours) *or* by continuous infusion at an average rate of 50–100 mg/hour over 24 hours, max. 2.4 g daily; CHILD, *by intramuscular injection or slow intravenous injection or infusion*, 20–30 mg/kg daily in divided doses

PoM **Cimetidine** (Non-proprietary)
Tablets, cimetidine 200 mg, net price 120-tab pack = £17.65; 400 mg, 60-tab pack = £18.70; 800 mg, 30-tab pack = £18.27
Available from APS, Ashbourne (Peptimax®), Cox, CP, Evans, Galen (Galenamet®), Kerfoot, Norton

PoM **Dyspamet**® (SK&F)
Chewtab® (chewable tablets), sugar-free, cimetidine 200 mg. Net price 120-tab pack = £16.73. Counselling, chew thoroughly
Suspension, sugar-free, cimetidine 200 mg/5 mL. Contains sorbitol 2.79 g/5 mL. Net price 600 mL = £21.89

PoM **Tagamet**® (SK&F)
Tablets, all green, f/c, cimetidine 200 mg, net price 120-tab pack = £17.80; 400 mg, 60-tab pack = £20.56; 800 mg, 30-tab pack = £20.56
Effervescent tablets, sugar-free, cimetidine 400 mg. Contains 7.7 mmol Na$^+$/tablet. Net price 60-tab pack = £18.69. Label: 13
Syrup, orange, cimetidine 200 mg/5 mL. Net price 600 mL = £25.90
Injection, cimetidine 100 mg/mL. Net price 2-mL amp = 30p
Intravenous infusion, cimetidine 4 mg/mL in sodium chloride intravenous infusion 0.9%. Net price 100-mL infusion bag = £1.86

Cimetidine with alginate
PoM **Algitec**® (SK&F)
Chewtab® (chewable tablets), off-white, cimetidine 200 mg, alginic acid 500 mg. Contains 2.05 mmol Na$^+$/tablet. Net price 120-tab pack = £22.49. Counselling, chew thoroughly
Suspension, cimetidine 100 mg, sodium alginate 250 mg/5 mL. Contains 1.43 mmol Na$^+$/5 mL. Net price 600 mL = £15.41
Dose: gastro-oesophageal reflux disease, 1 tablet chewed or 10 mL suspension 4 times daily (after meals and at bedtime), increased if necessary to 2 tablets or 20 mL suspension 4 times daily; to be taken for 4–8 weeks

FAMOTIDINE

Indications: see under Dose
Cautions: see under Cimetidine; does not inhibit hepatic microsomal drug metabolism
Side-effects: see under Cimetidine
Dose: benign gastric and duodenal ulceration, treatment, 40 mg at night for 4–8 weeks; maintenance, 20 mg at night
Reflux oesophagitis, 20–40 mg twice daily for 6–12 weeks
Zollinger–Ellison syndrome, 20 mg every 6 hours (higher dose in those who have previously been receiving another H$_2$-antagonist)

PoM **Pepcid**® (Morson)
Tablets, famotidine 20 mg (beige), net price 28-tab pack = £14.00; 40 mg (brown), 28-tab pack = £26.60

NIZATIDINE

Indications: see under Dose
Cautions: see under Cimetidine; does not inhibit hepatic microsomal drug metabolism
Side-effects: see under Cimetidine; sweating also reported; rare reports of gynaecomastia

Dose: benign gastric and duodenal ulceration, treatment, 300 mg at night *or* 150 mg twice daily for 4–8 weeks; maintenance, 150 mg at night for up to 1 year

Reflux oesophagitis, 150–300 mg twice daily for up to 12 weeks

PoM **Axid**® (Lilly)
Capsules, nizatidine 150 mg (pale yellow/dark yellow), net price 28-cap pack = £14.11; 300 mg (pale yellow/brown), 28-cap pack = £27.05

RANITIDINE

Indications: benign gastric and duodenal ulceration, stomal ulcer, reflux oesophagitis, Zollinger–Ellison syndrome, other conditions where reduction of gastric acidity is beneficial (see notes above and section 1.9.4)

Cautions: see under Cimetidine; does not significantly inhibit hepatic microsomal drug metabolism

Side-effects: see under Cimetidine; rare reports of breast swelling and tenderness in men

Dose: by mouth, 150 mg twice daily (morning and night), or for patients with gastric and duodenal ulceration 300 mg as a single daily dose at night, for 4 to 8 weeks, up to 6 weeks in chronic episodic dyspepsia, and up to 8 weeks in reflux oesophagitis and NSAID-associated ulceration in duodenal ulcer 300 mg can be given twice daily for 4 weeks to achieve a higher healing rate

Prophylaxis of NSAID-induced duodenal ulcer, 150 mg twice daily

Zollinger–Ellison syndrome, 150 mg 3 times daily increased if necessary to up to 6 g daily in divided doses

Maintenance, 150 mg at night

CHILD 8–18 years up to 150 mg twice daily

Gastric acid reduction (prophylaxis of acid aspiration) in obstetrics, *by mouth,* 150 mg at onset of labour, then every 6 hours; surgical procedures, *by intramuscular or slow intravenous injection,* 50 mg 45–60 minutes before induction (intravenous injection diluted to 20 mL and given over at least 2 minutes), or *by mouth,* 150 mg 2 hours before induction, and also, when possible on the preceding evening

By intramuscular injection, 50 mg every 6–8 hours

By slow intravenous injection, 50 mg diluted to 20 mL and given over at least 2 minutes; may be repeated every 6–8 hours

By intravenous infusion, 25 mg/hour for 2 hours; may be repeated every 6–8 hours

or, for prophylaxis of stress ulceration, following initial slow intravenous injection of 50 mg (as above) by *continuous infusion,* 125–250 micrograms/kg per hour

PoM **Zantac**® (Glaxo)
Tablets, f/c, ranitidine (as hydrochloride) 150 mg, net price 60-tab pack = £29.76; 300 mg, 30-tab pack = £27.43

Dispersible tablets, f/c, scored, sugar-free, ranitidine 150 mg (as hydrochloride). Net price 60-tab pack = £31.25. Label: 13

Effervescent tablets, pale yellow, ranitidine (as hydrochloride) 150 mg (contains 14.3 mmol Na$^+$/tablet), net price 60-tab pack = £31.25; 300 mg (contains 20.8 mmol Na$^+$/tablet), 30-tab pack = £31.25. Label: 13

Syrup, sugar-free, ranitidine (as hydrochloride) 75 mg/5 mL. Net price 300 mL = £22.32

Injection, ranitidine 25 mg (as hydrochloride)/mL. Net price 2-mL amp = 64p

1.3.2 Selective antimuscarinics

Pirenzepine is a selective antimuscarinic drug which inhibits gastric acid and pepsin secretion with fewer peripheral side-effects than the drugs in section 1.2. As it does not cross the blood-brain barrier it is unlikely to have central effects. It is as effective as H$_2$-receptor antagonists in healing *gastric and duodenal ulcers* and may also be useful in maintenance treatment. It has also been used in conjunction with H$_2$-receptor antagonists in resistant cases.

PIRENZEPINE

Indications: benign gastric and duodenal ulceration

Side-effects: occasionally dry mouth and visual disturbances; agranulocytosis and thrombocytopenia have been reported

Dose: 50 mg twice daily, increased if necessary to a max. of 150 mg daily in 3 divided doses, for 4–6 weeks, or in resistant cases for up to 3 months. Doses should preferably be taken 30 minutes before meals

PoM **Gastrozepin**® (Boots)
Tablets, scored, pirenzepine hydrochloride, equivalent to anhydrous pirenzepine hydrochloride, 50 mg. Net price 60 = £24.60. Label: 22

1.3.3 Chelates and complexes

Tripotassium dicitratobismuthate is a bismuth chelate effective in healing *gastric and duodenal ulcers.* It may act by a direct toxic effect on gastric *Helicobacter (Campylobacter) pylori,* or by stimulating mucosal prostaglandin or bicarbonate secretion. The healing tends to be longer lasting but relapse still occurs. The bismuth content is low but absorption has been reported; encephalopathy (described with older high-dose bismuth preparations) has not been reported. As the elixir, which has a pungent ammoniacal odour, is likely to adhere to food rather than to the surface of the ulcer, patients should be advised to avoid food, antacids, and large quantities of milk when taking doses. Tablets are as effective as the liquid and more palatable.

Sucralfate is another effective treatment for *gastric and duodenal ulcers* and may act by protecting the mucosa from acid-pepsin attack. It is a complex of aluminium hydroxide and sulphated sucrose but has minimal antacid properties.

BISMUTH CHELATE

Indications: benign gastric and duodenal ulceration

Cautions: avoid in severe renal impairment; see also notes above; **interactions:** Appendix 1 (bismuth chelate)

Side-effects: may darken tongue and blacken faeces; nausea and vomiting reported

De-Nol® (Brocades)
Liquid, red, tripotassium dicitratobismuthate 120 mg/5 mL. Net price 560 mL = £14.65. Counselling, see below
Dose: adults, 10 mL twice daily *or* 5 mL 4 times daily; taken for 28 days, followed by further 28 days if necessary; maintenance not indicated but course may be repeated after interval of 1 month; CHILDREN, no longer recommended
COUNSELLING. Each dose to be diluted with 15 mL of water; twice daily dosage to be taken 30 minutes before breakfast and main evening meal; four times daily dosage to be taken as follows: one dose 30 minutes before breakfast, midday meal and main evening meal, and one dose 2 hours after main evening meal; milk should not be drunk by itself during treatment but small quantities may be taken in tea or coffee or on cereal; antacids should not be taken half an hour before or after a dose; may darken tongue and blacken faeces

De-Noltab® (Brocades)
Tablets, white, tripotassium dicitratobismuthate 120 mg. Net price 112-tab pack = £20.98. Counselling, see below
Dose: adults 2 tablets twice daily *or* 1 tablet 4 times daily; taken for 28 days followed by further 28 days if necessary; maintenance not indicated but course may be repeated after interval of 1 month; CHILD, not recommended
COUNSELLING. Each dose to be swallowed with a tumblerful of water then as above under De-Nol

SUCRALFATE

Indications: benign gastric and duodenal ulceration; chronic gastritis

Cautions: renal disease; **interactions:** Appendix 1 (sucralfate)

Side-effects: constipation; diarrhoea, nausea, indigestion, dry mouth, rash, pruritus, back pain, dizziness, insomnia, and vertigo; also gastric discomfort reported

Dose: 2 g twice daily (on rising and at bedtime) *or* 1 g 4 times daily 1 hour before meals and at bedtime, taken for up to 6 weeks or in resistant cases 12 weeks; max. 8 g daily
Prophylaxis of stress ulceration (suspension), 1 g 6 times daily (max. 8 g daily)
COUNSELLING. Tablets may be dispersed in 10–15 mL of water; antacids should not be taken half an hour before or after a dose

PoM **Antepsin®** (Wyeth)
Tablets, scored, sucralfate 1 g. Net price 20 = £2.50. Label: 5, counselling, see dose above
Suspension, sucralfate, 1 g/5 mL. Net price 560 mL = £14.00. Label: 5, counselling, antacids

1.3.4 Prostaglandin analogues

Misoprostol, a synthetic analogue of prostaglandin E_1 (alprostadil) inhibits gastric acid secretion promoting *gastric and duodenal ulcer healing*. It can protect against *NSAID-associated gastric ulcers* but not dyspepsia.

MISOPROSTOL

Indications: see notes above and under Dose

Cautions: conditions where hypotension might precipitate severe complications (e.g. cerebrovascular disease, cardiovascular disease)

Contra-indications: pregnancy or planning pregnancy (increases uterine tone)

Side-effects: diarrhoea (may be severe, reduced by giving single doses not exceeding 200 micrograms and by avoiding magnesium-containing antacids); also reported: abdominal pain, dyspepsia, flatulence, nausea and vomiting, abnormal vaginal bleeding (including intermenstrual bleeding, menorrhagia, and postmenopausal bleeding)

Dose: benign gastric and duodenal ulceration and NSAID-associated ulceration, 800 micrograms daily (in 2–4 divided doses) with breakfast (or main meals) and at bedtime; treatment should be continued for at least 4 weeks and may be continued for up to 8 weeks if required
Prophylaxis of NSAID-induced gastric ulcer, 200 micrograms 2–4 times daily according to condition of patient

PoM **Cytotec®** (Searle)
Tablets, scored, misoprostol 200 micrograms. Net price 56-tab pack = £13.00; 112-tab pack = £26.00

With naproxen
Section 10.1.1.

1.3.5 Proton pump inhibitors

Omeprazole inhibits gastric acid by blocking the hydrogen-potassium adenosine triphosphatase enzyme system (the 'proton pump') of the gastric parietal cell. It is an effective treatment for *gastric and duodenal ulcers* and particularly for *erosive oesophagitis*.

OMEPRAZOLE

Indications: see under Dose

Cautions: exclude malignancy; avoid in pregnancy and breast-feeding; **interactions:** Appendix 1 (omeprazole)

Side-effects: diarrhoea, headache (both may be severe); also nausea, constipation, and flatulence; skin reactions (some serious), photosensitivity reported; muscle and joint pain, blurred vision, peripheral oedema, gynaecomastia, loss of taste, stomatitis, gastro-intestinal candidiasis and blood disorders also reported; reversible mental confusion, agitation, depression and hallucinations have been noted in the severely ill

Dose: benign gastric and duodenal ulcers (including those complicating NSAID therapy) 20 mg daily for 4 weeks in duodenal ulceration or 8 weeks in gastric ulceration; in severe cases increase to 40 mg daily; long-term use not recommended

Zollinger–Ellison syndrome, initially 60 mg once daily; usual range 20–120 mg daily (above 80 mg in 2 divided doses)

Healing of reflux oesophagitis, 20 mg daily for 4 weeks, followed by a further 4–8 weeks if not fully healed; 40 mg daily has been given for 8 weeks in reflux oesophagitis refractory to other treatment; may be continued at 20 mg daily

PoM **Losec**® (Astra)
Capsules, pink/brown, enclosing e/c granules, omeprazole 20 mg, net price 28-cap pack = £36.36 (also 5-cap pack, hosp. only). Label: 25

1.3.6 Other ulcer-healing drugs

Carbenoxolone, a synthetic derivative of glycyrrhizinic acid (a constituent of liquorice) is effective in *gastric ulcer*; it is also effective in *duodenal ulcer* if released at the site of the lesion. However, side-effects (commonly sodium and water retention and occasionally hypokalaemia) may cause or exacerbate hypertension, oedema, cardiac failure, and muscle weakness. For these reasons other drugs are preferred; if used regular monitoring of weight, blood pressure, and electrolytes is advisable during treatment. Carbenoxolone may act by protecting the mucosal barrier from acid–pepsin attack and increasing mucosal mucin production.

Deglycyrrhizinised liquorice is free from the above side-effects but is of doubtful efficacy.

CARBENOXOLONE SODIUM
Indications: benign gastric and duodenal ulceration in young and middle-aged patients
Cautions: cardiac disease, hypertension, impaired hepatic and renal function; elderly (see under preparations); not recommended in children. See also notes above. Potassium supplements and thiazides may be necessary; interactions: Appendix 1 (carbenoxolone)
Contra-indications: hypokalaemia, pregnancy; avoid use with spironolactone and amiloride
Side-effects: sodium and water retention leading to oedema, alkalosis, hypertension, hypokalaemia

PoM **Biogastrone**® (Sanofi Winthrop)
Tablets, scored, carbenoxolone sodium 50 mg. Net price 100-tab pack = £22.77. Label: 21
Dose: for gastric ulceration, 2 tablets 3 times daily after meals for 1 week, then 1 tablet 3 times daily for 6–12 weeks; not recommended under 16 years or over 65 years

Compound preparation
PoM **Pyrogastrone**® (Sanofi Winthrop)
Tablets, chewable, carbenoxolone sodium 20 mg, alginic acid 600 mg, dried aluminium hydroxide 240 mg, magnesium trisilicate 60 mg, sodium bicarbonate 210 mg (Na^+ 2.6 mmol/tablet). Net price 100-tab pack = £25.49. Label: 21, 24
Liquid, carbenoxolone sodium 10 mg, dried aluminium hydroxide 150 mg (Na^+ 0.85 mmol, K^+ 1.5 mmol)/5 mL when reconstituted with water. Net price 500 mL = £12.71. Label: 21
Dose: for oesophageal inflammation and ulceration, 1 tablet, chewed, 3 times daily after meals, and 2 at night, for 6–12 weeks or 10 mL liquid 3 times daily after meals and 20 mL at night, for 6–12 weeks; not recommended for children or for adults over 75 years

LIQUORICE, DEGLYCYRRHIZINISED
Indications: benign gastric and duodenal ulceration

Caved-S® (Tillotts)
Tablets, brown, deglycyrrhizinised liquorice 380 mg, aluminium hydroxide mixture 100 mg, bismuth subnitrate 100 mg, magnesium carbonate 200 mg, sodium bicarbonate 100 mg. Net price 20 = £1.25. Label: 24
Dose: benign gastric and duodenal ulceration, treatment, 2 tablets chewed 3 times daily (for duodenal ulceration increased if necessary to 6 times daily); maintenance, 1 tablet chewed 3 times daily (gastric ulceration), 2 tablets chewed 3 times daily (duodenal ulceration); CHILD no longer recommended
Note. Caved-S® tablets now contain bismuth subnitrate; long-term use should be avoided, see also section 1.1.3

1.4 Antidiarrhoeal drugs

The **first line** of treatment in acute diarrhoea, as in gastro-enteritis, is prevention or treatment of fluid and electrolyte depletion. This is particularly important in infants and in frail and elderly patients. Clinical signs of severe dehydration require immediate admission to hospital and urgent replacement of fluid and electrolytes. For details of **oral rehydration therapy** and of preparations available, see section 9.2.1.2.

Antidiarrhoeal drugs are of secondary value in the treatment of diarrhoea, may have undesirable side-effects, and may distract from giving fluids.

Antispasmodics (section 1.2) are occasionally of value in treating abdominal cramp associated with diarrhoea but they should not be used for primary treatment. Antispasmodics and antiemetics should be **avoided** in young children with gastro-enteritis as they are rarely effective and have troublesome side-effects.

Antibiotics and sulphonamides are generally unnecessary in simple gastro-enteritis, even when a bacterial cause is suspected, because the complaint will usually resolve quickly without such treatment, and infective diarrhoeas in the UK are often caused by viral infections. Systemic bacterial infection does, however, need appropriate systemic treatment. **Erythromycin** (see section 5.1.5) or **ciprofloxacin** (see section 5.1.12) can be used for treating enteritis caused by *Campylobacter* spp. For drugs for shigellosis and salmonellosis, see section 5.1, table 1. The general use of sulphonamides in treating diarrhoea of travellers is inadvisable because of the risks of rash and agranulocytosis.

36 Chapter 1: Gastro-intestinal system

Poorly absorbed drugs such as dihydrostreptomycin, neomycin, and sulphaguanidine should be **avoided** altogether in gastro-intestinal infection. They prolong rather than shorten the time taken to control diarrhoea by causing masked bacterial diarrhoea, carrier states, or pseudomembranous colitis. Clioquinol should be avoided as it is neurotoxic; both it and lactobacillus preparations are valueless.

1.4.1 Adsorbents and bulk-forming drugs

Adsorbents such as kaolin are **not** recommended for *acute diarrhoeas*. Bulk-forming drugs, such as ispaghula, methylcellulose, and sterculia (see section 1.6.1) are useful in controlling faecal consistency in ileostomy and colostomy, and in controlling diarrhoea associated with diverticular disease.

KAOLIN, LIGHT
Indications: diarrhoea but see notes above
Cautions: **interactions:** Appendix 1 (antacids and adsorbents)

Kaolin Mixture (BP)
(Kaolin Oral Suspension)
Oral suspension, light kaolin or light kaolin (natural) 20%, and 5% each of light magnesium carbonate and sodium bicarbonate in a suitable vehicle with a peppermint flavour. Extemporaneous preparations should be prepared according to the following formula: light kaolin or light kaolin (natural) 2 g, light magnesium carbonate 500 mg, sodium bicarbonate 500 mg, concentrated peppermint emulsion 0.25 mL, double-strength chloroform water 5 mL, water to 10 mL. It should be recently prepared, unless the kaolin has been sterilised. Net price 200 mL = 19p
Dose: 10–20 mL every 4 hours

Kaopectate® (Upjohn)
Mixture, sugar-free, kaolin 1.03 g/5 mL. Net price 100 mL = 94p
Dose: 10–30 mL every 4 hours; CHILD not recommended therefore no dose stated

KLN® (Ashe)
Mixture, kaolin 1.15 g, pectin 57.5 mg, sodium citrate 17.25 mg/5 mL. Net price 100 mL = £1.12
Dose: CHILD not recommended therefore no dose stated

1.4.2 Antimotility drugs

In *acute diarrhoeas* antimotility drugs have a very limited role as adjuncts to fluid and electrolyte replacement (see section 9.2.1.2); they are **not** recommended for acute diarrhoeas in young children.

For comments on their role in *chronic diarrhoeas* see section 1.5.

CODEINE PHOSPHATE
Indications: see notes above
Cautions; Contra-indications; Side-effects: see section 4.7.2; not recommended for children; tolerance and dependence may occur with prolonged use; **interactions:** Appendix 1 (opioid analgesics)
Dose: see under Preparations below

PoM **Codeine Phosphate Tablets,** codeine phosphate 15 mg, net price 20 = 38p; 30 mg, 20 = 39p; 60 mg, 20 = £1.24. Label: 2
Dose: 30 mg 3–4 times daily (range 15–60 mg); CHILD not recommended
Note. Travellers needing to take codeine phosphate tablets abroad may require a doctor's letter explaining why they are necessary.

PoM **Diarrest®** (Galen)
Liquid, yellow, codeine phosphate 5 mg, dicyclomine hydrochloride 2.5 mg, potassium chloride 40 mg, sodium chloride 50 mg, sodium citrate 50 mg/5 mL. For diarrhoea, vomiting, and cramp. Net price 200 mL = £3.34
Dose: 20 mL 4 times daily with water; CHILD 4–5 years 5 mL, 6–9 years 10 mL, 10–13 years 15 mL but see cautions and notes above.

Kaodene® (Boots)
Mixture, codeine phosphate 10 mg, light kaolin 3 g/10 mL. Net price 250 mL = 98p
Dose: 20 mL 3–4 times daily; CHILD over 5 years 10 mL but see cautions and notes above

CO-PHENOTROPE
A mixture of diphenoxylate hydrochloride and atropine sulphate in the mass proportions 100 parts to 1 part respectively
Indications: adjunct to rehydration in acute diarrhoea (but see notes above); chronic mild ulcerative colitis
Cautions; Contra-indications; Side-effects: see notes above and under Codeine Phosphate; young children are particularly susceptible to OVERDOSAGE and symptoms may be delayed so that observation is needed for at least 48 hours after ingestion; in addition the presence of subclinical doses of atropine may give rise to the side-effects of atropine in susceptible individuals or in overdosage

PoM **Lomotil®** (Gold Cross)
Tablets, co-phenotrope 2.5/0.025 (diphenoxylate hydrochloride 2.5 mg, atropine sulphate 25 micrograms). Net price 20 = £1.96
Dose: initially 4 tablets, followed by 2 tablets every 6 hours until diarrhoea controlled; CHILD 4–8 years 1 tablet 3 times daily, 9–12 years 1 tablet 4 times daily, 13–16 years 2 tablets 3 times daily, but see also notes above

Liquid, red, sugar-free, co-phenotrope 2.5/0.025 (diphenoxylate hydrochloride 2.5 mg, atropine sulphate 25 micrograms)/5 mL. Net price 100 mL = £3.73
Dose: initially 20 mL, followed by 10 mL every 6 hours until diarrhoea controlled; CHILD 4–8 years 5 mL 3 times daily, 9–12 years 5 mL 4 times daily, 13–16 years 10 mL 3 times daily, but see also notes above
Note. Co-phenotrope 2.5/0.025 tablets are also available from Mepra-pharm (Diarphen®)

LOPERAMIDE HYDROCHLORIDE
Indications: adjunct to rehydration in acute diarrhoea in adults and children over 4 years (but see notes above); chronic diarrhoea in adults only
Cautions; Contra-indications: see notes above and under Codeine Phosphate (except dependence)

Side-effects: abdominal cramps and skin reactions, including urticaria reported; paralytic ileus and abdominal bloating also reported
Dose: acute diarrhoea, 4 mg initially followed by 2 mg after each loose stool for up to 5 days; usual dose 6–8 mg daily; max. 16 mg daily; CHILD 4–8 years 1 mg 4 times daily for up to *3 days only*, 9–12 years 2 mg 4 times daily for up to 5 days
Chronic diarrhoea in adults, initially, 4–8 mg daily in divided doses, subsequently adjusted according to response and given in 2 divided doses for maintenance

PoM[1] **Loperamide** (Non-proprietary)
Capsules, loperamide hydrochloride 2 mg. Net price 30 = £2.21

PoM[1] **Imodium**® (Janssen)
Capsules, green/grey, loperamide hydrochloride 2 mg. Net price 30 = £2.17
Syrup, red, sugar-free, loperamide hydrochloride 1 mg/5 mL. Net price 100 mL = £1.90

1. Loperamide can be sold to the public, for adults and children over 12 years, provided it is licensed and labelled for the treatment of acute diarrhoea; proprietary brands (Arret® capsules and adult syrup and Diocalm Ultra® capsules) are on sale to the public

MORPHINE
Indications: see notes above
Cautions; Contra-indications; Side-effects: see notes above and under Codeine Phosphate, sedation and the risk of dependence are greater

Kaolin and Morphine Mixture (BP)
(Kaolin and Morphine Oral Suspension)
Oral suspension, light kaolin or light kaolin (natural) 20%, sodium bicarbonate 5%, and chloroform and morphine tincture 4% in a suitable vehicle. Extemporaneous preparations should be prepared according to the following formula: light kaolin or light kaolin (natural) 2 g, sodium bicarbonate 500 mg, chloroform and morphine tincture 0.4 mL, water to 10 mL. It should be recently prepared, unless the kaolin has been sterilised. Contains 550 to 800 micrograms of anhydrous morphine/10 mL.
Dose: 10 mL every 4 hours in water

1.5 Treatment of chronic diarrhoeas

Once tumours are ruled out individual complaints need specific treatment including dietary manipulation as well as drug treatment and the maintenance of a liberal fluid intake.

IRRITABLE BOWEL SYNDROME. This can present with pain, constipation, or diarrhoea, all of which may benefit from a high-fibre diet with bran or other agents which increase stool bulk (section 1.6.1) if necessary. In some patients there may be important psychological aggravating factors which respond to reassurance. Antimotility drugs such as **loperamide** may sometimes be necessary but prolonged use may aggravate the condition (section 1.4.2). Opioids such as codeine are better avoided because of the risk of dependence. Antispasmodics (section 1.2) may relieve the pain.

MALABSORPTION SYNDROMES. Individual conditions need specific treatment and also general nutritional consideration. Thus coeliac disease (gluten enteropathy) usually needs a gluten-free diet (Appendix 7) and pancreatic insufficiency needs pancreatin supplements (section 1.9.4).

ULCERATIVE COLITIS. For *acute attacks* topical **corticosteroid** treatment such as prednisolone enemas or suppositories for localised rectal disease will induce remission; foam preparations are especially useful where patients have difficulty retaining liquid enemas. More extensive disease requires oral corticosteroid treatment and severe extensive or fulminant disease needs hospital admission and intravenous corticosteroid administration.
Sulphasalazine, a chemical combination of sulphapyridine and 5-aminosalicylic acid ('5-ASA') is useful in mild symptomatic disease requiring oral treatment; it is also available as suppositories for rectal disease. Activity resides in the 5-aminosalicylic acid moiety; sulphapyridine acts only as a carrier to the colonic site of action (but it still causes side-effects). Newer alternatives include **mesalazine** (5-aminosalicylic acid itself, in a modified-release tablet) and **olsalazine** (2 molecules of 5-aminosalicylic acid bonded together, separating in the lower bowel). The sulphonamide-related side-effects of suphasalazine (rashes, blood disorders, azoospermia, and lupoid syndromes) are lacking from mesalazine and olsalazine, but they retain side-effect profiles associated with the 5-aminosalicylic acid moiety (watery diarrhoea, salicylate hypersensitivity, and interstitial nephritis).
Corticosteroids are unsuitable for *maintenance treatment* because of side-effects. Sulphasalazine, mesalazine, and olsalazine all have value in preventing relapse and choice is related in part to their different side-effects. In resistant cases **azathioprine** (see section 8.2.1), 2 mg/kg daily, given under close supervision may be helpful.
Laxatives are required to facilitate bowel movement when proctitis is present but a high-fibre diet and bulk-forming drugs such as **methylcellulose** are more useful in adjusting faecal consistency (section 1.6.1).
Antimotility drugs such as codeine and loperamide should not be used in severe colitis as they can precipitate paralytic ileus and megacolon. They have limited value in mild disease, but treatment of the inflammation is more logical. For similar reasons antispasmodics should **not** be used in ulcerative colitis.

CROHN'S DISEASE. Treatment particularly of colonic disease is similar to that for ulcerative colitis. In small bowel disease **sulphasalazine** is of doubtful value. **Oral corticosteroids** (e.g. prednisolone) suppress inflammation, and **metronidazole** may be beneficial possibly through antibacterial activity. Other antibacterials should

38 Chapter 1: Gastro-intestinal system

be given if specifically indicated and for managing bacterial overgrowth in the small bowel.

In both colitis and Crohn's disease general nutritional care and appropriate supplements are essential.

Cholestyramine and **aluminium hydroxide mixture** (section 1.1.1), bind unabsorbed bile salts and provide symptomatic relief of diarrhoea following ileal disease or resection, in bacterial colonisation of the small bowel, and in post-vagotomy diarrhoea.

PSEUDOMEMBRANOUS COLITIS. This is due to colonisation of the colon with *Clostridium difficile* which may develop after antibiotic therapy. It is usually of acute onset, but may run a chronic course; it is a particular hazard of clindamycin and lincomycin but few antibiotics are free of this side-effect. Oral **vancomycin** (see section 5.1.7) or **metronidazole** (see section 5.1.11) are used as specific treatment; vancomycin may be preferred for very sick patients.

DIVERTICULAR DISEASE. This is treated with a high-fibre diet, **bran supplements**, and **bulk-forming drugs**. **Antispasmodics** may provide symptomatic relief when colic is a problem (section 1.2). **Antibiotics** should be used only when the diverticula in the intestinal wall become infected. **Antimotility** drugs which slow intestinal motility, e.g. codeine, diphenoxylate, and loperamide could possibly exacerbate the symptoms of diverticular disease and are **contra-indicated**.

AMINOSALICYLATES

SULPHASALAZINE

Indications: induction and maintenance of remission in ulcerative colitis; treatment of active Crohn's disease (for use in rheumatoid arthritis see section 10.1.3)
Cautions: pregnancy; hepatic and renal disease; G6PD deficiency (including breast-feeding of affected infants); slow acetylator status; withdraw treatment if blood disorders, hypersensitivity reactions, or other serious disorders occur; upper gastro-intestinal side-effects become common with doses over 4 g daily; blood counts, liver-function tests, and rheumatoid arthritis, see section 10.1.3
Contra-indications: salicylate and sulphonamide hypersensitivity; porphyria (see section 9.8.2)
Side-effects: nausea, vomiting, epigastric discomfort, headache, rashes; *occasionally:* fever, minor haematological abnormalities such as Heinz-body anaemia, reversible neutropenia, folate deficiency; reversible azoospermia; *rarely:* pancreatitis, hepatitis, exacerbation of colitis, thrombocytopenia, agranulocytosis, Stevens–Johnson syndrome, neurotoxicity, photosensitisation, lupus erythematosus-like syndrome, and pneumonitis; proteinuria, crystalluria, haematuria, and nephrotic syndrome; urine may be coloured orange; some soft contact lenses may be stained

Dose: by mouth, acute attack 1–2 g 4 times daily (but see **cautions**) until remission occurs (if necessary corticosteroids may also be given), reducing to a maintenance dose of 500 mg 4 times daily; CHILD over 2 years, acute attack 40–60 mg/kg daily, maintenance dose 20–30 mg/kg daily

By rectum, in suppositories, alone or in conjunction with oral treatment 0.5–1 g morning and night after a bowel movement. As an enema, 3 g at night, retained for at least 1 hour

PoM **Sulphasalazine** (Non-proprietary)
Tablets, sulphasalazine 500 mg. Net price 100 = £7.95. Label: 14, counselling, lenses see above
Available from Cox, Norton

PoM **Salazopyrin**® (Kabi Pharmacia)
Tablets, orange-brown, scored, sulphasalazine 500 mg. Net price 20 = £1.41. Label: 14, counselling, lenses see above

EN-tablets® (= tablets e/c), yellow, f/c, sulphasalazine 500 mg. Net price 125-tab pack = £12.75. Label: 5, 14, 25, counselling, lenses see above

Suspension, yellow, sulphasalazine 250 mg/5 mL. Net price 500 mL = £16.86. Label: 14, counselling, lenses see above

Suppositories, brown, sulphasalazine 500 mg. Net price 10 = £2.95; 50 = £14.02. Label: 14, counselling, lenses see above

Retention enema, sulphasalazine 3 g in 100-mL single-dose disposable packs fitted with a nozzle. Net price 7 × 100 mL = £12.75. Label: 14, counselling, lenses see above

MESALAZINE

Indications: maintenance of remission in ulcerative colitis and treatment of mild to moderate exacerbations
Cautions: elderly; pregnancy and breast-feeding
Contra-indications: salicylate hypersensitivity; renal impairment (nephrotoxic)
Side-effects: nausea, diarrhoea, and abdominal pain; headache; exacerbation of symptoms of colitis; rarely reversible pancreatitis, hepatitis, and interstitial nephritis; leucopenia, neutropenia, and thrombocytopenia reported; myocarditis also reported
Dose: see under preparations, below

PoM **Asacol**® (SK&F)
Tablets, red, e/c, mesalazine 400 mg. Net price 120-tab pack = £34.30. Label: 5, 25
Dose: acute attack, 6 tablets daily in divided doses; maintenance 3–6 tablets daily in divided doses

Suppositories, mesalazine 250 mg, net price 20 = £6.50; 500 mg, 10 = £6.50
Dose: 3–6 suppositories of 250 mg (max. 3 suppositories of 500 mg) daily in divided doses, with last dose at bedtime

---

Abbreviations and symbols, see inside front cover   Prices are **net**, see p. 1

1.5 Treatment of chronic diarrhoeas

PoM **Pentasa**® (Brocades)
Tablets, m/r, enclosing coated granules, mesalazine 250 mg. Net price 200-tab pack = £32.28. Label: 25
Dose: maintenance of remission 2 tablets 3 times daily
Retention enema, mesalazine 1 g in 100-mL single-dose bottle. Net price 7 × 100 mL = £19.45
Dose: 100 mL enema at bedtime

PoM **Salofalk**® (Thames)
Tablets, e/c, yellow, mesalazine 250 mg. Net price 100-tab pack = £17.50. Label: 5, 25
Dose: acute attack, 6 tablets daily in 3 divided doses; maintenance 3–6 tablets daily in divided doses

OLSALAZINE SODIUM
Indications: treatment of acute mild ulcerative colitis and maintenance of remission
Cautions: elderly; pregnancy and breast-feeding
Contra-indications: salicylate hypersensitivity; renal impairment
Side-effects: watery diarrhoea, abdominal cramps, headache, nausea, dyspepsia, arthralgia, and rash; rarely reversible pancreatitis
Dose: acute attack, 1 g daily in divided doses increased if necessary over 1 week to max. 3 g daily (max. single dose 1 g)
Maintenance, 500 mg twice daily

PoM **Dipentum**® (Kabi Pharmacia)
Capsules, brown, olsalazine sodium 250 mg. Net price 20 = £4.78. Label: 21

ANION-EXCHANGE RESINS

CHOLESTYRAMINE
Indications: diarrhoea associated with Crohn's disease, ileal resection, vagotomy, diabetic vagal neuropathy, and radiation; pruritus in liver disease, and hypercholesterolaemia, see section 2.12
Cautions; Contra-indications; Side-effects: see section 2.12
Dose: diarrhoea, after initial introduction over 3–4 week period, 12–24 g daily mixed with water, in single or divided doses, subsequently adjusted as required; max. 36 g daily
COUNSELLING. Other drugs should be taken at least 1 hour before or 4–6 hours after cholestyramine to reduce possible interference with absorption

Preparations: section 2.12

CORTICOSTEROIDS

HYDROCORTISONE
Indications: inflammation associated with colitis, proctitis
Cautions; Contra-indications; Side-effects: systemic absorption may occur, see section 6.3.3; prolonged use should be avoided; avoid use of enemas and rectal foams in obstruction, bowel perforation, and extensive fistulas; contra-indicated in untreated infection
Dose: rectal, see under Preparations

PoM **Hydrocortisone Suppositories**, hydrocortisone or hydrocortisone acetate 25 mg in theobroma oil or other suitable basis. Net price 12 = £4.31
Dose: proctitis, 1 suppository inserted night and morning after a bowel movement

PoM **Colifoam**® (Stafford-Miller)
Foam in aerosol pack, hydrocortisone acetate 10%. Net price 25 g (= 14 applications) with applicator = £7.25
Dose: initially 1 metered application (125 mg hydrocortisone acetate) inserted into the rectum once or twice daily for 2–3 weeks, then once on alternate days

PREDNISOLONE
Indications: induction and maintenance of remission in ulcerative colitis, and Crohn's disease; other indications, see section 6.3.3
Cautions; Contra-indications; Side-effects: see under Hydrocortisone and section 6.3.3
Dose: by mouth, initial dose 40 mg daily, in single or divided doses, until remission occurs, followed by reducing doses
By rectum, see under Preparations

Oral preparations, see section 6.3.4.

Rectal preparations
PoM **Predenema**® (Pharmax)
Retention enema, prednisolone 20 mg (as sodium metasulphobenzoate) in 100-mL single-dose disposable pack. Net price 10 (standard tube) = £7.72, 7 (long tube) = £9.26
Dose: initially 1 enema at bedtime for 2–4 weeks, extending course if good response obtained

PoM **Predfoam**® (Pharmax)
Foam in aerosol pack, prednisolone 20 mg (as metasulphobenzoate sodium)/metered application. Net price 25 g (14 applications) with disposable applicators = £7.25
Dose: 1 metered application (containing 20 mg prednisolone) inserted into the rectum once or twice daily for 2 weeks, continued for further 2 weeks if good response

PoM **Predsol**® (Evans)
Retention enema, prednisolone 20 mg (as sodium phosphate) in 100-mL single-dose disposable packs fitted with a nozzle. Net price 7 = £5.24
Dose: initially 1 enema at bedtime for 2–4 weeks, extending course if good response obtained
Suppositories, prednisolone 5 mg (as sodium phosphate). Net price 10 = £1.00
Dose: proctitis and rectal complications of Crohn's disease, 1 suppository inserted night and morning after a bowel movement

CROMOGLYCATE

SODIUM CROMOGLYCATE
Indications: food allergy (in conjunction with dietary restriction)
Side-effects: occasional nausea, rashes, and joint pain

Dose: 200 mg 4 times daily before meals; CHILD 2–14 years 100 mg; capsules may be swallowed whole or the contents dissolved in hot water and diluted with cold water before taking. May be increased if necessary after 2–3 weeks to a max. of 40 mg/kg daily and then reduced according to the response

PoM **Nalcrom**® (Fisons)
Capsules, sodium cromoglycate 100 mg. Net price 100 = £13.73. Label: 22, counselling, see dose above

1.6 Laxatives

1.6.1 Bulk-forming drugs
1.6.2 Stimulant laxatives
1.6.3 Faecal softeners
1.6.4 Osmotic laxatives

Misconceptions about bowel habits have led to excessive laxative use. Abuse may lead to hypokalaemia and an atonic non-functioning colon. Simple constipation is usually relieved by increasing the intake of dietary fibre. The use of laxatives in children is undesirable and the introduction of fruit purée into the diet may be sufficient to regulate bowel action. In infants constipation is often remedied by adjustment of the diet.

Laxatives should generally be **avoided** except where straining will exacerbate a condition (such as angina) or increase the risk of rectal bleeding as in haemorrhoids. Laxatives are also of value in *drug-induced constipation*, for the expulsion of *parasites* after anthelmintic treatment, and to clear the alimentary tract before *surgery and radiological procedures*.

The laxatives that follow have been divided into 4 main groups (sections 1.6.1–1.6.4). This simple classification disguises the fact that some laxatives have a complex action.

1.6.1 Bulk-forming drugs

These relieve constipation by increasing faecal mass which stimulates peristalsis, but patients should be told that the full effect may take some days to develop. They are useful in the management of patients with *colostomy*, *ileostomy*, *haemorrhoids*, *anal fissure*, *chronic diarrhoea associated with diverticular disease*, *irritable bowel syndrome*, and *ulcerative colitis* (section 1.5). Adequate fluid intake must be maintained to avoid intestinal obstruction. Unprocessed wheat **bran**, taken with food or fruit juice, is a most effective bulk-forming preparation. Finely ground bran, though more palatable, has poorer water-retaining properties, but can be taken as bran bread or biscuits in appropriately increased quantities. Oat bran is also used.

Methylcellulose, **ispaghula**, and **sterculia** are useful in patients who cannot tolerate bran. Methylcellulose also acts as a faecal softener.

BRAN
Indications: see notes above
Cautions; Contra-indications; Side-effects: see under Ispaghula Husk. Calcium and iron absorption may be impaired. Avoid in gluten enteropathies and coeliac disease
Dose: see preparations below
COUNSELLING. Preparations that swell in contact with liquid should always be carefully swallowed with water and should not be taken immediately before going to bed

NHS **Fybranta**® (Norgine)
Tablets, brown, bran 2 g. Net price 20 = 46p. Label: 24, 27, counselling, see above
Dose: 1–3 tablets chewed and swallowed with water 3–4 times daily, preferably with meals

NHS **Proctofibe**® (Roussel)
Tablets, beige, f/c, fibrous grain extract 375 mg, fibrous citrus extract 94 mg. Net price 20 = 56p. Counselling, see above
Dose: ADULTS and CHILD over 3 years 4–12 tablets daily in divided doses swallowed with plenty of water *or* crushed and dispersed in water

Trifyba® (Sanofi)
Powder, wheat fibre 80%. Net price 56 sachets containing 3.5 g = £3.36. Counselling, see below
Dose: 1 sachet 2–3 times daily added to food; CHILD half to one sachet 1–2 times daily added to food
COUNSELLING. At least one glass of water or other liquid should be drunk with the meal

ISPAGHULA HUSK
Indications: see notes above
Cautions: adequate fluid intake should be maintained to avoid intestinal obstruction
Contra-indications: intestinal obstruction, colonic atony, faecal impaction
Side-effects: flatulence, abdominal distension
Dose: see preparations below
COUNSELLING. Preparations that swell in contact with liquid should always be carefully swallowed with water and should not be taken immediately before going to bed

Fybogel® (R&C)
Granules, buff or orange, effervescent, sugar- and gluten-free, ispaghula husk 3.5 g/sachet. Net price 60 sachets (plain or orange flavoured) = £4.24. Label: 13, counselling, see above
Note. Contains potassium approx. 7 mmol/sachet
Dose: 1 sachet in water twice daily preferably after meals; CHILD ½–1 level 5-mL spoonful

Isogel® (Charwell)
Granules, pink, sugar-free, ispaghula husk 90%. Net price 200 g = £1.51. Label: 13, counselling, see above
Dose: constipation, 2 teaspoonfuls in water once or twice daily, preferably at mealtimes; CHILD 1 teaspoonful
Diarrhoea (section 1.4.1), 1 teaspoonful 3 times daily

Metamucil® (Proctor & Gamble)
Powder, buff, ispaghula husk 49%, gluten-free. Net price 200 g = 80p. Label: 13, counselling, see above
Dose: one 5-mL spoonful 1–3 times daily in 150 mL water; CHILD 6–12 years 2.5–5 mL

1.6 Laxatives

Regulan® (Proctor & Gamble)
Powder, beige, effervescent, ispaghula husk 3.6 g/6.4-g sachet (gluten-free). Net price 30 sachets = £2.49. Label: 13, counselling, see above
Note. Contains potassium 6.4 mmol/sachet
Dose: 1 sachet in 150 mL water 1–3 times daily; CHILD 6–12 years 2.5–5 mL

METHYLCELLULOSE

Indications: see notes above
Cautions; Contra-indications; Side-effects: see under Ispaghula Husk
Dose: see preparations below
COUNSELLING. Preparations that swell in contact with liquid should always be carefully swallowed with water and should not be taken immediately before going to bed

Celevac® (Monmouth)
Tablets, pink, methylcellulose '450' 500 mg. Net price 112-tab pack = 93p. Counselling, see above and dose
Dose: 3–6 tablets twice daily. In constipation the dose should be taken with at least 300 mL of water. In diarrhoea, ileostomy, and colostomy control, minimise liquid intake for 30 minutes before and after the dose

STERCULIA

Indications: see notes above
Cautions; Contra-indications; Side-effects: see under Ispaghula Husk
COUNSELLING. Preparations that swell in contact with liquid should always be carefully swallowed with water and should not be taken immediately before going to bed

[1]Normacol® (Norgine)
Granules, coated, sterculia 62%. Net price 100 g = £1.13; 60 × 7-g sachets = £4.77. Label: 25, 27, counselling, see above
Dose: 1–2 heaped 5-mL spoonfuls, or the contents of 1–2 sachets, washed down without chewing with plenty of liquid once or twice daily after meals; CHILD 6–12 years half adult dose
1. Formerly Normacol Special

[2]Normacol Plus® (Norgine)
Granules, brown, coated, sterculia 62%, frangula (standardised) 8%. Net price 200 g = £2.43; 60 sachets = £5.11. Label: 25, 27, counselling, see above
Dose: constipation and after haemorrhoidectomy, 1–2 heaped 5-mL spoonfuls or the contents of 1–2 sachets washed down without chewing with plenty of liquid once or twice daily after meals
2. Formerly Normacol Standard

1.6.2 Stimulant laxatives

The recognised stimulant laxatives include **bisacodyl** and members of the **anthraquinone** group, e.g. senna. **Docusate** sodium probably acts both as a stimulant and as a softening agent. **Danthron** has limited indications (see below) because *rodent* studies indicate potential carcinogenic risk. Powerful stimulants such as **cascara** and **castor oil** are obsolete.

Stimulant laxatives increase intestinal motility and often cause abdominal cramp. They should not be used in intestinal obstruction, and prolonged use can precipitate the onset of an atonic non-functioning colon and hypokalaemia. They should preferably be avoided in children.

Glycerol suppositories act as a rectal stimulant by virtue of the mildly irritant action of glycerol.

Soft soap is a more severe irritant; the use of soft soap enema should be **avoided**, expecially in pregnancy, as it may inflame the colonic mucosa.

The **parasympathomimetics** bethanechol, distigmine, neostigmine, and pyridostigmine (see sections 7.4.1 and 10.2.1) enhance parasympathetic activity in the gut and increase intestinal motility. They are rarely used for their gastro-intestinal effects. Organic obstruction of the gut must first be excluded and they should be used with caution in bowel anastomosis.

Oxyphenisatin is indicated for diagnostic procedures or surgery only, since it causes hepatitis in chronic use.

BISACODYL

Indications: see under Dose; tablets act in 10–12 hours; suppositories act in 20–60 minutes
Cautions; Contra-indications; Side-effects: see notes on stimulant laxatives; tablets, griping; suppositories, local irritation
Dose: *by mouth* for constipation, 5–10 mg at night; occasionally necessary to increase to 15–20 mg; CHILD 5 mg
By rectum in suppositories for constipation, 10 mg in the morning; CHILD 5 mg
Before radiological procedures and surgery, 10 mg by mouth at bedtime for 2 days before examination and, if necessary, a 10-mg suppository 1 hour before examination.

Bisacodyl (Non-proprietary)
Tablets, e/c, bisacodyl 5 mg. Net price 20 = 26p. Label: 5, 25
Suppositories, bisacodyl 10 mg. Net price 12 = 99p
Paediatric suppositories, bisacodyl 5 mg. Net price 5 = 65p
Note. The brand name NHS Dulco-Lax® (Boehringer Ingelheim) is used for bisacodyl tablets, net price 20 = 84p; suppositories, 20 = £2.20; paediatric suppositories, 5 = 65p

DANTHRON

Indications: only for: constipation in geriatric practice; prophylaxis and treatment of analgesic-induced constipation in terminally ill patients of all ages; constipation in cardiac failure and coronary thrombosis (conditions in which bowel movement must be free of strain); acts within 6–12 hours
Cautions; Contra-indications; Side-effects: see notes on stimulant laxatives; urine may be coloured red; avoid prolonged contact with skin (as in incontinent patients) since irritation and excoriation may occur; avoid in pregnancy and breast-feeding; *rodent* studies indicate potential carcinogenic risk
Dose: see next page

Cautionary label wordings, see inside back cover Prices are **net**, see p. 1

Co-danthramer

PoM Co-danthramer (Non-proprietary)

Suspension, co-danthramer 25/200 in 5 mL (danthron 25 mg, poloxamer '188' 200 mg/5 mL). Label: 14 (urine red)

Dose: 5–10 mL; CHILD 2.5–5 mL (restricted indications, see notes above)

Note. The brand name NHS Codalax® (Napp) is used for co-danthramer 25/200 in 5 mL suspension, net price 300 mL = £9.32, 1 litre = £28.91

Strong suspension, co-danthramer 75/1000 in 5 mL (danthron 75 mg, poloxamer '188' 1 g/5 mL). Label: 14 (urine red)

Dose: 2.5–5 mL (restricted indications, see notes above)

Note. The brand name NHS Codalax Forte® (Napp) is used for co-danthramer 75/1000 in 5 mL suspension, net price 300 mL = £14.00, 1 litre = £46.33

PoM Co-danthrusate (Non-proprietary)

Capsules, co-danthrusate 50/60 (danthron 50 mg, docusate sodium 60 mg). Label: 14 (urine red)

Dose: 1–3 capsules, usually at bedtime; CHILD 6–12 years 1 capsule

Note. The brand name NHS Normax® (Evans) is used for co-danthrusate 50/60 capsules, net price 63-cap pack = £9.20

DOCUSATE SODIUM
(Dioctyl Sodium Sulphosuccinate)

Indications: constipation (oral preparations act within 1–2 days); adjunct in abdominal radiological procedures

Cautions; Contra-indications; Side-effects: see notes on stimulant laxatives; rectal preparations not indicated if haemorrhoids or anal fissure

Dose: by mouth, constipation, up to 500 mg daily in divided doses; initial doses should be large and gradually reduced; CHILD over 6 months 12.5–25 mg 3 times daily
With barium meal, 400 mg

Dioctyl® (Medo)

Tablets, yellow, f/c, docusate sodium 100 mg. Net price 100 = £2.76

Oral solution 1%, sugar-free, docusate sodium 50 mg/5 mL. Net price 300-mL pack = £2.25

Paediatric oral solution, sugar-free, docusate sodium 12.5 mg/5 mL. Net price 125-mL pack = 73p

Rectal preparations

Fletchers' Enemette® (Pharmax)

Enema, docusate sodium 90 mg, glycerol 3.78 g, macrogol 2.25 g, sorbic acid 5 mg/5 mL. Net price 5-mL unit = 31p

Dose: ADULT and CHILD over 3 years, 5-mL unit when required

Norgalax Micro-enema® (Norgine)

Enema, docusate sodium 120 mg in 10-g single-dose disposable packs. Net price 10-g unit = 66p

Dose: ADULT and CHILD over 12 years, 10-g unit

GLYCEROL
(Glycerin)

Indications: constipation
Dose: see below

Glycerol Suppositories (BP)
(Glycerin Suppositories)

Suppositories, gelatin 140 mg, glycerol 700 mg, purified water to 1 g. Net price 12 = 42p (infant), 47p (child), 55p (adult)

Dose: 1 suppository moistened with water before use. The usual sizes are for *infants* small (1-g mould), *children* medium (2-g mould), *adults* large (4-g mould)

OXYPHENISATIN

Indications: see under Dose
Cautions; Contra-indications; Side-effects: see notes on stimulant laxatives; avoid repeated use owing to liver toxicity

Veripaque® (Sanofi-Winthrop)

Enema, powder for reconstitution, oxyphenisatin 50 mg in 3 g. Net price 1 vial = £1.90

Dose: by rectum before diagnostic procedures or surgery, oxyphenisatin 50 mg dissolved in 2 litres of water given over 5–8 minutes
Adjuvant to barium enema, oxyphenisatin 50 mg mixed thoroughly with 2 litres of barium sulphate enema

SENNA

Indications: constipation; bowel evacuation before abdominal radiological procedures, endoscopy, and surgery; acts in 8–12 hours

Cautions; Contra-indications; Side-effects: see notes on stimulant laxatives

Senna Tablets, total sennosides 7.5 mg. Net price 20 = 30p

Dose: 2–4 tablets, usually at night; initial dose should be low then gradually increased; CHILD over 6 years, half adult dose

Note. The brand name NHS Senokot® (see below) is used for Senna tablets

[1]**Manevac®** (Galen)

Granules, coated, senna fruit 12.4%, ispaghula 54.2%. Net price 250 g = £3.14. Label: 25, 27, counselling, see Ispaghula Husk

Dose: 1–2 level 5-mL spoonfuls with water or warm drink after supper and, if necessary, before breakfast *or* every 6 hours in resistant cases for 1–3 days; CHILD 5–12 years 1 level 5-mL spoonful daily

1. Formerly Agiolax®

Senokot® (R&C)

NHS *Tablets*, brown, total sennosides (calculated as sennoside B) 7.5 mg. Net price 20 = 30p

Dose: 2–4 tablets, usually at bedtime; initial dose should be low then gradually increased; CHILD over 6 years, half adult dose

Note. For Senokot tablets on general sale to the public the maximum recommended dose is 2 tablets.

Granules, brown, total sennosides (calculated as sennoside B) 15 mg/5 mL or 5.5 mg/g (one 5-mL spoonful = 2.7 g). Net price 100 g = £1.89

Dose: 5–10 mL, usually at bedtime; CHILD over 6 years 2.5–5 mL

Syrup, brown, total sennosides (calculated as sennoside B) 7.5 mg/5 mL. Net price 100 mL = £1.30

Dose: 10–20 mL, usually at bedtime; CHILD 2–6 years 2.5–5 mL, over 6 years 5–10 mL

SODIUM PICOSULPHATE
Indications: constipation, bowel evacuation before abdominal radiological procedures, endoscopy, and surgery
Cautions; Contra-indications; Side-effects: see notes on stimulant laxatives
Dose: see below

Sodium Picosulphate Elixir, sodium picosulphate 5 mg/5 mL. Acts within 10–14 hours. Net price 100 mL = £1.38
Dose: 5–15 mL at night; CHILD 2–5 years 2.5 mL, 5–10 years 2.5–5 mL
Note. The brand name NHS Laxoberal® (Windsor) is used for sodium picosulphate elixir 5 mg/5 mL

Picolax® (Nordic)
Oral powder, sugar-free, sodium picosulphate 10 mg/sachet, with magnesium citrate (for bowel evacuation before radiological procedures, endoscopy, and surgery). Net price 2 sachets = 59p. Label: 10, patient information leaflet, 13, counselling, see below
Dose: ADULT and CHILD over 9 years, 1 sachet in water in morning (before 8 a.m.) and a second in afternoon (between 2 and 4 p.m.) of day preceding procedures; CHILD 1–2 years quarter sachet morning and afternoon, 2–4 years half sachet morning and afternoon, 4–9 years 1 sachet morning and half sachet afternoon
Acts within 3 hours of first dose
COUNSELLING. Patients should be warned that heat is generated on addition to water; for this reason the powder should be added initially to 30 mL (2 tablespoonfuls) of water; after 5 minutes (when reaction complete) the solution should be further diluted to 150 mL (about a tumblerful)

OTHER STIMULANT LAXATIVES

Unstandardised preparations of cascara, frangula, rhubarb, and senna should be **avoided** as their laxative action is unpredictable. Aloes, colocynth, and jalap should be **avoided** as they have a drastic purgative action. Phenolphthalein should be **avoided** as it may cause rashes. Its laxative effects may continue for several days because of enterohepatic recycling; alkaline urine may be coloured pink.

NHS **Alophen®** (W-L)
Pills, brown, f/c, aloin 15 mg, phenolphthalein 30 mg. Net price 50 pills = £1.52. Label: 14 (alkaline urine pink)
Dose: 1–3 pills, usually at bedtime

NHS **Kest®** (Torbet)
Tablets, magnesium sulphate 300 mg, phenolphthalein 50 mg. Net price 50 = 94p. Label: 14 (alkaline urine pink)
Dose: 1 tablet with water at bedtime and 2 tablets in the morning

1.6.3 Faecal softeners

Liquid paraffin, the classical lubricant, has disadvantages (see below). Bulk laxatives (section 1.6.1) and non-ionic surfactant 'wetting' agents e.g. docusate sodium (section 1.6.2) also have softening properties. Such drugs are useful for oral administration in the management of haemorrhoids and anal fissure; glycerol suppositories (section 1.6.2) are useful for rectal use.

Enemas containing **arachis oil** lubricate and soften impacted faeces and promote a bowel movement.

CSM recommendations

Preparations containing liquid paraffin for use as laxatives should no longer be available directly to the public and restrictions should be placed on over-the-counter sales through pharmacies:
pack size be limited to 160 mL;
be indicated only for symptomatic relief of constipation;
be contra-indicated for children under 3 years of age;
prolonged used not advised;
package labels to state 'repeated use is not recommended' and 'consult your doctor if laxatives are needed every day, if you have persistent abdominal pain or have a condition which makes swallowing difficult'.

ARACHIS OIL
Indications: see notes above
Dose: see below

Fletchers' Arachis Oil Retention Enema® (Pharmax)
Enema, arachis oil in 130-mL single-dose disposable packs. Net price 130 mL = £1.04
Dose: to soften impacted faeces, 130 mL; the enema should be warmed before use

LIQUID PARAFFIN
Indications: constipation but see CSM warning above
Cautions: avoid prolonged use
Side-effects: anal seepage of paraffin and consequent anal irritation after prolonged use, granulomatous reactions caused by absorption of small quantities of liquid paraffin (especially from the emulsion), lipoid pneumonia, and interference with the absorption of fat-soluble vitamins
Dose: 10–30 mL but see CSM warning above

Liquid Paraffin Oral Emulsion (BP)
(Liquid Paraffin Emulsion)
Oral emulsion, liquid paraffin 5 mL, vanillin 5 mg, chloroform 0.025 mL, benzoic acid solution 0.2 mL, methylcellulose-20 200 mg, saccharin sodium 500 micrograms, water to 10 mL
Dose: 10–30 mL at night when required

NHS **Petrolagar®** (Whitehall)
Emulsion, sugar-free, liquid paraffin 7%, light liquid paraffin 18%. Net price 100 mL = 61p
Dose: 10 mL morning and night or after meals

With phenolphthalein
NHS **Agarol®** (W-L)
Mixture, sugar-free, phenolphthalein 66 mg, liquid paraffin 1.6 mL, agar 10 mg/5 mL. Net price 100 mL = 87p. Label: 14 (urine pink)
Dose: 5–15 mL, usually at bedtime; CHILD not recommended

1.6.4 Osmotic laxatives

These act by retaining fluid in the bowel by osmosis or by changing the pattern of water distribution in the faeces.

Saline purgatives such as **magnesium hydroxide** are commonly abused but are satisfactory for occasional use; adequate fluid intake should be maintained. **Magnesium salts** are useful where rapid bowel evacuation is required. **Sodium salts** should be avoided as they may give rise to sodium and water retention in susceptible individuals. **Phosphate enemas** are useful in bowel clearance before radiology, endoscopy, and surgery.

Lactulose is a semi-synthetic disaccharide which is not absorbed from the gastro-intestinal tract. It produces an osmotic diarrhoea of low faecal pH, and discourages the proliferation of ammonia-producing organisms. It is therefore useful in the treatment of *hepatic encephalopathy*. **Lactitol** is a similar disaccharide.

LACTITOL

Indications; Contra-indications; Side-effects: see under Lactulose

Dose: constipation, initially 20 g daily in a single dose with morning or evening meal, subsequently adjusted to produce one stool daily (dose of 10 g daily may be sufficient); CHILD 1–6 years 2.5–5 g, 6–12 years 5–10 g, 12–16 years 10–20 g daily, subsequently adjusted to produce one stool daily

Hepatic encephalopathy, 500–700 mg/kg daily in 3 divided doses with meals, subsequently adjusted to produce 2 soft stools daily

COUNSELLING. Powder should be mixed with food or liquid and one to two glasses of liquid should be drunk with the meal

▼ PoM **Lactitol** (Non-proprietary)
Powder, lactitol 10 g/sachet. Net price 20-sachet pack = £2.31; 50-sachet pack = £5.77. Counselling, see above
Available from Zyma

LACTULOSE

Indications: constipation (may take up to 48 hours to act), hepatic encephalopathy (portal systemic encephalopathy)

Contra-indications: galactosaemia, intestinal obstruction

Side-effects: flatulence, cramps, and abdominal discomfort

Dose: expressed in terms of the elixir containing lactulose 3.35 g/5 mL
Constipation, initially 15 mL twice daily, gradually reduced according to patient's needs; CHILD under 1 year 2.5 mL, 1–5 years 5 mL, 6–12 years 10 mL twice daily, gradually reduced
Hepatic encephalopathy, 30–50 mL 3 times daily, subsequently adjusted to produce 2–3 soft stools daily

Lactulose (Non-proprietary)
Solution, lactulose 3.35 g/5 mL with other ketoses. Net price 200-mL pack = £1.55
Note. The brand name NHS Duphalac® (Duphar) is used for Lactulose solution; net price 200-mL pack = £1.54

MAGNESIUM SALTS

Indications; Dose: see under preparations

Cautions: renal impairment (risk of magnesium accumulation); hepatic impairment (see Appendix 2); elderly and debilitated; see also notes above; **interactions:** Appendix 1 (magnesium salts)

Contra-indications: acute gastro-intestinal conditions

Side-effects: colic

Magnesium citrate
Citramag® (Bioglan)
Powder, effervescent, providing when dissolved in water magnesium citrate 17.7 g/sachet. Net price 10-sachet pack = £9.70. Label 10, patient information leaflet, 13, counselling, see below
Dose: bowel evacuation before radiological examination and surgery, 1 sachet dissolved in 200 mL water and taken at about 8 p.m. on evening before procedure
COUNSELLING. The patient information leaflet advises that hot water is needed to make the solution and that effervescence should be allowed to subside (should be prepared at 6 p.m. for 8 p.m. dose); high fluid, low residue diet on day before procedure; on day of procedure water only should be taken until completed

Magnesium hydroxide
Magnesium Hydroxide Mixture (BP)
(Cream of Magnesia)
An aqueous suspension containing about 8% of hydrated magnesium oxide. Do not store in a cold place
Dose: constipation, 25–50 mL when required

Magnesium hydroxide with liquid paraffin (see also CSM recommendations on previous page)
Liquid Paraffin and Magnesium Hydroxide Emulsion (BP)
Oral emulsion, 25% dispersion of liquid paraffin in an aqueous suspension containing 6% of hydrated magnesium oxide
Dose: constipation, 5–20 mL when required

Magnesium sulphate
Magnesium Sulphate (Epsom salts). Label: 13, 23
Dose: rapid bowel evacuation (acts in 2–4 hours) 5–10 g in a tumblerful of water preferably before breakfast

Fletchers' Magnesium Sulphate Retention Enema® (Pharmax)
Enema, magnesium sulphate 50%, in 130-mL single-dose disposable packs. Net price 130 mL = 56p (hosp. only)
Dose: 130 mL, as an adjunct in neurosurgery to lower cerebrospinal fluid pressure

PHOSPHATES (RECTAL)

Indications: rectal use in constipation; bowel evacuation before abdominal radiological procedures, endoscopy, and surgery

Cautions: see notes above

Contra-indications: acute gastro-intestinal conditions
Dose: see below

¹Carbalax® (Pharmax)
Suppositories, sodium acid phosphate 1.72 g in an effervescent basis. Net price 12 = £2.30
Dose: constipation, 1 suppository, inserted 30 minutes before evacuation is required; moisten with water before use; CHILD, not recommended
1. Formerly Beogex

Fletchers' Phosphate Enema® (Pharmax)
Enema, sodium acid phosphate 12.8 g, sodium phosphate 10.24 g, purified water, freshly boiled and cooled, to 128 mL (corresponds to Phosphates Enema Formula B). Net price 128 mL with standard tube = 44p, with long rectal tube = 62p
Dose: 128 mL; CHILD, over 3 years, reduced according to body weight (under 3 years not recommended)

SODIUM CITRATE (RECTAL)
Indications: rectal use in constipation
Cautions: see notes above
Contra-indications: acute gastro-intestinal conditions
Dose: see below

Micolette Micro-enema® (Cusi)
Enema, sodium citrate 450 mg, sodium lauryl sulphoacetate 45 mg, glycerol 625 mg, together with citric acid, potassium sorbate, and sorbitol in a viscous solution, in 5-mL single-dose disposable packs with nozzle. Net price 5 mL = 33p
Dose: ADULT and CHILD over 3 years, 5–10 mL

Micralax Micro-enema® (Evans)
Enema, sodium citrate 450 mg, sodium alkylsulphoacetate 45 mg, sorbic acid 5 mg, together with glycerol and sorbitol in a viscous solution in 5-mL single-dose disposable packs with nozzle. Net price 5 mL = 45p
Dose: ADULT and CHILD over 3 years, 5 mL

Relaxit Micro-enema® (Kabi Pharmacia)
Enema, sodium citrate 450 mg, sodium lauryl sulphate 75 mg, sorbic acid 5 mg, together with glycerol and sorbitol in a viscous solution in 5-mL single-dose disposable packs with nozzle. Net price 5 mL = 15p
Dose: ADULT and CHILD over 3 years, 5 mL

BOWEL CLEANSING SOLUTIONS

Bowel cleansing solutions are used before colonic surgery, colonoscopy, or barium enema to ensure the bowel is free of solid contents. They are **not** treatments for constipation.
Indications: see above
Cautions: pregnancy; ulcerative colitis; impaired gag reflex; unconscious or semiconscious or possibility of regurgitation or aspiration; prevent absorption of oral medication
Contra-indications: gastro-intestinal obstruction, gastric retention, perforated bowel; toxic colitis, toxic megacolon or ileus; weight less than 20 kg

Side-effects: nausea, bloating, abdominal cramps (usually transient—reduced by taking more slowly); rarely vomiting, anal irritation; urticaria, rhinorrhoea and dermatitis reported

PoM Bowel Cleansing Solutions
Oral powder, macrogol 3350 or 4000 (polyethylene glycol 3350 or 4000) 59 g, anhydrous sodium sulphate 5.685 g, sodium bicarbonate 1.685 g, sodium chloride 1.465 g, potassium chloride 743 mg/sachet. Label: 10, counselling
Four sachets when reconstituted with water to 4 litres provides an iso-osmotic solution for bowel cleansing before surgery, colonoscopy or radiological procedures
Dose: by *mouth*, 240 mL (1 tumblerful) of reconstituted solution every 10–15 minutes, or by nasogastric tube 20–30 mL/minute, until 4 litres have been consumed or watery stools are free of solid matter (usually 3 litres). First bowel movement occurs after approximately 1 hour
COUNSELLING. Advise patient to take at least 2 hours after and preferably 3–4 hours after food; more palatable if chilled; do not add flavouring or other ingredients; drink each portion as rapidly as possible
After reconstitution the solution should be kept in a refrigerator and discarded if unused after 48 hours
Available from Norgine (*Klean-Prep*®), net price 4 sachets (to provide 4 litres) = £8.60

1.7 Preparations for haemorrhoids

1.7.1 Soothing preparations
1.7.2 Compound preparations with corticosteroids
1.7.3 Rectal sclerosants

Anal and perianal pruritus, soreness, and excoriation are best treated by application of bland ointments, suppositories, and dusting-powders (section 1.7.1). These conditions occur commonly in patients suffering from haemorrhoids, fistulas, and proctitis. Careful local toilet as well as adjustment of the diet to avoid hard stools, and bulk-forming materials such as bran (section 1.6.1) and a high residue diet are also helpful. In proctitis these measures may supplement treatment with corticosteroids or sulphasalazine (see section 1.5).

When necessary topical preparations containing **local anaesthetics** (section 1.7.1) or **corticosteroids** (section 1.7.2) are used provided perianal thrush has been excluded. Perianal thrush is best treated with **nystatin** by mouth and by local application (see sections 5.2, 7.2.2, and 13.10.2).

1.7.1 Soothing preparations

Bland soothing preparations containing mild astringents such as bismuth subgallate, zinc oxide, and hamamelis may give symptomatic relief in haemorrhoids. Many proprietary preparations also contain lubricants, vasoconstrictors, or mild antiseptics.

Prolonged application of preparations containing **resorcinol** should be **avoided** because it may interfere with thyroid function. Heparinoids are claimed to promote the resorption of local oedema and extravasated blood.

Local anaesthetics are used to relieve pain associated with *haemorrhoids*, and *pruritus ani* but good evidence is lacking. Lignocaine ointment (see section 15.2) is used before emptying the bowel to relieve pain associated with *anal fissure*. Alternative local anaesthetics include amethocaine, cinchocaine, and pramoxine, but they are more irritant.

Local anaesthetics should be used for short periods only (no longer than 2 weeks) since they may cause sensitisation of the anal skin.

ADMINISTRATION. Unless otherwise indicated a suppository is usually inserted into the rectum night and morning and after a bowel movement. Rectal ointments and creams are applied night and morning and after a bowel movement, externally or by rectum using a rectal nozzle.
Note. Local anaesthetic ointments can be absorbed through the rectal mucosa therefore excessive application should be avoided, particularly in infants and children.

Bismuth Subgallate Suppositories, Compound, bismuth subgallate 200 mg, castor oil 60 mg, resorcinol 60 mg, zinc oxide 120 mg, in theobroma oil or other suitable basis. Net price 12 = £1.82

Hamamelis and Zinc Oxide Suppositories. Usual strength hamamelis dry extract 200 mg, zinc oxide 600 mg. Net price 12 = £2.35

Anacal® (Panpharma)
Rectal ointment, laureth '9' 5%, a heparinoid 0.2%. Net price 30 g (with rectal nozzle) = £3.04
Apply 1–4 times daily
Suppositories, laureth '9' 50 mg, a heparinoid 4 mg. Net price 10 = £1.70
Insert 1 suppository once or twice daily

Anodesyn® (Crookes)
Ointment, ephedrine hydrochloride 0.25%, lignocaine hydrochloride 0.5%, allantoin 0.5%. Net price 25 g = £1.16
Suppositories, ephedrine hydrochloride 5.1 mg, lignocaine hydrochloride 10.25 mg, allantoin 10.25 mg. Net price 12 = £1.22

Anusol® (W-L)
Cream, bismuth oxide 2.14%, Peru balsam 1.8%, zinc oxide 10.75%. Net price 23 g (with rectal nozzle) = £1.34
Ointment, bismuth oxide 0.875%, bismuth subgallate 2.25%, zinc oxide 10.75%, Peru balsam 1.875%. Net price 25 g (with rectal nozzle) = £1.34
Suppositories, bismuth oxide 24 mg, bismuth subgallate 59 mg, Peru balsam 49 mg, zinc oxide 296 mg. Net price 12 = £1.18

1.7.2 Compound preparations with corticosteroids

Corticosteroids are often combined with antibiotics, local anaesthetics, and soothing agents. They are suitable for occasional short-term use after exclusion of infections, such as herpes simplex; see section 13.4 for general comments on topical corticosteroids.

Antibiotics may do little more than encourage the growth of resistant bacteria and should be avoided. See section 1.7.1 for comment on local anaesthetics.

PoM **Anugesic-HC**® (P-D)
Cream, benzyl benzoate 1.2%, bismuth oxide 0.875%, hydrocortisone acetate 0.5%, Peru balsam 1.85%, pramoxine hydrochloride 1%, zinc oxide 12.35%. Net price 30 g (with rectal nozzle) = £6.19
Apply night and morning and after a bowel movement; do not use for longer than 7 days
Suppositories, benzyl benzoate 33 mg, bismuth oxide 24 mg, bismuth subgallate 59 mg, hydrocortisone acetate 5 mg, Peru balsam 49 mg, pramoxine hydrochloride 27 mg, zinc oxide 296 mg. Net price 12 = £2.64
Insert 1 suppository night and morning and after a bowel movement; do not use for longer than 7 days

PoM **Anusol-HC**® (P-D)
Ointment, benzyl benzoate 1.25%, bismuth oxide 0.875%, bismuth subgallate 2.25%, hydrocortisone acetate 0.25%, Peru balsam 1.875%, zinc oxide 10.75%. Net price 30 g (with rectal nozzle) = £5.81
Apply night and morning and after a bowel movement; do not use for longer than 7 days
Suppositories, benzyl benzoate 33 mg, bismuth oxide 24 mg, bismuth subgallate 59 mg, hydrocortisone acetate 10 mg, Peru balsam 49 mg, zinc oxide 296 mg. Net price 12 = £2.64
Additives: include tartrazine lake
Insert 1 suppository night and morning and after a bowel movement; do not use for longer than 7 days

PoM **Betnovate**® (Glaxo)
Rectal ointment, betamethasone valerate 0.05%, lignocaine hydrochloride 2.5%, phenylephrine hydrochloride 0.1%. Net price 30 g (with applicator) = £1.50
Apply 2–3 times daily until inflammation subsides then once daily, externally or by rectum; do not use for longer than 7 days

PoM **Proctofoam HC**® (Stafford-Miller)
Foam in aerosol pack, hydrocortisone acetate 1%, pramoxine hydrochloride 1%. Net price 24-g pack (approx. 40 applications) with applicator = £4.83
Dose: haemorrhoids and proctitis, 1 applicatorful (4–6 mg hydrocortisone acetate, 4–6 mg pramoxine hydrochloride) by rectum 2–3 times daily and after a bowel movement

PoM **Proctosedyl**® (Roussel)
Ointment, cinchocaine hydrochloride 0.5%, hydrocortisone 0.5%. Net price 30 g = £6.65 (with cannula)
Apply morning and night and after a bowel movement, externally or by rectum
Suppositories, cinchocaine hydrochloride 5 mg, hydrocortisone 5 mg. Net price 12 = £3.00
Insert 1 suppository night and morning and after a bowel movement

1.8 Stoma care

Prescribing for patients with stoma calls for special care. The following is a brief account of some of the main points to be borne in mind.

Enteric-coated and *modified-release* preparations are **unsuitable**, particularly in patients with ileostomies, as there may not be sufficient release of the active ingredient.

Laxatives. Enemas and washouts should **not** be prescribed for patients with ileostomies as they may cause rapid and severe dehydration.

Colostomy patients may suffer from constipation and whenever possible should be treated by increasing fluid intake or dietary fibre. **Bulk-forming laxatives** (section 1.6.1) should be tried. If they are insufficient, as small a dose as possible of senna (section 1.6.2) should be used. Preparations such as X-Prep® should be avoided when preparing patients for radiological procedures as they may cause severe dehydration with nausea, vomiting, and griping.

Antidiarrhoeals. Drugs such as **loperamide**, **codeine phosphate**, or **co-phenotrope** (diphenoxylate with atropine) are effective. Bulk-forming drugs (section 1.6.1) may be tried but it is often difficult to adjust the dose appropriately.

Antibiotics should **not** be given for an episode of acute diarrhoea.

Antacids. The tendency to diarrhoea from magnesium salts or constipation from aluminium salts may be increased in these patients.

Diuretics should be used with caution in patients with ileostomies as they may become excessively dehydrated and potassium depletion may easily occur. It is usually advisable to use a **potassium-sparing** diuretic (see section 2.2.3).

Digoxin. Patients with a stoma are particularly susceptible to hypokalaemia if on digoxin therapy and potassium supplements or a potassium-sparing diuretic may be advisable (for comment see section 9.2.1.1).

Potassium supplements. Liquid formulations are preferred to modified-release formulations (see above).

Analgesics. Opioid analgesics (see section 4.7.2) may cause troublesome constipation in colostomy patients. When a non-opioid analgesic is required **paracetamol** is usually suitable but anti-inflammatory analgesics may cause gastric irritation and bleeding.

Iron preparations may cause loose stools and sore skin in these patients. If this is troublesome and if iron is definitely indicated one of the intramuscular iron preparations (see section 9.1.1.2) should be used. Modified-release preparations should be **avoided** for the reasons given above.

Patients are usually given advice about the use of *cleansing agents*, *protective creams*, *lotions*, *deodorants*, or *sealants* whilst in hospital, either by the surgeon or by the health authority stoma care nurses. Voluntary organisations offer help and support to patients with stoma.

PoM **Scheriproct**® (Schering Health Care)
Ointment, cinchocaine hydrochloride 0.5%, prednisolone hexanoate 0.19%. Net price 30 g = £4.41
Apply twice daily for 5–7 days (3–4 times daily on 1st day if necessary), then once daily for a few days after symptoms have cleared
Suppositories, cinchocaine hydrochloride 1 mg, prednisolone hexanoate 1.3 mg. Net price 12 = £2.08
Insert 1 suppository daily after a bowel movement, for 5–7 days (in severe cases initially 2–3 times daily)

PoM **Ultraproct**® (Schering Health Care)
Ointment, cinchocaine hydrochloride 0.5%, fluocortolone hexanoate 0.095%, fluocortolone pivalate 0.092%. Net price 30 g (with rectal nozzle) = £4.57
Apply twice daily for 5–7 days (3–4 times daily on 1st day if necessary), then once daily for few days after symptoms have cleared
Suppositories, cinchocaine hydrochloride 1 mg, fluocortolone hexanoate 630 micrograms, fluocortolone pivalate 610 micrograms. Net price 12 = £2.15
Insert 1 suppository daily after a bowel movement, for 5–7 days (in severe cases initially 2–3 times daily) then 1 suppository every other day for 1 week

PoM **Uniroid**® (Unigreg)
Ointment, cinchocaine hydrochloride 0.5%, hydrocortisone 0.5%, neomycin sulphate 3400 units, polymyxin B sulphate 6250 units/g. Net price 15 g (with applicator) = £2.77
Apply 3 times daily, preferably after a bowel movement, externally or by rectum; do not use for longer than 7 days
Suppositories, cinchocaine hydrochloride 5 mg, hydrocortisone 5 mg, neomycin sulphate 6800 units, polymyxin B sulphate 12 500 units. Net price 10 = £2.09
Insert 1 suppository 3 times daily, preferably after a bowel movement; do not use for longer than 7 days

PoM **Xyloproct**® (Astra)
Ointment (water-miscible), aluminium acetate 3.5%, hydrocortisone acetate 0.275%, lignocaine 5%, zinc oxide 18%. Net price 30 g (with applicator) = £3.48
Apply several times daily
Suppositories, aluminium acetate 50 mg, hydrocortisone acetate 5 mg, lignocaine 60 mg, zinc oxide 400 mg. Net price 10 = £1.63
Insert 1 suppository at night and after a bowel movement

1.7.3 Rectal sclerosants

Oily phenol injection is used to inject haemorrhoids particularly when unprolapsed.

PHENOL

Indications: see notes above
Side-effects: irritation, tissue necrosis

Oily Phenol Injection, (BP), phenol 5% in a suitable fixed oil. Net price 2-mL amp = 71p; 5-mL amp = £2.08; 25-mL vial = £5.00
Dose: 2–3 mL into the submucosal layer at the base of the pile; several injections may be given at different sites, max. total injected 10 mL at any one time

Chapter 1: Gastro-intestinal system

STOMA APPLIANCES AND ASSOCIATED PRODUCTS

For **urostomy** pouches see section 7.5

It is **not** necessary to state an **order number** on a prescription for one of these products provided the **full details** as given in the BNF are included on the **prescription**.

CLOSED POUCHES

Closed pouches are suitable for patients with a **colostomy** and well-formed stools

Body's Care range
Rubber bags screwcap (Body's Care)
  Black butyl, one-piece closed pouch. Net price 1 day pouch = £23.25; 1 night pouch = £27.12
  White rubber, one-piece closed pouch. Net price 1 day pouch = £12.92; 1 night pouch = £14.89
Rubber bags spout (Body's Care)
  Black butyl, one-piece closed pouch. Net price 1 day pouch or night pouch = £24.55
  White rubber, one-piece closed pouch. Net price 1 day pouch or night pouch = £11.62

Cambmac range
Dansac® (Cambmac)
  Combi Colo F, one-piece pouch with filter, opaque or clear. Net price 100 pouches (standard pouch: 25, 30, 38, 44, 50, or 63mm holes; small pouch: 25, 30, or 38 mm holes) = £139.70
  CombiMicro C + S, one-piece pouch with porous adhesive, filter, skin barrier ring, and fabric backing, opaque or clear. Net price 50 pouches (25, 32, 38, 44, 50, 63 mm or cut-to-fit holes) = £58.54
  Mini Petit C, one-piece pouch with porous adhesive skin protector, fabric backing, and filter, opaque. Net price 30 pouches (cut-to-fit) = £51.71
  Standard Colo, one-piece pouch with filter, clear. Net price 100 pouches (22, 30, 32, or 38 mm holes) = £125.48
  Supersquare System, two-piece pouch with filter, opaque or clear. Net price 100 (standard or small) pouches to fit 50 mm base plate = £121.33; 100 (standard) pouches to fit 80 mm base plate = £153.88; base plate 10 (100 mm × 100 mm) = £26.51; 10 (125 mm × 125 mm) = £48.98

CliniMed range
Biopore® (CliniMed)
  One-piece pouch with porous adhesive and filter, white/clear. Net price 50 pouches (25, 30, 35, 40, 45, 50 mm holes) = £58.75
Biotrol® (CliniMed)
  Colo S, one-piece pouch with skin protector adhesive, white. Net price 30 pouches (25, 30, 35, 40, 45, 50, or 60 mm holes) = £55.50
  Elite Closed, covered one-piece pouch with skin protector adhesive and filter, white or skin-tone. Net price 30 pouches (25, 30, 35, 40, 45, 50, 60, 70 mm or cut-to-fit holes) = £60.30; transparent (cut-to-fit holes) 30 pouches = £57.35
  Integrale, one-piece pouch with skin protector adhesive and filter, white. Net price 30 pouches (25, 30, 35, 40, 45, 50, 60, 70 mm or cut-to-fit holes) = £60.30
  Preference Closed, fabric covered one-piece pouch with skin protector adhesive, porous adhesive collar, and filter, white or skin-tone. Net price 30 pouches (25, 30, 35, 40, 45, 50, 60 mm or cut-to-fit holes) = £56.00

Coloplast range
Comfort® (Coloplast)
  Extra, one-piece closed pouch. Net price, No. 1 (24 mm hole), 100 pouches = £76.00; No. 2 (30 or 40 mm holes), 100 = £92.00; No. 3, 30 mm hole, 100 = £111.00, 50 mm hole, 100 = £112.00
  Regular, one-piece closed pouch. Net price, No. 1 (24 mm hole), 100 pouches = £64.00; No. 2 (30 mm hole), 100 = £76.00; No. 3 (30 mm hole), 100 = £91.00; No. 5 (24 mm hole), 100 = £85.00
Conseal® **System** (Coloplast)
  Two-piece pouch. Net price 30 bags (to fit 40 or 50 mm base plates) = £31.80; base plate (40 or 50 mm) 5 = £11.80; colostomy plug (40 × 35 or 45 mm, 50 × 35 or 45 mm) 10 = £10.60; discharge bag (40 or 50 mm) 50 = £2.50
K-Flex® (Coloplast)
  One-piece closed pouch with karaya skin protector and filter. Net price 30 pouches (clear: 10, 30, or 40 mm holes; opaque: 30 or 40 mm holes) = £57.90
mc2000® (Coloplast)
  One-piece closed pouch with double seal and filter, opaque or clear. Net price 30 pouches (25, 30, 35, 40, 45, 50, 55, or 60 mm holes) = £60.00
mc2002® (Coloplast)
  Two-piece pouch with filter, opaque or clear. Net price 30 pouches (to fit 40 or 60 mm base plates) = £33.90; base plate (40 mm × 15 or 25 mm, 60 × 35 or 45 mm) 5 = £12.50; belt plate (40 or 60 mm) 10 = £5.00
pc3000® (Coloplast)
  One-piece pouch, opaque or clear. Net price 30 pouches (25, 30, 35, 40, 45, 50, or 55 mm holes; 25 mm can be cut to fit up to 60 mm) = £56.40
Perfect® (Coloplast)
  One-piece pouch, opaque or clear. Net price 30 pouches (30 or 40 mm hole) = £56.40

ConvaTec range
Colodress® (ConvaTec)
  Colodress, one-piece closed pouch with textured backing, opaque beige. Net price 30 pouches (19, 32, 38, 45, or 50 mm holes; 19 mm can be cut to fit) = £54.75
  Colodress Plus, one-piece closed pouch with single-release paper and filter. Net price 30 pouches (opaque or clear: 19, 25, 32, 38, 45, 50, or 64 mm holes; opaque: 19 mm can be cut to fit) = £54.75; Mini pouches, 30 pouches (19, 25, 32, 38, or 45 mm holes) = £51.73
Surgicare System® **2** (ConvaTec)
  System 2, two-piece closed pouch, white. Net price 30 pouches (to fit 38, 45, 57, or 70 mm flanges) = £27.34
  System 2 Combihesive, two-piece closed pouch with textured backing, beige. Net price 30 pouches (to fit 38, 45, 57, or 70 mm flanges) = £27.34; with filter, 30 pouches = £28.24; Mini pouches, 20 pouches (to fit 32, 38, 45, or 57 mm flanges) = £15.48

De Puy range
Schacht® (De Puy)
  Colostomy bag (= pouch), one-piece closed bag. Net price 100 pouches = £32.30
  Colostomy appliance. Net price 1 appliance = £27.85
Slimline® (De Puy)
  Colostomy appliance. Net price 1 appliance = £30.25

Hollister range
Classic (Hollister)
  All with 25, 32, 38, 44, 51, 64, or 76 mm holes
  Adhesive (series 217), one-piece closed pouch with adhesive and filter, clear. Net price 50 pouches = £56.20
  Karaya seal (series 716), one-piece pouch with karaya skin protector (without filter), must be worn with belt, clear. Net price 30 pouches = £47.80
  Karaya seal with filter (series 211), one-piece closed pouch with karaya skin protector and filter, must be worn with belt, opaque. Net price 30 pouches = £47.80

1.8 Stoma care

Karaya 5® Seal (series 331 and 332), one-piece closed pouch with porous adhesive, karaya skin protector seal, and filter, may be worn with belt, opaque or clear. Net price 30 pouches = £57.95

Microporous adhesive (series 314), one-piece compact closed pouch with porous adhesive and filter, may be worn with belt, clear. Net price 50 pouches = £60.82

Premium® (Hollister)
All with 25, 32, 38, 44, 51, 64, or 76 mm holes
Karaya 5® Seal (series 355 and 353), one-piece closed pouch with porous adhesive, karaya skin protector and filter, may be worn with belt, opaque or clear. Net price 15 pouches = £29.30

Synthetic Seal (series 354 and 356), one-piece closed pouch with porous adhesive, synthetic skin protector seal and filter, opaque or clear. Net price 15 pouches = £30.55

HolliGard® (Hollister)
All with 25, 32, 38, 44, 51, 64, or 76 mm holes
Microporous adhesive (series 411), one-piece closed pouch with porous adhesive, HolliGard® seal and filter, may be worn with belt, opaque. Net price 30 pouches = £60.87

Without adhesive (series 416), one-piece closed pouch with HolliGard® seal and filter, must be worn with belt, clear. Net price 30 pouches = £55.19

Guardian® (Hollister)
All with 38, 51, or 64 mm holes
Guardian (series 451 and 450), two-piece closed pouch with filter, opaque or clear. Net price 15 pouches = £13.73

Guardian mini-pouch (series 452), two-piece compact closed pouch with filter, opaque or clear. Net price 15 pouches = £13.46

Flanges. Net price 'F' floating flange (25, 38, 51, 64, or 102 mm) 5 = £11.17; 'S' stationary flange (25, 38, 51, or 64 mm) 5 = £10.98

Stoma cap, with filter, opaque. Net price 30 (38, 51 or 64 mm) = £25.46

Belt adaptor. Net price 10 = £7.80.

Rüsch range
Ostopore® (Rüsch)
Colo AV-opaque, one-piece closed pouch with adhesive and vent. Net price 30 pouches (25, 32, 38, or 45 mm holes) with 2 belt flanges = £39.00

Colo KAV-opaque, one-piece closed pouch with karaya seal skin protector, adhesive, and vent. Net price 30 pouches (25, 32, 38, 45, or 51 mm holes) with 5 belt flanges = £53.10

Colo KAV-transparent, one-piece closed pouch with karaya seal skin protector, adhesive, and vent. Net price 30 pouches (32, 38, 45, or 51 mm holes) with 30 belt flanges = £67.80

Rubber bags (Rüsch)
White rubber, one-piece closed pouch with spout outlet. Net price (both 19, 25, or 28 mm holes), 1 day pouch = £10.64; 1 night pouch = £11.48

Translet® (Rüsch)
Premier colostomy set, 1 adhesive ring with 6 bags. Net price 15 (27, 40, or 57 mm hole) = £59.25; spare bags 10 (18 or 28 cm length) = £4.54; adhesive rings or microporous spare adhesive rings (27, 40, or 57 mm) 5 = £6.08

Royal colostomy set, 1 adhesive ring and 6 odourproof bags. Net price 15 (27, 40, or 57 mm) = £82.50; spare bags (18 or 28 cm length) 10 = £7.28

Salts range
NHS Cohflex® (Salts)
Closed, one-piece pouch with single-release paper, wafer, and filter, fabric front and back, opaque. Net price 30 pouches (all may be cut to fit; 30, 40, 50, 60 mm or 10–60 mm cut-to-fit holes) = £60.34

Coloset® (Salts)
Closed, one-piece pouch. Net price 30 pouches (medium: 713655) = £13.29; (small: 713656) = £8.75; (large: 713658) = £11.02; (medium: 713659) = £10.06

Eakin® (Salts)
Closed, one-piece pouch, white or clear. 32, 45, or 64 mm holes, net price 20 pouches = £37.01; 90 mm hole, 20 pouches = £46.05

Kombo® (Salts)
Kombo closed, one-piece pouch with karaya skin protector seal and adhesive, clear. Net price (30, 40, 50, or 60 mm holes), 30 pouches = £53.51; with filter, 30 pouches = £63.80

Palex® (Salts)
BCLF bag (= pouch), one-piece closed pouch with CL resin seal, porous adhesive, and filter. Net price 30 pouches (25, 32, 38, 44, 51, 64 mm or cut-to-fit holes) = £54.06

BCLF Petite mini bag (= pouch), one-piece closed pouch with CL resin seal, porous adhesive, and filter. Net price 30 pouches (25, 32, 38, 44 mm or cut-to-fit holes) = £47.70

Simplicity® (Salts)
Closed, two-piece closed pouch, clear or pink, medium. Net price, clear (40, 50, 60, or 70 mm) 30 = £14.08; pink (40, 50, or 60 mm holes) 30 = £13.94; flange, standard (30, 40, 50, or 60 mm hole) 5 = £2.55; flange with cohesive washer (30, 40, or 50 mm) 5 = £11.44

Simplicity 1® (Salts)
Closed, one-piece pouch with porous adhesive, skin protector seal, and filter, fabric front and back. Net price 30 pouches (all may be cut to fit; opaque: 30, 40, 50, or 60 mm holes; opaque or clear: cut-to-fit holes) = £60.34

Paediatric, closed one-piece pouch with single-release paper, porous adhesive, clear. Net price 30 pouches (13 mm cut-to-fit hole) = £39.29

Simplicity 2® (Salts)
Closed, two-piece closed pouch (may also be applied directly to skin). Net price 30 pouches (40, 50, 60, or 70 mm holes, also 30 mm only for direct application to skin) = £30.20; flange (30, 40, 50, or 60 mm) 5 = £12.62

Solo® (Salts)
Solo closed, one-piece closed pouch with single-release paper, and adhesive flange, clear. Net price (30, 40, 50, or 60 mm holes), 30 pouches = £16.78; with filter, 30 pouches = £25.34

Supasac® (Salts)
Closed, one-piece pouch. Net price 30 pouches (medium) = £20.73

Shannon range
Colostomy (Shannon)
Adhesive appliance. Net price, 1 appliance (TJS 948B) = £44.19

Appliance. Net price, 1 appliance (TJS 962) = £15.39

Day bag (= pouch). Net price 1 pouch, TJS 948f = £20.27; TJS 948j = £23.19

Disposable bag (= pouch). Net price TJS 948g, 100 pouches = £10.04

Night bag (= pouch). Net price 1 pouch, TJS 948e = £23.19; TJS 948k = £25.29

Outfit. Net price 1 TJS 948A = £68.43, 1 TJS 948NA = £66.27; 1 TJS 948T = £36.29

Easychange® (Shannon)
Appliance. Net price 1 appliance = £4.06

Spare bag (= pouch). Net price 100 pouches = £40.50

Shannon
Disposable bag (= pouch), closed pouches with plasters. Net price 12 pouches = £5.55

Elastic necks. Net price 50 pouches = £20.25

Cautionary label wordings, see inside back cover   Prices are **net**, see p. 1

Shaw range
Hainsworth® (Shaw)
Hainsworth bag (= pouch), one-piece closed pouch. Net price (both 25, 32, 38, or 51 mm holes), 20 pouches with body mould adhesive = £34.50; 20 pouches with Healwell® adhesive = £18.10

Shaw (Shaw)
Colostomy outfit, comprising, 4-inch wide elastic belt with groinstrap (26 to 42-inch), 1 flange and 100 colostomy pouches. Net price one NSI 6 outfit with 11 × 6inch pouches = £31.95; one NSI 7 outfit with 12 × 8-inch pouches = £32.60; one NSI 8 outfit with 11 × 6-inch pouches = £34.95
Double seal, one-piece closed pouch. Net price 100 11 × 6-inch pouches = £8.25; 100 12 × 8-inch pouches = £9.05
Stick-on bag (pouch), one-piece closed pouch with plasters. Net price 10 pouches = £6.90

Simcare range
Adhesive (Simcare)
Stomabag, one-piece closed pouch with adhesive, opaque. Net price (25, 32, 38, 44, 51, or 64 mm holes), 90 pouches = £105.30; with filter, 90 pouches = £118.35

Beta® (Simcare)
Closed, two-piece pouch with filter. Net price, 1 kit comprising 30 pouches and 8 Seel-a-peel sheets (100 × 100 mm) = £44.16; 90 spare pouches = £121.57

Chiron® (Simcare)
Adhesive appliance with spout bag. Net price 1 appliance (Mk I and Mk II) = £58.87
Clearseal bag (= pouch), one-piece closed pouch. Net price 10 pouches (305 × 127 mm: 22 mm hole) = £12.41
Closed bag, one-piece pouch. Net price 10 pouches (305 × 127 mm or 230 × 127 mm: 38 mm hole) = £12.41
Disposal bag (= pouch), one-piece closed pouch. Net price 10 pouches (305 × 102 mm or 305 × 127 mm: 19 mm hole) = £8.27
Reinforced, one-piece disposable pouch. Net price 10 pouches = £12.41

Chironseal® (Simcare)
Closed bag (= pouch), one-piece closed pouch. Net price 10 pouches (305 × 102, 305 × 127, 230 × 127, or 305 × 150 mm: 22 or 38 mm holes) = £9.30; 10 pouches (305 × 205 or 305 × 255 mm: 22 or 38 mm hole) = £10.69
Reinforced, one-piece disposable closed pouch. Net price 10 pouches (305 × 102 mm: 25 or 38 mm holes or 305 × 127 mm: 38 mm hole) = £12.41

EC1® (Simcare)
Colo Classic, one-piece closed pouch with wafer, comfort backing, and filter, opaque or clear. Net price 30 pouches (25, 32, 38, 44, 51, 64 mm or 15–44 mm cut-to-fit holes) = £58.53

Omni® (Simcare)
Closed, one-piece pouch with wafer, porous adhesive, filter. Net price 30 pouches (opaque: 25, 32, 38, 44, or 51 mm; opaque or clear: 15–44 mm cut-to-fit holes) = £59.39

Redifit® (Simcare)
Continuation bag (= pouch), one-piece closed pouch with karaya skin protector, may be worn with belt, opaque. Net price 20 pouches (32, 38, 44, 51, 64, or 75 mm holes) = £59.96
Non-adhesive bag (= pouch), one-piece closed pouch, must be worn with belt. Net price 20 pouches with karaya skin protector (opaque: 44 or 51 mm holes; clear: 44, 51, or 64 mm holes) = £59.96; without karaya, 20 pouches (opaque, 38 mm hole) = £45.30

Rediseal®
Small bag (= pouch), one-piece PVC compact closed pouch, opaque. Net price 10 pouches (38, 44, or 51 mm holes) = £11.71

Symphony® (Simcare)
WC Disposable, one-piece closed pouch with wafer and filter. Net price 30 pouches (opaque or clear: 25, 32, 38, 44, or 51 mm holes; opaque: 15–44 mm cut-to-fit holes) = £62.16

Simpla range
Phoenix® (Simpla)
Closed, one-piece closed pouch. Net price (both 32, 40, or 45 mm holes) 100 pouches = £134.46; 100 casual pouches = £125.08

Sassco® (Simpla)
Closed, one-piece closed pouch. Net price 100 pouches (32, 40, or 45 mm holes) = £128.07

Simplaseel® (Simpla)
Closed, one-piece closed pouch. Net price 30 pouches (26, 32, 40, 45, 50 mm or cut-to-fit holes) = £61.56; 30 casual pouches (32, 40, or 45 mm holes) = £57.27

Ward range
Ward
Disposable bag (= pouch), one-piece closed pouch. Net price 10 pouches (12 × 4-inch) with 4 × 3-inch plasters =£7.17; 10 pouches (12 × 5-inch) with 4 × 4-inch plasters = £7.17
Celluloid colostomy cup, with sponge or solid rim. Net price 1 (small, medium, or large) cup = £29.75; with belt fitting, 1 cup = £33.95; 1 pouch with mount outlet = £12.36

Welland range
Welland® (Welland)
Colostomy bag (= pouch), one-piece closed pouch with wafer and filter, opaque or clear. Net price 30 pouches (25, 32, 38, 44, 51, 60 mm or cut-to-fit holes) = £49.35
Softback colostomy bag, one-piece closed pouch with wafer, filter, and soft backing, opaque or clear. Net price 30 pouches (10, 25, 32, 38, 44, 51, 60 mm or cut-to-fit holes) = £50.65

DRAINABLE POUCHES

Drainable pouches are suitable for patients with an **ileostomy** or a **colostomy** with fluid effluent

Body's Care range
Rubber bags screwcap (Body's Care)
Black butyl, one-piece pouch. Net price 1 day pouch = £23.25; 1 night pouch = £27.12
White rubber, one-piece pouch. Net price 1 day pouch = £12.92; 1 night pouch = £14.89

Rubber bags spout (Body's Care)
Black butyl, one-piece pouch. Net price 1 day or night pouch = £24.55
White rubber, one-piece pouch. Net price 1 day pouch = £11.62; 1 night pouch = £11.62

Bullen range
Lenbul® (Bullen)
Bag, with one-piece flange. Net price 1 pouch (25 or 51 mm holes) = £26.52; 1 lightweight pouch (25 or 51 mm hole) = £1.53
Day bag (= pouch), one-piece pouch. Net price 1 pouch with screwcap outlet = £11.56; 1 pouch with screwcap outlet and larger opening = £12.00; 1 pouch with metal strip = £13.87; 1 pouch with tap outlet = £13.42
Night bag (= pouch), one-piece pouch. Net price 1 pouch with screwcap outlet = £12.73; 1 pouch with screwcap outlet and larger opening = £13.21; 1 pouch with metal strip = £13.87; 1 pouch with tap outlet = £15.34

LOP-F7® (Bullen)
Ileostomy appliance. Net price 1 appliance = £37.20

1.8 Stoma care

OPR-F® (Bullen)
Ileostomy appliance. Net price 1 appliance = £77.59
SR-F® (Bullen)
Ileostomy set. Net price 1 set = £53.47

Cambmac range
Dansac® (Cambmac)
Combi D + A, one-piece pouch with adhesive and karaya skin protector, opaque. Net price 30 pouches (19, 22, 25, 32, 38, 50, or 63 mm holes) = £70.46
Combi Ileo F, one-piece pouch, opaque. Net price 100 pouches (standard: 22 or 30 mm holes; small: 19 or 25 mm holes) = £155.35
CombiMicro D + S, one-piece pouch with porous adhesive, skin barrier ring, and fabric backing. Net price 30 pouches (25, 32, 38, 44, 50, 63 mm or cut-to-fit holes), opaque = £62.32; clear, 30 pouches = £58.80
Mini Infant, one-piece pouch with skin barrier ring and fabric backing, clear. Net price 30 pouches (cut-to-fit holes) = £51.03; 30 pouches (cut-to-fit holes), opaque or clear = £62.32
Infant, one-piece pouch, opaque or clear. Net price 30 pouches (cut-to-fit holes) = £51.03
Mini Petit D, one-piece pouch with skin barrier ring and fabric backing, opaque or clear. Net price 30 pouches (cut-to-fit holes) = £53.76
Supersquare System, two-piece pouch, opaque or clear. Net price 30 standard or small pouches to fit 50 mm base plate = £35.18; 30 standard pouches to fit 80 mm base plate = £50.82

CliniMed range
Biotrol® (CliniMed)
Elite, fabric covered one-piece pouch with skin protector adhesive and clamp closure, white or skin-tone. Net price 30 pouches (20, 25, 30, 35, 40, 45, 50, 60, 70 mm or cut-to-fit holes) = £61.70; 30 clear pouches (cut-to-fit holes) = £58.75
Ileo S, one-piece pouch with skin protector adhesive, white. Net price 30 pouches (20, 25, 30, 35, 40, 45, 50, 60, 70 mm or cut-to-fit holes) = £61.70
Post-op, one-piece pouch with skin protector adhesive, for temporary or permanent colostomies or ileostomies, clear. Net price (cut-to-fit holes) small, 30 pouches = £62.40; large, 30 pouches = £88.10
Preference, fabric covered one-piece pouch with skin protector adhesive, porous adhesive collar, skin-tone. Net price 30 pouches (20, 25, 30, 35, 40, 45, 50, 60 mm or cut-to-fit holes) = £61.70

Coloplast range
Ileo B® (Coloplast)
One-piece pouch with zinc oxide adhesive, clear or white. Net price 100 pouches (20 mm hole) = £138.00
Mini, one-piece compact pouch with zinc oxide adhesive, white. Net price 100 pouches (20 mm hole) = £137.00
K-Flex® (Coloplast)
One-piece pouch with karaya skin protector, clear. Net price 30 pouches (10 or 40 mm holes) = £64.20
mc2000® (Coloplast)
One-piece pouch with double seal, opaque or clear. Net price 30 pouches (20, 25, 30, 35, 40, 45, 50, 55, 60 mm holes or clear pouch with cut-to-fit hole) = £63.60
Mini, one-piece compact pouch, opaque. Net price 30 pouches (20, 25, 30, 35, or 40 mm holes) = £60.00
mc2002® (Coloplast)
Two-piece pouch, opaque or clear. Net price 30 pouches (to fit 40 or 60 mm base plates) = £37.50
Post-op, two-piece pouch, clear. Net price, to fit 70 mm base plate, 10 bags with clip = £15.30; to fit 100 mm base plate, 10 bags with clip = £20.10

pc3000® (Coloplast)
One-piece pouch, opaque or clear. Net price 30 pouches (20, 25, 30, 35, 40, 45, 50, 55, or 60 mm holes; 20 mm can be cut to fit up to 60 mm) = £56.40
Mini starter hole, one-piece pouch. Net price 30 pouches = £51.30
Sterile post-op bag, one-piece pouch. Net price 100 pouches (2200) = £207.00; (2202) = £135.00

ConvaTec range
Ileodress® (ConvaTec)
Ileodress, one-piece pouch with textured backing. Net price 10 standard pouches with clip (opaque or clear: 19, 38, 45, 50, or 64 mm holes; 19 mm can be cut to fit; opaque only: 25 and 32 mm holes) = £18.64; 10 small pouches with clip, opaque (19, 25, 32, 38, 45, 50, or 64 mm holes; 19 mm can be cut to fit) = £18.25
Ileodress Plus, one-piece pouch with single-release paper. Net price 10 standard pouches with clip (opaque or clear: 19, 38, 45, 50, or 64 mm holes; 19 mm can be cut to fit; opaque only: 25 and 32 mm holes) = £18.64
Little Ones® (ConvaTec)
Paediatric, one-piece pouch. Net price 15 pouches (8 mm cut-to-fit hole) = £25.65
Surgicare System® 2 (ConvaTec)
System 2, two-piece pouches, white. Net price 10 pouches with clip (to fit 32, 38, 45, 57, or 70 mm flanges) = £9.27
System 2 Combihesive, two-piece pouches with textured backing. Net price 10 standard or small pouches with clip, beige (to fit 32, 38, 45, 57, or 70 mm flanges) = £9.35; 10 standard pouches with clip, clear, to fit 45, 57, or 70 mm flanges = £9.35; to fit 100 mm flanges = £16.53

De Puy range
Raymed® (De Puy)
Butyl day bag (= pouch), one-piece pouch. Net price 1 pouch with screwcap outlet = £22.60; 1 pouch with tap outlet = £23.75
Schacht® (De Puy)
Ileostomy, one-piece pouches. Net price 50 pouches = £19.80
Ileostomy appliance, odourproof. Net price 1 appliance = £29.25

Drew range
Drew
Ileostomy bag (= pouch), one-piece pouch. Net price 50 D1/1 pouches = £59.48; 50 D1/6 pouches = £42.46
Ileostomy appliance. Net price 1 appliance (D1/1) = £31.27; 1 appliance (D1/6) = £26.79

Hollister range
Classic (Hollister)
Karaya seal (series 721), one-piece pouch with karaya skin protector seal, must be worn with belt, clear. Net price 30 pouches with 1 clamp (25, 32, 38, 44, 51, 64, or 76 mm hole) = £58.89
Karaya 5® transparent, one-piece pouch with karaya skin protector seal, may be worn with belt. 30- or 40-cm clear pouch with microporous adhesive (series 322 and 327), net price 30 pouches with 1 clamp (25, 32, 38, 44, 51, 64, or 76 mm hole) = £67.70; 30-cm pouches with regular adhesive (series 722) = £67.70
Karaya 5® opaque, one-piece pouch with karaya skin protector seal and porous adhesive, may be worn with belt. Net price 30 pouches with 1 clamp, 23-cm pouches (series 313: 25, 32, 38, 44, or 51 mm holes) = £67.70; 30-cm pouches (series 311: 25, 32, 38, 44, 51, 64, or 76 mm holes) = £65.19
Karaya 5® seal (series 360), one-piece pouch with porous adhesive and karaya skin protector seal, clear. Net price 15 pouches (25, 32, 38, 44, 51, 64, or 76 mm holes) with 1 clamp = £33.22

Cautionary label wordings, see inside back cover

Prices are **net**, see p. 1

Chapter 1: Gastro-intestinal system

Loop ostomy bag (= pouch). Net price 20 pouches (3.5 or 4.5 inch) = £58.56
Loop ostomy gasket. Net price 10 (3.5 or 4.5 inch) = £58.56)

Guardian® (Hollister)
All with 25, 38, 51, or 64 mm holes
Guardian (series 461 and 460), two-piece pouch, opaque or clear. Net price 10 pouches with 1 clamp = £9.15; larger pouch to fit 102-mm flange, 10 pouches (clear) with 1 clamp = £19.83
Guardian mini-pouch, two-piece compact pouch, opaque. Net price (series 464), 10 pouches = £9.00; NHS with inner film and replaceable filter (series 463), 10 pouches with pack of filters and 1 clamp
NHS *With replaceable filter* (series 462), two-piece pouch with inner film and replaceable filter, clear. 10 pouches with pack of filters and 1 clamp

Premium® (Hollister)
Karaya 5® seal with filter (series 366), one-piece pouch with porous adhesive, karaya skin protector seal, and replaceable filter, may be worn with belt, clear. Net price 15 pouches (25, 32, 38, 44, 51, or 64 mm holes) with 1 clamp and filter elements = £36.96
Synthetic seal (series 364), one-piece pouch with porous adhesive and synthetic skin protector seal, clear. Net price 15 pouches (25, 32, 38, 44, 51, or 64 mm holes) with 1 clamp = £33.22

Rüsch range
Birkbeck® (Rüsch)
Rubber, one-piece pouch, black or pink. Net price (both 19, 38, or 54 mm holes), 1 day pouch = £23.76; 1 night pouch = £27.17
Disposable, one-piece plastic pouch. Net price 100 pouches = £14.37
Ileostomy appliance. Net price 1 appliance "A" (19, 38, or 54 mm) = £82.95; 1 appliance "B" (19, 38, or 54 mm) = £53.52

Ostopore® (Rüsch)
Ileo KAV-opaque, one-piece pouch with karaya seal skin protector, adhesive, and vent, opaque. Net price 30 pouches (25, 32, or 38 mm holes) with 30 belt flanges and 10 clips = £59.40

Rubber bags (Rüsch)
White rubber, one-piece pouch. Net price, 1 day pouch (38, 44, or 51 mm holes) = £10.64; 1 screwcap pouch (38 mm hole) = £11.48; 1 pouch with vent (38 mm hole) = £12.72
White rubber child bag (= pouch), one-piece pouch. Net price (both 19, 25, or 28 mm holes), 1 day pouch = £10.25; 1 night pouch = £12.55
Latex rubber, one-piece pouch. Net price 1 day pouch (38, 44, or 51 mm holes) = £11.00; 1 night pouch (19, 25, or 28 mm holes) = £12.15

Salts range
NHS Cohflex® (Salts)
Drainable, one-piece pouch with single-release paper, wafer, and fabric front and back. Net price 30 pouches with integral closure clip (opaque: 30, 40, 50, or 60 mm, all may be cut to fit; clear: 10–60 mm cut-to-fit hole) = £59.94
Paediatric drainable, one-piece small pouch with single-release paper, wafer, and fabric backing, opaque/clear. Net price 30 pouches with integral closure clip (10–50 mm cut-to-fit hole) = £49.64

Eakin® (Salts)
Drainable, one-piece pouch, white or clear. Net price 20 small or large pouches (32, 45, or 64 mm holes) = £42.77; 20 wide pouches, clear (90 mm hole) = £103.02
Fistula, one-piece pouch. Net price 10 large pouches = £98.26; starter, 20 small pouches = £88.97, 20 medium pouches = £115.08

Light White (Salts)
Drainable, one-piece pouch, white. Net price 30 large, small, or medium pouches (all 25, 32, or 38 mm holes) = £42.76
Drainable self-adhesive, one-piece pouch with adhesive, white. Net price 30 pouches (large: 25, 32, 38, or 44 mm holes; small and medium: 25, 32, or 38 mm holes) = £48.52

Koenig Rutzen® screwcap (Salts)
All with screwcap outlet
Black butyl all rubber, one-piece pouch. Net price 1 pouch (large: 25, 29, 32, 35, 38, 44, or 51 mm holes; small: 25, 32, 38, 44, or 51 mm) = £26.25; with bridge (soft-face Maggie Bag), 1 pouch (large: 25, 32, 38, 44, or 51 mm holes; small: 25, 32, or 38 mm) = £35.21
Black butyl reinforced, one-piece pouch. Net price 1 large or small pouch (both 25, 32, or 38 mm holes) = £35.21; with bridge (hard-face Maggie Bag), 1 pouch (large: 25, 32, 38, 44, or 51 mm holes; small: 25, 32, or 38 mm) = £39.09

Koenig Rutzen® spout (Salts)
All with spout outlet
Black butyl all rubber, one-piece pouch. Net price 1 large or small pouch (both 25, 32, 38, 44, or 51 mm holes) = £19.82; with bridge, 1 pouch (large: 25, 32, 38, 44, or 51 mm holes; small: 25, 32, or 38 mm) = £25.69
Black butyl reinforced, one-piece pouch. Net price 1 large or small pouch (25, 32, or 38 mm holes) = £26.64; with bridge, 1 pouch (large: 25, 32, 38, 44, or 51 mm holes; small: 25, 32, or 38 mm) = £32.81

Kombo® (Salts)
Kombo drainable, one-piece pouch with karaya skin protector seal and adhesive, clear. Net price 30 pouches (30, 40, 50, 60, or 80 mm holes) = £51.26; with filter, 30 pouches = £61.55

Rubber bags (Salts)
All must be used with flange
Black butyl screw, one-piece bag with screwcap outlet. Net price 1 large or small pouch = £25.96
Black butyl spout, one-piece bag with spout outlet. Net price 1 large or small pouch = £18.73
White screw, one-piece bag with screwcap outlet. Net price 1 large or small pouch = £8.66
White spout, one-piece bag with spout outlet. Net price 1 large or small pouch = £7.33

Salger® (Salts)
Drainable, one-piece pouch. Net price 10 pouches (40 or 57 mm holes) = £9.98

Simplicity® (Salts)
Drainable, two-piece pouch, clear. Net price 30 230 × 137-mm pouches (40, 50, or 60 mm holes) = £16.05
Post-op, two-piece pouch. Net price 30 300 × 125-mm pouches (40, 50, or 60 mm holes) = £13.94

Simplicity 1® (Salts)
Drainable, one-piece pouch with porous adhesive and skin protector seal, fabric front and back. Net price 30 pouches with integral closure clip (opaque: 30, 40, 50, or 60 mm, all may be cut to fit; opaque or clear: 10–60 mm cut-to-fit hole) = £62.93
Paediatric drainable, one-piece pouch with porous adhesive and skin protector seal, clear. Net price 30 pouches (cut-to-fit hole) = £39.29
Post-op, one-piece pouch with single-release paper and wafer, clear. Net price 10 pouches (both cut-to-fit holes), small = £50.65; large = £69.55

Simplicity 2® (Salts)
Drainable, two-piece pouch (may also be applied directly to skin). Net price 15 pouches (40, 50, 60, or 70 mm holes, also 30 mm only for direct application to skin) = £16.76
Post-op, two-piece pouch (may also be applied directly to skin). Net price 30 pouches (40, 50, 60, or 70 mm holes, also 30 mm only for direct application to skin) = £33.10

1.8 Stoma care

Transverse, two-piece pouch (may also be applied directly to skin). Net price 10 pouches (cut-to-fit hole) = £37.63; 5 flanges = £18.40

Solo® (Salts)
Drainable, one-piece pouch with single-release paper and adhesive, clear. Net price 30 pouches (30, 40, 50, 60 or 80 mm holes) = £19.93; with filter, 30 pouches = £25.13

NHS United® (Salts)
Soft & Secure drainable, one-piece pouch, opaque or clear. Net price 10 pouches (38, 45, or 57 mm holes) = £8.47

Shaw range
Ileostomy outfit, with 5 inch wide elastic web belt. Net price 1 outfit (26–42 inch) = £49.15

Hainsworth® (Shaw)
Drainable bag, one-piece pouch with adhesive. Net price 20 pouches (0.875, 1, 1.25, or 1.5 inch holes) = £34.50

Rubber bags (Shaw)
Black screwcap, one-piece pouch with screwcap outlet. Net price (both 19, 38 or 54 mm holes), 1 day pouch = £19.40; 1 night pouch = £20.65

Simcare range
Adhesive (Simcare)
Stomabag, one-piece pouch with adhesive, opaque. Net price 60 pouches (19, 25, 32, 38, 51 mm or cut-to-fit holes) = £76.99

Beta® (Simcare)
Post-op, two-piece large capacity pouch. Net price (cut-to-fit hole), 4 pouches with 1 wire closure = £26.94, 20 pouches with 20 wire closures = £39.34

Cavendish® (Simcare)
Odourproof, one-piece pouch. Net price (all 25, 32, or 38 mm holes), 10 opaque pouches with non-adhesive flange = £26.71; 10 opaque pouches with adhesive flange = £32.17; 10 clear PVC pouches = £26.88

Chiron® **screwcap** (Simcare)
All with screwcap outlet
Butyl rubber day bag (= pouch), one-piece pouch, black. Net price 1 pouch (38, 44, or 51 mm hole) = £27.38
Butyl rubber night bag (= pouch), one-piece pouch, black. Net price 1 pouch (38 or 44 mm holes) = £32.86
Latex rubber day bag (= pouch), one-piece pouch. Net price 1 pouch (38 mm hole) = £13.70
Latex rubber night bag (= pouch), one-piece pouch. Net price 1 pouch (38 mm hole) = £18.14
White rubber day bag (= pouch), one-piece pouch. Net price 1 pouch (38, 44, or 51 mm) = £15.76, child-size pouch (38 mm hole) = £13.70; body-size outlet, 1 pouch (38 mm hole) = £15.76, child-size pouch (38 mm hole) = £12.46
White rubber night bag (= pouch), one-piece pouch. Net price 1 pouch (38 or 51 mm hole) = £18.14; body-size outlet, 1 pouch (38 mm hole) = £15.07

Chiron® **spout** (Simcare)
White rubber bag (= pouch), one-piece pouch. Net price 1 day pouch (38 mm hole) = £13.55; 1 night pouch (38 mm hole) = £14.72

EC1® (Simcare)
Ileo classic, one-piece pouch with wafer and comfort backing, opaque. Net price 30 pouches with 1 clamp (19, 25, 32, 38, 44 mm or 10–44 mm cut-to-fit holes) = £61.31
Mini classic, one-piece compact pouch with wafer and comfort backing, opaque or clear. Net price 30 pouches with 1 clamp (10–44 mm cut-to-fit holes) = £61.31
Post-op classic, one-piece pouch with wafer and comfort backing, clear. Net price 30 pouches with 1 clamp, 10–64 mm cut-to-fit holes = £63.24; 10–90 mm cut-to-fit holes = £89.49

Omni® (Simcare)
Drainable, one-piece pouch with porous adhesive wafer and replaceable filter. Net price 20 pouches (opaque: 25, 32, 38, 44 mm; opaque or clear: 10–44 mm cut-to-fit hole) = £40.85; NHS opaque (10–90 mm cut-to-fit hole) = £48.43

Redifit® (Simcare)
Opaque, one-piece pouch with karaya skin protector, may be worn with belt. Net price 20 pouches with 2 closure clips (25, 32, 38, 44, 51, or 64 mm holes) = £59.97; small outline pouches, 20 pouches with 2 closure clips (25, 32, or 38 mm) = £59.97
Clear fronted, one-piece pouch with karaya skin protector, may be worn with belt. Net price 20 pouches with 2 closure clips (25, 32, 44, 51, or 64 mm holes) = £59.97

Simpla range
Sassco® (Simpla)
Ileostomy bag (= pouch), one-piece pouch. Net price 100 pouches (26 or 32 mm holes) = £147.03

Simplaseel® (Simpla)
Drainable bag (= pouch), one-piece pouch, opaque. Net price 30 pouches (26, 32, 40, 45, or 50 mm holes) = £62.52
Post-op drainable bag (= pouch), one-piece pouch. Net price 10 pouches = £33.89
Paediatric drainable bag (= pouch), one-piece pouch. Net price 30 pouches = £54.83

Steeper range
Rubber bags® (Steeper)
Bag, rubber. Net price 1 pouch, spring-in-neck, with vulcanite screw outlets (small) = £11.99, (medium) = £16.62, (large) = £17.02; 1 pouch, complete with collar = £19.69; 1 pouch, with tap outlet and skirt = £2.39
Night bag (= pouch), shaped rubber with long vertical spring vulcanite screw outlet. Net price 1 pouch = £18.63

Donald Rose® (Steeper)
Bag (= pouch), with celluloid collars, solid, flat or fluid rims. Net price 1 pouch = £18.14
Ileostomy appliance. Net price 1 appliance (first stage) = £44.39; 1 appliance (second stage) = £43.90; 1 appliance (new improved) = £46.60

Ward range
Rubber bags (Ward)
Black rubber bag (= pouch), one-piece pouch with screwcap outlet. Net price (19, 35, or 54 mm hole), 1 day pouch = £14.94; 1 night pouch = £15.60
White rubber ileostomy bag (= pouch) with flange, pouch with St. Mark's flange. Net price 1 pouch = £22.65
White rubber ileostomy bag (= pouch), one-piece pouch. Net price 1 day pouch (screwcap or spout outlet) = £10.20; 1 night pouch (screwcap or spout outlet) = £11.49; tap outlet, 1 day pouch = £14.95; 1 night pouch = £16.64
White rubber transverse ileostomy bag (= pouch), one-piece pouch. Net price 1 pouch = £23.93

Welland range
Welland® (Welland)
Ileostomy bag (= pouch), one-piece pouch with wafer, opaque or clear. Net price 30 pouches (25, 32, 38, 44, 51 mm or cut-to-fit holes) = £49.00
Softback ileostomy bag (= pouch), one-piece with wafer and soft backing, opaque or clear. Net price 30 pouches (25, 32, 38, 44, 51 mm or cut-to-fit holes) = £52.00
Mini-bag, one-piece with wafer, clear. Net price (both cut-to-fit holes), 30 pouches = £48.50; with soft backing, 30 pouches = £50.50
Oval drainable, one-piece pouch with wafer, opaque. Net price (both cut-to-fit holes), 30 pouches = £53.00; with soft backing, 30 pouches = £55.00
Oval post-op, one-piece pouch with wafer, clear. Net price (both cut-to-fit holes), 30 pouches = £53.00; with soft backing, 30 pouches = £55.00

Chapter 1: Gastro-intestinal system

ADHESIVE PREPARATIONS, ADHESIVE REMOVERS AND DEODORANTS

Adhesive preparations
Dow Corning DC 355® (Dow Corning)
Medical adhesive brushable. Net price 20-mL bottle (with brush) = £2.92
Dow Corning B Spray® (Dow Corning)
Spray adhesive. Net price 206-g aerosol spray = £9.64
Hollister® (Hollister)
Medical adhesive spray (with silicones). Net price 170-g aerosol spray = £12.10
Latex adhesive solution (Salt)
Net price per tube = £1.70. Label: 15

Adhesive removers
Dow Corning B Remover® (Dow Corning)
Adhesive remover spray. Net price 227-g aerosol spray = £7.59
Hollister® (Hollister)
Adhesive remover spray. Net price 170-g spray = £10.13
Salts 'SPR' Plaster Remover (Rezolve®) (Salts)
Adhesive remover spray. Net price 70-g aerosol spray = £2.53. Label: 15

Deodorants
Atmocol® is used as a deodorising spray when emptying the appliance. The other deodorants listed are placed in the appliance.

Atmocol® (DePuy)
Aerosol deodorant. Net price 1 unit (400 sprays) = £1.90
Chironair Odour Control Liquid® (Simcare)
Deodorant solution. Net price 113 g = £4.79
Colostomy Plus® (Shannon)
Deodorant. Net price 1 unit = £2.46
Day-drop® (Loxley)
Deodorant solution. Net price 7.5 mL = 89p; 15 mL = £1.48
Dor® (Simpla)
Deodorant solution. Net price 7 mL = £1.55
Forest Breeze® (Shaw)
Deodorant. Net price 1 unit = £2.73
Limone® (CliniMed)
Deodorant spray. Net price 50 mL = £3.60
Nilodor® (Cussons)
Deodorant solution. Net price (with dropper) 7.5 mL = £1.60
Ostobon® (Coloplast)
Deodorant powder. Net price 22 g = £3.39
Saltair No-Roma® (Salts)
Deodorant solution. Net price 30 mL = £2.02; 300 mL = £6.59
Stomogel® (DePuy)
Deodorant gel. Net price 50 g = £2.60
Sween® (Bullen & Smears)
Deodorant. Net price 15 mL = £3.80
Translet Plus One® (Rüsch)
Deodorant solution for men. Net price 7 mL = £2.77
Translet Plus Two® (Rüsch)
Deodorant solution for women. Net price 7 mL = £2.77

ADHESIVE DEVICES AND RINGS

Bullen range
Adhesive plaster, double-sided. Net price 10 zinc oxide plasters 3.5 × 3.5 inch = £3.72, 4 × 4 inch = £4.59, 5 × 5 inch = £7.76; 10 acrylic base plasters 3.5 × 3.5 inch = £3.45, 4 × 4 inch = £4.43, 5 × 5 inch = £7.46
Flange retention strips. Net price 50 strips 4 × 1 inch = £1.66, 4 × 2 inch = £2.24

3M range
Stomaseal® (3M)
Adhesive discs. Net price 12 discs (10 cm diameter) = £3.81

Rüsch range
Ostomy plasters, double-sided. Net price 25 plasters (25 mm hole, or no hole) = £7.50

Salts range
Kidney seals. Net price 10 = £3.80
Reliaseal® (Salts)
Adhesive discs, double-sided, round, hypo-allergic. Net price 10 discs (13, 19, 22, 25, 29, 32, or 38 mm) = £14.54
Transacryl® (Salts)
Adhesive plasters, double-sided. Net price 10 plasters (25, 32, or 38 mm) = £4.83
Zopla® (Salts)
Adhesive plasters, double-sided. Net price (both 25, 32, or 38 mm) 10 square plasters = £3.63; 10 round plasters = £4.21

Shannon range
Adhesive plasters, double-sided. Net price 25 plasters = £13.66
Rings. Net price 5 rubber retaining rings = £5.46; 1 plastic locking ring = £2.03
Easychange® (Shannon)
Adhesive plasters, with rings (spare). Net price 5 plasters = £5.40

Shaw range
Adhesive plasters, double-sided, hole cut-to-size. Net price 10 plasters, 4 × 4 inch = £6.15; 5 × 5 inch = £6.35

Simcare range
Adhesive discs, double-sided. Net price 10 discs (76 mm diameter: 19 or 25 mm opening; 90 mm diameter: 32 or 38 mm opening) = £3.76
Rings, elastic, for use with spout bags. Net price 3 rings = £1.86
Carshalton® (Simcare)
Adhesive plasters. Net price both (25, 32, or 38 mm) 10 acrylic plasters = £3.99; 10 zinc oxide plasters = £6.31
Chiron® (Simcare)
Adhesive plasters, double-sided. Net price 10 plasters (90 mm square: 19 or 35 mm hole) = £5.11, (102 mm square: 19 or 35 mm hole) = £5.86, (127 mm square: 19 or 35 mm hole) = £6.47, (150 mm square and 102 × 76 mm: both 19 mm hole) = £7.22, (90 and 102 mm square: both 25 mm hole) = £7.22, (125 mm square: 25 mm hole) = £7.92
Clearseal plasters. Net price 10 plasters (100 mm square: 19 or 35 mm hole) = £5.86
Kidney seals, adhesive flange retaining strips. Net price 10 strips (small or large) = £4.10

Ward range
Adhesive plasters, double-sided with opening. Net price 10 plasters = £3.64

BAG CLOSURES

Clamps
Available from *CliniMed* (Biotrol® for post-op or for drainage pouches, 1 clamp = 88p), *Hollister* (for drainable pouches, 1 clamp = 89p, 20 = £14.73; for Premium® pouches, 1 clamp = 93p, 20 = £15.60), *Simcare* (10 clamps = £7.08; Carshalton®, 5 clamps = £8.39), *Simpla* (for Ileo® pouches, 20 clamps = £4.89)

1.8 Stoma care

Clips
Available from *ConvaTec* (10 beige clips = £2.43; for Surgicaire System® 2, 10 white clips = £2.43, *Drew* (10 clips = 18p), *DePuy* (for Stomastar® drainable, 10 = £5.85), *Salts* (5 clips = £1.62), *Shaw* (1 clip = 65p), *Simcare* (for odourproof pouches, 10 = £5.41)

Closing Tape
Available from *Shannon* (1 reel = £1.47)

Fastening Ring
Rubber pouch fastening ring. Available from *Shaw* (1 ring = 95p)

Ties
Available from *ConvaTec* (50 soft wire ties = £4.50)

BAG COVERS

Body's Care
Bag cover, cloth. Net price 1 cover = £3.60

Bullen
Bag cover, cloth, for day or night bags. Net price 1 cover = £7.49

CliniMed
Bag cover, cloth for Biotrol® pouches. Net price 5 covers = £6.98

Coloplast
Bag cover, cloth for closed or drainable MC2000® or MC2002® pouches (white or flesh), for MC2000® mini pouches (decorated: white or flesh), for Ileo B® standard pouches, or for URO2002® pouches (white). Net price 5 covers = £19.00

ConvaTec
Bag cover, cloth for Surgicaire System® 2. Net price 3 covers (for 32/38 mm Mini pouches: 45/57 mm pouches, or large urostomy pouches) = £5.64; 3 covers (for standard drainable pouches, urostomy pouches, small closed 38/45 mm pouches: small drainable pouches, combihesive closed pouches, medium closed pouches: 57 and 70 mm) = £5.96

Drew
Bag cover, cotton. Net price 1 cover = £1.29

Hollister
Bag cover, non-woven. Net price 5 covers (for closed or non-drainable pouch) = £3.72

Nationwide Ostomy
Ostocover® *bag cover*, cloth, white or coloured. Net price 3 covers = £6.60

Rüsch
Bag cover, cloth for Ostopore® pouches. Net price 5 covers (small or large) = £16.40

Salts
Bag covers, cotton, appliance to be stated. Net price 1 cover = £3.15. Cloth, for Eakin® pouches, 1 cover small or large (both 32, 45 or 64 mm) = £3.84

Shaw
Bag covers, cloth. Net price 1 day pouch cover, cotton = £4.15; lycra = £4.40. 1 night cover, cotton = £4.40; lycra = £4.75

Simcare
Bag cover. Net price 1 day or night cotton pouch cover = £9.44; 5 stomabag covers (white or coloured) = £20.87; for Redifit® pouches, 1 cotton cover (25 and 32 mm, 38, 44, and 51 mm, 64, and 75 mm holes) = £6.49; for Symphony® pouches, 5 polyethylene covers = £3.71

Simpla
Bag cover, cotton, for Colo® pouch. Net price 5 covers, normal = £8.87, casual = £8.81; for Ileo® pouch, 5 covers = £9.15

Steeper
Bag cover, white linen. Net price 1 cover = £5.98

Welland
Bag shields, spunbonded polypropylene. Net price 10 shields (small: 25–44 mm; large: 10, 51, or 60 mm) = £2.70

BELTS

Body's Care
Belts. Net price 3-inch belt = £12.18: 3-inch one-piece belt, = £15.89; 4-inch one-piece belt = £16.05; 1-inch web and elastic with button and buckle fastening = £6.77; 2-inch belt = £8.00; 3-inch belt = £9.22: 1 girdle and panti-brief with hole for stoma and suspenders or understrap = £39.40; 1 St Mark's (male or female) = £46.95; 1 St Mark's Coutilostomy = £31.82

Bullen
Belts. Net price 1.5-inch belt with aluminium retaining shield (small, medium, or large) = £8.87: 1.5-inch elastic belt with wire or plastic ring retainer (wire; small, medium, or large) = £9.05; 4-inch belt (wire; small, medium, or large) = £13.26; 1-inch elastic belt with plastic ring shield = £9.58: 1 waterproof canvas retaining shield (small, medium, or large) = £14.32; 1 St Mark's = £37.16

Cambmac
Belt with plates for Dansac® pouches. Net price 1 belt plus 5 plates (19–44 mm or 50–63 mm) = £30.08

CliniMed
Waist belt for Biotrol® pouches. Net price 1 belt = £3.55

Coloplast
Belts. For Ileo B® pouches, net price 1 belt = £6.27 or for K-Flex® pouches, 1 belt = £4.78

ConvaTec
Belt, for Surgicaire System® 2. Net price 1 belt = £2.43

DePuy
Belts. Net price 1 ostomy girdle or panty girdle (white or skin colour) = £28.90; 1 4-inch nightbelt with waterproof backing = £9.25; for Schacht® pouches, 1 36-inch belt = £5.05; or for Slimline® pouches, 1 belt with beltplate = £11.60

Drew
Belts. Net price 1 waistband with metal ends = £2.52, with plastic ends = £7.86; 1 day belt = £18.41; 1 night belt = £12.52; 1 × 4 inch belt (deep stoma hole) = £6.00; stoma/bones = £6.59

Ellis Son & Passmore
Belt. Net price 1 night colostomy belt (Clifton®) = £11.42; 1 St Mark's = £28.70, 1 shield = £9.37

Hollister
Belt. Net price 1 adjustable ostomy belt (small, medium, or large) = £5.68; 10 = £47.30

Peacock
Belts. Net price 1 St Mark's belt = £38.15

Rüsch
Belts. Net price 5 elastic waistbands (Birkbeck®) = £31.29; 5 elastic waistbands with shields = £41.16; 5 retaining rings (19, 38, or 54 mm) = £7.81. 5 narrow or normal width belts (Ostopore®), waist: 17–34 inch or 28–56 inch) = £26.15. White rubber belting 28 mm = £3.42/metre, 72 mm = £7.07/metre. White sausage belt per metre = £7.04. 1 waist and support strap = £5.84

Sallis
Belts. Net price 1 night belt, 14a = £5.58; 14b = £8.87; 14c = £4.63; 1 day belt, 15a = £24.43; 15b = £6.82. 1 zipped pocket (to fit 15a, 15b and 16) = £4.15; 1 St Mark's = £22.40, 1 shield = £8.10

Salts
Belts. Net price 25 mm elastic belt (single), with 2 loops (standard 35 inch or extra-large 42 inch) = £2.91; with suspender ends = £2.91; double elastic with 4 loops = £4.06; with waterproof panel 102 mm = £11.79, 150 mm = £14.39; with 4 loops and retaining ring = £15.72. 1 rubber belt with straps and buckles = £4.89; with 2 fastening studs = £3.36. 25 mm button belt with or without loop = £2.91. 1 baby lycra belt = £11.61; with Velcro fastening (standard 35 inch or extra-large 42 inch) = £2.96. 1 colostomy belt = £61.23. 1 ileostomy girdle (Saltair®) = £39.11; 1 ileostomy elastic night belt

Chapter 1: Gastro-intestinal system

(Saltair®) = £11.66. For Eakin® pouches, 1 elastic belt (small or large) = £3.01. For Salger® pouches, 1 elastic adjustable belt with or without Velcro fastening = £2.94

Shannon
Belt. Net price 1 elastic belt with shield and Velcro fastening = £6.77; with button and buckle fastening = £4.08

Shaw
Belts, colostomy, all made to measure. Net price 4 inch elastic web belt = £11.50; with under-strap or suspenders, 6 inch = £15.45, 8 inch = £22.25; with lace fastenings, 6 inch = £21.00; 8 inch = £26.45; 10 inch = £25.15; 12 inch = £27.65; 14 inch (made to measure) = £28.20; with zip panel, 10 inch = £31.80; 12 inch = £33.65; 14 inch = £35.25; elastic with nylon fronts, 10 inch = £29.55; 12 inch = £30.55; 14 inch = £33.00. 1 inch adjustable colostomy/ileostomy belt = £6.70; 4 inch (3 sections) = £16.90; 6 inch (3 sections) = £21.40. 1 colostomy night belt (net or rayon, no hole, for use with dressing pad), = £12.40. 4 inch ostomy belt with groin strap = £13.20; with lace fastenings = £14.00; with wire spring = £12.90; double zip panel = £6.70

Simcare
Belts. Net price 25 mm web and elastic belt (WL002 range) = £8.59; 51 mm = £10.02; 75 mm = £11.44; (WL008) 25 mm = £9.39; 1 belt, child (25 mm) = £7.22, 38 mm = £10.07. 1 web end belt with buckle (short) = £5.80. 1 narrow belt (flange diameter: 32, 38, or 51 mm) = £17.86. 1 Leno belt (white with Velcro fastening, flange diameter: 38 mm) = £17.86. 1 Redifit adjustable belt (small, medium, or large) = £7.22. 1 non-slip belt = £14.72; 1 elastic non-slip belt = £10.07. 1 rubber belt ('sausage' or tubular) = £18.75; 1 narrow belt = £5.45. 1 two-way stretch night belt (small, medium, large, or extra-large) = £20.12. 1 stoma belt (small: 17–26 inch or medium: 26–43 inch) = £4.77. 1 Carshalton® belt (small, medium, or large) = £7.62

Simpla
Belt. Net price 1 belt/collar = £3.40

Steeper
Belts. Made to measure, all sizes. Net price 1 day belt = £37.76; 1 night belt = £27.80. 1 nylon elastic colostomy belt, with hook and eye fastening and 2 pairs or suspenders or understraps = £39.00. 1 two-way stretch pull-on elastic belt = £10.61; 1 adjustable belt with buckle fastening and celluloid hook ends = £8.04; 1 belt with double waistband and cellulosed hook ends = £8.04. 1 rubber adjustable belt with window = £10.72. 1 wide rubberised ileostomy belt with 2 straps and buttonholed ends for use with ileostomy boxes or with celluoid hook ends for use with ileostomy bags = £22.15. 1 belt with understraps or suspenders = £24.91. 1 window = £4.15. 1 colostomy belt, with 2 pairs or understraps or suspenders (Gabriel®) = £44.08

Ward
Belts. Net price 1 web and elastic belt with button and buckle fastening, (1 inch) = £6.35; 2 inch = £8.17; 3 inch = £9.30. 1 colostomy/ileostomy bath belt = £14.57. 1 plastic elastic belt with hook end = £8.85

FILTERS AND BRIDGES

Filters
Available from *CliniMed* (Biotrol®, 50 filters = £10.10), *Coloplast* (Filtrodor®, 50 filters = £16.50; Maclet®, 20 filter washers = £23.00), *ConvaTec* (Surgicaire System® 2 for closed pouches, 30 filters = £7.02), *Cuxson* (50 patches = £2.75), *Hollister* (replacement filter elements for series 366 drainable bags, 20 = £2.52, 100 = £12.62), *Simcare* (for Beta® and mini bags, 20 = £6.08; Doublesure®, 10 filters = £2.89)

Bridges
Available from *Salts* (20 metal bridges ready fixed to lightweight and LWU disposable bags = £7.72; 30 bridges for use with other disposable bags = £11.59), *Simcare* (20 bridges = £2.58)

FLANGES

Body's Care
Flanges. Net price 1 St Mark's soft rubber = £10.99

Bullen
Flanges. Net price 1 lightweight, plastic flange (small, medium, or large) = £3.42. 1 flange for Lenbul® pouches (1 inch diameter, 2 inch base) = £8.42; 1.5 inch diameter, 3 inch base £12.42; 2 inch diameter, 4 inch base = £14.50

DePuy
Flanges. Net price 1 Ileo B® standard rubber flange (0.75, 1, 1.25, 1.375, 1.5 inch) = £8.00. For Schacht® pouches, 1 flange (with locking ring) = £5.10; 1 ileo flange (with locking ring) = £5.10. For Slimline® pouches, 1 padded flange = £4.00

Drew
Flange. Net price 1 kapok flange (1–1.5 inch) = £13.48

Rüsch
Flange. Net price 2 Birkbeck® white rubber flanges (75 mm base, 16 mm deep, 20 mm diameter); 90 mm base, 16 mm deep, 38 mm diameter; 110 mm base, 16 mm deep, 58 mm diameter = £19.92; in two rubbers with hard centre (76 mm base, 10 or 16 mm deep, 32 or 38 mm diameter), 2 flanges = £29.86; 76 mm base, 13 or 16 mm deep, 25 mm diameter, 2 flanges = £29.86; 102 mm base, 16 mm deep, 44 or 51 mm diameter = £29.86: in soft honey coloured rubber (51 or 76 mm base, 13 mm deep, 25 mm diameter) = £17.41; (76 mm base, 10 or 16 mm deep, 32 or 38 mm diameter) = £17.41; 102 mm base, 16 mm deep, 44 or 51 mm diameter = £17.41; with diaphragm, cowl, or dressing retainer at extra cost = £2.88: black, firm rubber (51 mm base, 13 mm deep, 25 mm diameter) = £19.92; (76 mm base, 10 or 16 mm deep, 32 or 38 mm diameter) = £19.92; 102 mm base, 16 mm deep, 44 or 51 mm diameter = £19.92

Salts
Flange. Net price 1 flange (SF1, soft rubber, 25 mm) = £6.13; SF2, semi-rigid, 25 mm = £9.70; SF3, hard rubber, 25 mm = £7.00; SF4, soft rubber, 38 mm = £6.13; SF5, semi-rigid, 38 mm = £10.50; SF6, semi-rigid, hard rubber = £7.00; SF7, soft rubber, 51 mm = £7.71; SF8R, flexible, recessed, 32 mm = £9.70. 1 baby flange with diaphragm (19 mm) = £8.15. 1 Latex® foam diaphragm flange = £34.33; 1 sheath for use with flange = £5.72. For Salger® pouches, 1 polythene flange (40 or 57 mm) = £1.73

Shannon
Flange ring. Net price 1 = £2.04

Shaw
Flange. Net price 1 rubber, adhesive = £4.80; rubber, non-stick = £5.90; with diaphragm = £7.60; non-stick inner diaphragm £2.30; 1 colostomy rubber foam facepiece (face hole diameter: 1.75, 2. 2.5, or 3 inch) = £8.85

Simcare
Flange. Net price 1 rubber flange (16 mm deep, 38 mm diameter) = £13.62; double base hole (38 mm diameter) = £18.05; blue rubber (51 mm base, 13 mm deep, 25 mm diameter or 76 mm base, 10 or 16 mm deep, 38 mm diameter) = £12.31; blue and brown, (76 mm base, 13 mm deep, 25 mm diameter; 10 or 16 mm deep, 38 mm diameter) = £17.89. 1 belt flange (19, 25, 32, 38, 44, 51, or 64 mm) = 22p. For Chiron® pouches, 1 flange (10 or 16 mm deep, 38 mm

1.8 Stoma care

diameter) = £13.62; 13 mm deep, 25 mm diameter = £13.62; 16 mm deep, 32 mm diameter = £13.62; plastic without diaphragm (13 mm deep, 32 or 38 mm diameter) = £6.81. For Redifit® pouches, 1 belt flange = 54p; (1 flange (51 mm base, 13 mm deep, 25 mm diameter, 76 mm base: 13 mm deep, 25 mm diameter; 10 or 16 mm deep, 32 mm diameter; 10 or 16 mm deep, 38 mm diameter; 102 mm base: 16 mm deep, 44 or 51 mm diameter) = £11.60: with dressing retainer or with 16 mm canopy, 38 mm = £14.51

Ward
Flange. Net price 1 plastic/rubber air-filled flange = £14.45; 1 St Mark's standard = £9.49; 1 St Mark's with diaphragm = £11.58

IRRIGATION AND WASH-OUT APPLIANCES

Available from *Astra Meditec* (Medena® 5 ileostomy catheters = £4.15), *Cambmac* (1 water container = £14.54; 1 clamp = £6.30; 1 cone = £9.34; 1 brush = £1.58; 1 tube = £1.10; 1 belt = £30.08; Irradrain® with ring holder for silicone ring, 20 = £18.59 or adhesive, 20 = £18.59; silicone ring, 1 = £3.73; *CliniMed* (Biotrol®, 50 irrigation sleeves = £32.40 or 1 cone = £2.30), *Coloplast* (30 disposable sleeves (1540 or 1560) = £27.30; 1 colotip = £5.16; 1 irrigator bag = £9.75; 1 supporting plate = £4.90; 1 irrigation belt = £4.78), *Hollister* (irrigation drain for use with Guardian® Two-Piece system, 5 (flange: 38, 51, 64, or 102 mm) = £5.50; 1 stoma cone/irrigator kit = £16.61; 20 irrigator drains = £23.24; 10 replacement cones = £58.91; 1 = £7.20; 1 stoma lubricant = £4.08), *Ward* (1 wash-out cup = £23.40; 1 cap = £1.25; 1 belt = £6.77; 1 tube = £4.41)

PRESSURE PLATES, SHIELDS

Available from *Body's Care* (St Mark's, 4 inch shield = £6.58; with rubber ring = £7.68), *Coloplast* (1 supporting plate = £4.90), *DePuy* (5 slimline rubber retaining rings = £2.75), *Drew* pressure plate (oval or round) = £2.58; pressure plate (4 slot) = £3.87; *Salts* (plastic retaining shield, single = £2.73, double = £4.21, large = £4.21; S S Wire retaining ring, large = £2.73, medium = £2.60, small = £2.53; light white anti-sag ring = £1.09, for belt use = £1.23, for velcro belt fastening = £1.40; convex plate for light white bag (32, 38, or 44 mm), 5 = £11.72; pressure plate for Kombo®, Simplicity®, or Solo® pouches (30, 40, 50, or 60 mm) = £1.70; Eakin® support frame (32, 45, 64, or 90 mm) = £1.11, *Shannon* (faceplate = £6.90), *Simcare* (plastic pressure plates, Surrey model: 25 or 32 mm or Standard model with attached flange for use with lightweight bags: 25, 32, or 38 mm = £6.13; stainless wire pressure frame, hook, lug, to fit 25, 32, 38, 44, or 51 mm flange) = £7.48; cotton facepiece = £18.60; pressure plates (25, 32, or 38 mm) = £4.24, *Ward* (celluloid colostomy cup with sponge or solid rim, small, medium, or large = £29.75, with sponge rubber or solid rim, belt fitting = £33.95; St Mark's shield, celluloid with 4 studs = £6.47)

SKIN PROTECTIVES, FILLERS, CLEANSERS

Balspray® (Bullen)
Aerosol. Net price 1 unit = £6.42
Bullen Karaya Gum Powder® (Bullen)
Powder. Net price 70 g = £4.14
Cambmac® (Cambmac)
Karaya paste. Net price 50 g = £2.18
Soft paste. Net price 50 g = £2.60

Chiron® (Simcare)
Barrier cream (with antiseptic). Net price 52 g = £4.12
CliniShield Barrier Wipes® (CliniMed)
Barrier wipes. Net price 50 = £10.35
Comfeel® (Coloplast)
Barrier cream. Net price 60 g = £3.30
Protective film. Net price 30 sachets = £7.80; applicator = £3.64
Derma-gard® (Simcare)
Protective skin wipes. Net price 50 = £12.07
Hollister® (Hollister)
Karaya paste. Net price 128 g = £6.00
Do not apply to severely excoriated skin
Karaya powder. Net price 71 g = £7.12
Skin gel. Net price 28 g = £5.21. Label: 15
Do not apply to severely excoriated skin
Orabase® (ConvaTec)
Paste, see section 12.3.1
Orahesive® (ConvaTec)
Powder (with adherent properties), see section 12.3.1
Saltair® (Salts)
Karaya gum powder. Net price per puffer pack = £3.81
Ostomy cleansing soap (soap spirit). Net price 110-mL = £2.29
Skin prep wipes. Net price 50 = £12.47
Simcare® (Simcare)
Karaya gel. Net price 35 g = £4.94
Karaya gum powder. Net price 100 g = £5.81
Karaya gum sheet. Net price 1 = £5.82
Simpla® (Simpla)
Gel. Net price 35 g = £5.44
Stomahesive® (ConvaTec)
Paste. Net price 60 g = £5.79. For filling and sealing skin creases
Stomobar® (DePuy)
Barrier cream. Net price 20 g = £1.90
Stomosol® (DePuy)
Deodorising antiseptic liquid. Dilute before use. Net price 200 mL = £4.12
Skin shield. Net price 50 = £7.45
Translet® (Rüsch)
Barrier cream. Net price 51 g = £2.64
Wipes. Net price 30 = £5.24
United Skin Barrier Paste® (Salt)
Paste. Net price 70 g = £5.78

SKIN PROTECTORS

Bullen
Karaya gum washers, regular or extra hard. Net price 10 washers (2 inch diameter: 2 × 0.875 inch or 2 × 1.125 inch hole) = £11.24; 2.5 inch diameter: regular 2.5 × 1.25 inch or extra hard 2.5 × 1.5 inch hole = £13.03; 3 inch diameter: 3 × 0.875 inch, 3 × 1.125 inch, 3 × 1.5 inch, or 3 × 2 inch hole = £14.94

Cambmac
Karaya rings. Net price 25 rings (22, 25, 32, 38, 50 or 63 mm) = £34.65

CliniMed
Biotrol® skin protectors. Net price 20 × 20 cm, 5 = £34.00; 10 × 10 cm or 10 cm diameter, 10 = £14.20

Coloplast
Protectives. Net price 10 non-sterile sheets (10 × 10 cm) = £17.60; 5 (15 × 15 cm) = £20.40; 5 (20 × 20 cm) = £37.10; 30 rings (10, 15, 20, 25, 30, 40, 50 mm) = £29.40

ConvaTec
Wafers. Net price 5 Stomahesive® wafers (100 × 100 mm) = £8.63; 3 (200 × 200 mm) = £21.06; 10 Varihesive® wafers (100 × 100 mm) = £7.40

DePuy
Schachtrings. Net price 10 foam, colostomy or ileostomy rings = £7.50

Cautionary label wordings, see inside back cover   Prices are **net**, see p. 1

Chapter 1: Gastro-intestinal system

Drew
Washers. Net price 20 K Seal® karaya gum washers (small) = £8.53; large = £9.71
Hollister
Skin barrier. Net price 5 Hollister® skin barriers (4 × 4 inch) = £9.02; 5 (8 × 8 inch) = £27.33
Salts
Protectors. Net price 10 karaya gum washers (small) = £6.54; 10 (large) = £10.65; 5 foam cushions (25, 32, 38, or 51 mm) = £2.16; 5 dri pads (40 mm) = £2.19; 20 Cohesive® washers (small: 50 mm) = £27.69; 10 (large: 95 mm) = £18.32; 10 Realistic® washers (13, 19, 22, 25, 29, 32, or 38 mm) = £13.32; 1 Saltair® twinpack (small) = £8.00; large = £11.20; 10 foam seals (as in twin packs) = £1.64; 5 United® skin barrier wafers (10 × 10 cm) = £8.68; 3 = £20.43; for Salger® pouches, 5 karaya washers with foam (40 or 57 mm) = £11.34
Shannon
Protectors. Net price 1 foam sponge ring = 67p; 10 Kaygee® washers (2.5 inch base: 0.875 or 1.125 inch hole or 2.75 inch base: 0.875 or 1.375 inch hole) = £6.05
Shaw
Protectors. Net price 5 Body Mould® squares (1, 1.25, or 1.5 inch hole) = £8.90; 10 washers (1 or 1.25 inch hole) = £8.20; 5 rings (1, 1.25, or 1.5 inch hole) = £8.20; 12 Healwell® squares (1, 1.25 or 1.5 inch hole) = £8.40; 12 rings (1, 1.25 or 1.5 inch hole) = £7.25; 12 rings (5 × 5 inch: 1, 1.25 or 1.5 inch hole) = £10.19
Simcare
Protectors. Net price 5 foam pads, white (76 mm diameter: 25 mm hole) = £3.94; 76 mm diameter: 29, 32, or 38 mm hole or 90 mm diameter: 32 or 38 mm = £5.39; black (25 mm hole) = £5.05; 1 karaya gum sheet (300 × 100 mm) = £5.82; 20 rings (19, 25, 32, 38, or 44 mm) = £19.39; karaya rings (19, 25, 32, 38, or 51 mm) = £21.20; 10 Down's® adhesive karaya gum washers (51 mm base: 22 or 29 mm hole) = £9.44; 70 mm base: 22 or 29 mm hole = £11.64; 10 Redifit® karaya gum washers (25, 32, 38, 44, or 51 mm) = £11.64; 20 Seel-a-peel® squares (100 mm sq) = £33.17; 5 squares (150 mm sq) = £20.43
Simpla
Wafers. Net price 10 Simplaseel® wafers (100 × 100 mm) = £15.58

STOMA CAPS AND DRESSINGS

Available from *Bullen* (1 stoma cap = £4.02), *Cambmac* (50 Dansac® Mini caps (30 or 44 mm) = £46.52), *Coloplast* (100 Colocap® stomacaps = £92.00), *ConvaTec* (Colodress®, 30 stoma caps (19 mm hole cut-to-size) = £28.08, *Hollister* (50 stoma caps (51 or 76 mm) = £48.87), *Salts* (Palex® mini, 30 stoma caps = £25.97; 30 stoma caps for Simplicity 1® pouches = £29.26), *Simcare* (20 leisure pouches = £19.65), *Steeper* (1 celluloid colostomy shield, 10 cm with 4 studs = £4.35; 12 waterproof material squares for use with colostomy dressings (16.5 × 16.5 cm) = £2.93; 1 celluloid colostomy cup with solid rim and 4 studs = £18.54; 1 celluloid cup with 4 studs and chute = £22.31; 1 zip fastener fitted to colostomy belt = £7.29; 1 waterproof front fitted to colostomy belt = £6.01; 1 pair woven understraps with buttonholed ends = £2.79; 1 sq yd waterproof material = £2.84; 1 Donald Rose® ileostomy/colostomy bath belt with internal chamber for dressings and stud fastenings for adjustment = £18.07)

TUBING

Available from *Hollister* (10 urostomy drain tubes = £20.60; 8 tubes for fitting to Lo-Profile® urostomy bags = £19.16; for Premium® urostomy pouches, 10 drain tube adaptors = £16.41), *Salts* (2 night tube adaptors = 82p), *Simcare* (for Carshalton® urostomy pouches, 10 connectors = £3.40), *Steeper* (1 metal spring tubing clip = £2.03)

1.9 Drugs affecting intestinal secretions

1.9.1 Drugs acting on the gall bladder
1.9.2 Drugs which increase gastric acidity
1.9.3 Aprotinin
1.9.4 Pancreatin

1.9.1 Drugs acting on the gall bladder

The bile acids **chenodeoxycholic** or **ursodeoxycholic acid** are used in selected patients to dissolve cholesterol gallstones as an alternative to surgery. They are only suitable for patients who have mild symptoms, unimpaired gall bladder function, and small or medium sized radiolucent stones; they are not suitable for radio-opaque stones, which are unlikely to be dissolved. Patients should preferably be supervised in hospital because radiological monitoring is required. Long-term prophylaxis may be needed after complete dissolution of the gallstones has been confirmed (preferably with cholecystograms and ultrasound on two separate occasions) as gallstones may recur in up to 25% of patients within one year of stopping treatment.

Dehydrocholic acid is used to improve biliary drainage by stimulating the secretion of thin watery bile. It is given after surgery of the biliary tract to flush the common duct and drainage tube and wash away small calculi obstructing flow through the common bile duct but its value has not been established.

A **terpene** mixture (Rowachol®) also raises biliary cholesterol solubility. It is less effective than the bile acids but may be a useful adjunct.

CHENODEOXYCHOLIC ACID

Indications; Cautions: see notes above
Contra-indications: do not use when stones are radio-opaque, in pregnancy, in non-functioning gall bladders, in chronic liver disease, and inflammatory diseases of the small intestine and colon
Side-effects: diarrhoea particularly initially with high dosage (reduce dose for few days), pruritus, minor hepatic abnormalities and transient rise in serum transaminases
Dose: 10–15 mg/kg daily as a single dose at bedtime *or* in divided doses for 3–24 months, depending on size of stone; treatment is continued for 3 months after stones dissolve

PoM **Chendol**® (CP)
Capsules, orange/white, chenodeoxycholic acid 125 mg. Net price 224-cap pack = £48.50
Tablets, orange, f/c, scored, chenodeoxycholic acid 250 mg. Net price 112-tab pack = £47.50

1.9 Drugs affecting intestinal secretions

PoM Chenofalk® (Thames)
Capsules, chenodeoxycholic acid 250 mg. Net price 60 = £22.50
Additives: include gluten

PoM Lithofalk® (Thames)
Tablets, scored, chenodeoxycholic acid 250 mg, ursodeoxycholic acid 250 mg. Net price 60-tab pack = £49.95
Dose: 2 tablets (patients over 80 kg, 3 tablets) daily as a single dose at bedtime for 6–24 months, discontinuing treatment after 12 months if no reduction in size of stone; treatment is continued for 4–12 weeks after stones dissolved

---

DEHYDROCHOLIC ACID
Indications: see notes above
Contra-indications: complete mechanical biliary obstruction and occlusive hepatitis, chronic liver disease
Dose: 250–750 mg, 3 times daily
Cholecystography, 500–750 mg every 4 hours for 12 hours before and after the examination

Dehydrocholic Acid (Non-proprietary)
Tablets, dehydrocholic acid 250 mg. Net price 20 = £8.44

URSODEOXYCHOLIC ACID
Indications; Cautions; Contra-indications: see under Chenodeoxycholic Acid
Side-effects: see under Chenodeoxycholic Acid; diarrhoea occurs rarely; liver changes have not been reported
Dose: 8–12 mg/kg (obese patients up to 15 mg/kg) daily as a single dose at bedtime or in divided doses, for up to 2 years; treatment is continued for 3–4 months after stones dissolve

PoM Destolit® (Merrell)
Tablets, scored, ursodeoxycholic acid 150 mg. Net price 60 = £19.40. Label: 21
PoM Ursofalk® (Thames)
Capsules, ursodeoxycholic acid 250 mg. Net price 60 = £31.50. Label: 21
Additives: include gluten

With chenodeoxycholic acid
See under Chenodeoxycholic acid

OTHER PREPARATIONS FOR BILIARY DISORDERS

PoM Rowachol® (Monmouth)
Capsules, green, e/c, borneol 5 mg, camphene 5 mg, cineole 2 mg, menthol 32 mg, menthone 6 mg, pinene 17 mg in olive oil. Net price 50-cap pack = £7.54. Label: 22
Dose: 1–2 capsules 3 times daily before food
Interactions: Appendix 1 (*Rowachol®*)

1.9.2 Drugs which increase gastric acidity

Muripsin® is used in achlorhydria and hypochlorhydria but is of uncertain value; it replaced dilute hydrochloric acid.

Muripsin® (Norgine)
Tablets, orange, f/c, glutamic acid hydrochloride 500 mg: 1 tablet ≈ 1 mL dilute hydrochloric acid. Net price 50 = £5.28. Label: 21
Dose: 1–2 tablets with meals

1.9.3 Aprotinin
Now in section 2.11.

1.9.4 Pancreatin

Supplements of pancreatin are given by mouth to compensate for reduced or absent exocrine secretion in cystic fibrosis, and following pancreatectomy, total gastrectomy, or chronic pancreatitis. They assist the digestion of starch, fat, and protein.

Pancreatin is inactivated by gastric acid therefore pancreatin preparations are best taken with food (or immediately before or after food). Gastric acid secretion may be reduced by giving cimetidine or ranitidine an hour beforehand (section 1.3). Concurrent use of antacids also reduces gastric acidity. The newer enteric-coated preparations such as Creon®, Nutrizym GR®, and Pancrease® deliver a higher enzyme concentration in the duodenum (providing the granules are swallowed whole without chewing).

Since pancreatin is also inactivated by heat, excessive heat should be avoided if preparations are mixed with liquids or food; the resulting mixtures should not be kept for more than one hour.

Dosage is adjusted according to size, number, and consistency of stools, so that the patient thrives; extra allowance may be needed if snacks are taken between meals.

Pancreatin may irritate the skin around mouth and anus, particularly if preparations are retained in the mouth or dosage is excessive. Hypersensitivity reactions occur occasionally and may affect those handling the powder.

For reference to acetylcysteine in cystic fibrosis, see Acetylcysteine Granules (section 3.7).

PANCREATIN
Indications; Cautions; Side-effects: see above
Dose: see below

Creon® (Duphar)
Capsules, brown/yellow, enclosing buff-coloured e/c granules of pancreatin, providing: protease 210 units, lipase 8000 units, amylase 9000 units. Net price 100 = £13.33. Counselling, see dose
Dose: initially 1–2 capsules with meals either taken whole or contents mixed with fluid or soft food (then swallowed immediately without chewing); usual range 5–15 capsules daily

Capsules '25000', orange/yellow, enclosing brown-coloured e/c pellets of pancreatin, providing: protease 1000 units, lipase 25 000 units, amylase 18 000 units. Net price 50-cap pack = £19.50. Counselling, see dose

Dose: initially 1 capsule with meals either taken whole or contents mixed with fluid or soft food (then swallowed immediately without chewing); dosage adjusted according to response

Nutrizym® GR (Merck)
Capsules, green/orange, enclosing e/c pellets of pancreatin, providing minimum of: protease 650 units, lipase 10 000 units, amylase 10 000 units. Net price 100 = £12.52. Counselling, see dose

Dose: 1–2 capsules with meals swallowed whole or contents sprinkled on soft food (then swallowed immediately without chewing); dosage may be increased in severe cases

Pancrease® (Cilag)
Capsules, enclosing e/c beads of pancreatin, providing minimum of: protease 330 units, lipase 5000 units, amylase 2900 units. Net price 100 = £17.07. Counselling, see dose

Dose: 1–2 (occasionally 3) capsules during each meal and 1 capsule with snacks swallowed whole or contents sprinkled on liquid or soft food (then swallowed immediately without chewing)

Pancrex® (Paines & Byrne)
Granules, pancreatin, providing minimum of: protease 300 units, lipase 5000 units, amylase 4000 units/g. Net price 100 g = £7.15, 500 g = £28.61. Label: 25, counselling, see dose

Dose: 5–10 g 4 times daily with meals washed down or mixed with liquid

Pancrex V® (Paines & Byrne)
Capsules, pancreatin, providing minimum of: protease 430 units, lipase 8000 units, amylase 9000 units. Net price 100 = £4.29. Counselling, see dose

Dose: up to 1 year 1–2 capsules mixed with feeds; adults and children over 1 year 2–6 capsules 4 times daily with meals, swallowed whole or sprinkled on food

Capsules '125', pancreatin, providing minimum of: protease 160 units, lipase 2950 units, amylase 3300 units. Net price 50 = £1.63. Counselling, see dose

Dose: NEONATE 1–2 capsules with feeds

Tablets, e/c, s/c, pancreatin, providing minimum of: protease 110 units, lipase 1900 units, amylase 1700 units. Net price 100 = £1.43. Label: 5, 25, counselling, see dose

Dose: 5–15 tablets 4 times daily before meals

Tablets forte, e/c, s/c, pancreatin, providing minimum of: protease 330 units, lipase 5600 units, amylase 5000 units. Net price 100 = £3.72. Label: 5, 25, counselling, see dose

Dose: 6–10 tablets 4 times daily before meals

Powder, pancreatin, providing minimum of: protease 1400 units, lipase 25 000 units, amylase 30 000 units/g. Net price 100 g = £9.75, 250 g = £20.76. Counselling, see dose

Dose: 0.5–2 g 4 times daily washed down or mixed with liquid

2: Drugs used in the treatment of diseases of the
CARDIOVASCULAR SYSTEM

In this chapter, drug treatment is discussed under the following headings:

2.1 Positive inotropic drugs
2.2 Diuretics
2.3 Anti-arrhythmic drugs
2.4 Beta-adrenoceptor blocking drugs
2.5 Antihypertensive therapy
2.6 Nitrates and calcium-channel blockers
2.7 Sympathomimetics
2.8 Anticoagulants and Protamine
2.9 Antiplatelet drugs
2.10 Fibrinolytic drugs
2.11 Antifibrinolytic drugs and haemostatics
2.12 Lipid-lowering drugs
2.13 Local sclerosants

2.1 Positive inotropic drugs

2.1.1 Cardiac glycosides
2.1.2 Phosphodiesterase inhibitors

Positive inotropic drugs increase the force of contraction of the myocardium; for sympathomimetics with inotropic activity see section 2.7.1.

2.1.1 Cardiac glycosides

The principal actions of the cardiac glycosides are an increase in the force of myocardial contraction and a reduction in the conductivity of the heart. They are most useful in the treatment of *supraventricular tachycardias*, especially for controlling ventricular response in atrial fibrillation. *Heart failure* may also be improved, even in patients in sinus rhythm, because of changes in the availability of intracellular calcium; this action is relatively unimportant, however, compared with effects that can be achieved with diuretics and vasodilators. Except when needed to maintain satisfactory rhythm, cardiac glycosides can often be withdrawn from patients with heart failure that is well controlled, without clinical deterioration. In the elderly who are particularly susceptible to digitalis toxicity, cardiac glycosides should be used with special care in the management of heart failure without atrial fibrillation.

Loss of appetite, nausea, and vomiting are common toxic effects; sinus bradycardia, atrioventricular block, ventricular extrasystoles, and sometimes ventricular tachycardia or atrial tachycardia with block also occur—especially in the presence of underlying conducting system defects or myocardial disease. These unwanted effects depend both on the plasma concentrations of the drugs and on the sensitivity of the conducting system or myocardium, which is often increased in heart disease. Thus, no one plasma concentration can indicate toxicity reliably but the likelihood increases progressively through the range 1.5 to 3 micrograms/litre for digoxin; higher steady-state concentrations must certainly be avoided. Measurements of plasma concentration are not necessary, however, unless problems occur during maintenance treatment. Hypokalaemia predisposes to toxicity, therefore diuretics used with digoxin should either be potassium sparing or should be given with potassium supplements.

Renal function is the most important determinant of digoxin dosage, whereas elimination of digitoxin depends on metabolism by the liver. Toxicity can often be managed by discontinuing therapy and correcting hypokalaemia if appropriate; serious manifestations require urgent specialist management. Digoxin-specific antibody fragments are available for reversal of life-threatening overdosage (see next page).

Digoxin is the glycoside most commonly used. In patients with *mild failure* a loading dose is not required, and a satisfactory plasma concentration can be achieved over a period of about a week, using a dose of 125 to 250 micrograms twice a day which may then be reduced having special regard to renal function. Because it has a long half-life maintenance doses need only be given once daily (but higher doses should be divided to avoid nausea). For management of *atrial fibrillation* the maintenance dose can usually be governed by ventricular response which should not be allowed to fall below 60 beats per minute except in special and recognised circumstances, e.g. with the concomitant administration of beta-blockers.

When *very rapid control* is needed, digoxin may be given intravenously in a digitalising dose of 0.75 to 1 mg, preferably as an infusion (suggested volume 50 mL) over two or more hours, followed by normal maintenance therapy. The intramuscular route is not recommended, except when other methods of administration are not available.

Digitoxin has a long half-life and maintenance doses, again, need only be given once daily.

CHILDREN. The dose is based on body-weight; they require a relatively larger dose of digoxin than adults.

DIGOXIN

Indications: heart failure, supraventricular arrhythmias (particularly atrial fibrillation)
Cautions: recent infarction, hypothyroidism; reduce dose in the elderly and in renal impairment; avoid hypokalaemia; **interactions:** Appendix 1 (cardiac glycosides)
Contra-indications: supraventricular arrhythmias caused by Wolff-Parkinson-White syndrome
Side-effects: anorexia, nausea, vomiting, diarrhoea, abdominal pain; visual disturbances, headache, fatigue, drowsiness, confusion, delirium, hallucinations; arrhythmias, heart block; see also notes above

Cautionary label wordings, see inside back cover   Prices are **net**, see p. 1

Dose: by mouth, rapid digitalisation, 1–1.5 mg in divided doses over 24 hours; less urgent digitalisation, 250–500 micrograms daily (higher dose divided)
Maintenance, 62.5–500 micrograms daily (higher dose divided) according to renal function and, in atrial fibrillation, on heart-rate response; usual range, 125–250 micrograms daily (elderly 125 micrograms)
For intravenous doses, see notes above
Note. For plasma concentration monitoring blood should ideally be taken at least 6 hours after a dose

PoM **Digoxin** (Non-proprietary)
Tablets, digoxin 62.5 micrograms, net price 20 = 9p; 125 micrograms, 20 = 6p; 250 micrograms, 20 = 9p
Injection, digoxin 250 micrograms/mL, see Lanoxin®
Paediatric injection, digoxin 100 micrograms/mL (hosp. only, available from Boots)
PoM **Lanoxin**® (Wellcome)
Tablets, digoxin 125 micrograms, net price 20 = 32p; 250 micrograms (scored), 20 = 28p
Injection, digoxin 250 micrograms/mL. Net price 2-mL amp = 65p

PoM **Lanoxin-PG**® (Wellcome)
Tablets, blue, digoxin 62.5 micrograms. Net price 20 = 32p
Elixir, yellow, digoxin 50 micrograms/mL. Do not dilute, measure with pipette. Net price 60 mL = £5.23. Counselling, use of pipette

DIGITOXIN

Indications: heart failure, supraventricular arrhythmias (particularly atrial fibrillation)
Cautions; Contra-indications; Side-effects: see under Digoxin
Dose: maintenance, 50–200 micrograms daily

PoM **Digitoxin** (Evans)
Tablets, digitoxin 100 micrograms, net price 20 = 50p

DIGOXIN-SPECIFIC ANTIBODY

PoM **Digibind**® (Wellcome)
Injection, powder for preparation of infusion, digoxin-specific antibody fragments (F(ab)) 40 mg. Net price per vial = £87.44
For reversal of life-threatening manifestations of intoxication by digoxin; although designed specifically to treat digoxin overdose has successfully reversed digitoxin overdose

2.1.2 Phosphodiesterase inhibitors

Enoximone and milrinone are selective phosphodiesterase inhibitors which exert most of their effect on the myocardium. Sustained haemodynamic benefit has been observed after administration, but as yet there is no conclusive evidence of any beneficial effect on survival.

ENOXIMONE

Indications: congestive heart failure where cardiac output reduced and filling pressures increased
Cautions: heart failure associated with hypertrophic cardiomyopathy, stenotic or obstructive valvular disease or other outlet obstruction; monitor blood pressure, heart rate, ECG, central venous pressure, fluid and electrolyte status, platelet count, hepatic enzymes; reduce dose in renal impairment; avoid extravasation
Side-effects: ectopic beats; less frequently ventricular tachycardia or supraventricular arrhythmias (more likely in patients with pre-existing arrhythmias); hypotension; also headache, insomnia, nausea and vomiting, diarrhoea; occasionally, chills, oliguria, fever, urinary retention; upper and lower limb pain
Dose: by slow intravenous injection (rate not exceeding 12.5 mg/minute), diluted before use, initially 0.5–1 mg/kg, then 500 micrograms/kg every 30 minutes until satisfactory response or total of 3 mg/kg given; maintenance, initial dose of up to 3 mg/kg may be repeated every 3–6 hours as required
By intravenous infusion, initially 90 micrograms/kg/minute over 10–30 minutes, followed by continuous or intermittent infusion of 5–20 micrograms/kg/minute
Total dose over 24 hours should not normally exceed 24 mg/kg

PoM **Perfan**® (Merrell)
Injection, enoximone 5 mg/mL. For dilution before use. Net price 20-mL amp = £15.40
Note. Plastic apparatus should be used; crystal formation if glass used

MILRINONE

Indications: short-term treatment of severe congestive heart failure unresponsive to conventional maintenance therapy (not immediately after myocardial infarction); acute heart failure, including low output states, following heart surgery
Cautions; Side-effects: see under Enoximone; also correct hypokalaemia, monitor renal function, chest pain reported
Dose: by slow intravenous injection (over 10 minutes), 50 micrograms/kg followed by *intravenous infusion* at a rate of 375–750 nanograms/kg/minute, usually for up to 12 hours following surgery or for 48–72 hours in congestive heart failure; max. daily dose 1.13 mg/kg

PoM **Primacor**® (Sanofi Winthrop)
Injection, milrinone (as lactate) 1 mg/mL. For dilution before use. Net price 10-mL amp = £16.22

2.2 Diuretics

2.2.1 Thiazides and related diuretics
2.2.2 Loop diuretics
2.2.3 Potassium-sparing diuretics
2.2.4 Potassium-sparing diuretics with other diuretics
2.2.5 Osmotic diuretics
2.2.6 Mercurial diuretics
2.2.7 Carbonic anhydrase inhibitors
2.2.8 Diuretics with potassium

Thiazides (section 2.2.1) are used to relieve oedema due to *heart failure* and, in lower doses, to reduce *blood pressure*.

Loop diuretics (section 2.2.2) are used in pulmonary oedema due to *left ventricular failure* and in patients with *longstanding heart failure* who no longer respond to thiazides.

Combination diuretic therapy may be effective in patients with oedema resistant to treatment with one diuretic. For example, a loop diuretic may be combined with a potassium-sparing diuretic (section 2.2.3).

The combination of a thiazide with spironolactone is of value in *less severe heart failure* when hypokalaemia is difficult to counter or when any degree of hypokalaemia should be avoided, as in patients with a continuing tendency to life-threatening ventricular arrhythmias.

THE ELDERLY. Diuretics are overprescribed in old age and the elderly are particularly susceptible to many of their side-effects. They should not be used on a long-term basis to treat simple gravitational oedema (which will usually respond to increased movement, raising the legs, and support stockings).

POTASSIUM LOSS. Hypokalaemia may occur with both thiazide and loop diuretics. It is dangerous in severe coronary artery disease and in patients also being treated with cardiac glycosides. Often the use of potassium-sparing diuretics (section 2.2.3) avoids the need to take potassium supplements.

In hepatic failure hypokalaemia caused by diuretics can precipitate encephalopathy, particularly in alcoholic cirrhosis; diuretics may also increase the risk of hypomagnesaemia in alcoholic cirrhosis, leading to arrhythmias.

Potassium supplements are seldom necessary when thiazides are used in the routine treatment of hypertension. For further comment see section 9.2.1.1.

2.2.1 Thiazides and related diuretics

Thiazides and related compounds are moderately potent diuretics; they inhibit sodium reabsorption at the beginning of the distal convoluted tubule. They act within 1 to 2 hours of oral administration and most have a duration of action of 12 to 24 hours; they are usually administered early in the day so that the diuresis does not interfere with sleep.

In the management of *hypertension* a low dose of a thiazide, e.g. bendrofluazide 2.5 mg daily, produces a maximal or near-maximal blood pressure lowering effect, with very little biochemical disturbance. Higher doses cause more marked changes in plasma potassium, uric acid, glucose, and lipids, with no advantage in blood pressure control, and should not be used. Optimum doses for the control of *heart failure* may be larger, and long-term effects are of less importance.

Bendrofluazide is widely used for mild or moderate heart failure when the patient is not desperately ill and severe pulmonary oedema is not present. It is also used for hypertension—alone in the treatment of mild hypertension or with other drugs in more severe hypertension.

Chlorthalidone, a thiazide-related compound, has a longer duration of action than the thiazides and may be given on alternate days to control oedema. It is also useful if acute retention is liable to be precipitated by a more rapid diuresis or if patients dislike the altered pattern of micturition promoted by diuretics.

Other thiazides do not offer any significant advantage over those mentioned above, and newer ones are more expensive than the longer-established thiazides.

Metolazone is particularly effective when combined with a loop diuretic (even in renal failure); profound diuresis may occur therefore the patient should be monitored carefully.

Xipamide resembles chlorthalidone structurally, and is more potent than the other thiazides.

Indapamide is also chemically related to chlorthalidone. It is claimed to lower blood pressure with less metabolic disturbance, particularly less aggravation of diabetes mellitus.

BENDROFLUAZIDE

Indications: oedema, hypertension

Cautions: may cause hypokalaemia, aggravates diabetes and gout; pregnancy (see also Appendix 4) and breast-feeding; renal and hepatic impairment (avoid if severe, see Appendixes 2 and 3); see also notes above; **interactions:** Appendix 1 (diuretics)

Contra-indications: hypercalcaemia, severe renal and hepatic impairment, Addison's disease, porphyria (see section 9.8.2)

Side-effects: impotence (reversible on withdrawal of treatment), hypokalaemia (see also notes above), hypomagnesaemia, hyponatraemia, hypercalcaemia, hypochloraemic alkalosis, hyperuricaemia, gout, hyperglycaemia, and increases in plasma cholesterol concentration; less commonly rashes, photosensitivity, neutropenia, and thrombocytopenia (when given in late pregnancy neonatal thrombocytopenia has been reported)

Dose: oedema, initially 5–10 mg in the morning, daily *or* on alternate days; maintenance 2.5–10 mg 1–3 times weekly

Hypertension, 2.5 mg in the morning; higher doses rarely necessary (see notes above)

PoM Bendrofluazide (Non-proprietary)
Tablets, bendrofluazide 2.5 mg, net price 20 = 13p; 5 mg, 20 = 5p
Available from APS, Berk (Berkozide®), Boots (Aprinox®), Cox, CP, Evans (including Neo-NaClex®, 5 mg only), Kerfoot, Leo (Centyl®)

BENZTHIAZIDE

Cautions; Contra-indications; Side-effects: see under Bendrofluazide

Preparation
Ingredient of Dytide® (section 2.2.4)

CHLOROTHIAZIDE

Indications: oedema, hypertension
Cautions; Contra-indications; Side-effects: see under Bendrofluazide
Dose: oedema, initially 0.5–1 g 1–2 times daily; maintenance 0.5–1 g daily, on alternate days, or less frequently
Hypertension, 0.5–1 g daily in single or divided doses

PoM Saluric® (MSD)
Tablets, scored, chlorothiazide 500 mg. Net price 20 = 46p

CHLORTHALIDONE

Indications: oedema, hypertension; diabetes insipidus (see section 6.5.2)
Cautions; Contra-indications; Side-effects: see under Bendrofluazide
Dose: oedema, initially 50 mg in the morning *or* 100–200 mg on alternate days, reduced for maintenance if possible
Hypertension, 25 mg, increased to 50 mg if necessary, in the morning

PoM Hygroton® (Geigy)
Tablets, yellow, scored, chlorthalidone 50 mg, net price 28-tab pack = £1.19

CLOPAMIDE

Cautions; Contra-indications; Side-effects: see under Bendrofluazide

Preparation
Ingredient of Viskaldix® (see under Pindolol, section 2.4)

CYCLOPENTHIAZIDE

Indications: oedema, hypertension
Cautions; Contra-indications; Side-effects: see under Bendrofluazide
Dose: oedema, initially 0.5–1 mg in the morning; maintenance 500 micrograms on alternate days
Hypertension, 250–500 micrograms in the morning
Max. 1.5 mg daily

PoM Navidrex® (Ciba)
Tablets, scored, cyclopenthiazide 500 micrograms. Net price 28-tab pack = 50p
Additives: include gluten

HYDROCHLOROTHIAZIDE

Indications: oedema, hypertension
Cautions; Contra-indications; Side-effects: see under Bendrofluazide
Dose: oedema, initially 50–100 mg daily; maintenance 25–50 mg on alternate days
Hypertension, 25 mg daily, can be increased to 50–100 mg daily if necessary

PoM Esidrex® (Ciba)
Tablets, both scored, hydrochlorothiazide 25 mg, net price 20 = 57p; 50 mg, 20 = £1.05
Additives: include gluten

PoM HydroSaluric® (MSD)
Tablets, both scored, hydrochlorothiazide 25 mg, net price 20 = 29p; 50 mg, 20 = 54p

HYDROFLUMETHIAZIDE

Indications: oedema, hypertension
Cautions; Contra-indications; Side-effects: see under Bendrofluazide
Dose: oedema, initially 50–200 mg in the morning; maintenance 25–50 mg on alternate days
Hypertension, 25–50 mg daily

PoM Hydrenox® (Boots)
Tablets, hydroflumethiazide 50 mg. Net price 20 = 38p

INDAPAMIDE

Indications: hypertension
Cautions: renal impairment (stop if deterioration); monitor plasma potassium and urate concentrations in elderly, hyperaldosteronism, gout, or with concomitant cardiac glycosides; hyperparathyroidism (discontinue if hypercalcaemia); pregnancy and breast-feeding; **interactions:** Appendix 1 (diuretics)
Contra-indications: recent cerebrovascular accident, severe hepatic impairment
Side-effects: hypokalaemia, headache, dizziness, fatigue, muscular cramps, nausea, anorexia, diarrhoea, constipation, dyspepsia, rashes (erythema multiforme, epidermal necrolysis reported); rarely orthostatic hypotension, metabolic alkalosis, hyperglycaemia, increased plasma urate concentrations, paraesthesia, photosensitivity, impotence, renal impairment, reversible acute myopia; diuresis with doses above 2.5 mg daily
Dose: 2.5 mg daily in the morning

PoM Natrilix® (Servier)
Tablets, pink, s/c, indapamide 2.5 mg. Net price 30-tab pack = £5.96, 60-tab pack = £11.72
Note. Tablets containing indapamide 2.5 mg also available from Ashbourne (Indaxa 2.5®)

MEFRUSIDE

Indications: oedema, hypertension
Cautions; Contra-indications; Side-effects: see under Bendrofluazide
Dose: initially 25–50 mg in the morning, increased to 75–100 mg for oedema; maintenance 25 mg daily *or* on alternate days

2.2 Diuretics

PoM **Baycaron**® (Bayer)
Tablets, scored, mefruside 25 mg. Net price 20 = £1.41

METHYCLOTHIAZIDE
Indications: oedema, hypertension
Cautions; Contra-indications; Side-effects: see under Bendrofluazide
Dose: 2.5–5 mg in the morning, increased to 10 mg daily if required

PoM **Enduron**® (Abbott)
Tablets, pink, scored, methyclothiazide 5 mg. Net price 20 = 41p

METOLAZONE
Indications: oedema, hypertension
Cautions; Contra-indications; Side-effects: see under Bendrofluazide; also profound diuresis on concomitant administration with frusemide (monitor patient carefully)
Dose: see preparations below

PoM **Metenix 5**® (Hoechst)
Tablets, blue, metolazone 5 mg. Net price 20 = £1.75
Dose: oedema, 5–10 mg in the morning, increased if necessary to 20 mg daily in resistant oedema, max. 80 mg daily
Hypertension, initially 5 mg in the morning; maintenance 5 mg on alternate days

Low dose
Note. Xuret® brand of metolazone has a much lower dose than other brands of metolazone. It must therefore be prescribed by brand name and is not interchangeable with other brands of metolazone

PoM **Xuret**® (Galen)
Tablets, metolazone 500 micrograms. Net price 56-tab pack = £6.08
Dose: mild to moderate hypertension, 1 tablet daily in the morning; increased if necessary to 2 tablets daily

POLYTHIAZIDE
Indications: oedema, hypertension
Cautions; Contra-indications; Side-effects: see under Bendrofluazide
Dose: usually 1–4 mg daily; in hypertension 500 micrograms daily may be adequate

PoM **Nephril**® (Pfizer)
Tablets, scored, polythiazide 1 mg. Net price 28-tab pack = 79p

XIPAMIDE
Indications: oedema, hypertension
Cautions; Contra-indications: see under Bendrofluazide
Side-effects: slight gastro-intestinal disturbances; mild dizziness

Dose: oedema, initially 40 mg in the morning, increased to 80 mg in resistant cases; maintenance 20 mg in the morning
Hypertension, usual dose 20 mg in the morning (may be increased to 40 mg if necessary, but not if other antihypertensive therapy being given)

PoM **Diurexan**® (ASTA Medica)
Tablets, scored, xipamide 20 mg. Net price 14-tab pack = £1.97

2.2.2 Loop diuretics

These drugs inhibit resorption from the ascending loop of Henle in the renal tubule and are powerful diuretics. Hypokalaemia may develop, and care is needed to avoid hypotension. If there is an enlarged prostate, urinary retention may occur; this is less likely if small doses and less potent diuretics are used initially.

Frusemide and **bumetanide** are similar in activity; both act within 1 hour of oral administration and diuresis is complete within 6 hours so that, if necessary, they can be given twice in one day without interfering with sleep. Following intravenous administration they have a peak effect within 30 minutes. The degree of diuresis associated with these drugs is dose related. In patients with impaired renal function very large doses may occasionally be needed; in such doses both drugs can cause deafness and bumetanide can cause myalgia.

Ethacrynic acid has a similar onset and duration of action. Gastro-intestinal side-effects are more severe and deafness may occur in patients with renal failure, especially when it is given intravenously.

Piretanide is the newest member of this group; it has properties similar to those of frusemide and bumetanide, but is promoted for the treatment of hypertension.

FRUSEMIDE
Indications: oedema, oliguria due to renal failure
Cautions: pregnancy (see also Appendix 4); may cause hypokalaemia and hyponatraemia; aggravates diabetes mellitus and gout; liver failure, prostatic enlargement; **interactions:** Appendix 1 (diuretics)
Contra-indications: precomatose states associated with liver cirrhosis; porphyria (see section 9.8.2)
Side-effects: hyponatraemia, hypokalaemia (see also section 2.2), hypochloraemic alkalosis, increased calcium excretion, hypotension; less commonly nausea, gastro-intestinal disturbances, hyperuricaemia and gout; hyperglycaemia (less common than with thiazides); temporary increase in plasma cholesterol and triglyceride concentrations; rarely rashes and bone marrow depression (withdraw treatment), pancreatitis (with large parenteral doses), tinnitus and deafness (usually with large parenteral doses and rapid administration and in renal impairment)

Cautionary label wordings, see inside back cover

Prices are **net**, see p. 1

Dose: by mouth, oedema, initially 40 mg in the morning; maintenance 20 mg daily *or* 40 mg on alternate days, increased in resistant oedema to 80 mg daily; CHILD 1–3 mg/kg daily
Oliguria, initially 250 mg daily; if necessary larger doses, increasing in steps of 250 mg, may be given every 4–6 hours to a max. of a single dose of 2 g (rarely used)
By intramuscular injection or slow intravenous injection (rate not exceeding 4 mg/minute), initially 20–50 mg; CHILD 0.5–1.5 mg/kg to a max. daily dose of 20 mg
By intravenous infusion (by syringe pump if necessary), in oliguria, initially 250 mg over 1 hour (rate not exceeding 4 mg/minute), if satisfactory urine output not obtained in the subsequent hour further 500 mg over 2 hours, then if no satisfactory response within subsequent hour, further 1 g over 4 hours, if no response obtained dialysis probably required; effective dose (up to 1 g) can be repeated every 24 hours

PoM **Frusemide** (Non-proprietary)
Tablets, frusemide 20 mg, net price 20 = 29p; 40 mg, 20 = 8p; 500 mg, 20 = £5.99
Various strengths available from APS, Ashbourne (Frumax®), Berk (Dryptal®), Cox, CP (including Rusyde®), Evans, Kerfoot, Norton
Oral solutions, sugar-free, frusemide 1 mg/mL available as Lasix® paediatric liquid; frusemide 4 mg, 8 mg, and 10 mg/mL available from RP Drugs (special order)
Injection, frusemide 10 mg/mL, net price 2-mL amp = 27p
Available from Evans (also 5-mL amp)

PoM **Lasix**® (Hoechst)
Tablets, all scored, frusemide 20 mg, net price 28-tab pack = 84p; 40 mg, 28-tab pack = £1.22; 500 mg (yellow), 20 = £11.74
Paediatric liquid, sugar-free, frusemide 1 mg/mL when reconstituted with purified water, freshly boiled and cooled, net price 150 mL = £1.13
Injection, frusemide 10 mg/mL, net price 2-mL amp = 26p; 5-mL amp = 54p; 25-mL amp = £2.27
Note. Large volume frusemide injections also available from IMS (Min-I-Jet®)

BUMETANIDE
Indications: oedema, oliguria due to renal failure
Cautions; Contra-indications: see under Frusemide (but has been used in porphyria, see section 9.8.2)
Side-effects: see under Frusemide; also myalgia
Dose: by mouth, 1 mg in the morning, repeated after 6–8 hours if necessary; severe cases, increased up to 5 mg or more daily
ELDERLY, 500 micrograms daily may be sufficient
By intravenous injection, 1–2 mg, repeated after 20 minutes; when *intramuscular injection* considered necessary, 1 mg initially then adjusted according to response
By intravenous infusion, 2–5 mg over 30–60 minutes

PoM **Burinex**® (Leo)
Tablets, both scored, bumetanide 1 mg, net price 20 = £1.14; 5 mg, 20 = £8.01
Liquid, green, sugar-free, bumetanide 1 mg/5 mL. Net price 150 mL = £3.41
Injection, bumetanide 500 micrograms/mL. Net price 2-mL amp = 41p; 4-mL amp = 71p; 10-mL amp = £1.49

ETHACRYNIC ACID
Indications: oedema, oliguria due to renal failure
Cautions; Contra-indications; Side-effects: see under Frusemide and notes above; gastro-intestinal disturbances more severe; also pain on injection
Dose: by mouth, initially 50 mg daily after breakfast; effective initial range of 50–150 mg daily (max. 400 mg) can often be reduced for maintenance and given on alternate days (daily doses above 50 mg divided)
By slow intravenous injection or infusion, 50 mg, increased to 100 mg if necessary

PoM **Edecrin**® (MSD)
Tablets, scored, ethacrynic acid 50 mg. Net price 20 = 75p. Label: 21
Injection, powder for reconstitution, ethacrynic acid (as sodium salt). Net price 50-mg vial = £1.05

PIRETANIDE
Indications: hypertension
Cautions: causes hypokalaemia, monitor plasma electrolytes in hepatic and renal impairment; prostatism; **interactions:** Appendix 1 (diuretics)
Contra-indications: severe electrolyte imbalance, hypovolaemia
Side-effects: rarely nausea, vomiting, diarrhoea, rashes; myalgia after high doses
Dose: 6–12 mg in the morning with food

PoM **Arelix**® (Hoechst)
Capsules, m/r, green/orange, enclosing yellow pellets, piretanide 6 mg. Net price 28-cap pack = £3.70. Label: 21

2.2.3 Potassium-sparing diuretics

Amiloride and **triamterene** on their own are weak diuretics. They cause retention of potassium and are therefore used as an alternative to giving potassium supplements with thiazide or loop diuretics. (See section 2.2.4 for compound preparations with thiazides or loop diuretics.)

Spironolactone is also a potassium-sparing diuretic, and potentiates thiazide or loop diuretics by antagonising aldosterone. It is of value in the treatment of the oedema of cirrhosis of the liver and is effective in oedema of heart failure, particularly when congestion has caused hepatic engorgement.

Spironolactone is also used in primary hyperaldosteronism (Conn's syndrome).

Potassium canrenoate has similar uses to spironolactone, but can be given parenterally. It is metabolised to canrenone, which is also a metabolite of spironolactone.

Potassium supplements must **not** be given with potassium-sparing diuretics.

AMILORIDE HYDROCHLORIDE

Indications: oedema, potassium conservation with thiazide and loop diuretics
Cautions: pregnancy; diabetes mellitus; elderly; **interactions:** Appendix 1 (diuretics)
Contra-indications: hyperkalaemia, renal failure
Side-effects: include gastro-intestinal disturbances, dry mouth, rashes, confusion, orthostatic hypotension, hyperkalaemia, hyponatraemia
Dose: alone, initially 10 mg daily *or* 5 mg twice daily, adjusted according to response; max. 20 mg daily
With other diuretics, congestive heart failure and hypertension, initially 5–10 mg daily
Cirrhosis with ascites, initially 5 mg daily

PoM **Amiloride** (Non-proprietary)
Tablets, amiloride hydrochloride 5 mg, net price 20 = £1.36
Available from APS, Ashbourne (Amilospare®), Berk (Berkamil®), Cox, CP, Evans, Kerfoot, Norton
Oral solution, sugar-free, amiloride hydrochloride 5 mg/5 mL available from RP Drugs (special order)
PoM **Midamor**® (Morson)
Tablets, yellow, amiloride hydrochloride 5 mg. Net price 20 = £1.46

Compound preparations with thiazides or loop diuretics, see section 2.2.4

TRIAMTERENE

Indications: oedema, potassium conservation with thiazide and loop diuretics
Cautions; Contra-indications: see under Amiloride Hydrochloride; monitor plasma urea and potassium, particularly in the elderly and in renal impairment; also may cause blue fluorescence of urine
Side-effects: include gastro-intestinal disturbances, dry mouth, rashes; slight decrease in blood pressure, hyperkalaemia; photosensitivity and blood disorders also reported; triamterene found in kidney stones
Dose: initially 150–250 mg daily, reducing to alternate days after 1 week; taken in divided doses after breakfast and lunch; lower initial dose when given with other diuretics
COUNSELLING. Urine may look slightly blue in some lights

PoM **Dytac**® (SK&F)
Capsules, maroon, triamterene 50 mg. Net price 30-cap pack = £1.94. Label: 14 (see above), 21

Compound preparations with thiazides or loop diuretics, see section 2.2.4

ALDOSTERONE ANTAGONISTS

POTASSIUM CANRENOATE

Indications: oedema associated with secondary aldosteronism, liver failure, chronic decompensated heart disease
Cautions; Contra-indications: see under Spironolactone; also contra-indicated in hyponatraemia
Side-effects: nausea and vomiting, particularly after high doses; hyperkalaemia, especially in renal impairment; pain and irritation at injection site
Dose: by *slow intravenous injection or intravenous infusion*, 200–400 mg daily (exceptionally 800 mg)

PoM **Spiroctan-M**® (Boehringer Mannheim)
Injection, potassium canrenoate 20 mg/mL. Net price 10-mL amp = 72p

SPIRONOLACTONE

Indications: oedema and ascites in cirrhosis of the liver, malignant ascites, nephrotic syndrome, congestive heart failure; primary aldosteronism
Cautions: potential human metabolic products carcinogenic in *rodents*; elderly; hepatic and renal impairment (avoid if severe); **interactions:** Appendix 1 (diuretics)
Contra-indications: hyperkalaemia, severe renal impairment; pregnancy and breast-feeding; Addison's disease; porphyria (see section 9.8.2)
Side-effects: gastro-intestinal disturbances, gynaecomastia; hyperkalaemia
Dose: 100–200 mg daily, increased to 400 mg if required; CHILD 3 mg/kg daily in divided doses

PoM **Spironolactone** (Non-proprietary)
Tablets, spironolactone 25 mg, net price 20 = 54p; 50 mg, 20 = £2.40; 100 mg, 20 = £2.20
Available from APS, Ashbourne (Spirospare®), Berk (Spirolone®), Cox, CP, Evans, Kerfoot, Lagap (Laractone®), Norton
Oral suspensions, sugar-free, spironolactone 5, 10, 25, and 50 mg/5 mL available from RP Drugs (special order)
PoM **Aldactone**® (Searle)
Tablets, all f/c, spironolactone 25 mg (buff), net price 20 = £1.80; 50 mg (off-white), 20 = £3.59; 100 mg (buff), 20 = £7.18
PoM **Spiroctan**® (Boehringer Mannheim)
Tablets, both s/c, spironolactone 25 mg (blue, contains tartrazine), net price 20 = £1.48; 50 mg (green), 20 = £2.84
Capsules, green, spironolactone 100 mg. Net price 28-cap pack = £7.75

Compound preparations with thiazides or loop diuretics, see section 2.2.4

2.2.4 Potassium-sparing diuretics with other diuretics

Although it is preferable to prescribe thiazides and potassium-sparing diuretics separately, the use of fixed combinations may be justified if compliance is a problem. For **interactions**, see Appendix 1 (diuretics).

Amiloride with thiazides

PoM Co-amilozide (Non-proprietary)
Tablets, co-amilozide 5/50 (amiloride hydrochloride 5 mg, hydrochlorothiazide 50 mg). Net price 20 = £1.21
Available from APS, Ashbourne (Amilmaxco 5/50®), Baker Norton (Amilco®), Cox, CP, Evans, Kerfoot, Schwarz (Hypertane 50®), Shire (Vasetic®)
Dose: 1–2 tablets, increased if necessary to max. of 4, daily
Tablets, co-amilozide 2.5/25 available as Moduret 25®

PoM Moduret 25® (Du Pont)
Tablets, off-white, co-amilozide 2.5/25 (amiloride hydrochloride 2.5 mg, hydrochlorothiazide 25 mg). Net price 28-tab pack = £2.08
Dose: 1–4 tablets, increased if necessary to a max. of 8, daily

PoM Moduretic® (Du Pont)
Tablets, peach, scored, co-amilozide 5/50 (amiloride hydrochloride 5 mg, hydrochlorothiazide 50 mg). Net price 30 = £2.70
Dose: 1–2 tablets, increased if necessary to a max. of 4, daily
Oral solution, co-amilozide 5/50 (amiloride hydrochloride 5 mg, hydrochlorothiazide 50 mg/5 mL). Do not dilute. Net price 200 mL = £4.95
Dose: as for tablets above (5 mL = 1 tablet)

PoM Navispare® (Ciba)
Tablets, f/c, orange, amiloride 2.5 mg, cyclopenthiazide 250 micrograms. Net price 28-tab pack = £1.79
Dose: 1–2 tablets in the morning

Amiloride with loop diuretics

PoM Burinex A® (Leo)
Tablets, ivory, scored, amiloride hydrochloride 5 mg, bumetanide 1 mg. Net price 28-tab pack = £3.28
Dose: 1–2 tablets daily

PoM Frumil® (Rhône-Poulenc Rorer)
LS tablets, orange, co-amilofruse 2.5/20 (amiloride hydrochloride 2.5 mg, frusemide 20 mg). Net price 28-tab pack = £3.25, 56-tab pack = £6.37
Dose: 1 tablet in the morning
Tablets, orange, scored, co-amilofruse 5/40 (amiloride hydrochloride 5 mg, frusemide 40 mg). Net price 28-tab pack = £3.97, 56-tab pack = £7.77
Dose: 1–2 tablets in the morning
Forte tablets, orange, scored, co-amilofruse 10/80 (amiloride hydrochloride 10 mg, frusemide 80 mg). Net price 28-tab pack = £7.38, 56-tab pack = £14.47
Dose: 1 tablet daily in the morning

PoM Lasoride® (Hoechst)
Tablets, yellow, co-amilofruse 5/40 (amiloride hydrochloride 5 mg, frusemide 40 mg). Net price 28-tab pack = £3.33
Dose: 1–2 tablets in the morning

Triamterene with thiazides
COUNSELLING. Urine may look slightly blue in some lights

PoM Dyazide® (SK&F)
Tablets, peach, scored, triamterene 50 mg, hydrochlorothiazide 25 mg. Net price 30-tab pack = £2.36. Label: 14 (see above), 21
Dose: hypertension, 1 tablet daily after breakfast; oedema, 2 tablets daily (1 after breakfast and 1 after midday meal) increased to 3 daily if necessary (2 after breakfast and 1 after midday meal); usual maintenance, 1 daily or 2 on alternate days; max. 4 daily
Note. Tablets containing triamterene 50 mg and hydrochlorothiazide 25 mg are also available from Ashbourne (TriamaxCo®), Norton (Triamco®)

PoM Dytide® (SK&F)
Capsules, clear/maroon, triamterene 50 mg, benzthiazide 25 mg. Net price 30-cap pack = £2.08. Label: 14 (see above), 21
Dose: oedema, initially 3 capsules daily (2 after breakfast and 1 after midday meal) for 1 week then 1 or 2 on alternate days

PoM Kalspare® (Cusi)
LS tablets, peach, f/c, triamterene 50 mg, chlorthalidone 25 mg. Net price 28-tab pack = £2.95. Label: 14 (see above), 21
Dose: 1–2 tablets in the morning
Tablets, orange, f/c, scored, triamterene 50 mg, chlorthalidone 50 mg. Net price 28-tab pack = £3.27. Label: 14 (see above), 21
Dose: 1–2 tablets in the morning

Triamterene with loop diuretics
COUNSELLING. Urine may look slightly blue in some lights

PoM Frusene® (CP)
Tablets, yellow, scored, triamterene 50 mg, frusemide 40 mg. Net price 56-tab pack = £5.39. Label: 14 (see above), 21
Dose: 1–2 tablets daily

Spironolactone with thiazides

PoM Aldactide 25® (Gold Cross)
Tablets, buff, f/c, co-flumactone 25/25 (hydroflumethiazide 25 mg, spironolactone 25 mg). Net price 20 = £3.07
Dose: congestive heart failure, initially 4 tablets daily; range 1–8 daily

PoM Aldactide 50® (Gold Cross)
Tablets, buff, f/c, co-flumactone 50/50 (hydroflumethiazide 50 mg, spironolactone 50 mg). Net price 20 = £5.79
Dose: congestive heart failure, initially 2 tablets daily; range 1–4 daily

Spironolactone with loop diuretics

PoM Lasilactone® (Hoechst)
Capsules, blue/white, spironolactone 50 mg, frusemide 20 mg. Net price 28-cap pack = £5.04
Dose: resistant oedema, 1–4 capsules daily

2.2.5 Osmotic diuretics

Osmotic diuretics are rarely used in heart failure as they may acutely expand the blood volume. **Mannitol** is used in cerebral oedema—a typical dose is 1 g/kg as a 20% solution given by rapid intravenous infusion.

MANNITOL

Indications: see notes above
Cautions: extravasation causes inflammation and thrombophlebitis
Contra-indications: congestive cardiac failure, pulmonary oedema
Side-effects: chills, fever
Dose: by intravenous infusion, diuresis, 50–200 g over 24 hours, preceded by a test dose of 200 mg/kg by slow intravenous injection
Cerebral oedema, see notes above

PoM **Mannitol** (Non-proprietary)
Intravenous infusion, mannitol 10%, 20%, and 25%
Available from Baxter (10% and 20%) and IMS (Min-I-Jet® Mannitol 25%)

2.2.6 Mercurial diuretics

They are effective diuretics but are now little used because of their nephrotoxicity. Mersalyl **must** be given by intramuscular injection; intravenous use may cause severe hypotension and sudden death.

MERSALYL

Indications: oedema unresponsive to other diuretics
Cautions: recent myocardial infarction, treatment with cardiac glycosides, frequent extrasystoles
Contra-indications: renal impairment; pregnancy; porphyria (see section 9.8.2)
Side-effects: gastro-intestinal disturbances, allergic reactions

PoM **Mersalyl Injection**, mersalyl sodium 100 mg, theophylline 50 mg/mL
Dose: by deep intramuscular injection, 0.5–2 mL

2.2.7 Carbonic anhydrase inhibitors

Acetazolamide and dichlorphenamide are weak diuretics, and are little used for their diuretic effect. They inhibit the formation of aqueous fluid, and are used in glaucoma (see section 11.6). Although acetazolamide is used as a prophylactic measure for mountain sickness it is not a substitute for acclimatisation.

2.2.8 Diuretics with potassium

Many patients on diuretics do not need potassium supplements (see section 9.2.1.1). For many of those who do, the amount of potassium ion in combined preparations may not be enough, and for this reason their use is to be discouraged.

Diuretics with potassium and potassium-sparing diuretics should **not** usually be given together.

COUNSELLING. Modified-release potassium tablets should be swallowed whole with plenty of fluid during meals while sitting or standing

PoM **Burinex K**® (Leo)
Tablets, bumetanide 500 micrograms, potassium 7.7 mmol for modified release. Net price 20 = 85p. Label: 25, 27, counselling, see above

PoM **Centyl K**® (Leo)
Tablets, green, bendrofluazide 2.5 mg, potassium 7.7 mmol for modified release. Net price 20 = 58p. Label: 25, 27, counselling, see above

PoM **Diumide-K Continus**® (ASTA Medica)
Tablets, f/c, white/orange, frusemide 40 mg, potassium 8 mmol for modified release. Net price 30-tab pack = £2.02. Label: 25, 27, counselling, see above

PoM **Hygroton-K**® (Geigy)
Tablets, red, s/c, chlorthalidone 25 mg, potassium 6.7 mmol for modified release. Net price 20 = 48p. Label: 25, 27, counselling, see above
Additives: include gluten and azo dyes

PoM **Lasikal**® (Hoechst)
Tablets, white/yellow, f/c, frusemide 20 mg, potassium 10 mmol for modified release. Net price 20 = £1.09. Label: 25, 27, counselling, see above

PoM **Lasix + K**® (Hoechst)
Calendar pack, 30 white scored tablets, frusemide 40 mg; 60 m/r yellow tablets, potassium chloride (potassium 10 mmol). Net price = £3.05. Label: 25, 27, counselling, see above

PoM **Neo-NaClex-K**® (Goldshield)
Tablets, pink/white, f/c, bendrofluazide 2.5 mg, potassium 8.4 mmol for modified release. Net price 20 = 24p. Label: 25, 27, counselling, see above

2.3 Anti-arrhythmic drugs

2.3.1 Management of arrhythmias
2.3.2 Drugs for arrhythmias

2.3.1 Management of arrhythmias

Management of an arrhythmia, apart from the treatment of associated heart failure, requires precise diagnosis of the type of arrhythmia, and electrocardiography is essential.

Ectopic beats. If spontaneous with a normal heart, these rarely require treatment beyond reassurance. If they are particularly troublesome, beta-blockers are sometimes effective and may be safer than other suppressant drugs.

Atrial fibrillation. The ventricular rate can be controlled with digoxin (section 2.1.1).

Atrial flutter. The ventricular rate can often be controlled with digoxin. Reversion to sinus rhythm (if indicated) is best achieved by appropriately synchronised d.c. shock, rather than by drug therapy. If the arrhythmia is long-standing a period of treatment with anticoagulants should be considered before cardioversion to avoid the complication of emboli.

Paroxysmal supraventricular tachycardia. In most patients this remits spontaneously or can be returned to sinus rhythm by reflex vagal stimulation with respiratory manoeuvres, prompt squatting, or pressure over one carotid sinus (**important:** pressure over carotid sinus should be restricted to monitored patients, it can be dangerous in recent ischaemia, digitalis toxicity, or the elderly).

Cautionary label wordings, see inside back cover

Prices are **net**, see p. 1

If vagal stimulation fails, digitalisation or intravenous administration of a beta-blocker may be effective. Intravenous administration of verapamil is useful for patients without myocardial or valvular disease (**important**: never in patients recently treated with beta-blockers, see section 2.3.2). For arrhythmias that are poorly tolerated, synchronised d.c. shock usually provides rapid relief.

In cases of paroxysmal supraventricular tachycardia with block, digitalis toxicity should be suspected. In addition to stopping administration of the cardiac glycoside and giving potassium supplements, intravenous administration of a beta-blocker or phenytoin may be useful. Specific digoxin antibody is available if the toxicity is considered life-threatening (section 2.1.1).

Acute arrhythmias after myocardial infarction. It is best to do nothing in patients with a paroxysmal tachycardia or rapid irregularity of the pulse until an ECG record is obtainable. If the condition of the patient is such that death due to the arrhythmia seems possible 100 mg of lignocaine should be given intravenously. Bradycardia, particularly if complicated by hypotension, should be treated with atropine sulphate, given intravenously in an initial dose of 300 micrograms, increasing to 1 mg if necessary.

Ventricular tachycardia. Drug treatment is used both for the treatment of ventricular tachycardia and for prophylaxis of recurrent attacks that merit suppression. Ventricular tachycardia requires treatment most commonly in the acute stage of myocardial infarction, but the likelihood of this and other life-threatening arrhythmias diminishes sharply over the first 24 hours after the attack, especially in patients without heart failure or shock. Lignocaine is the preferred drug for emergency use. Other drugs are best administered under specialist supervision. Very rapid ventricular tachycardia causes profound circulatory collapse and should be treated urgently with d.c. shock.

CAUTIONS. The negative inotropic effects of anti-arrhythmic drugs tend to be additive therefore special care should be taken if two or more are used, especially in impaired myocardial function. Most or all drugs that are effective in countering arrhythmias can also provoke them in some circumstances; moreover, hypokalaemia enhances the arrhythmogenic (pro-arrhythmic) effect of many drugs.

SUPRAVENTRICULAR ARRHYTHMIAS

Oral administration of a **cardiac glycoside** (such as digoxin, section 2.1.1) is the treatment of choice in slowing ventricular response in cases of atrial fibrillation and atrial flutter. Intravenous digoxin, preferably infused slowly, is occasionally required if the ventricular rate needs rapid control. Ouabain acts more quickly but may be difficult to obtain since it is not on the UK market.

Verapamil (section 2.6.2) is usually effective for supraventricular tachycardias. An initial intravenous dose may be followed by oral treatment; hypotension may occur with larger doses. It should not be used for tachyarrhythmias where the QRS complex is wide (i.e. broad complex) unless a supraventricular origin has been established beyond reasonable doubt. It is also contra-indicated in atrial fibrillation with pre-excitation (e.g. Wolff-Parkinson-White syndrome). It should not be used in children with arrhythmias without specialist advice; some supraventricular arrhythmias in childhood can be accelerated by verapamil with dangerous consequences.

> Verapamil should not be injected into patients recently treated with **beta-blockers** because of the risk of hypotension and asystole. It has been suggested that when verapamil injection has been given first, an interval of 30 minutes before giving a beta-blocker is sufficient but this too is open to doubt.
>
> It may even be hazardous to give verapamil and a beta-blocker together by mouth (should only be contemplated if myocardial function well preserved).

2.3.2 Drugs for arrhythmias

Anti-arrhythmic drugs can be classified clinically into those that act on supraventricular arrhythmias (e.g. verapamil), those that act on both supraventricular and ventricular arrhythmias (e.g. quinidine), and those that act on ventricular arrhythmias (e.g. lignocaine).

They can also be classified according to their effects on the electrical behaviour of myocardial cells during activity (termed 'action potential'):

Class Ia, b, c	Membrane stabilising drugs (e.g. quinidine, lignocaine, flecainide respectively)
Class II	Beta-blockers
Class III	Amiodarone, Bretylium, and Sotalol (also Class II)
Class IV	Calcium-channel blockers (includes verapamil but not the nifedipine group)

This latter classification (the Vaughan Williams classification) is of less clinical significance.

ADENOSINE

Indications: rapid reversion to sinus rhythm of paroxysmal supraventricular tachycardias, including those associated with accessory pathways (e.g. Wolff-Parkinson-White syndrome); aid to diagnosis of broad or narrow complex supraventricular tachycardias

Cautions: atrial fibrillation or flutter with accessory pathway (increased conduction down anomalous pathway may develop); asthma; **interactions:** Appendix 1 (adenosine)

Contra-indications: second- or third-degree atrio-ventricular block and sick sinus syndrome (unless pacemaker fitted)

Side-effects: include transient facial flush, dyspnoea, choking sensation, nausea, light-headedness; severe bradycardia reported (requiring temporary pacing); ECG may show transient rhythm disturbances

2.3 Anti-arrhythmic drugs

Dose: by rapid intravenous injection into large peripheral vein, 3 mg over 2 seconds with cardiac monitoring; if necessary followed by 6 mg after 1–2 minutes, and then by 12 mg after a further 1–2 minutes

▼ PoM **Adenocor**® (Sanofi Winthrop)
Injection, adenosine 3 mg/mL in physiological saline. Net price 2-mL vial = £4.15 (hosp. only)

CARDIAC GLYCOSIDES
Section 2.1.1

VERAPAMIL
Section 2.6.2

SUPRAVENTRICULAR AND VENTRICULAR ARRHYTHMIAS

Amiodarone is used in the treatment of tachycardia associated with the Wolff-Parkinson-White syndrome. It may only be used for the treatment of other arrhythmias when other drugs are ineffective or contra-indicated and should be initiated only under hospital or specialist supervision. These include paroxysmal supraventricular, nodal and ventricular tachycardias, atrial fibrillation and flutter, and ventricular fibrillation. Since amiodarone has a very long half-life it only needs to be given once daily (but high doses may cause nausea unless divided). It may be given by intravenous infusion as well as by mouth, and has the advantage of causing little or no myocardial depression. Unlike oral amiodarone, intravenous amiodarone may act relatively rapidly.

Most patients taking amiodarone develop corneal microdeposits (reversible on withdrawal of treatment); these rarely interfere with vision, but drivers may be dazzled by headlights at night. Because of the possibility of phototoxic reactions, patients should be advised to shield the skin from light and to use a wide-spectrum sunscreen such as RoC Total Sunblock® (section 13.8.1) to protect against both long ultraviolet and visible light.

Amiodarone contains iodine and can cause disorders of thyroid function; both hypothyroidism and hyperthyroidism may occur. Thyroid function tests which rely on plasma concentrations of thyroxine alone, rather than on both thyroxine and tri-iodothyronine, may be spuriously elevated, but where doubt exists amiodarone should be withdrawn. Monitoring of tri-iodothyronine (T3) concentrations about every six months may give early warning of amiodarone-related thyrotoxicosis (which can be very refractory to treatment).

Pneumonitis should always be suspected if new or progressive shortness of breath or cough develops. Fresh neurological symptoms should raise the possibility of peripheral neuropathy (although this is rare).

Beta-blockers act as anti-arrhythmic drugs principally by attenuating the effects of the sympathetic system on automaticity and conductivity within the heart, for details see section 2.4.

Disopyramide may be given by intravenous injection to control arrhythmias after myocardial infarction (including those not responding to lignocaine), but it impairs cardiac contractility. Oral administration of disopyramide is useful but it has an antimuscarinic effect which limits its use in patients with glaucoma or prostatic hypertrophy.

Flecainide is a newer drug in the same general class as lignocaine. It may be of value for serious symptomatic ventricular arrhythmias. It may also be indicated for junctional re-entry tachycardias. Preliminary results with paroxysmal atrial fibrillation are promising, but as with quinidine it may precipitate serious arrhythmias in a small minority of patients (including those with otherwise normal hearts).

Procainamide can be given by intravenous injection to control ventricular arrhythmias, but prolonged oral use can cause a syndrome resembling systemic lupus erythematosus.

Quinidine may be effective in suppressing supraventricular and ventricular arrhythmias. It may itself precipitate rhythm disorders, and is best used on specialist advice; it can cause hypersensitivity reactions and gastro-intestinal upsets.

AMIODARONE HYDROCHLORIDE
Indications: see notes above (should be initiated in hospital)
Cautions: liver-function and thyroid-function tests required in long-term therapy; interferes with tests of thyroid function; heart failure; renal impairment; elderly; severe bradycardia and conduction disturbances in excessive dosage; intravenous use may cause moderate and transient fall in blood pressure (circulatory collapse precipitated by rapid administration or overdosage); **interactions:** Appendix 1 (amiodarone)
Contra-indications: sinus bradycardia, sino-atrial heart block; unless pacemaker fitted avoid in severe conduction disturbances or sinus node disease; avoid intravenous use in severe respiratory failure, circulatory collapse, severe arterial hypotension, congestive heart failure; thyroid dysfunction; pregnancy and breast-feeding; iodine sensitivity; porphyria (see section 9.8.2)
Side-effects: reversible corneal microdeposits (sometimes with night glare), rarely impaired vision due to optic neuritis; peripheral neuropathy and myopathy (usually reversible on withdrawal), bradycardia and conduction disturbances (see Cautions); phototoxicity and rarely persistent slate-grey skin discoloration (see also notes); hypothyroidism, hyperthyroidism, diffuse pulmonary alveolitis and fibrosis, hepatitis; rarely nausea, vomiting, metallic taste, tremor, nightmares, vertigo, headache, sleeplessness, fatigue, benign raised intracranial pressure, epididymitis; ataxia, rashes (including exfoliative dermatitis), vasculitis, blood disorders, increased prothrombin time reported; anaphylaxis on rapid injection, also bronchospasm or apnoea in respiratory failure

Dose: by mouth, 200 mg 3 times daily for 1 week reduced to 200 mg twice daily for a further week; maintenance, usually 200 mg daily or the minimum required to control the arrhythmia
By intravenous infusion via caval catheter, 5 mg/kg over 20–120 minutes with ECG monitoring; max. 1.2 g in 24 hours

Note. In extreme emergency only, may be given *by slow intravenous injection* of 150–300 mg in 10–20 mL glucose 5% over at least 3 minutes with ECG monitoring (usually in intensive care unit); do not repeat for at least 15 minutes

PoM **Cordarone X**® (Sanofi Winthrop)
Tablets, both scored, amiodarone hydrochloride 100 mg, net price 28-tab pack = £5.13; 200 mg, 28-tab pack = £8.40. Label: 11
Note. Tablets containing amiodarone hydrochloride 100 mg and 200 mg available from Cox, Generics
Injection, amiodarone hydrochloride 50 mg/mL. Net price 3-mL amp = £1.54. For dilution and use as an infusion

DISOPYRAMIDE

Indications: ventricular arrhythmias, especially after myocardial infarction; supraventricular arrhythmias
Cautions: glaucoma; heart failure (avoid if severe); prostatic enlargement; hepatic and renal impairment; elderly; pregnancy; **interactions:** Appendix 1 (disopyramide)
Contra-indications: second- and third-degree heart block and sinus node dysfunction (unless pacemaker fitted); cardiogenic shock; severe uncompensated heart failure
Side-effects: myocardial depression, hypotension, atrioventricular block; antimuscarinic effects include dry mouth, blurred vision, urinary retention
Dose: by mouth, 300–800 mg daily in divided doses
By slow intravenous injection, 2 mg/kg over at least 5 minutes to a max. of 150 mg, with ECG monitoring, followed immediately *either* by 200 mg *by mouth*, then 200 mg every 8 hours for 24 hours *or* 400 micrograms/kg/hour *by intravenous infusion*; max. 300 mg in first hour and 800 mg daily

PoM **Disopyramide** (Non-proprietary)
Capsules, disopyramide 100 mg, net price 20 = £1.60; 150 mg, 20 = £2.68
Available from APS, CP (100 mg), Kerfoot (100 mg), Monmouth (Isomide® 100 mg), Norton (100 mg)

PoM **Rythmodan**® (Roussel)
Capsules, disopyramide 100 mg (green/beige), net price 84-cap pack = £7.52; 150 mg, 84-cap pack = £11.27
Injection, disopyramide 10 mg (as phosphate)/mL, net price 5-mL amp = 70p

Modified release
PoM **Dirythmin SA**® (Astra)
Durules® (= tablets, m/r), f/c, disopyramide 150 mg (as phosphate). Net price 20 = £2.53. Label: 25
Dose: 300 mg every 12 hours; max. 900 mg daily

PoM **Rythmodan Retard**® (Roussel)
Tablets, m/r, scored, f/c, disopyramide 250 mg (as phosphate). Net price 56-tab pack = £16.24. Label: 25
Dose: 250–375 mg every 12 hours
Note. Modified-release capsules containing disopyramide 250 mg (as phosphate) also available from Monmouth (Isomide® CR)

FLECAINIDE ACETATE

Indications: (should be initiated in hospital) *tablets and injection:* AV nodal reciprocating tachycardia, Wolff-Parkinson-White syndrome and similar conditions with accessory pathway and anterograde or retrograde conduction, paroxysmal atrial fibrillation in patients with disabling symptoms (arrhythmias of recent onset will respond more readily); *tablets only:* symptomatic sustained ventricular tachycardia, premature ventricular contractions and/or non-sustained ventricular tachycardia causing disabling symptoms in patients resistant to or intolerant of other therapy; *injection only:* ventricular tachyarrhythmias resistant to other treatment
Cautions: patients with pacemakers (especially those who may be pacemaker dependent because stimulation threshold may rise appreciably); avoid in sinus node dysfunction, atrial conduction defects, second-degree or greater AV block, bundle branch block or distal block unless pacing rescue available; atrial fibrillation following heart surgery; elderly; hepatic and renal impairment (see Appendixes 2 and 3); pregnancy (toxicity in *animal* studies); **interactions:** Appendix 1 (flecainide)
Contra-indications: heart failure; history of myocardial infarction and either asymptomatic ventricular ectopics or asymptomatic non-sustained ventricular tachycardia; long-standing atrial fibrillation where no attempt has been made to convert to sinus rhythm; haemodynamically significant valvular heart disease
Side-effects: dizziness, visual disturbances (corneal deposits reported); arrhythmogenic (pro-arrhythmic) effect; rarely nausea and vomiting; reversible increases in liver enzymes, jaundice; ataxia, peripheral neuropathy and ataxia, pulmonary fibrosis, pneumonitis also reported
Dose: by mouth, ventricular arrhythmias, 100 mg twice daily; max. 400 mg daily (usually reserved for rapid control or in heavily built patients), reduced after 3–5 days if possible; elderly 100 mg twice daily, reduced after 1 week if possible
Supraventricular arrhythmias, 50 mg twice daily, increased if required to max. 300 mg daily; elderly 50 mg twice daily, reduced after 1 week if possible
By slow intravenous injection, 2 mg/kg over 10–30 minutes, max. 150 mg, with ECG monitoring; followed if required by *infusion* at a rate of 1.5 mg/kg/hour for 1 hour, subsequently reduced to 100–250 micrograms/kg/hour for up to 24 hours; max. cumulative dose in first 24

hours, 600 mg; transfer to *oral* treatment, as above

PoM **Tambocor**® (3M)
Tablets, scored, flecainide acetate 100 mg. Net price 60-tab pack = £19.98
Injection, flecainide acetate 10 mg/mL. Net price 15-mL amp = £4.25

PROCAINAMIDE HYDROCHLORIDE
Indications: ventricular arrhythmias, especially after myocardial infarction; atrial tachycardia
Cautions: elderly; hepatic and renal impairment, asthma, myasthenia gravis; **interactions:** Appendix 1 (procainamide)
Contra-indications: heart block, heart failure, hypotension
Side-effects: nausea, diarrhoea, rashes, fever, myocardial depression, heart failure, lupus erythematosus-like syndrome, agranulocytosis after prolonged treatment
Dose: by mouth, ventricular arrhythmias, up to 50 mg/kg daily in divided doses, preferably controlled by measurement of plasma concentration (dosage intervals can range from 3–6 hours); atrial arrhythmias, higher doses may be required
By slow intravenous injection, rate not exceeding 50 mg/minute, 100 mg with ECG monitoring, repeated at 5-minute intervals until arrhythmia controlled; max. 1 g
By intravenous infusion, 500–600 mg over 25–30 minutes with ECG monitoring, followed by maintenance at rate of 2–6 mg/minute, then if necessary oral treatment as above, starting 3–4 hours after infusion

PoM **Pronestyl**® (Squibb)
Tablets, scored, procainamide hydrochloride 250 mg. Net price 20 = 94p
Injection, procainamide hydrochloride 100 mg/mL. Net price 10-mL vial = £1.90

Modified release
PoM **Procainamide Durules**® (Astra)
Tablets, m/r, yellow, procainamide hydrochloride 500 mg. Net price 20 = £1.46. Label: 25
Dose: 1–1.5 g every 8 hours

QUINIDINE
Indications: suppression of supraventricular tachycardias and ventricular arrhythmias (see notes above)
Cautions: 200-mg test dose to detect hypersensitivity reactions; **interactions:** Appendix 1 (quinidine)
Contra-indications: heart block
Side-effects: see under Procainamide Hydrochloride; also ventricular arrhythmias, thrombocytopenia, haemolytic anaemia; rarely granulomatous hepatitis; also cinchonism (see Quinine, section 5.4.1) with tinnitus, visual disturbances, headache, hot and flushed skin, confusion, vertigo, vomiting, and abdominal pain

Dose: by mouth, quinidine sulphate 200–400 mg 3–4 times daily
Note. Quinidine sulphate 200 mg ≡ quinidine bisulphate 250 mg

PoM **Quinidine Sulphate** (Non-proprietary)
Tablets, quinidine sulphate 200 mg, net price 20 = £1.31; 300 mg, 20 = £1.76
Available from CP, Evans (300 mg)

Modified release
PoM **Kiditard**® (Delandale)
Capsules, m/r, blue, quinidine bisulphate 250 mg. Net price 20 = £4.05. Label: 25
Dose: 500 mg every 12 hours, adjusted as required
PoM **Kinidin Durules**® (Astra)
Tablets, m/r, f/c, quinidine bisulphate 250 mg. Net price 20 = £2.15. Label: 25
Dose: 500 mg every 12 hours, adjusted as required

VENTRICULAR ARRHYTHMIAS

Bretylium is only used as an anti-arrhythmic drug in resuscitation. It is given both intramuscularly and intravenously but can cause severe hypotension, particularly after intravenous administration; nausea and vomiting can occur with either route. The intravenous route should only be used in emergency when there is doubt about absorption because of inadequate circulation.

Lignocaine is relatively safe when used by slow intravenous injection and should be considered first for emergency use. Though effective in suppressing ventricular tachycardia and reducing the risk of ventricular fibrillation following myocardial infarction, it has not been shown convincingly to reduce mortality when used prophylactically in this condition. In patients with cardiac or hepatic failure doses may need to be reduced to avoid convulsions, depression of the central nervous system, or depression of the cardiovascular system.

Mexiletine may be given as a slow intravenous injection if lignocaine is ineffective; it has a similar action. Adverse cardiovascular and central nervous system effects may limit the dose tolerated; nausea and vomiting may prevent an effective dose being given by mouth.

Phenytoin by slow intravenous injection is sometimes useful in ventricular arrhythmias particularly those caused by cardiac glycosides.

Propafenone is a newer drug for the prophylaxis and treatment of ventricular arrhythmias and is undergoing evaluation in some supraventricular arrhythmias. For CSM advice on avoidance in obstructive airways disease, see next page.

Tocainide is an analogue of lignocaine; because of a high incidence of blood disorders its use is limited to treatment of life-threatening symptomatic ventricular tachyarrhythmias associated with severely compromised left ventricular function in patients who do not respond to other therapy or for whom other therapy is contra-indicated.

BRETYLIUM TOSYLATE
Indications: ventricular arrhythmias resistant to other treatment
Cautions: do not give noradrenaline or other sympathomimetic amines; may exacerbate ventricular arrhythmias due to cardiac glycosides; **interactions:** Appendix 1 (bretylium)
Contra-indications: phaeochromocytoma
Side-effects: hypotension, nausea and vomiting
Dose: by intramuscular injection, 5 mg/kg repeated after 6–8 hours if necessary
By slow intravenous injection, 5–10 mg/kg over 8–10 minutes with blood pressure and ECG monitoring; may be repeated after 1–2 hours to a total dosage of 30 mg/kg (initial dose being diluted to 10 mg/mL in glucose 5% or sodium chloride intravenous infusion)
Maintenance 5–10 mg/kg *by intramuscular injection* every 6–8 hours *or* 1–2 mg/minute *by intravenous infusion*

PoM **Bretylate**® (Wellcome)
Injection, bretylium tosylate 50 mg/mL. Net price 10-mL amp = £19.81
PoM **Min-I-Jet**® **Bretylium Tosylate** (IMS)
Injection, bretylium tosylate 50 mg/mL. Net price 10-mL disposable syringe = £25.16

LIGNOCAINE HYDROCHLORIDE
Indications: ventricular arrhythmias, especially after myocardial infarction
Cautions: lower doses in congestive cardiac failure, in hepatic failure, and following cardiac surgery; **interactions:** Appendix 1 (lignocaine)
Contra-indications: sino-atrial disorders, all grades of atrioventricular block, severe myocardial depression; porphyria (see section 9.8.2)
Side-effects: confusion, convulsions
Dose: by intravenous injection, in patients without gross circulatory impairment, 100 mg as a bolus over a few minutes, followed by *infusion* of 2–4 mg/minute

PoM **Lignocaine in Glucose Injection,** lignocaine hydrochloride 0.1% (1 mg/mL) and 0.2% (2 mg/mL) in glucose intravenous infusion 5%. 500-mL containers
Available from Baxter
PoM **Min-I-Jet**® **Lignocaine** (IMS)
Injection, lignocaine hydrochloride 1% (10 mg/mL), net price 10-mL disposable syringe = £3.10; 2% (20 mg/mL), 5-mL disposable syringe = £2.84
PoM **Select-A-Jet**® **Lignocaine** (IMS)
Injection, lignocaine hydrochloride 20% (200 mg/mL). To be diluted before use. Net price 5-mL vial = £4.26
PoM **Xylocard**® (Astra)
Injection 100 mg, lignocaine hydrochloride (anhydrous) 20 mg/mL. Net price 5-mL syringe = £1.65
Intravenous infusion, lignocaine hydrochloride (anhydrous) 200 mg/mL. To be diluted before use. Net price 5-mL syringe (1 g) = £2.01; 10-mL syringe (2 g) = £2.35

MEXILETINE HYDROCHLORIDE
Indications: ventricular arrhythmias, especially after myocardial infarction
Cautions: hepatic impairment; close monitoring on initiation of therapy (including ECG, blood pressure, etc.); **interactions:** Appendix 1 (mexiletine)
Contra-indications: bradycardia, heart block
Side-effects: bradycardia, hypotension, confusion, convulsions, psychiatric disorders, dysarthria, nystagmus, tremor; jaundice, hepatitis, and blood disorders reported
Dose: by mouth, initial dose 400 mg (may be increased to 600 mg if opioid analgesics also given), followed after 2 hours by 200–250 mg 3–4 times daily
By intravenous injection, 100–250 mg at a rate of 25 mg/minute with ECG monitoring followed by *infusion* of 250 mg as a 0.1% solution over 1 hour, 125 mg/hour for 2 hours, then 500 micrograms/minute

PoM **Mexitil**® (Boehringer Ingelheim)
Capsules, mexiletine hydrochloride 50 mg (purple/red), net price 20 = 91p; 200 mg (red), 20 = £2.18
Injection, mexiletine hydrochloride 25 mg/mL. Net price 10-mL amp = £1.36
PoM **Mexitil PL**® (Boehringer Ingelheim)
Perlongets® (= capsules, m/r, each enclosing 5 miniature tablets), turquoise/scarlet, mexiletine hydrochloride 360 mg. Net price 56-cap pack = £10.98. Label: 25
Dose: 1 capsule twice daily

PHENYTOIN SODIUM
Indications: arrhythmias, see notes above; for use in epilepsy, see section 4.8.1
Cautions; Contra-indications; Side-effects: see section 4.8.2
Dose: arrhythmias, *by intravenous injection* via caval catheter, 3.5–5 mg/kg at a rate not exceeding 50 mg/minute, with blood pressure and ECG monitoring; repeat once if necessary

Preparations: see section 4.8.2

PROPAFENONE HYDROCHLORIDE
Indications: ventricular arrhythmias
Cautions: heart failure; hepatic and renal impairment; elderly; pacemaker patients; pregnancy; **CSM** advises great caution in obstructive airways disease owing to beta-blocking activity (contra-indicated if severe); **interactions:** Appendix 1 (propafenone)
Contra-indications: uncontrolled congestive heart failure, cardiogenic shock (except arrhythmia induced), severe bradycardia, uncontrolled electrolyte disturbances, severe obstructive pulmonary disease, marked hypotension; myasthenia gravis; unless adequately paced avoid in sinus node dysfunction, atrial conduction defects, second degree or greater atrioventricular block, bundle branch block or distal block

Side-effects: constipation, blurred vision, dry mouth (due to antimuscarinic action); dizziness, nausea and vomiting, fatigue, bitter taste, diarrhoea, headache, and allergic skin reactions reported; postural hypotension, particularly in elderly; bradycardia, sino-atrial, atrioventricular, or intraventricular blocks; arrhythmogenic (pro-arrhythmic) effect; rarely cholestasis, blood disorders, lupus syndrome, seizures

Dose: 70 kg and over, initially 150 mg 3 times daily after food under direct hospital supervision with ECG monitoring and blood pressure control, increased at intervals of at least 3 days to 300 mg twice daily and, if necessary, to max. 300 mg 3 times daily; under 70 kg, reduce dose ELDERLY may respond to lower doses

PoM **Arythmol**® (Knoll)
Tablets, both f/c, propafenone hydrochloride 150 mg, net price 90-tab pack = £19.98; 300 mg (scored), 60-tab pack = £19.98. Label: 21, 25

TOCAINIDE HYDROCHLORIDE

Indications: ventricular arrhythmias (restricted use—see notes above)

Cautions: weekly blood counts essential for first 12 weeks, then monthly; severe hepatic or renal impairment; elderly; uncompensated heart failure, bradycardia and hypotension; pregnancy (toxicity in *animal* studies); **interactions:** Appendix 1 (tocainide)

Contra-indications: second-degree or greater AV block (unless paced)

Side-effects: CNS effects including tremor, dizziness, convulsions, paraesthesia; gastro-intestinal effects including nausea and vomiting; abnormal liver-function tests; fever and rash (including Stevens-Johnson syndrome and exfoliative dermatitis); lupus erythematosus-like syndrome, pulmonary fibrosis; interstitial pneumonitis; fibrosing alveolitis, agranulocytosis, aplastic anaemia, and thrombocytopenia—see also notes above; psychiatric disorders reported

Dose: 1.2 g daily in 3 divided doses; max. 2.4 g daily

PoM **Tonocard**® (Astra)
Tablets, yellow, f/c, tocainide hydrochloride 400 mg, net price 20 = £3.35

2.4 Beta-adrenoceptor blocking drugs

Beta-adrenoceptor blocking drugs (beta-blockers) block the beta-adrenoreceptors in the heart, peripheral vasculature, bronchi, pancreas, and liver.

Many beta-blockers are now available and in general they are all equally effective. There are, however, differences between them which may affect choice in treating particular diseases or individual patients.

Intrinsic sympathomimetic activity (ISA, partial agonist activity) represents the capacity of beta-blockers to stimulate as well as to block adrenergic receptors. **Oxprenolol, pindolol,** and **acebutolol** have intrinsic sympathomimetic activity; they tend to cause less bradycardia than the other beta-blockers and may also cause less coldness of the extremities.

Some beta-blockers are *lipid soluble* and some are *water soluble*. **Atenolol, nadolol,** and **sotalol** are the most water-soluble; they are less likely to enter the brain, and may therefore cause less sleep disturbance and nightmares. Water-soluble beta-blockers are excreted by the kidneys; they accumulate in renal impairment and dosage reduction is therefore often necessary.

Some beta-blockers have a *relatively short duration of action* and have to be given twice or three times daily. Many of these are, however, available in modified-release formulations so that in general it is not necessary to give beta-blockers more often than once daily for hypertension. For angina twice-daily treatment may sometimes be needed even with a modified-release formulation.

All beta-blockers *slow the heart* and may induce myocardial depression and precipitate heart failure. They should not therefore be given to patients who have incipient cardiac failure or those with second- or third-degree heart block. **Sotalol** may prolong the QT interval, and has occasionally caused life-threatening ventricular arrhythmias (**important:** particular care should be taken to avoid hypokalaemia in patients taking sotalol).

Beta-blockers may *precipitate asthma* and this effect can be dangerous. Some, such as **atenolol, betaxolol, bisoprolol, metoprolol,** and (to a lesser extent) **acebutolol**, have less effect on the beta$_2$ (bronchial) receptors and are, therefore, relatively *cardioselective*, but they are **not** *cardiospecific*. They have a lesser effect on airways resistance but are not free of this side-effect. Patients who have a tendency towards obstructive airways disease must be treated with great caution and may require to take increased doses of their beta$_2$-stimulants (e.g. salbutamol) to overcome the effect of blockade of the bronchial adrenoceptors.

> **CSM advice.** Beta-blockers, even those with apparent cardioselectivity, should not be used in patients with asthma or a history of obstructive airways disease, unless no alternative treatment is available. In such cases the risk of inducing bronchospasm should be appreciated and appropriate precautions taken.

Beta-blockers are also associated with *fatigue, coldness of the extremities* (may be less common with those with ISA, see above), and *sleep disturbances with nightmares* (may be less common with the water-soluble ones, see above).

Beta-blockers can lead to a small deterioration of *glucose tolerance* in diabetics; they also interfere with metabolic and autonomic responses to hypoglycaemia. Their use is not contra-indicated in diabetics, but cardioselective beta-blockers (see above) may be preferable and they should be avoided altogether in those with frequent episodes of hypoglycaemia.

Labetalol combines alpha- and beta-receptor blocking activity. The alpha-blocking activity in the peripheral vessels *lowers peripheral resistance*. **Celiprolol** is a relatively cardioselective beta-blocker with additional partial beta$_2$-agonist activity, and the latter property again lowers peripheral resistance. There is no evidence that these drugs have important advantages over other beta-blockers in the treatment of hypertension.

HYPERTENSION

Beta-blockers are effective *antihypertensives* but their mode of action is not understood; they reduce cardiac output, alter baroceptor reflex sensitivity, and block peripheral adrenoceptors. Some beta-blockers depress plasma renin secretion. It is possible that a central effect may also explain their mode of action. Blood pressure can usually be controlled with relatively few side-effects. In general the dose of beta-blocker does not have to be as high as originally thought. The maximum dose of **oxprenolol** and **propranolol** necessary is probably 320 mg daily. **Atenolol** can usually be given in a dose of 50 mg daily and it is no longer considered necessary to increase to 100 mg.

Combined thiazide/beta-blocker preparations may help compliance but combined preparations should only be used when blood pressure is not adequately controlled by a thiazide or a beta-blocker alone. Beta-blockers reduce, but do not abolish, the tendency for diuretics to cause hypokalaemia.

Beta-blockers can be used to control the pulse rate in patients with *phaeochromocytoma*. However, they should never be used alone as beta-blockade without concurrent alpha-blockade may lead to a hypertensive crisis. For this reason phenoxybenzamine should always be used together with the beta-blocker.

ANGINA

Beta-blockers improve exercise tolerance and relieve symptoms in patients with *angina*; this effect is caused by their reduction of cardiac work. As with hypertension there is no good evidence of the superiority of any one drug, although occasionally a patient will respond better to one beta-blocker than to another. There is some evidence that sudden withdrawal may cause an exacerbation of angina therefore gradual reduction of dose is preferable when beta-blockers are to be stopped. There is a risk of precipitating heart failure when beta-blockers and verapamil are used together in established ischaemic heart disease (**important**: see section 2.3.2).

MYOCARDIAL INFARCTION

Several studies have shown that some beta-blockers can cause a reduction in the recurrence rate of *myocardial infarction*. However, pre-existing heart failure, hypotension, bradyarrhythmias, and obstructive airways disease render this group of drugs unsuitable in some patients who have recovered from a myocardial infarction. **Atenolol** and **metoprolol** may reduce early mortality after intravenous and subsequent oral administration in the acute phase, while **timolol** and **propranolol** have protective value when started in the early convalescent phase. The evidence relating to other beta-blockers is less convincing; some have not been tested in trials of secondary protection. It is also not known whether the protective effect of beta-blockers continues after two years; it is possible that sudden cessation may cause a rebound worsening of myocardial ischaemia.

ARRHYTHMIAS

Beta-blockers act as *anti-arrhythmic drugs* principally by attenuating the effects of the sympathetic system on automaticity and conductivity within the heart. Some have additional anti-arrhythmic properties. They may be used in conjunction with digoxin to control the ventricular response in atrial fibrillation, especially in patients with thyrotoxicosis. Beta-blockers are also useful in the management of supraventricular tachycardias, and are used to control those following myocardial infarction, see above.

THYROTOXICOSIS

Beta-blockers are used in pre-operative preparation for thyroidectomy. Administration of propranolol can reverse clinical features of *thyrotoxicosis* within 4 days. Routine tests of increased thyroid function remain unaltered. The thyroid gland is rendered less vascular thus making surgery easier (see section 6.2.2).

OTHER USES

Beta-blockers have been used to alleviate some symptoms of *anxiety*; probably patients with palpitations, tremor, and tachycardia respond best. (See also sections 4.1.2 and 4.9.3.) Beta-blockers are also used in the *prophylaxis of migraine* (see section 4.7.4.2). Beta-blockers are used topically in the management of *glaucoma* (see section 11.6).

PROPRANOLOL HYDROCHLORIDE
Indications: see under Dose
Cautions: late pregnancy and breast-feeding (see also Appendices 4 and 5); avoid abrupt withdrawal in angina; reduce oral dose of propranolol in liver disease; liver function deteriorates in portal hypertension; reduce initial dose in renal impairment; diabetes; myasthenia gravis; see also notes above; **interactions:** Appendix 1 (beta-blockers), **important:** verapamil interaction, see also section 2.3.2
Contra-indications: asthma or history of obstructive airways disease (see CSM advice on previous page), uncontrolled heart failure, sick sinus syndrome, second or third degree heart block, cardiogenic shock
Side-effects: bradycardia, heart failure, bronchospasm, peripheral vasoconstriction, gastro-intestinal disturbances, fatigue, sleep disturbances; rare reports of rashes and dry eyes (reversible on withdrawal)
Dose: by mouth, hypertension, initially 80 mg twice daily, increased at weekly intervals as required; maintenance 160–320 mg daily
Portal hypertension, initially 40 mg twice daily, increased to 80 mg twice daily according to heart-rate; max. 160 mg twice daily
Phaeochromocytoma (only with an alpha-blocker), 60 mg daily for 3 days before surgery; 30 mg daily in patients unsuitable for surgery
Angina, initially 40 mg 2–3 times daily; maintenance 120–240 mg daily
Arrhythmias, hypertrophic obstructive cardiomyopathy, anxiety tachycardia, and thyrotoxicosis, 10–40 mg 3–4 times daily
Anxiety with symptoms such as palpitations, sweating, tremor, 40 mg twice daily, increased to 3 times daily if necessary
Prophylaxis after infarction, 40 mg 4 times daily for 2–3 days, then 80 mg twice daily, beginning 5 to 21 days after infarction
Migraine prophylaxis and essential tremor, initially 40 mg 2–3 times daily; maintenance 80–160 mg daily
By intravenous injection, arrhythmias and thyrotoxic crisis, 1 mg over 1 minute; if necessary repeat at 2-minute intervals; max. 10 mg (5 mg in anaesthesia)
Note. Excessive bradycardia can be countered with intravenous injection of atropine sulphate 0.6–2.4 mg in divided doses of 600 micrograms

PoM **Propranolol** (Non-proprietary)
Tablets, propranolol hydrochloride 10 mg, net price 20 = 5p; 40 mg, 20 = 8p; 80 mg, 20 = 15p; 160 mg, 20 = 26p. Label: 8
Available from APS (Apsolol®), Ashbourne (Propanix®), Berk (Berkolol®), Cox, CP (Cardinol®), DDSA (Angilol®), Evans, Kerfoot, Norton
Oral suspensions, propranolol hydrochloride 5 mg/5 mL and 50 mg/5 mL available from RP Drugs (special order)

PoM **Inderal**® (ICI)
Tablets, all pink, f/c, propranolol hydrochloride 10 mg, net price 20 = 18p; 40 mg, 20 = 49p; 80 mg, 20 = 80p. Label: 8
Injection, propranolol hydrochloride 1 mg/mL, net price 1-mL amp = 22p

Modified release
PoM **Half-Inderal LA**® (ICI)
Capsules, m/r, lavender/pink, propranolol hydrochloride 80 mg. Net price 28-cap pack = £5.04. Label: 8, 25
PoM **Inderal-LA**® (ICI)
Capsules, m/r, lavender/pink, propranolol hydrochloride 160 mg. Net price 28-cap pack = £6.84. Label: 8, 25
Note. Modified-release capsules containing propranolol hydrochloride 160 mg also available from Ashbourne (Propanix SR®), CP (Sloprolol®), Lagap (Bedranol SR®), Monmouth (Betadur CR®), Tillomed (Beta-Prograne®)

With diuretic
PoM **Inderetic**® (ICI)
Capsules, propranolol hydrochloride 80 mg, bendrofluazide 2.5 mg. Net price 20 = £2.00. Label: 8
Dose: hypertension, 1 capsule twice daily
PoM **Inderex**® (ICI)
Capsules, pink/grey, propranolol hydrochloride 160 mg (m/r), bendrofluazide 5 mg. Net price 28-cap pack = £7.72. Label: 8, 25
Dose: hypertension, 1 capsule daily

ACEBUTOLOL
Indications: see under Dose
Cautions; Contra-indications; Side-effects: see under Propranolol Hydrochloride
Dose: hypertension, initially 400 mg once daily *or* 200 mg twice daily, increased after 2 weeks to 400 mg twice daily if necessary
Angina, initially 400 mg once daily *or* 200 mg twice daily; 300 mg 3 times daily in severe angina; up to 1.2 g daily has been used
Arrhythmias, 0.4–1.2 g daily in 2–3 divided doses

PoM **Sectral**® (Rhône-Poulenc Rorer)
Capsules, acebutolol (as hydrochloride) 100 mg (buff/white), net price 84-cap pack = £7.14; 200 mg (buff/pink), 56-cap pack = £9.16. Label: 8
Tablets, f/c, acebutolol 400 mg (as hydrochloride). Net price 28-tab pack = £8.88. Label: 8

With diuretic
PoM **Secadrex**® (Rhône-Poulenc Rorer)
Tablets, f/c, acebutolol 200 mg (as hydrochloride), hydrochlorothiazide 12.5 mg. Net price 28-tab pack = £8.39. Label: 8
Dose: hypertension, 1 tablet daily, increased to 2 daily as a single dose if necessary

ATENOLOL
Indications: see under Dose
Cautions; Contra-indications; Side-effects: see under Propranolol Hydrochloride; reduce dose in renal impairment (25-mg tablets available)
Dose: by mouth,
Hypertension, 50 mg daily (higher doses no longer considered necessary)
Angina, 100 mg daily in 1 or 2 doses
Arrhythmias, 50–100 mg daily
By intravenous injection, arrhythmias, 2.5 mg at a rate of 1 mg/minute, repeated at 5-minute intervals to a max. of 10 mg
   Note. Excessive bradycardia can be countered with intravenous injection of atropine sulphate 0.6–2.4 mg in divided doses of 600 micrograms
By intravenous infusion, arrhythmias, 150 micrograms/kg over 20 minutes, repeated every 12 hours if required
Early intervention within 12 hours of infarction, 5–10 mg *by slow intravenous injection*, then *by mouth* 50 mg after 15 minutes, 50 mg after 12 hours, then 100 mg daily

PoM **Atenolol** (Non-proprietary)
Tablets, atenolol 50 mg, net price 28-tab pack = £4.82; 100 mg, 28-tab pack = £6.82. Label: 8
Available from APS, Ashbourne (Atenix®), Berk (Antipressan®), Cox, CP (Totamol®), Evans, Kerfoot, Norton, Shire (Vasaten®)
PoM **Tenormin**® (Stuart)
'25' *tablets*, f/c, atenolol 25 mg. Net price 28-tab pack = £4.31. Label: 8
LS tablets, orange, f/c, scored, atenolol 50 mg. Net price 28-tab pack = £5.49. Label: 8
Tablets, orange, f/c, scored, atenolol 100 mg. Net price 28-tab pack = £6.98. Label: 8
Syrup, sugar-free, atenolol 25 mg/5 mL. Net price 300 mL = £8.35. Label: 8
Injection, atenolol 500 micrograms/mL. Net price 10-mL amp = £1.03 (hosp. only)

With diuretic
PoM **Co-tenidone** (Non-proprietary)
Tablets, co-tenidone 50/12.5 (atenolol 50 mg, chlorthalidone 12.5 mg), net price 28-tab pack = £5.27; co-tenidone 100/25 (atenolol 100 mg, chlorthalidone 25 mg), 28-tab pack = £7.50. Label: 8
Available from Ashbourne (AtenixCo®), Cox, Kerfoot
Dose: hypertension, 1 tablet daily (but see also under Dose above)
PoM **Kalten**® (Stuart)
Capsules, red/ivory, atenolol 50 mg, co-amilozide 2.5/25 (anhydrous amiloride hydrochloride 2.5 mg, hydrochlorothiazide 25 mg). Net price 28-cap pack = £7.49. Label: 8
Dose: hypertension, 1 capsule daily
PoM **Tenoret 50**® (Stuart)
Tablets, brown, f/c, co-tenidone 50/12.5 (atenolol 50 mg, chlorthalidone 12.5 mg). Net price 28-tab pack = £5.85. Label: 8
Dose: hypertension, 1 tablet daily

PoM **Tenoretic**® (Stuart)
Tablets, brown, f/c, co-tenidone 100/25 (atenolol 100 mg, chlorthalidone 25 mg). Net price 28-tab pack = £8.33. Label: 8
Dose: hypertension, 1 tablet daily (but see also under Dose above)

With calcium-channel blocker
Note. Only indicated when calcium-channel blocker or beta-blocker alone proves inadequate
PoM **Beta-Adalat**® (Bayer)
Capsules, reddish-brown, atenolol 50 mg, nifedipine 20 mg (m/r). Net price 28-cap pack = £10.90. Label: 8, 25
Dose: hypertension, 1 capsule daily, increased if necessary to twice daily; elderly, 1 daily
Angina, 1 capsule twice daily
PoM **Tenif**® (Stuart)
Capsules, reddish-brown, atenolol 50 mg, nifedipine 20 mg (m/r). Net price 28-cap pack = £10.90. Label: 8, 25
Dose: hypertension, 1 capsule daily, increased if necessary to twice daily; elderly, 1 daily
Angina, 1 capsule twice daily

BETAXOLOL HYDROCHLORIDE
Indications: hypertension
Cautions; Contra-indications; Side-effects: see under Propranolol; renal impairment
Dose: 20 mg daily (elderly patients 10 mg), increased to 40 mg if required

PoM **Kerlone**® (Lorex)
Tablets, f/c, scored, betaxolol hydrochloride 20 mg. Net price 28-tab pack = £7.70. Label: 8

BISOPROLOL FUMARATE
Indications: hypertension, angina
Cautions; Contra-indications; Side-effects: see under Propranolol Hydrochloride; reduce dose in hepatic and renal impairment
Dose: usual dose 10 mg daily (5 mg may be adequate in some patients); max. recommended dose 20 mg daily

PoM **Emcor**® (Merck)
LS Tablets, yellow, f/c, scored, bisoprolol fumarate 5 mg. Net price 28-tab pack = £7.98. Label: 8
Tablets, orange, f/c, scored, bisoprolol fumarate 10 mg. Net price 28-tab pack = £8.96. Label: 8
PoM **Monocor**® (Cyanamid)
Tablets, both f/c, bisoprolol fumarate 5 mg (pink), net price 28-tab pack = £7.98; 10 mg, 28-tab pack = £8.96. Label: 8

CARTEOLOL HYDROCHLORIDE
Indications: angina
Cautions; Contra-indications; Side-effects: see under Propranolol Hydrochloride
Dose: 10 mg daily; if necessary increased gradually to 30 mg daily

PoM **Cartrol**® (Sanofi Winthrop)
Tablets, carteolol hydrochloride 10 mg. Net price 28-tab pack = £5.60. Label: 8

2.4 Beta-adrenoceptor blocking drugs

CELIPROLOL HYDROCHLORIDE
Indications: mild to moderate hypertension
Cautions: pregnancy, breast-feeding; avoid abrupt withdrawal; hepatic and renal impairment (avoid if severe); **interactions**: Appendix 1 (beta-blockers)
Contra-indications: as for Propranolol Hydrochloride; also severe renal impairment
Side-effects: headache, dizziness, fatigue, nausea and somnolence; rarely bradycardia
Dose: 200 mg once daily in the morning, increased to 400 mg once daily if necessary

▼ PoM **Celectol**® (Rhône-Poulenc Rorer)
Tablets, f/c, yellow, scored, celiprolol hydrochloride 200 mg. Net price 28-tab pack = £9.80. Label: 8, 22

ESMOLOL HYDROCHLORIDE
New preparation, see p. xii

LABETALOL HYDROCHLORIDE
Indications: hypertension (including hypertension in pregnancy, hypertension with angina, and hypertension following acute myocardial infarction); hypertensive crisis (but see section 2.5); controlled hypotension in surgery
Cautions: late pregnancy, breast-feeding; avoid abrupt withdrawal; stop and do not restart if liver damage occurs; interferes with laboratory tests for catecholamines; **interactions**: Appendix 1 (beta-blockers)
Contra-indications: as for Propranolol Hydrochloride; also liver disease
Side-effects: postural hypotension (avoid upright position during and for 3 hours after intravenous administration), tiredness, weakness, headache, rashes, scalp tingling, difficulty in micturition, epigastric pain, nausea, vomiting; liver damage (see Cautions); rarely lichenoid rash
Dose: by mouth, initially 100 mg (50 mg in elderly) twice daily with food, increased at intervals of 14 days to usual dose of 200 mg twice daily; up to 800 mg daily in 2 divided doses (3–4 divided doses if higher); max. 2.4 g daily
By intravenous injection, 50 mg over at least 1 minute, repeated after 5 minutes if necessary; max. 200 mg
Note. Excessive bradycardia can be countered with intravenous injection of atropine sulphate 0.6–2.4 mg in divided doses of 600 micrograms
By intravenous infusion, 2 mg/minute; usual range 50–200 mg, higher doses in phaeochromocytoma
Hypertension of pregnancy, 20 mg/hour, doubled every 30 minutes; usual max. 160 mg/hour
Hypertension following infarction, 15 mg/hour, gradually increased to max. 120 mg/hour

PoM **Labetalol Hydrochloride** (Non-proprietary)
Tablets, all f/c, labetalol hydrochloride 100 mg, net price 20 = £1.46; 200 mg, 20 = £2.32; 400 mg, 20 = £3.70. Label: 8, 21
Available from APS, Cox, CP, Evans (100 mg, 200 mg), Kerfoot, Lagap (Labrocol®), Norton

PoM **Trandate**® (DF)
Tablets, all orange, f/c, labetalol hydrochloride 50 mg, net price 56-tab pack = £5.05; 100 mg, 56-tab pack = £5.56; 200 mg, 56-tab pack = £9.02; 400 mg, 20 = £4.26. Label: 8, 21
Injection, labetalol hydrochloride 5 mg/mL. Net price 20-mL amp = £2.83

METOPROLOL TARTRATE
Indications: see under Dose
Cautions; Contra-indications; Side-effects: see under Propranolol Hydrochloride; reduce dose in hepatic and renal impairment
Dose: by mouth, hypertension, initially 100 mg daily, maintenance 100–200 mg daily in 1–2 doses
Angina, 50–100 mg 2–3 times daily
Arrhythmias, usually 50 mg 2–3 times daily; up to 300 mg daily in divided doses if necessary
Migraine prophylaxis, 100–200 mg daily in divided doses
Thyrotoxicosis, 50 mg 4 times daily
By intravenous injection, arrhythmias, up to 5 mg at rate 1–2 mg/minute, repeated after 5 minutes if necessary, total dose 10–15 mg
Note. Excessive bradycardia can be countered with intravenous injection of atropine sulphate 0.6–2.4 mg in divided doses of 600 micrograms
In surgery, 2–4 mg *by slow intravenous injection* at induction or to control arrhythmias developing during anaesthesia; 2-mg doses may be repeated to a max. of 10 mg
Early intervention within 12 hours of infarction, 5 mg *by intravenous injection* every 2 minutes to a max. of 15 mg, followed after 15 minutes by 50 mg *by mouth* every 6 hours for 48 hours; maintenance 200 mg daily in divided doses

PoM **Metoprolol Tartrate** (Non-proprietary)
Tablets, metoprolol tartrate 50 mg, net price 20 = 94p; 100 mg, 20 = £1.75. Label: 8
Available from APS, Ashbourne (Mepranix®), Cox, Evans, Kerfoot, Norton

PoM **Betaloc**® (Astra)
Tablets, both scored, metoprolol tartrate 50 mg, net price 20 = 94p; 56-tab pack = £2.90; 100 mg, 20 = £1.71. Label: 8
Injection, metoprolol tartrate 1 mg/mL. Net price 5-mL amp = 45p

PoM **Lopresor**® (Geigy)
Tablets, both f/c, scored, metoprolol tartrate 50 mg (pink), net price 56-tab pack = £3.26; 100 mg (blue), 56-tab pack = £6.06. Label: 8

Modified release
PoM **Betaloc-SA**® (Astra)
Durules® (= tablets, m/r), metoprolol tartrate 200 mg. Net price 28-tab pack = £6.51. Label: 8, 25
Dose: 200–400 mg daily

PoM Lopresor SR® (Geigy)
Tablets, m/r, yellow, f/c, metoprolol tartrate 200 mg. Net price 28-tab pack = £7.42. Label: 8, 25
Dose: 200–400 mg daily

With diuretic
PoM Co-Betaloc® (Astra)
Tablets, scored, metoprolol tartrate 100 mg, hydrochlorothiazide 12.5 mg. Net price 28-tab pack = £6.65. Label: 8
Dose: hypertension, 1–3 tablets daily in single or divided doses

PoM Co-Betaloc SA® (Astra)
Tablets, yellow, f/c, metoprolol tartrate 200 mg (m/r), hydrochlorothiazide 25 mg. Net price 28-tab pack = £8.20. Label: 8, 25
Dose: hypertension, 1 tablet daily

PoM Lopresoretic® (Geigy)
Tablets, f/c, scored, metoprolol tartrate 100 mg, chlorthalidone 12.5 mg. Net price 56-tab pack = £7.47. Label: 8
Dose: hypertension, 1–2 tablets in the morning; max. 3–4 daily in single or divided doses

NADOLOL
Indications: see under Dose
Cautions; Contra-indications; Side-effects: see under Propranolol Hydrochloride; reduce dose in renal impairment
Dose: hypertension, 80 mg daily, increased at weekly intervals if required; max. 240 mg daily
Angina, 40 mg daily, increased at weekly intervals if required; usual max. 160 mg daily
Arrhythmias, initially 40 mg daily, increased to 160 mg if required; reduce to 40 mg if bradycardia occurs
Migraine prophylaxis, initially 40 mg daily, increased by 40 mg at weekly intervals; usual maintenance dose 80–160 mg daily
Thyrotoxicosis, 80–160 mg daily

PoM Corgard® (Squibb)
Tablets, both blue, nadolol 40 mg, net price 28-tab pack = £3.86; 80 mg, 28-tab pack = £5.59. Label: 8

With diuretic
PoM Corgaretic 40® (Squibb)
Tablets, scored, nadolol 40 mg, bendrofluazide 5 mg. Net price 28-tab pack = £6.07. Label: 8
Dose: hypertension, 1–2 tablets daily

PoM Corgaretic 80® (Squibb)
Tablets, scored, nadolol 80 mg, bendrofluazide 5 mg. Net price 28-tab pack = £8.69. Label: 8
Dose: hypertension, 1–2 tablets daily

OXPRENOLOL HYDROCHLORIDE
Indications: see under Dose
Cautions; Contra-indications; Side-effects: see under Propranolol Hydrochloride
Dose: hypertension, initially 80 mg twice daily, increased as required at weekly intervals; max. 480 mg daily
Angina, 40–160 mg 3 times daily
Arrhythmias, initially 20–40 mg 3 times daily, increased as necessary
Anxiety symptoms (short-term use), initially 40 mg twice daily, increased if necessary to 160 mg daily in divided doses

PoM Oxprenolol (Non-proprietary)
Tablets, all coated, oxprenolol hydrochloride 20 mg, net price 20 = 30p; 40 mg, 20 = 43p; 80 mg, 20 = 71p; 160 mg, 20 = £1.38. Label: 8
Available from APS (Apsolox®, 80-mg tablets contain tartrazine), Cox, Evans, Kerfoot

PoM Trasicor® (Ciba)
Tablets, all f/c, oxprenolol hydrochloride 20 mg (contain gluten), net price 20 = 58p; 40 mg (contain gluten), 20 = 96p; 80 mg (beige), 56-tab pack = £4.10; 160 mg (orange), 56-tab pack = £7.38. Label: 8

Modified release
PoM Slow-Trasicor® (Ciba)
Tablets, m/r, f/c, oxprenolol hydrochloride 160 mg. Net price 28-tab pack = £6.50. Label: 8, 25
Dose: 160–480 mg daily
Note. Modified-release tablets containing oxprenolol hydrochloride 160 mg also available from Ashbourne (Oxyprenix SR®), Norton

With diuretic
PoM Trasidrex® (Ciba)
Tablets, red, s/c, co-prenozide 160/0.25 (oxprenolol hydrochloride 160 mg (m/r), cyclopenthiazide 250 micrograms). Net price 28-tab pack = £6.73. Label: 8, 25
Dose: hypertension, 1 tablet daily, increased to 2 daily as a single dose; max. 3 daily

PENBUTOLOL SULPHATE
Indications: hypertension
Cautions; Contra-indications; Side-effects: see under Propranolol Hydrochloride
Dose: see below

With diuretic
PoM Lasipressin® (Hoechst)
Tablets, yellow-white, f/c, scored, penbutolol sulphate 40 mg, frusemide 20 mg. Net price 30-tab pack = £8.49. Label: 8
Dose: hypertension, 1 tablet daily, increased to twice daily if necessary

PINDOLOL
Indications: see under Dose
Cautions; Contra-indications; Side-effects: see under Propranolol Hydrochloride; reduce dose in renal impairment
Dose: hypertension, initially 5 mg 2–3 times daily *or* 15 mg once daily, increased as required at weekly intervals; max. 45 mg daily
Angina, 2.5–5 mg up to 3 times daily

PoM **Visken**® (Sandoz)
Tablets, both scored, pindolol 5 mg, net price 100-tab pack = £7.46; 15 mg, 30-tab pack = £6.71. Label: 8

With diuretic
PoM **Viskaldix**® (Sandoz)
Tablets, scored, pindolol 10 mg, clopamide 5 mg. Net price 28-tab pack = £5.72. Label: 8
Dose: hypertension, 1 tablet daily in the morning, increased if necessary to 2 daily; max. 3 daily

SOTALOL HYDROCHLORIDE
Indications: see under Dose
Cautions; Contra-indications; Side-effects: see under Propranolol Hydrochloride; reduce dose in renal impairment; occasionally causes atypical ventricular arrhythmias (torsade de pointes)—special need to avoid hypokalaemia if given with thiazide or loop diuretic (also stop if severe or persistent diarrhoea etc.)
Dose: by mouth, hypertension and angina, initially 80 mg twice daily *or* 160 mg once daily; maintenance 160 mg daily, increased to 400–600 mg daily if necessary
Arrhythmias, 120–240 mg daily in single or divided doses
Thyrotoxicosis, 120–240 mg daily in single or divided doses
Prophylaxis after infarction, 320 mg daily, starting 5–14 days after infarction
By slow intravenous injection, arrhythmias, 20–60 mg over 2–3 minutes with ECG monitoring, repeated if necessary with 10-minute intervals between injections; up to 100 mg over 3 minutes or longer
Note. Excessive bradycardia can be countered with intravenous injection of atropine sulphate 0.6–2.4 mg in divided doses of 600 micrograms

PoM **Beta-Cardone**® (Evans)
Tablets, all scored, sotalol hydrochloride 40 mg (green), net price 20 = 79p; 80 mg (pink), 20 = £1.17; 200 mg, 30-tab pack = £4.15. Label: 8
PoM **Sotacor**® (Bristol-Myers)
Tablets, sotalol hydrochloride 80 mg (pink), net price 28-tab pack = £3.49; 160 mg (blue), 28-tab pack = £6.89. Label: 8
Injection, sotalol hydrochloride 10 mg/mL. Net price 4-mL amp = £1.76

With diuretic
Note. Increased risk of hypokalaemia if combined with thiazide or loop diuretic (see Cautions above)
PoM **Sotazide**® (Bristol-Myers)
Tablets, blue, sotalol hydrochloride 160 mg, hydrochlorothiazide 25 mg. Net price 28-tab pack = £7.12. Label: 8
Dose: hypertension, 1 tablet daily, increased to 2 daily if necessary
PoM **Tolerzide**® (Bristol-Myers)
Tablets, lilac, sotalol hydrochloride 80 mg, hydrochlorothiazide 12.5 mg. Net price 28-tab pack = £4.05. Label: 8
Dose: hypertension, 1 tablet daily

TIMOLOL MALEATE
Indications: see under Dose
Cautions; Contra-indications; Side-effects: see under Propranolol Hydrochloride
Dose: hypertension, initially 5 mg twice daily *or* 10 mg once daily; max. 60 mg daily
Angina, initially 5 mg 2–3 times daily, maintenance 15–45 mg daily
Prophylaxis after infarction, initially 5 mg twice daily, increased after 2 days to 10 mg twice daily, starting 7 to 28 days after infarction
Migraine prophylaxis, 10–20 mg daily

PoM **Betim**® (Leo)
Tablets, scored, timolol maleate 10 mg. Net price 20 = £1.75. Label: 8
PoM **Blocadren**® (MSD)
Tablets, blue, scored, timolol maleate 10 mg. Net price 20 = £2.12. Label: 8

With diuretic
PoM **Moducren**® (Morson)
Tablets, blue, scored, timolol maleate 10 mg, co-amilozide 2.5/25 (amiloride hydrochloride 2.5 mg, hydrochlorothiazide 25 mg). Net price 28-tab pack = £8.00. Label: 8
Dose: hypertension, 1–2 tablets daily as a single dose
PoM **Prestim**® (Leo)
Tablets, scored, timolol maleate 10 mg, bendrofluazide 2.5 mg. Net price 20 = £2.79. Label: 8
Dose: hypertension, 1–2 tablets daily; max. 4 daily
PoM **Prestim Forte**® (Leo)
Tablets, scored, timolol maleate 20 mg, bendrofluazide 5 mg. Net price 20 = £5.88. Label: 8
Dose: hypertension, ½–2 tablets daily in single or divided doses

2.5 Antihypertensive therapy

2.5.1 Vasodilator antihypertensive drugs
2.5.2 Centrally acting antihypertensive drugs
2.5.3 Adrenergic neurone blocking drugs
2.5.4 Alpha-adrenoceptor blocking drugs
2.5.5 Angiotensin-converting enzyme inhibitors
2.5.6 Ganglion blocking drugs
2.5.7 Tyrosine hydroxylase inhibitors

Antihypertensive therapy has improved the outlook for patients with high blood pressure by decreasing the frequency of stroke, heart failure, and renal failure; treatment also reduces the incidence of coronary events. The recommendations of the British Hypertension Society are that, in general, patients whose diastolic pressure averages 110 mmHg or higher when measured on three separate occasions, or 100 to 109 mmHg when measured repeatedly over 4 to 6 months, should receive antihypertensive therapy. Below that level the benefits of therapy are unproven. The usual aim should be to reduce the diastolic blood pressure preferably to below 90 mmHg and certainly below 100 mmHg. The quality of control of blood pressure at follow-up is an important predictor of outcome, and efficient long-term care is necessary.

Malignant (or accelerated) hypertension or very severe hypertension (diastolic blood pressure >140 mmHg) requires urgent treatment in hospital but is not an indication for parenteral antihypertensive therapy. Normally treatment should be by mouth with a beta-blocker (atenolol or labetalol) or a calcium-channel blocker (nifedipine). Within the first 24 hours the diastolic blood pressure should be reduced to 100–110 mmHg. Over the next two or three days blood pressure should be normalised by using beta-blockers, calcium-channel blockers, diuretics, vasodilators, or angiotensin-converting enzyme inhibitors. Very rapid falls in blood pressure can cause reduced cerebral perfusion leading to cerebral infarction and blindness, a reduction in renal perfusion causing a deterioration in renal function, and myocardial ischaemia. Parenteral antihypertensive drugs are, therefore, hardly ever necessary.

On the rare occasions when a parenteral antihypertensive is necessary, sodium nitroprusside by infusion is the drug of choice.

In moderate to severe hypertension (diastolic blood pressure >110 mmHg) or in patients with vascular complications, antihypertensive drugs are best added 'stepwise' until control has been achieved; an attempt can then be made to 'step down' treatment under supervision. In mild uncomplicated hypertension (diastolic blood pressure <110 mmHg), drugs may be substituted rather than added. The strategy for reducing blood pressure is probably best as follows:

1. *Non-drug treatment*—obesity, high alcohol intake, and high salt intake may elevate blood pressure and these should be corrected.
2. *Diuretic therapy*—any thiazide will be effective, e.g. bendrofluazide 2.5 mg/day (section 2.2.1). The optimum dose of a thiazide used to treat hypertension is the lowest possible dose; higher doses do not have a major additional anti-hypertensive effect, but do cause more metabolic side-effects. Potassium supplements are seldom necessary but plasma potassium concentration should be checked 3 to 4 weeks after starting treatment. Potassium-sparing diuretics (amiloride or triamterene) are usually not necessary in the routine treatment of hypertension, unless hypokalaemia develops.
3. *Beta-adrenoceptor blocking drugs* (section 2.4) should be used in combination with a thiazide where they are not effective alone.
4(a). *Calcium-channel blockers*—calcium-channel blockers such as nifedipine, nicardipine, and verapamil have antihypertensive efficacy broadly similar to that of thiazides or beta-blockers. Minor side-effects are more common, and their safety during long-term treatment is less well established; they should therefore be considered for hypertension only when thiazides and beta-blockers are contra-indicated, not tolerated, or fail to control blood pressure. There are important differences between verapamil and dihydropyridine calcium-channel blockers such as nifedipine and nicardipine (see section 2.6.2).
4(b). *ACE inhibitors* (section 2.5.5)—all ACE inhibitors may cause a precipitate drop in blood pressure in patients with renal impairment and/or receiving diuretic therapy; they should be given in low initial doses and where possible diuretic therapy should be omitted for a few days before starting. About 20% of women and 10% of men receiving an ACE inhibitor develop a persistent dry cough.
5. *Other drugs*—Vasodilators (hydralazine, minoxidil, diazoxide), alpha-adrenoceptor blocking drugs (prazosin, terazosin, doxazosin), and centrally acting drugs (methyldopa, reserpine) are generally reserved for patients whose blood pressure is not controlled by, or who have contra-indications to, the drugs already mentioned.

SYSTOLIC HYPERTENSION. Isolated systolic hypertension (systolic blood pressure >160 mmHg, diastolic <90 mmHg) is associated with an increased risk of stroke and coronary events, particularly in those over 60 years of age. Systolic blood pressure averaging 160 mmHg or higher over 3 to 6 months observation (despite appropriate non-drug treatment) should be lowered in those over 60 years, even if diastolic hypertension is absent. The regimen proven effective is a low dose of a thiazide, with addition of a beta-blocker when necessary. It is not clear whether isolated systolic hypertension should be treated in younger subjects, but benefits of treatment are likely to be smaller than in older patients.

HYPERTENSION IN PREGNANCY. It is important to control blood pressure in pregnancy. High blood pressure may be due to pre-existing essential hypertension or to pre-eclampsia. Oral methyldopa is safe in pregnancy. Beta-blockers are effective and safe in the third trimester but may cause intra-uterine growth retardation when used from earlier in pregnancy. Hydralazine by mouth is useful as second-line therapy; intravenous injection can be used to control hypertensive crises associated with *eclampsia*.

HYPERTENSION IN THE ELDERLY. Antihypertensive therapy reduces the incidence of cardiovascular complications substantially in elderly hypertensive subjects. The benefit is evident up to at least 85 years of age, and it is probably inappropriate to apply a strict age limit when coming to a decision on drug therapy. Elderly subjects who have a good outlook for longevity from other points of view should have their blood pressure lowered if they are hypertensive. The criteria for treatment are diastolic blood pressure averaging 100 mmHg or higher *or* systolic averaging 160 mmHg or higher over 3 to 6 months observation (despite appropriate non-drug treatment). A low dose of a thiazide is the clear drug of first choice, with addition of a beta-blocker when necessary.

2.5 Antihypertensive therapy

2.5.1 Vasodilator antihypertensive drugs

These are potent drugs, especially when used in combination with a beta-blocker and a thiazide.

Diazoxide is diabetogenic and is not used by mouth, except in very severe hypertension; it can be used by intravenous injection in hypertensive emergencies.

Hydralazine given by mouth is a useful adjunct to other treatment, but when used alone causes tachycardia and fluid retention. Side-effects can be few if the dose is kept below 100 mg daily, but systemic lupus erythematosus should be suspected if there is unexplained weight loss, arthritis, or any other unexplained ill health.

Sodium nitroprusside is given by intravenous infusion to control severe hypertensive crises.

Minoxidil should be reserved for the treatment of severe hypertension resistant to other drugs. Vasodilatation is accompanied by increased cardiac output and tachycardia and the patients develop fluid retention. For this reason a beta-blocker and a diuretic (usually frusemide, in high dosage) are mandatory. Hypertrichosis is troublesome and renders this drug unsuitable for women.

Prazosin and **terazosin** (section 2.5.4) have alpha-blocking and vasodilator properties.

DIAZOXIDE

Indications: acute treatment of severe hypertension associated with renal disease (but see section 2.5); hypoglycaemia, see section 6.1.4

Cautions: ischaemic heart disease, pregnancy, labour, impaired renal function; **interactions:** Appendix 1 (diazoxide)

Side-effects: tachycardia, hyperglycaemia, sodium and water retention

Dose: by rapid intravenous injection (less than 30 seconds), 1–3 mg/kg to max. single dose of 150 mg (see below); may be repeated after 5–15 minutes if required

Note. Single doses of 300 mg have been associated with angina and with myocardial and cerebral infarction

PoM Eudemine® (Evans)
Injection, diazoxide 15 mg/mL. Net price 20-mL amp = £2.70

HYDRALAZINE HYDROCHLORIDE

Indications: moderate to severe hypertension, with beta-blocker and thiazide; hypertensive crisis (but see section 2.5)

Cautions: reduce initial dose in renal impairment; coronary artery disease (may provoke angina, avoid after myocardial infarction until stabilised), cerebrovascular disease; over-rapid blood pressure reduction is occasionally encountered even with low parenteral doses; pregnancy, breast-feeding; **interactions:** Appendix 1 (hydralazine)

Contra-indications: idiopathic systemic lupus erythematosus, severe tachycardia, high output heart failure, myocardial insufficiency due to mechanical obstruction, cor pulmonale, dissecting aortic aneurysm; porphyria (see section 9.8.2)

Side-effects: tachycardia, fluid retention, nausea, and vomiting; headache; systemic lupus erythematosus-like syndrome after long-term therapy with over 100 mg daily (or less in women) (see also notes above); rarely rashes, fever, changes in blood count, peripheral neuritis

Dose: by mouth, 25 mg twice daily, increased to a max. of 50 mg twice daily (see notes above)

By slow intravenous injection, 5–10 mg over 20 minutes; may be repeated after 20–30 minutes (see Cautions)

By intravenous infusion, initially 200–300 micrograms/minute; maintenance usually 50–150 micrograms/minute

PoM Hydralazine (Non-proprietary)
Tablets, hydralazine hydrochloride 25 mg, net price 20 = 30p; 50 mg, 20 = 60p

PoM Apresoline® (Ciba)
Tablets, both s/c, hydralazine hydrochloride 25 mg (yellow), net price 20 = 36p; 50 mg (violet), 20 = 70p
Additives: include gluten

Injection, powder for reconstitution, hydralazine hydrochloride. Net price 20-mg amp = 32p

MINOXIDIL

Indications: severe hypertension, in addition to a diuretic and a beta-blocker

Cautions: see notes above; angina; after myocardial infarction (until stabilised); lower doses in dialysis patients; pregnancy; **interactions:** Appendix 1 (minoxidil)

Contra-indications: phaeochromocytoma; porphyria (see section 9.8.2)

Side-effects: sodium and water retention; weight gain, peripheral oedema, tachycardia, hypertrichosis; reversible rise in creatinine and blood urea nitrogen; occasionally, gastro-intestinal disturbances, breast tenderness, rashes

Dose: initially 5 mg daily, in 1–2 doses, increased by 5–10 mg every 3 or more days; max. usually 50 mg daily

PoM Loniten® (Upjohn)
Tablets, all scored, minoxidil 2.5 mg, net price 20 = £2.47; 5 mg, 20 = £4.40; 10 mg, 20 = £8.52

SODIUM NITROPRUSSIDE

Indications: hypertensive crisis (but see section 2.5); controlled hypotension in surgery; acute or chronic heart failure

Cautions: hypothyroidism, severe renal impairment, impaired cerebral circulation, elderly; monitor plasma-cyanide concentration; **interactions:** Appendix 1 (nitroprusside)

Contra-indications: severe hepatic impairment; vitamin B$_{12}$ deficiency; Leber's optic atrophy; compensatory hypertension

Side-effects: headache, dizziness, nausea, retching, abdominal pain, perspiration, palpitations, apprehension, retrosternal discomfort—reduce infusion rate

Cautionary label wordings, see inside back cover

Prices are **net**, see p. 1

Dose: hypertensive crisis, in patients not already receiving antihypertensives, *by intravenous infusion*, 0.3–1 micrograms/kg/minute initially, then adjusted; usual range 0.5–6 micrograms/kg/minute (20–400 micrograms/minute); max. 8 micrograms/kg/minute; lower doses for patients already being treated with antihypertensives

Lower doses should also be employed for controlled hypotension in surgery (max. 1.5 micrograms/kg/minute)

Heart failure, *by intravenous infusion*, initially 10–15 micrograms/minute, increased every 5–10 minutes as necessary; usual range 10–200 micrograms/minute; max. 280 micrograms/minute (4 micrograms/kg/minute)

PoM **Sodium Nitroprusside** (Non-proprietary)
Intravenous solution, sodium nitroprusside 10 mg/mL. For dilution and use as an infusion. 5-mL vial
Available from David Bull, CP

PoM **Nipride**® (Roche)
Infusion, sodium nitroprusside 50-mg amp (with solvent for reconstitution). Net price = £4.00

2.5.2 Centrally acting antihypertensive drugs

This group includes methyldopa and clonidine and is largely falling from use.

Methyldopa, however, has the advantage of being safe in asthmatics, in heart failure, and in pregnancy. Side-effects are minimised if the daily dose is kept below 1 g.

Clonidine has the disadvantage that sudden withdrawal may cause a hypertensive crisis.

Reserpine and rauwolfia are no longer used in Britain.

CLONIDINE HYDROCHLORIDE

Indications: hypertension (for use in migraine, see section 4.7.4.2)
Cautions: must be withdrawn gradually to avoid hypertensive crisis; Raynaud's syndrome or other occlusive peripheral vascular disease; history of depression; avoid in porphyria (see section 9.8.2); **interactions:** Appendix 1 (clonidine)
DRIVING. Drowsiness may affect performance of skilled tasks (e.g. driving); effects of alcohol may be enhanced
Side-effects: dry mouth, sedation, depression, fluid retention, bradycardia, Raynaud's phenomenon, headache, dizziness, euphoria, nocturnal unrest, rash, nausea, constipation, rarely impotence
Dose: by mouth, 50–100 micrograms 3 times daily, increased every second or third day; max. daily dose usually 1.2 mg
By slow intravenous injection, 150–300 micrograms; max. 750 micrograms in 24 hours

PoM **Catapres**® (Boehringer Ingelheim)
Tablets, both scored, clonidine hydrochloride 100 micrograms, net price 84-tab pack = £5.39; 300 micrograms, 84-tab pack = £12.56. Label: 3, 8
Injection, clonidine hydrochloride 150 micrograms/mL. Net price 1-mL amp = 27p

PoM **Dixarit**® (migraine), see section 4.7.4.2

Modified release
PoM **Catapres**® **Perlongets** (Boehringer Ingelheim)
Capsules, m/r, red/yellow, clonidine hydrochloride 250 micrograms. Net price 56-cap pack = £12.74. Label: 3, 8, 25
Dose: usually 1 capsule in the evening; 2–3 capsules daily (1 morning and 1–2 evening) if necessary

METHYLDOPA

Indications: hypertension, in conjunction with diuretic; hypertensive crisis when immediate effect not necessary
Cautions: positive direct Coombs' test in up to 20% of patients (may affect blood cross-matching); interference with laboratory tests; reduce initial dose in renal impairment; blood counts and liver-function tests advised; **interactions:** Appendix 1 (methyldopa)
DRIVING. Drowsiness may affect performance of skilled tasks (e.g. driving); effects of alcohol may be enhanced
Contra-indications: history of depression, active liver disease, phaeochromocytoma; porphyria (see section 9.8.2)
Side-effects: dry mouth, sedation, depression, drowsiness, diarrhoea, fluid retention, failure of ejaculation, liver damage, haemolytic anaemia, systemic lupus erythematosus-like syndrome, parkinsonism, rashes, nasal stuffiness
Dose: by mouth, 250 mg 2–3 times daily, gradually increased at intervals of 2 or more days; max. daily dose 3 g
ELDERLY 125 mg twice daily initially, gradually increased; max. daily dose 2 g
By intravenous infusion, methyldopate hydrochloride 250–500 mg, repeated after 6 hours if required

PoM **Methyldopa** (Non-proprietary)
Tablets, coated, methyldopa (anhydrous) 125 mg, net price 20 = 43p; 250 mg, 20 = 68p; 500 mg, 20 = £1.38. Label: 3, 8
Available from APS, Ashbourne (Metalpha®), Berk (Dopamet®), Cox, CP, Evans, Kerfoot

PoM **Aldomet**® (MSD)
Tablets, all yellow, f/c, methyldopa (anhydrous) 125 mg, net price 20 = 77p; 250 mg, 20 = £1.19; 500 mg, 20 = £2.34. Label: 3, 8
Suspension, methyldopa 250 mg/5 mL. Net price 200 mL = £3.96. Label: 3, 8
Injection, methyldopa hydrochloride 50 mg/mL. Net price 5-mL amp = £2.31

With diuretic
PoM **Hydromet**® (MSD)
Tablets, pink, f/c, methyldopa (anhydrous) 250 mg, hydrochlorothiazide 15 mg. Net price 20 = £1.52. Label: 3, 8

2.5.3 Adrenergic neurone blocking drugs

These drugs prevent the release of noradrenaline from postganglionic adrenergic neurones. Guanethidine also depletes the nerve endings of nor-

2.5 Antihypertensive therapy

adrenaline. These drugs do not control supine blood pressure and may cause postural hypotension. For this reason they have largely fallen from use, but they may be necessary in combination with other therapy in resistant hypertension.

GUANETHIDINE MONOSULPHATE

Indications: moderate to severe hypertension that has failed to respond adequately to other antihypertensives, in conjunction with a diuretic or a vasodilator antihypertensive
Cautions: postural hypotension may cause falls in elderly; coronary or cerebral arteriosclerosis, asthma, history of peptic ulceration; pregnancy; **interactions:** Appendix 1 (adrenergic neurone blockers)
Contra-indications: phaeochromocytoma, renal failure, heart failure
Side-effects: postural hypotension, failure of ejaculation, fluid retention, nasal congestion, headache, diarrhoea, drowsiness
Dose: by mouth, 10 mg daily, increased by 10 mg at weekly intervals; usual daily dose 25–50 mg
By intramuscular injection, 10–20 mg, repeated after 3 hours if required

PoM **Ismelin**® (Ciba)
Tablets, guanethidine monosulphate 10 mg, net price 20 = 46p; 25 mg (pink), 20 = £1.03
Additives: include gluten
Injection, guanethidine monosulphate 10 mg/mL. Net price 1-mL amp = 23p

BETHANIDINE SULPHATE

Indications; Cautions; Contra-indications; Side-effects: see under Guanethidine Monosulphate (except diarrhoea)
Dose: 10 mg (elderly 5 mg) 3 times daily after food, increased by 5 mg at intervals; max. daily dose 200 mg

PoM **Bendogen**® (Lagap)
Tablets, scored, bethanidine sulphate 10 mg, net price 20 = £1.20. Label: 21

DEBRISOQUINE

Indications; Cautions; Contra-indications; Side-effects: see under Guanethidine Monosulphate (except diarrhoea)
Dose: 10 mg 1–2 times daily, increased by 10 mg every 3 days; usual range 20–60 mg daily (120 mg or higher in severe hypertension)

PoM **Declinax**® (Roche)
Tablets, both scored, debrisoquine (as sulphate) 10 mg, net price 100-tab pack = £3.87; 20 mg (blue), 100-tab pack = £5.60

2.5.4 Alpha-adrenoceptor blocking drugs

Prazosin has post-synaptic alpha-blocking and vasodilator properties and rarely causes tachycardia. It may, however, cause a rapid reduction in blood pressure after the first dose and should be introduced with caution. **Doxazosin** and **terazosin** have properties similar to those of prazosin.

Phenoxybenzamine and **indoramin** are alpha-blockers which are effective agents, but have many side-effects. Phenoxybenzamine is used with a beta-blocker in the short-term management of severe hypertensive episodes associated with phaeochromocytoma; it is also used in the management of severe shock unresponsive to conventional therapy.

Phentolamine is used rarely as a suppression test for phaeochromocytoma.

PROSTATIC HYPERTROPHY. Both prazosin and indoramin are also indicated for benign prostatic hypertrophy (see below and also section 7.4.1).

DOXAZOSIN

Indications: hypertension, if necessary in conjunction with thiazide or beta-blocker
Cautions: care with initial dose (postural hypotension); **interactions:** Appendix 1 (alpha-blockers)
Side-effects: postural hypotension (rarely associated with fainting); dizziness, vertigo, headache, fatigue, asthenia, oedema
Dose: 1 mg daily, increased after 1–2 weeks to 2 mg daily, and thereafter to 4 mg daily, if necessary; max. 16 mg daily

PoM **Cardura**® (Invicta)
Tablets, doxazosin (as mesylate) 1 mg, net price 28-tab pack = £9.60; 2 mg, 28-tab pack = £12.80; 4 mg, 28-tab pack = £16.00

INDORAMIN

Indications: see preparations below
Cautions: avoid alcohol (enhances rate and extent of absorption); control incipient heart failure with diuretics and digoxin; hepatic or renal impairment; elderly patients; Parkinson's disease; epilepsy (convulsions in *animal* studies); history of depression; **interactions:** Appendix 1 (alpha-blockers)
DRIVING. Drowsiness may affect performance of skilled tasks (e.g. driving); effects of alcohol may be enhanced
Contra-indications: established heart failure; patients receiving MAOIs
Side-effects: sedation; also dizziness, depression, failure of ejaculation, dry mouth, nasal congestion, extrapyramidal effects, weight gain
Dose: see preparations below

PoM **Baratol**® (Monmouth)
Tablets, both f/c, indoramin (as hydrochloride) 25 mg (blue), net price 20 = £2.15; 50 mg (green, scored), 20 = £3.80. Label: 2
Dose: hypertension, usually in conjunction with thiazide or beta-blocker, initially 25 mg twice daily, increased by 25–50 mg daily at intervals of 2 weeks; max. daily dose 200 mg in 2–3 divided doses

Cautionary label wordings, see inside back cover   Prices are **net**, see p. 1

Prostatic hypertrophy
PoM Doralese® (Bencard)
Tablets, yellow, f/c, indoramin 20 mg. Net price 60-tab pack = £8.40. Label: 2
Dose: benign prostatic hypertrophy, 20 mg twice daily; increased if necessary by 20 mg every 2 weeks to max. 100 mg daily in divided doses; ELDERLY, 20 mg at night may be adequate
Note. Not licensed for treatment of hypertension

PHENOXYBENZAMINE HYDROCHLORIDE

Indications: phaeochromocytoma (see notes above)
Cautions: elderly patients; congestive heart failure; severe or ischaemic heart disease (avoid for 3–4 weeks after myocardial infarction; marked arteriosclerosis (avoid if history of cerebrovascular accident); renal impairment; carcinogenic in *animals*; pregnancy; avoid in porphyria (see section 9.8.2); avoid infusion in hypovolaemia; avoid extravasation (irritant to tissues)
Side-effects: postural hypotension with dizziness and marked compensatory tachycardia, lassitude, nasal congestion, miosis, inhibition of ejaculation; rarely gastro-intestinal disturbances; decreased sweating and dry mouth after intravenous infusion; idiosyncratic profound hypotension within few minutes of starting infusion
Dose: by mouth, phaeochromocytoma, 10 mg daily, increased by 10 mg daily; usual dose 1–2 mg/kg daily in 2 divided doses

PoM Dibenyline® (SK&F)
Capsules, red/white, phenoxybenzamine hydrochloride 10 mg. Net price 30-cap pack = £3.19
Injection concentrate, phenoxybenzamine hydrochloride 50 mg/mL. To be diluted before use. 2-mL amp (hosp. only)
Dose: by intravenous infusion (preferably through large vein), phaeochromocytoma and adjunct in severe shock, 1 mg/kg daily in 200 mL physiological saline over at least 2 hours; do not repeat within 24 hours (intensive care facilities needed)
CAUTION. Owing to risk of contact sensitisation doctors, nurses, and other health workers should avoid contamination of hands

PHENTOLAMINE MESYLATE

Indications: hypertensive crises due to phaeochromocytoma or interaction of foods with MAOIs, diagnosis of phaeochromocytoma; clonidine withdrawal; acute left ventricular failure
Cautions: monitor blood pressure (avoid in hypotension), heart rate
Side-effects: hypotension, tachycardia, dizziness; nausea, diarrhoea, nasal congestion
Dose: by intravenous injection, 5–10 mg repeated if necessary
By intravenous infusion, 5–60 mg over 10–30 minutes at a rate of 0.2–2 mg/minute

PoM Rogitine® (Ciba)
Injection, phentolamine mesylate 10 mg/mL. Net price 1-mL amp = 27p

PRAZOSIN HYDROCHLORIDE

Indications: see under Dose
Cautions: first dose may cause collapse due to hypotension (therefore should be taken on retiring to bed); elderly; reduce initial dose in renal impairment; **interactions:** Appendix 1 (alpha-blockers)
Side-effects: postural hypotension, drowsiness, weakness, dizziness, headache, lack of energy, nausea, palpitations; urinary frequency, incontinence reported
Dose: hypertension, 500 micrograms 2–3 times daily, the initial dose on retiring to bed at night (to avoid collapse, see Cautions); increased to 1 mg 2–3 times daily after 3–7 days; further increased if necessary to max. 20 mg daily
Congestive heart failure, 500 micrograms 2–4 times daily (initial dose at bedtime, see above), increasing to 4 mg daily in divided doses; maintenance 4–20 mg daily (but rarely used)
Raynaud's syndrome, initially 500 micrograms twice daily (initial dose at bedtime, see above); maintenance 1–2 mg twice daily
Benign prostatic hypertrophy, initially 500 micrograms twice daily for 3–7 days (initial dose at bedtime, see above), dose subsequently adjusted according to response; usual maintenance (and max.) 2 mg twice daily

PoM Hypovase® (Invicta)
Tablets, prazosin hydrochloride 500 micrograms, net price 56-tab pack = £2.41; 1 mg (orange, scored), 56-tab pack = £3.10; 2 mg (scored), 56-tab pack = £4.21; 5 mg (scored), 56-tab pack = £9.07; starter pack of 8 × 500-microgram tabs and 32 × 1-mg tabs = £2.90. Label: 3, counselling, see dose above
Note. Prazosin tablets also available from Ashbourne (Alphavase®), Norton

TERAZOSIN

Indications: mild to moderate hypertension
Cautions: first dose may cause collapse due to hypotension (within 30–90 minutes, therefore should be taken on retiring to bed) (may also occur with rapid dose increase); **interactions:** Appendix 1 (alpha-blockers)
Side-effects: dizziness, lack of energy, peripheral oedema; urinary frequency reported
Dose: 1 mg at bedtime (compliance with bedtime dose important to avoid collapse, see Cautions); dose doubled after 7 days if necessary; usual maintenance dose 2–10 mg daily; more than 20 mg daily rarely improves efficacy

PoM Hytrin® (Abbott)
Tablets, terazosin (as hydrochloride) 2 mg (yellow), net price 28-tab pack = £12.87; 5 mg (tan), 28-tab pack = £19.37; 10 mg (blue), 28-tab pack = £27.27; starter pack of 7 × 1-mg tabs and 21 × 2-mg tabs = £13.33. Label: 3, counselling, see dose above

2.5.5 Angiotensin-converting enzyme inhibitors
(ACE inhibitors)

Angiotensin-converting enzyme inhibitors inhibit the conversion of angiotensin I to angiotensin II. They are effective and generally well tolerated, but experience is limited as regards long-term use.

They should therefore be considered for *hypertension* only when thiazides and beta-blockers are contra-indicated, not tolerated, or fail to control blood pressure. All may cause very rapid falls of blood pressure in some patients. Therefore where possible diuretic therapy should be stopped for a few days before initiating therapy and the first dose should preferably be given at bedtime.

ACE inhibitors have a valuable role in *heart failure* when used as an adjunct to diuretics and, where appropriate, digoxin. They have been shown to improve the prognosis substantially, and in this respect are superior to regimens such as modified-release nitrates with hydralazine. Introduction of an ACE inhibitor should be considered when heart failure is not completely controlled by frusemide 80 mg daily (or an equivalent dose of another loop diuretic). To avoid dangerous hyperkalaemia, any potassium-sparing diuretic should be omitted from the diuretic regimen before introducing an ACE inhibitor, changing to the loop diuretic alone; potassium supplements should also be discontinued. Profound first-dose hypotension is common (and potentially serious) when ACE inhibitors are introduced to patients with heart failure receiving loop diuretics. Temporary withdrawal of the loop diuretic reduces the risk, but may cause severe rebound pulmonary oedema. The ACE inhibitor should therefore be started at a very low dosage (e.g. captopril 6.25 mg), with the patient recumbent and under close supervision, and with facilities available to treat profound hypotension. Treatment should therefore generally be initiated under hospital supervision.

RENAL IMPAIRMENT. ACE inhibitors occasionally cause impairment of renal function which may progress and become severe. At particular risk are those with pre-existing renal disease or impairment, the elderly, and those with bilateral renal artery stenosis (or stenosis of the artery supplying a single functioning kidney). Concomitant treatment with NSAIDs increases the risk of renal damage, and potassium-sparing diuretics or use of potassium-containing salt substitutes increase the risk of hyperkalaemia. Renal function and electrolytes should be checked before starting an ACE inhibitor, and monitored during treatment.

ACE inhibitors should be used with **particular caution** in patients with peripheral vascular disease or generalised atherosclerosis, as such patients may have clinically silent renovascular disease.

COMBINATION PRODUCTS. A number of products incorporating an ACE inhibitor with a thiazide diuretic are now available. Use of these combination products should be reserved for patients whose blood pressure has not responded to a thiazide diuretic or an ACE inhibitor alone (see also comments above).

CAPTOPRIL

Indications: mild to moderate essential hypertension alone or with thiazide therapy and severe hypertension resistant to other treatment (but see cautions and notes above); congestive heart failure (adjunct)

Cautions: diuretics (**important:** see notes above); first doses may cause hypotension especially in patients taking diuretics, on a low-sodium diet, on dialysis, or dehydrated; monitor renal function before and during treatment; reduce dose or **avoid** in renal impairment (white cell counts and urinary protein estimations needed); see also notes above; in dialysis patients avoid combination of ACE inhibitor therapy with use of high-flux polyacrylonitrile membranes (anaphylactoid reactions reported); **interactions:** Appendix 1 (ACE inhibitors)

Contra-indications: hypersensitivity to ACE inhibitors; known or suspected renovascular disease, aortic stenosis or outflow tract obstruction; pregnancy (see Appendix 4); porphyria (see section 9.8.2)

Side-effects: persistent dry cough, throat discomfort, voice changes; loss of taste, sore mouth, abdominal pain, rash, angioedema, hypotension (see Cautions); proteinuria, thrombocytopenia, neutropenia, agranulocytosis, hyperkalaemia (all more common in renal impairment); increases in liver enzymes, liver damage, and cholestatic jaundice reported; renal impairment, see notes above

Dose: hypertension, used alone, initially 12.5 mg twice daily; if used in addition to diuretic (see notes), in elderly, or in renal impairment, initially 6.25 mg twice daily (first dose at bedtime); usual maintenance dose 25 mg twice daily; max. 50 mg twice daily (rarely 3 times daily in severe hypertension)

Heart failure (adjunct), initially 6.25–12.5 mg under close hospital supervision; usual maintenance dose 25 mg 2–3 times daily

PoM **Capoten**® (Squibb)
Tablets, captopril 12.5 mg (scored), net price 100 = £18.86; 25 mg, 56-tab pack = £12.03, 90-tab pack = £19.34; 50 mg (scored), 56-tab pack = £20.50, 90-tab pack = £32.95 (also available as Acepril®)

With diuretic
Note. For mild to moderate hypertension in patients stabilised on the individual components in the same proportions
PoM **Capozide**® (Squibb)
LS tablets, scored, captopril 25 mg, hydrochlorothiazide 12.5 mg. Net price 28-tab pack = £11.25
Tablets, scored, captopril 50 mg, hydrochlorothiazide 25 mg. Net price 28-tab pack = £16.07 (also available as Acezide®)

CILAZAPRIL

Indications: essential hypertension where standard therapy ineffective or inappropriate because of adverse effects (but see cautions and notes above)

Cautions; Contra-indications: see under Captopril and notes above

Side-effects: see under Enalapril

Dose: initially, 1 mg once daily; usual range 2.5–5 mg once daily; if used in addition to diuretic (see notes) or in elderly, initially 500 micrograms once daily; if patient also has congestive heart failure, initially 500 micrograms once daily under close hospital supervision

Note. If possible discontinue diuretic for 2–3 days beforehand (see also notes above)

▼ PoM **Vascace**® (Roche)

Tablets, all f/c, cilazapril 250 micrograms (pink), net price 28-tab pack = £3.87; 500 micrograms (white), 28-tab pack = £4.10; 1 mg (yellow), 28-tab pack = £7.06; 2.5 mg (pink), 28-tab pack = £10.67

ENALAPRIL MALEATE

Indications: all grades of essential hypertension (but see cautions and notes above); congestive heart failure (adjunct)

Cautions; Contra-indications: see under Captopril and notes above

Side-effects: persistent dry cough, throat discomfort, voice changes; dizziness, headache, fatigue, weakness, hypotension (see Cautions), change of taste, nausea, diarrhoea, muscle cramps, rash, and angioedema; rarely pancreatitis; renal impairment, see notes above

Dose: hypertension, used alone, initially 5 mg daily; if used in addition to diuretic (see notes), in elderly patients, or in renal impairment, initially 2.5 mg daily; usual maintenance dose 10–20 mg daily; max. 40 mg daily

Heart failure (adjunct), initially 2.5 mg daily under close hospital supervision; usual maintenance 10–20 mg daily

PoM **Innovace**® (MSD)

Tablets, enalapril maleate 2.5 mg, net price 50 = £10.00; 5 mg (scored), 28-tab pack = £7.86, 50 = £14.03; 10 mg (red), 28-tab pack = £11.03, 50 = £19.69; 20 mg (peach), 28-tab pack = £13.10, 50 = £23.40

With diuretic

Note. For mild to moderate hypertension in patients stabilised on the individual components in the same proportions

PoM **Innozide**® (MSD)

Tablets, yellow, scored, enalapril maleate 20 mg, hydrochlorothiazide 12.5 mg. Net price 28-tab pack = £14.56

FOSINOPRIL

Indications: essential hypertension where standard therapy ineffective or inappropriate because of adverse effects (but see cautions and notes above)

Cautions; Contra-indications: see under Captopril and notes above

Side-effects: see under Enalapril; upper respiratory symptoms; palpitations, chest pain, paraesthesia, pruritus also reported

Dose: initially 10 mg daily; usual maintenance 20 mg daily; max. 40 mg daily

Note. If used in addition to diuretic, discontinue diuretic several days before and resume after about 4 weeks if blood pressure inadequately controlled (if diuretic therapy cannot be stopped careful medical supervision for several hours)

▼ PoM **Staril**® (Squibb)

Tablets, fosinopril sodium 10 mg, net price 28-tab pack = £12.04; 20 mg, 28-tab pack = £21.00

LISINOPRIL

Indications: all grades of essential hypertension (but see cautions and notes above); congestive heart failure (adjunct)

Cautions; Contra-indications: see under Captopril and notes above

Side-effects: see under Enalapril; palpitations also reported

Dose: hypertension, initially 2.5 mg daily; usual maintenance dose 10–20 mg daily; max. 40 mg daily

Note. In hypertension discontinue diuretic for 2–3 days beforehand and resume later if required (see also notes above)

Heart failure (adjunct), initially 2.5 mg daily under close hospital supervision; usual maintenance dose 5–20 mg daily

PoM **Carace**® (Morson)

Tablets, lisinopril 2.5 mg (blue), net price 50 = £15.30; 5 mg (scored), 28-tab pack = £10.14; 10 mg (yellow, scored), 28-tab pack = £12.13; 20 mg (orange, scored), 28-tab pack = £20.30

PoM **Zestril**® (ICI)

Tablets, lisinopril (as dihydrate) 2.5 mg, net price 28-tab pack = £7.84; 5 mg (pink, scored), 28-tab pack = £9.83; 10 mg (pink), 28-tab pack = £12.13; 20 mg (red), 28-tab pack = £20.96

With diuretic

Note. For mild to moderate hypertension in patients stabilised on the individual components in the same proportions

PoM **Carace Plus**® (Morson)

Tablets, yellow, scored, lisinopril 20 mg, hydrochlorothiazide 12.5 mg. Net price 28-tab pack = £17.36, 56-tab pack = £34.72

PoM **Zestoretic**® (ICI)

Tablets, lisinopril 20 mg, hydrochlorothiazide 12.5 mg. Net price 28-tab pack = £17.36

PERINDOPRIL

Indications: essential hypertension where standard therapy is ineffective or inappropriate because of adverse effects (but see cautions and notes above); congestive heart failure (adjunct)

Cautions; Contra-indications: see under Captopril and notes above

Side-effects: see under Enalapril; abdominal pain, mood and sleep disturbances also reported
Dose: hypertension, initially 2 mg daily; usual maintenance dose 4–8 mg once daily; max. 8 mg daily
Note. In hypertension discontinue diuretic 3 days beforehand and resume later if required (see also notes above)
Heart failure (adjunct), initial dose 2 mg in the morning under close hospital supervision; usual maintenance 4 mg daily

PoM **Coversyl**® (Servier)
Tablets, perindopril tert-butylamine 2 mg, net price 30-tab pack = £9.45; 4 mg (scored), 30-tab pack = £13.00. Label: 22

QUINAPRIL

Indications: all grades of essential hypertension where standard therapy ineffective or inappropriate because of adverse effects (but see cautions and notes above); congestive heart failure (adjunct)
Cautions; Contra-indications: see under Captopril and notes above
Side-effects: see under Enalapril; rhinitis, sinusitis, pharyngitis, dyspepsia, abdominal pain, back pain, vomiting, chest pain, insomnia, paraesthesia, nervousness also reported
Dose: hypertension, initially 5 mg daily; with a diuretic, in elderly, or in renal impairment initially 2.5 mg daily; usual maintenance dose 20–40 mg daily in single or 2 divided doses; up to 80 mg daily has been given
Heart failure (adjunct), initial dose 2.5 mg under close hospital supervision; usual maintenance 10–20 mg daily in 2 divided doses; up to 40 mg daily has been given

PoM **Accupro**® (P-D)
Tablets, all brown, f/c, quinapril 5 mg, net price 28-tab pack = £9.82; 10 mg, 28-tab pack = £10.07; 20 mg, 28-tab pack = £10.32

RAMIPRIL

Indications: mild to moderate essential hypertension where standard therapy ineffective or inappropriate because of adverse effects (but see cautions and notes above)
Cautions; Contra-indications: see under Captopril and notes above
Side-effects: see under Enalapril; also abdominal pain, vomiting; increases in blood urea nitrogen and serum creatinine (particularly in renal impairment)
Dose: initially 1.25 mg daily, increased at intervals of 1–2 weeks; usual range 2.5–5 mg daily; max. 10 mg daily
Note. Discontinue diuretic for 2–3 days beforehand and resume later if required (see also notes above)

PoM **Tritace**® (Astra, Hoechst)
Capsules, ramipril 1.25 mg (yellow/white), net price 28-cap pack = £5.44; 2.5 mg (orange/white), 28-cap pack = £7.70; 5 mg (red/white), 28-cap pack = £9.79

2.5.6 Ganglion-blocking drugs

Trimetaphan is used to provide controlled hypotension in surgery.

TRIMETAPHAN CAMSYLATE

Indications: see notes above
Cautions: hepatic or renal impairment, diabetes mellitus, elderly, cerebral or coronary vascular disease, adrenal insufficiency, Addison's disease, CNS degenerative disease
Contra-indications: severe arteriosclerosis, severe cardiac disease, pyloric stenosis, pregnancy
Side-effects: tachycardia and respiratory depression (particularly with muscle relaxants); constipation, increased intra-ocular pressure, pupillary dilatation
Dose: by intravenous infusion, 3–4 mg/minute initially, then adjusted according to response

PoM **Arfonad**® (Cambridge)
Injection, trimetaphan camsylate 50 mg/mL. Net price 5-mL amp = £3.12. For dilution and use as an infusion

2.5.7 Tyrosine hydroxylase inhibitor

Metirosine inhibits the enzyme tyrosine hydroxylase, and hence the synthesis of catecholamines. It is used in the pre-operative management of phaeochromocytoma, and long term in patients unsuitable for surgery; an alpha-adrenoceptor blocking drug (e.g. phenoxybenzamine) may also be required. Metirosine should **not** be used to treat essential hypertension.

METIROSINE

Indications: see notes above
Cautions: maintain high fluid intake and adequate blood volume; may impair ability to drive or operate machinery; **interactions:** Appendix 1 (metirosine)
Side-effects: sedation; extrapyramidal symptoms; diarrhoea (may be severe); hypersensitivity reactions
Dose: initially 250 mg 4 times daily, increased to max. of 4 g daily in divided doses; doses of 2–3 g daily should be given for 5–7 days before surgery

PoM **Demser**® (MSD)
Capsules, blue, metirosine 250 mg (hosp. only). Label: 2

2.6 Nitrates and other vasodilators, and calcium-channel blockers

- 2.6.1 Nitrates
- 2.6.2 Calcium-channel blockers
- 2.6.3 Peripheral vasodilators
- 2.6.4 Cerebral vasodilators

Most patients with *angina pectoris* are treated with beta-blockers (section 2.4) or calcium-channel blockers (section 2.6.2). However, short-acting nitrates (section 2.6.1) retain an important role both for prophylactic use before exertion and for chest pain occurring at rest. Nitrates are sometimes used as sole therapy, especially in elderly patients with infrequent symptoms.

Vasodilators are known to act in *heart failure* either by:

arteriolar dilatation which reduces both peripheral vascular resistance and left ventricular pressure at systole and results in improved cardiac output, *or*

venous dilatation which results in dilatation of capacitance vessels, increase of venous pooling, and diminution of venous return to the heart (decreasing left ventricular end-diastolic pressure).

For a comment on the role of ACE inhibitors in heart failure, see section 2.5.5.

Glyceryl trinitrate or isosorbide dinitrate may be tried by *intravenous injection* when the sublingual form is ineffective in patients with chest pain due to myocardial infarction or severe ischaemia. Intravenous injections are also useful in the treatment of acute left ventricular failure.

TOLERANCE. Some patients on long-acting or transdermal nitrates rapidly develop tolerance (with reduced therapeutic effects). Reduction of blood-nitrate concentrations to low levels for 4 to 8 hours each day usually maintains effectiveness in such patients. If tolerance is suspected after the use of transdermal patches they should be removed for several consecutive hours in each 24 hours; in the case of modified-release tablets of isosorbide dinitrate (and conventional formulations of isosorbide mononitrate), the second of the two daily doses can be given after about 8 hours rather than after 12 hours. Conventional formulations of isosorbide mononitrate should not usually be given more than twice daily unless small doses are used; modified-release formulations of isosorbide mononitrate should only be given once daily.

2.6.1 Nitrates

Sublingual **glyceryl trinitrate** is one of the most effective drugs for providing rapid symptomatic relief of angina, but its effect lasts only for 20 to 30 minutes. Though a potent coronary vasodilator, its principal benefit follows from a reduction in venous return which reduces left ventricular work. Unwanted effects such as flushing, headache, and postural hypotension may limit therapy, especially when angina is severe or when patients are unusually sensitive to the effects of nitrates; the 300-microgram tablet is often appropriate when glyceryl trinitrate is first used. Duration of action may be prolonged by *modified-release* preparations. The *aerosol spray* provides an alternative method of rapid relief of symptoms for those who find difficulty in dissolving sublingual preparations. The *percutaneous* preparations may be useful in the prophylaxis of angina for patients who suffer attacks at rest, especially at night.

Isosorbide dinitrate is active *sublingually* and is a more stable preparation for those who only require nitrates infrequently. It is also effective by mouth for prophylaxis; although the effect is slower in onset, it may persist for several hours. Duration of action of up to 12 hours is claimed for *modified-release* preparations. The activity of isosorbide dinitrate may depend on the production of active metabolites, the most important of which is isosorbide mononitrate. **Isosorbide mononitrate** itself is also available for angina prophylaxis, though the advantages over isosorbide dinitrate have not yet been firmly established.

GLYCERYL TRINITRATE

Indications: prophylaxis and treatment of angina; left ventricular failure

Cautions: hypotensive conditions (avoid intravenous); tolerance (see notes above); **interactions:** Appendix 1 (glyceryl trinitrate)

Contra-indications: marked anaemia, head trauma, cerebral haemorrhage, closed-angle glaucoma

Side-effects: throbbing headache, flushing, dizziness, postural hypotension, tachycardia

Dose: sublingually, 0.3–1 mg, repeated as required

By mouth, 2.6–6.4 mg as modified-release tablets, 2–3 times daily

By intravenous infusion, 10–200 micrograms/minute

Short-acting tablets and sprays
Glyceryl Trinitrate (Non-proprietary)
Sublingual tablets, glyceryl trinitrate 300 micrograms, net price 100 = £1.05; 500 micrograms, 100 = 44p; 600 micrograms, 100 = 67p. Label: 16

Note. Glyceryl trinitrate tablets should be supplied in glass containers of not more than 100 tablets, closed with a foil-lined cap, and containing no cotton wool wadding; they should be discarded after 8 weeks in use

Coro-Nitro Spray® (Boehringer Mannheim)
Aerosol spray, glyceryl trinitrate 400 micrograms/metered dose. Net price 200-dose unit = £3.36

Dose: treatment or prophylaxis of angina, spray 1–2 doses under tongue and then close mouth
Caution: flammable

2.6 Nitrates and calcium-channel blockers

Glytrin Spray® (Sanofi Winthrop)
Aerosol spray, glyceryl trinitrate 400 micrograms/metered dose. Net price 200-dose unit = £3.28. Label: 10 patient leaflet
Dose: treatment or prophylaxis of angina, spray 1–2 doses under tongue and then close mouth
Caution: flammable

GTN 300 mcg (Martindale)
Sublingual tablets, glyceryl trinitrate 300 micrograms. Net price 100 = £1.29. Label: 16

Nitrolingual Spray® (Lipha)
Aerosol spray, glyceryl trinitrate 400 micrograms/metered dose. Net price 200-dose unit = £4.36
Dose: treatment or prophylaxis of angina, spray 1–2 doses under tongue and then close mouth
Caution: flammable

Modified-release tablets
Nitrocontin Continus® (ASTA Medica)
Tablets, m/r, both pink, glyceryl trinitrate 2.6 mg, net price 20 = 67p; 6.4 mg, 20 = 88p. Label: 25

Suscard® (Pharmax)
Buccal tablets, m/r, glyceryl trinitrate 1 mg, net price 20 = £1.95; 2 mg, 20 = £2.91; 3 mg, 20 = £4.08; 5 mg, 20 = £5.72. Counselling below
Dose: treatment of angina, 2 mg as required (1 mg in sensitive patients), increased to 3 mg if necessary; prophylaxis 1–3 mg 3 times daily; 5 mg in severe angina
Unstable angina (adjunct), up to 5 mg with ECG monitoring
Congestive heart failure, 5 mg 3 times daily, increased to 10 mg 3 times daily in severe cases
Acute heart failure, 5 mg repeated until symptoms abate
ADMINISTRATION. Tablets are placed between upper lip and gum, and left to dissolve

Sustac® (Pharmax)
Tablets, m/r, all pink, glyceryl trinitrate 2.6 mg, net price 20 = £1.21; 6.4 mg, 20 = £1.74; 10 mg, 20 = £2.43. Label: 25
Dose: severe angina, 10 mg 3 times daily

Parenteral preparations
Note. Glass or polyethylene apparatus is preferable; loss of potency will occur if PVC is used

PoM **Glyceryl Trinitrate** (Non-proprietary)
Injection, glyceryl trinitrate 5 mg/mL. To be diluted before use. Net price 5-mL amp = £6.00; 10-mL amp = £12.00
Available from David Bull

PoM **Nitrocine**® (Schwarz)
Injection, glyceryl trinitrate 1 mg/mL. To be diluted before use or given undiluted with syringe pump. Net price 10-mL amp = £9.45; 50-mL bottle = £22.15

PoM **Nitronal**® (Lipha)
Injection, glyceryl trinitrate 1 mg/mL. To be diluted before use or given undiluted with syringe pump. Net price 5-mL vial = £2.20; 50-mL vial = £18.00

PoM **Tridil**® (Du Pont)
Injection, to be diluted before use, glyceryl trinitrate 500 micrograms/mL, net price 10-mL amp = £4.50; 5 mg/mL, 10-mL amp = £21.88, 10-mL amp with polyethylene giving set = £24.98

Transdermal preparations
Deponit® (Schwarz)
'5' patch, self-adhesive, transparent, releasing glyceryl trinitrate approx. 5 mg/24 hours when in contact with skin. Net price 30 = £19.25. Label: 10 patient information leaflet, counselling, see administration below
'10' patch, self-adhesive, transparent, releasing glyceryl trinitrate approx. 10 mg/24 hours when in contact with skin. Net price 30 = £21.19. Label: 10 patient information leaflet, counselling, see administration below
ADMINISTRATION: prophylaxis of angina, apply one '5' or one '10' patch to lateral chest wall; replace every 24 hours, siting replacement patch on different area; see also notes above

Nitro-Dur® (Schering-Plough)
Patch '0.1 mg/h', self-adhesive, buff, releasing glyceryl trinitrate approx. 2.5 mg/24 hours when in contact with skin. Net price 28 = £16.14. Label: 10 patient information leaflet, counselling, see administration below
Patch '0.2 mg/h', self-adhesive, buff, releasing glyceryl trinitrate approx. 5 mg/24 hours when in contact with skin. Net price 28 = £17.92. Label: 10 patient information leaflet, counselling, see administration below
Patch '0.4 mg/h', self-adhesive, buff, releasing glyceryl trinitrate approx. 10 mg/24 hours when in contact with skin. Net price 28 = £19.84. Label: 10 patient information leaflet, counselling, see administration below
Patch '0.6 mg/h', self-adhesive, buff, releasing glyceryl trinitrate approx. 15 mg/24 hours. Net price 28 = £21.83. Label: 10 patient information leaflet, counselling, see administration below
ADMINISTRATION: prophylaxis of angina, apply one '0.2 mg/h' patch to chest or outer upper arm; replace every 24 hours, siting replacement patch on different area: adjust dose according to response

Percutol® (Cusi)
Ointment, glyceryl trinitrate 2%. Net price 30 g = £6.14. Counselling, see administration below
ADMINISTRATION: prophylaxis of angina, ½–2 inches of ointment measured on to Applirule, which is applied to body (usually chest, arm, or thigh) without rubbing in, and secured with a dressing; repeat every 3–4 hours or as required
Note. 1 inch of ointment contains glyceryl trinitrate 16.64 mg

Transiderm-Nitro® (Geigy)
'5' patch, self-adhesive, pink, releasing glyceryl trinitrate approx. 5 mg/24 hours when in contact with skin. Net price 30 = £15.95. Label: 10 patient information leaflet, counselling, see administration below
'10' patch, self-adhesive, pink, releasing glyceryl trinitrate approx. 10 mg/24 hours when in contact with skin. Net price 30 = £17.54. Label: 10 patient information leaflet, counselling, see administration below

ADMINISTRATION: prophylaxis of angina, apply one '5' or one '10' patch to lateral chest wall; replace every 24 hours, siting replacement patch on different area; max. two '10' patches daily; see also notes above
Prophylaxis of phlebitis and extravasation ('5' patch only), see literature

ISOSORBIDE DINITRATE

Indications: prophylaxis and treatment of angina; left ventricular failure
Cautions; Contra-indications; Side-effects: see under Glyceryl Trinitrate
Dose: sublingually, 5–10 mg
By mouth, daily in divided doses, angina 30–120 mg, left ventricular failure 40–160 mg, up to 240 mg if required
By intravenous infusion, 2–10 mg/hour

Short-acting tablets
Isosorbide Dinitrate (Non-proprietary)
Tablets, isosorbide dinitrate 10 mg, net price 20 = 24p; 20 mg, 20 = 70p
Available from Cox, Evans, Hillcross, Kerfoot, Norton

Cedocard® (Tillotts)
Cedocard-5 tablets (sublingual), isosorbide dinitrate 5 mg. Net price 60-tab pack = £1.55
Cedocard-10 tablets, pink, scored, isosorbide dinitrate 10 mg. Net price 100-tab pack = £1.70
Cedocard-20 tablets, blue, scored, isosorbide dinitrate 20 mg. Net price 100-tab pack = £3.25
Cedocard-40 tablets, green, scored, isosorbide dinitrate 40 mg. Net price 120-tab pack = £9.05

Isordil® (Monmouth)
Tablets (sublingual), pink, isosorbide dinitrate 5 mg. Net price 20 = 23p. Label: 26
Tablets, both scored, isosorbide dinitrate 10 mg, net price 20 = 23p; 30 mg, 20 = 54p

Sorbichew® (Stuart)
Tablets (chewable), green, scored, isosorbide dinitrate 5 mg. Net price 20 = 31p. Label: 24

Sorbitrate® (Stuart)
Tablets, both scored, isosorbide dinitrate 10 mg (yellow), net price 20 = 29p; 20 mg (blue), 20 = 43p

Vascardin® (Nicholas)
Tablets, scored, isosorbide dinitrate 10 mg (as diluted isosorbide dinitrate), net price 20 = 28p

Modified-release preparations
Cedocard Retard® (Tillotts)
Retard-20 tablets, m/r, yellow, scored, isosorbide dinitrate 20 mg. Net price 60-tab pack = £5.71. Label: 25
Dose: prophylaxis of angina, 1 tablet every 12 hours
Retard-40 tablets, m/r, orange-red, scored, isosorbide dinitrate 40 mg. Net price 60-tab pack = £11.37. Label: 25
Dose: prophylaxis of angina, 1–2 tablets every 12 hours

Isoket Retard® (Schwarz)
Retard-20 tablets, m/r, yellow, scored, isosorbide dinitrate 20 mg. Net price 50-tab pack = £3.24. Label: 25
Retard-40 tablets, m/r, orange, scored, isosorbide dinitrate 40 mg. Net price 50-tab pack = £7.99. Label: 25
Dose: prophylaxis of angina, 20–40 mg every 12 hours

Isordil Tembids® (Monmouth)
Capsules, m/r, blue/clear, isosorbide dinitrate 40 mg. Net price 20 = £1.28. Label: 25
Dose: prophylaxis of angina, 1 capsule 2–3 times daily

Soni-Slo® (Lipha)
Capsules, m/r, pink/clear, enclosing off-white pellets, isosorbide dinitrate 20 mg. Net price 20 = £1.19. Label: 25
Capsules, m/r, yellow/clear, enclosing off-white pellets, isosorbide dinitrate 40 mg. Net price 20 = £1.40. Label: 25
Dose: prophylaxis of angina, 40–120 mg daily in divided doses

Sorbid SA® (Stuart)
Sorbid-20 SA capsules, m/r, red/yellow, isosorbide dinitrate 20 mg. Net price 56-cap pack = £3.59. Label: 25
Dose: prophylaxis of angina, 1–2 capsules twice daily
Sorbid-40 SA capsules, m/r, red/clear, isosorbide dinitrate 40 mg. Net price 56-cap pack = £5.13. Label: 25
Dose: prophylaxis of angina, 1–2 capsules twice daily

Parenteral preparations
PoM Cedocard IV® (Tillotts)
Injection, isosorbide dinitrate 1 mg/mL. To be diluted before use. Net price 10-mL amp = £4.33; 50-mL infusion bottle = £21.50; 100-mL infusion bottle = £29.69
Note. Glass or polyethylene infusion apparatus is preferable; loss of potency if PVC used

PoM Isoket® (Schwarz)
Injection 0.05%, isosorbide dinitrate 500 micrograms/mL. To be diluted before use or given undiluted with syringe pump. Net price 50-mL bottle = £11.50
Injection 0.1%, isosorbide dinitrate 1 mg/mL. To be diluted before use. Net price 10-mL amp = £4.33; 50-mL bottle = £21.50; 100-mL bottle = £29.69
Note. Glass or polyethylene infusion apparatus is preferable; loss of potency if PVC used

ISOSORBIDE MONONITRATE

Indications: prophylaxis and treatment of angina; adjunct in congestive heart failure
Cautions; Contra-indications; Side-effects: see under Glyceryl Trinitrate
Dose: initially 20 mg 2–3 times daily *or* 40 mg twice daily (10 mg twice daily in those who have not previously received nitrates); up to 120 mg daily in divided doses if required

Isosorbide Mononitrate (Non-proprietary)
Tablets, isosorbide mononitrate 10 mg, net price 20 = £1.10; 20 mg, 20 = £1.40; 40 mg, 20 = £2.69. Label: 25
Various strengths available from APS, Ashbourne (Isib®), Cox, CP, Evans, Kerfoot, Lagap, Norton

2.6 Nitrates and calcium-channel blockers

Elantan® (Schwarz)
Elantan 10 tablets, scored, isosorbide mononitrate 10 mg. Net price 50-tab pack = £3.33. Label: 25
PoM *Elantan 20 tablets*, scored, isosorbide mononitrate 20 mg. Net price 50-tab pack = £4.34. Label: 25
PoM *Elantan 40 tablets*, scored, isosorbide mononitrate 40 mg. Net price 50-tab pack = £7.07. Label: 25

Ismo® (Boehringer Mannheim)
Ismo 10 tablets, isosorbide mononitrate 10 mg. Net price 20 = £1.16. Label: 25
Ismo 20 tablets, isosorbide mononitrate 20 mg. Net price 60-tab pack = £5.10. Label: 25
Starter pack, 8 tablets, isosorbide mononitrate 10 mg; 60 tablets, scored, isosorbide mononitrate 20 mg. Net price = £5.52. Label: 25
Ismo 40 tablets, isosorbide mononitrate 40 mg. Net price 20 = £2.79. Label: 25

Isotrate® (Bioglan)
Tablets, isosorbide mononitrate 20 mg. Net price 60-tab pack = £4.60. Label: 25

Monit® (Stuart)
Tablets, scored, isosorbide mononitrate 20 mg. Net price 56-tab pack = £4.78. Label: 25

Monit LS® (Stuart)
Tablets, isosorbide mononitrate 10 mg. Net price 56-tab pack = £3.74. Label: 25

Mono-Cedocard® (Tillotts)
Mono-Cedocard 10 tablets, orange, scored, isosorbide mononitrate 10 mg. Net price 60-tab pack = £3.77. Label: 25
Mono-Cedocard 20 tablets, scored, isosorbide mononitrate 20 mg. Net price 100-tab pack = £7.00. Label: 25
Mono-Cedocard 40 tablets, scored, isosorbide mononitrate 40 mg. Net price 60-tab pack = £9.35. Label: 25

Modified release
Elantan LA® (Schwarz)
Elantan LA25 capsules, m/r, light pink/dark pink, enclosing white micropellets, isosorbide mononitrate 25 mg. Net price 28-cap pack = £7.00. Label: 25
Dose: prophylaxis of angina, 1 capsule in the morning, increased if necessary to 2 capsules
Elantan LA50 capsules, m/r, pink/dark pink, enclosing white micropellets, isosorbide mononitrate 50 mg. Net price 28-cap pack = £11.30. Label: 25
Dose: prophylaxis of angina, 1 capsule daily in the morning

PoM **Imdur®** (Astra)
Durules® (= tablets m/r), yellow, f/c, scored, isosorbide mononitrate 60 mg. Net price 28-tab pack = £11.43. Label: 25
Dose: prophylaxis of angina, 1 tablet in the morning (half a tablet if headache occurs), increased to 2 tablets if required

Ismo Retard® (Boehringer Mannheim)
Tablets, m/r, s/c, isosorbide mononitrate 40 mg. Net price 28-tab pack = £10.50. Label: 25
Dose: prophylaxis of angina, 1 tablet daily in the morning

[1]**MCR-50®** (Tillotts)
Capsules, m/r, containing white micropellets, isosorbide mononitrate 50 mg. Net price 28-cap pack = £11.30. Label: 25
Dose: prophylaxis of angina, 1 capsule in the morning, increased to 2 capsules if required
1. Full product name Mono Cedocard Retard-50

Monit SR® (Stuart)
Tablets, m/r, s/c, isosorbide mononitrate 40 mg. Net price 28-tab pack = £10.50. Label: 25
Dose: prophylaxis of angina, 1 tablet daily in the morning

PENTAERYTHRITOL TETRANITRATE
Indications: prophylaxis of angina
Cautions; Contra-indications; Side-effects: see under Glyceryl Trinitrate
Dose: see below

Mycardol® (Sanofi Winthrop)
Tablets, scored, pentaerythritol tetranitrate 30 mg. Net price 20 = 89p. Label: 22
Dose: 2 tablets 3–4 times daily

2.6.2 Calcium-channel blockers

Calcium-channel blockers (less correctly called 'calcium-antagonists') interfere with the inward displacement of calcium ions through the slow channels of active cell membranes. They influence the myocardial cells, the cells within the specialised conducting system of the heart, and the cells of vascular smooth muscle. Thus, myocardial contractility may be reduced, the formation and propagation of electrical impulses within the heart may be depressed, and coronary or systemic vascular tone may be diminished. They should usually be avoided in heart failure because they may further depress cardiac function and cause clinically significant deterioration.

Calcium-channel blockers differ in their predeliction for the various possible sites of action therefore their therapeutic effects are disparate, with much greater variation than those of beta-blockers. There are important differences between verapamil and the dihydropyridine calcium-channel blockers, nifedipine, nicardipine and isradipine.

Verapamil is used for the treatment of *angina, hypertension*, and *arrhythmias* (section 2.3.2). It reduces cardiac output, slows the heart rate, and may impair atrioventricular conduction. It may precipitate heart failure, exacerbate conduction disorders, and cause hypotension at high doses and should **not** be used with beta-blockers (see section 2.3.2). Constipation is the most common side-effect.

Nifedipine relaxes vascular smooth muscle and dilates coronary and peripheral arteries. It has more influence on vessels and less on the myocardium than does verapamil, and unlike verapamil has no anti-arrhythmic activity. It rarely precipitates heart failure because any negative inotropic effect is offset by a reduction in left ventricular work. **Nicardipine** has similar effects to those of nifedipine and may produce less reduction of myocardial contractility. **Amlodipine** and **felodipine** also resemble nifedipine and nicardipine in their effects and do not reduce myocardial contractility. They have a longer duration of action and can be given once daily. Nifedipine, nicardipine, and amlodipine are used for the treatment of angina or hypertension. All are valuable in forms of *angina associated with coronary vasospasm*; they are useful as adjuncts to beta-blockers for patients with severe symptoms, and as alternative treatment for those who are intolerant of beta-blockers. Side-effects associated with vasodilatation such as flushing and headache (which become less obtrusive after a few days), and ankle swelling (which does not respond to diuretics) are common.

Isradipine has similar effects to those of nifedipine and nicardipine; it is only indicated for *hypertension*.

Nimodipine is related to nifedipine but the smooth muscle relaxant effect preferentially acts on cerebral arteries. Its use if confined to prevention of *vascular spasm following subarachnoid haemorrhage*.

Diltiazem is effective in most forms of *angina*; the longer-acting formulation is also used for *hypertension*. It may be used in patients for whom beta-blockers are contra-indicated or ineffective. It has a less negative inotropic effect than verapamil and significant myocardial depression occurs rarely. Nevertheless because of the risk of bradycardia it should be used with caution in association with beta-blockers.

WITHDRAWAL. There is some evidence that sudden withdrawal of calcium-channel blockers may be associated with an exacerbation of angina.

AMLODIPINE BESYLATE

Indications: hypertension, prophylaxis of angina
Cautions: pregnancy; hepatic impairment; **interactions:** Appendix 1 (calcium-channel blockers)
Side-effects: headache, oedema, fatigue, nausea, flushing, dizziness
Dose: hypertension or angina, initially 5 mg once daily; max. 10 mg daily

PoM **Istin**® (Pfizer)
Tablets, amlodipine (as besylate) 5 mg. Net price 28-tab pack = £11.85; 10 mg, 28-tab pack = £17.70

DILTIAZEM HYDROCHLORIDE

Indications: prophylaxis and treatment of angina; hypertension (longer-acting formulation)
Cautions: reduce dose in hepatic and renal impairment; heart failure or significantly impaired left ventricular function, mild bradycardia (avoid if severe), first degree AV block, or prolonged PR interval; **interactions:** Appendix 1 (calcium-channel blockers)
Contra-indications: severe bradycardia, second- or third-degree heart block (unless pacemaker fitted), sick sinus syndrome; pregnancy (toxicity in *animal* studies), left ventricular failure; porphyria (see section 9.8.2)
Side-effects: bradycardia, sino-atrial block, atrio-ventricular block, hypotension, malaise, headache, hot flushes, gastro-intestinal disturbances, ankle oedema; rarely rashes (toxic erythema reported); hepatitis and depression reported
Dose: angina, 60 mg 3 times daily (elderly initially twice daily); increased if necessary to 360 mg daily (max. 480 mg daily)
Longer-acting formulations, see below

PoM **Diltiazem** (Non-proprietary)
Tablets, m/r, diltiazem hydrochloride 60 mg. Net price 100 = £15.00. Label: 25
Available from APS, Ashbourne (Angiozem®), Berk, Cox, CP, Evans, Kerfoot, Norton, Thames (Britiazim®)

PoM **Adizem-60**® (Napp)
Tablets, m/r, f/c, diltiazem hydrochloride 60 mg. Net price 100-tab pack = £15.77. Label: 25

PoM **Tildiem**® (Lorex)
Tablets, m/r, off-white, diltiazem hydrochloride 60 mg. Net price 100 = £15.00. Label: 25

Longer acting
Note. To avoid confusion between these different formulations of diltiazem tablets, prescribers should specify the brand to be dispensed

PoM **Adizem-SR**® (Napp)
Tablets, m/r, f/c, diltiazem hydrochloride 120 mg. Net price 56-tab pack = £18.60. Label: 25
Dose: prophylaxis of angina, 1 tablet twice daily; max. 2 twice daily
Note. Not appropriate for the elderly or those with hepatic or renal impairment

PoM **Tildiem Retard**® (Lorex)
Tablets, m/r, diltiazem hydrochloride 90 mg, net price 56-tab pack = £11.34; 120 mg, 56-tab pack = £12.60. Label: 25
Dose: mild to moderate hypertension, initially 120 mg twice daily (elderly once daily); up to 360 mg daily may be required (elderly 240 mg daily)
Angina, initially 120 mg twice daily (elderly, dose form not appropriate for initial dose titration); up to 480 mg daily in divided doses may be required (elderly up to 240 mg daily)

FELODIPINE

Indications: hypertension
Cautions: withdraw if ischaemic pain occurs; hepatic impairment; breast-feeding; **interactions:** Appendix 1 (calcium-channel blockers)
Contra-indications: pregnancy
Side-effects: flushing, headache, palpitations, dizziness, fatigue, gravitational oedema, rash and pruritus, gum hyperplasia
Dose: initially 5 mg daily in the morning; usual maintenance 5–10 mg once daily; doses above 20 mg daily rarely needed

▼ PoM **Plendil**® (Astra)
Tablets, both m/r, f/c, felodipine 5 mg, net price 28-tab pack = £8.12; 10 mg, 28-tab pack = £10.92. Label: 25

2.6 Nitrates and calcium-channel blockers

ISRADIPINE
Indications: hypertension
Cautions: tight aortic stenosis, sick sinus syndrome (if pacemaker not fitted); reduce dose in hepatic or renal impairment; pregnancy (may prolong labour); **interactions:** Appendix 1 (calcium-channel blockers)
Side-effects: headache, flushing, dizziness, tachycardia and palpitations, localised peripheral oedema; hypotension uncommon; rarely weight gain, fatigue, abdominal discomfort, rashes
Dose: 2.5 mg twice daily (1.25 mg twice daily in elderly, hepatic or renal impairment); increased if necessary after 3–4 weeks to 5 mg twice daily (exceptionally up to 10 mg twice daily); maintenance 2.5 or 5 mg once daily may be sufficient

▼ PoM **Prescal**® (Ciba)
Tablets, yellow, scored, isradipine 2.5 mg. Net price 56-tab pack = £11.39

NICARDIPINE HYDROCHLORIDE
Indications: prophylaxis and treatment of angina; mild to moderate hypertension
Cautions: withdraw if ischaemic pain occurs or existing pain worsens within 30 minutes of initiating treatment or increasing dose; congestive heart failure or significantly impaired left ventricular function; elderly; hepatic or renal impairment; **interactions:** Appendix 1 (calcium-channel blockers)
Contra-indications: advanced aortic stenosis; pregnancy
Side-effects: dizziness, headache, peripheral oedema, flushing, palpitations, nausea; also gastro-intestinal disturbances, drowsiness, insomnia, tinnitus, hypotension, rashes, salivation, frequency of micturition
Dose: initially 20 mg 3 times daily, increased to 30 mg 3 times daily (usual range 60–120 mg daily); patients with hypertension controlled on 20–30 mg 3 times daily can be given 30–40 mg twice daily

PoM **Cardene**® (Syntex)
Capsules, nicardipine hydrochloride 20 mg (blue/white), net price 20 = £3.04; 30 mg (blue/pale blue), 56-cap pack = £9.89

NIFEDIPINE
Indications: prophylaxis and treatment of angina; hypertension; Raynaud's phenomenon
Cautions: withdraw if ischaemic pain occurs or existing pain worsens shortly after initiating treatment; heart failure or significantly impaired left ventricular function; severe hypotension; reduce dose in hepatic impairment; diabetes mellitus; may inhibit labour; breast-feeding; **interactions:** Appendix 1 (calcium-channel blockers)
Contra-indications: cardiogenic shock; pregnancy (toxicity in *animal* studies); porphyria (see section 9.8.2)
Side-effects: headache, flushing, dizziness, lethargy; also gravitational oedema, rash, nausea, increased frequency of micturition, eye pain, gum hyperplasia; depression reported; telangiectasia reported
Dose: see preparations below

PoM **Adalat**® (Bayer)
Capsules, both orange, nifedipine 5 mg, net price 20 = £1.63; 10 mg, 20 = £2.44. Label: 21, counselling, see dose
Dose: angina and Raynaud's phenomenon, initially 10 mg (elderly 5 mg) 3 times daily with or after food; usual maintenance 5–20 mg 3 times daily; for immediate effect in angina bite into capsule and retain liquid in mouth or swallow (evidence points to more rapid action if contents swallowed)
Note. Nifedipine capsules also available from APS, Ashbourne (Angiopine®), Cox, CP, Eastern (Calcilat®), Evans, Kerfoot, Norton

PoM **Adalat**® IC (Bayer)
Coronary injection, nifedipine 100 micrograms/mL. Net price 2-mL pre-filled syringe = £7.43
Note. Use polyethylene catheters only
Dose: for treatment of coronary spasm during coronary angiography and balloon angioplasty, 100–200 micrograms via coronary catheter over 90–120 seconds (with monitoring of blood pressure and pulse); reduce dose in severe stenosis; lasts 15 minutes; do not exceed total of six 200-microgram injections in 3 hours

Modified release
Note. To avoid confusion between these different formulations of nifedipine, precribers should specify the brand to be dispensed

PoM **Adalat**® LA (Bayer)
LA 30 tablets, m/r, pink, nifedipine 30 mg. Net price 28-tab pack = £11.76. Label: 25
LA 60 tablets, m/r, pink, nifedipine 60 mg. Net price 28-tab pack = £15.40. Label: 25
Dose: mild to moderate hypertension, 30 mg once daily, increased if necessary; max. 90 mg once daily

PoM **Adalat**® Retard (Bayer)
Retard 10 tablets, m/r, pink, nifedipine 10 mg. Net price 56-tab pack = £8.34. Label: 21, 25
Retard 20 tablets, m/r, pink, nifedipine 20 mg. Net price 20 = £3.86. Label: 21, 25
Dose: hypertension and angina prophylaxis, 20 mg twice daily with or after food (initial titration 10 mg twice daily); usual maintenance 10–40 mg twice daily

PoM **Coracten**® (Evans)
Capsules, both m/r, nifedipine 10 mg (grey/pink, enclosing yellow pellets), net price 60-cap pack = £7.15; 20 mg (pink/brown, enclosing yellow pellets), 60-cap pack = £10.43. Label: 25
Dose: hypertension and angina prophylaxis, one 20-mg capsule every 12 hours, adjusted within range 10–40 mg every 12 hours

Cautionary label wordings, see inside back cover   Prices are **net**, see p. 1

Chapter 2: Cardiovascular system

PoM Nifensar XL® (Rhône-Poulenc Rorer)
Tablets, m/r, yellow, nifedipine 20 mg. Net price 28-tab pack = £7.56. Label: 21, 25
Dose: mild to moderate hypertension, initially 40 mg once daily (initially 20 mg in elderly not previously treated with nifedipine, or in renal impairment); usual maintenance dose 20–40 mg daily; max. 100 mg daily

With atenolol
Section 2.4

NIMODIPINE

Indications: prevention and treatment of ischaemic neurological deficits following subarachnoid haemorrhage
Cautions: cerebral oedema or severely raised intracranial pressure; avoid concomitant administration of nimodipine tablets and infusion, other calcium-channel blockers, or beta-blockers; impaired renal function or nephrotoxic drugs; pregnancy; **interactions:** Appendix 1 (calcium-channel blockers)
Side-effects: hypotension, variation in heart-rate, flushing, headache, gastro-intestinal disorders, nausea, and feeling of warmth; transient increase in liver enzymes after intravenous administration
Dose: prevention, *by mouth*, 60 mg every 4 hours (total daily dose 360 mg), starting within 4 days of subarachnoid haemorrhage and continued for 21 days
Treatment, *by intravenous infusion* via central catheter, 1 mg/hour initially, increased after 2 hours to 2 mg/hour, providing no severe decrease in blood pressure; patients with unstable blood pressure or weighing less than 70 kg, 500 micrograms/hour initially or less if necessary; treatment should start as soon as possible and should continue for at least 5 days (max. 14 days); in the event of surgical intervention during treatment continue for at least 5 days after

PoM Nimotop® (Bayer)
Tablets, yellow, f/c, nimodipine 30 mg. Net price 100-tab pack = £35.30
Intravenous infusion, nimodipine 200 micrograms/mL; also contains ethanol 20% and macrogol '400' 17%. Net price 50-mL vial (with polyethylene infusion catheter) = £13.24; 250-mL bottle = £66.20
Note. Polyethylene or polypropylene apparatus should be used; PVC should be avoided

VERAPAMIL HYDROCHLORIDE

Indications: see under Dose
Cautions: first-degree heart block; acute phase of myocardial infarction (avoid if bradycardia, hypotension, left ventricular failure); patients taking beta-blockers (**important:** see section 2.3.2—both oral and intravenous routes); reduce dose in hepatic impairment; children, specialist advice only (see section 2.3.2); pregnancy and breast-feeding; **interactions:** Appendix 1 (calcium-channel blockers)

Contra-indications: hypotension, bradycardia, second- and third-degree heart block, sick sinus syndrome, cardiogenic shock, sino-atrial block; history of heart failure or significantly impaired left ventricular function, even if controlled by therapy; atrial flutter or fibrillation complicating Wolff-Parkinson-White syndrome; porphyria (see section 9.8.2)
Side-effects: constipation; less commonly nausea, vomiting, flushing, headache, dizziness, fatigue, ankle oedema; rarely reversible impairment of liver function; rarely gynaecomastia and gingival hyperplasia after long-term treatment; after intravenous administration, hypotension, bradycardia, heart block, ventricular fibrillation, and asystole
Dose: by mouth, supraventricular arrhythmias, 40–120 mg 3 times daily
Angina, 80–120 mg 3 times daily
Hypertension, 240–480 mg daily in 2–3 divided doses
By slow intravenous injection over 2 minutes (3 minutes in elderly), 5–10 mg (preferably with ECG monitoring); in paroxysmal tachy-arrhythmias a further 5 mg after 5–10 minutes if required

PoM Verapamil (Non-proprietary)
Tablets, coated, verapamil hydrochloride 40 mg, net price 20 = 89p; 80 mg, 20 = £1.78; 120 mg, 20 = £2.72; 160 mg, 20 = £3.28
Various strengths available from APS, Berk (Berkatens®), Cox, CP, Cusi (Geangin®), Evans, Kerfoot, Norton
Oral solution, sugar-free, verapamil hydrochloride 40 mg/5 mL available from RP Drugs (special order)

PoM Cordilox® (Baker Norton)
Tablets, all yellow, f/c, verapamil hydrochloride 40 mg, net price 20 = 89p; 80 mg, 20 = £1.78; 120 mg, 20 = £2.72; 160 mg, 56-tab pack = £13.10
Injection, verapamil hydrochloride 2.5 mg/mL, net price 2-mL amp = £1.11

PoM Securon® (Knoll)
Tablets, f/c, verapamil hydrochloride 40 mg, net price 100 = £4.69; 80 mg, 100 = £9.38; 120 mg, 56-tab pack = £7.87, 100 = £14.05; 160 mg, 56-tab pack = £10.49, 100 = £18.73
Injection, verapamil hydrochloride 2.5 mg/mL. Net price 2-mL syringe = £1.11

PoM Securon SR® (Knoll)
Tablets, m/r, pale green, f/c, verapamil hydrochloride 240 mg. Net price 28-tab pack = £10.92. Label: 25
Dose: hypertension, 1 tablet daily, increased to twice daily if necessary (new patients, initial dose ½ tablet); angina, 1 tablet twice daily (may sometimes be reduced to once daily)

PoM Univer® (Rhône-Poulenc Rorer)
Capsules, all m/r, verapamil hydrochloride 120 mg (yellow/dark blue), net price 28-cap pack = £7.00; 180 mg (yellow), 56-cap pack = £16.92; 240 mg (yellow/dark blue), 28-cap pack = £11.42. Label: 25
Dose: hypertension, 240 mg daily, max. 480 mg daily (new patients, initial dose 120 mg); angina, 360 mg daily, max. 480 mg daily

2.6.3 Peripheral vasodilators and related drugs

Most serious peripheral disorders, such as *intermittent claudication*, are now known to be due to occlusion of vessels, either by spasm or sclerotic plaques; use of vasodilators may increase blood flow at rest, but no controlled studies have shown any improvement in walking distance or sustained increase in muscle blood flow during exercise. Rest pain is rarely affected.

Management of *Raynaud's syndrome* includes avoidance of exposure to cold and stopping smoking. More severe symptoms may require vasodilator treatment, which is most often successful in primary Raynaud's syndrome. Nifedipine (section 2.6.2), prazosin (section 2.5.4) and thymoxamine have all been shown to be beneficial; cyclandelate, naftidrofuryl, nicotinic acid derivatives, and oxpentifylline are not established as being effective.

CHILBLAINS. Vasodilator therapy is not established as being effective for chilblains (see section 13.14).

CINNARIZINE

Indications: peripheral vascular disease, Raynaud's syndrome
Cautions; Side-effects: see section 4.6
Dose: initially, 75 mg 3 times daily; maintenance, 75 mg 2–3 times daily

Stugeron Forte® (Janssen)
Capsules, orange/ivory, cinnarizine 75 mg. Net price 20 = £1.61. Label: 2
Stugeron® see section 4.6

NICOTINIC ACID DERIVATIVES

Indications: peripheral vascular disease (for hyperlipidaemia, see section 2.12)
Side-effects: flushing, dizziness, nausea, vomiting, hypotension (more frequent with nicotinic acid than derivatives); occasional diabetogenic effect reported with nicotinic acid and nicotinyl alcohol

Bradilan® see section 2.12
Hexopal® (Sanofi Winthrop)
Tablets, scored, inositol nicotinate 500 mg. Net price 20 = £4.17
Dose: 1 g 3 times daily, increased to 4 g daily if required
Tablets forte, scored, inositol nicotinate 750 mg. Net price 112-tab pack = £34.89
Dose: 1.5 g twice daily
Suspension, sugar-free, inositol nicotinate 1 g/5 mL. Net price 300 mL = £21.39
Dose: as for tablets (above)

Ronicol® (Roche)
Tablets, scored, nicotinyl alcohol 25 mg (as tartrate). Net price 20 = 37p
Dose: 25–50 mg 4 times daily
Timespan® (= tablets m/r), red, s/c, nicotinyl alcohol 150 mg (as tartrate). Net price 20 = £1.58. Label: 25
Dose: 150–300 mg twice daily

OXPENTIFYLLINE

Indications: peripheral vascular disease
Cautions: hypotension, coronary artery disease; avoid in porphyria (see section 9.8.2)
Side-effects: gastro-intestinal disturbances, dizziness, headache; rarely flushing, tachycardia
Dose: 400 mg 2–3 times daily

PoM **Trental**® (Hoechst)
Tablets, m/r, pink, s/c, oxpentifylline 400 mg. Net price 90-tab pack = £17.24. Label: 21, 25

THYMOXAMINE

Indications: primary Raynaud's syndrome (short-term treatment)
Cautions: diabetes mellitus
Side-effects: nausea, diarrhoea, flushing, headache, dizziness
Dose: initially 40 mg 4 times daily, increased to 80 mg 4 times daily if poor initial response; discontinue after 2 weeks if no response

PoM **Opilon**® (P-D)
Tablets, yellow, f/c, thymoxamine 40 mg (as hydrochloride). Net price 120-tab pack = £28.00. Label: 21

OTHER PREPARATION USED IN PERIPHERAL VASCULAR DISEASE

Rutosides (oxerutins, Paroven®) are not vasodilators and are not generally regarded as effective preparations as capillary sealants or for the treatment of cramps.

Paroven® (Zyma)
Capsules, yellow, oxerutins 250 mg. Net price 20 = £2.34. Label: 21. For relief of symptoms of oedema associated with chronic venous insufficiency

2.6.4 Cerebral vasodilators

These drugs are claimed to improve mental function. Some improvements in performance of psychological tests have been reported but the drugs have not been shown clinically to be of much benefit in dementia.

CO-DERGOCRINE MESYLATE

A mixture in equal proportions of dihydroergocornine mesylate, dihydroergocristine mesylate, and (in the ratio 2:1) α- and β-dihydroergocryptine mesylates
Indications: adjunct in elderly patients with mild to moderate dementia
Cautions: severe bradycardia
Side-effects: gastro-intestinal disturbances, flushing, headache, rash, nasal congestion; postural hypotension in hypertensive patients
Dose: 1.5 mg 3 times daily *or* 4.5 mg once daily

PoM **Hydergine**® (Sandoz)
Tablets, co-dergocrine mesylate 1.5 mg (scored), net price 20 = £2.21; 4.5 mg, 28-tab pack = £11.06. Label: 22

CYCLANDELATE

Indications: cerebral and peripheral vascular disease
Contra-indications: acute phase of cerebrovascular accident and myocardial infarction
Side-effects: nausea, flushing, dizziness with high doses
Dose: 400 mg 3–4 times daily

Cyclobral® (Norgine)
Capsules, pink/brown, cyclandelate 400 mg. Net price 20 = £2.36

NAFTIDROFURYL OXALATE

Indications: cerebral and peripheral vascular disease
Contra-indications: parenteral administration in atrioventricular block
Side-effects: nausea, epigastric pain, rash
Dose: see below

PoM **Praxilene**® (Lipha)
Capsules, pink, naftidrofuryl oxalate 100 mg. Net price 84-cap pack = £8.60. Label: 25, 27
Dose: peripheral vascular disease, 100–200 mg 3 times daily; cerebral vascular disease, 100 mg 3 times daily
Injection forte, naftidrofuryl oxalate 20 mg/mL. Net price 10-mL amp = £1.10
Dose: peripheral vascular disease only, by intravenous or intra-arterial infusion, 200 mg over at least 90 minutes, twice daily

2.7 Sympathomimetics

2.7.1 Inotropic sympathomimetics
2.7.2 Vasoconstrictor sympathomimetics

The properties of sympathomimetics vary according to whether they act on alpha or on beta adrenergic receptors. Adrenaline acts on both alpha and beta receptors and increases both heart rate and contractility (beta$_1$ effects); it can cause peripheral vasodilation (a beta$_2$ effect) or vasoconstriction (an alpha effect).

In *cardiac arrest* adrenaline 1 in 10 000 (1 mg per 10 mL) is recommended in a dose of 10 mL by central intravenous injection. The procedure for cardiopulmonary resuscitation is given in the algorithm (see next page) which reflects the revised recommendations of the Resuscitation Council (UK).

IMPORTANT. For *acute anaphylaxis* use **intramuscular route** (for dose, see p. 131).

ADRENALINE

Indications and Dose: see notes above
Cautions: ischaemic heart disease, diabetes mellitus, hyperthyroidism, hypertension; **interactions:** Appendix 1 (sympathomimetics)
Side-effects: anxiety, tremor, tachycardia, headache, cold extremities; in overdosage arrhythmias, cerebral haemorrhage, pulmonary oedema

PoM **Adrenaline Injection**, adrenaline 1 in 10000 (adrenaline 100 micrograms/mL as acid tartrate). 10-mL amp.
Available from Martindale and Penn (special order); also from IMS (Min-I-Jet® Adrenaline 3- and 10-mL disposable syringes)
Note. Adrenaline Injection BP is 1 in 1000 (adrenaline 1 mg/mL, as acid tartrate), see p. 131

2.7.1 Inotropic sympathomimetics

The cardiac stimulants **dobutamine** and **dopamine** act on beta$_1$ receptors in cardiac muscle, and increase contractility with little effect on rate; they are used in cardiogenic shock. Dosage of dopamine is critical since although low doses induce vasodilatation and increase renal perfusion, higher doses (more than 5 micrograms per kg per minute) lead to vasoconstriction and may exacerbate heart failure.

Xamoterol also acts on beta$_1$ receptors but being a partial agonist it provokes only a modest stimulatory response at rest. **Important:** for CSM restriction limiting xamoterol to **mild heart failure only**, owing to deterioration in patients with moderate to severe heart failure, see p. 100.

Dopexamine acts on beta$_2$ receptors in cardiac muscle to produce its positive inotropic effect; and on peripheral dopamine receptors to increase renal perfusion; it is reported not to induce vasoconstriction.

Isoprenaline is less selective and increases both heart rate and contractility; it may prevent Stokes-Adams attacks, but insertion of a pacemaker is preferable. It is now only used as a short-term emergency treatment of heart block or severe bradycardia.

DOBUTAMINE HYDROCHLORIDE

Indications: inotropic support in infarction, cardiac surgery, cardiomyopathies, septic shock, and cardiogenic shock
Cautions: severe hypotension complicating cardiogenic shock
Side-effects: tachycardia and marked increase in systolic blood pressure indicate overdosage
Dose: by intravenous infusion, 2.5–10 micrograms/kg/minute, adjusted according to response

PoM **Dobutrex**® (Lilly)
Strong sterile solution, dobutamine (as hydrochloride) 12.5 mg/mL. For dilution and use as an intravenous infusion. Net price 20-mL vial = £13.92

DOPAMINE HYDROCHLORIDE

Indications: cardiogenic shock in infarction or cardiac surgery
Cautions: correct hypovolaemia; low dose in shock due to acute myocardial infarction—see notes above

CARDIOPULMONARY RESUSCITATION

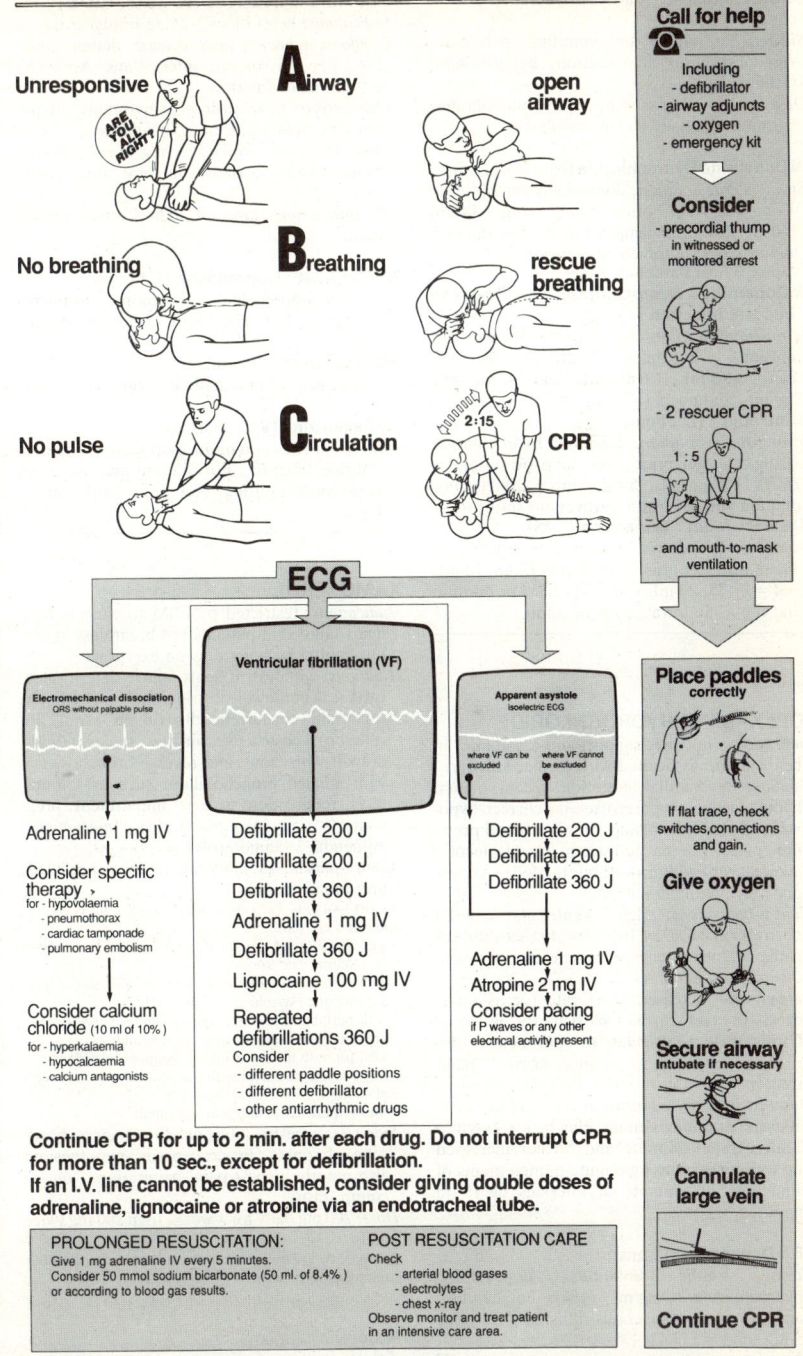

Unresponsive — ARE YOU ALL RIGHT?

Airway — open airway

No breathing

Breathing — rescue breathing

No pulse

Circulation — CPR (2:15)

Call for help
Including
- defibrillator
- airway adjuncts
- oxygen
- emergency kit

Consider
- precordial thump in witnessed or monitored arrest

- 2 rescuer CPR (1:5)

- and mouth-to-mask ventilation

ECG

Electromechanical dissociation
QRS without palpable pulse

- Adrenaline 1 mg IV
- Consider specific therapy for
  - hypovolaemia
  - pneumothorax
  - cardiac tamponade
  - pulmonary embolism
- Consider calcium chloride (10 ml of 10%) for
  - hyperkalaemia
  - hypocalcaemia
  - calcium antagonists

Ventricular fibrillation (VF)

- Defibrillate 200 J
- Defibrillate 200 J
- Defibrillate 360 J
- Adrenaline 1 mg IV
- Defibrillate 360 J
- Lignocaine 100 mg IV
- Repeated defibrillations 360 J
  Consider
  - different paddle positions
  - different defibrillator
  - other antiarrhythmic drugs

Apparent asystole
isoelectric ECG

where VF can be excluded / where VF cannot be excluded

- Defibrillate 200 J
- Defibrillate 200 J
- Defibrillate 360 J

- Adrenaline 1 mg IV
- Atropine 2 mg IV
- Consider pacing if P waves or any other electrical activity present

Continue CPR for up to 2 min. after each drug. Do not interrupt CPR for more than 10 sec., except for defibrillation.
If an I.V. line cannot be established, consider giving double doses of adrenaline, lignocaine or atropine via an endotracheal tube.

PROLONGED RESUSCITATION:	POST RESUSCITATION CARE
Give 1 mg adrenaline IV every 5 minutes. Consider 50 mmol sodium bicarbonate (50 ml of 8.4%) or according to blood gas results.	Check - arterial blood gases - electrolytes - chest x-ray Observe monitor and treat patient in an intensive care area.

Place paddles correctly

If flat trace, check switches, connections and gain.

Give oxygen

Secure airway
Intubate if necessary

Cannulate large vein

Continue CPR

The Resuscitation Council (UK)

Reproduced with permission of the Resuscitation Council (UK), charts available from Laerdal Medical Ltd

Contra-indications: tachyarrhythmia, phaeochromocytoma

Side-effects: nausea and vomiting, peripheral vasoconstriction, hypotension, hypertension, tachycardia

Dose: by intravenous infusion, 2–5 micrograms/kg/minute initially (see notes above)

PoM **Dopamine Hydrochloride** (Non-proprietary)
Strong sterile solution, dopamine hydrochloride 40 mg/mL, net price 5-mL amp = £4.56; 160 mg/mL, 5-mL amp = £18.29. For dilution and use as an intravenous infusion
Available from David Bull, Evans

PoM **Dopamine Hydrochloride in Dextrose (Glucose) Injection** (Abbott)
Intravenous infusions (in glucose 5% intravenous infusion), dopamine hydrochloride 800 micrograms/mL, 1.6 mg/mL, and 3.2 mg/mL. 250-mL containers (all hosp. only)

PoM **Intropin**® (Du Pont)
Strong sterile solution, dopamine hydrochloride 40 mg/mL, net price 5-mL amp or syringe = £4.80; 160 mg/mL, 5-mL amp = £19.20. For dilution and use as an intravenous infusion

PoM **Select-A-Jet**® **Dopamine** (IMS)
Strong sterile solution, dopamine hydrochloride 40 mg/mL. Net price 5-mL vial = £3.88; 10-mL vial = £7.75; 20-mL vial = £11.63. For dilution and use as an intravenous infusion.

DOPEXAMINE HYDROCHLORIDE

Indications: inotropic support and vasodilator in heart failure associated with cardiac surgery

Cautions: myocardial infarction, recent angina, hypokalaemia, hyperglycaemia; correct hypovolaemia before starting, monitor blood pressure, pulse, plasma potassium, blood glucose; avoid abrupt withdrawal; interactions: Appendix 1 (sympathomimetics)

Contra-indications: left ventricular outlet obstruction such as hypertrophic cardiomyopathy or aortic stenosis; phaeochromocytoma, thrombocytopenia

Side-effects: increased heart rate (occasionally excessive tachycardia, particularly in atrial fibrillation), ventricular ectopic beats; also reported: nausea, vomiting, anginal pain, tremor

Dose: by intravenous infusion via caval catheter, 500 nanograms/kg/minute, may be increased to 1 microgram/kg/minute and further increased up to 6 micrograms/kg/minute in increments of 1 microgram/kg/minute at intervals of 10–15 minutes

▼ PoM **Dopacard**® (Fisons)
Strong sterile solution, dopexamine hydrochloride 10 mg/mL (1%). For dilution and use as an intravenous infusion. Net price 5-mL amp = £19.42
Note. Contact with metal in infusion apparatus should be minimised

ISOPRENALINE HYDROCHLORIDE

Indications: heart block, severe bradycardia

Cautions: ischaemic heart disease, diabetes mellitus, hyperthyroidism; **interactions:** Appendix 1 (sympathomimetics)

Side-effects: tachycardia, arrhythmias, hypotension, sweating, tremor, headache

Dose: by mouth, initially 30 mg every 6 hours, range 90–840 mg daily (but oral route rarely used)
By intravenous infusion, 0.5–10 micrograms/minute

PoM **Min-I-Jet**® **Isoprenaline** (IMS)
Injection, isoprenaline hydrochloride 20 micrograms/mL. Net price 10-mL disposable syringe = £3.55

PoM **Saventrine**® (Pharmax)
Tablets, isoprenaline hydrochloride 30 mg. Net price 20 = £1.72

PoM **Saventrine IV**® (Pharmax)
Strong sterile solution, isoprenaline hydrochloride 1 mg/mL. For dilution and use as an intravenous infusion. Net price 2-mL amp = 45p

XAMOTEROL

Indications: restricted by CSM to chronic mild heart failure (in patients not breathless at rest but limited by symptoms on exertion)

Cautions: withdraw if heart failure deteriorates; cardiac outflow obstruction, arrhythmias (maintain concurrent digoxin in atrial fibrillation), obstructive airways disease (withdraw if worsening, and reverse bronchospasm with inhaled bronchodilator such as salbutamol), reduce dose in renal impairment; pregnancy (toxicity in *animal* studies); **interactions:** Appendix 1 (xamoterol)

Contra-indications: moderate to severe heart failure; breast-feeding

HEART FAILURE. Patients in whom xamoterol is contra-indicated are those:
 who are short of breath or fatigued at rest or limited on minimal exercise;
 with resting tachycardia (>90 beats per minute) or hypotension (systolic BP<100 mmHg);
 with peripheral oedema, raised jugular venous pressure, enlarged liver, or third heart sound;
 with (or with history of) acute pulmonary oedema;
 who require treatment with frusemide in dose in excess of 40 mg daily (or equivalent);
 who require ACE inhibitor treatment

Side-effects: gastro-intestinal disturbances, headache, dizziness, bronchospasm, hypotension; also reported: chest pain, palpitations, muscle cramp, rashes

Dose: 200 mg daily for 1 week, then 200 mg twice daily

IMPORTANT. Treatment should be started in hospital after full assessment of severity of heart failure by exercise test

PoM **Corwin**® (Stuart)
Tablets, yellow, f/c, xamoterol (as fumarate) 200 mg. Net price 56-tab pack = £26.60

2.7.2 Vasoconstrictor sympathomimetics

Vasoconstrictor sympathomimetics raise blood pressure transiently by acting on alpha-adrenergic receptors to constrict peripheral vessels. They are sometimes used as an emergency method of elevating blood pressure. They may also be used in general and spinal anaesthesia to control blood pressure.

The danger of vasoconstrictors is that although they raise blood pressure they do so at the expense of perfusion of vital organs such as the kidney. Further, in many patients with shock the peripheral resistance is already high, and to raise it further is unhelpful. Thus the use of vasoconstrictors in the treatment of shock is to be generally **deprecated**. The use of plasma substitutes, or of inotropic agents such as dopamine or dobutamine (section 2.7.1) is more appropriate. Treatment of the underlying condition is obviously important.

Spinal and epidural anaesthesia may result in sympathetic block with resultant hypotension. Management may include intravenous fluids (which are also given prophylactically in obstetrics), oxygen, elevation of the legs, and injection of a pressor drug such as ephedrine or methoxamine. As well as constricting peripheral vessels ephedrine also accelerates the heart rate (by acting on beta receptors). Use is made of this dual action of **ephedrine** to manage associated bradycardia (although intravenous injection of atropine sulphate 400 to 600 micrograms may also be required if bradycardia persists). When the hypotension occurs in association with tachycardia the pure alpha-adrenergic stimulant action of **methoxamine** is more appropriate.

EPHEDRINE HYDROCHLORIDE

Indications: see under Dose
Cautions: hyperthyroidism, diabetes mellitus, ischaemic heart disease, hypertension, elderly; may cause acute retention in prostatic hypertrophy; **interactions:** Appendix 1 (sympathomimetics)
Side-effects: tachycardia, anxiety, restlessness, insomnia; also tremor, arrhythmias, dry mouth, cold extremities; acute retention in prostatic hypertrophy
Dose: reversal of hypotension from spinal or epidural anaesthesia, *by slow intravenous injection* of a solution containing ephedrine hydrochloride 3 mg/mL, 3–6 mg repeated every 3–4 minutes to max. 30 mg (but more than 9 mg rarely required)
  Prevention of hypotension from spinal anaesthesia, *by intramuscular injection,* 15–30 mg

PoM **Ephedrine Hydrochloride** (Non-proprietary)
Injection, ephedrine hydrochloride 30 mg/mL. For dilution before intravenous administration. 1-mL amp

METARAMINOL

Indications: acute hypotension
Cautions; Contra-indications: see under Noradrenaline Acid Tartrate
Side-effects: tachycardia, arrhythmias, reduced renal blood flow
Dose: by intravenous infusion, 15–100 mg in 500 mL, adjusted according to response

PoM **Aramine**® (MSD)
Injection, metaraminol 10 mg (as tartrate)/mL. Net price 1-mL amp = 48p

METHOXAMINE HYDROCHLORIDE

Indications: hypotension in anaesthesia
Cautions: hyperthyroidism; pregnancy; **interactions:** Appendix 1 (sympathomimetics)
Contra-indications: severe coronary or cardiovascular disease
Side-effects: headache, hypertension, bradycardia
Dose: by intramuscular injection, 5–20 mg
  By slow intravenous injection, 5–10 mg (rate 1 mg/minute)

PoM **Vasoxine**® (Wellcome)
Injection, methoxamine hydrochloride 20 mg/mL. Net price 1-mL amp = 52p

NORADRENALINE ACID TARTRATE

Indications: acute hypotension, cardiac arrest
Cautions: extravasation at injection site may cause necrosis; **interactions:** Appendix 1 (sympathomimetics)
Contra-indications: myocardial infarction, pregnancy
Side-effects: headache, palpitations, bradycardia
Dose: by intravenous infusion, of a solution containing noradrenaline acid tartrate 8 micrograms/mL (equivalent to noradrenaline base 4 micrograms/mL) at an initial rate of 2 to 3 mL/minute, adjusted according to response
  By rapid intravenous or intracardiac injection, 0.5 to 0.75 mL of a solution containing noradrenaline acid tartrate 200 micrograms/mL (equivalent to noradrenaline base 100 micrograms/mL)

PoM **Levophed**® (Sanofi Winthrop)
Strong sterile solution, noradrenaline acid tartrate 2 mg/mL (equivalent to noradrenaline base 1 mg/mL). For dilution and use as an intravenous infusion. Net price 2-mL amp = 95p; 4-mL amp = £1.39
Special injection, noradrenaline acid tartrate 200 micrograms/mL (equivalent to noradrenaline base 100 micrograms/mL). Net price 2-mL amp = 92p

PHENYLEPHRINE HYDROCHLORIDE

Indications: acute hypotension
Cautions; Contra-indications: see under Noradrenaline Acid Tartrate; also contra-indicated in severe hypertension and hyperthyroidism

Side-effects: hypertension with headache, palpitations, vomiting; tachycardia or reflex bradycardia; tingling and coolness of skin
Dose: by subcutaneous or intramuscular injection, 5 mg
By slow intravenous injection, 100–500 micrograms
By intravenous infusion, 5–20 mg in 500 mL, adjusted according to response

PoM **Phenylephrine Injection 1%** (Boots)
Injection, phenylephrine hydrochloride 10 mg/mL. 1-mL amp

2.8 Anticoagulants and protamine

2.8.1 Parenteral anticoagulants
2.8.2 Oral anticoagulants
2.8.3 Protamine sulphate

The main use of anticoagulants is to prevent thrombus formation or extension of an existing thrombus in the slower-moving venous side of the circulation, where the thrombus consists of a fibrin web enmeshed with platelets and red cells. They are therefore widely used in the prevention and treatment of *deep-vein thrombosis in the legs.*

Anticoagulants are of less use in preventing thrombus formation in arteries, for in faster-flowing vessels thrombi are composed mainly of platelets with little fibrin. They are used to prevent thrombi forming on *prosthetic heart valves.*

2.8.1 Parenteral anticoagulants

Heparin is given to initiate anticoagulation and is rapidly effective. As its effects are short-lived it is best given by continuous intravenous infusion; it is preferably not given by intermittent intravenous injection. Oral anticoagulants are started at the same time, and the heparin infusion withdrawn after 3 days.

If oral anticoagulants cannot be given and heparin is continued, its dose is adjusted after determination of the activated partial thromboplastin time.

If haemorrhage occurs it is usually sufficient to withdraw heparin, but if rapid reversal of the effects of heparin is required, protamine sulphate is a specific antidote (section 2.8.3).

For the prophylaxis of thrombosis in patients undergoing heart surgery or haemodialysis full therapeutic doses of heparin are given for the duration of the procedure. Low-dose heparin by subcutaneous injection is widely advocated to prevent postoperative deep-vein thrombosis and pulmonary embolism in 'high risk' patients, i.e. those with obesity, malignant disease, previous history of thrombosis, or in older patients. Laboratory monitoring is not required with this regimen.

There is evidence that **low molecular weight heparins** are as effective and as safe as unfractionated heparin in the prevention of venous thrombo-embolism. They have a longer duration of action than unfractionated heparin; once-daily dosage means that they are convenient to use.

> **CSM advice.** Platelet counts should be measured in patients under heparin treatment for longer than 5 days and the treatment should be stopped immediately in those who develop thrombocytopenia.

HEPARIN

Indications: treatment of thrombo-embolic disorders such as deep-vein thrombosis and pulmonary embolism; prophylaxis after myocardial infarction; prevention of postoperative thrombosis and thrombo-embolic events in susceptible patients
Cautions: pregnancy; **interactions:** Appendix 1 (heparin)
Contra-indications: haemophilia and other haemorrhagic disorders, thrombocytopenia, peptic ulcer, cerebral aneurysm, severe hypertension, severe liver disease, recent surgery of eye or nervous system, hypersensitivity to heparin
Side-effects: haemorrhage, thrombocytopenia (see CSM advice above), hypersensitivity reactions; osteoporosis after prolonged use, alopecia
Dose: by intravenous injection, loading dose of 5000 units followed by continuous *infusion* of 1000–2000 units/hour (approx. 14–28 units/kg/hour) adjusted daily by laboratory monitoring *or* 5000–10 000 units by *intravenous injection* every 4 hours (but *continuous intravenous infusion* preferred, see notes above)
By subcutaneous injection, prophylaxis of deep-vein thrombosis, 5000 units 2 hours before surgery, then every 8–12 hours until patient is ambulant; in pregnancy (with monitoring), 10 000 units every 12 hours (important: not intended to cover prevention of prosthetic heart valve thrombosis in pregnancy which calls for separate specialist management)
Treatment of deep-vein thrombosis, initially 10 000–20 000 units every 12 hours *or* 250 units/kg (2500 units/10 kg) every 12 hours, adjusted daily by laboratory monitoring
Note. The above doses do not apply to the low molecular weight heparins (see below)

Intravenous preparations
PoM **Heparin Injection** (heparin sodium)
1000 units/mL, net price 1-mL amp = 21p; 5-mL amp = 69p; 5-mL vial = 54p
5000 units/mL, net price 1-mL amp = 33p; 5-mL amp = 98p; 5-mL vial = £1.46
10 000 units/mL, net price 1-mL amp = 45p
25 000 units/mL, net price 1-mL amp = 86p; 5-mL vial = £6.43
PoM **Monoparin**® (CP)
Injection, heparin sodium (mucous) 1000 units/mL, net price 1-mL amp = 17p; 5-mL amp = 46p; 10-mL amp = 66p; 5000 units/mL, 1-mL amp = 32p; 5-mL amp = 98p; 25 000 units/mL, 1-mL amp = £1.27

2.8 Anticoagulants and protamine

PoM **Multiparin**® (CP)
Injection, heparin sodium (mucous) 1000 units/mL, net price 5-mL vial = 45p; 5000 units/mL, 5-mL vial = £1.32; 25 000 units/mL, 5-mL vial = £5.41

PoM **Pump-Hep**® (Leo)
Intravenous infusion, heparin sodium (mucous) 1000 units/mL. Net price 5-mL amp = 40p; 10-mL amp = 66p; 20-mL amp = 98p
Dose: by continuous infusion pump, 20 000–40 000 units daily

PoM **Unihep**® (Leo)
Injection, heparin sodium (mucous) 1000 units/mL, net price 1-mL amp = 14p; 5000 units/mL, 1-mL amp = 27p; 10 000 units/mL, 1-mL amp = 45p; 25 000 units/mL, 1-mL amp = £1.07

Subcutaneous preparations

PoM **Heparin Injection** (heparin sodium or heparin calcium)
25 000 units/mL (subcutaneous). Net price 0.2-mL amp = 41p

PoM **Calciparine**® (Sanofi Winthrop)
Injection (subcutaneous), heparin calcium 25 000 units/mL. Net price 0.2-mL syringe = 70p; 0.5-mL syringe = £1.50; 0.8-mL amp or syringe = £1.80

PoM **Minihep**® (Leo)
Injection (subcutaneous), heparin sodium 25 000 units/mL. Net price 0.2-mL amp = 42p

PoM **Minihep Calcium**® (Leo)
Injection (subcutaneous), heparin calcium 25 000 units/mL. Net price 0.2-mL amp = 45p

PoM **Monoparin**® (CP)
Injection (subcutaneous), heparin sodium (mucous) 25 000 units/mL. Net price 0.2-mL amp = 37p

PoM **Monoparin Calcium**® (CP)
Injection (subcutaneous), heparin calcium 25 000 units/mL. Net price 0.2 mL amp = 52p

PoM **Uniparin**® (CP)
Injection (subcutaneous), heparin sodium 25 000 units/mL. Net price 0.2-mL syringe = 60p; 0.4-mL syringe (Uniparin Forte) = £1.30

PoM **Uniparin Calcium**® (CP)
Injection (subcutaneous), heparin calcium 25 000 units/mL. Net price 0.2-mL syringe = 60p; 0.5-mL syringe = £1.45

LOW MOLECULAR WEIGHT HEPARINS

▼ PoM **Clexane**® (Rhône-Poulenc Rorer)
Injection, enoxaparin (low molecular weight heparin) 100 mg/mL. Net price 0.2-mL syringe (20 mg) = £3.64; 0.4-mL syringe (40 mg) = £4.85
Prophylaxis of deep-vein thrombosis, *by subcutaneous injection*, *moderate risk*, 20 mg (2000 units) 1–2 hours before surgery then 20 mg (2000 units) every 24 hours for 7–10 days; *high risk*, 40 mg (4000 units) 12 hours before surgery then 40 mg (4000 units) every 24 hours for 7–10 days
Prevention of clotting in extracorporeal circulation (consult data sheet)

▼ PoM **Fragmin**® (Kabi Pharmacia)
Injection, dalteparin sodium (low molecular weight heparin) 2500 units/mL, net price 4-mL amp = £5.50; 10 000 units/mL, 1-mL amp = £5.50; 12 500 units/mL, 0.2-mL syringe = £2.60; 25 000 units/mL, 0.2-mL syringe = £3.70
Prophylaxis of deep-vein thrombosis, *by subcutaneous injection*, *moderate risk*, 2500 units 1–2 hours before surgery then 2500 units every 24 hours for 5 days; *high risk*, 2500 units 1–2 hours before surgery, then 2500 units 12 hours later, then 5000 units every 24 hours for 5 days
Prevention of clotting in extracorporeal circulation (consult data sheet)

HEPARIN FLUSHES

For maintaining catheter patency sodium chloride injection 0.9% is as effective as heparin flushes for up to 48 hours, and is therefore recommended for cannulas intended to be in place for 48 hours or less. Heparin flushes are recommended for cannulas intended to be in place for longer than 48 hours.

PoM **Hep-Flush**® (Leo)
Solution, heparin sodium 100 units/mL. Net price 2-mL amp = 26p; 10-mL vial = £1.30
To maintain patency of catheters, cannulas, etc., 200 units flushed through every 4–8 hours. Not for therapeutic use

PoM **Heplok**® (Leo)
Solution, heparin sodium 10 units/mL. Net price 5-mL amp = 30p
To maintain patency of catheters, cannulas, etc., 10–50 units flushed through every 4 hours. Not for therapeutic use

PoM **Hepsal**® (CP)
Solution, heparin sodium 10 units/mL. Net price 5-mL amp = 22p
To maintain patency of catheters, cannulas, etc., 50 units flushed through every 4 hours or as required. Not for therapeutic use

Ancrod reduces plasma fibrinogen by cleavage of fibrin but is not in common use.

ANCROD

Indications: deep-vein thrombosis, prevention of post-operative thrombosis ('named patient' basis only)
Cautions; Contra-indications; Side-effects: see under Heparin; resistance may develop; avoid administration with dextrans
Dose: by intravenous infusion, 2–3 units/kg over 4–12 hours (usually 6–8 hours), then *by infusion or slow intravenous injection*, 2 units/kg every 12 hours
By subcutaneous injection, prophylaxis of deep-vein thrombosis, 280 units immediately after surgery, then 70 units daily for 4 days (fractured femur) or 8 days (hip replacement)
Note. The initial infusion must be given slowly, as there is a risk of massive intravascular formation of unstable fibrin. Response can be monitored by observing clot size after the blood has been allowed to stand for about 2 hours, the aim being to predict a dose that produces a 2–3 mm clot. Alternatively, plasma-fibrinogen concentrations can be measured directly.

The major complication of ancrod is haemorrhage, and since it takes 12 to 24 hours for haemostatic fibrinogen concentrations to be restored after stopping administration it may be necessary to give ancrod antivenom (Arvin® Antidote, available from Armour) as an antidote (0.2-mL test dose subcutaneously followed by 0.8 mL intramuscularly, and 30 minutes later 1 mL intravenously). The antivenom may cause anaphylaxis (adrenaline etc. should be available, for details see Allergic Emergencies, section 3.4.3). As an alternative to the antivenom reconstituted freeze-dried fibrinogen may be given, or if this is not available one litre of fresh frozen plasma.

PoM Arvin® (Knoll)
Injection, ancrod 70 units/mL. 1-mL amp (available only on 'named patient' basis)

Epoprostenol (prostacyclin) can be given to inhibit platelet aggregation during renal dialysis either alone or with heparin. Since its half-life is only about 3 minutes it must be given by continuous intravenous infusion. It is a potent vasodilator and therefore its side-effects include flushing, headache, and hypotension.

EPOPROSTENOL
Indications: see notes above
Cautions: anticoagulant monitoring required when given with heparin
Side-effects: see notes above; also bradycardia, pallor, sweating with higher doses
Dose: see manufacturer's literature

PoM Flolan® (Wellcome)
Infusion, powder for reconstitution, epoprostenol (as sodium salt). Net price 500-microgram vial (with diluent) = £103.86

2.8.2 Oral anticoagulants

Oral anticoagulants antagonise the effects of vitamin K, and take at least 48 to 72 hours for the anticoagulant effect to develop fully; if an immediate effect is required, heparin must be given concomitantly.

The main indication for oral anticoagulant therapy is *deep-vein thrombosis*. Patients with *pulmonary embolism* should also be treated, as should those with *atrial fibrillation who are at risk of embolisation*, and those with *mechanical heart valve prostheses* (to prevent emboli developing on the valves); antiplatelet drugs may also be useful in these patients.

Oral anticoagulants should not be used in cerebral thrombosis or peripheral arterial occlusion, but may be of value in patients with *transient brain ischaemic attacks* whether due to carotid or vertebrobasilar arterial disease; if these patients also have severe hypertension anticoagulants are contra-indicated, and antiplatelet drugs are an alternative (section 2.9).

Warfarin is the drug of choice; **nicoumalone** and **phenindione** are seldom used.

Whenever possible, the base-line prothrombin time should be determined before the initial dose is given.

A typical induction dose of warfarin is 10 mg[1] daily for 2 days (but this should be tailored to individual requirement). The subsequent maintenance dose depends upon the prothrombin time (reported as INR[2]); the currently recommended therapeutic ranges are:
INR 2–2.5 for prophylaxis of deep-vein thrombosis including surgery on high-risk patients;
INR 2–3 for prophylaxis in hip surgery and fractured femur operations, for treatment of deep-vein thrombosis, pulmonary embolism, systemic embolism, prevention of venous thromboembolism in myocardial infarction, mitral stenosis with embolism, transient ischaemic attacks, atrial fibrillation, and tissue prosthetic heart valves;
INR 3–4.5 for recurrent deep-vein thrombosis and pulmonary embolism, arterial disease including myocardial infarction, and mechanical prosthetic heart valves.

It is essential that the INR be determined:
daily or on alternate days in early days of treatment, *then*
at longer intervals (depending on response) *then*
up to every 8 weeks

The daily maintenance dose[3] of warfarin is usually 3 to 9 mg (taken at the **same time** each day).

The main adverse effect of all oral anticoagulants is haemorrhage. Omission of dosage with checking of the INR is essential. The following recommendations of the British Society for Haematology are based on the result of the INR and the clinical state:
Life-threatening haemorrhage—immediately give phytomenadione (vitamin K₁) 5 mg by slow intravenous injection and a concentrate of factors II, IX, X (with factor VII concentrate if available). If no concentrate is available, fresh frozen plasma should be infused (approximately 1 litre for an adult) but this may not be as effective
Less severe haemorrhage e.g. haematuria and epistaxis—withhold warfarin for one or more days and consider giving phytomenadione (vitamin K₁) 0.5–2 mg[4] by slow intravenous injection
INR 4.5–7 without haemorrhage—withhold warfarin for 1 or 2 days then review
INR > 7 without haemorrhage—withhold warfarin and consider giving phytomenadione (vitamin K₁) 500 micrograms by slow intravenous injection
Unexpected bleeding at therapeutic levels[5]—investigate possibility of underlying cause e.g. unexpected renal or alimentary tract pathology

---

1. Less than 10 mg if base-line prothrombin time prolonged, if liver-function tests abnormal, or if patient in cardiac failure, on parenteral feeding, less than average body weight, or over 80 years of age.
2. The International Normalised Ratio (INR) has now replaced the British Ratio (BR).
3. Change in patient's clinical condition, particularly associated with liver disease, intercurrent illness, or drug administration, necessitates more frequent testing. See also **interactions**, Appendix 1 (warfarin). Major changes in diet (especially involving vegetables) may also affect warfarin control.
4. Usually 1 mg adequate and should be given if INR greater than desired; higher doses will prevent oral anticoagulants from acting for several days or even weeks.
5. Should always be investigated regardless of INR since even if patients over-anticoagulated bleeding generally has an additional underlying cause.

PREGNANCY. Oral anticoagulants are weakly teratogenic and should not be given in the first trimester of pregnancy. Women at risk of pregnancy should be warned of this danger. Also, oral anticoagulants cross the placenta with risk of placental or fetal haemorrhage; they should therefore not be given during the last few weeks of pregnancy.

Anticoagulant treatment booklets must be carried by patients, and are available from:

England:	Scottish Office
DH Stores	Health Department
No. 2 Site,	Room 64
Heywood Stores,	St. Andrew's House
Manchester Rd	Edinburgh EH1 3DH
Heywood	Northern Ireland Office
Lancs OL10 2PZ	Central Services Agency
Wales:	27 Adelaide St
Room 106	Belfast BT2 8FH
Royal Pharmaceutical Society	
of Great Britain	

Booklets giving advice for patients on anticoagulant treatment may be given to patients at the discretion of the doctor or pharmacist.

WARFARIN SODIUM
Indications: prophylaxis of embolisation in rheumatic heart disease and atrial fibrillation; prophylaxis after insertion of prosthetic heart valve; prophylaxis and treatment of venous thrombosis and pulmonary embolism; transient ischaemic attacks
Cautions: hepatic or renal disease, recent surgery; **interactions:** Appendix 1 (warfarin)
Contra-indications: pregnancy (see notes above), peptic ulcer, severe hypertension, bacterial endocarditis
Side-effects: haemorrhage
Dose: see notes above

PoM **Marevan**® (Evans)
Tablets, brown, scored, warfarin sodium 1 mg. Net price 20 = 9p. Label: 10 anticoagulant card
Tablets, blue, scored, warfarin sodium 3 mg. Net price 20 = 10p. Label: 10 anticoagulant card
Tablets, pink, scored, warfarin sodium 5 mg. Net price 20 = 16p. Label: 10 anticoagulant card

PoM **Warfarin WBP** (Boehringer Ingelheim)
Tablets, brown, scored, warfarin sodium 1 mg. Net price 20 = 9p. Label: 10 anticoagulant card
Tablets, blue, scored, warfarin sodium 3 mg. Net price 20 = 10p. Label: 10 anticoagulant card
Tablets, pink, scored, warfarin sodium 5 mg. Net price 20 = 16p. Label: 10 anticoagulant card

NICOUMALONE
Indications: prophylaxis of embolisation in rheumatic heart disease and atrial fibrillation; prophylaxis after insertion of prosthetic heart valve; prophylaxis and treatment of venous thrombosis and pulmonary embolism; transient ischaemic attacks
Cautions; Contra-indications; Side-effects: see under Warfarin Sodium; avoid breast-feeding
Dose: 8–12 mg on 1st day; 4–8 mg on 2nd day; maintenance dose usually 1–8 mg daily

PoM **Sinthrome**® (Geigy)
Tablets, nicoumalone 1 mg. Net price 20 = 15p. Label: 10 anticoagulant card
Tablets, scored, nicoumalone 4 mg. Net price 20 = 31p. Label: 10 anticoagulant card

PHENINDIONE
Indications: prophylaxis of embolisation in rheumatic heart disease and atrial fibrillation; prophylaxis after insertion of prosthetic heart valve; prophylaxis and treatment of venous thrombosis and pulmonary embolism
Cautions; Contra-indications; Side-effects: see under Warfarin Sodium; also hypersensitivity reactions including rashes, fever, leucopenia, agranulocytosis, diarrhoea, renal and hepatic damage; urine coloured pink; avoid breast-feeding; **interactions:** Appendix 1 (phenindione)
Dose: 200 mg on 1st day; 100 mg on 2nd day; maintenance dose usually 50–150 mg daily

PoM **Dindevan**® (Evans)
Tablets, phenindione 10 mg, net price 20 = 26p; 25 mg (green), 20 = 36p; 50 mg, 20 = 46p. Label: 10 anticoagulant card, 14 (urine pink)

2.8.3 Protamine sulphate
Although protamine sulphate is used to counteract overdosage with heparin, if used in excess it has an anticoagulant effect.

PROTAMINE SULPHATE
Indications; Cautions: see above
Side-effects: flushing, hypotension, bradycardia
Dose: by slow intravenous injection, 1 mg neutralises 100 units heparin (mucous) or 80 units heparin (lung) when given within 15 minutes; if longer time, less protamine required as heparin rapidly excreted; max. 50 mg

PoM **Protamine Sulphate** (Non-proprietary)
Injection, protamine sulphate 10 mg/mL. Net price 5-mL amp = 98p; 10-mL amp = £1.75
Available from Boots, CP (Prosulf®), Evans

2.9 Antiplatelet drugs
By decreasing platelet aggregation, these drugs may inhibit thrombus formation on the arterial side of the circulation, where thrombi are formed by platelet aggregation and anticoagulants have little effect. Antiplatelet drugs have little effect in venous thromboembolism. **Dipyridamole** is used by mouth as an adjunct to oral anticoagulation for prophylaxis of thromboembolism associated with prosthetic heart valves.

Encouraging results have been obtained using **aspirin** 300 mg daily for the *secondary* prevention of thrombotic cerebrovascular or cardiovascular disease; studies are still needed to determine whether lower doses (such as 75 mg daily or 300 mg on alternate days) might not be equally (or more) effective. Aspirin has also been shown to reduce mortality when given in a dose of 150 mg daily for a month after myocardial infarction. Low doses of aspirin (such as 75 or 100 mg daily) are also given following bypass surgery. Physicians in the USA have demonstrated that 325 mg on alternate days can have a *primary* preventive action for myocardial infarction but further analysis is awaited before aspirin can be recommended for routine use in primary prevention.

For use of epoprostenol, see section 2.8.1.

ASPIRIN (antiplatelet)

Indications: prophylaxis of cerebrovascular disease or myocardial infarction (see notes above)

Cautions: asthma; uncontrolled hypertension; pregnancy (but see Appendix 4); **interactions:** Appendix 1 (aspirin)

Contra-indications: children under 12 years and in breast-feeding (Reye's syndrome, see section 4.7.1); active peptic ulceration; haemophilia and other bleeding disorders

Side-effects: bronchospasm; gastro-intestinal haemorrhage (occasionally major), also other haemorrhage (e.g. subconjunctival)

Dose: see notes above

Aspirin (Non-proprietary)
Dispersible tablets, aspirin 75 mg, net price 20 = 10p; 300 mg, see section 4.7.1. Label: 13, 21, 32

Angettes 75® (Bristol-Myers)
Tablets, aspirin 75 mg. Net price 56-tab pack = £1.88. Label: 32

Caprin (Nicholas): see section 4.7.1

Nu-Seals Aspirin 300 mg: see section 4.7.1

Platet® (Nicholas)
Tablets, effervescent, aspirin 100 mg, net price 30-tab pack = 99p; 300 mg, 30-tab pack = £1.13. Label: 13, 32

DIPYRIDAMOLE

Indications: see notes above

Cautions: rapidly worsening angina, aortic stenosis, recent myocardial infarction; may exacerbate migraine, hypotension; **interactions:** Appendix 1 (dipyridamole)

Side-effects: nausea, diarrhoea, throbbing headache, hypotension

Dose: by mouth, 300–600 mg daily in 3–4 divided doses before food

By intravenous injection, diagnostic only, see manufacturer's literature

PoM **Dipyridamole** (Non-proprietary)
Tablets, coated, dipyridamole 25 mg, net price 20 = 74p; 100 mg, 20 = £1.89. Label: 22
Available from APS, Ashbourne (Cerebrovase®), Berk, Cox, Evans, Kerfoot, Norton, Shire (Vasyrol®)

PoM **Persantin®** (Boehringer Ingelheim)
Tablets, both s/c, dipyridamole 25 mg (orange), net price 84-tab pack = £3.17; 100 mg, 84-tab pack = £8.84. Label: 22
Injection, dipyridamole 5 mg/mL. Net price 2-mL amp = 10p

2.10 Fibrinolytic drugs

Fibrinolytic drugs act as thrombolytics by activating plasminogen to form plasmin, which degrades fibrin and so breaks up thrombi.

Streptokinase is used in the treatment of *life-threatening venous thrombosis,* and in *pulmonary embolism,* but treatment must be started rapidly.

Urokinase is currently used for *thrombolysis in the eye* and in *arteriovenous shunts.* It has the advantage of being non-immunogenic.

The value of thrombolytic drugs for the treatment of *myocardial infarction* has recently been established. **Streptokinase, alteplase,** and **anistreplase** have all been shown to reduce mortality when given by the intravenous route; evidence on comparative efficacy is incomplete. The potential for benefit lessens as the delay from the onset of major symptoms increases, but the value of treatment within the first 12 hours is reasonably well established. Knowledge of the role of adjuvant therapy is also incomplete, but in the case of streptokinase the reduction in mortality by aspirin has been shown to be additive whilst immediate heparin is necessary to obtain full efficacy from alteplase. Thrombolytic drugs are indicated for any patient with acute myocardial infarction for whom the benefit is believed to outweigh the risk of treatment. Trials have shown that the benefit is greatest in those with ECG changes that include ST segment elevation and in those with anterior infarction. Patients should not be excluded on account of age alone because mortality in this group is high and the percentage reduction in mortality is the same as in younger patients.

CAUTIONS. Risk of bleeding from venepuncture or invasive procedures, any external chest compression, pregnancy, possibility of pre-existing thrombus as in abdominal aneurysm or enlarged left atrium with atrial fibrillation (risk of dissolution of clot and subsequent embolisation), recent or concurrent anticoagulant therapy.

CONTRA-INDICATIONS. Recent haemorrhage, trauma, or surgery (including dental extraction), coagulation defects, bleeding diatheses, history of cerebrovascular disease especially recent events or with any residual disability, recent symptoms of possible peptic ulceration, heavy vaginal bleeding, severe hypertension, pulmonary disease with cavitation, acute pancreatitis, diabetic retinopathy, severe liver disease, oesophageal varices. In the case of streptokinase or anistreplase, previous allergic reactions to either drug, or therapy with either drug from 5 days to 12 months previously.

SIDE-EFFECTS. Side-effects of thrombolytics are mainly nausea and vomiting and bleeding. Bleeding is usually limited to the site of injection, but intracerebral haemorrhage or bleeding from other sites may occur. Serious bleeding calls for discontinuation of the thrombolytic and may require administration of coagulation factors and antifibrinolytic drugs (aprotinin or tranexamic acid).

2.11 Antifibrinolytic drugs and haemostatics

Streptokinase and anistreplase may cause allergic reactions and anaphylaxis has been reported (for details of management see Allergic Emergencies, section 3.4.3).

ALTEPLASE
(rt-PA, tissue-type plasminogen activator)
Indications: acute myocardial infarction (see notes above)
Cautions; Contra-indications; Side-effects: see notes above
Dose: by intravenous injection, 10 mg over 1–2 minutes, followed by *intravenous infusion* of 50 mg over 1 hour, then 40 mg over the subsequent 2 hours (total dose 100 mg over 3 hours); treatment should be initiated within 6 hours; patients weighing less than 67 kg should receive a total dose of 1.5 mg/kg according to the above schedule

PoM **Actilyse**® (Boehringer Ingelheim)
Injection, powder for reconstitution, alteplase 20 mg (11.6 mega units)/vial, net price per vial (with diluent and transfer device) = £200.00; 50 mg (29 mega units)/vial, pack of 2 vials (with diluent, transfer device, and infusion bag) = £816.00

ANISTREPLASE
(APSAC)
Indications: acute myocardial infarction (see notes above)
Cautions; Contra-indications; Side-effects: see notes above
Dose: by intravenous injection, 30 units over 4–5 minutes; treatment should be initiated as soon as possible and preferably within 6 hours

PoM **Eminase**® (Beecham)
Injection, powder for reconstitution, anistreplase. Net price 30-unit vial = £495.00

STREPTOKINASE
Indications: deep-vein thrombosis, pulmonary embolism, acute arterial thromboembolism, thrombosed arteriovenous shunts; acute myocardial infarction (see notes above)
Cautions; Contra-indications; Side-effects: see notes above
Dose: by intravenous infusion, 250 000 units over 30 minutes, then 100 000 units every hour for up to 24–72 hours according to condition (see data sheet)
Myocardial infarction, 1 500 000 units over 60 minutes followed by aspirin 150 mg daily *by mouth* for at least 4 weeks (see data sheet)

PoM **Kabikinase**® (Kabi Pharmacia)
Injection, powder for reconstitution, streptokinase; net price 100 000-unit vial = £7.50; 250 000-unit vial = £15.00; 600 000-unit vial = £34.20; 1.5 million-unit vial = £85.00

PoM **Streptase**® (Hoechst)
Injection, powder for reconstitution, streptokinase; net price 250 000-unit vial = £15.36; 750 000-unit vial = £40.26; 1.5 million-unit vial = £80.52 (hosp. only)

UROKINASE
Indications: thrombosed arteriovenous shunts and intravenous cannulas; thrombolysis in the eye; deep-vein thrombosis, pulmonary embolism, peripheral vascular occlusion
Cautions; Contra-indications; Side-effects: see notes above
Dose: by instillation into arteriovenous shunt, 5000–37 500 International units in 2–3 mL sodium chloride intravenous infusion 0.9%
By intravenous infusion, 4400 International units/kg over 10 minutes, then 4400 units/kg/hour for 12 hours in pulmonary embolism or 12–24 hours in deep-vein thrombosis; for bolus injection for pulmonary embolism consult data sheet
Peripheral vascular occlusion, consult data sheet
Intra-ocular administration, 5000–37 500 International units in 2 mL sodium chloride intravenous infusion 0.9%

PoM **Ukidan**® (Serono)
Injection, powder for reconstitution, urokinase; net price 5000 International unit vial = £6.71; 25 000 International unit vial = £23.58; 100 000 International unit vial = £60.00

PoM **Urokinase** (Leo)
Injection, powder for reconstitution, urokinase; net price 5 000 International unit vial = £9.75; 25 000 International unit vial = £27.79

2.11 Antifibrinolytic drugs and haemostatics

Fibrin dissolution can be impaired by the administration of **tranexamic acid**, which inhibits plasminogen activation and fibrinolysis. It may be useful when haemorrhage cannot be staunched, e.g. in prostatectomy, dental extraction in haemophiliacs, or menorrhagia; it may also be used in hereditary angioedema and in streptokinase overdose.

Desmopressin (see section 6.5.2) is used in the management of mild to moderate haemophilia.

Aprotinin is a proteolytic enzyme inhibitor acting on plasmin and kallidinogenase (kallikrein). It is indicated for patients at high risk of major blood loss during and after open heart surgery with extracorporeal circulation and for patients in whom optimal blood conservation during open heart surgery is an absolute priority; it is also indicated for the treatment of life-threatening haemorrhage due to hyperplasminaemia (occasionally observed during the mobilisation and dissection of malignant tumours, in acute promyelocytic leukaemia, and following thrombolytic therapy).

Cautionary label wordings, see inside back cover

Ethamsylate reduces capillary bleeding in the presence of a normal number of platelets. It does not act by fibrin stabilisation, but probably by correcting abnormal platelet adhesion.

APROTININ

Indications: see notes above
Side-effects: occasionally hypersensitivity reactions and localised thrombophlebitis
Dose: by slow intravenous injection or infusion
Open heart surgery, loading dose, 2 000 000 units (200 mL) after induction of anaesthesia and before sternotomy, *by slow intravenous injection* initially 50 000 units (5 mL) over several minutes (to detect allergy), remainder *by intravenous infusion* over 20 minutes; maintenance dose, *by intravenous infusion* 500 000 units (50 mL) every hour until end of operation (or early postoperative period in septic endocarditis); pump prime, 2 000 000 units (200 mL) in priming volume of extracorporeal circuit; in septic endocarditis 3 000 000 units (300 mL) added to pump prime
Hyperplasminaemia, *by slow intravenous injection or by infusion* initially, 500 000 units (50 mL) to 1 000 000 units (100 mL) at max. rate 10 mL/min; followed if necessary by 200 000 units (20 mL) every hour until bleeding stops

PoM **Trasylol**® (Bayer)
Injection, aprotinin 10 000 kallikrein inactivator units/mL. Net price 50-mL vial = £20.53
Note. Aprotinin injection containing 10 000 kallikrein inactivator units/mL also available from Paines & Byrne

ETHAMSYLATE

Indications: see under preparations
Contra-indications: porphyria (see section 9.8.2)
Side-effects: nausea, headache, rashes
Dose: see below

PoM **Dicynene**® (Delandale)
Tablets, scored, ethamsylate 500 mg, net price 100-tab pack = £20.12
Dose: short-term treatment of blood loss in menorrhagia, 500 mg 4 times daily during menstruation
Injection, ethamsylate 125 mg/mL. Net price 2-mL amp = 74p
Dose: prophylaxis and treatment of periventricular haemorrhage in low birth-weight infants, by intramuscular or intravenous injection, 12.5 mg/kg every 6 hours
IMPORTANT. The ampoules currently available contain a total of 250 mg in 2 mL volume therefore **small fraction only** required for neonatal use

TRANEXAMIC ACID

Indications: see notes above
Cautions: reduce dose in renal impairment; massive haematuria (avoid if risk of ureteric obstruction); regular eye examinations and liver function tests in long-term treatment of hereditary angioedema

Contra-indications: thromboembolic disease
Side-effects: nausea, vomiting, diarrhoea (reduce dose); giddiness on rapid intravenous injection
Dose: by mouth, 1–1.5 g 2–4 times daily
By slow intravenous injection, 1 g 3 times daily

PoM **Cyklokapron**® (Kabi Pharmacia)
Tablets, f/c, scored, tranexamic acid 500 mg. Net price 60-tab pack = £12.96
Syrup, tranexamic acid 500 mg/5 mL. Net price 300 mL = £15.60
Injection, tranexamic acid 100 mg/mL. Net price 5-mL amp = £1.35

BLOOD PRODUCTS

FACTOR VIII FRACTION, DRIED

(Human Antihaemophilic Fraction, Dried)
A concentrate prepared from pooled plasma from suitable human donors
Indications: control of haemorrhage in haemophilia A
Cautions: intravascular haemolysis after large or frequently repeated doses in patients with blood groups A, B, or AB
Side-effects: allergic reactions including chills, fever; hyperfibrinogenaemia occurred after massive doses with earlier products but less likely since fibrinogen content has now been substantially reduced
Available from Alpha (Profilate-SD®), Armour (Monoclate-P®), BPL (8SM®, 8Y®), SNBTS

FACTOR VIII INHIBITOR BYPASSING FRACTION

Preparations with factor VIII inhibitor bypassing activity are prepared from human plasma
Human Factor VIII Inhibitor Bypassing Fraction (*Feiba Immuno*, Immuno) is used in patients with factor VIII inhibitors
Note. A porcine preparation of antihaemophilic factor for patients with inhibitors to human factor VIII is available from Porton (Hyate C®)

FACTOR IX FRACTION, DRIED

Factor IX fraction is prepared from pooled human plasma and may also contain clotting factors II, VII, and X.
Indications: congenital factor IX deficiency (haemophilia B)
Cautions: risk of thrombosis
Contra-indications: disseminated intravascular coagulation
Side-effects: allergic reactions, including chills, fever
Available as: *Dried Factor IX Fraction, Heat-Treated* (BPL); *Human Factor IX Concentrate* (SNBTS)

FRESH FROZEN PLASMA

Fresh frozen plasma is prepared from the supernatant liquid obtained by centrifugation of one donation of whole blood.

Indications: to replace coagulation factors or other plasma proteins where their concentration or functional activity is critically reduced, e.g. to reverse warfarin effect

Cautions: avoid in circulatory overload; need for compatibility

Side-effects: allergic reactions including chills, fever, bronchospasm; adult respiratory distress syndrome

Available from Regional Blood Transfusion Services and BPL

2.12 Lipid-lowering drugs

There are a number of common conditions, some familial, in which there are very high plasma concentrations of cholesterol, or triglycerides, or both. There is evidence that therapy which lowers low density lipoprotein (LDL) cholesterol and raises high density lipoprotein (HDL) cholesterol reduces the progression of coronary atherosclerosis and may even induce regression. Lipid-lowering drugs should be reserved for patients with coronary heart disease and those at high risk of developing coronary heart disease on account of multiple risk factors or severe hyperlipidaemia inadequately controlled by a modified fat diet. Any drug therapy must be combined with strict adherence to diet, maintenance of near-ideal body weight and, if appropriate, reduction of blood pressure and cessation of smoking.

Severe hyperlipidaemia often requires combinations of lipid-lowering drugs such as an anion-exchange resin with a fibrate, an HMG CoA reductase inhibitor, or nicotinic acid. Combinations of HMG CoA reductase inhibitors with nicotinic acid or a fibrate carry an increased risk of side-effects and should be used with great caution.

ANION-EXCHANGE RESINS

Cholestyramine and **colestipol** are anion-exchange resins used in the management of hypercholesterolaemia. They act by binding bile acids, preventing their reabsorption; this promotes hepatic conversion of cholesterol into bile acids; the resultant increased LDL-receptor activity of liver cells increases the breakdown of LDL-cholesterol. Thus both compounds effectively reduce LDL-cholesterol but can aggravate hypertriglyceridaemia.

COUNSELLING. Other drugs should be taken at least 1 hour before or 4–6 hours after cholestyramine or colestipol to reduce possible interference with absorption

CHOLESTYRAMINE

Indications: hyperlipidaemias, particularly type IIa, in patients who have not responded adequately to diet and other appropriate measures; primary prevention of coronary heart disease in men aged 35–59 years with primary hypercholesterolaemia who have not responded to diet and other appropriate measures; pruritus associated with partial biliary obstruction and primary biliary cirrhosis; diarrhoeal disorders, see section 1.5

Cautions: supplements of fat-soluble vitamins and of folic acid may be required with high doses, particularly in children; pregnancy and breast-feeding; **interactions:** Appendix 1 (cholestyramine and colestipol)

Contra-indications: complete biliary obstruction

Side-effects: nausea and vomiting, constipation or diarrhoea, heartburn, flatulence, abdominal discomfort; on prolonged use, increased bleeding tendency (due to hypoprothrombinaemia associated with vitamin K deficiency)

Dose: lipid reduction (after initial introduction over 3–4 weeks) 8–24 g daily in water in single or up to 4 divided doses; up to 36 g daily if necessary

Pruritus, 4–8 g daily in water

PoM **Questran**® (Bristol-Myers)
Powder, orange, cholestyramine (anhydrous) 4 g/sachet. Net price 168-sachet pack = £70.21. Label: 13, counselling, avoid other drugs at same time (see notes above)

PoM **Questran A**® (Bristol-Myers)
Powder, orange, cholestyramine (anhydrous) 4 g/sachet, with aspartame. Net price 168-sachet pack = £73.72. Label: 13, counselling, avoid other drugs at same time (see notes above)

COLESTIPOL HYDROCHLORIDE

Indications: hyperlipidaemias, particularly type IIa, in patients who have not responded adequately to diet and other appropriate measures

Cautions; Contra-indications; Side-effects: see under Cholestyramine

Dose: 5 g 1–2 times daily in liquid increased if necessary at intervals of 1–2 months to max. of 30 g daily (in single or 2 divided doses)

PoM **Colestid**® (Upjohn)
Granules, yellow, colestipol hydrochloride. Net price 30 × 5-g sachets = £12.54. Label: 13, counselling, avoid other drugs at same time (see notes above)

CLOFIBRATE GROUP

Clofibrate, **bezafibrate**, **fenofibrate**, and **gemfibrozil** can be regarded as broad-spectrum lipid-modulating agents in that although their main action is to decrease serum triglycerides they also tend to reduce LDL-cholesterol and to raise HDL-cholesterol.

All can cause a myositis-like syndrome, especially in patients with impaired renal function. In addition, clofibrate predisposes to gallstones by increasing biliary cholesterol excretion; it is therefore only indicated in patients who have had a cholecystectomy.

BEZAFIBRATE

Indications: hyperlipidaemias of types IIa, IIb, III, IV and V in patients who have not responded adequately to diet and other appropriate measures
Cautions: renal impairment (avoid if severe); **interactions:** Appendix 1 (clofibrate group)
Contra-indications: severe renal or hepatic impairment, hypoalbuminaemia, primary biliary cirrhosis, gall bladder disease, nephrotic syndrome, pregnancy
Side-effects: nausea, abdominal discomfort; rarely myositis-like syndrome, pruritus, urticaria, impotence; headache reported
Dose: 200 mg 3 times daily with or after food; may be reduced to 200 mg twice daily in hypertriglyceridaemia

PoM **Bezalip**® (Boehringer Mannheim)
Tablets, f/c, bezafibrate 200 mg. Net price 20 = £2.11. Label: 21

PoM **Bezalip-Mono**® (Boehringer Mannheim)
Tablets, m/r, f/c, bezafibrate 400 mg. Net price 28-tab pack = £8.72. Label: 21, 25
Dose: 1 tablet daily in the evening

CLOFIBRATE

Indications: hyperlipidaemias of types IIb, III, IV and V in patients who have not responded adequately to diet and other appropriate measures (but see also notes above)
Cautions; Contra-indications: see under Bezafibrate and notes above
Side-effects: see under Bezafibrate; also cholesterol cholelithiasis
Dose: over 65 kg, 2 g daily (50–65 kg, 1.5 g daily) in 2 or 3 divided doses

PoM **Atromid-S**® (ICI)
Capsules, red, clofibrate 500 mg. Net price 100-cap pack = £4.18. Label: 21

FENOFIBRATE

Indications: hyperlipidaemias of types IIa, IIb, III, IV, and V in patients who have not responded adequately to diet and other appropriate measures
Cautions: see under Bezafibrate
Contra-indications: severe renal or hepatic impairment, existing gall bladder disease, pregnancy
Side-effects: see under Bezafibrate
Dose: initially 300 mg daily in divided doses with food, adjusted according to response within range 200–400 mg daily; CHILD 5 mg/kg daily

PoM **Lipantil**® (Fournier)
Capsules, fenofibrate 100 mg. Net price 84-cap pack = £19.80. Label: 21

GEMFIBROZIL

Indications: hyperlipidaemias of types IIa, IIb, III, IV and V in patients who have not responded adequately to diet and other appropriate measures; primary prevention of coronary heart disease in men aged 40–55 years with hyperlipidaemias that have not responded to diet and other appropriate measures
Cautions: lipid profile, blood counts, and liver-function tests before initiating long-term treatment; renal impairment; annual eye examinations; **interactions:** Appendix 1 (clofibrate group)
Contra-indications: alcoholism, hepatic impairment, gallstones; pregnancy
Side-effects: gastro-intestinal disturbances; pruritus, urticaria, rash, headache, dizziness, blurred vision, painful extremities; rarely myalgia; impotence reported
Dose: 1.2 g daily, usually in 2 divided doses; range 0.9–1.5 g daily

PoM **Lopid**® (P-D)
'300' *capsules*, white/maroon, gemfibrozil 300 mg. Net price 100-cap pack = £24.96
'600' *tablets*, f/c, gemfibrozil 600 mg. Net price 56-tab pack = £27.96

NICOTINIC ACID GROUP

The value of **nicotinic acid** and **nicofuranose** is limited by their side-effects, especially vasodilatation. In doses of 1.5 to 3 g daily they lower both cholesterol and triglyceride concentrations by inhibiting synthesis; they also increase HDL-cholesterol. **Acipimox** seems to have fewer side-effects but may be less effective in its lipid-modulating capabilities.

ACIPIMOX

Indications: hyperlipidaemias of types IIa, IIb, and IV in patients who have not responded adequately to diet and other appropriate measures
Cautions: renal impairment
Contra-indications: peptic ulcer; pregnancy
Side-effects: vasodilatation, flushing, itching, rashes, erythema; occasionally, heartburn, epigastric pain, nausea, diarrhoea, headache, malaise
Dose: usually 500–750 mg daily in divided doses

PoM **Olbetam**® (Farmitalia Carlo Erba)
Capsules, brown/pink, acipimox 250 mg. Net price 100-cap pack = £44.00. Label: 21

NICOFURANOSE
Indications: see notes above (for use in peripheral vascular disease, see section 2.6.3)
Cautions; Side-effects: see under Nicotinic Acid, but prostaglandin-mediated symptoms less severe
Dose: 500 mg 3 times daily, gradually increased if necessary to 1 g 3 times daily

Bradilan® (Napp)
Tablets, e/c and s/c, nicofuranose 250 mg. Net price 20 = £1.55. Label: 5, 25

NICOTINIC ACID
Indications: see notes above
Cautions: diabetes mellitus, gout, liver disease, peptic ulcer
Contra-indications: pregnancy, breast-feeding
Side-effects: flushing, dizziness, headache, palpitations, pruritus (prostaglandin-mediated symptoms can be reduced by low initial doses taken with meals, or by taking aspirin 300 mg 30 minutes before the dose—needed in only a very small proportion of patients); nausea, vomiting; rarely impaired liver function and rashes
Dose: initially 100–200 mg 3 times daily (see above), gradually increased over 2–4 weeks to 1–2 g 3 times daily

Nicotinic Acid Tablets, nicotinic acid 50 mg, net price 20 = 14p. Label: 21

FISH OILS
A fish-oil preparation (Maxepa®), rich in omega-3 marine triglycerides, is useful in the treatment of severe hypertriglyceridaemia; however, it can sometimes aggravate hypercholesterolaemia.

OMEGA-3 MARINE TRIGLYCERIDES
Indications: reduction of plasma triglycerides in patients with severe hypertriglyceridaemia judged to be at special risk of ischaemic heart disease and/or pancreatitis, in conjunction with dietary and other methods (see notes above)
Side-effects: occasional nausea and belching
Dose: see under preparations below

Maxepa® (Innovex)
Capsules, 1 g (approx. 1.1 mL) concentrated fish oils of composition below. Net price 200-cap pack = £28.57. Label: 21
Dose: 5 capsules twice daily with food
Liquid, golden-coloured, concentrated fish oils containing, as percentage of total fatty acid composition, eicosapentaenoic acid 18% w/w, docosahexaenoic acid 12% w/w. Vitamin A content less than 100 units/g, vitamin D content less than 10 units/g. Net price 150 mL = £21.43. Label: 21
Dose: 5 mL twice daily with food

Cautionary label wordings, see inside back cover

OTHER DRUGS

Probucol decreases both LDL- and HDL-cholesterol; despite the latter effect it appears to promote resolution of xanthomata. Moreover, its antioxidant properties may decrease the atherogenicity of LDL.

Simvastatin and **pravastatin** belong to a new class of drugs which competitively inhibit 3-hydroxy-3-methylglutaryl coenzyme A (HMG CoA) reductase, an enzyme that catalyses a step in cholesterol synthesis, especially in the liver. They are more potent than anion-exchange resins in lowering LDL-cholesterol but less effective than the clofibrate group in reducing triglycerides and raising HDL-cholesterol. The main side-effect is reversible myositis, which is rare except in patients also receiving cyclosporin, nicotinic acid, or gemfibrozil (careful monitoring of liver function and creatine phosphokinase should be performed if these drugs are used with an HMG CoA reductase inhibitor).

PROBUCOL
Indications: see notes above
Cautions: ECG before treatment in patients with recent myocardial damage, ventricular arrhythmias; avoid pregnancy during and for 6 months after stopping treatment
Contra-indications: breast-feeding
Side-effects: generally mild and transient and mainly consist of gastro-intestinal effects such as nausea, vomiting, flatulence, diarrhoea, abdominal pain; ventricular arrhythmias and angioedema rarely reported
Dose: 500 mg twice daily with food

PoM **Lurselle®** (Merrell)
Tablets, scored, probucol 250 mg. Net price 120-tab pack = £13.40. Label: 21

PRAVASTATIN
Indications: primary hypercholesterolaemia (hyperlipidaemia type IIa), in patients intolerant of or not responsive to other therapy, with cholesterol concentration above 7.8 mmol/litre
Cautions; Contra-indications; Side-effects: as for Simvastatin; **interactions:** Appendix 1 (pravastatin)
Dose: usual range 10–40 mg once daily at night, adjusted at intervals of not less than 4 weeks

▼ PoM **Lipostat®** (Squibb)
Tablets, both pink, pravastatin sodium 10 mg, net price 28-tab pack = £16.18; 20 mg, 28-tab pack = £31.09

SIMVASTATIN

Indications: primary hypercholesterolaemia (hyperlipidaemia type IIa) in patients with cholesterol concentration of 6.5 mmol/litre or greater and resistant to dietary control

Cautions: monitor liver function before and during treatment; history of liver disease (avoid if active); high alcohol intake; avoid pregnancy during and for 1 month after treatment; advise patients to report muscle pain; **interactions:** Appendix 1 (simvastatin)

Contra-indications: active liver disease; pregnancy (toxicity in *animal* studies) and breast-feeding; porphyria (see section 9.8.2)

Side-effects: constipation, flatulence, headache, nausea, dyspepsia, abdominal pain, diarrhoea, fatigue, insomnia, rash, rhabdomyolysis, hepatitis reported; raised creatine phosphokinase concentrations (discontinue if markedly raised or myopathy diagnosed); angioedema reported

Dose: 10 mg daily at night, adjusted at intervals of not less than 4 weeks; usual range 10–40 mg once daily at night

PoM **Zocor**® (MSD)
Tablets, both f/c, simvastatin 10 mg (peach), net price 28-tab pack = £18.29; 20 mg (tan), 28-tab pack = £31.09

2.13 Local sclerosants

Ethanolamine oleate and sodium tetradecyl sulphate are used in sclerotherapy of varicose veins, and phenol is used in haemorrhoids (see section 1.7.3).

ETHANOLAMINE OLEATE

Indications: sclerotherapy of varicose veins

Cautions: extravasation may cause necrosis of tissues

Contra-indications: inability to walk, acute phlebitis, oral contraceptive use, obese legs

Side-effects: allergic reactions (including anaphylaxis)

PoM **Ethanolamine Oleate Injection,** ethanolamine oleate 5%. Net price 5-mL amp = 97p
Available from Evans

Dose: by slow injection into empty isolated segment of vein, 2–5 mL divided between 3–4 sites; repeated at weekly intervals

SODIUM TETRADECYL SULPHATE

Indications: sclerotherapy of varicose veins

Cautions; Contra-indications; Side-effects: see under Ethanolamine Oleate

PoM **STD**® (STD Pharmaceutical)
Injection, sodium tetradecyl sulphate 0.5%, net price 2-mL amp = £1.10; 1%, 2-mL amp = £1.19; 3%, 2-mL amp = £1.36, 5-mL vial = £2.45

Dose: by slow injection into empty isolated segment of vein, 0.1–1 mL according to site and condition being treated (consult manufacturer's literature)

3: Drugs used in the treatment of diseases of the
RESPIRATORY SYSTEM

In this chapter, drug treatment is described under the following headings:
- 3.1 Bronchodilators
- 3.2 Corticosteroids
- 3.3 Cromoglycate and related therapy
- 3.4 Antihistamines, hyposensitisation, and allergic emergencies
- 3.5 Respiratory stimulants and surfactants
- 3.6 Oxygen
- 3.7 Mucolytics
- 3.8 Aromatic inhalations
- 3.9 Antitussives
- 3.10 Systemic nasal decongestants

The initial treatment of exacerbations of chronic bronchitis and bacterial pneumonia is indicated in section 5.1 (Table 1) and the treatment of tuberculosis is discussed in section 5.1.9.

3.1 Bronchodilators

- 3.1.1 Adrenoceptor stimulants
- 3.1.2 Antimuscarinic bronchodilators
- 3.1.3 Theophylline
- 3.1.4 Compound bronchodilator preparations
- 3.1.5 Peak flow meters and inhaler devices

3.1.1 Adrenoceptor stimulants (sympathomimetics)

- 3.1.1.1 Selective beta$_2$-adrenoceptor stimulants
- 3.1.1.2 Other adrenoceptor stimulants

Most *mild to moderate* attacks of asthma respond rapidly to aerosol administration of a selective beta$_2$-adrenoceptor stimulant such as salbutamol or terbutaline (section 3.1.1.1). In *frequently occurring moderate* asthma the introduction of a corticosteroid by inhalation (section 3.2), sodium cromoglycate (section 3.3), or oral theophylline (section 3.1.3) may stabilise the asthma and avoid the use of oral corticosteroids. However in *more severe attacks* a short course of an oral corticosteroid may be necessary to bring the asthma under control (section 3.2).

Treatment of patients with *severe acute asthma* or airways obstruction (see also below) is safer in hospital where oxygen and resuscitation facilities are immediately available.

Patients with *chronic bronchitis* and *emphysema* are often described as having irreversible airways obstruction, but they usually respond partially to the beta$_2$-adrenoceptor stimulant drugs or to the antimuscarinic drug ipratropium (section 3.1.2).

CHOICE OF DRUG. The **selective beta$_2$-adrenoceptor stimulants** (selective beta$_2$-agonists) (section 3.1.1.1) such as salbutamol or terbutaline (preferably given by aerosol inhalation) are the safest and most effective beta-stimulants.

There is some evidence that patients who use beta$_2$-adrenoceptor stimulants on an 'as required' basis show a greater improvement in their asthma than those using them on a regular basis. For patients who require beta$_2$-adrenoceptor stimulants more than once or twice daily, preventative treatment with an inhaled corticosteroid, sodium cromoglycate, or nedocromil should be tried.

There are some differences between the various selective beta$_2$-adrenoceptor stimulant drugs. **Salbutamol** and **terbutaline** are available in the widest range of formulations. **Rimiterol** has a shorter duration of action than salbutamol, terbutaline and fenoterol. **Fenoterol** may be less beta$_2$-selective than salbutamol. The dose or frequency of administration of beta$_2$-adrenoceptor stimulants can often be reduced by concurrent treatment with prophylactic drugs such as corticosteroid inhalations (section 3.2) or sodium cromoglycate (section 3.3).

Salmeterol is a longer-acting beta$_2$-adrenoceptor stimulant that has recently been introduced for twice daily administration; it is not suitable for the relief of an acute attack (a short-acting beta$_2$-stimulant such as salbutamol should be used). Salmeterol should be added to existing corticosteroid therapy and **not** replace it.

CHOICE OF FORMULATION. The *pressurised aerosol inhaler* is an effective and convenient method of administration for mild to moderate airways obstruction. The duration of action of an aerosol inhaler depends on the drug and the dose administered. With recommended doses rimiterol will usually last for 1 to 2 hours, salbutamol, terbutaline and fenoterol for 3 to 5 hours, and salmeterol for around 12 hours. Aerosol inhalation is preferred because it provides relief more rapidly and causes fewer side-effects (such as tremor and nervous tension) than tablets; the drug is delivered directly to the bronchi and is therefore effective in smaller doses.

Patients should be given careful instruction on the use of their pressurised aerosol inhalers and it is important to check that they continue to use them correctly as inadequate technique may be mistaken for drug failure. In particular, it should be emphasised that they must inhale slowly and hold their breath for 10 seconds after inhalation. Most patients can be successfully taught to use pressurised aerosol inhalers but some patients, particularly the elderly, the arthritic, and small children are unable to use them; some patients are unable to synchronise their breathing with the administration of aerosol. For such patients a variety of *spacing devices* (see section 3.1.5) is now available. Alternatively *dry powder inhalers*, which are activated by the patient's inspiration, are of value; some dry powder inhalations occasionally cause coughing.

Cautionary label wordings, see inside back cover

The **dose** should be stated **explicitly** in terms of the number of inhalations at one time, the frequency, and the maximum number of inhalations allowed in 24 hours. High doses of beta$_2$-stimulants can be dangerous in some patients. Excessive use is usually an indication of **inadequately treated** asthma and should be treated with preventative medication such as an inhaled corticosteroid. Patients should be advised to seek medical advice when they fail to obtain their usual degree of symptomatic relief as this usually indicates a worsening of the asthma and may require alternative medication. When patients with asthma **are not adequately controlled** with inhalation of a beta$_2$-stimulant once or twice daily, **addition of a prophylactic drug** such as a corticosteroid inhalation should be considered; this is more convenient for the patient than higher doses of beta$_2$-stimulants and usually provides better overall control.

Respirator solutions of salbutamol and terbutaline are increasingly used for the treatment of *acute asthma* both in hospital and in general practice; a respirator solution of fenoterol is also available. They are administered over a period of about 15 minutes from a nebuliser, usually driven from an oxygen cylinder in hospital. An electrical compressor is most suitable for domiciliary use but these are costly and not currently prescribable under the NHS. Patients with a severe attack of asthma should have oxygen if possible during nebulisation since beta-adrenoceptor stimulants can cause an increase in arterial hypoxaemia. For patients with *chronic bronchitis and hypercapnia*, however, oxygen can be dangerous, and the nebuliser should be driven by air. The dose prescribed by nebuliser is substantially higher than that prescribed by metered dose inhaler. For example, a 2.5-mL Ventolin Nebule® contains 2.5 mg of salbutamol, which is equivalent to 25 puffs from the aerosol inhaler. Patients should therefore be warned that it is dangerous to exceed the stated dose and that if they fail to respond to the usual dose of their respirator solution they should call for help.

Oral preparations are available for patients who cannot manage the inhaled route. They are sometimes used for children, though the inhaled route is better and most children can use one or other of the inhalation devices available. They have a slower onset but a slightly more prolonged action than the aerosol inhalers. The *modified-release* preparations may be of value in patients with *nocturnal asthma* as an alternative to the modified-release theophylline preparations (section 3.1.3).

Intravenous, and occasionally *subcutaneous*, injections of salbutamol and terbutaline are given for severe bronchospasm.

EMERGENCY TREATMENT OF SEVERE ACUTE ASTHMA. Severe asthma can be fatal and **must** be treated promptly and energetically. It is characterised by persistent dyspnoea poorly relieved by bronchodilators, restlessness, exhaustion, a high pulse rate (usually over 110/minute), often pulsus paradoxus of over 10 mmHg, and a very low peak expiratory flow. The respiration is so shallow that wheezing may be absent. Such patients should be given a large dose of a **corticosteroid** (see section 6.3.4)—for adults hydrocortisone 200 mg (preferably as sodium succinate) intravenously or prednisolone 40 mg by mouth, children half these doses. They should also be given a beta$_2$-selective adrenoceptor stimulant such as **salbutamol** or **terbutaline** by nebuliser with oxygen if available.

If there is little response the following additional treatment should be considered: **ipratropium** by nebuliser (section 3.1.2), **aminophylline** by slow intravenous injection, if the patient has not already been receiving theophylline (section 3.1.3), or change of administration of the beta$_2$-selective adrenoceptor stimulant to the intravenous route.

Further treatment of these patients is safer in hospital where resuscitation facilities are immediately available. Treatment should **never** be delayed for investigations, patients should **never** be sedated, and the possibility of a pneumothorax should also be remembered.

If the patient deteriorates despite appropriate pharmacological treatment, intermittent positive pressure ventilation may be needed temporarily.

CSM advice. Potentially serious hypokalaemia may result from beta$_2$-adrenoceptor stimulant therapy. Particular caution is required in severe asthma, as this effect may be potentiated by concomitant treatment with theophylline and its derivatives, corticosteroids, and diuretics, and by hypoxia. Plasma potassium concentrations should therefore be monitored in severe asthma.

CHILDREN. Selective beta$_2$-adrenoceptor stimulants are useful even in children under the age of 18 months. They are most effective by the inhaled route, but an inhalation device may be needed (with the technique carefully checked). They are also effective by mouth. In severe attacks nebulisation using a selective beta$_2$-adrenoceptor stimulant or ipratropium is advisable.

PREGNANCY AND BREAST-FEEDING. It is particularly important that asthma should be well-controlled during pregnancy; where this is achieved asthma has no important effects on pregnancy, labour, or the fetus.

Inhalation has particular advantages as a means of drug administration during pregnancy because the therapeutic action can be achieved without the need for plasma concentrations liable to have a pharmacological effect on the fetus.

Severe exacerbations of asthma can have an adverse effect on pregnancy and should be treated promptly with conventional therapy, including oral or parenteral administration of corticosteroids and nebulisation of a selective beta$_2$-adrenoceptor stimulant; prednisolone is the preferred corticosteroid for oral administration since placental transfer is slower than with some others.

3.1 Bronchodilators

Although theophylline has been given without adverse effects during pregnancy or breast-feeding there have been occasional reports of toxicity in the fetus and neonate.

See also under Prescribing in Pregnancy (Appendix 4) and Prescribing during Breast-feeding (Appendix 5).

3.1.1.1 SELECTIVE BETA$_2$-ADRENOCEPTOR STIMULANTS

SALBUTAMOL

Indications: asthma and other conditions associated with reversible airways obstruction; premature labour, see section 7.1.2

Cautions: hyperthyroidism, myocardial insufficiency, arrhythmias, hypertension, pregnancy (but appropriate to use, see notes above), elderly patients; intravenous administration to diabetics (monitor blood glucose; ketoacidosis reported); see also notes above; **interactions:** Appendix 1 (sympathomimetics, beta$_2$)

Side-effects: fine tremor (usually hands), nervous tension, headache, peripheral vasodilatation, tachycardia (seldom troublesome when given by aerosol inhalation); hypokalaemia after high doses (**CSM** recommends monitor plasma-potassium in severe asthma, see opposite); hypersensitivity reactions including paradoxical bronchospasm, urticaria, and angioedema reported; slight pain on intramuscular injection

Dose: by mouth, 4 mg (elderly and sensitive patients initially 2 mg) 3–4 times daily; max. single dose 8 mg (but unlikely to provide much extra benefit or to be tolerated); CHILD under 2 years 100 micrograms/kg 4 times daily; 2–6 years 1–2 mg 3–4 times daily, 6–12 years 2 mg

By subcutaneous or intramuscular injection, 500 micrograms, repeated every 4 hours if necessary

By slow intravenous injection, 250 micrograms, repeated if necessary

By intravenous infusion, initially 5 micrograms/minute, adjusted according to response and heart-rate usually in range 3–20 micrograms/minute, or more if necessary

By aerosol inhalation, acute and intermittent episodes of wheezing and asthma, 100–200 micrograms (1–2 puffs); CHILD 100 micrograms (1 puff)

Prophylaxis in exercise-induced bronchospasm, 200 micrograms (2 puffs); CHILD 100 micrograms (1 puff)

Chronic maintenance therapy, 200 micrograms (2 puffs) 3–4 times daily; CHILD 100 micrograms (1 puff) 3–4 times daily, increased to 200 micrograms (2 puffs) if necessary

By inhalation of a powder (Rotacaps®, Ventodisks®), acute and intermittent episodes of wheezing and asthma, 200–400 micrograms; CHILD 200 micrograms

Prophylaxis in exercise-induced bronchospasm (*powder*), 400 micrograms; CHILD 200 micrograms

Chronic maintenance therapy (*powder*), 400 micrograms 3–4 times daily; CHILD 200 micrograms 3–4 times daily

Note. Bioavailability appears to be lower, so recommended doses for dry powder inhalers are twice those in a metered inhaler

By inhalation of nebulised solution, chronic bronchospasm unresponsive to conventional therapy and severe acute asthma, 2.5 mg, repeated up to 4 times daily, increased to 5 mg if necessary; in refractory patients with severe acute asthma up to 10 mg if side-effects permit; CHILD 2.5 mg, increased to 5 mg if required

---

When a patient with asthma is not adequately controlled with a beta$_2$-stimulant inhaled once or twice daily, addition of a prophylactic drug such as a corticosteroid should be considered. For further details see p. 114.

Oral

PoM **Salbutamol** (Non-proprietary)

Tablets, salbutamol (as sulphate) 2 mg, net price 20 = 17p; 4 mg, 20 = 35p

Available from APS, Cox, CP, Evans, Kerfoot, Norton, Tillotts (Salbuvent®)

Syrup, salbutamol (as sulphate) 2 mg/5 mL, net price 150 mL = 67p

Available from Tillotts (Salbuvent®)

PoM **Ventolin**® (A&H)

Tablets, both pink, scored, salbutamol (as sulphate), 2 mg, net price 20 = 22p; 4 mg, 20 = 43p

CR Tablets, modified-release, salbutamol (as sulphate) 4 mg, net price 56-tab pack = £10.00; 8 mg, 56-tab pack = £12.00. Label: 25, 27

Dose: 8 mg twice daily; CHILD 3–12 years 4 mg twice daily

Syrup, sugar-free, salbutamol 2 mg (as sulphate)/5 mL. Net price 150 mL = 67p

PoM **Volmax**® (DF)

Tablets, modified-release, salbutamol (as sulphate) 4 mg, net price 56-tab pack = £10.00; 8 mg, 56-tab pack = £12.00. Label: 25

Dose: 8 mg twice daily; CHILD 3–12 years 4 mg twice daily

Parenteral

PoM **Salbuvent**® (Tillotts)

Injection, salbutamol (as sulphate) 500 micrograms/mL. Net price 1-mL amp = 43p

Solution for intravenous infusion, salbutamol (as sulphate) 1 mg/mL. Dilute before use. Net price 5-mL amp = £3.08

PoM **Ventolin**® (A&H)

Injection, salbutamol 50 micrograms (as sulphate)/mL. Net price 5-mL amp = 57p

Injection, salbutamol 500 micrograms (as sulphate)/mL. Net price 1-mL amp = 43p

Solution for intravenous infusion, salbutamol 1 mg (as sulphate)/mL. Dilute before use. Net price 5-mL amp = £3.08

Inhalation

COUNSELLING. Advise patients not to exceed prescribed dose and to follow manufacturer's directions

PoM **Salbutamol** (Non-proprietary)

Aerosol inhalation, salbutamol 100 micrograms/metered inhalation, net price 200-dose unit = £2.08

Available from APS, Ashbourne (Maxivent®), Cox, CP, Evans, Kerfoot, 3M (Salbulin®), Norton, Tillotts (Salbuvent®)

PoM **Aerolin® Autohaler**[1] (3M)

Aerosol inhalation, salbutamol 100 micrograms (as sulphate)/metered inhalation. Net price 200-dose breath-actuated unit = £11.00; also 100-dose unit = £5.25 (hosp. only)

[1] replaces *Aerolin Auto*

PoM **Ventodisks®** (A&H)

Dry powder for inhalation, disks containing 8 blisters of salbutamol (as sulphate) 200 micrograms/blister, net price pack of 14 disks with Disk-haler® = £7.11; 14-disk refill = £6.54; 400 micrograms/blister, pack of 14 disks with Diskhaler® = £12.02; 14-disk refill = £11.45

PoM **Ventolin®** (A&H)

Aerosol inhalation, salbutamol 100 micrograms/metered inhalation. Net price 200-dose unit = £2.62

Nebules® (for use with nebuliser), salbutamol 0.1% (1 mg/mL, as sulphate), net price 2.5 mL (2.5 mg) = 19p; 0.2% (2 mg/mL), 2.5 mL (5 mg) = 38p. May be diluted with physiological saline

Note. Salbutamol 0.1% (1 mg/mL, as sulphate) also available for nebulisation in 2.5-mL unit doses as Steri-Neb Salamol® (Baker Norton)

Respirator solution (for use with a nebuliser or ventilator), salbutamol 0.5% (5 mg/mL, as sulphate). Net price 20 mL = £2.71. May be diluted with physiological saline

Rotacaps® (dry powder for inhalation), salbutamol (as sulphate), 200 micrograms (light-blue/clear), net price 20 = £1.06; 400 micrograms (dark-blue/clear), 20 = £1.79

Note. Capsules containing 200 or 400 micrograms salbutamol (as sulphate) as dry powder for inhalation also available as Salbutamol Cyclocaps® (Goldshield); only for use with Cyclohaler®

Inhaler devices
See section 3.1.5

TERBUTALINE SULPHATE

Indications; Cautions; Side-effects: see under Salbutamol; premature labour, see section 7.1.2

Dose: by mouth, 5 mg 2–3 times daily; CHILD under 3 years 750 micrograms 3 times daily, 3–7 years 0.75–1.5 mg 3 times daily, 7–15 years 1.5–3 mg 3 times daily (as syrup) *or* 2.5 mg 2–3 times daily (as tablets)

By subcutaneous, intramuscular, or slow intravenous injection, 250–500 micrograms up to 4 times daily; CHILD 2–15 years 10 micrograms/kg to a max. of 300 micrograms

By continuous intravenous infusion as a solution containing 3–5 micrograms/mL, 1.5–5 micrograms/minute for 8–10 hours; reduce dose for children

By aerosol inhalation, acute and maintenance treatment, adults and children 250–500 micrograms (1–2 puffs) repeated after 6 hours if necessary; not more than 8 inhalations should be necessary in any 24 hours

By inhalation of powder (Turbohaler®), 500 micrograms (1 inhalation) as required; not more than 4 inhalations in any 24 hours

By inhalation of nebulised solution, 5–10 mg 2–4 times daily; additional doses may be necessary in severe acute asthma; CHILD, up to 3 years 2 mg, 3–6 years 3 mg; 6–8 years 4 mg, over 8 years 5 mg, 2–4 times daily

---

When a patient with asthma is not adequately controlled with a beta$_2$-stimulant inhaled once or twice daily, addition of a prophylactic drug such as a corticosteroid should be considered. For further details see p. 114.

Oral and parenteral

PoM **Bricanyl®** (Astra)

Tablets, scored, terbutaline sulphate 5 mg. Net price 20 = 71p

Syrup, sugar-free, terbutaline sulphate 1.5 mg/5 mL. Net price 300 mL = £2.24

Injection, terbutaline sulphate 500 micrograms/mL. Net price 1-mL amp = 28p; 5-mL amp = £1.30

PoM **Bricanyl SA®** (Astra)

Tablets, m/r, terbutaline sulphate 7.5 mg. Net price 20 = £1.59. Label: 25

Dose: 7.5 mg twice daily

PoM **Monovent®** (Lagap)

Syrup, terbutaline sulphate 1.5 mg/5 mL. Net price 300 mL = £2.20

Inhalation

PoM **Bricanyl®** (Astra)

COUNSELLING. Advise patients not to exceed prescribed dose and to follow manufacturer's directions; little sensation associated with use of Turbohaler®

Aerosol inhalation, terbutaline sulphate 250 micrograms/metered inhalation. Net price 400-dose unit = £5.31; 400-dose unit with Spacer inhaler (collapsible extended mouthpiece) = £7.21; 400-dose refill cannister for use with Nebuhaler or Spacer inhaler = £5.21

Turbohaler® (= breath-actuated dry powder inhaler), terbutaline sulphate 500 micrograms/inhalation. Net price 100-dose unit = £8.94

Respules® (= single-dose units for nebulisation), terbutaline sulphate 2.5 mg/mL. Net price 20 × 2-mL units = £3.76

Respirator solution (for use with a nebuliser or ventilator), terbutaline sulphate 10 mg/mL. Net price 10 mL = £1.35. Before use dilute with sterile physiological saline

Inhaler devices
See section 3.1.5

FENOTEROL HYDROBROMIDE

Indications: reversible airways obstruction
Cautions; Side-effects: see under Salbutamol
Dose: acute and episodic bronchospasm, *by aerosol inhalation*, 100–200 micrograms (1–2 puffs Berotec '100') 1–3 times daily; not more than 200 micrograms (2 puffs Berotec '100') every 6 hours; max. 800 micrograms daily; CHILD 6–12 years 100 micrograms (1 puff Berotec '100') 1–3 times daily; not more than 200 micrograms (2 puffs Berotec '100') every 6 hours; max. 800 micrograms daily
Persistent bronchospasm not adequately controlled by Berotec '100', *by aerosol inhalation*, 200–400 micrograms (1–2 puffs Berotec '200') 1–3 times daily; not more than 400 micrograms (2 puffs Berotec '200') every 6 hours; max. 1.6 mg daily; CHILD under 16 years, not recommended
By inhalation of nebulised solution, 0.5–1.25 mg up to 4 times daily, dilution adjusted to equipment and length of administration; exceptionally 2.5–5 mg may be given under strict medical supervision; CHILD 6–14 years, up to 1 mg 3 times daily
Note. The above doses of fenoterol represent revised recommendations following evidence that fenoterol is effective at doses lower than those recommended previously. The CSM has advised that patients already receiving fenoterol should have their dosage regimens reviewed

> When a patient with asthma is not adequately controlled with a beta$_2$-stimulant inhaled once or twice daily, addition of a prophylactic drug such as a corticosteroid should be considered. For further details see p. 114.

PoM **Berotec**® (Boehringer Ingelheim)
COUNSELLING. Advise patients not to exceed prescribed dose and to follow manufacturer's directions
'100' aerosol inhalation, fenoterol hydrobromide 100 micrograms/metered inhalation. Net price 200-dose unit = £2.36
'200' aerosol inhalation, fenoterol hydrobromide 200 micrograms/metered inhalation. Net price 200-dose unit = £2.78
Note. Only for persistent bronchospasm inadequately controlled by Berotec '100'
Nebuliser solution, fenoterol hydrobromide 0.5% (5 mg/mL, 20 drops ≈1 mL). Net price 20 mL (with dropper) = £1.76. For use with nebuliser or ventilator; if dilution is necessary, use only sterile sodium chloride 0.9% solution

PIRBUTEROL

Indications: reversible airways obstruction
Cautions; Side-effects: see under Salbutamol
Dose: *by mouth*, 10–15 mg 3–4 times daily
By aerosol inhalation, intermittent episodes, prophylaxis in exercise-induced bronchospasm, 200–400 micrograms (1–2 puffs) repeated after 4 hours if necessary; max. 2.4 mg (12 puffs) daily
Chronic maintenance, 400 micrograms (2 puffs) 3–4 times daily or in severe bronchospasm every 4 hours; max. 2.4 mg (12 puffs) daily

PoM **Exirel**® (3M)
Capsules, pirbuterol (as hydrochloride) 10 mg (turquoise/olive), net price 90-cap pack = £2.14; 15 mg (turquoise/beige), 90-cap pack = £3.20
Aerosol inhalation, pirbuterol 200 micrograms (as acetate)/metered inhalation. Net price 200-dose unit = £2.86
COUNSELLING. Advise patients not to exceed prescribed dose and to follow manufacturer's directions

REPROTEROL HYDROCHLORIDE

Indications: reversible airways obstruction
Cautions; Side-effects: see under Salbutamol
Dose: *by aerosol inhalation*, intermittent episodes and prophylaxis in exercise-induced bronchospasm, 0.5–1 mg (1–2 puffs) repeated after 3–6 hours if necessary; CHILD 6–12 years 500 micrograms (1 puff)
Chronic maintenance therapy, 1 mg (2 puffs) 3 times daily; CHILD 6–12 years 500 micrograms (1 puff) 3 times daily

PoM **Bronchodil**® (ASTA Medica)
Aerosol inhalation, reproterol hydrochloride 500 micrograms/metered inhalation. Net price 400-dose unit = £6.84
COUNSELLING. Advise patients not to exceed prescribed dose and to follow manufacturer's directions

RIMITEROL HYDROBROMIDE

Indications: reversible airways obstruction (particularly when short action required)
Cautions; Side-effects: see under Salbutamol
Dose: *by aerosol inhalation*, adults and children 200–600 micrograms (1–3 puffs); should not be repeated in less than 30 minutes; max. 8 doses daily

PoM **Pulmadil**® (3M)
COUNSELLING. Advise patients not to exceed prescribed dose and to follow manufacturer's directions
Aerosol inhalation, rimiterol hydrobromide 200 micrograms/metered inhalation. Net price 300-dose unit = £6.32
Auto aerosol inhalation, rimiterol hydrobromide 200 micrograms/metered inhalation. Net price 300-dose cartridge in breath-actuated unit = £7.93; replacement cartridge = £6.32

SALMETEROL

Indications: long-term regular treatment of reversible airways obstruction in asthma (including nocturnal and exercise-induced) and chronic bronchitis
Note. CSM has emphasised that salmeterol is not for immediate relief of acute attacks and that existing corticosteroid therapy should not be reduced or withdrawn
Cautions; Side-effects: see under Salbutamol and notes above; significant incidence of paradoxical bronchospasm
Dose: *by inhalation*, 50 micrograms (2 puffs or 1 blister) twice daily; up to 100 micrograms (4 puffs or 2 blisters) twice daily in more severe airways obstruction

▼ PoM **Serevent**® (A&H)
Aerosol inhalation, salmeterol (as xinafoate (= hydroxynaphthoate)) 25 micrograms/metered inhalation, net price 120-inhalation unit = £28.60
Powder for inhalation, disks containing 4 blisters of salmeterol (as xinafoate (= hydroxynaphthoate)) 50 micrograms/blister, net price pack of 14 disks with Diskhaler® = £29.97; 14-disk refill = £29.40

TULOBUTEROL HYDROCHLORIDE
Indications: reversible airways obstruction
Cautions: see under Salbutamol; also mild renal impairment (avoid if severe)
Contra-indications: moderate to severe renal impairment; acute liver failure, chronic liver disease
Side-effects: see under Salbutamol
Dose: 2 mg twice daily; increased if necessary to 2 mg 3 times daily; CHILD over 10 years, 1–2 mg twice daily

▼ PoM **Brelomax**® (Abbott)
Tablets, scored, tulobuterol hydrochloride 2 mg. Net price 60-tab pack = £13.00

3.1.1.2 OTHER ADRENOCEPTOR STIMULANTS

These preparations (including the partially selective orciprenaline) are now regarded as less suitable and less safe for use as bronchodilators than the selective beta$_2$-adrenoceptor stimulants, as they are more likely to cause arrhythmias and other side-effects. They should be avoided whenever possible
Adrenaline injection (1 in 1000) is used in the emergency treatment of acute allergic and anaphylactic reactions (section 3.4.3).

EPHEDRINE HYDROCHLORIDE
Indications: reversible airways obstruction, but see notes above
Cautions: hyperthyroidism, diabetes mellitus, ischaemic heart disease, hypertension, renal impairment, elderly; may cause acute retention in prostatic hypertrophy; interaction with MAOIs a disadvantage; **interactions:** Appendix 1 (sympathomimetics)
Side-effects: tachycardia, anxiety, restlessness, insomnia common; also tremor, arrhythmias, dry mouth, cold extremities
Dose: 3 times daily, 15–60 mg; CHILD 3 times daily, up to 1 year 7.5 mg, 1–5 years 15 mg, 6–12 years 30 mg (not recommended, see above)

PoM [1]**Ephedrine Hydrochloride** (Non-proprietary)
Tablets, ephedrine hydrochloride 15 mg, net price 20 = 6p; 30 mg, 20 = 10p; 60 mg, 20 = 26p
Elixir, ephedrine hydrochloride 15 mg/5 mL in a suitable flavoured vehicle, containing alcohol 12%. Net price 100 mL = 49p
1. For exemptions see *Medicines, Ethics and Practice*, No. 8, London, Pharmaceutical Press, 1992 (and subsequent editions as available)

CAM® (Rybar)
Mixture, sugar-free, ephedrine hydrochloride 4 mg/5 mL. Net price 150 mL = £1.59
Dose: 20 mL 3–4 times daily; CHILD 3 months–2 years 2.5 mL, 2–4 years 5 mL, 5–12 years 10 mL, 3 times daily (but not recommended, see notes above)

ISOPRENALINE SULPHATE
Indications: reversible airways obstruction, but see notes above
Cautions; Side-effects: see under Salbutamol (section 3.1.1.1) and notes above

PoM **Medihaler-iso**® (3M)
Aerosol inhalation, isoprenaline sulphate 80 micrograms/metered inhalation. Net price 400-dose vial = £2.73
Note. Not recommended therefore no dose stated

PoM **Medihaler-iso Forte**® (3M)
Aerosol inhalation, isoprenaline sulphate 400 micrograms/metered inhalation. Net price 400-dose vial = £3.17
Note. Not recommended therefore no dose stated

ORCIPRENALINE SULPHATE
Indications: reversible airways obstruction, but see notes above
Cautions; Side-effects: see under Salbutamol (section 3.1.1.1) and notes above
Dose: by mouth, 20 mg 4 times daily; CHILD up to 1 year 5–10 mg 3 times daily, 1–3 years 5–10 mg 4 times daily, 3–12 years 40–60 mg daily in divided doses (but not recommended, see notes above)
By aerosol inhalation, 750–1500 micrograms (1–2 puffs) repeated if necessary after not less than 30 minutes to a max. of 9 mg (12 puffs) daily; CHILD up to 6 years 750 micrograms (1 puff) up to 4 times daily, 6–12 years 750–1500 micrograms (1–2 puffs) up to 4 times daily (but not recommended, see notes above)

PoM **Alupent**® (Boehringer Ingelheim)
Tablets, scored, orciprenaline sulphate 20 mg. Net price 112-tab pack = £4.26
Syrup, sugar-free, orciprenaline sulphate 10 mg/5 mL. Net price 100 mL = 69p
Aerosol inhalation, orciprenaline sulphate 750 micrograms/metered inhalation. Net price 300-dose vial with mouthpiece = £3.22; refill vial = £2.66
COUNSELLING. Advise patients not to exceed prescribed dose and to follow manufacturer's directions

3.1.2 Antimuscarinic bronchodilators

These drugs have traditionally been regarded as more effective in relieving bronchoconstriction associated with chronic bronchitis. **Ipratropium** may provide some bronchodilation in patients with chronic bronchitis who fail to respond to the selective beta$_2$-adrenoceptor stimulants (section 3.1.1.1). Unlike the older antimuscarinic drugs, side-effects are rare and it does not increase sputum viscosity or affect mucociliary clearance of sputum. The aerosol inhalation has a slower onset of action than that of the beta$_2$-adrenoceptor stimulants, with a maximum effect 30–60 minutes after use; its duration of action is longer than that of beta$_2$-adrenoceptor stimulants following

3.1 Bronchodilators

inhalation and bronchodilatation can usually be maintained with treatment three times a day.

Oxitropium has been introduced recently and has a similar duration of action to that of ipratropium.

IPRATROPIUM BROMIDE
Indications: reversible airways obstruction, particularly in chronic bronchitis
Cautions: glaucoma (standard doses unlikely to be harmful but see also under nebuliser, below); prostatic hypertrophy; pregnancy
Side-effects: dry mouth occasionally reported; rarely urinary retention, constipation
Dose: see below

PoM **Atrovent**® (Boehringer Ingelheim)
COUNSELLING. Advise patient not to exceed prescribed dose and to follow manufacturer's directions
Aerosol inhalation, ipratropium bromide 20 micrograms/metered inhalation. Net price 200-dose unit = £4.21
Dose: by aerosol inhalation, 20–40 micrograms (1–2 puffs), in early treatment up to 80 micrograms (4 puffs) at a time, 3–4 times daily; CHILD up to 6 years 20 micrograms (1 puff) 3 times daily, 6–12 years 20–40 micrograms (1–2 puffs) 3 times daily

Forte aerosol inhalation, ipratropium bromide 40 micrograms/metered inhalation. Net price 200-dose unit = £4.91
Dose: by aerosol inhalation 40 micrograms (1 puff), in early treatment 80 micrograms (2 puffs), 3–4 times daily; CHILD 6–12 years 40 micrograms (1 puff) 3 times daily

Nebuliser solution, isotonic, ipratropium bromide 250 micrograms/mL (0.025%); net price 10 × 1-mL unit-dose vials (preservative-free) = £3.20; 10 × 2-mL vials = £3.76. If dilution is necessary use only sterile sodium chloride solution 0.9%
Dose: reversible airways obstruction, *by inhalation of nebulised solution*, 100–500 micrograms (0.4–2 mL of a 0.025% solution) up to 4 times daily; CHILD 3–14 years 100–500 micrograms up to 3 times daily. Dilution of solution is adjusted according to equipment and length of administration
Note. Because paradoxical bronchospasm has occurred, first dose should be inhaled under medical supervision.
GLAUCOMA. Acute angle closure glaucoma has been reported in patients given nebulised ipratropium, particularly when used in association with nebulised salbutamol. Special caution is needed and care should be taken to avoid escape from mask to patient's eyes.

PoM **Rinatec**® nasal spray, see section 12.2.2

OXITROPIUM BROMIDE
Indications: reversible airways obstruction, particularly in chronic bronchitis
Cautions; Side-effects: see under Ipratropium Bromide; rarely blurring of vision
Dose: by aerosol inhalation, 200 micrograms (2 puffs) 2–3 times daily

▼ PoM **Oxivent**® (Boehringer Ingelheim)
Aerosol inhalation, oxitropium bromide 100 micrograms/metered inhalation. Net price 200-dose unit = £12.98
COUNSELLING. Advise patient not to exceed prescribed dose and to follow manufacturer's directions

3.1.3 Theophylline

Theophylline is used for the relief of *bronchospasm*. It may have an additive effect when used in conjunction with small doses of beta$_2$-adrenoceptor stimulants; the combination may increase the risk of side-effects, including hypokalaemia (for CSM advice see p. 114).

Theophylline is metabolised in the liver and there is considerable variation in its half-life in healthy non-smokers, which is even more marked in smokers, in patients with hepatic impairment or heart failure, or if other drugs are taken concurrently. The half-life is *increased* in heart failure, cirrhosis, viral infections, and by drugs such as cimetidine, ciprofloxacin, erythromycin, and oral contraceptives. The half-life is *decreased* in smokers and in heavy drinkers, and by drugs such as phenytoin, carbamazepine, rifampicin, and barbiturates. For other interactions of theophylline see Appendix 1.

These differences in half-life are important because theophylline has a narrow margin between the therapeutic and toxic dose. In most subjects *plasma concentrations* of between 10 and 20 mg/litre are required for satisfactory bronchodilatation. Side-effects can occur with concentrations below 20 mg/litre and are common at concentrations above 30–40 mg/litre.

Theophylline modified-release preparations are usually able to produce adequate plasma concentrations for up to 12 hours. When given as a single dose at night they have a useful role in controlling *nocturnal asthma* and *early morning wheezing*. There is no evidence that **choline theophyllinate** (a derivative of theophylline) is better tolerated than the modified-release preparations. The use of *rapid-release* oral theophylline preparations has declined because of the high incidence of side-effects associated with rapid absorption.

Theophylline is given by injection as **aminophylline**, a mixture of theophylline with ethylenediamine, which is 20 times more soluble than theophylline alone. Aminophylline must be given by **very slow** intravenous injection; it is too irritant for intramuscular use. Theophylline is also available for slow intravenous injection as a mixture with lysine.

Intravenous aminophylline is of established value in the treatment of *severe attacks of asthma* and is still preferred by many prescribers to intravenous treatment with the selective beta$_2$-adrenoceptor stimulants (section 3.1.1.1). Measurement of *plasma concentrations* may be helpful, and is **essential** if aminophylline is to be given to patients who have been taking oral theophylline preparations, as serious side-effects such as convulsions and arrhythmias can occasionally occur

Cautionary label wordings, see inside back cover

before the appearance of other symptoms of toxicity.

Aminophylline injection was formerly also used in the treatment of left ventricular failure but has been superseded for this purpose by diuretics (see sections 2.2.1 and 2.2.2) and the opioid analgesics (see section 4.7.2). However, it may have a role in patients with heart failure who are also suffering from asthma and bronchitis, where opioids are contra-indicated, though care is needed in those with increased myocardial excitability.

Aminophylline was formerly available for *rectal administration* as suppositories but these caused proctitis and showed an unpredictable response; there was a particular risk of toxicity in children.

THEOPHYLLINE

Indications: reversible airways obstruction, severe acute asthma

Cautions: see notes above; also liver disease, epilepsy, pregnancy and breast-feeding, cardiac disease, elderly, fever; **CSM** advice on hypokalaemia risk, p. 114; avoid in porphyria (see section 9.8.2); **interactions:** Appendix 1 (theophylline)

Side-effects: tachycardia, palpitations, nausea, gastro-intestinal disturbances, headache, insomnia, arrhythmias, and convulsions especially if given rapidly by intravenous injection; overdosage: see Emergency Treatment of Poisoning, p. 20

Dose: see below

Note. Plasma theophylline concentration for optimum response 10–20 mg/litre (55–110 micromol/litre); narrow margin between therapeutic and toxic dose, see also notes above

Biophylline® (Delandale)
Syrup, yellow, sugar-free, theophylline hydrate 125 mg (as sodium glycinate)/5 mL. Net price 250 mL = £3.77 (includes 2.5-mL measure). Label: 21
Dose: 125–250 mg 3–4 times daily; CHILD 2–6 years 62.5 mg, 7–12 years 62.5–125 mg, 3–4 times daily

PoM **Labophylline**® (LAB)
Injection, theophylline 20 mg/mL, lysine 12.2 mg/mL. Net price 10-mL amp = 31p
Dose: in patients not previously treated with xanthines, *by slow intravenous injection* (over 20 minutes) initially 200 mg, *or by intravenous infusion* 4 mg/kg; maintenance if required, 500 micrograms/kg/hour for 12 hours, then 400 micrograms/kg/hour; CHILD *by slow intravenous injection* (over 20 minutes) 4 mg/kg initially

Nuelin® (3M)
Tablets, scored, theophylline 125 mg. Net price 90-tab pack = £3.39. Label: 21
Dose: 125 mg 3–4 times daily after food, increased to 250 mg if required; CHILD 7–12 years 62.5–125 mg 3–4 times daily

Liquid, brown, theophylline 60 mg (as sodium glycinate)/5 mL. Net price 200 mL = £2.02. Label: 21
Dose: 120–240 mg 3–4 times daily after food; CHILD 2–6 years 60–90 mg, 7–12 years 90–120 mg, 3–4 times daily

Modified release
Note. The Council of the Royal Pharmaceutical Society of Great Britain advises pharmacists that if a general practitioner prescribes a modified-release, oral theophylline preparation without specifying a brand name, the pharmacist should contact the prescriber and agree the brand to be dispensed. Additionally, it is essential that a patient discharged from hospital should be maintained on the brand on which that patient was stabilised as an inpatient.

Biophylline® (Delandale)
Tablets, m/r, both scored, theophylline 350 mg, net price 56-tab pack = £5.44; 500 mg, 56-tab pack = £7.44. Label: 25
Dose: over 70 kg, 500 mg every 12 hours; under 70 kg and elderly, 350 mg every 12 hours

Lasma® (Pharmax)
Tablets, m/r, scored, theophylline 300 mg. Net price 20 = £1.94. Label: 25
Dose: 300 mg every 12 hours (increased after 1 week to 450 mg every 12 hours in patients over 70 kg); adjust dose by 150-mg increments as required
Total daily dose may be given as single dose at night when nocturnal symptoms predominate (daytime symptoms then controlled with inhaled bronchodilators)

Nuelin SA® (3M)
Tablets, m/r, theophylline 175 mg. Net price 60-tab pack = £3.13. Label: 25
Dose: 175–350 mg every 12 hours; CHILD over 6 years 175 mg every 12 hours

Nuelin SA 250® (3M)
Tablets, m/r, scored, theophylline 250 mg. Net price 60-tab pack = £4.39. Label: 25
Dose: 250–500 mg every 12 hours; CHILD over 6 years 125–250 mg every 12 hours

Pro-Vent® (Wellcome)
Capsules, m/r, white/clear, theophylline 300 mg. Net price 20 = £2.13. Label: 25
Dose: 300 mg every 12 hours, an additional 300 mg may be taken daily (night *or* morning) if plasma concentrations inadequate

Slo-Phyllin® (Lipha)
Capsules, m/r, white/clear, enclosing white pellets, theophylline 60 mg. Net price 56-cap pack = £2.02. Label: 25 *or* counselling, see below
Capsules, m/r, brown/clear, enclosing white pellets, theophylline 125 mg. Net price 56-cap pack = £2.55. Label: 25 *or* counselling, see below
Capsules, m/r, blue/clear, enclosing white pellets, theophylline 250 mg. Net price 56-cap pack = £3.18. Label: 25 *or* counselling, see below
Dose: 250–500 mg every 12 hours; CHILD, every 12 hours, 2–6 years 60–120 mg, 7–12 years 125–250 mg
COUNSELLING. Swallow whole with fluid *or* swallow enclosed granules with soft food (e.g. yoghurt)

Theo-Dur® (Astra)
Tablets, m/r, both scored, theophylline 200 mg, net price 20 = £1.24; 300 mg, 20 = £1.80. Label: 25
Dose: every 12 hours; CHILD up to 35 kg 100 mg, over 35 kg 200 mg, every 12 hours

3.1 Bronchodilators

Uniphyllin Continus® (Napp)
Tablets, m/r, both scored, theophylline 300 mg, net price 56-tab pack = £5.50; 400 mg, 56-tab pack = £7.51. Label: 25
Dose: 200 mg every 12 hours increased after 1 week to 300 mg every 12 hours; over 70 kg 300 mg every 12 hours increased after 1 week to 400 mg every 12 hours
May be appropriate to give larger evening or morning dose to achieve optimum therapeutic effect when symptoms most severe; in patients whose night- or daytime symptoms persist despite other therapy, who are not currently receiving theophylline, total daily requirement may be added as single evening or morning dose
Paediatric tablets, m/r, scored, theophylline 200 mg. Net price 56-tab pack = £3.61. Label: 25
Dose: CHILD over 5 years, maintenance, 9 mg/kg twice daily

Phyllocontin Continus® (Napp)
Tablets, m/r, yellow, f/c, aminophylline 225 mg. Net price 60-tab pack = £3.40. Label: 25
Dose: 1 tablet twice daily initially, increased after 1 week to 2 tablets twice daily
Forte tablets, m/r, yellow, f/c, aminophylline 350 mg. Net price 60-tab pack = £6.00. Label: 25
Note. Forte tablets are for smokers and other patients with decreased theophylline half-life (see notes above)
Paediatric tablets, m/r, yellow, aminophylline 100 mg. Net price 50-tab pack = £1.86. Label: 25
Dose: CHILD over 3 years, 6 mg/kg twice daily initially, increased after 1 week to 12 mg/kg twice daily
Note. Modified-release tablets containing aminophylline 225 mg and 350 mg also available from Ashbourne (Amnivent®)

AMINOPHYLLINE
Note: Aminophylline is a stable mixture or combination of theophylline and ethylenediamine; the ethylenediamine confers greater solubility in water
Indications: reversible airways obstruction, severe acute asthma
Cautions; Side-effects: see under Theophylline; also allergy to ethylenediamine can cause urticaria, erythema, and exfoliative dermatitis
Dose: see below
Note. Plasma theophylline concentration for optimum response 10–20 mg/litre (55–110 micromol/litre); narrow margin between therapeutic and toxic dose, see also notes above

Aminophylline (Non-proprietary)
Tablets, aminophylline 100 mg, net price 20 = 92p. Label: 21
Dose: by mouth, 100–300 mg, 3–4 times daily, after food
PoM *Injection*, aminophylline 25 mg/mL, net price 10-mL amp = 71p
Available from Evans, IMS (Min-I-Jet®)
Dose: by slow intravenous injection (over 20 minutes), 250–500 mg (5 mg/kg) when necessary; maintenance, if required, in patients not previously treated with theophylline, 500 micrograms/kg/hour *by slow intravenous infusion*
CHILD, *by slow intravenous injection* (over 20 minutes), 5 mg/kg; maintenance, if required, in patients not previously treated with theophylline, 6 months–9 years 1 mg/kg/hour, 10–16 years 800 micrograms/kg/hour *by slow intravenous infusion*

Modified release (see advice on p. 120)
Pecram® (Zyma)
Tablets, m/r, yellow, aminophylline hydrate 225 mg. Net price 20 = £1.02. Label: 25
Dose: 1 tablet twice daily initially, increased if necessary to 2 tablets twice daily (steady-state concentrations usually reached after 3–4 days)

CHOLINE THEOPHYLLINATE
Indications: reversible airways obstruction
Cautions; Side-effects: see under Theophylline
Dose: by mouth, 100–400 mg 2–4 times daily preferably after food; CHILD, 3 times daily, 3–5 years 62.5–125 mg, 6–12 years 100 mg
Note. Plasma theophylline concentration for optimum response 10–20 mg/litre (55–110 micromol/litre); narrow margin between therapeutic and toxic dose, see also notes above

Choledyl® (P-D)
Tablets, both compression coated, choline theophyllinate 100 mg (pink), net price 100-tab pack = £2.20; 200 mg (yellow), 100-tab pack = £3.00
Syrup, yellow, choline theophyllinate 62.5 mg/5 mL. Net price 200 mL = £2.57

Modified release (see advice on p. 120)
Sabidal SR 270® (Zyma)
Tablets, m/r, light yellow, choline theophyllinate 424 mg. Net price 20 = £1.54. Label: 25
Dose: 1 tablet twice daily initially, increased after 3 days to 1 in the morning and 2 at night

3.1.4 Compound bronchodilator preparations

Most compound bronchodilator preparations have no place in the management of patients with airways obstruction.

In general, patients are best treated with single-ingredient preparations, such as a selective beta$_2$-adrenoceptor stimulant (section 3.1.1.1) or ipratropium bromide (section 3.1.2), so that the dose of each drug can be adjusted. This flexibility is lost with combinations, although those in which both components are effective may occasionally have a role when compliance is a problem.

Cautionary label wordings, see inside back cover

Prices are **net**, see p. 1

PoM Duovent® (Boehringer Ingelheim)
Aerosol inhalation, fenoterol hydrobromide 90 micrograms, ipratropium bromide 36 micrograms/metered inhalation. Net price 200-dose unit with mouthpiece = £5.28 (extension tube also available)
Dose: 1–2 puffs 3–4 times daily; CHILD over 6 years 1 puff 3 times daily

With theophylline
Note. Compound theophylline preparations on sale to the public include Do-Do® tablets (theophylline, ephedrine, caffeine), Franolyn Expect® (theophylline, ephedrine, guaiphenesin)

PoM Franol® (Sanofi Winthrop)
Tablets, ephedrine hydrochloride 11 mg, theophylline 120 mg. Net price 100-tab pack = £5.42. Label: 21
Dose: 1 tablet 3 times daily; an additional tablet may be taken at bedtime for nocturnal attacks

PoM Franol Plus® (Sanofi Winthrop)
Tablets, ephedrine sulphate 15 mg, theophylline 120 mg. Net price 20 = £1.50. Label: 21
Dose: 1 tablet 3 times daily; an additional tablet may be taken at bedtime for nocturnal attacks

3.1.5 Peak flow meters and inhaler devices

PEAK FLOW METERS

Measurement of peak flow is particularly helpful for patients who are 'poor perceivers' and hence slow to detect deterioration in their asthma, and for those with moderate or severe asthma. Patients can also be encouraged to adjust some of their own treatment (within specified limits) according to changes in peak flow rate.

Mini-Wright® (Clement Clarke)
Peak flow meter, standard (60 to 800 litres/minute), net price = £6.39, low range (30 to 370 litres/minute) = £6.39, replacement universal mouthpiece = 38p

Vitalograph Pulmo-Aide® (DeVilbiss)
Peak flow meter, standard (50 to 750 litres/minute), net price = £5.99, low range (25 to 280 litres/minute) = £5.99, replacement mouthpiece = 40p

Wright® (Ferraris)
Pocket peak flow meter, standard (75–800 litres/minute), net price = £5.85, low range (50–400 litres/minute) = £5.85, replacement mouthpiece adult = 38p, paediatric = 38p

INHALER DEVICES

A variety of spacing devices is now available for use with metered dose inhalers. By providing a space between inhaler and mouth, they reduce the velocity of the aerosol and subsequent impaction on the oropharynx; in addition they allow more time for evaporation of the propellent so that a larger proportion of the particles can be inhaled and deposited in the lungs; also co-ordination of inspiration with actuation of the aerosol is less important. They range from the Bricanyl Spacer® (for terbutaline), a collapsible extended mouthpiece, to larger spacing devices with a one-way valve (Nebuhaler®, Rondo®, Volumatic®). Spacing devices are particularly useful for patients with poor inhalation technique, for children, for patients requiring higher doses, for nocturnal asthma, and for patients prone to develop candidiasis with inhaled corticosteroids.

Cyclohaler® (Goldshield)
Breath actuated device for use with Salbutamol Cyclocaps. Net price = 78p

NHS Haleraid® (Glaxo)
Device to place over standard inhalers as aid to operation by patients with impaired strength in hands (e.g. with arthritis). Net price = 80p

Nebuhaler® (Astra)
Device, fitted with plastic cone and one-way valve. For use with Bricanyl and Pulmicort refill canisters. Net price = £4.75

Rondo® (Tillotts)
Spacer device for use with Salbuvent. Net price = £2.75

Rotahaler® (A&H)
Breath actuated device for use with Rotacaps. Net price = 78p

Spinhaler®, see section 3.3

Volumatic® (A&H)
Inhaler, large-volume device. For use with Ventolin, Becotide, Becloforte, and Ventide inhalers. Net price = £2.75

3.2 Corticosteroids

Corticosteroids have been used in asthma for many years, and the use of inhaled corticosteroids has increased so that they are now recommended for prophylactic treatment when patients are using a beta$_2$-stimulant more than once or twice daily. They have many fewer side-effects than those associated with systemic administration (see section 6.3.3).

Corticosteroids are usually of no benefit in patients with chronic bronchitis and emphysema; some patients with asthma, however, may be clinically indistinguishable from those with chronic bronchitis except that they will respond to a trial course of corticosteroids.

The action of corticosteroids is not fully understood but they probably reduce bronchial mucosal inflammation, and hence reduce oedema and secretion of mucus into the airway.

INHALATION. Corticosteroid *aerosol inhalations* must be used regularly to obtain maximum benefit; alleviation of symptoms usually occurs 3 to 7 days after initiation. **Beclomethasone dipropionate** and **budesonide** appear to be equally effective. If a beta$_2$-adrenoceptor stimulant is to be taken at the same time as an inhaled corticosteroid it should be taken first to help increase the penetration of the inhaled corticosteroid.

Patients who have been taking long-term oral corticosteroids can often be transferred to inhalation but the transfer must be done slowly, with gradual reduction in dose of oral corticosteroid, and at a time when the asthma is well controlled.

3.2 Corticosteroids

High-dose aerosol inhalers are available for patients who only have a partial response to standard inhalers. The maximum doses for high-dose corticosteroid inhalers are associated with some adrenal suppression (see section 6.3.3), therefore patients on high doses should be given a 'steroid card' and may need corticosteroid cover during an episode of stress (e.g. an operation). Systemic therapy may also be necessary during episodes of infection or increased bronchoconstriction where higher doses are needed and access of inhaled drug to small airways may be reduced; patients may need a reserve supply of tablets.

Although inhaled corticosteroids have considerably fewer systemic effects than oral corticosteroids, recent evidence has shown that effects on bone metabolism can be detected following inhalation of the higher doses of beclomethasone and budesonide. Although there is no firm evidence that this may lead to increased osteoporosis in the future, it is sensible to ensure that the dose of inhaled corticosteroid is no higher than necessary to keep a patient's asthma under good control. The dose can therefore be reduced cautiously when the asthma has been well controlled for a few weeks as long as the patient knows that it is necessary to reinstate it should their asthma deteriorate or the peak flow rate fall.

Corticosteroids are better inhaled from aerosol inhalers using 'spacer devices' (e.g. Nebuhaler® or Volumatic®). These increase airway deposition and reduce oropharyngeal deposition, resulting in a marked reduction in the incidence of candidiasis and reducing systemic absorption (so that there is less adrenal suppression); these devices are bulky, but most patients only need to use them morning and night.

Dry powder inhalers (Becotide Rotacaps®) which are actuated by the patient's inhalation may be tried in patients who are unable to use the aerosol inhalers.

Suspensions for nebulisation are now also available. Beclomethasone dipropionate suspension for nebulisation (Becotide®) is relatively inefficient because of its poor solubility; only a small amount is nebulised in 15 minutes. A spacing device will allow a larger amount to be administered more effectively and can be used by some children as young as 2 years. Budesonide suspension for nebulisation (Pulmicort Respules®) is also now available.

ORAL. *Acute attacks* of asthma should be treated with short courses of oral corticosteroids starting with a high dose, e.g. prednisolone 30 to 40 mg daily for a few days, gradually reduced once the attack has been controlled. Patients whose asthma has deteriorated rapidly usually respond quickly to corticosteroids, which can then be tailed down over a few days; more gradual reduction is necessary in those whose asthma has deteriorated gradually.

For use of corticosteroids in the emergency treatment of *severe acute asthma* see section 3.1.1.

In *chronic continuing asthma*, when the response to other anti-asthma drugs has been relatively small, continued administration of oral corticosteroids may be necessary; in such cases high doses of inhaled corticosteroids should be continued so that oral requirements are reduced to a minimum. Oral corticosteroids should normally be taken as a single dose in the morning to reduce the disturbance to circadian cortisol secretion. Dosage should always be titrated to the lowest dose which controls symptoms. Regular monitored peak flow measurements often help both patient and doctor to adjust the dose optimally. Prednisolone is available as tablets of 1 mg as well as 5 mg, and the smaller tablets may conveniently be used to adjust the maintenance dosage to the minimum necessary.

Alternate-day administration has not been very successful in the management of asthma and patients tend to deteriorate during the second 24 hours. If an attempt is made to introduce this pulmonary function should be monitored carefully over the 48 hours.

BECLOMETHASONE DIPROPIONATE

Indications: prophylaxis of asthma especially if not fully controlled by bronchodilators or cromoglycate

Cautions: see notes above; also active or quiescent tuberculosis; may need to reinstate systemic therapy during periods of stress or when airways obstruction or mucus prevent drug access to smaller airways

Side-effects: see notes above; also hoarseness and candidiasis of mouth or throat (usually only with large doses—reduced by using spacer, see notes above, and responds to antifungal lozenges, see section 12.3.2, without discontinuation of therapy—rinsing the mouth with water after inhalation of a dose may also be helpful)

Dose: see preparations below

Standard-dose inhalers
PoM **AeroBec®** (3M)
 AeroBec 50 Autohaler® (aerosol inhalation), beclomethasone dipropionate 50 micrograms/metered inhalation, net price 200-inhalation breath-actuated unit = £11.00. Label: 8, counselling, dose
 AeroBec 100 Autohaler® (aerosol inhalation), beclomethasone dipropionate 100 micrograms/metered inhalation, net price 200-inhalation breath-actuated unit = £13.50. Label: 8, counselling, dose
 Dose: by aerosol inhalation, 200 micrograms twice daily *or* 100 micrograms 3–4 times daily (in more severe cases initially 600–800 micrograms daily); CHILD 50–100 micrograms 2–4 times daily

Chapter 3: Respiratory system

PoM Becodisks® (A&H)
Dry powder for inhalation, disks containing 8 blisters of beclomethasone dipropionate 100 micrograms/blister, net price pack of 14 disks with Diskhaler® = £10.99, 14-disk refill = £10.42;
200 micrograms/blister, pack of 14 disks with Diskhaler® = £20.90, 14-disk refill = £20.33;
400 micrograms/blister, pack of 7 disks with Diskhaler® = £20.90, 7-disk refill = £20.33. Label: 8, counselling, dose
Dose: by inhalation of powder, 400 micrograms twice daily *or* 200 micrograms 3–4 times daily; CHILD 100 micrograms 2–4 times daily *or* 200 micrograms twice daily

PoM Becotide Inhaler® (A&H)
Becotide-50 aerosol inhalation, beclomethasone dipropionate 50 micrograms/metered inhalation. Net price 200-dose unit = £5.56. Label: 8, counselling, dose
Becotide-100 aerosol inhalation, beclomethasone dipropionate 100 micrograms/metered inhalation. Net price 200-dose unit = £10.56. Label: 8, counselling, dose
Becotide-200 aerosol inhalation, beclomethasone dipropionate 200 micrograms/metered inhalation. Net price 200-dose unit = £20.07. Label: 8, counselling, dose
Note. Becotide-200 not indicated for children
Dose: by aerosol inhalation, 200 micrograms twice daily *or* 100 micrograms 3–4 times daily (in more severe cases initially 600–800 micrograms daily); CHILD 50–100 micrograms 2–4 times daily *or* 100–200 micrograms twice daily

PoM Becotide Rotacaps® (A&H)
Rotacaps® (dry powder for inhalation), buff/clear, beclomethasone dipropionate 100 micrograms. Net price 100-cap pack = £7.56. Label: 8, counselling, dose
Rotacaps® (dry powder for inhalation), brown/clear, beclomethasone dipropionate 200 micrograms. Net price 100-cap pack = £14.35. Label: 8, counselling, dose
Rotacaps® (dry powder for inhalation), dark brown/clear, beclomethasone dipropionate 400 micrograms. Net price 100-cap pack = £27.27. Label: 8, counselling, dose
Dose: by inhalation of powder, 200 micrograms 3–4 times daily *or* 400 micrograms twice daily; CHILD 100 micrograms 2–4 times daily *or* 200 micrograms twice daily

PoM Becotide for Nebulisation® (A&H)
Suspension for nebulisation, beclomethasone dipropionate 50 micrograms/mL. Net price 10 mL = £2.50. For use with respirator or nebuliser. May be diluted up to 50% with sterile physiological saline
Dose: by inhalation of nebulised suspension, CHILD up to 1 year 50 micrograms 2–4 times daily; 1–12 years 100 micrograms 2–4 times daily, adjusted according to response
Note. Unsuitable for adults because of large volumes required

High-dose inhalers
Note. High-dose inhalers not indicated for children

PoM AeroBec Forte® (3M)
Aerosol inhalation, beclomethasone dipropionate 250 micrograms/metered inhalation, net price 200-inhalation breath-actuated unit (Autohaler®) = £25.10. Label: 8, counselling, dose, 10 steroid card
Dose: by aerosol inhalation, 500 micrograms twice daily *or* 250 micrograms 4 times daily; if necessary may be increased to 500 micrograms 4 times daily

PoM Becloforte® (A&H)
Aerosol inhalation, beclomethasone dipropionate 250 micrograms/metered inhalation. Net price 200-dose unit = £23.10; net price Becloforte® VM (2 Becloforte® inhalers with Volumatic®) = £46.20. Label: 8, counselling, dose, 10 steroid card
Dose: by aerosol inhalation, 500 micrograms (2 puffs) twice daily *or* 250 micrograms (1 puff) 4 times daily; if necessary may be increased to 500 micrograms 3–4 times daily
Dry powder for inhalation, disks containing 8 blisters for beclomethasone dipropionate 400 micrograms/blister, net price 14 disks with Diskhaler® = £39.70; 14-disk refill = £39.13. Label: 8, counselling, dose, 10 steroid card
Dose: by inhalation of powder, 400 micrograms twice daily; if necessary may be increased to 800 micrograms twice daily

Compound preparations
Not recommended, see section 3.3

PoM Ventide® (A&H)
Aerosol inhalation, beclomethasone dipropionate 50 micrograms, salbutamol 100 micrograms/metered inhalation. Net price 200-dose unit = £8.02. Label: 8, counselling, dose
Dose: maintenance, 2 puffs 3–4 times daily; CHILD 1–2 puffs 2–4 times daily
Paediatric Rotacaps®, light grey/clear, beclomethasone dipropionate 100 micrograms, salbutamol (as sulphate) 200 micrograms. Net price 100 = £12.59. Label: 8, counselling, dose
Dose: by inhalation of powder, 1 Paediatric Rotacap® 2–4 times daily
Rotacaps®, dark grey/clear, beclomethasone dipropionate 200 micrograms, salbutamol (as sulphate) 400 micrograms. Net price 100 = £22.83. Label: 8, counselling, dose
Dose: by inhalation of powder, 1 Rotacap® 3–4 times daily

Inhaler devices
See section 3.1.5

BUDESONIDE

Indications; Cautions; Side-effects: see under Beclomethasone Dipropionate
Dose: see preparations

PoM Pulmicort Inhaler® (Astra)
LS aerosol inhalation, budesonide 50 micrograms/metered inhalation. Net price 200-dose unit with standard or Spacer inhaler =

£6.66; 200-dose refill for use with Nebuhaler or Spacer inhaler = £4.66. Label: 8, counselling, dose

Aerosol inhalation, budesonide 200 micrograms/metered inhalation. Net price 200-dose unit with standard or Spacer inhaler = £19.00; 200-dose refill for use with Nebuhaler or Spacer inhaler = £17.00; 100-dose unit with standard and Spacer inhaler = £8.16 (hosp. only); 100-dose refill = £8.66 (hosp. only). Label: 8, counselling, dose, 10 steroid card

Turbohaler® (= breath-actuated dry powder inhaler), budesonide 100 micrograms/inhalation, net price 200-dose unit = £18.50; 200 micrograms/inhalation, 100-dose unit = £18.50; 400 micrograms/inhalation, 50-dose unit =£18.50. Label: 8, counselling, dose, 10 steroid card

Note. Little sensation associated with use

Dose: by aerosol inhalation, 200 micrograms twice daily; may be reduced in well-controlled asthma to not less than 200 micrograms daily; in severe asthma dose may be increased to 1.6 mg daily; CHILD 50–200 micrograms twice daily; in severe asthma may be increased to 400 micrograms twice daily

PoM **Pulmicort Respules**® (Astra)

Repsules® (= single-dose units for nebulisation), budesonide 250 micrograms/mL, net price 20 × 2-mL unit = £32.00; 500 micrograms/mL, 20 × 2-mL unit = £44.64. May be diluted up to 50% with sterile physiological saline. Label: 8, counselling, dose, 10 steroid card

Dose: by inhalation of nebulised suspension, when starting treatment, during periods of severe asthma, and while reducing or discontinuing oral corticosteroids, 1–2 mg twice daily (may be increased further in very severe asthma); CHILD 3 months–12 years, 0.5–1 mg twice daily

Maintenance, usually half above doses

Inhaler devices
See section 3.1.5

3.3 Cromoglycate and related therapy

Regular inhalation of sodium cromoglycate can reduce the incidence of attacks of asthma and allow dosage reduction of bronchodilators and oral corticosteroids. In general, prophylaxis with sodium cromoglycate is less effective in adults than prophylaxis with corticosteroid inhalations (see section 3.2) but the fact that in the long term corticosteroid inhalations may be associated with more side-effects needs to be borne in mind. Sodium cromoglycate is of no value in the treatment of acute attacks of asthma.

Sodium cromoglycate is of value in the prevention of exercise-induced asthma, a single dose being inhaled half-an-hour beforehand.

The mode of action of sodium cromoglycate is not completely understood but it prevents release of pharmacological mediators of bronchospasm by stabilising mast-cell membranes. It is of particular value in asthma with an allergic basis, but, in practice, it is difficult to predict who will benefit, therefore it is reasonable to try it for a 4-week period in any patient whose asthma is poorly controlled with bronchodilators. Children seem to respond better than adults. Dose frequency is adjusted according to response but is usually 4 times a day initially; this may subsequently be reduced.

If inhalation of the dry powder form of sodium cromoglycate causes bronchospasm a selective beta$_2$-adrenoceptor stimulant such as salbutamol or terbutaline should be inhaled a few minutes beforehand. The nebuliser solution is useful for patients who cannot manage the dry powder inhaler or the aerosol.

Nedocromil has a pharmacological action similar to that of sodium cromoglycate.

Ketotifen is an antihistamine with an action said to resemble that of sodium cromoglycate. It has not fulfilled its early promise.

SODIUM CROMOGLYCATE

Indications: prophylaxis of asthma

Side-effects: coughing, transient bronchospasm, and throat irritation due to inhalation of powder (see also notes above)

Dose: see below

COUNSELLING. Regular use is necessary .

PoM **Intal**® (Fisons)

Aerosol inhalation, sodium cromoglycate 5 mg/metered inhalation. Net price 112-dose unit = £15.97. Label: 8

Dose: by aerosol inhalation, adults and children, 10 mg (2 puffs) 4 times daily initially, increased in severe cases or during periods of risk to 6–8 times daily; additional doses may also be taken before exercise; maintenance 5 mg (1 puff) 4 times daily

Note. Sodium cromoglycate 5 mg/metered inhalation also available from Ashbourne (Glycavent®), Baker Norton (Cromogen®)

Autohaler® (= breath-actuated inhaler), sodium cromoglycate 5 mg/metered inhalation. Net price 112-dose unit = £21.84. Label: 8

Dose: as for Aerosol inhalation above

Spincaps®, yellow/clear, sodium cromoglycate 20 mg. Net price 112-cap pack = £12.05. Label: 8

Dose: by inhalation of powder, adults and children, 20 mg 4 times daily, increased in severe cases to 8 times daily

Spinhaler insufflator® (for use with Intal and Intal Compound Spincaps). Net price = £1.94

Nebuliser solution, sodium cromoglycate 10 mg/mL. Net price 2-mL amp = 28p. For use with power-operated nebuliser

Dose: by inhalation of nebulised solution, adults and children, 20 mg 4 times daily, increased in severe cases to 6 times daily

Note. Sodium cromoglycate 10 mg/mL also available for nebulisation in 2-mL unit doses as Steri-Neb Cromogen® (Baker Norton)

PoM **Intal Compound**® (Fisons)
Spincaps®, orange/clear, isoprenaline sulphate 100 micrograms, sodium cromoglycate 20 mg. Net price 112-cap pack = £9.54. Label: 8
Note. The compound inhalation of sodium cromoglycate with isoprenaline is not recommended; not only has isoprenaline a less selective action but the inhalation is liable to be used inappropriately for relief of bronchospasm rather than for its prophylactic effect

KETOTIFEN
Indications: see notes above
Cautions: previous anti-asthmatic treatment should be continued for a minimum of 2 weeks after initiation of ketotifen treatment; **interactions:** Appendix 1 (antihistamines)
DRIVING. Drowsiness may affect performance of skilled tasks (e.g. driving); effects of alcohol enhanced
Side-effects: dry mouth, sedation
Dose: 1–2 mg twice daily with food; initial treatment in readily sedated patients 0.5–1 mg at night; CHILD over 2 years 1 mg twice daily

PoM **Zaditen**® (Sandoz)
Capsules, ketotifen 1 mg (as hydrogen fumarate). Net price 60-cap pack = £8.35. Label: 2, 8, 21
Tablets, off-white, scored, ketotifen 1 mg (as hydrogen fumarate). Net price 60-tab pack = £8.35. Label: 2, 8, 21
Elixir, sugar-free, ketotifen 1 mg (as hydrogen fumarate)/5 mL. Net price 150 mL = £4.94. Label: 2, 8, 21

NEDOCROMIL SODIUM
Indications: prophylaxis of asthma
Side-effects: see under Sodium Cromoglycate; also headache, nausea (both mild and transient); bitter taste (masked by mint flavour)
Dose: by aerosol inhalation, 4 mg (2 puffs) twice daily, increased to 4 times daily if necessary; CHILD under 12 years, not yet recommended

PoM **Tilade Mint**® (Fisons)
Aerosol inhalation, nedocromil sodium 2 mg/metered inhalation. Net price 2 × 56-puff mint-flavoured units = £18.65. Label: 8

3.4 Antihistamines, hyposensitisation, and allergic emergencies

3.4.1 Antihistamines
3.4.2 Hyposensitisation
3.4.3 Allergic emergencies

For the treatment of asthma see sections 3.1.1 and 3.2. For the treatment of hay fever by nasal application of corticosteroids and prophylaxis with sodium cromoglycate see section 12.2. For eye preparations see section 11.4. For the treatment of allergic skin conditions with topical corticosteroid preparations see section 13.4.

3.4.1 Antihistamines
All antihistamines are of potential value in the treatment of *nasal allergies*, particularly seasonal (hay fever), and may be of some value in *vasomotor rhinitis*. They reduce rhinorrhoea and sneezing but are usually less effective for nasal congestion.

Oral antihistamines are also of some value in preventing *urticaria* and are used to treat *allergic rashes, pruritus,* and *insect bites and stings*; they are also used in *drug allergies*. Injections of chlorpheniramine or promethazine are used as an adjunct to adrenaline in the emergency treatment of *angioedema* and *anaphylaxis* (section 3.4.3).

There is no evidence that any one of the older, sedative antihistamines is superior to any other and patients vary widely in their responses. They differ somewhat in duration of action and incidence of side-effects (drowsiness and antimuscarinic effects). Most are relatively short-acting but some, (e.g. promethazine) act for up to 12 hours. They all cause sedation but **promethazine, trimeprazine,** and **dimenhydrinate** may be more sedating whereas **chlorpheniramine, cyclizine,** and **mequitazine** may be less so.

Acrivastine, astemizole, cetirizine, loratadine, and **terfenadine** are newer antihistamines; they are a very major advance over the older antihistamines. They cause less sedation and psychomotor impairment because they only penetrate the blood brain barrier to a slight extent (and for this reason do not alleviate pruritus of non-allergic origin). Astemizole has a relatively slow onset of action and is more appropriate for use on a regular basis than when symptoms occur. The drug interactions described in Appendix 1 apply to a lesser extent to the non-sedative antihistamines, and they do not appear to potentiate the effects of alcohol.

DISADVANTAGES OF ANTIHISTAMINES. With most of the older antihistamines drowsiness is a serious disadvantage; patients should be warned that their ability to drive or operate machinery may be impaired, and that the effects of alcohol may be increased. Other side-effects include headache, psychomotor impairment, antimuscarinic effects such as urinary retention, dry mouth, blurred vision, and gastro-intestinal disturbances; occasional rashes and photosensitivity reactions have been reported; paradoxical stimulation may rarely occur, especially in high dosage or in children. Antihistamines should be used with caution in epilepsy, prostatic hypertrophy, glaucoma, and hepatic disease. Most antihistamines should be avoided in porphyria, but chlorpheniramine and cyclizine have been used (see section 9.8.2).
Interactions: Appendix 1 (antihistamines). **Pregnancy** and **breast-feeding:** Appendixes 4 and 5 (antihistamines).

NON-SEDATIVE ANTIHISTAMINES

DRIVING. Although drowsiness is rare, nevertheless patients should be advised that it can occur and may affect performance of skilled tasks (e.g. driving); excess alcohol should be avoided.

ACRIVASTINE

Indications: symptomatic relief of allergy such as hay fever, urticaria
Cautions: see notes above; pending specific studies avoid in renal impairment
Side-effects: see notes above; incidence of sedation and antimuscarinic effects low
Dose: 8 mg 3 times daily; CHILD under 12 years, not yet recommended

PoM **Semprex**® (Wellcome)
Capsules, acrivastine 8 mg. Net price 84-cap pack = £5.92. Counselling, driving

ASTEMIZOLE

Indications: symptomatic relief of allergy such as hay fever, urticaria
Cautions: see notes above; pregnancy (toxicity at high doses in *animal* studies)
Side-effects: see notes above; weight gain occurs infrequently; incidence of sedation and antimuscarinic effects low; ventricular arrhythmias have followed excessive dosage
Dose: 10 mg daily (must **not** be exceeded); CHILD 6–12 years, 5 mg daily (must **not** be exceeded)

PoM [1]**Hismanal**® (Janssen)
Tablets, scored, astemizole 10 mg. Net price 30-tab pack = £5.70. Counselling, driving
Suspension, sugar-free, astemizole 5 mg/5 mL. Net price 200 mL = £5.80. Counselling, driving
1. Can be sold to the public provided it is licensed and labelled for the treatment of hay fever in adults and children over 12 years; a proprietary brand of astemizole tablets (Pollon-eze®) is on sale to the public

CETIRIZINE

Indications: symptomatic relief of allergy such as hay fever, urticaria
Cautions: see notes above; halve dose in renal impairment; incidence of sedation and antimuscarinic effects low
Side-effects: see notes above
Dose: 10 mg daily *or* 5 mg twice daily; CHILD under 12 years, not yet recommended

PoM **Zirtek**® (UCB Pharma)
Tablets, f/c, scored, cetirizine hydrochloride 10 mg. Net price 30-tab pack = £8.95. Counselling, driving

LORATADINE

Indications: symptomatic relief of allergy such as hay fever; urticaria
Cautions; Side-effects: see notes above; incidence of sedation and antimuscarinic effects low; pregnancy (toxicity at high doses in *animals*)
Dose: 10 mg daily; CHILD 2–12 years, under 30 kg 5 mg daily, over 30 kg 10 mg daily

PoM **Clarityn**® (Schering-Plough)
Tablets, scored, loratadine 10 mg. Net price 30-tab pack = £7.76. Counselling, driving
Syrup, yellow, loratadine 5 mg/5 mL. Net price 100 mL = £7.76

TERFENADINE

Indications: symptomatic relief of allergy such as hay fever, urticaria
Cautions: see notes above; **interactions:** Appendix 1 (antihistamines)
Side-effects: see notes above; incidence of sedation and antimuscarinic effects low; hair loss reported; ventricular arrhythmias (torsade de pointes) have followed excessive dosage, see also Arrhythmias below
ARRHYTHMIAS. Company has commented on rare hazardous arrhythmias associated with terfenadine particularly in association with increased blood concentrations. Company advises: *not to exceed* recommended dose, *to avoid* in significant hepatic impairment, *to avoid* concomitant administration of drugs that inhibit metabolism (in particular, ketoconazole and erythromycin and other macrolides)
Dose: 60 mg twice daily *or* 120 mg in the morning; CHILD 3–6 years 15 mg twice daily; 6–12 years 30 mg twice daily

Triludan® (Merrell)
Tablets, scored, terfenadine 60 mg. Net price 60-tab pack = £5.80. Counselling, driving
Forte tablets, terfenadine 120 mg. Net price 7-tab pack = £2.02; 30-tab pack = £5.80. Counselling, driving
Suspension, sugar-free, terfenadine 30 mg/5 mL. Net price 200 mL = £4.24. Counselling, driving
Note. A proprietary brand of terfenadine (Seldane®) is on sale to the public

SEDATIVE ANTIHISTAMINES

DRIVING. Drowsiness may affect performance of skilled tasks (e.g. driving); effects of alcohol enhanced.

AZATADINE MALEATE

Indications: symptomatic relief of allergy such as hay fever, urticaria
Cautions; Side-effects: see notes above
Dose: 1 mg, increased if necessary to 2 mg, twice daily; CHILD 1–6 years 250 micrograms twice daily, 6–12 years 0.5–1 mg twice daily

Optimine® (Schering-Plough)
Tablets, scored, azatadine maleate 1 mg. Net price 56-tab pack = £4.48. Label: 2
Syrup, azatadine maleate 500 micrograms/5 mL. Net price 120 mL = £1.43. Label: 2

BROMPHENIRAMINE MALEATE

Indications: symptomatic relief of allergy such as hay fever, urticaria
Cautions; Side-effects: see notes above
Dose: 4–8 mg 3–4 times daily; CHILD up to 3 years 0.4–1 mg/kg daily in 4 divided doses, 3–6 years 2 mg 3–4 times daily, 6–12 years 2–4 mg 3–4 times daily

Dimotane® (Wyeth)
Tablets, peach, scored, brompheniramine maleate 4 mg. Net price 20 = 59p. Label: 2
Elixir, yellow-green, brompheniramine maleate 2 mg/5 mL. Net price 100 mL = 71p. Label: 2

Dimotane LA® (Wyeth)
Tablets, m/r, peach, s/c, brompheniramine maleate 12 mg. Net price 20 = 89p. Label: 2, 25
Dose: 12–24 mg twice daily; CHILD 6–12 years 12 mg at bedtime, increased if necessary to 12 mg twice daily

CHLORPHENIRAMINE MALEATE

Indications: symptomatic relief of allergy such as hay fever, urticaria; emergency treatment of anaphylactic reactions (section 3.4.3)
Cautions; Side-effects: see notes above. Injections may be irritant and cause transitory hypotension or CNS stimulation
Dose: by mouth, 4 mg every 4–6 hours, max. 24 mg daily; CHILD 1–2 years 1 mg twice daily, 2–5 years 1 mg every 4–6 hours, max. 6 mg daily, 6–12 years 2 mg every 4–6 hours, max. 12 mg daily
By subcutaneous or intramuscular injection, 10–20 mg, repeated if required; max. 40 mg in 24 hours
By slow intravenous injection over 1 minute, 10–20 mg diluted in syringe with 5–10 mL blood

Chlorpheniramine (Non-proprietary)
Tablets, chlorpheniramine maleate 4 mg. Net price 20 = 9p. Label: 2
Available from Cox

Piriton® (A&H)
Tablets, ivory, chlorpheniramine maleate 4 mg. Net price 20 = 19p. Label: 2
Syrup, chlorpheniramine maleate 2 mg/5 mL. Net price 150 mL = 57p. Label: 2
PoM *Injection*, chlorpheniramine maleate 10 mg/mL. Net price 1-mL amp = 12p

CLEMASTINE

Indications: symptomatic relief of allergy such as hay fever, urticaria
Cautions; Side-effects: see notes above
Dose: 1 mg twice daily; CHILD 1–3 years 250–500 micrograms twice daily; 3–6 years 500 micrograms twice daily; 6–12 years 0.5–1 mg twice daily; CHILD under 1 year, no longer recommended

Tavegil® (Sandoz)
Tablets, scored, clemastine 1 mg (as hydrogen fumarate). Net price 50-tab pack = £2.10. Label: 2
Elixir, sugar-free, clemastine 500 micrograms (as hydrogen fumarate)/5 mL. Net price 150 mL = 98p. Label: 2
Note. A proprietary brand of clemastine hydrogen fumarate (Aller-Eze®) is on sale to the public

CYPROHEPTADINE HYDROCHLORIDE

Indications: symptomatic relief of allergy such as hay fever, urticaria
Cautions; Side-effects: see notes above; may cause weight gain
Dose: allergy, usual dose 4 mg 3–4 times daily; usual range 4–20 mg daily, max. 32 mg daily; CHILD 2–6 years 2 mg 2–3 times daily, max. 12 mg daily; 7–14 years 4 mg 2–3 times daily, max. 16 mg daily
Migraine, 4 mg with a further 4 mg after 30 minutes if necessary; maintenance, 4 mg every 4–6 hours
Stimulation of appetite—not recommended therefore no dose stated

Periactin® (MSD)
Tablets, scored, cyproheptadine hydrochloride 4 mg. Net price 20 = 57p. Label: 2
Syrup, yellow, cyproheptadine hydrochloride 2 mg/5 mL. Net price 200 mL = £1.27. Label: 2

DIMENHYDRINATE

See section 4.6

DIMETHINDENE MALEATE

Indications: symptomatic relief of allergy such as hay fever, urticaria
Cautions; Side-effects: see notes above

Fenostil Retard® (Zyma)
Tablets, m/r, greyish-white, dimethindene maleate 2.5 mg. Net price 20 = 57p. Label: 2, 25
Dose: 2.5 mg twice daily

DIPHENHYDRAMINE HYDROCHLORIDE

Indications: symptomatic relief of allergy such as hay fever
Cautions; Side-effects: see notes above

Preparations
Ingredient of compound cough preparations (section 3.9.2)

DIPHENYLPYRALINE HYDROCHLORIDE

Indications: symptomatic relief of allergy such as hay fever, urticaria
Cautions; Side-effects: see notes above

Histryl® (SK&F)
Spansule® (= capsules m/r), pink/clear, enclosing pink and white pellets, diphenylpyraline hydrochloride 5 mg. Net price 30-cap pack = £1.79. Label: 2, 25
Dose: 5–10 mg twice daily
Paediatric Spansule® (= capsules m/r), pink/clear, enclosing pink and white pellets, diphenylpyraline hydrochloride 2.5 mg. Net price 30-cap pack = £1.36. Label: 1, 25
Dose: CHILD over 7 years 2.5 mg twice daily

HYDROXYZINE HYDROCHLORIDE
Indications: pruritus, anxiety (short-term)
Cautions; Side-effects: see notes above
Dose: pruritus, initially 25 mg at night increased if necessary to 25 mg 3–4 times daily; CHILD 6 months–6 years initially 5–15 mg daily increased if necessary to 50 mg daily in divided doses; over 6 years initially 15–25 mg daily increased if necessary to 50–100 mg daily in divided doses
Anxiety (adults only), 50–100 mg 4 times daily

PoM **Atarax**® (Pfizer)
Tablets, both s/c, hydroxyzine hydrochloride 10 mg (orange), net price 84-tab pack = £1.52; 25 mg (green), 28-tab pack = £1.02. Label: 2
Syrup, hydroxyzine hydrochloride 10 mg/5 mL. Net price 150-mL pack = 85p. Label: 2

PoM **Ucerax**® (UCB Pharma)
Tablets, f/c, scored, hydroxyzine hydrochloride 25 mg, net price 25-tab pack = £1.77. Lable: 2
Syrup, hydroxyzine hydrochloride 10 mg/5 mL. Net price 200-mL pack = £1.96. Label: 2

KETOFIFEN
See section 3.3

MEBHYDROLIN
Indications: symptomatic relief of allergy such as hay fever, urticaria
Cautions: see notes above
Side-effects: see notes above; also very rarely granulocytopenia or agranulocytosis
Dose: ADULT and CHILD over 10 years, 50–100 mg 3 times daily

PoM **Fabahistin**® (Bayer)
Tablets, orange, s/c, mebhydrolin 50 mg. Net price 20 = 68p. Label: 2

MEQUITAZINE
Indications: symptomatic relief of allergy such as hay fever, urticaria
Cautions; Side-effects: see notes above
Dose: 5 mg twice daily; CHILD under 12 years, not yet recommended

PoM **Primalan**® (Rhône-Poulenc Rorer)
Tablets, mequitazine 5 mg. Net price 56-tab pack = £5.00. Label: 2

OXATOMIDE
Indications: symptomatic relief of allergy such as hay fever, food allergy, urticaria
Cautions; Side-effects: see notes above; drowsiness most common; increased appetite with weight gain may occur above 120 mg daily
Dose: 30 mg twice daily after food, increased if necessary to 60 mg twice daily; ELDERLY 30 mg twice daily; CHILD 5–14 years 15–30 mg twice daily

PoM **Tinset**® (Janssen)
Tablets, scored, oxatomide 30 mg. Net price 25-tab pack = £4.90. Label: 2, 21

PHENINDAMINE TARTRATE
Indications: symptomatic relief of allergy such as hay fever, urticaria
Cautions; Side-effects: see notes above; may cause mild CNS stimulation
Dose: 25–50 mg 1–3 times daily; CHILD over 10 years 25 mg 1–3 times daily

Thephorin® (Sinclair)
Tablets, s/c, phenindamine tartrate 25 mg. Net price 50-tab pack = £2.42. Label: 2

PHENIRAMINE MALEATE
Indications: symptomatic relief of allergy such as hay fever, urticaria
Cautions; Side-effects: see notes above

Daneral SA® (Hoechst)
Tablets, m/r, pink, s/c, pheniramine maleate 75 mg. Net price 30-tab pack = £2.61. Label: 2, 25
Dose: 75–150 mg at night or 75 mg night and morning

PROMETHAZINE HYDROCHLORIDE
Indications: symptomatic relief of allergy such as hay fever, urticaria, emergency treatment of anaphylactic reactions (section 3.4.3)
For use in premedication see section 15.1.4.1; sedation see section 4.1.1
Cautions; Side-effects: see notes above; intramuscular injection may be painful
Dose: by mouth, 25 mg at night increased to 50 mg if necessary *or* 10–20 mg 2–3 times daily; CHILD 1–5 years 5–15 mg daily (1–2 years on doctor's advice only), 5–10 years 10–25 mg daily
By deep intramuscular injection, 25–50 mg; max. 100 mg; CHILD 5–10 years 6.25–12.5 mg
By slow intravenous injection in emergencies, 25–50 mg, max. 100 mg, as a solution containing 2.5 mg/mL in water for injections

Phenergan® (Rhône-Poulenc Rorer)
Tablets, both blue, f/c, promethazine hydrochloride 10 mg, net price 56-tab pack = £1.03; 25 mg, 56-tab pack = £1.53. Label: 2
Elixir, golden, promethazine hydrochloride 5 mg/5 mL. Net price 100 mL = £1.15. Label: 2
PoM *Injection*, promethazine hydrochloride 25 mg/mL. Net price 1-mL amp = 28p; 2-mL amp = 34p
Note. A proprietary brand of promethazine hydrochloride tablets 20 mg (Sominex®) is on sale to the public for the treatment of occasional insomnia in adults

PROMETHAZINE THEOCLATE
See section 4.6

TRIMEPRAZINE TARTRATE

Indications: urticaria and pruritus; premedication, see section 15.1.4.1
Cautions; Side-effects: see notes above
Dose: 10 mg 2–3 times daily, in severe cases up to max. 100 mg daily has been used; ELDERLY 10 mg 1–2 times daily; CHILD over 2 years 2.5–5 mg 3–4 times daily

PoM **Vallergan**® (Rhône-Poulenc Rorer)
Tablets, blue, f/c, trimeprazine tartrate 10 mg. Net price 28-tab pack = £1.06. Label: 2
Syrup, straw coloured, trimeprazine tartrate 7.5 mg/5 mL. Net price 100 mL = £1.96. Label: 2
Syrup forte, trimeprazine tartrate 30 mg/5 mL. Net price 100 mL = £2.48. Label: 2
Note. For use of Forte Syrup see section 15.1.4.2

TRIPROLIDINE HYDROCHLORIDE

Indications: symptomatic relief of allergy such as hay fever, urticaria
Cautions; Side-effects: see notes above
Dose: see preparation

Pro-Actidil® (Wellcome)
Tablets, m/r, white/pink/blue, triprolidine hydrochloride 10 mg. Net price 20 = £5.48. Label: 2, 25
Dose: 10 mg early evening or 5–6 hours before retiring increased to 20 mg daily if symptoms very severe; CHILD under 12 years not recommended

3.4.2 Hyposensitisation

Except for wasp and bee sting allergy the value of specific hyposensitisation is uncertain; administration of allergen extract desensitising vaccines is associated with a significant risk of anaphylaxis, see CSM warning below. Most atopic (allergic) patients are sensitive to a wide range of allergens hence hyposensitisation with an extract of a single allergen is usually no more than partially successful.

Diagnostic skin tests are unreliable and can only be used in conjunction with a detailed history of allergen exposure.

CSM Warning. The CSM has warned that since 1980, in the UK alone, 11 patients, most of whom were young, have died from anaphylaxis caused by allergen extract desensitising vaccines; patients with asthma appear to be particularly susceptible. The CSM is not aware of such problems when these allergens are used for diagnostic purposes (skin testing). Although some vaccines can prevent anaphylactic reactions (e.g. to bee stings) the effectiveness of the others is controversial. The CSM therefore recommends that it is important for doctors to balance carefully the known risks of desensitising vaccines against potential benefits before embarking on treatment. *Such treatment should only be carried out where facilities for full cardiorespiratory resuscitation are immediately available, and patients should be kept under medical observation for at least 2 hours after treatment.*

For details of the management of anaphylactic shock, see section 3.4.3.

ALLERGEN EXTRACT VACCINES

Each set usually contains vials for the administration of graded amounts to patients undergoing hyposensitisation. Maintenance sets containing vials at the highest strength are also available. Manufacturer's literature must be consulted for details of allergens, vial strengths, and administration

Indications: hypersensitivity to one or more common allergens (see notes above)
Cautions: see notes above including CSM warning; manufacturers recommend that patients should be warned not to eat a heavy meal before the injection
Contra-indications: pregnancy, febrile conditions, acute asthma
Side-effects: allergic reactions, especially in small children
Dose: by *subcutaneous injection*, see manufacturer's literature; very sensitive patients may be given an antihistamine tablet one hour before the injection

Pollen allergy (hay fever) preparations
PoM **Spectralgen Single Species**® (Kabi Pharmacia)
Prepared from Timothy grass. Net price treatment set = £59.29
PoM **Spectralgen 4 Grass Mix**® (Kabi Pharmacia)
Prepared from 4 varieties of common grasses. Net price treatment set = £64.99
PoM **Spectralgen 3 Tree Mix**® (Kabi Pharmacia)
Prepared from 3 varieties of common trees. Net price treatment set = £63.06

Wasp and bee venom allergy preparations
PoM **Pharmalgen**® (Kabi Pharmacia)
Bee venom extract (*Apis mellifera*) or wasp venom extract (*Vespula* spp.). Net price treatment set = £45.50 (bee), £55.80 (wasp).

3.4.3 Allergic emergencies

Anaphylactic shock requires prompt energetic treatment of laryngeal oedema, bronchospasm, and hypotension. It is relatively uncommon and is usually precipitated by blood products, vaccines, insect stings, and certain drugs such as antibiotics, iron injections, anti-inflammatory analgesics, heparin, hyposensitising (allergen) preparations, and neuromuscular blocking drugs. It is more likely to occur after parenteral administration and atopic individuals are particularly susceptible.

First-line treatment includes restoration of blood pressure, laying the patient flat, raising the feet, and administration of **adrenaline*** injection. This is given **intramuscularly** in a dose of 0.5–1 mg (0.5–1 mL adrenaline injection 1 in 1000), repeated every 10 minutes, according to blood pressure and pulse, until improvement occurs. Antihistamines, e.g. **chlorpheniramine**, given by slow intravenous injection (section 3.4.1), are a useful adjunctive treatment. This is given after adrenaline injection and continued for 24 to 48 hours to prevent relapse.

* In patients on non-cardioselective beta-blockers severe anaphylaxis may not respond to adrenaline injection, calling for addition of salbutamol by intravenous injection

Continuing deterioration requires further treatment including intravenous fluids (see section 9.2.2), intravenous aminophylline (section 3.1.3) or a nebulised beta$_2$-adrenoceptor stimulant (such as salbutamol or terbutaline, section 3.1.1.1), oxygen, assisted respiration, and possibly emergency tracheotomy.

Intravenous **corticosteroids** are of secondary value in anaphylatic shock as their onset of action is delayed for several hours but they should be used to prevent further deterioration in severely affected patients (see section 6.3.4).

Some patients with severe allergy to insect stings are encouraged to carry pre-filled adrenaline syringes for emergency administration during periods of risk; adrenaline inhalations (Medihaler-epi®) are much less effective.

Angioedema is dangerous when it affects respiration. If obstruction is present, adrenaline injection should be given as described above; antihistamine injections are also helpful but corticosteroids are of secondary value (see also above). Tracheal intubation as well as other measures may be necessary. The administration of C$_1$ esterase inhibitor (in fresh frozen plasma or in partially purified form) may terminate acute attacks of *hereditary angioedema*, but is not practical for long-term prophylaxis.

ADRENALINE

Indications: emergency treatment of acute anaphylaxis; cardiopulmonary resuscitation, section 2.7

Cautions: hyperthyroidism, diabetes mellitus, ischaemic heart disease, hypertension, elderly patients; **interactions:** Appendix 1 (sympathomimetics)

Side-effects: anxiety, tremor, tachycardia, arrhythmias, dry mouth, cold extremities

Dose: acute anaphylaxis, *by intramuscular injection*, see table below:

IMPORTANT. Intravenous route is for cardiac resuscitation **only** (see section 2.7)

Volume of adrenaline injection 1 in 1000 (1 mg/mL) for intramuscular injection in anaphylactic shock	
Age	Volume of adrenaline 1 in 1000
Under 1 year	0.05 mL
1 year	0.1 mL
2 years	0.2 mL[1]
3–4 years	0.3 mL[1]
5 years	0.4 mL[1]
6–12 years	0.5 mL[1]
Adult	0.5–1 mL

These doses may be repeated every 10 minutes, according to blood pressure and pulse, until improvement occurs (may be repeated several times).

1. Suitable for robust children in these age groups; for underweight children use half these doses.

PoM **Adrenaline Injection, BP**, adrenaline 1 in 1000 (adrenaline 1 mg/mL as acid tartrate). Net price 0.5-mL amp = 31p; 1-mL amp = 31p
Available from Boots, Evans, Hillcross, Martindale
Note. For 1 in 10000 strength, see section 2.7

PoM **Min-I-Jet® Adrenaline** (IMS)
Injection, adrenaline 1 in 1000 (1 mg/mL as hydrochloride). Net price 0.5-mL = £3.81; 1-mL = £3.26 (both disposable syringe)
Injection, adrenaline 1 in 10000, see section 2.7

Inhalation
PoM **Medihaler-epi®** (3M)
Aerosol inhalation, adrenaline acid tartrate 280 micrograms/metered inhalation. Net price 400-inhalation unit = £2.73
Dose: by aerosol inhalation, adjunct to anaphylaxis treatment only, min. of 20 puffs

3.5 Respiratory stimulants and surfactants

3.5.1 Respiratory stimulants
3.5.2 Respiratory surfactants

3.5.1 Respiratory stimulants

Respiratory stimulants (analeptic drugs) have a limited place in the treatment of ventilatory failure in patients with chronic obstructive airways disease. They are effective only when given by intravenous injection or infusion and have a short duration of action. Their use has largely been replaced by ventilatory support. However, occasionally when the latter is contra-indicated and in patients with hypercapnic respiratory failure who are becoming drowsy or comatose, respiratory stimulants in the short term may arouse patients sufficiently to co-operate and clear their secretions.

Respiratory stimulants may be harmful in respiratory failure since they stimulate non-respiratory as well as respiratory muscles. They should only be given under **expert supervision** in hospital and must be combined with active physiotherapy. There is at present no oral respiratory stimulant available for long-term use in chronic respiratory failure.

Doxapram is given by continuous intravenous infusion in an initial dosage of 2 mg per minute. Frequent arterial blood gas studies and pH measurements are necessary during treatment to ensure the correct dosage.

Nikethamide and ethamivan were formerly used as respiratory stimulants but are no longer recommended; the effective doses were close to those causing toxic effects, especially convulsions. Respiratory stimulants such as ethamivan and nikethamide have no place whatsoever in the management of asphyxia in the newborn.

DOXAPRAM HYDROCHLORIDE

Indications: ventilatory failure (see notes above)
Cautions: epilepsy, hepatic impairment; see also notes above; **interactions:** Appendix 1 (doxapram)
Contra-indications: severe hypertension, status asthmaticus, coronary artery disease, thyrotoxicosis
Side-effects: increase in blood pressure and heart rate, dizziness, perineal warmth

Dose: by intravenous infusion, 1.5–4 mg per minute according to patient's response
By intravenous injection over at least 30 seconds, 1–1.5 mg/kg repeated if necessary at intervals of 1 hour
Postoperative respiratory depression, see section 15.1.7

PoM **Dopram**® (Wyeth)
Injection, doxapram hydrochloride 20 mg/mL. Net price 5-mL amp = £2.14
Intravenous infusion, doxapram hydrochloride 2 mg/mL in glucose 5%. Net price 500-mL bottle = £22.34

NIKETHAMIDE
Indications: not recommended, see notes above
Cautions: see notes above, severe hypertension
Contra-indications: respiratory failure due to neurological disease or drug overdose; status asthmaticus, coronary artery disease, thyrotoxicosis; porphyria (see section 9.8.2)
Side-effects: nausea, restlessness, convulsions, dizziness, tremor, vasoconstriction, arrhythmias
Dose: by slow intravenous injection, 0.5–1 g but not recommended see notes above

PoM **Nikethamide Injection**, nikethamide 250 mg/mL. Net price 2-mL amp = £2.45 (hosp. only)

ETHAMIVAN
Indications; Cautions; Contra-indications; Side-effects: see under Nikethamide and notes above
Dose: by intravenous injection, 100 mg, but not recommended see notes above

PoM **Clairvan**® (Sinclair)
Injection, ethamivan 50 mg/mL (5%). Net price 2-mL amp = £3.05

3.5.2 Respiratory surfactants

COLFOSCERIL PALMITATE
Indications: newborn babies with birthweight of 700 g or more undergoing mechanical ventilation for respiratory distress syndrome, whose heart rate and arterial oxygenation are continuously monitored
Cautions: continuous monitoring required to avoid hyperoxaemia (due to rapid improvement in arterial oxygen concentration)
Side-effects: may increase incidence of pulmonary haemorrhage; obstruction of endotracheal tube by mucous secretions
Dose: by endotracheal tube, 67.5 mg/kg; if still intubated, may be repeated after 12 hours

▼ PoM **Exosurf Neonatal**® (Wellcome)
Suspension, colfosceril palmitate 108 mg for reconstitution with 8 mL water for injections (when reconstituted, contains 67.5 mg/5 mL). Net price per vial = £314.29

3.6 Oxygen

Oxygen should be regarded as a drug. It is prescribed for hypoxaemic patients to increase alveolar oxygen tension and decrease the work of breathing necessary to maintain a given arterial oxygen tension. The concentration depends on the condition being treated; an inappropriate concentration may have serious or even lethal effects.

High concentration oxygen therapy, with concentrations of up to 60% for short periods, is safe in conditions such as pneumonia, pulmonary thromboembolism, and fibrosing alveolitis. In such conditions low arterial oxygen (P_aO_2) is usually associated with low or normal arterial carbon dioxide (P_aCO_2), therefore there is little risk of hypoventilation and carbon dioxide retention.

In severe acute asthma, the arterial carbon dioxide (P_aCO_2) is usually subnormal but as asthma deteriorates may rise steeply (particularly in children). These patients usually require high concentrations of oxygen and if the arterial carbon dioxide (P_aCO_2) remains high despite other treatment intermittent positive pressure ventilation needs to be considered urgently. Where facilities for blood gas measurements are not immediately available, for example while transferring the patient to hospital, 35% to 50% oxygen delivered through a conventional mask is recommended. Exceptionally, asthma is diagnosed in patients with a long history of chronic bronchitis and probable respiratory failure; in these patients a lower concentration (24% to 28%) may be needed to limit oxygen-induced reduction of respiratory drive.

Low concentration oxygen therapy (controlled oxygen therapy) is reserved for patients with ventilatory failure due to chronic obstructive airways disease or other causes. The concentration should not exceed 28% and in some patients a concentration above 24% may be excessive. The aim is to provide the patient with just enough oxygen to improve hypoxaemia without worsening pre-existing carbon dioxide retention and respiratory acidosis. Treatment should be initiated in hospital as repeated blood gas measurements are required to estimate the correct concentration.

DOMICILIARY OXYGEN. Oxygen should only be prescribed for patients in the home after careful evaluation in hospital by respiratory experts; it should never be prescribed on a placebo basis.

Patients should be **advised of the fire risks** when receiving oxygen therapy.

OXYGEN CYLINDERS

Oxygen is occasionally prescribed for *intermittent* use for episodes of hypoxaemia of short duration, for example asthma. It is important, however, that the patient does not rely on oxygen instead of obtaining medical help or taking more specific treatment.

Alternatively, intermittent oxygen may be prescribed for patients with advanced irreversible respiratory disorders to increase mobility and capacity for exercise and to ease discomfort, for example in chronic obstructive bronchitis, emphysema, widespread fibrosis, and primary or thromboembolic pulmonary hypertension. Appropriate patients may be prescribed portable equipment through the hospital service, refillable from cylinders in the home.

Under the NHS oxygen may be supplied by chemist contractors as cylinders. Oxygen flow can be adjusted as the cylinders are equipped with an oxygen flow meter with 'medium' (2 litres/minute) and 'high' (4 litres/minute) settings. The FHSAs have lists of pharmacy contractors who provide domiciliary oxygen services.

Patients are supplied with either constant or variable performance masks. The Intersurgical 010 28% or Ventimask Mk 4 28% are constant performance masks and provide a nearly constant supply of oxygen (28%) over a wide range irrespective of the patient's breathing pattern. The variable performance masks include the Intersurgical 005 Mask, the MC Mask, and the Venticaire mask; the concentration of oxygen supplied to the patient varies with the rate of flow of oxygen and also with the patient's breathing pattern.

OXYGEN CONCENTRATORS

Long-term administration of oxygen (at least 15 hours daily) may prolong survival in patients with severe chronic obstructive airways disease with cor pulmonale.

Department of Health guidelines suggest that this treatment should be provided for patients who fulfil the following criteria:

$P_aO_2 < 7.3$ kPa; $P_aCO_2 > 6$ kPa;
$FEV_1 < 1.5$ litre and $FVC < 2$ litre

The measurements should be stable on two occasions at least three weeks apart after the patient has received appropriate bronchodilator therapy.

Less information is available on long-term oxygen in patients with a similar degree of hypoxaemia and airflow obstruction but no hypercapnia; the Department of Health suggests that these patients should not be denied this form of treatment but the effects of long-term therapy have not yet been assessed completely.

Increased respiratory depression from low concentrations of oxygen is seldom a problem in patients with stable respiratory failure although it may occur during exacerbations; patients and relatives should be warned to call for medical help if drowsiness or confusion occur.

Oxygen concentrators are more economical for patients requiring oxygen for long periods, and in England and Wales are now prescribable on the NHS on a regional tendering basis (see below). A concentrator was formerly only provided for a patient who required oxygen for 15 hours a day but it has been found to be cost-effective to provide one for a patient requiring it for 8 hours a day (or 21 cylinders per month).

Cautionary label wordings, see inside back cover

PRESCRIBING ARRANGEMENTS FOR OXYGEN CONCENTRATORS

Prescribe concentrator and accessories (face mask, nasal cannula, and humidifier) on form FP10. Specify amount of oxygen required (hours per day) and flow rate. If required, prescribe back-up oxygen set and cylinder at same time. Inform patient that the supplier will be in contact to make arrangements and that the prescription form is to be given to the person who installs the concentrator.

Inform supplier by telephone (see table below) that a concentrator has been prescribed. The supplier will send written confirmation of the order to the prescriber, the patient, and the FHSA.

Follow the same procedure if a back-up oxygen set and cylinder are required later.

FHSA regional group	Supplier
Eastern North Western London North Wales West Midlands	DeVilbiss Health Care Ltd *to order:* Dial 100 *and ask for:* Freephone Oxygen Concentrator
London South (includes Kent, Surrey, and Sussex)	Omnicare Health Group Ltd *to order:* Dial 100 *and ask for:* Freephone Omnicare Oxygen
Northern South Western Yorkshire (South and West) and Humberside	Oxygen Therapy Co Ltd *to order:* Dial 0800 373580

In **Scotland** refer the patient for assessment by a respiratory consultant. If the need for a concentrator is confirmed the consultant will arrange for the provision of a concentrator through the Common Services Agency.

3.7 Mucolytics

Mucolytics are often prescribed to facilitate expectoration by reducing sputum viscosity in chronic asthma and bronchitis. Few patients, however, have been shown to derive much benefit from them although they do render sputum less viscid. Steam inhalation with postural drainage, is good expectorant therapy in bronchiectasis and some chronic bronchitics.

ACETYLCYSTEINE

Indications: reduction of sputum viscosity
Side-effects: occasional gastro-intestinal irritation, headache, urticaria, tinnitus, and sensitivity
Dose: adults and children over 6 years, 200 mg in water 3 times daily, usually for 5–10 days but if necessary may be extended to 6 months or longer; CHILD up to 2 years 200 mg daily, 2–6 years 200 mg twice daily

Prices are **net**, see p. 1

NHS * PoM **Acetylcysteine Granules,** acetylcysteine 200 mg/sachet. Net price 30 sachets = £5.75. Label: 13
* except for abdominal complications associated with cystic fibrosis and endorsed 'SLS' ('S2B' in Scotland)
Note. The brand name NHS Fabrol® (Zyma) is used for acetylcysteine granules

CARBOCISTEINE
Indications: reduction of sputum viscosity
Side-effects: occasional gastro-intestinal irritation, rashes
Dose: 750 mg 3 times daily initially, then 1.5 g daily in divided doses; CHILD 2–5 years 62.5–125 mg 4 times daily, 6–12 years 250 mg 3 times daily

NHS *PoM **Carbocisteine Capsules,** carbocisteine 375 mg. Net price 30-cap pack = £3.20
NHS *PoM **Carbocisteine Syrup,** carbocisteine 125 mg/5 mL, net price 300 mL = £3.50; 250 mg/5 mL, 300 mL = £4.50
* except, for patients under the age of 18 years, any condition which, through damage or disease, affects the airways and has required a tracheostomy and endorsed 'SLS' ('S2B' in Scotland)
Note. The brand name NHS Mucodyne® (Rhône-Poulenc Rorer) is used for carbocisteine preparations; capsules and 250 mg/5 mL strength of syrup contain tartrazine

METHYLCYSTEINE HYDROCHLORIDE
Indications: reduction of sputum viscosity
Dose: 100–200 mg 3–4 times daily before meals reduced to 200 mg twice daily after 6 weeks; CHILD over 5 years 100 mg 3 times daily
Prophylaxis, 100–200 mg 2–3 times every other day during winter months

NHS **Visclair**® (Sinclair)
Tablets, yellow, s/c, e/c, methylcysteine hydrochloride 100 mg. Net price 20 = £3.43. Label: 5, 22, 25

3.8 Aromatic inhalations

Inhalations containing volatile substances such as eucalyptus oil are traditionally used and although the vapour may contain little of the additive it encourages deliberate inspiration of warm moist air which is often comforting in bronchitis; boiling water should not be used owing to the risk of scalding. Inhalations are also used for the relief of nasal obstruction in acute rhinitis or sinusitis.

CHILDREN. The use of strong aromatic decongestants (applied as rubs or to pillows) is not advised for infants under the age of 3 months. Mothers with young infants in whom nasal obstruction with mucus is a problem can readily be taught appropriate techniques of suction aspiration.

Benzoin Tincture, Compound, BP, Friars' Balsam, balsamic acids approx. 4.5%. Label: 15
Directions for use: add one teaspoonful to a pint of hot, **not** boiling, water and inhale the vapour

NHS **Menthol and Benzoin Inhalation, BP,** menthol 2 g, benzoin inhalation to 100 mL. Label: 15
Directions for use: add one teaspoonful to a pint of hot, **not** boiling, water and inhale the vapour

Menthol and Eucalyptus Inhalation, BP 1980, menthol 2 g, eucalyptus oil 10 mL, light magnesium carbonate 7 g, water to 100 mL
Directions for use: add one teaspoonful to a pint of hot, **not** boiling, water and inhale the vapour

NHS **Karvol**® (Crookes)
Inhalation capsules, menthol 35.33 mg, with chlorbutol, pine oils, terpineol, and thymol. Net price 10 = 86p
Directions for use: inhale vapour from contents of 1 capsule expressed into handkerchief or a pint of hot, **not** boiling, water; avoid in infants under 3 months

3.9 Antitussives

3.9.1 Cough suppressants
3.9.2 Expectorant, demulcent, and compound cough preparations

3.9.1 Cough suppressants

The drawbacks of prescribing cough suppressants are rarely outweighed by the benefits of treatment and only occasionally are they useful, as, for example, if sleep is disturbed by a dry cough. Cough suppressants may cause sputum retention and this may be harmful in patients with chronic bronchitis and bronchiectasis.

Opioid cough suppressants such as codeine, dextromethorphan, and pholcodine are seldom sufficiently potent to be effective in severe cough; all tend to cause constipation.

Sedative antihistamines, such as diphenhydramine, are used as the cough suppressant component of many compound cough preparations on sale to the public; all tend to cause drowsiness which may reflect their main mode of action.

CHILDREN. The use of cough suppressants containing codeine or similar opioid analgesics is not generally recommended in children and should be avoided altogether in those under 1 year of age.

CODEINE PHOSPHATE
Indications: dry or painful cough
Cautions: asthma; hepatic and renal impairment; history of drug abuse; see also notes above and section 4.7.2; **interactions:** Appendix 1 (opioid analgesics)
Contra-indications: liver disease, ventilatory failure
Side-effects: constipation, in large doses respiratory depression

PoM[1] **Codeine Linctus, BP,** codeine phosphate 15 mg/5 mL. Net price 100 mL = 35p (diabetic, 63p)
Dose: 5–10 mL 3–4 times daily; CHILD 5–12 years, 2.5–5 mL
Available from APS, Evans, Galen (Galcodine®, sugar-free), Kerfoot

1. Can be sold to the public provided the maximum single dose does not exceed 5 mL

3.9 Antitussives

Note. Addendum 1991 to BP 1988 directs that when Diabetic Codeine Linctus is prescribed, Codeine Linctus formulated with a vehicle appropriate for administration to diabetics, whether or not labelled 'Diabetic Codeine Linctus', shall be dispensed or supplied

Codeine Linctus, Paediatric, BP, codeine phosphate 3 mg/5 mL. Net price 100 mL = 18p
Dose: CHILD 1–5 years 5 mL 3–4 times daily
Available from Evans, Galen (Galcodine®, sugar-free)
Note. Sugar-free versions are available
Paediatric Codeine Linctus may be prepared extemporaneously by diluting Codeine Linctus with a suitable vehicle in accordance with the manufacturer's instructions

DEXTROMETHORPHAN
Indications: dry or painful cough
Cautions; Contra-indications; Side-effects: see under Codeine Phosphate

Preparations
Ingredient of compound cough preparations (section 3.9.2)
Note. A proprietary brand of dextromethorphan modified-release capsules (NHS Coughcaps®) is on sale to the public

ISOAMINILE CITRATE
Indications: dry or painful cough
Cautions: see notes above
Side-effects: occasionally constipation, dizziness, nausea
Dose: see below

PoM **Isoaminile Linctus,** isoaminile citrate 40 mg/5 mL. Net price 150 mL = £1.88
Dose: 5 mL 3–5 times daily; CHILD, 2.5–5 mL
The brand name NHS Dimyril® (Fisons) is used for isoaminile linctus

PHOLCODINE
Indications: dry or painful cough
Cautions; Contra-indications; Side-effects: see under Codeine Phosphate

Pholcodine Linctus, BP, pholcodine 5 mg/5 mL in a suitable flavoured vehicle, containing citric acid monohydrate 1%. Net price 100 mL = 29p
Dose: 5–10 mL 3–4 times daily; CHILD 5–12 years 2.5–5 mL
Available from APS, Boehringer Ingelheim (Pavacol-D®, sugar-free), Evans, Galen (Galenphol®, sugar-free), Kerfoot, Medo (NHS Pholcomed D®, sugar-free)

Pholcodine Linctus, Strong, BP, pholcodine 10 mg/5 mL in a suitable flavoured vehicle, containing citric acid monohydrate 2%. Net price 100 mL = 49p
Dose: 5 mL 3–4 times daily
Available from APS, Evans, Kerfoot, Medo (NHS Pholcomed Diabetic Forte®, sugar-free)

Galenphol® (Galen)
Paediatric linctus, orange, sugar-free, pholcodine 2 mg/5 mL. Diluent as above. Net price 100 mL = 17p
Dose: CHILD 1–5 years 5 mL 3 times daily; 6–12 years 5–10 mL
Note. A proprietary brand of pholcodine pastilles (NHS Pholcomed®) is on sale to the public

TERMINAL CARE

Diamorphine and methadone are available in linctuses to control distressful cough in terminal lung cancer although morphine is now preferred (see Terminal Care, p. 12). In other circumstances they are contra-indicated because they induce sputum retention and ventilatory failure as well as causing opioid dependence.

DIAMORPHINE HYDROCHLORIDE
Indications: cough in terminal disease
Cautions; Contra-indications; Side-effects: see notes in section 4.7.2; more potent than morphine
Dose: see below

CD **Diamorphine Linctus, BPC 1973,** diamorphine hydrochloride 3 mg, oxymel 1.25 mL, glycerol 1.25 mL, compound tartrazine solution 0.06 mL, syrup to 5 mL. It should be recently prepared. Label: 2
Dose: 2.5–10 mL every 4 hours

METHADONE HYDROCHLORIDE
Indications: cough in terminal disease
Cautions; Contra-indications; Side-effects: see notes in section 4.7.2; longer-acting than morphine therefore effects may be cumulative
Dose: see below

CD **Methadone Linctus,** methadone hydrochloride 2 mg/5 mL in a suitable vehicle with a tolu flavour. Label: 2
Dose: 2.5–5 mL every 4–6 hours, reduced to twice daily on prolonged use

MORPHINE HYDROCHLORIDE
Indications: cough in terminal disease (see also p. 12)
Cautions; Contra-indications; Side-effects: see notes in section 4.7.2
Dose: initially 5 mg every 4 hours

Preparations
See section 4.7.2

3.9.2 Expectorant, demulcent, and compound cough preparations

Expectorants are claimed to promote expulsion of bronchial secretions but there is no evidence that any drug can specifically facilitate expectoration. The assumption that sub-emetic doses of expectorants, such as ammonium chloride, ipecacuanha, and squill promote expectoration is a myth. However, a simple expectorant mixture may serve a useful placebo function and has the advantage of being inexpensive.

Demulcent cough preparations contain soothing substances such as syrup or glycerol and certainly some patients believe that such preparations relieve a dry irritating cough. Preparations such as **simple linctus** have the advantage of being harmless and inexpensive; **paediatric simple**

136 Chapter 3: Respiratory system

linctus is particularly useful in children, but it has a high sugar content.

Compound cough preparations are on sale to the public; the rationale for some is dubious.

CHILDREN. The use of cough suppressants containing codeine or similar opioid analgesics is not generally recommended in children and should be avoided altogether in those under 1 year of age.

NHS **Ammonia and Ipecacuanha Mixture, BP,** ammonium bicarbonate 200 mg, liquorice liquid extract 0.5 mL, ipecacuanha tincture 0.3 mL, concentrated camphor water 0.1 mL, concentrated anise water 0.05 mL, double-strength chloroform water 5 mL, water to 10 mL. It should be recently prepared
Dose: 10–20 mL 3–4 times daily

NHS **Ammonium Chloride and Morphine Mixture, BP,** ammonium chloride 300 mg, ammonium bicarbonate 200 mg, chloroform and morphine tincture 0.3 mL, liquorice liquid extract 0.5 mL, water to 10 mL. It should be recently prepared. Contains 500 micrograms of anhydrous morphine in 10 mL
Dose: 10–20 mL 3–4 times daily

NHS **Ipecacuanha and Morphine Mixture BP, 1980,** ipecacuanha tincture 0.2 mL, chloroform and morphine tincture 0.4 mL, liquorice liquid extract 1 mL, water to 10 mL. It should be recently prepared. 10 mL contains 700 micrograms of anhydrous morphine
Dose: 10 mL 3–4 times daily

Simple Linctus, BP, citric acid monohydrate 125 mg, concentrated anise water 0.05 mL, chloroform spirit 0.3 mL, amaranth solution 0.075 mL, syrup to 5 mL. Net price 100 mL = 16p
Dose: 5 mL 3–4 times daily

Simple Linctus, Paediatric, BP, simple linctus 1.25 mL, syrup to 5 mL. Net price 100 mL = 17p
Dose: CHILD, 5–10 mL 3–4 times daily

NHS **Squill Linctus, Opiate, BP,** Gee's Linctus, equal volumes of camphorated opium tincture, squill oxymel, and tolu syrup. It contains 800 micrograms of anhydrous morphine in 5 mL
Dose: 5 mL 3–4 times daily

Tolu Linctus, Compound, Paediatric, citric acid monohydrate 30 mg/5 mL in a suitable vehicle with a tolu flavour
Dose: CHILD, 5–10 mL 3–4 times daily

NHS **Actifed Compound Linctus**® (Wellcome)
Linctus, dextromethorphan hydrobromide, pseudoephedrine hydrochloride, triprolidine hydrochloride. Net price 100 mL = £1.23; 200 mL = £1.98. Label: 2

NHS **Actifed Expectorant**® (Wellcome)
Elixir, guaiphenesin, pseudoephedrine hydrochloride, triprolidine hydrochloride. Net price 100 mL = £1.23; 200 mL = £1.98. Label: 2

NHS **Benylin Chesty Cough Linctus**[1]® (W-L)
Syrup, diphenhydramine hydrochloride, ammonium chloride, menthol. Net price 125 mL = £1.44; 300 mL = £2.85. Label: 2
1. Has replaced Benylin Expectorant

NHS **Benylin Childrens Cough Linctus**[2]® (W-L)
Syrup, diphenhydramine hydrochloride, menthol. Net price 125 mL = £1.32. Label: 1
2. Has replaced Benylin Paediatric

NHS **Benylin with Codeine**® (W-L)
Syrup, codeine phosphate, diphenhydramine hydrochloride, menthol, sodium citrate. Net price 300 mL = £3.24. Label: 2

NHS **Benylin Dry Cough Linctus**[3]® (W-L)
Syrup, diphenhydramine hydrochloride, dextromethorphan hydrobromide, menthol. Net price 125 mL = £1.37. Label: 2
3. Has replaced Benylin Fortified

NHS **Benylin Mentholated Linctus**® (W-L)
Syrup, diphenhydramine hydrochloride, dextromethorphan hydrobromide, pseudoephedrine hydrochloride, menthol. Net price 125 mL = £1.37. Label: 2

NHS **Copholco**® (Fisons)
Linctus, pholcodine, cineole, menthol, terpin hydrate. Net price 100 mL = £1.05

NHS **Davenol**® (Whitehall)
Linctus, carbinoxamine maleate, ephedrine hydrochloride, pholcodine. Net price 100 mL = 46p. Label: 2

NHS **Dimotane Expectorant**® (Whitehall)
Elixir, brompheniramine maleate, guaiphenesin, pseudoephedrine hydrochloride. Net price 100 mL = £1.31. Label: 2

NHS **Dimotane Co**® (Whitehall)
Elixir, brompheniramine maleate, codeine phosphate, pseudoephedrine hydrochloride. Net price 100 mL = £1.31. Label: 2

NHS **Dimotane Co Paediatric**® (Whitehall)
Elixir, brompheniramine maleate, codeine phosphate, pseudoephedrine hydrochloride. Net price 100 mL = £1.28. Label: 1

NHS **Expulin**® (Galen)
Linctus, chlorpheniramine maleate, pseudoephedrine hydrochloride, pholcodine, menthol. Net price 100 mL = £1.14. Label: 2
Paediatric linctus, chlorpheniramine maleate, pholcodine, menthol. Net price 100 mL = £1.10. Label: 1

NHS **Guanor Expectorant**® (RP Drugs)
Syrup, ammonium chloride, diphenhydramine hydrochloride, menthol, sodium citrate. Net price 200 mL = £1.25. Label: 2

NHS **Histalix**® (Wallace Mfg)
Syrup, ammonium chloride, diphenhydramine hydrochloride, menthol, sodium citrate. Net price 150 mL = £1.14. Label: 2

NHS **Phensedyl**® (Rhône-Poulenc Rorer)
Linctus, codeine phosphate, promethazine hydrochloride. Net price 100 mL = £1.43. Label: 2

NHS **Sudafed Expectorant**® (Wellcome)
Syrup, guaiphenesin, pseudoephedrine hydrochloride. Net price 100 mL = £1.23

NHS **Sudafed Linctus**® (Wellcome)
Linctus, dextromethorphan hydrobromide, pseudoephedrine hydrochloride. Net price 100 mL = £1.23. Label: 2

NHS **Tancolin**® (Ashe)
Linctus (paediatric), ascorbic acid, citric acid, dextromethorphan hydrobromide, glycerol, sodium citrate. Net price 100 mL = £1.22

NHS **Terpoin**® (Hough)
Elixir, codeine phosphate with cineole and menthol. Net price 225 mL = £3.28

NHS **Tixylix**® (Intercare)
Linctus, pholcodine (as citrate), promethazine hydrochloride. Net price 100 mL = £1.28. Label: 1 *or* 2

3.10 Systemic nasal decongestants

These preparations are of doubtful value but unlike the preparations for local application (see section 12.2.2) they do not give rise to rebound nasal congestion. They contain sympathomimetics, and should therefore be **avoided** in

3.10 Systemic nasal decongestants

patients with hypertension, hyperthyroidism, coronary heart disease, or diabetes, and in patients taking monoamine-oxidase inhibitors; **interactions:** Appendix 1 (sympathomimetics). Many of the preparations also contain antihistamines which may cause drowsiness and affect ability to drive or operate machinery.

NHS **Actifed**® (Wellcome)
Tablets, pseudoephedrine hydrochloride, triprolidine hydrochloride. Net price 12-tab pack = 94p. Label: 2
Syrup, pseudoephedrine hydrochloride, triprolidine hydrochloride. Net price 100 mL = £1.11. Label: 2

Dimotane Plus® (Wyeth)
Liquid, brown, sugar-free, brompheniramine maleate 4 mg, pseudoephedrine hydrochloride 30 mg/5 mL. Net price 100 mL = 81p. Label: 2
Dose: 10 mL 3 times daily; CHILD 2–6 years 2.5 mL, 6–12 years 5 mL
Paediatric liquid, brown, sugar-free, brompheniramine maleate 2 mg, pseudoephedrine hydrochloride 15 mg/5 mL. Net price 100 mL = 74p. Label: 1
Dose: CHILD 2–6 years 5 mL, 6–12 years 10 mL, 3 times daily

PoM **Dimotane**® **Plus LA** (Wyeth)
Tablets, m/r, f/c, brompheniramine maleate 12 mg, pseudoephedrine hydrochloride 120 mg. Net price 56-tab pack = £3.09. Label: 2, 25
Dose: 1 tablet twice daily

NHS **Dimotapp**® (Whitehall)
Elixir, brompheniramine maleate, phenylephrine hydrochloride, phenylpropanolamine hydrochloride. Net price 100 mL = £1.19. Label: 2
Paediatric elixir, brompheniramine maleate, phenylephrine hydrochloride, phenylpropanolamine hydrochloride. Net price 100 mL = £1.13. Label: 1

NHS **Dimotapp LA**® (Whitehall)
Tablets, brompheniramine maleate, phenylephrine hydrochloride, phenylpropanolamine hydrochloride. Net price 30 = £2.45. Label: 2, 25, counselling, gluten

NHS **Eskornade**® (SK&F)
Spansule® (= capsules m/r), diphenylpyraline hydrochloride, phenylpropanolamine hydrochloride. Net price 30-cap pack = £3.02. Label: 2, 25
Syrup, diphenylpyraline hydrochloride, phenylpropanolamine hydrochloride. Net price 150 mL = £3.11. Label: 2

NHS **Expurhin**® (Galen)
Paediatric linctus, chlorpheniramine maleate, ephedrine hydrochloride, menthol. Net price 100 mL = £1.10. Label: 1

Galpseud® (Galen)
Tablets, pseudoephedrine hydrochloride 60 mg. Net price 20 = 72p
Dose: 1 tablet 3 times daily
Linctus, orange, sugar-free, pseudoephedrine hydrochloride 30 mg/5 mL. Net price 100 mL = 57p
Dose: 10 mL 3 times daily; CHILD 2–6 years 2.5 mL, 6–12 years 5 mL

Haymine® (Pharmax)
Tablets, m/r, yellow, chlorpheniramine maleate 10 mg, ephedrine hydrochloride 15 mg. Net price 30-tab pack = £2.79. Label: 2, 25
Dose: 1 tablet 1–2 times daily

Sudafed® (Wellcome)
Tablets, red, f/c, pseudoephedrine hydrochloride 60 mg. Net price 20 = £1.17
Dose: 1 tablet 3 times daily
Elixir, pink, pseudoephedrine hydrochloride 30 mg/5 mL. Net price 100 mL = 94p
Dose: 10 mL 3 times daily; CHILD 2–5 years 2.5 mL, 6–12 years 5 mL

Sudafed Plus® (Wellcome)
Tablets, pseudoephedrine hydrochloride 60 mg, triprolidine hydrochloride 2.5 mg. Net price 100-tab pack = £6.49. Label: 2
Dose: 1 tablet 3 times daily
Syrup, yellow, pseudoephedrine hydrochloride 30 mg, triprolidine hydrochloride 1.25 mg/5 mL. Net price 100 mL = £1·06. Label: 2
Dose: 10 mL 3 times daily; CHILD 2–5 years 2.5 mL 3 times daily, 6–12 years 5 mL 3 times daily

PoM **Sudafed SA**® (Wellcome)
Capsules, m/r, red/clear, pseudoephedrine hydrochloride 120 mg. Net price 20 = £1.44. Label: 25
Dose: 1 capsule every 12 hours

NHS **Sudafed-Co**® (Wellcome)
Tablets, paracetamol, pseudoephedrine hydrochloride. Net price 12-tab pack = 99p

NHS **Triogesic**® (Beecham)
Tablets, paracetamol, phenylpropanolamine hydrochloride. Net price 30-tab pack = £1.77

NHS **Triominic**® (Beecham)
Tablets, pheniramine maleate, phenylpropanolamine hydrochloride. Net price 30-tab pack = £1.77. Label: 2

NHS **Uniflu with Gregovite C**® (Unigreg)
Tablets, composite pack of pairs of tablets: Uniflu *tablets*, caffeine, codeine phosphate, diphenhydramine hydrochloride, paracetamol, phenylephrine hydrochloride; Gregovite C *tablets*, ascorbic acid. Net price 6 of each tablet = £1.38; or 12 of each tablet = £2.30. Label: 2
Dose: 1 of each tablet every 6 hours

Cautionary label wordings, see inside back cover

Prices are **net**, see p. 1

4: Drugs acting on the
CENTRAL NERVOUS SYSTEM

In this chapter, drug treatments are discussed under the following headings:

- **4.1** Hypnotics and anxiolytics
- **4.2** Drugs used in psychoses and related disorders
- **4.3** Antidepressant drugs
- **4.4** Central nervous stimulants
- **4.5** Appetite suppressants
- **4.6** Drugs used in nausea and vertigo
- **4.7** Analgesics
- **4.8** Antiepileptics
- **4.9** Drugs used in parkinsonism and related disorders
- **4.10** Drugs used in substance dependence

4.1 Hypnotics and anxiolytics

- **4.1.1** Hypnotics
- **4.1.2** Anxiolytics
- **4.1.3** Barbiturates

Most anxiolytics ('sedatives') will induce sleep when given in large doses at night and most hypnotics will sedate when given in divided doses during the day. Prescribing of these drugs is widespread but dependence (either physical or psychological) and tolerance to their effects occurs. This may lead to difficulty in withdrawing the drug after the patient has been taking it regularly for more than a few weeks (see Dependence and Withdrawal, below). Hypnotics and anxiolytics should not therefore be prescribed indiscriminately and should, instead, be reserved for short courses to alleviate acute conditions after causal factors have been established.

Prescribing of more than one anxiolytic or hypnotic at the same time is **not** recommended. It may constitute a hazard and there is no evidence that side-effects are minimised.

Benzodiazepines are the most commonly used anxiolytics and hypnotics; they act at benzodiazepine receptors which are associated with gamma-aminobutyric acid (GABA) receptors. Barbiturates (section 4.1.3) are no longer recommended.

Benzodiazepines have fewer side-effects than barbiturates and are much less dangerous in overdosage. They are also less likely to interact with other drugs because, unlike barbiturates, they do not induce liver microsomal enzymes.

A paradoxical increase in hostility and aggression may be reported by patients taking benzodiazepines. The effects range from talkativeness and excitement, to aggressive and antisocial acts. Adjustment of the dose (up or down) usually attenuates the impulses. Increased anxiety and perceptual disorders are other paradoxical effects. Increased hostility and aggression after barbiturates and alcohol usually indicates intoxication.

DEPENDENCE AND WITHDRAWAL. The benzodiazepine withdrawal syndrome may not develop until up to 3 weeks after stopping a long-acting benzodiazepine, but may occur within a few hours in the case of a short-acting one. It is characterised by insomnia, anxiety, loss of appetite and body weight, tremor, perspiration, tinnitus, and perceptual disturbances. These symptoms may be similar to the original complaint and encourage further prescribing; some symptoms may continue for weeks or months after stopping benzodiazepines entirely.

Withdrawal of a benzodiazepine should be gradual as abrupt withdrawal may produce confusion, toxic psychosis, convulsions, or a condition resembling delirium tremens.

DRIVING. Hypnotics and anxiolytics may impair judgement and increase reaction time, and so affect ability to drive or operate machinery; they increase the effects of alcohol. Moreover the hangover effects of a night dose may impair driving on the following day.

BENZODIAZEPINE WITHDRAWAL

A suggested protocol for patients unable to reduce existing benzodiazepine[1]:
1. Transfer patient to equivalent daily dose of diazepam[2] preferably taken at night
2. Reduce diazepam dose in fortnightly steps of 2 or 2.5 mg; if withdrawal symptoms occur, maintain this dose until symptoms improve
3. Reduce dose further, if necessary in smaller fortnightly steps[3]; it is better to reduce too slowly rather than too quickly
4. Stop completely; time needed for withdrawal can vary from about 4 weeks to a year or more

Counselling may help; beta-blockers should **only** be tried if other measures fail; antidepressants should **only** be used if clinical depression present; **avoid** antipsychotics (which may aggravate withdrawal symptoms)

---

1. Existing benzodiazepines can be withdrawn in steps of about $\frac{1}{8}$ (range $\frac{1}{10}$–$\frac{1}{4}$) of daily dose every fortnight
2. Approximate equivalent doses, diazepam 5 mg
   - ≡ chlordiazepoxide 15 mg
   - ≡ lorazepam 500 micrograms
   - ≡ nitrazepam 5 mg
   - ≡ oxazepam 15 mg
   - ≡ temazepam 10 mg
   - ≡ triazolam 125–250 micrograms
3. Steps may be adjusted according to initial dose and duration of treatment and can range from diazepam 500 micrograms ($\frac{1}{4}$ of a 2-mg tablet) to 2.5 mg

> **CSM advice.**
> 1. Benzodiazepines are indicated for the short-term relief (two to four weeks only) of anxiety that is severe, disabling or subjecting the individual to unacceptable distress, occurring alone or in association with insomnia or short-term psychosomatic, organic or psychotic illness.
> 2. The use of benzodiazepines to treat short-term 'mild' anxiety is inappropriate and unsuitable.
> 3. Benzodiazepines should be used to treat insomnia only when it is severe, disabling, or subjecting the individual to extreme distress.

4.1.1 Hypnotics

Before a hypnotic is prescribed the cause of the insomnia should be established and, where possible, underlying factors should be treated. However, it should be noted that some patients have unrealistic sleep expectations, and others understate their alcohol consumption which is often the cause of the insomnia.

Transient insomnia may occur in those who normally sleep well and may be due to extraneous factors such as noise, shift work, and jet lag. If a hypnotic is indicated one that is rapidly eliminated should be chosen, and only one or two doses should be given.

Short-term insomnia is usually related to an emotional problem or serious medical illness. It may last for a few weeks, and may recur; a hypnotic can be useful but should not be given for more than three weeks (preferably only one week). Intermittent use is desirable with omission of some doses. A rapidly eliminated drug is generally appropriate.

Chronic insomnia is rarely benefited by hypnotics and is more often due to mild dependence caused by injudicious prescribing. Psychiatric disorders such as anxiety, depression, and abuse of drugs and alcohol are common causes. Sleep disturbance is very common in depressive illness and early wakening is often a useful pointer. The underlying psychiatric complaint should be treated, adapting the drug regimen to alleviate insomnia. For example, amitriptyline, prescribed for depression, will also help to promote sleep if it is taken at night. Other causes of insomnia include daytime cat-napping and physical causes such as pain, pruritus, and dyspnoea.

Hypnotics should **not** be prescribed indiscriminately and routine prescribing is undesirable. Ideally, they should be reserved for short courses in the acutely distressed. Tolerance to their effects develops within 3 to 14 days of continuous use and long-term efficacy cannot be assured. A major drawback of long-term use is that withdrawal causes rebound insomnia and precipitates a withdrawal syndrome (section 4.1).

Where prolonged administration is unavoidable hypnotics should be discontinued as soon as feasible and the patient warned that sleep may be disturbed for a few days before normal rhythm is re-established; broken sleep with vivid dreams and increased REM (rapid eye movement) may persist for several weeks. This represents a mild form of dependence even if clinical doses are used.

CHILDREN. The prescribing of hypnotics to children, except for occasional use such as for night terrors and somnambulism (sleep-walking), is not justified.

ELDERLY. Hypnotics should be avoided in the elderly, who are at risk of becoming ataxic and confused and so liable to fall and injure themselves.

BENZODIAZEPINES

Benzodiazepines used as hypnotics include **nitrazepam**, **flunitrazepam**, and **flurazepam** which have a prolonged action and may give rise to residual effects on the following day; repeated doses tend to be cumulative.

Loprazolam, **lormetazepam**, and **temazepam** act for a shorter time and they have little or no hangover effect. Withdrawal phenomena however are more common with the short-acting benzodiazepines.

Benzodiazepine anxiolytics such as **diazepam** given as a single dose at night may also be used as hypnotics.

For general guidelines on benzodiazepine prescribing see section 4.1.2 and for benzodiazepine withdrawal see section 4.1.

NITRAZEPAM

Indications: insomnia (short-term use)

Cautions: respiratory disease, muscle weakness, history of drug abuse, marked personality disorder, pregnancy, breast-feeding; reduce dose in elderly and debilitated, and in hepatic and renal impairment; avoid prolonged use (and abrupt withdrawal thereafter); **interactions:** Appendix 1 (benzodiazepines)
  DRIVING. Drowsiness may persist the next day and affect performance of skilled tasks (e.g. driving); effects of alcohol enhanced

Contra-indications: respiratory depression; acute pulmonary insufficiency; phobic or obsessional states, chronic psychosis; porphyria (see section 9.8.2)

Side-effects: drowsiness and lightheadedness the next day; confusion and ataxia (especially in the elderly); dependence; see also under Diazepam (section 4.1.2); overdosage: see Emergency Treatment of Poisoning, p. 19.

Dose: 5–10 mg at bedtime; ELDERLY (or debilitated) 2.5–5 mg

PoM **Nitrazepam** (Non-proprietary)
Tablets, nitrazepam 5 mg, net price 20 = 7p. Label: 19
Available from APS, Cox, CP, DDSA (NHS Remnos®), Evans, Kerfoot, Roche (NHS Mogadon®), Unigreg (NHS Unisomnia®)
Oral suspension, nitrazepam 2.5 mg/5 mL. Net price 150 mL = £3.74. Label: 19
Available from Norgine (NHS Somnite®)
NHS *Capsules,* nitrazepam 5 mg. Net price 20 = £1·04. Label: 19
Available from Roche (NHS Mogadon®)

FLUNITRAZEPAM

Indications: insomnia (short-term use)
Cautions; Contra-indications; Side-effects: see under Nitrazepam
Dose: 0.5–1 mg at bedtime; max. 2 mg; ELDERLY (or debilitated) 500 micrograms (max. 1 mg)

NHS PoM **Rohypnol**® (Roche)
Tablets, purple, f/c, scored, flunitrazepam 1 mg. Net price 30-tab pack = £3.66. Label: 19

FLURAZEPAM

Indications: insomnia (short-term use)
Cautions; Contra-indications; Side-effects: see under Nitrazepam
Dose: 15–30 mg at bedtime; ELDERLY 15 mg

NHS PoM **Dalmane**® (Roche)
Capsules, flurazepam (as hydrochloride), 15 mg (grey/yellow), net price 30-cap pack = £2.42; 30 mg (black/grey), 30-cap pack = £3.12. Label: 19

LOPRAZOLAM

Indications: insomnia (short-term use)
Cautions; Contra-indications; Side-effects: see under Nitrazepam
Dose: 1 mg at bedtime, increased to 1.5 or 2 mg if required; ELDERLY (or debilitated) 0.5–1 mg

PoM **Loprazolam** (Non-proprietary)
Tablets, loprazolam 1 mg (as mesylate). Net price 28-tab pack = £1.35. Label: 19
Available from Roussel (previously known as NHS Dormonoct®)

LORMETAZEPAM

Indications: insomnia (short-term use)
Cautions; Contra-indications; Side-effects: see under Nitrazepam; shorter acting
Dose: 0.5–1.5 mg at bedtime; ELDERLY (or debilitated) 500 micrograms

PoM **Lormetazepam** (Non-proprietary)
Tablets, lormetazepam 500 micrograms, net price 20 = 53p; 1 mg, 20 = 93p. Label: 19
Available from APS, Cox, Wyeth

TEMAZEPAM

Indications: insomnia (short-term use); see also section 15.1.4.1 for peri-operative use
Cautions; Contra-indications; Side-effects: see under Nitrazepam; shorter acting
Dose: 10–30 mg (severe insomnia, up to 40–60 mg) at bedtime; ELDERLY (or debilitated) 5–15 mg

PoM **Temazepam** (Non-proprietary)
Gel-filled capsules (soft gelatin), temazepam 10 mg, net price 20 = 48p; 15 mg, 20 = 62p; 20 mg, 20 = 84p; 30 mg, 20 = £1.24. Label: 19
Available from APS, Berk, Cox, CP, Evans, Farmitalia Carlo Erba, Kerfoot, Norton, Wyeth; the name NHS Temazepam Gelthix® is used for some gel-filled capsules
Note. Gel-filled capsules may be subject to abuse

Tablets, temazepam 10 mg, net price 20 = 48p; 20 mg, 20 = 84p. Label: 19
Oral solution, temazepam 10 mg/5 mL, net price 300 mL = £8.35. Label: 19

CHLORAL AND DERIVATIVES

Chloral hydrate and chloral derivatives are useful hypnotics for children (but see notes above). There is no convincing evidence that they are particularly useful in the elderly. **Triclofos sodium** causes fewer gastro-intestinal upsets than chloral hydrate.

CHLORAL HYDRATE

Indications: insomnia (short-term use)
Cautions: respiratory disease, history of drug abuse, marked personality disorder, pregnancy, breast-feeding; reduce dose in elderly and debilitated; avoid prolonged use (and abrupt withdrawal thereafter); avoid contact with skin and mucous membranes; **interactions:** Appendix 1 (chloral)
DRIVING. Drowsiness may persist the next day and affect performance of skilled tasks (e.g. driving); effects of alcohol enhanced
Contra-indications: severe cardiac disease, gastritis, marked hepatic or renal impairment
Side-effects: gastric irritation; *occasionally:* rashes, headache, ketonuria, excitement, delirium; dependence and renal damage on prolonged use
Dose: insomnia, 0.5–1 g (max. 2 g) with plenty of water at bedtime; CHILD 30–50 mg/kg up to a max. single dose of 1 g

PoM **Chloral Mixture** (BP)
(Chloral Oral Solution)
Mixture, chloral hydrate 10% in a suitable vehicle. Extemporaneous preparations should be recently prepared according to the following formula: chloral hydrate 1 g, syrup 2 mL, water to 10 mL. Net price 100 mL = 17p. Label: 19, 27
Dose: 5–20 mL; CHILD 1–5 years 2.5–5 mL, 6–12 years 5–10 mL, taken well diluted with water at bedtime

PoM **Chloral Elixir, Paediatric** (BP)
(Chloral Oral Solution, Paediatric)
Elixir, chloral hydrate 4% in a suitable vehicle with a blackcurrant flavour. Extemporaneous preparations should be recently prepared according to the following formula: chloral hydrate 200 mg, water 0.1 mL, blackcurrant syrup 1 mL, syrup to 5 mL. Net price 100 mL = 30p. Label: 1, 27
Dose: up to 1 year 5 mL, taken well diluted with water at bedtime

PoM **Noctec**® (Squibb)
Capsules, red, chloral hydrate 500 mg. Net price 50-cap pack = £1.90. Label: 19, 27
Dose: 1–2 capsules with plenty of water at bedtime (max. 4 capsules); CHILD not recommended

4.1 Hypnotics and anxiolytics

PoM **Welldorm**® (S&N Pharm.)
Tablets, blue-purple, f/c, chloral betaine 707 mg (≡chloral hydrate 414 mg). Net price 30-tab pack = £2.54. Label: 19, 27
Dose: 1–2 tablets with water or milk at bedtime, max. 5 tablets (2 g chloral hydrate) daily
Elixir, red, chloral hydrate 143 mg/5 mL. Net price 150-mL pack = £2.68. Label: 19, 27
Dose: 15–45 mL (0.4–1.3 g chloral hydrate) with water or milk, at bedtime, max. 70 mL (2 g chloral hydrate) daily; CHILD 1–1.75 mL/kg (30–50 mg/kg chloral hydrate), max. 35 mL (1 g chloral hydrate) daily
Note. Previous formulations of Welldorm® Tablets and Elixir contained dichloralphenazone

TRICLOFOS SODIUM

Indications: insomnia (short-term use)
Cautions; Contra-indications; Side-effects: see under Chloral Hydrate; less gastric irritation
Dose: see under preparation below

PoM **Triclofos** (Non-proprietary)
Elixir, triclofos sodium 500 mg/5 mL. Net price 100 mL = £6.10. Label: 19
Dose: 10–20 mL (1–2 g triclofos sodium) at bedtime; CHILD up to 1 year 1–2.5 mL (100–250 mg triclofos sodium), 1–5 years 2.5–5 mL (250–500 mg triclofos sodium), 6–12 years 5–10 mL (0.5–1 g triclofos sodium)

OTHER HYPNOTICS

Chlormethiazole may be a useful hypnotic for elderly patients because of its freedom from hangover but, as with all hypnotics, routine administration is undesirable and dependence occurs occasionally. It is used in the treatment of acute withdrawal symptoms in alcohol dependence but to minimise the risk of dependence administration should be limited to 9 days under inpatient supervision.

Promethazine is popular for use in children (but see notes above).

Zopiclone is a newly introduced hypnotic; although not a benzodiazepine it acts on the same receptors as benzodiazepines. As with other hypnotics it should not be used for long-term treatment.

Alcohol is a poor hypnotic as its diuretic action interferes with sleep during the latter part of the night. With chronic use, alcohol disturbs sleep patterns and causes insomnia; **interactions**: Appendix 1 (alcohol).

CHLORMETHIAZOLE

Indications: see under Dose; also status epilepticus (section 4.8.2), sedation during regional anaesthesia (section 15.1.4.1); eclampsia (see data sheet)
Cautions: cardiac and respiratory disease (confusional state may indicate hypoxia); history of drug abuse; marked personality disorder; pregnancy and breast-feeding; elderly (excessive sedation with higher doses); hepatic impairment (especially if severe since sedation can mask hepatic coma); renal impairment; avoid prolonged use (and abrupt withdrawal thereafter); **interactions**: Appendix 1 (chlormethiazole)
SPECIAL CAUTIONS FOR INTRAVENOUS INFUSION. Resuscitation facilities must be available; maintain clear airway (risk of mechanical obstruction in deep sedation); *rapid infusion* to be given only under direct medical supervision (risk of apnoea and hypotension—special care in those susceptible to cerebral or cardiac complications, e.g. the elderly); during *continuous infusion* sleep induced may lapse into deep unconsciousness and patient must be kept under close and constant observation; *prolonged infusion* may lead to accumulation and delay recovery, may also cause electrolyte imbalance (infusion does not contain electrolytes)
DRIVING. Drowsiness may persist the next day and affect performance of skilled tasks (e.g. driving); effects of alcohol enhanced
Contra-indications: acute pulmonary insufficiency; alcohol-dependent patients who continue to drink
Side-effects: nasal congestion and irritation (with sneezing), conjunctival irritation, headache; gastro-intestinal disturbances; rarely, paradoxical excitement, confusion, dependence; on *intravenous infusion*, localised thrombophlebitis, tachycardia and transient fall in blood pressure (apnoea and hypotension on rapid infusion, see Cautions)
Dose: *by mouth*, severe insomnia in the elderly (short-term use), 1–2 capsules (*or* 5–10 mL syrup) at bedtime
Restlessness and agitation in the elderly, 1 capsule (*or* 5 mL syrup) 3 times daily
Alcohol withdrawal, initially 2–4 capsules, if necessary repeated after some hours;
day 1 (first 24 hours), 9–12 capsules in 3–4 divided doses;
day 2, 6–8 capsules in 3–4 divided doses;
day 3, 4–6 capsules in 3–4 divided doses; then gradually reduced over days 4–6; total treatment for not more than 9 days
Note. For an equivalent therapeutic effect 1 capsule ≡ 5 mL syrup
By intravenous infusion, acute alcohol withdrawal, when oral administration not practicable, as a 0.8% solution, initially 3–7.5 mL (24–60 mg)/minute until shallow sleep induced (from which patient can be easily awakened) then reduced to 0.5–1 mL (4–8 mg)/minute to achieve lowest possible rate to maintain shallow sleep and adequate spontaneous respiration; urgent deep sedation (direct medical supervision only) 40–100 mL (320–800 mg) over 3–5 minutes then reduced to maintenance as indicated above
IMPORTANT. See special cautions for intravenous infusion under Cautions (above).

PoM **Heminevrin**® (Astra)
Capsules, grey-brown, chlormethiazole base 192 mg in an oily basis. Net price 60 = £4.45. Label: 19

Syrup, sugar-free, chlormethiazole edisylate 250 mg/5 mL. Net price 300-mL pack = £3.72. Label: 19

Intravenous infusion 0.8%, chlormethiazole edisylate 8 mg/mL. Net price 500-mL bottle = £5.25

PROMETHAZINE HYDROCHLORIDE
Indications: night sedation and insomnia (short-term use); other indications, see sections 3.4.1, 4.6, 15.1.4.1
Cautions; Side-effects: see section 3.4.1
Dose: by mouth, 25 mg at bedtime increased to 50 mg if necessary; CHILD 1–5 years 15–20 mg (1–2 years on doctors advice only), 5–10 years 20–25 mg, at bedtime

Preparations
See section 3.4.1

ZOPICLONE
Indications: insomnia (short-term use)
Cautions: hepatic impairment; pregnancy and breast-feeding; elderly; history of drug abuse, psychiatric illness; avoid prolonged use (and abrupt withdrawal thereafter); **interactions:** Appendix 1 (zopiclone)
DRIVING. Drowsiness may persist the next day and affect performance of skilled tasks (e.g. driving); effects of alcohol enhanced
Side-effects: bitter or metallic taste; gastro-intestinal disturbances including nausea and vomiting; irritability, confusion, depressed mood; drowsiness, dizziness, lightheadedness, and incoordination on the next day; dependence; rarely urticaria and rashes; hallucinations, amnesia, and behavioural disturbances (including aggression) reported
Dose: 7.5 mg at bedtime increased to 15 mg in severe insomnia; ELDERLY initially 3.75 mg at bedtime

PoM **Zimovane**® (Rhône-Poulenc Rorer)
Tablets, f/c, scored, zopiclone 7.5 mg. Net price 28-tab pack = £27.44. Label: 19

4.1.2 Anxiolytics

Benzodiazepine anxiolytics can be effective in alleviating definite anxiety states and they are widely prescribed. Although there has been a tendency to prescribe these drugs to almost anyone with stress-related symptoms, unhappiness, or minor physical disease, their use in many situations is unjustified. In particular, they should not be used to treat depression, phobic or obsessional states, or chronic psychosis. In bereavement, psychological adjustment may be inhibited by benzodiazepines. In children anxiolytic treatment should be used only to relieve acute anxiety (and related insomnia) caused by fear e.g. before surgery.

Anxiolytic treatment should be limited to the lowest possible dose for the shortest possible time (see CSM advice, section 4.1). Dependence is particularly likely in patients with a history of alcohol or drug abuse and in patients with marked personality disorders.

Anxiolytics, particularly the benzodiazepines, have been termed 'minor tranquillisers'. This term is misleading because not only do they differ markedly from the antipsychotic drugs ('major tranquillisers') but their use is by no means minor. Antipsychotics, in low doses, are also sometimes used in severe anxiety for their sedative action but long-term use should be avoided in view of a possible risk of tardive dyskinesia (section 4.2.1).

BENZODIAZEPINES

Benzodiazepines are indicated for the short-term relief of severe anxiety but long-term use should be avoided (see notes above). Diazepam, alprazolam, bromazepam, chlordiazepoxide, clobazam, clorazepate, and medazepam have a sustained action. Shorter-acting compounds such as **lorazepam** and **oxazepam** may be preferred in patients with hepatic impairment but they carry a greater risk of withdrawal symptoms.

Diazepam or lorazepam are very occasionally administered intravenously for the control of panic attacks. This route is the most rapid but the procedure is not without risk (section 4.8.2) and should be used only when alternative measures have failed. The intramuscular route has no advantage over the oral route.

For guidelines on benzodiazepine withdrawal, see section 4.1.

DIAZEPAM
Indications: short-term use in anxiety or insomnia, adjunct in acute alcohol withdrawal; status epilepticus see section 4.8.2; muscle spasm see section 10.2.2; peri-operative use see section 15.1.4.1
Cautions: respiratory disease, muscle weakness, history of drug abuse, marked personality disorder, pregnancy, breast-feeding; reduce dose in elderly and debilitated, and in hepatic and renal impairment; avoid prolonged use (and abrupt withdrawal thereafter); special precautions for intravenous injection (section 4.8.2); **interactions:** Appendix 1 (benzodiazepines)
DRIVING. Drowsiness may affect performance of skilled tasks (e.g. driving); effects of alcohol enhanced
Contra-indications: respiratory depression; acute pulmonary insufficiency; phobic or obsessional states, chronic psychosis; porphyria (but see section 9.8.2)
Side-effects: drowsiness and lightheadedness the next day; confusion and ataxia (especially in the elderly); amnesia may occur; dependence; *occasionally:* headache, vertigo, hypotension, salivation changes, gastro-intestinal disturbances, rashes, visual disturbances, changes in libido, urinary retention; blood disorders

4.1 Hypnotics and anxiolytics 143

and jaundice reported; on intravenous injection, pain, thrombophlebitis, and rarely apnoea or hypotension; overdosage: see Emergency Treatment of Poisoning, p. 19.

Dose: by mouth, anxiety, 2 mg 3 times daily increased if necessary to 15–30 mg daily in divided doses; ELDERLY (or debilitated) half adult dose

Insomnia associated with anxiety, 5–15 mg at bedtime

CHILD night terrors and somnambulism, 1–5 mg at bedtime

By intramuscular injection or slow intravenous injection (at a rate of not more than 5 mg/minute), for severe anxiety, control of acute panic attacks, and acute alcohol withdrawal, 10 mg, repeated if necessary after 4 hours

Note. Only use intramuscular route when oral and intravenous routes not possible

By intravenous infusion—section 4.8.2

By rectum as rectal solution, for acute anxiety and agitation, adults and children over 3 years 10 mg (elderly 5 mg), repeated after 5 minutes if necessary; CHILD 1–3 years, 5 mg

PoM **Diazepam** (Non-proprietary)
Tablets, diazepam 2 and 5 mg, net price (both), 20 = 2p; 10 mg, 20 = 5p. Label: 2 *or* 19
Available from APS, Berk (NHS Atensine®), Cox, DDSA (NHS Tensium®), Evans, Kerfoot, Rima (NHS Rimapam®), Roche (NHS Valium®)
Oral solution, diazepam 2 mg/5 mL, net price 100 mL = £1.54. Label: 2 *or* 19
Available from Cox, Lagap, Roche (NHS Valium®)
NHS *Strong oral solution*, diazepam 5 mg/5 mL, net price 100-mL pack = £3.30. Label: 2 *or* 19
Available from Lagap
Injection (solution), diazepam 5 mg/mL. Do not dilute (except for intravenous infusion). Net price 2-mL amp = 30p
Available from CP, Roche (Valium®)
Injection (emulsion), diazepam 5 mg/mL. For intravenous injection or infusion. Net price 2-mL amp = 69p
Available from Dumex (Diazemuls®)
Rectal tubes (= rectal solution), diazepam 2 mg/mL, net price 5 × 2.5-mL (5 mg) tubes = £5.78; 4 mg/mL, 5 × 2.5-mL (10 mg) tubes = £7.37
Available from CP (Stesolid®)
Suppositories, diazepam 10 mg, net price 5 = £1.08. Label: 2 *or* 19
Available from Sinclair

ALPRAZOLAM

Indications: anxiety (short-term use)
Cautions; Contra-indications; Side-effects: see under Diazepam
Dose: 250–500 micrograms 3 times daily (elderly or debilitated 250 micrograms 2–3 times daily), increased if necessary to a total of 3 mg daily

NHS PoM **Xanax**® (Upjohn)
Tablets, both scored, alprazolam 250 micrograms, net price 60-tab pack = £2.75; 500 micrograms (pink), 60-tab pack = £5.27. Label: 2

BROMAZEPAM

Indications: anxiety (short-term use)
Cautions; Contra-indications; Side-effects: see under Diazepam
Dose: 3–18 mg daily in divided doses; ELDERLY (or debilitated) half adult dose; max. (in exceptional circumstances in hospitalised patients) 60 mg daily in divided doses

NHS PoM **Lexotan**® (Roche)
Tablets, both scored, bromazepam 1.5 mg (lilac), net price 60-tab pack = £4.90; 3 mg (pink), 60-tab pack = £6.22. Label: 2

CHLORDIAZEPOXIDE

Indications: anxiety (short-term use), adjunct in acute alcohol withdrawal
Cautions; Contra-indications; Side-effects: see under Diazepam
Dose: anxiety, 10 mg 3 times daily increased if necessary to 60–100 mg daily in divided doses; ELDERLY (or debilitated) half adult dose
Note. The doses stated above refer equally to chlordiazepoxide and to its hydrochloride

PoM **Chlordiazepoxide Capsules**, chlordiazepoxide hydrochloride 5 mg, net price 20 = 28p; 10 mg, 20 = 35p. Label: 2
Available from APS, Cox, DDSA (NHS Tropium®), Kerfoot, Norton, Roche (NHS Librium®)
PoM **Chlordiazepoxide Hydrochloride Tablets**, chlordiazepoxide hydrochloride 5 mg, net price 20 = 20p; 10 mg, 20 = 22p; 25 mg, 20 = 44p. Label: 2
PoM **Chlordiazepoxide Tablets**, chlordiazepoxide 5 mg, net price 20 = 28p; 10 mg, 20 = 35p; 25 mg, 20 = 78p. Label: 2
Available from Roche (NHS Librium®)

CLOBAZAM

Indications: anxiety (short-term use); adjunct in epilepsy
Cautions; Contra-indications; Side-effects: see under Diazepam
Dose: anxiety, 20–30 mg daily in divided doses or as a single dose at bedtime, increased in severe anxiety (in hospital patients) to a max. of 60 mg daily in divided doses; ELDERLY (or debilitated) 10–20 mg daily
Epilepsy, 20–30 mg daily; max. 60 mg daily; CHILD over 3 years, not more than half adult dose

NHS ¹PoM **Clobazam** (Non-proprietary)
Capsules, clobazam 10 mg. Net price 30-cap pack = £2.60. Label: 2 *or* 19
1. except for epilepsy and endorsed 'SLS' ('S2B' in Scotland)
Note. The brand name NHS Frisium® (Hoechst) is used for clobazam capsules

Cautionary label wordings, see inside back cover
Prices are **net**, see p. 1

CLORAZEPATE DIPOTASSIUM

Indications: anxiety (short-term use)
Cautions; Contra-indications; Side-effects: see under Diazepam
Dose: 7.5–22.5 mg daily in 2–3 divided doses *or* a single dose of 15 mg at bedtime; ELDERLY (or debilitated) half adult dose

NHS PoM **Tranxene**® (Boehringer Ingelheim)
Capsules, clorazepate dipotassium 7.5 mg (maroon/grey), net price 20-cap pack = £1.97; 15 mg (pink/grey), 20-cap pack = £2.08. Label: 2 *or* 19

LORAZEPAM

Indications: short-term use in anxiety or insomnia; status epilepticus (section 4.8.2); peri-operative (section 15.1.4.1)
Cautions; Contra-indications; Side-effects: see under Diazepam; short acting
Dose: by mouth, anxiety, 1–4 mg daily in divided doses; ELDERLY (or debilitated) half adult dose
Insomnia associated with anxiety, 1–2 mg at bedtime
By intramuscular or slow intravenous injection, acute panic attacks, 25–30 micrograms/kg, repeated every 6 hours if necessary
Note. Only use intramuscular route when oral and intravenous routes not possible

PoM **Lorazepam** (Non-proprietary)
Tablets, lorazepam 1 mg, net price 20 = 24p; 2.5 mg, 20 = 38p. Label: 2 *or* 19
Available from APS, Cox, CP, Evans, Kerfoot, Lagap, Norton, Wyeth (NHS Ativan®)
Injection, lorazepam 4 mg/mL. Net price 1-mL amp = 40p.
For intramuscular injection it should be diluted with an equal volume of water for injections or physiological saline (but only use when oral and intravenous routes not possible)
Available from Wyeth (Ativan®)

MEDAZEPAM

Indications: anxiety (short-term use)
Cautions; Contra-indications; Side-effects: see under Diazepam
Dose: anxiety, 15–30 mg daily in divided doses, increased in severe anxiety to max. 40 mg daily in divided doses; ELDERLY (or debilitated) half adult dose

NHS PoM **Nobrium**® (Roche)
Capsules, orange/yellow, medazepam 5 mg, net price 20 = 62p. Label: 2

OXAZEPAM

Indications: anxiety (short-term use)
Cautions; Contra-indications; Side-effects: see under Diazepam; short acting
Dose: anxiety, 15–30 mg (elderly or debilitated 10–20 mg) 3–4 times daily
Insomnia associated with anxiety, 15–25 mg (max. 50 mg) at bedtime

PoM **Oxazepam** (Non-proprietary)
Tablets, oxazepam 10 mg, net price 20 = 24p; 15 mg, 20 = 27p; 30 mg, 20 = 33p. Label: 2
Available from APS, Berk, Cox, CP, Kerfoot, Norton, Wyeth

OTHER DRUGS FOR ANXIETY

Buspirone is a new drug for the treatment of anxiety; it is thought to act at specific serotonin ($5HT_{1A}$) receptors. Response to treatment may take up to 2 weeks. It does not alleviate the symptoms of benzodiazepine withdrawal. Therefore a patient taking a benzodiazepine still needs to have the benzodiazepine withdrawn gradually; it is advisable to do this before starting buspirone. The dependence and abuse liability of buspirone has not yet been established.

Meprobamate is **less effective** than the benzodiazepines, more hazardous in overdosage, and can also induce dependence.

Beta-blockers (e.g. propranolol, oxprenolol) (see section 2.4) do not affect psychological symptoms, such as worry, tension, and fear, but they do reduce autonomic symptoms, such as palpitations, sweating, and tremor; they do not reduce non-autonomic symptoms, such as muscle tension. Beta-blockers are therefore indicated for patients with predominantly somatic symptoms; this, in turn, may prevent the onset of worry and fear. Patients with predominantly psychological symptoms may obtain no benefit.

BUSPIRONE HYDROCHLORIDE

Indications: anxiety (short-term use)
Cautions: does not alleviate benzodiazepine withdrawal (see notes above); history of hepatic or renal impairment; **interactions:** Appendix 1 (buspirone)
DRIVING. May affect performance of skilled tasks (e.g. driving); effects of alcohol may be enhanced
Contra-indications: epilepsy, severe hepatic or renal impairment, pregnancy and breast-feeding
Side-effects: nausea, dizziness, headache, nervousness, lightheadedness, excitement; rarely tachycardia, palpitations, chest pain, drowsiness, confusion, dry mouth, fatigue, and sweating
Dose: initially 5 mg 2–3 times daily, increased as necessary every 2–3 days; usual range 15–30 mg daily in divided doses; max. 45 mg daily (30 mg in elderly)

PoM **Buspar**® (Bristol-Myers)
Tablets, buspirone hydrochloride 5 mg, net price 126-tab pack = £40.32; 10 mg, 100-tab pack = £48.00. Counselling, driving

CHLORMEZANONE

Indications: short-term use in anxiety or insomnia; muscle spasm (but see section 10.2.2)
Cautions: respiratory disease, muscle weakness, history of drug abuse, marked personality disorder, pregnancy, breast-feeding; reduce dose

in elderly and debilitated, and in hepatic and renal impairment; avoid prolonged use (and abrupt withdrawal thereafter); **interactions:** Appendix 1 (chlormezanone)
DRIVING. Drowsiness may persist the next day and affect performance of skilled tasks (e.g. driving); effects of alcohol enhanced

Contra-indications: acute pulmonary insufficiency; respiratory depression; porphyria (see section 9.8.2)

Side-effects: drowsiness and lethargy, dizziness, nausea, headache, dry mouth, rashes, dependence; cholestatic jaundice reported

Dose: 200 mg 3–4 times daily *or* 400 mg at bedtime; elderly patients half adult dose

PoM Trancopal® (Sanofi Winthrop)
Tablets, yellow, chlormezanone 200 mg. Net price 60 = £5.73. Label: 2 *or* 19

HYDROXYZINE HYDROCHLORIDE
See section 3.4.1

MEPROBAMATE

Indications: short-term use in anxiety, but see notes above

Cautions: respiratory disease, muscle weakness, epilepsy (may induce seizures), history of drug abuse, marked personality disorder, pregnancy; elderly and debilitated; hepatic and renal impairment; avoid prolonged use, abrupt withdrawal may precipitate convulsions; **interactions:** Appendix 1 (meprobamate)
DRIVING. Drowsiness may affect performance of skilled tasks (e.g. driving); effects of alcohol enhanced

Contra-indications: acute pulmonary insufficiency; respiratory depression; porphyria (see section 9.8.2); breast-feeding

Side-effects: see under Diazepam, but the incidence is greater and drowsiness is the most common side-effect. Also gastro-intestinal disturbances, hypotension, paraesthesia, weakness, CNS effects which include headache, paradoxical excitement, disturbances of vision; rarely agranulocytosis and rashes

Dose: 400 mg 3–4 times daily; elderly patients half adult dose or less

CD Equanil® (Wyeth)
Tablets, meprobamate 200 mg, net price 20 = 15p; 400 mg (scored), 20 = 22p. Label: 2

4.1.3 Barbiturates

The intermediate-acting **barbiturates** only have a place in the treatment of severe intractable insomnia in patients already taking barbiturates; they should be avoided in the elderly. The long-acting barbiturates, phenobarbitone and methylphenobarbitone, are of value in epilepsy (section 4.8.1) but their use as sedatives is unjustified. The very short-acting barbiturates, methohexitone and thiopentone, are used in anaesthesia (see section 15.1.1).

BARBITURATES
Indications: severe intractable insomnia in patients already taking barbiturates
Cautions: avoid use where possible; dependence and tolerance readily occur; abrupt withdrawal may precipitate a serious withdrawal syndrome (rebound insomnia, anxiety, tremor, dizziness, nausea, convulsions, delirium, and death); repeated doses are cumulative and may lead to excessive sedation; caution in respiratory disease, renal disease, hepatic impairment; **interactions:** Appendix 1 (barbiturates and primidone)
DRIVING. Drowsiness may persist the next day and affect performance of skilled tasks (e.g. driving); effects of alcohol enhanced

Contra-indications: insomnia caused by pain; porphyria (see section 9.8.2), pregnancy, breast-feeding; avoid in children, young adults, elderly and debilitated patients, also patients with a history of drug or alcohol abuse

Side-effects: hangover with drowsiness, dizziness, ataxia, respiratory depression, hypersensitivity reactions, headache, particularly in elderly; paradoxical excitement and confusion occasionally precede sleep; overdosage: see Emergency Treatment of Poisoning, p. 19

Dose: see under preparations below

CD Amytal® (Lilly)
Tablets, amylobarbitone 50 mg, net price 20 = 28p. Label: 19
Dose: 100–200 mg at bedtime

CD Sodium Amytal® (Lilly)
Capsules, both blue, amylobarbitone sodium 60 mg, net price 20 = 46p; 200 mg, 20 = 91p. Label: 19
Dose: 60–200 mg at bedtime
Injection, powder for reconstitution, amylobarbitone sodium. Net price 500-mg vial = £10.00
Dose: by deep intramuscular injection into large muscle, preferably gluteal, (max. 5 mL at any one site) or by slow intravenous injection (max. 50 mg/minute), 0.25–1 g; max. single dose, intramuscular 500 mg, intravenous 1 g
Note. For specialised use in procedures in expert epilepsy centres only

CD Soneryl® (Rhône-Poulenc Rorer)
Tablets, pink, scored, butobarbitone 100 mg. Net price 56-tab pack = 73p. Label: 19
Dose: 100–200 mg at bedtime

Quinalbarbitone
Note. Quinalbarbitone has been transferred from schedule 3 to schedule 2 of the Misuse of Drugs Regulations 1985; receipt and supply must therefore be recorded in the CD register.

CD Seconal Sodium® (Lilly)
Capsules, both orange, quinalbarbitone sodium 50 mg, net price 20 = 85p; 100 mg, 20 = £1.29. Label: 19
Dose: 50–100 mg at bedtime

CD Tuinal® (Lilly)
Capsules, orange/blue, a mixture of amylobarbitone sodium 50 mg, quinalbarbitone sodium 50 mg. Net price 20 = 54p. Label: 19
Dose: 1–2 capsules at bedtime
Note. Only one strength available therefore prescriptions need only specify 'Tuinal capsules'

4.2 Drugs used in psychoses and related disorders

4.2.1 Antipsychotic drugs
4.2.2 Antipsychotic depot injections
4.2.3 Antimanic drugs

4.2.1 Antipsychotic drugs

Antipsychotic drugs are also known as 'neuroleptics' and (misleadingly) as 'major tranquillisers'. Antipsychotic drugs generally tranquillise without impairing consciousness and without causing paradoxical excitement but they should not be regarded merely as tranquillisers. For conditions such as schizophrenia the tranquillising effect is of secondary importance.

In the short term they are used to quieten disturbed patients whatever the underlying psychopathology, which may be brain damage, mania, toxic delirium, agitated depression, or acute behavioural disturbance.

They are used to alleviate severe anxiety but this too should be a short-term measure. Some antipsychotic drugs (e.g. chlorpromazine, thioridazine, flupenthixol) also have an antidepressant effect while others may exacerbate depression (e.g. fluphenazine, pimozide, pipothiazine).

SCHIZOPHRENIA. Antipsychotic drugs relieve florid psychotic symptoms such as thought disorder, hallucinations, and delusions, and prevent relapse. Although they are usually less effective in apathetic withdrawn patients, they sometimes appear to have an activating influence. For example, chlorpromazine may restore an acutely ill schizophrenic to normal activity and social behaviour who was previously withdrawn or even mute and akinetic. Patients with acute schizophrenia generally respond better than those with chronic symptoms.

Long-term treatment of a patient with a definite diagnosis of schizophrenia may be necessary even after the first episode of illness in order to prevent the manifest illness from becoming chronic. Withdrawal of drug treatment requires careful surveillance because the patient who appears well on medication may suffer a disastrous relapse if treatment is withdrawn inappropriately. In addition the need for continuation of treatment may not become immediately evident because relapse is often delayed for several weeks after cessation of treatment.

Antipsychotic drugs are considered to act by interfering with dopaminergic transmission in the brain by blocking dopamine receptors and may give rise to the extrapyramidal effects described below, and also to hyperprolactinaemia. Antipsychotic drugs also affect cholinergic, alpha-adrenergic, histaminergic, and serotonergic receptors.

SIDE-EFFECTS. Extrapyramidal symptoms are the most troublesome. They are caused most frequently by the piperazine phenothiazines (fluphenazine, perphenazine, prochlorperazine, and trifluoperazine), the butyrophenones (benperidol, droperidol, haloperidol, and trifluperidol), and the depot preparations. They are easy to recognise but cannot be accurately predicted because they depend partly on the dose and partly on the type of drug, and on patient susceptibility. They consist of parkinsonian symptoms (including tremor) which may occur gradually, dystonia (abnormal face and body movements) which may appear after only a few doses, akathisia (restlessness) which may resemble an exacerbation of the condition being treated, and tardive dyskinesia (which usually takes longer to develop).

Parkinsonian symptoms remit if the drug is withdrawn and may be suppressed by the administration of **antimuscarinic** drugs (section 4.9.2). Routine administration of such drugs is **not** justified as not all patients are affected and because tardive dyskinesia may be unmasked or worsened by them. Furthermore, these drugs are sometimes abused for their mood-altering effects. Tardive dyskinesia is of particular concern because it may be irreversible on withdrawing therapy and treatment may be ineffective. It occurs fairly frequently in patients (especially the elderly) on long-term therapy and with high dosage, and the treatment of such patients must be carefully and regularly reviewed. Tardive dyskinesia may also occur occasionally after short-term treatment with low dosage.

Hypotension and interference with temperature regulation are dose-related side-effects and are liable to cause dangerous falls and hypothermia in the elderly; very serious consideration should be given before prescribing these drugs for patients over 70 years of age.

Neuroleptic malignant syndrome (hyperthermia, fluctuating level of consciousness, muscular rigidity and autonomic dysfunction with pallor, tachycardia, labile blood pressure, sweating, and urinary incontinence) is a rare but potentially fatal side-effect of some drugs. Drugs for which it has been reported in the UK include haloperidol, chlorpromazine, and flupenthixol decanoate. Discontinuation of drug therapy is essential as there is no proven effective treatment but bromocriptine and dantrolene have been used. The syndrome, which usually lasts for 5–10 days after drug discontinuation, may be unduly prolonged if depot preparations have been used.

Overdosage: see Emergency Treatment of Poisoning, p. 20.

CLASSIFICATION OF ANTIPSYCHOTICS. The **phenothiazine** derivatives can be divided into 3 main groups.

Group 1: chlorpromazine, methotrimeprazine, and promazine, generally characterised by pronounced sedative effects and moderate antimuscarinic and extrapyramidal side-effects.

Group 2: pericyazine, pipothiazine, and thioridazine, generally characterised by moderate sedative effects, marked antimuscarinic effects, but fewer extrapyramidal side-effects than groups 1 or 3.

Group 3: fluphenazine, perphenazine, prochlorperazine, and trifluoperazine, generally characterised by fewer sedative effects, fewer antimuscarinic effects, but more pronounced extrapyramidal side-effects than groups 1 and 2.

Drugs of other chemical groups tend to resemble the phenothiazines of *group 3*. They include the **butyrophenones** (benperidol, droperidol, haloperidol, and trifluperidol); **diphenylbutylpiperi-**

4.2 Drugs used in psychoses and related disorders

dines (fluspirilene and pimozide); **thioxanthenes** (flupenthixol and zuclopenthixol); **oxypertine**; and **loxapine**. Clozapine differs in that it is sedative with fewer extrapyramidal effects.

CHOICE. As indicated above, the various drugs differ somewhat in predominant actions and side-effects. Selection is influenced by the degree of sedation required and the patient's susceptibility to extrapyramidal side-effects. However, the differences between antipsychotic drugs are less important than the great variability in patient response; moreover, tolerance to these secondary effects usually develops.

Prescribing of more than one antipsychotic at the same time is **not** recommended; it may constitute a hazard and there is no significant evidence that side-effects are minimised.

Chlorpromazine is widely used. It has a marked sedating effect and is particularly useful for treating violent patients without causing stupor. Agitated states in the elderly can be controlled without confusion, a dose of 25 mg usually being adequate.

Flupenthixol and **pimozide** (see CSM advice p. 151) are less sedating than chlorpromazine.

Sulpiride is structurally distinct from other antipsychotic drugs. In high doses it controls florid positive symptoms, but in lower doses it has an alerting effect on apathetic withdrawn schizophrenics. **Remoxipride** is a new antipsychotic drug said to have a low level of extrapyramidal and sedative side-effects.

Fluphenazine, haloperidol, and **trifluoperazine** are also of value but their use is limited by the high incidence of extrapyramidal symptoms. Haloperidol may be preferred for the rapid control of hyperactive psychotic states.

Thioridazine is popular for treating the elderly as there is a reduced incidence of extrapyramidal symptoms.

Promazine is not sufficiently active by mouth to be used as an antipsychotic drug

Clozapine is indicated only for the treatment of schizophrenia in patients unresponsive to, or intolerant of, conventional antipsychotic drugs. It is less likely to cause tardive dyskinesia but as it can cause agranulocytosis, its use is restricted to patients registered with the Clozaril Patient Monitoring Service (see under Clozapine, below).

Loxapine causes relatively little sedation; in overdosage it has a high potential for serious neurological and cardiac toxicity.

OTHER USES. Nausea and vomiting (section 4.6), choreas, motor tics (section 4.9.3), and intractable hiccup (see under Chlorpromazine Hydrochloride and under Haloperidol). **Benperidol** is used in deviant antisocial sexual behaviour but its value is not established.

Equivalent doses of oral antipsychotics

These equivalences are intended **only** as an approximate guide; individual dosage instructions should **also** be checked; patients should be carefully monitored after **any** change in medication

Antipsychotic	Daily dose
Chlorpromazine	100 mg
Clozapine	50 mg
Haloperidol	2–3 mg[1]
Loxapine	10–20 mg
Pimozide	2 mg[2]
Sulpiride	200 mg
Thioridazine	100 mg
Trifluoperazine	5 mg

1. In specialist psychiatric units where very high doses are required the equivalent dose of haloperidol might be up to 10 mg
2. See also the CSM warning concerning pimozide dose, p. 151

WITHDRAWAL. Withdrawal of antipsychotic drugs after long-term therapy should always be gradual and closely monitored to avoid the risk of acute withdrawal syndromes or rapid relapse.

> DOSAGE. In some patients it is necessary to raise the dose of an antipsychotic drug above that which is normally recommended. This should be done with caution and under specialist supervision.
> *Once-daily dose.* After an initial period of stabilisation, in most patients, the long half-life of antipsychotic drugs allows the total daily dose to be given as a single dose.

CHLORPROMAZINE HYDROCHLORIDE

WARNING. Owing to the risk of contact sensitisation, pharmacists, nurses, and other health workers should avoid direct contact with chlorpromazine; tablets should not be crushed and solutions should be handled with care

Indications: see under Dose; antiemetic (in terminal illness), section 4.6; peri-operative use, see section 15.1.4.1

Cautions: cardiovascular and cerebrovascular disease, respiratory disease, phaeochromocytoma, parkinsonism, epilepsy, acute infections, pregnancy, breast-feeding, renal and hepatic impairment (avoid if severe), history of jaundice, leucopenia (blood counts if unexplained infections); hypothyroidism, myasthenia gravis, prostatic hypertrophy, closed-angle glaucoma; caution in elderly particularly in very hot or very cold weather; avoid abrupt withdrawal; patients should remain supine for 30 minutes after intramuscular injection; **interactions:** Appendix 1 (phenothiazines and other antipsychotics)

DRIVING. Drowsiness may affect performance of skilled tasks (e.g. driving); effects of alcohol enhanced

Contra-indications: coma caused by CNS depressants; bone-marrow depression; avoid in phaeochromocytoma

Side-effects: extrapyramidal symptoms (reversed by dose reduction or antimuscarinic drugs) and, on prolonged administration, occasionally tardive dyskinesia; hypothermia (occasionally pyrexia), drowsiness, apathy, pallor, nightmares, insomnia, depression, and, more rarely, agitation, EEG changes, convulsions; antimuscarinic symptoms such as dry mouth, nasal congestion, constipation, difficulty with micturition, and blurred vision; cardiovascular symptoms such as hypotension, tachycardia, and arrhythmias; ECG changes; endocrine effects such as menstrual disturbances, galactorrhoea, gynaecomastia, impotence, and weight gain; sensitivity reactions such as agranulocytosis, leucopenia, leucocytosis, and haemolytic anaemia, photosensitisation (more common with chlorpromazine than with other antipsychotics), contact sensitisation and rashes, jaundice and alterations in liver function; neuroleptic malignant syndrome; lupus erythematosus-like syndrome reported; with prolonged high dosage, corneal and lens opacities and purplish pigmentation of the skin, cornea, conjunctiva, and retina; intramuscular injection may be painful, cause hypotension and tachycardia (see Cautions), and give rise to nodule formation; overdosage: see Emergency Treatment of Poisoning, p. 20

Dose: by mouth,
Schizophrenia and other psychoses, mania, short-term adjunctive management of severe anxiety, psychomotor agitation, excitement, and violent or dangerously impulsive behaviour initially 25 mg 3 times daily (*or* 75 mg at night), adjusted according to response, to usual maintenance dose of 75–300 mg daily (but up to 1 g daily may be required in psychoses);
CHILD 1–5 years 500 micrograms/kg every 4–6 hours (max. 40 mg daily); 6–12 years third to half adult dose (max. 75 mg daily)
ELDERLY (or debilitated) third to half adult dose
Intractable hiccup, 25–50 mg 3–4 times daily
By deep intramuscular injection, (for relief of acute symptoms), 25–50 mg every 6–8 hours; CHILD, as dose by mouth
By rectum in suppositories, chlorpromazine 100 mg every 6–8 hours
Note. For equivalent therapeutic effect 100 mg chlorpromazine base given *rectally* as a suppository = 20–25 mg chlorpromazine hydrochloride *by intramuscular injection* = 40–50 mg of chlorpromazine base or hydrochloride *by mouth*

PoM **Chlorpromazine** (Non-proprietary)
Tablets, coated, chlorpromazine hydrochloride 10 mg, net price 20 = 12p; 25 mg, 20 = 14p; 50 mg, 20 = 26p; 100 mg, 20 = 46p. Label: 2
Available from APS, DDSA (Chloractil®), Norton
Elixir, chlorpromazine hydrochloride 25 mg/5 mL. Net price 100 mL = 26p. Label: 2
Injection, chlorpromazine hydrochloride 25 mg/mL, net price 1-mL amp = 21p; 2-mL amp = 28p
Suppositories, chlorpromazine 100 mg. Net price 10 = £1.91. Label: 2
Available from Penn (special order)

PoM **Largactil**® (Rhône-Poulenc Rorer)
Tablets, all off-white, f/c, chlorpromazine hydrochloride 10 mg. Net price 56-tab pack = 33p; 25 mg, 56-tab pack = 50p; 50 mg, 56-tab pack = £1.16; 100 mg, 56-tab pack = £2.16. Label: 2
Syrup, brown, chlorpromazine hydrochloride 25 mg/5 mL. Net price 100-mL pack = 59p. Label: 2
Suspension forte, orange, sugar-free, chlorpromazine hydrochloride 100 mg (as embonate)/5 mL. Net price 100-mL pack = £1.19. Label: 2
Injection, chlorpromazine hydrochloride 25 mg/mL. Net price 2-mL amp = 28p

BENPERIDOL
Indications: control of deviant antisocial sexual behaviour (but see notes above)
Cautions; Contra-indications; Side-effects: see under Haloperidol; avoid in children
Dose: 0.25–1.5 mg daily in divided doses, adjusted according to the response; ELDERLY (or debilitated) initially half adult dose

PoM **Anquil**® (Janssen)
Tablets, benperidol 250 micrograms. Net price 20 = £5.36. Label: 2

CLOZAPINE
Indications: schizophrenia in patients unresponsive to, or intolerant of, conventional antipsychotic drugs
Cautions: see under Chlorpromazine Hydrochloride; leucocyte and differential blood counts must be normal before treatment and must be monitored weekly for first 18 weeks then fortnightly; avoid drugs which depress leucopoiesis; withdraw treatment if leucocyte count falls below 3000/mm^3 or absolute neutrophil count falls below 1500/mm^3; patients should report any infections; avoid in children; **interactions**: Appendix 1 (clozapine)
Contra-indications: history of drug-induced neutropenia/agranulocytosis; bone marrow disorders; alcoholic and toxic psychoses; drug intoxication; coma or severe CNS depression; pregnancy and breast-feeding
Side-effects: see under Chlorpromazine Hydrochloride but more sedating and high incidence of antimuscarinic symptoms; extrapyramidal symptoms may occur less frequently; neutropenia and potentially fatal agranulocytosis, headache and dizziness, hypersalivation, urinary incontinence, myocarditis, and delirium; rarely circulatory collapse (but hypertension also reported)
Dose: initially 25–50 mg daily (elderly 25 mg), increased as necessary by 25–50 mg daily (elderly 25 mg) over 7–14 days to 300 mg daily in divided doses (larger dose at night; up to 200 mg daily may be given as a single dose at bedtime); usual antipsychotic dose 200–450 mg daily (max. 900 mg daily), and subsequently adjusted to usual maintenance of 150–300 mg daily

4.2 Drugs used in psychoses and related disorders

PoM **Clozaril**® (Sandoz)
Tablets, both yellow, scored, clozapine 25 mg, net price 84-tab pack = £38.50; 100 mg, 84-tab pack = £154.00 (hosp. only, patient, prescriber, and supplying pharmacist must be registered with the Sandoz Clozaril Patient Monitoring Service—takes several days to do this). Label: 2, 10 patient information leaflet

DROPERIDOL

Indications: see under Dose; peri-operative use, see section 15.1.4.1
Cautions; Contra-indications; Side-effects: see under Haloperidol
Dose: by mouth, tranquillisation and emergency control in mania, 5–20 mg repeated every 4–8 hours if necessary (elderly, initially half adult dose); CHILD, 0.5–1 mg daily
By intramuscular injection, up to 10 mg repeated every 4–6 hours if necessary (elderly, initially half adult dose); CHILD, 0.5–1 mg daily
By intravenous injection, 5–15 mg repeated every 4–6 hours if necessary (elderly, initially half adult dose)
Cancer chemotherapy-induced nausea and vomiting, *by intramuscular or intravenous injection*, 1–10 mg 30 minutes before starting therapy, followed by *continuous intravenous infusion* of 1–3 mg/hour *or* 1–5 mg *by intramuscular or intravenous injection* every 1–6 hours as necessary; CHILD *by intramuscular or intravenous injection*, 20–75 micrograms/kg

PoM **Droleptan**® (Janssen)
Tablets, yellow, scored, droperidol 10 mg. Net price 50-tab pack = £12.62. Label: 2
Oral liquid, sugar-free, droperidol 1 mg/mL. Net price 100-mL pack (with graduated cap) = £4.59; 500-mL pack = £21.79. Label: 2
Injection, droperidol 5 mg/mL. Net price 2-mL amp = 92p

FLUPENTHIXOL

Indications: schizophrenia and other psychoses, particularly with apathy and withdrawal but not mania or psychomotor hyperactivity; depression, section 4.3.4
Cautions; Contra-indications; Side-effects: see under Chlorpromazine Hydrochloride but less sedating; extrapyramidal symptoms more frequent (25% of patients); avoid in children, senile confusional states, excitable and overactive patients, and in porphyria (see section 9.8.2)
Dose: initially 3–9 mg twice daily adjusted according to the response; max. 18 mg daily

PoM **Depixol**® (Lundbeck)
Tablets, yellow, s/c, flupenthixol 3 mg (as dihydrochloride). Net price 20 = £2.59. Label: 2
Depot injection (flupenthixol decanoate): section 4.2.2
PoM **Fluanxol**® (depression), see section 4.3.4

FLUPHENAZINE HYDROCHLORIDE

Indications: see under Dose
Cautions; Contra-indications; Side-effects: see under Chlorpromazine Hydrochloride, but less sedating and fewer antimuscarinic or hypotensive symptoms; extrapyramidal symptoms, particularly dystonic reactions and akathisia, are more frequent; avoid in depression; avoid in children
Dose: schizophrenia and other psychoses, mania, initially 2.5–10 mg daily in 2–3 divided doses, adjusted according to response to 20 mg daily; doses above 20 mg daily (10 mg in elderly) only with special caution
Short-term adjunctive management of severe anxiety, psychomotor agitation, excitement, and violent or dangerously impulsive behaviour, initially 1 mg twice daily, increased as necessary to 2 mg twice daily

PoM **Moditen**® (Squibb)
Tablets, all s/c, fluphenazine hydrochloride 1 mg (pink), net price 20 = £1.09; 2.5 mg (yellow), 20 = £1.36; 5 mg, 20 = £1.82. Label: 2
Depot injections (fluphenazine decanoate): section 4.2.2

HALOPERIDOL

Indications: see under Dose; motor tics, section 4.9.3
Cautions; Contra-indications; Side-effects: see under Chlorpromazine Hydrochloride but less sedating, and fewer antimuscarinic or hypotensive symptoms; pigmentation and photosensitivity reactions rare. Extrapyramidal symptoms, particularly dystonic reactions and akathisia are more frequent especially in thyrotoxic patients. Rarely weight loss. Avoid in basal ganglia disease
Dose: by mouth,
Schizophrenia and other psychoses, mania, short-term adjunctive management of psychomotor agitation, excitement, and violent or dangerously impulsive behaviour, initially 1.5–20 mg daily in divided doses, gradually increased to 100 mg (and occasionally 200 mg) daily in severely disturbed patients; ELDERLY (or debilitated) initially half adult dose; CHILD initially 25–50 micrograms/kg daily to a max. of 10 mg; adolescents up to 30 mg daily (exceptionally 60 mg)
Short-term adjunctive management of severe anxiety, adults 500 micrograms twice daily
Intractable hiccup, 1.5 mg 3 times daily adjusted according to response
By intramuscular injection, 2–10 mg (increasing to 30 mg for emergency control) then 5 mg up to every hour if necessary (intervals of 4–8 hours may be satisfactory)
Nausea and vomiting, 1–2 mg

PoM **Haloperidol** (Non-proprietary)
Tablets, haloperidol 1.5 mg, net price 20 = 89p; 5 mg, 20 = £2.52; 10 mg, 20 = £4.71; 20 mg, 20 = £8.45. Label: 2

PoM Dozic® (RP Drugs)
Oral liquid, sugar-free, haloperidol 1 mg/mL, net price 100-mL pack (with pipette) = £5.00; 2 mg/mL, 100-mL pack (with pipette) = £5.10. Label: 2

PoM Haldol® (Janssen)
Tablets, both scored, haloperidol 5 mg (blue), net price 20 = £1.69; 10 mg (yellow), 20 = £3.30. Label: 2
Oral liquid, sugar-free, haloperidol 2 mg/mL. Net price 100-mL pack (with pipette) = £5.21. Label: 2
Oral liquid concentrate, sugar-free, haloperidol 10 mg/mL. Net price 100-mL pack = £22.84. Label: 2
Diluent purified water, freshly boiled and cooled, life of diluted concentrate 14 days. Alternatively, purified water, freshly boiled and cooled, containing 0.05% of methyl hydroxybenzoate and 0.005% of propyl hydroxybenzoate, life of diluted concentrate 2 months.
Injection, haloperidol 5 mg/mL. Net price 1-mL amp = 33p; 2-mL amp = 63p
Depot injection (haloperidol decanoate): section 4.2.2

PoM Serenace® (Baker Norton)
Capsules, green, haloperidol 500 micrograms. Net price 20 = 67p. Label: 2
Tablets, all scored, haloperidol 1.5 mg, net price 20 = £1.19; 5 mg (pink), 20 = £3.36; 10 mg (pale pink), 20 = £6.02; 20 mg (dark pink), 20 = £10.85. Label: 2
Oral liquid, sugar-free, haloperidol 2 mg/mL. Net price 100-mL pack = £8.99. Label: 2
Injection, haloperidol 5 mg/mL, net price 1-mL amp = 59p; 10 mg/mL, 2-mL amp = £2.03

LOXAPINE

Indications: acute and chronic psychoses
Cautions; Contra-indications: see under Chlorpromazine Hydrochloride
Side-effects: see under Chlorpromazine Hydrochloride; nausea and vomiting, weight gain or loss, dyspnoea, ptosis, hyperpyrexia, flushing and headache, paraesthesia, and polydipsia also reported; no endocrine effects yet reported; avoid in porphyria (see section 9.8.2)
Dose: initially 20–50 mg daily in 2 divided doses, increased as necessary over 7–10 days to 60–100 mg daily (max. 250 mg) in 2–4 divided doses, then adjusted to usual maintenance dose of 20–100 mg daily

PoM Loxapac® (Novex)
Capsules, loxapine (as succinate) 10 mg (yellow/green), net price 100-cap pack = £9.52; 25 mg (light green/dark green), 100-cap pack = £19.05; 50 mg (blue/dark green), 100-cap pack = £34.27. Label: 2

METHOTRIMEPRAZINE

Indications: see under Dose
Cautions; Contra-indications; Side-effects: see under Chlorpromazine Hydrochloride but more sedating; risk of postural hypotension particularly in patients over 50 years
Dose: by mouth, schizophrenia, initially 25–50 mg daily in divided doses increased as necessary; bedpatients initially 100–200 mg daily in 3 divided doses, increased if necessary to 1 g daily
Adjunctive treatment in terminal care (including management of pain and associated restlessness, distress, or vomiting), 12.5–50 mg every 4–8 hours
By intramuscular injection or by intravenous injection (after dilution with an equal volume of sodium chloride 0.9% injection), adjunct in terminal care, 12.5–25 mg (severe agitation up to 50 mg) every 6–8 hours if necessary
By continuous subcutaneous infusion, adjunct in terminal care (via syringe driver), 25–200 mg daily (over 24-hour period), diluted in a suitable volume of sodium chloride 0.9% injection

PoM Nozinan® (Rhône-Poulenc Rorer)
Tablets, scored, methotrimeprazine maleate 25 mg. Net price 20 = £2.11. Label: 2
Injection, methotrimeprazine hydrochloride 25 mg/mL. Net price 1-mL amp = £1.23

OXYPERTINE

Indications: see under Dose
Cautions; Contra-indications; Side-effects: see under Chlorpromazine Hydrochloride, but extrapyramidal symptoms may occur less frequently. With low doses agitation and hyperactivity occur and with high doses sedation. Occasionally photophobia may occur
Dose: schizophrenia and other psychoses, mania, short-term adjunctive management of psychomotor agitation, excitement, and violent or dangerously impulsive behaviour, initially 80–120 mg daily in divided doses adjusted according to the response; max. 300 mg daily
Short-term adjunctive management of severe anxiety, initially 10 mg 3–4 times daily preferably after food; max. 60 mg daily

PoM Oxypertine (Sanofi Winthrop)
Capsules, oxypertine 10 mg. Net price 20 = £1.93. Label: 2
Tablets, scored, oxypertine 40 mg. Net price 20 = £6.04. Label: 2
Note. The brand name Integrin® was formerly used for oxypertine preparations

PERICYAZINE

Indications: see under Dose
Cautions; Contra-indications; Side-effects: see under Chlorpromazine Hydrochloride, but more sedating; hypotension commonly occurs when treatment initiated
Dose: schizophrenia and other psychoses, initially 75 mg daily in divided doses increased at weekly intervals by steps of 25 mg according to response; usual max. 300 mg daily (elderly initially 15–30 mg daily).

Short-term adjunctive management of severe anxiety, psychomotor agitation, and violent or dangerously impulsive behaviour, initially 15–30 mg (elderly 5–10 mg) daily divided into 2 doses, taking the larger dose at bedtime, adjusted according to response
CHILD (severe mental or behavioural disorders only), initially, 500 micrograms daily for 10-kg child, increased by 1 mg for each additional 5 kg to max. total daily dose of 10 mg; dose may be gradually increased according to response but maintenance should not exceed twice initial dose

PoM **Neulactil**® (Rhône-Poulenc Rorer)
Tablets, all yellow, scored, pericyazine 2.5 mg, net price 84-tab pack = £1.87; 10 mg, 84-tab pack = £5.04; 25 mg, 50-tab pack = £8.29. Label: 2
Syrup forte, brown, pericyazine 10 mg/5 mL. Net price 100-mL pack = £2.45. Label: 2

PERPHENAZINE

Indications: see under Dose; anti-emetic, section 4.6
Cautions; Contra-indications; Side-effects: see under Chlorpromazine Hydrochloride, but less sedating; extrapyramidal symptoms, especially dystonia, more frequent, particularly at high dosage; avoid in children under 14 years; not indicated for agitation and restlessness in the elderly
Dose: schizophrenia and other psychoses, mania, short-term adjunctive management of severe anxiety, psychomotor agitation, excitement, and violent or dangerously impulsive behaviour, initially 4 mg 3 times daily adjusted according to the response; max. 24 mg daily; elderly quarter to half adult dose (but see Cautions)

PoM **Fentazin**® (Evans)
Tablets, both s/c, perphenazine 2 mg, net price 20 = 52p; 4 mg, 20 = 62p. Label: 2

PIMOZIDE

Indications: see under Dose
Cautions; Contra-indications; Side-effects: see under Chlorpromazine Hydrochloride, but less sedating; avoid in children; contra-indicated in breast-feeding; serious arrhythmias reported (contra-indicated if history of arrhythmias or pre-existing congenital QT prolongation); following reports of sudden unexplained death, the CSM recommends ECG before treatment in all patients, periodic ECGs at doses over 16 mg daily and review of need for pimozide if repolarisation changes or arrhythmias develop (close supervision and preferably dose reduction advised); concurrent cardioactive or antipsychotic drugs, or electrolyte disturbances (notably hypokalaemia) may predispose to cardiotoxicity

Dose: schizophrenia, initially 10 mg daily in acute conditions, adjusted according to response in increments of 2–4 mg at intervals of not less than 1 week; max. 20 mg daily; prevention of relapse, initially 2 mg daily (range 2–20 mg daily)
Monosymptomatic hypochondriacal psychosis, paranoid psychoses, initially 4 mg daily, adjusted according to response in increments of 2–4 mg at intervals of not less than 1 week; max. 16 mg daily
Mania, hypomania, short-term adjunctive management of excitement and psychomotor agitation, initially 10 mg daily adjusted according to response in increments of 2–4 mg at intervals of not less than 1 week; max. 20 mg daily
ELDERLY half usual starting dose

PoM **Orap**® (Janssen)
Tablets, all scored, pimozide 2 mg, net price 20 = £3.25; 4 mg (green), 20 = £6.29; 10 mg, 20 = £12.06. Label: 2

PROCHLORPERAZINE

Indications: see under Dose; anti-emetic, section 4.6
Cautions; Contra-indications; Side-effects: see under Chlorpromazine Hydrochloride, but less sedating; extrapyramidal symptoms, particularly dystonic reactions, more frequent; avoid in children (but see section 4.6 for use as anti-emetic)
Dose: by mouth, schizophrenia and other psychoses, mania, prochlorperazine maleate or mesylate, 12.5 mg twice daily for 7 days adjusted to usual dose of 75–100 mg daily according to response
Short-term adjunctive management of severe anxiety, 15–20 mg daily in divided doses; max. 40 mg daily
By deep intramuscular injection, psychoses, mania, prochlorperazine mesylate 12.5–25 mg 2–3 times daily
By rectum in suppositories, psychoses, mania, the equivalent of prochlorperazine maleate 25 mg 2–3 times daily

Preparations
Section 4.6

PROMAZINE HYDROCHLORIDE

Indications: see under Dose
Cautions; Contra-indications; Side-effects: see under Chlorpromazine Hydrochloride
Dose: by mouth, short-term adjunctive management of psychomotor agitation, 100–200 mg 4 times daily
Agitation and restlessness in elderly, 25–50 mg 4 times daily
By intramuscular injection, short-term adjunctive management of psychomotor agitation, 50 mg (25 mg in elderly or debilitated), repeated if necessary after 6–8 hours

PoM **Promazine** (Non-proprietary)
Tablets, coated, promazine hydrochloride 25 mg, 50 mg, and 100 mg. Label: 2
Available from Biorex

PoM **Sparine**® (Wyeth)
Suspension, yellow, promazine hydrochloride 50 mg (as embonate)/5 mL. Net price 150-mL pack = £1.08. Label: 2.
Note. Not recommended for children
Injection, promazine hydrochloride 50 mg/mL. Net price 1-mL amp = 26p

REMOXIPRIDE HYDROCHLORIDE

Indications: schizophrenia and other psychoses (except due to depressive illness)
Cautions; Contra-indications: see under Chlorpromazine Hydrochloride; avoid in children; *interactions*: Appendix 1 (remoxipride)
Side-effects: see under Chlorpromazine Hydrochloride but less sedating and extrapyramidal symptoms may occur less frequently; insomnia, concentration difficulties, anxiety, aggression, nausea, headache, and hypersalivation also reported
Dose: initially 300 mg daily (elderly 150 mg daily), adjusted according to response; usual range 150–450 mg daily (max. 600 mg daily); usual maintenance 150–300 mg daily

▼ PoM **Roxiam**® (Astra)
Capsules, both blue, m/r, remoxipride hydrochloride 150 mg, net price 28-cap pack = £12.80; 300 mg, 28-cap pack = £21.56. Label: 3, 25

SULPIRIDE

Indications: schizophrenia
Cautions; Contra-indications; Side-effects: see under Chlorpromazine Hydrochloride, but less sedating; structurally distinct from chlorpromazine hence not associated with jaundice or skin reactions; avoid in porphyria (see section 9.8.2) and breast-feeding; reduce dose (preferably avoid) in renal impairment
Dose: 200–400 mg twice daily; max. 800 mg daily in patients with predominantly negative symptoms, and 2.4 g daily in patients with mainly positive symptoms; ELDERLY, initially 100–200 mg

PoM **Dolmatil**® (Squibb)
Tablets, scored, sulpiride 200 mg. Net price 20 = £4.20. Label: 2

PoM **Sulpitil**® (Tillotts)
Tablets, scored, sulpiride 200 mg. Net price 28-tab pack = £5.75; 112-tab pack = £23.00. Label: 2

THIORIDAZINE

Indications: see under Dose
Cautions; Contra-indications; Side-effects: see under Chlorpromazine Hydrochloride, but less sedating and extrapyramidal symptoms and hypothermia rarely occur; more likely to induce hypotension. Pigmentary retinopathy (with reduced visual acuity, brownish colouring of vision, and impaired night vision) occurs rarely with high doses—on prolonged use examinations for eye defects are required; sexual dysfunction, particularly retrograde ejaculation, may occur; avoid in porphyria (see section 9.8.2)
Dose: schizophrenia and other psychoses, mania, 150–600 mg daily (initially in divided doses); max. 800 mg daily (hospital patients only) for up to 4 weeks
Short-term adjunctive management of psychomotor agitation, excitement, violent or dangerously impulsive behaviour, 75–200 mg daily
Short-term adjunctive management of severe anxiety, and agitation and restlessness in the elderly, 30–100 mg daily
CHILD (severe mental or behavioural problems only) under 5 years 1 mg/kg daily, 5–12 years 75–150 mg daily (in severe cases, up to 300 mg daily)

PoM **Thioridazine** (Non-proprietary)
Tablets, coated, thioridazine hydrochloride 25 mg, net price 20 = 31p; 50 mg, 20 = 58p; 100 mg, 20 = £1.10. Label: 2

PoM **Melleril**® (Sandoz)
Tablets, all f/c, thioridazine hydrochloride 10 mg, net price 20 = 23p; 25 mg, 20 = 32p; 50 mg, 20 = 61p; 100 mg, 20 = £1.16. Label: 2
Suspension 25 mg/5 mL, thioridazine 25 mg/5 mL. Net price 100 mL = 58p. Label: 2
Suspension 100 mg/5 mL, thioridazine 100 mg/5 mL. Net price 100 mL = £2.13. Label: 2
Note. These suspensions should not be diluted but the two preparations may be mixed with each other to provide intermediate doses
Syrup, orange, thioridazine 25 mg (as hydrochloride)/5 mL. Net price 100-mL pack = 62p. Label: 2

TRIFLUOPERAZINE

Indications: see under Dose; anti-emetic, section 4.6
Cautions; Contra-indications; Side-effects: see under Chlorpromazine Hydrochloride but less sedating, and hypotension, hypothermia, and antimuscarinic side-effects occur less frequently; extrapyramidal symptoms, particularly dystonic reactions and akathisia, are more frequent (particularly when the daily dose exceeds 6 mg); caution in children
Dose: *by mouth* (reduce initial doses in elderly by at least half)
Schizophrenia and other psychoses, short-term adjunctive management of psychomotor agitation, excitement, and violent or dangerously impulsive behaviour, initially 5 mg twice daily, *or* 10 mg daily in modified-release form, increased by 5 mg after 1 week, then at intervals of 3 days, according to the response; CHILD up to 12 years, initially up to 5 mg daily in divided doses, adjusted according to response, age, and body-weight

4.2 Drugs used in psychoses and related disorders

Short-term adjunctive management of severe anxiety, 2–4 mg daily in divided doses *or* 2–4 mg daily in modified-release form, increased if necessary to 6 mg daily; CHILD 3–5 years up to 1 mg daily, 6–12 years up to 4 mg daily
By deep intramuscular injection 1–3 mg daily in divided doses to max. 6 mg daily; CHILD 50 micrograms/kg daily in divided doses

PoM **Trifluoperazine** (Non-proprietary)
Tablets, coated, trifluoperazine (as hydrochloride) 1 mg, net price 20 = 37p; 5 mg, 20 = 52p. Label: 2

PoM **Stelazine**® (SK&F)
Tablets, both blue, s/c, trifluoperazine (as hydrochloride) 1 mg, net price 20 = 42p; 5 mg, 20 = 60p. Label: 2
Spansule® (= capsules m/r), all clear/yellow, enclosing dark blue, light blue, and white pellets, trifluoperazine (as hydrochloride) 2 mg, net price 60-cap pack = £2.71; 10 mg, 30-cap pack = £1.77; 15 mg, 30-cap pack = £2.66. Label: 2, 25
Syrup, yellow, sugar-free, trifluoperazine 1 mg (as hydrochloride)/5 mL. Net price 200-mL pack = £1.65. Label: 2
Liquid concentrate, yellow, sugar-free, trifluoperazine 10 mg (as hydrochloride)/mL for dilution before use. Net price 100 mL = £3.71 (hosp. only)
Diluent sorbitol solution (70%) or water containing benzoic acid 0.1%, life of diluted liquid 12 weeks.
Injection, trifluoperazine 1 mg (as hydrochloride)/mL. Net price 1-mL amp = 47p

TRIFLUPERIDOL

Indications: schizophrenia and other psychoses, particularly those with manic features
Cautions; Contra-indications; Side-effects: see under Haloperidol
Dose: initially 500 micrograms daily, adjusted by 500 micrograms every 3–4 days according to response; max. 6–8 mg daily; CHILD 5–12 years initially 250 micrograms daily, adjusted according to response; max. 2 mg daily; usual maintenance 1 mg daily

PoM **Triperidol**® (Lagap)
Tablets, both scored, trifluperidol 500 micrograms, net price 20 = £2.59; 1 mg, 20 = £2.69. Label: 2

ZUCLOPENTHIXOL ACETATE

Indications: short-term management of acute psychosis, mania, or exacerbations of chronic psychosis
Cautions; Contra-indications; Side-effects: see under Chlorpromazine Hydrochloride; avoid in porphyria (see section 9.8.2); treatment duration should not exceed 2 weeks
Dose: by deep intramuscular injection into the gluteal muscle or lateral thigh, 50–150 mg (elderly 50–100 mg), if necessary repeated after 2–3 days (1 additional dose may be needed 1–2 days after the first injection); max. cumulative dose 400 mg per course and max. 4 injections; if maintenance treatment necessary change to an oral antipsychotic 2–3 days after last injection, *or* to a longer acting antipsychotic depot injection given concomitantly with last injection of zuclopenthixol acetate

PoM **Clopixol Acuphase**® (Lundbeck)
Injection (oily), zuclopenthixol acetate 50 mg/mL. Net price 1-mL amp = £4.50; 2-mL amp = £9.01

ZUCLOPENTHIXOL DIHYDROCHLORIDE

Indications: schizophrenia and other psychoses, particularly when associated with agitated, aggressive, or hostile behaviour
Cautions; Contra-indications; Side-effects: see under Chlorpromazine Hydrochloride; should not be used in apathetic or withdrawn states; avoid in children and in porphyria (see section 9.8.2)
Dose: initially 20–30 mg daily in divided doses, increasing to a max. of 150 mg daily if necessary; usual maintenance dose 20–50 mg daily

PoM **Clopixol**® (Lundbeck)
Tablets, all f/c, zuclopenthixol (as dihydrochloride) 2 mg (pink), net price 20 = 61p; 10 mg (light brown), 20 = £1.50; 25 mg (brown), 20 = £3.00. Label: 2
Depot injection (zuclopenthixol decanoate): section 4.2.2

4.2.2 Antipsychotic depot injections

For maintenance therapy, long-acting depot injections of antipsychotic drugs are used because they are more convenient than oral preparations and ensure better patient compliance. However, they may give rise to a higher incidence of extrapyramidal reactions than oral preparations.

ADMINISTRATION. Depot antipsychotics are administered by deep intramuscular injection at intervals of 1 to 4 weeks. Patients should first be given a small test-dose as undesirable side-effects are prolonged. In general not more than 2–3 mL of oily injection should be administered at any one site.

Individual responses to neuroleptic drugs are very variable and to achieve optimum effect, dosage and dosage interval must be titrated according to the patient's response.

Equivalent doses of depot antipsychotics

Antipsychotic	Dose (mg)	Interval
Flupenthixol decanoate	40	2 weeks
Fluphenazine decanoate	25	2 weeks
Haloperidol (as decanoate)	100	4 weeks
Pipothiazine palmitate	50	4 weeks
Zuclopenthixol decanoate	200	2 weeks

These equivalences are intended **only** as an approximate guide; patients should be carefully monitored after **any** change in medication

CHOICE. There is no clear-cut division in the use of these drugs, but **zuclopenthixol** may be suitable for the treatment of agitated or aggressive patients whereas **flupenthixol** can cause over-excitement in such patients. **Fluspirilene** has a shorter duration of action than the other depot injections. The incidence of extrapyramidal reactions is similar for all these drugs.

CAUTIONS. Treatment requires careful monitoring for optimum effect; extrapyramidal symptoms occur frequently. When transferring from oral to depot therapy, dosage by mouth should be gradually phased out. Caution in arteriosclerosis.

CONTRA-INDICATIONS. Do not use in children, confusional states, coma caused by CNS depressants, parkinsonism, intolerance to antipsychotics.

SIDE-EFFECTS. Pain may occur at injection site and occasionally erythema, swelling, and nodules. For side-effects of specific antipsychotics see under the relevant monograph.

FLUPENTHIXOL DECANOATE

Indications: maintenance in schizophrenia and other psychoses

Cautions; Contra-indications; Side-effects: see under Chlorpromazine Hydrochloride (section 4.2.1) and notes above, but it may have a mood elevating effect; extrapyramidal symptoms usually appear 1–3 days after administration and continue for about 5 days but may be delayed; an alternative antipsychotic may be necessary if symptoms such as aggression or agitation appear; avoid in porphyria (see section 9.8.2)

Dose: by deep intramuscular injection into the gluteal muscle, test dose 20 mg, then after 5–10 days 20–40 mg repeated at intervals of 2–4 weeks, adjusted according to response; max. 400 mg weekly; usual maintenance dose 50 mg every 4 weeks to 300 mg every 2 weeks
ELDERLY initially quarter to half adult dose

PoM **Depixol**® (Lundbeck)
Injection (oily), flupenthixol decanoate 20 mg/mL. Net price 1-mL amp = £1.55; 1-mL syringe = £1.70; 2-mL amp = £2.60; 2-mL syringe = £2.75; 10-mL vial = £14.74

PoM **Depixol Conc.**® (Lundbeck)
Injection (oily), flupenthixol decanoate 100 mg/mL. Net price 0.5-mL amp = £3.49; 1-mL amp = £6.40; 5-mL vial = £28.27

PoM **Depixol Low Volume**® (Lundbeck)
Injection (oily), flupenthixol decanoate 200 mg/mL. Net price 1-mL amp = £19.90

FLUPHENAZINE DECANOATE

Indications: maintenance in schizophrenia and other psychoses

Cautions; Contra-indications; Side-effects: see under Chlorpromazine Hydrochloride (section 4.2.1) and notes above. Extrapyramidal symptoms usually appear a few hours after the dose has been administered and continue for about 2 days but may be delayed. Contra-indicated in severely depressed states

Dose: by deep intramuscular injection into the gluteal muscle, test dose 12.5 mg (6.25 mg in elderly), then after 4–7 days 12.5–100 mg repeated at intervals of 14–35 days, adjusted according to response

PoM **Modecate**® (Squibb)
Injection (oily), fluphenazine decanoate 25 mg/mL. Net price 0.5-mL amp = £1.45; 1-mL amp = £2.52; 1-mL syringe = £2.79; 2-mL amp = £4.97; 2-mL syringe = £5.05; 10-mL vial = £24.05

PoM **Modecate Concentrate**® (Squibb)
Injection (oily), fluphenazine decanoate 100 mg/mL. Net price 0.5-mL amp = £5.00; 1-mL amp = £9.77

FLUSPIRILENE

Indications: maintenance in schizophrenia
Cautions; Contra-indications; Side-effects: see under Chlorpromazine Hydrochloride (section 4.2.1) and notes above, but less sedating. Extrapyramidal symptoms usually appear 6–12 hours after the dose and continue for about 48 hours but may be delayed. Common side-effects are restlessness and sweating. With prolonged use, tissue damage (subcutaneous nodules) may occur at injection site

Dose: by deep intramuscular injection, 2 mg, increased by 2 mg at weekly intervals, according to response; usual maintenance dose 2–8 mg weekly; max. 20 mg weekly
ELDERLY initially quarter to half adult dose

PoM **Redeptin**® (SK&F)
Injection (aqueous suspension), fluspirilene 2 mg/mL. Net price 1-mL amp = 90p; 3-mL amp = £1.59; 6-mL vial = £2.76

HALOPERIDOL DECANOATE

Indications: maintenance in schizophrenia and other psychoses

Cautions; Contra-indications; Side-effects: see under Haloperidol (section 4.2.1) and notes above

Dose: by deep intramuscular injection into the gluteal muscle, haloperidol (as decanoate), initially 50 mg every 4 weeks, if necessary increasing after 2 weeks by 50-mg increments to 300 mg every 4 weeks; higher doses may be needed in some patients; ELDERLY, initially 12.5–25 mg every 4 weeks

PoM **Haldol Decanoate**® (Janssen)
Injection (oily), haloperidol (as decanoate) 50 mg/mL, net price 1-mL amp = £4.66; 100 mg/mL, 1-mL amp = £5.91

PIPOTHIAZINE PALMITATE

Indications: maintenance in schizophrenia and other psychoses

Cautions; Contra-indications; Side-effects: see under Chlorpromazine Hydrochloride (section 4.2.1) and notes above

Dose: by deep intramuscular injection into the gluteal muscle, test dose 25 mg, then a further 25–50 mg after 4–7 days, then adjusted according to response at intervals of 4 weeks; usual maintenance range 50–100 mg (max. 200 mg) every 4 weeks

ELDERLY initially 5–10 mg

PoM **Piportil Depot**® (Rhône-Poulenc Rorer)
Injection (oily), pipothiazine palmitate 50 mg/mL. Net price 1-mL amp = £6.28; 2-mL amp = £10.27

ZUCLOPENTHIXOL DECANOATE

Indications: maintenance in schizophrenia and other psychoses, particularly with aggression and agitation

Cautions; Contra-indications; Side-effects: see under Chlorpromazine Hydrochloride (section 4.2.1) and notes above, but less sedating; avoid in porphyria (see section 9.8.2)

Dose: by deep intramuscular injection into the gluteal muscle, test dose 100 mg, followed after 7–28 days by 100–200 mg or more, followed by 200–400 mg at intervals of 2–4 weeks, adjusted according to response; max. 600 mg weekly

PoM **Clopixol**® (Lundbeck)
Injection (oily), zuclopenthixol decanoate 200 mg/mL. Net price 1-mL amp = £3.01; 10-mL vial = £28.63

PoM **Clopixol Conc.**® (Lundbeck)
Injection (oily), zuclopenthixol decanoate 500 mg/mL. Net price 1-mL amp with needle = £7.25

4.2.3 Antimanic drugs

Drugs are used in mania both to control acute attacks and also to prevent their recurrence.

ANTIPSYCHOTIC DRUGS

In an acute attack of mania, treatment with an antipsychotic drug (section 4.2.1) is usually required because it may take a few days for lithium to exert its antimanic effect. Lithium may be given concurrently with the antipsychotic drug, and treatment with the antipsychotic gradually tailed off as lithium becomes effective. Alternatively, lithium therapy may be commenced once the patient's mood has been stabilised with the antipsychotic. Haloperidol may be preferred for rapid control of acute mania. However, high doses of haloperidol, fluphenazine, or flupenthixol may be hazardous when used with lithium; irreversible toxic encephalopathy has been reported.

LITHIUM

Lithium salts are used in the *prophylaxis and treatment of mania*, in the *prophylaxis of manic-depressive illness* (bipolar illness or bipolar depression) and in the *prophylaxis of recurrent depression* (unipolar illness or unipolar depression). Lithium is unsuitable for children.

The decision to give prophylactic lithium usually requires specialist advice, and must be based on careful consideration of the likelihood of recurrence in the individual patient, and the benefit weighed against the risks. In long-term use, therapeutic concentrations have been thought to cause histological and functional changes in the kidney. The significance of such changes is not clear but is of sufficient concern to discourage long-term use of lithium unless it is definitely indicated. Patients should therefore be maintained on lithium after 3–5 years only if, on assessment, benefit persists.

PLASMA CONCENTRATIONS. Lithium salts have a narrow therapeutic/toxic ratio and should therefore not be prescribed unless facilities for monitoring plasma concentrations are available. There seem few if any reasons for preferring one or other of the salts of lithium available. Doses are adjusted to achieve plasma concentrations of 0.4 to 1.0 mmol Li$^+$/litre (lower end of the range for maintenance therapy and elderly patients) on samples taken 12 hours after the preceding dose. It is important to determine the optimum range for each individual patient.

Overdosage, usually with plasma concentrations over 1.5 mmol Li$^+$/litre, may be fatal and toxic effects include tremor, ataxia, dysarthria, nystagmus, renal impairment, and convulsions. If these potentially hazardous signs occur, treatment should be stopped, plasma-lithium concentrations redetermined, and steps taken to reverse lithium toxicity. In mild cases withdrawal of lithium and administration of generous amounts of sodium and fluid will reverse the toxicity. Plasma concentrations in excess of 2.0 mmol Li$^+$/litre require emergency treatment as indicated under Emergency Treatment of Poisoning, p. 19. When toxic concentrations are reached there may be a delay of 1 or 2 days before maximum toxicity occurs.

INTERACTIONS. Lithium toxicity is made worse by sodium depletion, therefore concurrent use of diuretics (particularly thiazides) is hazardous and should be avoided. For other **interactions** with lithium, see Appendix 1 (lithium).

LITHIUM CARDS. A lithium treatment card available from pharmacies tells patients how to take lithium preparations, what to do if a dose is missed, and what side-effects to expect. It also explains why regular blood tests are important and warns that some medicines and illnesses can change lithium plasma concentrations.

The cards are available from NPA Services, 38–42 St Peter's St, St. Albans, Herts AL1 3NP.

Cautionary label wordings, see inside back cover

LITHIUM CARBONATE

Indications: treatment and prophylaxis of mania, manic-depressive illness, and recurrent depression (see also notes above); aggressive or self-mutilating behaviour

Cautions: measure plasma concentrations regularly (every 3 months on stabilised regimens), monitor thyroid function; maintain adequate sodium and fluid intake; avoid in renal impairment, cardiac disease, and conditions with sodium imbalance such as Addison's disease; reduction in dose or discontinuation may be necessary in diarrhoea, vomiting and intercurrent infection (especially when associated with profuse sweating); caution in pregnancy, breast-feeding, elderly patients (reduce dose), diuretic treatment, myasthenia gravis; surgery (see section 15.1); **interactions:** Appendix 1 (lithium)

Side-effects: gastro-intestinal disturbances, fine tremor, polyuria and polydipsia; also weight gain and oedema (may respond to dose reduction). Signs of lithium intoxication are blurred vision, increasing gastro-intestinal disturbances (anorexia, vomiting, diarrhoea), muscle weakness, increasing CNS disturbances (mild drowsiness and sluggishness increasing to giddiness with ataxia, coarse tremor, lack of co-ordination, dysarthria), and require withdrawal of treatment. With severe overdosage (plasma concentrations above 2 mmol/litre) hyperreflexia and hyperextension of limbs, convulsions, toxic psychoses, syncope, oliguria, circulatory failure, coma, and occasionally, death. Goitre, raised antidiuretic hormone concentration, hypothyroidism, hypokalaemia, ECG changes, exacerbation of psoriasis, and kidney changes may also occur. See also Emergency Treatment of Poisoning, p. 19

Dose: see under preparations below, adjusted to achieve a plasma concentration of 0.4–1.0 mmol Li$^+$/litre 12 hours after the preceding dose on the fourth or seventh day of treatment, then every week until dosage has remained constant for 4 weeks and every 3 months thereafter; doses are initially divided throughout the day, but once daily administration is preferred when plasma concentrations stabilised

PoM **Camcolit**® (Norgine)
Camcolit 250® *tablets*, f/c, scored, lithium carbonate 250 mg (6.8 mmol Li$^+$). Net price 20 = 59p. Label: 10 lithium card, counselling, see below
Camcolit 400® *tablets*, m/r, f/c, scored, lithium carbonate 400 mg (10.8 mmol Li$^+$). Net price 20 = 79p. Label: 10 lithium card, 25, counselling, see above
Dose (plasma monitoring, see above):
Treatment, initially 1.5–2 g daily (elderly, 0.5–1 g daily)
Prophylaxis, initially 0.5–1.2 g daily (elderly, 0.5–1 g daily)
Camcolit 250® should be given in divided doses, whereas Camcolit 400® may be given in single or divided doses

PoM **Liskonum**® (SK&F)
Tablets, m/r, f/c, scored, lithium carbonate 450 mg (12.2 mmol Li$^+$). Net price 60-tab pack = £2.82. Label: 10 lithium card, 25, counselling, see below
Dose (plasma monitoring, see above):
Treatment, initially 450–675 mg twice daily (elderly, initially 225 mg twice daily)
Prophylaxis, initially 450 mg twice daily (elderly, 225 mg twice daily)

PoM **Phasal**® (Lagap)
Tablets, m/r, lithium carbonate 300 mg (8.1 mmol Li$^+$). Net price 60-tab pack = £3.82. Label: 10 lithium card, 25, counselling, see below
Dose (plasma monitoring, see above):
Treatment, initially 600 mg twice daily (elderly, 0.5–1 g daily in divided doses)
Prophylaxis, initially 600 mg daily

PoM **Priadel**® (Delandale)
Tablets, both m/r, scored, lithium carbonate 200 mg (5.4 mmol Li$^+$), net price 20 = 42p; 400 mg (10.8 mmol Li$^+$), 20 = 62p. Label: 10 lithium card, 25, counselling, see below
Dose (plasma monitoring, see above):
Treatment and prophylaxis, initially 0.4–1.2 g daily as a single dose or in 2 divided doses (elderly or patients less than 50 kg, 400 mg daily)

Liquid, see under Lithium Citrate, below

COUNSELLING. Patients should maintain an adequate fluid intake and should avoid dietary changes which might reduce or increase sodium intake; lithium treatment cards are available from pharmacies (see above)
Note. **Different preparations vary widely in bioavailability**; a change in the preparation used requires the same precautions as initiation of treatment

---

LITHIUM CITRATE

Indications; Cautions; Side-effects: see under Lithium Carbonate and notes above
Dose: see under preparations below, adjusted to achieve plasma concentrations of 0.4–1.0 mmol Li$^+$/litre as described under Lithium Carbonate

PoM **Li-Liquid**® (RP Drugs)
Oral solution, sugar-free, lithium citrate 509 mg/5 mL (5.4 mmol Li$^+$/5 mL), yellow, net price 100-mL pack = £4.50; 1.018 g/5 mL (10.8 mmol Li$^+$/5 mL), orange, 100-mL pack = £9.00. Label: 10 lithium card, counselling, see above
Dose (plasma monitoring, see above):
Treatment and prophylaxis, initially 1.018–3.054 g daily in 2 divided doses (elderly or patients less than 50 kg, initially 509 mg twice daily)

PoM **Litarex**® (CP)
Tablets, m/r, lithium citrate 564 mg (6 mmol Li$^+$). Net price 20 = 72p. Label: 10 lithium card, 25, counselling, see above
Dose (plasma monitoring, see above):
Treatment and prophylaxis, initially 564 mg twice daily

PoM **Priadel**® (Delandale)
Liquid, yellow, sugar-free, lithium citrate 520 mg/5 mL (approx. 5.4 mmol Li$^+$/5 mL). Net price 150-mL pack = £6.75. Label: 10 lithium card, counselling, see above
Dose (plasma monitoring, see above):
Treatment and prophylaxis, initially 1.04–3.12 g daily in 2 divided doses (elderly or patients less than 50 kg, 520 mg twice daily)

CARBAMAZEPINE

Carbamazepine may be used for the prophylaxis of manic-depressive illness in patients unresponsive to lithium; it seems to be particularly effective in patients with rapid cycling manic-depressive illness (4 or more affective episodes per year).

CARBAMAZEPINE
Indications: prophylaxis of manic-depressive illness unresponsive to lithium; for use in epilepsy see section 4.8.1
Cautions; Contra-indications; Side-effects: see section 4.8.1
Dose: initially 400 mg daily in divided doses increased until symptoms controlled; usual range 400–600 mg daily; max. 1.6 g daily

Preparations
Section 4.8.1

4.3 Antidepressant drugs

4.3.1 Tricyclic and related antidepressant drugs
4.3.2 Monoamine-oxidase inhibitors (MAOIs)
4.3.3 Compound antidepressant preparations
4.3.4 Other antidepressant drugs

Tricyclic and related antidepressants (antidepressives) are the drugs of choice in the treatment of depressive illness, unless it is so severe that electroconvulsive therapy is immediately indicated. They are preferred to MAOIs because they are more effective antidepressants and do not show the dangerous interactions with some foods and drugs that are characteristic of the MAOIs. **Lithium** (section 4.2.3) has a mood-regulating action and is used in the treatment and prophylaxis of mania, manic depressive illness, and recurrent depression.

Prescribing more than one antidepressant of the tricyclic type at the same time is **not** recommended. It may constitute a hazard and there is no evidence that side-effects are minimised.

Mixtures of antidepressants with tranquillisers are in section 4.3.3; they are **not** recommended.

Other drugs used to treat depression are in section 4.3.4.

It should be noted that although anxiety is often present in depressive illness and may be the presenting symptom, the use of antipsychotics or anxiolytics may mask the true diagnosis. They should therefore be used with caution though they are useful adjuncts in agitated depression.

4.3.1 Tricyclic and related antidepressant drugs

The term 'tricyclic' is misleading as there are now 1-, 2-, and 4-ring structured drugs with broadly similar properties.

These drugs are most effective for treating moderate to severe *endogenous depression* associated with psychomotor and physiological changes such as loss of appetite and sleep disturbances; improvement in sleep is usually the first benefit of therapy. Since there may be an interval of 2 weeks before the antidepressant action takes place electroconvulsive treatment may be required in severe depression when delay is hazardous or intolerable.

Tricyclic antidepressants are also effective in the management of *panic disorder*.

Oral and facial pain may respond to a tricyclic antidepressant, particularly if associated with depression.

Some tricyclic antidepressants are used for the treatment of *nocturnal enuresis* in children, see section 7.4.2.

DOSAGE. About 10 to 20% of patients fail to respond to tricyclic and related antidepressant drugs and inadequate plasma concentrations may account for some of these failures. It is important to achieve plasma concentrations which are sufficiently high for effective treatment but not high enough to cause toxic effects. Low doses should be used for initial treatment in the **elderly** (see under Side-effects, below).

In most patients the long half-life of tricyclic antidepressant drugs allows **once-daily** administration, usually at night; the use of modified-release preparations is therefore unnecessary.

MANAGEMENT. The patient's condition must be checked frequently, especially in the early weeks of treatment, to detect any suicidal tendencies. Limited quantities of antidepressant drugs should be prescribed at any one time as they are dangerous in overdosage. Some of the newer drugs, for example mianserin and trazodone, seem less dangerous in overdose than the older tricyclics.

Treatment should be continued for 2 weeks before suppression of symptoms can be expected and thereafter should be maintained at the optimum level for at least another month before any attempt is made at dose reduction. Treatment should not be withdrawn prematurely, otherwise symptoms are likely to recur. The natural history of depressive illness suggests that remission usually occurs after 3 months to a year or more and some patients appear to benefit from maintenance therapy with about half the therapeutic dosage for several months to prevent relapse. In recurrent depression, prophylactic maintenance therapy may need to be continued for several years.

In patients who do not respond to antidepressants, the diagnosis, dosage, compliance, and possible continuation of psychosocial or physical aggravating causes should all be carefully reviewed; other drug treatment may be successful. The patient may respond to low-dose flupenthixol (Fluanxol®, section 4.3.4) or to MAOIs (section 4.3.2), but see **Interactions**, below.

WITHDRAWAL. Gastro-intestinal symptoms of nausea, vomiting, and anorexia, accompanied by headache, giddiness, 'chills', and insomnia, and sometimes by hypomania, panic-anxiety, and extreme motor restlessness may occur if an antidepressant (particularly an MAOI) is stopped suddenly after regular administration for 8 weeks or more. Reduction in dosage should preferably be carried out gradually over a period of about 4 weeks.

CHOICE. Antidepressant drugs can be roughly divided into those with additional sedative properties, e.g. **amitriptyline**, and those with less, e.g. **imipramine**. Agitated and anxious patients tend to respond best to the sedative compounds whereas withdrawn and apathetic patients will often obtain most benefit from less sedating compounds.

Antidepressants with **sedative** properties include amitriptyline, clomipramine, dothiepin, doxepin, maprotiline, mianserin, trazodone, and trimipramine.

Less sedative antidepressants include amoxapine, butriptyline, desipramine, imipramine, iprindole, lofepramine, nortriptyline, and viloxazine. Protriptyline has a **stimulant** action.

Amitriptyline may be given in divided doses or the entire daily dose may be given at night to promote sleep and avoid daytime drowsiness. **Imipramine** can also be given once daily but as it has a much less sedative action there is less need.

Imipramine and amitriptyline are well established and relatively safe and effective, but nevertheless have more marked antimuscarinic or cardiac side-effects than some of the newer compounds (**doxepin, lofepramine, mianserin, trazodone,** and **viloxazine**); this may be important in individual patients.

Amoxapine is related to the antipsychotic loxapine and its side-effects include tardive dyskinesia; overdosage has been associated with seizures.

SIDE-EFFECTS. Arrhythmias and heart block occasionally follow the use of tricyclic antidepressants, particularly amitriptyline, and may be a factor in the sudden death of patients with cardiac disease. They are also sometimes associated with convulsions and hepatic and haematological reactions. In particular, mianserin has been associated with haematological and hepatic reactions and maprotiline has been associated with convulsions. Patients being treated with these drugs therefore require careful supervision. In the case of **mianserin** a full **blood count** is recommended every 4 weeks during the first 3 months of treatment; subsequent clinical monitoring should continue and treatment should be stopped and a full blood count obtained if fever, sore throat, stomatitis, or other signs of infection develop.

Other side-effects of tricyclic and related antidepressants include drowsiness, dry mouth, blurred vision, constipation, and urinary retention (all attributed to antimuscarinic activity), and sweating. The patient should be encouraged to persist with treatment as some tolerance to these side-effects seems to develop. They are further reduced if low doses are given initially and then gradually increased.

This gradual introduction of treatment is particularly important in the elderly, who, because of the hypotensive effects of these drugs, are prone to attacks of dizziness or even syncope. The tricyclic and related antidepressants should be prescribed with caution in epilepsy as they lower the convulsive threshold.

Neuroleptic malignant syndrome (section 4.2.1) may, very rarely, arise in the course of antidepressant treatment.

Overdosage: see Emergency Treatment of Poisoning, p. 19.

INTERACTIONS. MAOIs should preferably not be started until at least a week after tricyclics and related antidepressants have been stopped; tricyclics and related antidepressants should not be given for 2 weeks after stopping MAOI treatment. For other tricyclic **interactions**, see Appendix 1 (antidepressants, tricyclic).

TRICYCLIC ANTIDEPRESSANTS

AMITRIPTYLINE HYDROCHLORIDE

Indications: depressive illness, particularly where sedation is required; nocturnal enuresis in children (see section 7.4.2)

Cautions: cardiac disease (particularly with arrhythmias, see contra-indications below), epilepsy, pregnancy and breast-feeding see appendixes 4 and 5, elderly, hepatic impairment, thyroid disease, psychoses (may aggravate mania), closed-angle glaucoma, urinary retention, concurrent electroconvulsive therapy. Avoid abrupt cessation of therapy. Also caution in anaesthesia (increased risk of arrhythmias and hypotension, see surgery section 15.1). See section 7.4.2 for nocturnal enuresis; **interactions:** Appendix 1 (antidepressants, tricyclic).

DRIVING. Drowsiness may affect performance of skilled tasks (e.g. driving); effects of alcohol enhanced

Contra-indications: recent myocardial infarction, heart block, mania; porphyria (see section 9.8.2)

Side-effects: dry mouth, sedation, blurred vision, constipation, nausea, difficulty with micturition (due to antimuscarinic action). Other common side-effects are cardiovascular (arrhythmias, postural hypotension, tachycardia, syncope, particularly with high doses), sweating, tremor, rashes, behavioural disturbances (particularly children), hypomania, confusion (particularly elderly), interference with sexual function, blood sugar changes; increased appetite and weight gain (occasionally weight loss). Less common, black tongue, paralytic ileus, convulsions, agranulocytosis, leucopenia, eosinophilia, purpura, thrombocytopenia, and jaundice; overdosage: see Emergency Treatment of Poisoning, p. 19

4.3 Antidepressant drugs

Dose: by mouth, initially 50–75 mg (elderly and adolescents 25–50 mg) daily in divided doses *or* as a single dose at bedtime increased gradually as necessary to max. 150–200 mg; usual maintenance 50–100 mg daily
Nocturnal enuresis, CHILD 7–10 years 10–20 mg, 11–16 years 25–50 mg at night; max. period of treatment (including gradual withdrawal) 3 months
By intramuscular or intravenous injection, 10–20 mg 4 times daily

PoM **Amitriptyline** (Non-proprietary)
Tablets, coated, amitriptyline hydrochloride 10 mg, net price 20 = 22p; 25 mg, 20 = 8p; 50 mg, 20 = 48p. Label: 2
Available from APS, Berk (Domical®), Cox, DDSA (Elavil®), Evans, Kerfoot

PoM **Lentizol**® (P-D)
Capsules, m/r, both enclosing white pellets, amitriptyline hydrochloride 25 mg (pink), net price 100-cap pack = £4.61; 50 mg (pink/red), 100-cap pack = £8.56. Label: 2, 25

PoM **Tryptizol**® (Morson)
Tablets, all f/c, amitriptyline hydrochloride 10 mg (blue), net price 20 = 22p; 25 mg (yellow), 20 = 46p; 50 mg (brown), 20 = 95p. Label: 2
Capsules, m/r, orange, amitriptyline hydrochloride 75 mg. Net price 20 = £1.78. Label: 2, 25
Mixture, pink, sugar-free, amitriptyline 10 mg (as embonate)/5 mL. Net price 200-mL pack = £1.87. Label: 2
Injection, amitriptyline hydrochloride 10 mg/mL. Net price 10-mL vial = 54p

AMOXAPINE

Indications: depressive illness
Cautions; Contra-indications; Side-effects: see under Amitriptyline Hydrochloride; tardive dyskinesia reported; menstrual irregularities, breast enlargement, and galactorrhoea reported in women
Dose: initially 100–150 mg daily in divided doses *or* as a single dose at bedtime increased as necessary to max. 300 mg daily; usual maintenance 150–250 mg daily
ELDERLY initially 25 mg twice daily increased as necessary after 5–7 days to max. 50 mg 3 times daily

PoM **Asendis**® (Novex)
Tablets, amoxapine 25 mg, net price 20 = £2.18; 50 mg (orange, scored), 20 = £3.63; 100 mg (blue, scored), 20 = £6.05; 150 mg (scored), 20 = £9.02. Label: 2

BUTRIPTYLINE

Indications: depressive illness
Cautions; Contra-indications; Side-effects: see under Amitriptyline Hydrochloride, but less sedating

Dose: 25 mg 3 times daily, increased gradually as necessary to max. 150 mg daily; usual maintenance dose 25 mg 3 times daily

PoM **Evadyne**® (Wyeth)
Tablets, orange, f/c, butriptyline (as hydrochloride) 25 mg, net price 100-tab pack = £3.87. Label: 2

CLOMIPRAMINE HYDROCHLORIDE

Indications: depressive illness, phobic and obsessional states; adjunctive treatment of cataplexy associated with narcolepsy
Cautions; Contra-indications; Side-effects: see under Amitriptyline Hydrochloride. Postural hypotension may occur on intravenous infusion
Dose: by mouth, initially 10 mg daily, increased gradually as necessary to 30–150 mg (elderly 75 mg) in divided doses *or* as a single dose at bedtime; max. 250 mg daily; usual maintenance 30–50 mg daily (severe cases 50–100 mg daily)
Phobic and obsessional states, initially 25 mg daily (elderly 10 mg daily) increased over 2 weeks to 100–150 mg daily
By intramuscular injection, initially 25–50 mg daily, increased by 25 mg daily to 100–150 mg daily
By intravenous infusion, initially to assess tolerance, 25–50 mg, then usually about 100 mg daily for 7–10 days

PoM **Clomipramine** (Non-proprietary)
Capsules, clomipramine hydrochloride 10 mg, net price 20 = 65p; 25 mg, 20 = £1.29; 50 mg, 20 = £2.45. Label: 2
Available from Cox, Generics, Hillcross, Norton

PoM **Anafranil**® (Geigy)
Capsules, clomipramine hydrochloride 10 mg (yellow/caramel), net price 84-cap pack = £2.76; 25 mg (orange/caramel), 84-cap pack = £5.43; 50 mg (blue/caramel), 56-cap pack = £6.89. Label: 2
Syrup, clomipramine hydrochloride 25 mg/5 mL. Net price 150-mL pack = £6.18. Label: 2
Injection, clomipramine hydrochloride 12.5 mg/mL. Net price 2-mL amp = 40p

PoM **Anafranil SR**® (Geigy)
Tablets, m/r, pink, f/c, clomipramine hydrochloride 75 mg. Net price 28-tab pack = £6.86. Label: 2, 25

DESIPRAMINE HYDROCHLORIDE

Indications: depressive illness
Cautions; Contra-indications; Side-effects: see under Amitriptyline Hydrochloride, but less sedating
Dose: 75 mg daily in divided doses *or* as a single dose at bedtime, increased as necessary to a max. of 200 mg
ELDERLY initially 25 mg daily

PoM **Pertofran**® (Ciba)
Tablets, pink, s/c, desipramine hydrochloride 25 mg. Net price 84-tab pack = £2.99. Label: 2

DOTHIEPIN HYDROCHLORIDE

Indications: depressive illness, particularly where sedation is required

Cautions; Contra-indications; Side-effects: see under Amitriptyline Hydrochloride

Dose: initially 75 mg (elderly 50–75 mg) daily in divided doses *or* as a single dose at bedtime, increased gradually as necessary to 150 mg daily (elderly 75 mg may be sufficient); up to 225 mg daily in some circumstances (e.g. hospital use)

PoM **Dothiepin** (Non-proprietary)
Capsules, dothiepin hydrochloride 25 mg, net price 20 = 95p. Label: 2
Available from APS, Ashbourne (Dothapax®), Berk (Prepadine®), Cox, Generics, Hillcross, Kerfoot, Norton
Tablets, dothiepin hydrochloride 75 mg, net price 28-tab pack = £3.43. Label: 2
Available from APS, Ashbourne (Dothapax®), Berk (Prepadine®), Cox, Generics, Hillcross, Kerfoot, Norton

PoM **Prothiaden**® (Boots)
Capsules, red/brown, dothiepin hydrochloride 25 mg. Net price 20 = £1.00. Label: 2
Tablets, red, s/c, dothiepin hydrochloride 75 mg. Net price 28-tab pack = £4.00. Label: 2

DOXEPIN

Indications: depressive illness, particularly where sedation is required

Cautions; Contra-indications; Side-effects: see under Amitriptyline Hydrochloride; avoid in breast-feeding (see Appendix 5)

Dose: initially 75 mg (elderly 10–50 mg) daily in 3 divided doses, increased gradually to max. 300 mg daily in divided doses; range 30–300 mg daily; up to 100 mg may be given as a single dose at bedtime

PoM **Sinequan**® (Pfizer)
Capsules, doxepin (as hydrochloride) 10 mg (orange), net price 56-cap pack = £1.10; 25 mg (orange/blue), 28-cap pack = 79p; 50 mg (blue), 28-cap pack = £1.30; 75 mg (yellow/blue), 28-cap pack = £2.06. Label: 2

IMIPRAMINE HYDROCHLORIDE

Indications: depressive illness; nocturnal enuresis in children (see section 7.4.2)

Cautions; Contra-indications; Side-effects: see under Amitriptyline Hydrochloride, but less sedating

Dose: initially up to 75 mg daily in divided doses increased gradually to 150–200 mg (up to 300 mg in hospital patients); up to 150 mg may be given as a single dose at bedtime; usual maintenance 50–100 mg daily; ELDERLY initially 10 mg daily, increased gradually to 30–50 mg daily
Nocturnal enuresis, CHILD 7 years 25 mg, 8–11 years 25–50 mg, over 11 years 50–75 mg at bedtime; max. period of treatment (including gradual withdrawal) 3 months

PoM **Imipramine** (Non-proprietary)
Tablets, coated, imipramine hydrochloride 10 mg, net price 20 = 15p; 25 mg, 20 = 14p. Label: 2

PoM **Tofranil**® (Geigy)
Tablets, both red-brown, s/c, imipramine hydrochloride 10 mg, net price 84-tab pack = £1.39; 25 mg, 84-tab pack = £2.65. Label: 2
Syrup, imipramine hydrochloride 25 mg/5 mL. Net price 150-mL pack = £2.70. Label: 2

LOFEPRAMINE

Indications: depressive illness

Cautions; Contra-indications; Side-effects: see under Amitriptyline Hydrochloride, but less sedating; hepatic disorders reported; contra-indicated in hepatic and severe renal impairment

Dose: 140–210 mg daily in divided doses

PoM **Gamanil**® (Merck)
Tablets, f/c, brown-violet, lofepramine 70 mg (as hydrochloride). Net price 56-tab pack = £9.97. Label: 2

NORTRIPTYLINE

Indications: depressive illness; nocturnal enuresis in children (see section 7.4.2)

Cautions; Contra-indications; Side-effects: see under Amitriptyline Hydrochloride but less sedating

Dose: initially 20–40 mg (elderly 30 mg) daily in single *or* divided doses, increased gradually as necessary to max. 100 mg daily; usual maintenance dose 30–75 mg daily
Nocturnal enuresis, CHILD 7 years 10 mg, 8–11 years 10–20 mg, over 11 years 25–35 mg, at night; max period of treatment (including gradual withdrawal) 3 months

PoM **Allegron**® (Dista)
Tablets, nortriptyline (as hydrochloride) 10 mg, net price 20 = 67p; 25 mg (orange, scored), 20 = £1.36. Label: 2

PoM **Aventyl**® (Lilly)
Capsules, both yellow/white, nortriptyline (as hydrochloride) 10 mg, net price 20 = 67p; 25 mg, 20 = £1.36. Label: 2

PROTRIPTYLINE HYDROCHLORIDE

Indications: depressive illness, particularly with apathy and withdrawal

Cautions; Contra-indications; Side-effects: see under Amitriptyline Hydrochloride but less sedating; anxiety, agitation, tachycardia, and hypotension more common; rashes associated with photosensitisation (avoid direct sunlight); daily dose above 20 mg in elderly (increased risk of cardiovascular side-effects)

Dose: initially 10 mg 3–4 times daily (elderly 5 mg 3 times daily initially) if insomnia, last dose not after 4 p.m.; usual range 15–60 mg daily

4.3 Antidepressant drugs 161

PoM **Concordin**® (MSD)
Tablets, both f/c, protriptyline hydrochloride 5 mg (pink), net price 20 = 44p; 10 mg, 20 = 65p. Label: 2, 11

TRIMIPRAMINE

Indications: depressive illness, particularly where sedation is required
Cautions; Contra-indications; Side-effects: see under Amitriptyline Hydrochloride
Dose: 50–75 mg daily as a single dose 2 hours before bedtime *or* as 25 mg midday and 50 mg evening, increased as necessary to max. of 300 mg daily; usual maintenance dose 75–150 mg daily
ELDERLY 10–25 mg 3 times daily initially, half adult maintenance dose may be sufficient

PoM **Surmontil**® (Rhône-Poulenc Rorer)
Capsules, green/white, trimipramine 50 mg (as maleate). Net price 28-cap pack = £4.63. Label: 2
Tablets, trimipramine (as maleate) 10 mg, net price 50-tab pack = £2.48; 25 mg, 50-tab pack = £4.12. Label: 2

RELATED ANTIDEPRESSANTS

IPRINDOLE

Indications: depressive illness
Cautions; Contra-indications; Side-effects: see under Amitriptyline Hydrochloride, but less sedating. Caution in liver disease; jaundice, although rare, may develop, usually in the first 21 days
Dose: initially 15–30 mg 3 times daily, increased gradually to max. 60 mg 3 times daily; usual maintenance 30 mg 3 times daily

PoM **Prondol**® (Wyeth)
Tablets, yellow, iprindole (as hydrochloride) 15 mg, net price 20 = 42p. Label: 2

MAPROTILINE HYDROCHLORIDE

Indications: depressive illness, particularly where sedation is required
Cautions; Contra-indications; Side-effects: see under Amitriptyline Hydrochloride, antimuscarinic effects may occur less frequently but rashes common and increased risk of convulsions at higher dosage; contra-indicated if history of epilepsy
Dose: initially 25–75 mg (elderly 30 mg) daily in 3 divided doses *or* as a single dose at bedtime, increased gradually as necessary to max. 150 mg daily

PoM **Ludiomil**® (Ciba)
Tablets, all f/c, maprotiline hydrochloride 10 mg (pale yellow), net price 20 = 60p; 25 mg (greyish-red), 20 = £1.10; 50 mg (light orange), 28-tab pack = £3.01; 75 mg (brownish-orange), 28-tab pack = £4.40. Label: 2
Additives: include gluten

MIANSERIN HYDROCHLORIDE

Indications: depressive illness, particularly where sedation is required
Cautions; Contra-indications; Side-effects: see under Amitriptyline Hydrochloride; leucopenia, agranulocytosis and aplastic anaemia (particularly in the elderly); jaundice; arthritis, arthralgia; influenza-like syndrome may occur; **blood counts needed, p. 158**
Fewer and milder antimuscarinic and cardiovascular effects; **interactions:** Appendix 1 (mianserin)
Dose: initially 30–40 mg (elderly 30 mg) daily in divided doses *or* as a single dose at bedtime, increased gradually as necessary; usual dose range 30–90 mg

PoM **Mianserin** (Non-proprietary)
Tablets, mianserin hydrochloride 10 mg, net price 20 = £1.36; 20 mg, 20 = £2.73; 30 mg, 20 = £4.04. Label: 2, 25
PoM **Bolvidon**® (Organon)
Tablets, all f/c, mianserin hydrochloride 10 mg, net price 20 = £1.16; 20 mg, 20 = £2.33; 30 mg, 20 = £3.49. Label: 2, 25
PoM **Norval**® (Bencard)
Tablets, all orange, f/c, mianserin hydrochloride 10 mg, net price 84-tab pack = £5.50; 20 mg, 28-tab pack = £3.66; 30 mg, 28-tab pack = £5.50. Label: 2, 25

TRAZODONE HYDROCHLORIDE

Indications: depressive illness, particularly where sedation is required
Cautions; Contra-indications; Side-effects: see under Amitriptyline Hydrochloride but fewer antimuscarinic and cardiovascular effects; rarely priapism; **interactions:** Appendix 1 (trazodone)
Dose: initially 150 mg (elderly 100 mg) daily in divided doses after food *or* as a single dose at bedtime; may be increased to 300 mg daily; hospital patients up to max. 600 mg daily in divided doses

PoM **Molipaxin**® (Roussel)
Capsules, trazodone hydrochloride 50 mg (violet/green), net price 84-cap pack = £17.30; 100 mg (violet/fawn), 56-cap pack = £20.38. Label: 2, 21
Tablets, pink, f/c, trazodone hydrochloride 150 mg. Net price 28-tab pack = £11.62. Label: 2, 21
Liquid, sugar-free, trazodone hydrochloride 50 mg/5 mL. Net price 150-mL pack = £7.74. Label: 2, 21
CR tablets, m/r, blue, f/c, trazodone hydrochloride 150 mg. Net price 28-tab pack = £11.62. Label: 2, 21, 25
Dose: initially 1 tablet daily (elderly, dose form not appropriate for initial dose titration), increased if necessary to 2 tablets daily (up to 4 tablets daily in hospital patients)

VILOXAZINE HYDROCHLORIDE

Indications: depressive illness

Cautions; Contra-indications; Side-effects: see under Amitriptyline Hydrochloride, but less sedating and antimuscarinic and cardiovascular side-effects are fewer and milder; nausea and headache may occur; **interactions:** Appendix 1 (viloxazine)

Dose: 300 mg daily (preferably as 200 mg in the morning and 100 mg at midday), increased gradually as necessary; max. 400 mg daily; last dose not later than 6 p.m.

ELDERLY 100 mg daily initially, half adult maintenance dose may be sufficient

PoM **Vivalan**® (ICI)
Tablets, f/c, viloxazine 50 mg (as hydrochloride). Net price 20 = £1.27. Label: 2

4.3.2 Monoamine-oxidase inhibitors (MAOIs)

Monoamine-oxidase inhibitors are used much less frequently than tricyclic and related antidepressants because of the dangers of dietary and drug interactions and the fact that it is easier to prescribe MAOIs when tricyclic antidepressants have been unsuccessful than vice versa. **Tranylcypromine**, is the most **hazardous** of the MAOIs because of its stimulant action. The drugs of choice are **phenelzine** or **isocarboxazid** which are less stimulant and therefore safer.

Phobic patients and depressed patients with atypical, hypochondriacal, or hysterical features are said to respond best to MAOIs. However, MAOIs should be tried in any patients who are refractory to treatment with other antidepressants as there is occasionally a dramatic response. Response to treatment may be delayed for 3 weeks or more and may take an additional 1 or 2 weeks to become maximal.

WITHDRAWAL. See section 4.3.1

INTERACTIONS. MAOIs inhibit monoamine oxidase, thereby causing an accumulation of amine neurotransmitters. The metabolism of some amine drugs such as indirect-acting sympathomimetics is also inhibited and their pressor action may be potentiated; the pressor effect of tyramine (in some foods) may also be dangerously potentiated.

Sympathomimetics are present in many proprietary cough mixtures and decongestant nasal drops. See Appendix 1 (MAOIs) and Treatment Card. These interactions may cause a dangerous rise in blood pressure. An early warning symptom may be a throbbing headache. The danger of interaction persists for up to 14 days after treatment with MAOIs is discontinued. Treatment cards which list the necessary precautions are distributed by the Royal Pharmaceutical Society and given to patients at pharmacies etc.

Other antidepressants should **not** be given to patients for 14 days after treatment with MAOIs has been discontinued. Some psychiatrists use selected tricyclics in conjunction with MAOIs but this is hazardous, indeed potentially lethal, except in experienced hands and there is no evidence that the combination is more effective than when either constituent is used alone. The combination of tranylcypromine with clomipramine is particularly **dangerous**.

MAOIs should preferably not be started until at least a week after tricyclics and related antidepressants have been stopped; they should not be started until 2 weeks after a serotonin uptake inhibitor antidepressant has been stopped (5 weeks in the case of fluoxetine).

For other interactions with monoamine-oxidase inhibitors including those with opioid analgesics (notably pethidine), see Appendix 1 (MAOIs).

Other MAOIs. Discontinue first MAOI for at least a week before starting another.

TREATMENT CARD

Carry this card with you at all times. Show it to any doctor who may treat you other than the doctor who prescribed this medicine, and to your dentist if you require dental treatment.

INSTRUCTIONS TO PATIENTS

Please read carefully

While taking this medicine and for 14 days after your treatment finishes you must observe the following simple instructions:–

1 Do not eat CHEESE, PICKLED HERRING OR BROAD BEAN PODS.

2 Do not eat or drink BOVRIL, OXO, MARMITE or ANY SIMILAR MEAT OR YEAST EXTRACT.

3 Eat only FRESH foods and avoid food that you suspect could be stale or 'going off'. This is especially important with meat, fish, poultry or offal. Avoid game.

4 Do not take any other MEDICINES (including tablets, capsules, nose drops, inhalations or suppositories) whether purchased by you or previously prescribed by your doctor, without first consulting your doctor or your pharmacist.

NB *Treatment for coughs and colds, pain relievers, tonics and laxatives are medicines.*

5 Avoid alcoholic drinks and de-alcoholised (low alcohol) drinks.

Keep a careful note of any food or drink that disagrees with you, avoid it and tell your doctor.

Report any unusual or severe symptoms to your doctor and follow any other advice given by him.

M.A.O.I. Prepared by The Pharmaceutical Society and the British Medical Association on behalf of the Health Departments of the United Kingdom.

Printed in the UK for HMSO 8217411/150M/9.89/4529
Revised Sep. 1989

PHENELZINE

Indications: depressive illness

Cautions: diabetes mellitus, cardiovascular disease, epilepsy, blood disorders, concurrent electroconvulsive therapy; avoid abrupt dis-

4.3 Antidepressant drugs

continuation of treatment; severe hypertensive reactions to certain drugs and foods (see Treatment Card); avoid in elderly and agitated patients; pregnancy and breast-feeding; surgery (see section 15.1); **interactions:** Appendix 1 (MAOIs)

DRIVING. Drowsiness may affect performance of skilled tasks (e.g. driving)

Contra-indications: hepatic impairment (see Appendix 2), cerebrovascular disease, phaeochromocytoma, porphyria (see section 9.8.2), children

Side-effects: adverse effects commonly associated with phenelzine and other MAOIs include postural hypotension and dizziness; other common side-effects include drowsiness, headache, weakness and fatigue, dryness of mouth, constipation and other gastro-intestinal disturbances, and oedema; agitation and tremors, nervousness, blurred vision, difficulty in micturition, sweating, convulsions, rashes, leucopenia, sexual disturbances, and weight gain with inappropriate appetite may also occur; psychotic episodes with hypomanic behaviour, confusion, and hallucinations, may be induced in susceptible persons; jaundice has been reported and, on rare occasions, fatal progressive hepatocellular necrosis; peripheral neuropathy may be due to pyridoxine deficiency

Dose: 15 mg 3 times daily, increased if necessary to 4 times daily after 2 weeks (hospital patients, max. 30 mg 3 times daily), then reduced gradually to lowest possible maintenance dose (15 mg on alternate days may be adequate)

PoM **Nardil**® (P-D)
Tablets, orange, f/c, phenelzine 15 mg (as sulphate). Net price 20 = £1.33. Label: 3, 10 MAOI card

ISOCARBOXAZID

Indications: depressive illness
Cautions; Contra-indications; Side-effects: see under Phenelzine
Dose: initially up to 30 mg daily in single or divided doses increased after 4 weeks if necessary to max. 60 mg daily for up to 6 weeks under close supervision only; then reduced to usual maintenance dose 10–20 mg daily (but up to 40 mg daily may be required)

PoM **Marplan**® (Cambridge)
Tablets, pink, scored, isocarboxazid 10 mg. Net price 50 = 98p. Label: 3, 10 MAOI card

TRANYLCYPROMINE

Indications: depressive illness
Cautions; Contra-indications; see under Phenelzine; also contra-indicated in hyperthyroidism

Side-effects: see under Phenelzine; insomnia if given in evening; hypertensive crises with throbbing headache requiring discontinuation of treatment occur more frequently than with other MAOIs; liver damage occurs less frequently than with phenelzine
Dose: initially 10 mg twice daily not later than 3 p.m., increasing the second daily dose to 20 mg after 1 week if necessary; doses above 30 mg daily under close supervision only; usual maintenance dose 10 mg daily

PoM **Parnate**® (SK&F)
Tablets, red, s/c, tranylcypromine 10 mg (as sulphate). Net price 20 = 91p. Label: 3, 10 MAOI card

4.3.3 Compound antidepressant preparations

The use of preparations listed below is **not** recommended because the dosage of the individual components should be adjusted separately. Whereas antidepressants are given continuously over several months, anxiolytics are prescribed on a short-term basis.

NHS PoM **Limbitrol**® (Roche)
'*5*' *Capsules*, pink/green, amitriptyline 12.5 mg (as hydrochloride), chlordiazepoxide 5 mg. Net price 20 = £1.15. Label: 2
'*10*' *Capsules*, pink/dark green, amitriptyline 25 mg (as hydrochloride), chlordiazepoxide 10 mg. Net price 20 = £1.67. Label: 2

PoM **Motipress**® (Squibb)
Tablets, yellow, s/c, fluphenazine hydrochloride 1.5 mg, nortriptyline 30 mg (as hydrochloride). Net price 28-tab pack = £2.90. Label: 2

PoM **Motival**® (Squibb)
Tablets, pink, s/c, fluphenazine hydrochloride 500 micrograms, nortriptyline 10 mg (as hydrochloride). Net price 20 = 70p. Label: 2

PoM **Parstelin**® (SK&F)
Tablets, green, s/c, tranylcypromine 10 mg (as sulphate), trifluoperazine 1 mg (as hydrochloride). Net price 20 = 93p. Label: 3, 10 MAOI card
Caution: contains MAOI

PoM **Triptafen**® (Evans)
Tablets, pink, s/c, amitriptyline hydrochloride 25 mg, perphenazine 2 mg. Net price 20 = 54p. Label: 2

PoM **Triptafen-M**® (Evans)
Tablets, pink, s/c, amitriptyline hydrochloride 10 mg, perphenazine 2 mg. Net price 20 = 48p. Label: 2

4.3.4 Other antidepressant drugs

FLUPENTHIXOL

The thioxanthene **flupenthixol** (Fluanxol®) has antidepressant properties, and low doses (1 to 3 mg daily) are given by mouth for this purpose. Its advantages over the tricyclic and related antidepressants are that, with the low doses employed, side-effects are fewer, and that overdosage is less toxic.

FLUPENTHIXOL

Indications: depressive illness (short-term use). For use in psychoses, see section 4.2.1

Cautions: cardiovascular disease (including cardiac disorders and cerebral arteriosclerosis), senile confusional states, parkinsonism, renal and hepatic disease; avoid in excitable and overactive patients; avoid in porphyria (see section 9.8.2); **interactions:** Appendix 1 (phenothiazines and other antipsychotics)
DRIVING. Drowsiness may affect performance of skilled tasks (e.g. driving); effects of alcohol enhanced

Side-effects: restlessness, insomnia; hypomania reported; rarely dizziness, tremor, visual disturbances, headache, hyperprolactinaemia, extrapyramidal symptoms

Dose: initially 1 mg (elderly 500 micrograms) in the morning, increased after 1 week to 2 mg (elderly 1 mg) if necessary. Max. 3 mg (elderly 2 mg) daily, doses above 2 mg (elderly 1 mg) being divided in 2 portions, second dose not after 4 p.m. Discontinue if no response after 1 week at maximum dosage
COUNSELLING. Although drowsiness may occur, can also have an alerting effect so should not be taken in the evening

PoM **Depixol**® (psychoses), see section 4.2.1
PoM **Fluanxol**® (Lundbeck)
Tablets, both red, s/c, flupenthixol (as dihydrochloride) 500 micrograms, net price 20 = £1.18; 1 mg, 60-tab pack = £7.16. Label: 2, counselling, administration

TRYPTOPHAN

Tryptophan appeared to benefit some patients when given alone or as adjunctive therapy but tryptophan products have been withdrawn following evidence of an association with the eosinophilia-myalgia syndrome; they remain available on a named-patient basis for patients for whom no alternative treatment is suitable.

SEROTONIN UPTAKE INHIBITORS

Fluvoxamine, fluoxetine, paroxetine, and **sertraline** selectively inhibit the re-uptake of serotonin (5-hydroxytryptamine, 5-HT); they appear to be effective antidepressants. They are less sedative than the tricyclics, with few antimuscarinic effects and with low cardiotoxicity. They do not cause weight gain. Gastro-intestinal side-effects (diarrhoea, nausea and vomiting) are dose-related; headache, restlessness and anxiety may also occur. As with the tricyclic antidepressants caution is necessary in epilepsy.

INTERACTIONS. MAOIs should preferably not be started until at least 2 weeks after a serotonin uptake inhibitor antidepressant has been stopped (5 weeks after stopping in the case of fluoxetine). Serotonin uptake inhibitor antidepressants should preferably not be started until at least 2 weeks after an MAOI has been stopped.
Other interactions, see Appendix 1.

FLUOXETINE HYDROCHLORIDE

Indications: see under Dose

Cautions: hepatic impairment, renal impairment (avoid if severe), epilepsy (avoid if poorly controlled), diabetes mellitus, pregnancy; long half-life (delayed response to dose change or cessation); rare reports of prolonged seizures with electroconvulsive therapy; **interactions:** Appendix 1 (antidepressants, serotonin uptake inhibitor)
DRIVING. May impair performance of skilled tasks (e.g. driving)

Contra-indications: breast-feeding

Side-effects: rash (discontinue treatment, may be associated with vasculitis, anaphylaxis, and pulmonary inflammation or fibrosis), nausea, vomiting, diarrhoea, anorexia with weight loss, headache, nervousness, insomnia, anxiety, tremor, dry mouth, dizziness, hypomania, drowsiness, convulsions, fever, sexual dysfunction, sweating; other side-effects reported are vaginal bleeding on withdrawal, hyperprolactinaemia, thrombocytopenia, altered platelet function and abnormal bleeding, confusion; rarely hyponatraemia

Dose: depressive illness, 20 mg daily
Bulimia nervosa, 60 mg daily

PoM **Prozac**® (Dista)
Capsules, green/off-white, fluoxetine hydrochloride 20 mg. Net price 30-cap pack = £32.05. Counselling, driving

FLUVOXAMINE MALEATE

Indications: depressive illness

Cautions: renal and hepatic impairment; pregnancy and breast-feeding; **interactions:** Appendix 1 (antidepressants, serotonin uptake inhibitor)
DRIVING. May impair performance of skilled tasks (e.g. driving); effects of alcohol enhanced

Contra-indications: history of epilepsy

Side-effects: nausea and vomiting, diarrhoea, drowsiness, dizziness, agitation, anxiety, headache, tremor; bradycardia; convulsions; rarely increase in liver enzymes with symptoms (discontinue)

Dose: 100–200 mg daily (up to 100 mg as single dose in evening); max. 300 mg daily

PoM **Faverin**® (Duphar)
Tablets, both yellow, e/c, fluvoxamine maleate 50 mg, net price 60-tab pack = £25.00; 100 mg, 30-tab pack = £25.00. Label: 5, 25, counselling, driving

PAROXETINE

Indications: depressive illness

Cautions: cardiac disease, epilepsy, hepatic or renal impairment, pregnancy, breast-feeding, history of mania; avoid abrupt withdrawal; **interactions:** Appendix 1 (antidepressants, serotonin uptake inhibitor)
DRIVING. May affect performance of skilled tasks (e.g. driving)

Side-effects: nausea, drowsiness, sweating, tremor, asthenia, dry mouth, insomnia, sexual dysfunction
Dose: usually 20 mg each morning, if necessary increased gradually in increments of 10 mg to max. 50 mg daily (elderly, 40 mg daily)

▼ PoM **Seroxat**® (SmithKline Beecham)
Tablets, both f/c, scored, paroxetine 20 mg (as hydrochloride), net price 30-tab pack = £33.90; 30 mg (blue), 30-tab pack = £50.85. Label: 21, 25, counselling, driving

SERTRALINE
Indications: depressive illness
Cautions: epilepsy (avoid if unstable); avoid in hepatic and renal impairment, and in electroconvulsive therapy; pregnancy and breast-feeding; **interactions:** Appendix 1 (antidepressants, serotonin uptake inhibitor)
DRIVING. May affect performance of skilled tasks (e.g. driving)
Side-effects: dry mouth, nausea, diarrhoea, delayed ejaculation, tremor, increased sweating, dyspepsia; rarely, increase in serum transaminases (discontinue)
Dose: initially 50 mg daily, increased if necessary by increments of 50 mg over several weeks to max. 200 mg daily, then reduced to usual maintenance of 50–100 mg daily; doses of 150 mg or greater should not be used for more than 8 weeks

▼ PoM **Lustral**® (Invicta)
Tablets, sertraline (as hydrochloride) 50 mg, net price 28-tab pack = £26.51; 100 mg, 28-tab pack = £39.77. Label: 21, counselling, driving

4.4 Central nervous stimulants

Central nervous system stimulants have very few indications and in particular, should **not** be used to treat depression, obesity, senility, debility, or for relief of fatigue.

Caffeine is a weak stimulant present in tea and coffee. It is included in some analgesic preparations (section 4.7.1.1) but does not contribute to their analgesic or anti-inflammatory effect. Over-indulgence may lead to a state of anxiety.

The **amphetamines** have a limited field of usefulness and their use should be **discouraged** as they may cause dependence and psychotic states.

Patients with narcolepsy may derive benefit from treatment with amphetamines.

Amphetamines have been advocated for the management of hyperactive children; beneficial effects have been described. However, they must be used very selectively as they retard growth and the effect of long-term therapy has not been evaluated.

Amphetamines have **no place** in the management of **depression** or **obesity**.

Pemoline is a weak central nervous system stimulant that has been advocated for the management of hyperactive children. The same general reservations apply as for amphetamines and treatment should be carried out only under specialist supervision.

DEXAMPHETAMINE SULPHATE
Indications: narcolepsy, adjunct in the management of hyperkinesia in children (under specialist supervision)
Cautions: mild hypertension (contra-indicated if moderate or severe); monitor growth in children; avoid abrupt withdrawal; **interactions:** Appendix 1 (sympathomimetics)
Contra-indications: cardiovascular disease or moderate to severe hypertension (caution if mild), hyperexcitable states, hyperthyroidism, history of drug abuse, glaucoma, extrapyramidal disorders, pregnancy and breast-feeding, porphyria (see section 9.8.2)
DRIVING. May affect performance of skilled tasks (e.g. driving); effects of alcohol unpredictable
Side-effects: insomnia, restlessness, irritability, nervousness, night terrors, euphoria, tremor, dizziness, headache; dependence, tolerance, sometimes psychosis; anorexia, gastro-intestinal symptoms, growth retardation in children; dry mouth, sweating, tachycardia, palpitations, increased blood pressure; rarely cardiomyopathy reported with chronic use; overdosage: see Emergency Treatment of Poisoning, p. 20
Dose: narcolepsy, 10 mg (elderly, 5 mg) daily in divided doses increased by 10 mg (elderly, 5 mg) daily at intervals of 1 week to a max. of 60 mg daily
Hyperkinesia, CHILD over 6 years 5–10 mg in the morning, increased if necessary by 5 mg at intervals of 1 week to usual max. 20 mg daily (older children have received max. 40 mg daily)

CD **Dexedrine**® (Evans)
Tablets, scored, dexamphetamine sulphate 5 mg. Net price 20 = 15p. Counselling, driving

PEMOLINE
Indications: adjunct in the management of hyperkinesia in children (under specialist supervision)
Cautions; Contra-indications; Side-effects: see under Dexamphetamine Sulphate; chorea, tics, mania, depression, neutropenia, and liver enzyme abnormalities also reported
Dose: CHILD over 6 years, initially 20 mg every morning increased by increments of 20 mg at intervals of 1 week to 60 mg every morning, followed, if no improvement, by gradual increase to max. 120 mg every morning

PoM **Volital**® (LAB)
Tablets, scored, pemoline 20 mg. Net price 25-tab pack = £1.40

STIMULANT WITH VITAMINS

Prolintane is contained in a preparation with vitamins; it is **not** recommended and is specifically **contra-indicated** in epilepsy and hyperthyroidism.

NHS PoM **Villescon**® (Boehringer Ingelheim)
Liquid, red, prolintane hydrochloride 2.5 mg/5 mL with vitamins B group and C. Net price 150-mL pack = 85p
Dose: 10 mL twice daily before 4 p.m. for 1–2 weeks but see notes above.

COCAINE

Cocaine is a drug of addiction which causes central nervous stimulation. Its clinical use is mainly as a topical local anaesthetic (see sections 11.7 and 15.2). It has been included in analgesic elixirs for the relief of pain in terminal care but this use is obsolete.

4.5 Appetite suppressants

4.5.1 Bulk-forming drugs
4.5.2 Centrally acting appetite suppressants

The development of obesity appears to be multifactorial. Aggravating factors may be depression or other psychosocial problems or drug treatment.

The main treatment of the obese patient is an appropriate diet, carefully explained to the patient, with support and encouragement from the doctor. Attendance at groups (for example 'weight-watchers') helps some individuals. Drugs can play only a limited role and should never be used as the sole element of treatment; their effects tend to be disappointing.

The use of diuretics is **not** appropriate for weight reduction.

4.5.1 Bulk-forming drugs

The most commonly used bulk-forming drug is **methylcellulose**. It is claimed to reduce intake by producing feelings of satiety but there is little evidence to support this claim.

METHYLCELLULOSE

Indications: obesity; other indications, see section 1.6.1
Cautions: maintain adequate fluid intake
Contra-indications: gastro-intestinal obstruction
Side-effects: flatulence, abdominal distension, intestinal obstruction
Dose: see under preparations below
COUNSELLING. Preparations that swell in contact with liquid should always be carefully swallowed with water and should not be taken immediately before going to bed

Celevac® (Boehringer Ingelheim)
Tablets, pink, methylcellulose '450' 500 mg. Net price 112-tab pack = 93p. Counselling, see above and dose
Dose: 3 tablets, chewed or crushed, with a tumblerful of liquid half an hour before food or when hungry

Nilstim® (De Witt)
Tablets, green, cellulose (microcrystalline) 220 mg, methylcellulose '2500' 400 mg. Net price 20 = 25p. Counselling, see above and dose
Dose: 2 tablets, chewed or crushed, with a tumblerful of liquid 15 minutes before the 2 main meals or when hungry

STERCULIA

Indications; Cautions; Contra-indications; Side-effects: see under Methylcellulose
Dose: see under preparation below

Prefil® (Norgine)
Granules, brown, coated, sterculia 55%. Net price 200 g = £2.27. Label: 22, 27, counselling, administration
Dose: two 5-mL spoonfuls followed by a tumblerful of liquid ½–1 hour before food, reduced in patients accustomed to a low-residue diet

4.5.2 Centrally acting appetite suppressants

Centrally acting appetite suppressants are of no real value in the treatment of obesity since they do not improve the long-term outlook. They are sympathomimetics and most have a pronounced stimulant effect on the central nervous system.

Use of the amphetamine-like drugs **diethylpropion**, **mazindol**, and **phentermine** is **not** justified as any possible benefits are outweighed by the risks involved; abuse, particularly of diethylpropion, is an increasing problem.

Although **fenfluramine** is also related to amphetamine, in standard doses it has a sedative rather than a stimulant effect. Nevertheless, abuse has occurred and abrupt withdrawal may induce depression. It should preferably be avoided but may be considered for short-term adjunctive treatment in selected patients with severe obesity, given close support and supervision. It should **not** be given to patients with a past history of epilepsy, drug abuse or psychiatric illness and is **not** recommended for periods of treatment beyond 3 months. It should **not** be used for cosmetic reasons in mild to moderate obesity.

Dexfenfluramine is the dextro isomer of fenfluramine.

Thyroid hormones have no place in the treatment of obesity except in hypothyroid patients.

CHILDREN. These drugs should be avoided in children because of the possibility of growth suppression.

DEXFENFLURAMINE HYDROCHLORIDE

Indications: see notes above
Cautions; Contra-indications; Side-effects: see under Fenfluramine Hydrochloride
Dose: 15 mg morning and evening, at mealtimes; max. period of treatment should not exceed 3 months

▼ PoM **Adifax**® (Servier)
Capsules, dexfenfluramine hydrochloride 15 mg, net price 60-cap pack = £8.29. Label: 2

DIETHYLPROPION HYDROCHLORIDE
Indications: see notes above
Cautions: severe hepatic or renal impairment; cardiovascular disease (avoid if severe), avoid in peptic ulceration, prostatic hypertrophy, depression; **interactions:** Appendix 1 (sympathomimetics)
DRIVING. May impair performance of skilled tasks (e.g. driving); effects of alcohol unpredictable
Contra-indications: glaucoma, hyperthyroidism, epilepsy, unstable personality, severe hypertension, history of drug abuse, porphyria (see section 9.8.2); pregnancy (congenital malformations reported) and breast-feeding; avoid in children and elderly
Side-effects: dry mouth, headache, rashes, dependence; less common, insomnia, increased nervousness, depression, psychosis, hallucinations, tachycardia, hypertension, constipation; rarely, gynaecomastia

CD **Apisate**® (Wyeth)
Tablets, m/r, yellow, diethylpropion hydrochloride 75 mg, thiamine hydrochloride 5 mg, pyridoxine hydrochloride 2 mg, riboflavine 4 mg, nicotinamide 30 mg. Net price 20 = 52p. Label: 25, counselling, driving
Dose: 1 tablet mid-morning; to reduce risk of dependence max. continuous period of treatment should not exceed 4–8 weeks (followed by similar period without treatment)

CD **Tenuate Dospan**® (Merrell)
Tablets, m/r, scored, diethylpropion hydrochloride 75 mg. Net price 30-tab pack = 96p. Label: 25, counselling, driving
Dose: 1 tablet mid-morning; to reduce risk of dependence max. continuous period of treatment should not exceed 8 weeks (followed by similar period without treatment)
Note. Brand name prescriptions for Tenuate Dospan must also specify the word 'tablets' (i.e. 'Tenuate Dospan Tablets').

FENFLURAMINE HYDROCHLORIDE
Indications: see notes above
Cautions: dependence reported, depression on sudden withdrawal; elderly; **interactions:** Appendix 1 (sympathomimetics)
DRIVING. Drowsiness may affect performance of skilled tasks (e.g. driving); effects of alcohol enhanced
Contra-indications: history of depressive illness, drug or alcohol abuse; personality disorders; epilepsy; pregnancy and breast-feeding; porphyria (see section 9.8.2); avoid in children
Side-effects: diarrhoea and other gastro-intestinal disturbances; drowsiness, dizziness, and lethargy; also dry mouth, headache, nervousness, irritability, sleep disturbances, depression, visual disorders, hypotension, urinary frequency, impotence and loss of libido; rarely rashes, blood disorders, pulmonary hypertension, schizophrenia-like reactions; neurotoxicity reported in *animal* studies
Dose: see below

PoM **Ponderax**® (Servier)
Pacaps® (= capsules m/r), clear/blue, enclosing white pellets, fenfluramine hydrochloride 60 mg. Net price 60-cap pack = £7.26. Label: 2, 25
Dose: 1 capsule daily; max. period of treatment should not exceed 3 months (see also notes above)

MAZINDOL
Indications: see notes above
Cautions; Contra-indications; Side-effects: see under Diethylpropion Hydrochloride
Dose: 2 mg after breakfast; to reduce the risk of dependence max. continuous period of treatment should not exceed 4–8 weeks (followed by similar period without treatment)

CD **Teronac**® (Sandoz)
Tablets, scored, mazindol 2 mg. Net price 30-tab pack = £3.02. Counselling, driving

PHENTERMINE
Indications: see notes above
Cautions; Contra-indications; Side-effects: see under Diethylpropion Hydrochloride
Dose: 15–30 mg before breakfast; to reduce risk of dependence max. continuous period of treatment should not exceed 4–8 weeks (followed by similar period without treatment)

CD **Duromine**® (3M)
Capsules, both m/r, phentermine (as resin complex) 15 mg (green/grey), net price 30-cap pack = £1.24; 30 mg (maroon/grey), 30-cap pack = £1.63. Label: 25, counselling, driving

CD **Ionamin**® (Lipha)
Capsules, both m/r, phentermine (as resin complex) 15 mg (grey/yellow), net price 20 = 99p; 30 mg (yellow), 20 = £1.26. Label: 25, counselling, driving

4.6 Drugs used in nausea and vertigo

Anti-emetics should be prescribed only when the cause of vomiting is known, particularly in children, otherwise the symptomatic relief that they produce may delay diagnosis. Anti-emetics are unnecessary and sometimes harmful when the cause can be treated, e.g. as in diabetic ketoacidosis, or in excessive digoxin or antiepileptic dosage.

If antinauseant drug treatment is indicated the choice of drug depends on the aetiology of vomiting.

VESTIBULAR DISORDERS

Anti-emetics may be required in motion sickness, Ménière's disease, positional vertigo, labyrinthitis, and operative manipulation of the otovestibular apparatus. **Hyoscine** and the **antihistamines**, which act on the vomiting centre, are the drugs of choice. If possible they should be administered prophylactically at least 30 minutes before the emetic stimulus. Patients should be **warned** that these compounds may cause drowsiness, impair driving performance, and enhance the effects of alcohol and central nervous depressants.

MOTION SICKNESS. The most effective drug for the prevention of motion sickness is **hyoscine**. Adverse effects (drowsiness, blurred vision, dry mouth, urinary retention) are more frequent than with the antihistamines but are not generally prominent at the doses employed.

Antihistamines such as cinnarizine, cyclizine, dimenhydrinate, and promethazine are slightly less effective but generally better tolerated. There is no evidence that one antihistamine is superior to another but their duration of action and incidence of adverse effects (drowsiness and antimuscarinic effects) differ. If a sedative effect is desired **promethazine** and **dimenhydrinate** are useful, but generally a less sedating antihistamine like **cyclizine** or **cinnarizine** is preferred. To prevent motion sickness the first dose is usually taken half an hour (2 hours for cinnarizine) before the start of the journey. **Metoclopramide** and the **phenothiazines** (except promethazine), which act selectively on the chemoreceptor trigger zone, are ineffective in motion sickness.

OTHER LABYRINTHINE DISORDERS. Vertigo and nausea associated with Ménière's disease and middle-ear surgery disorders may be difficult to treat. **Hyoscine, antihistamines**, and **phenothiazines** (such as prochlorperazine and thiethylperazine) are effective in the prophylaxis and treatment of such conditions. **Betahistine** and **cinnarizine** have been promoted as specific treatment for Ménière's disease. In the acute attack **cyclizine** or **prochlorperazine** may be given rectally or by intramuscular injection.

Treatment of vertigo in its chronic forms is seldom fully effective but antihistamines (such as dimenhydrinate) or phenothiazines (such as prochlorperazine) may help.

For advice to avoid the inappropriate prescribing of drugs (notably phenothiazines) for dizziness in the elderly, see Prescribing for the Elderly, p. 14.

VOMITING OF PREGNANCY

Nausea in the first trimester of pregnancy does **not** require drug therapy. On rare occasions if vomiting is severe, an antihistamine or a phenothiazine (promethazine or thiethylperazine) may be required. If symptoms have not settled in 24 to 48 hours then a specialist opinion should be sought.

SYMPTOMATIC RELIEF OF NAUSEA FROM UNDERLYING DISEASE

The **phenothiazines** are dopamine antagonists and act centrally by blocking the chemoreceptor trigger zone. In low doses they are the drugs of choice for the prophylaxis and treatment of nausea and vomiting associated with diffuse neoplastic disease, radiation sickness, and the emesis caused by drugs such as opioid analgesics, general anaesthetics, and cytotoxic drugs. Rectal or parenteral administration is required if the vomiting has already started. **Prochlorperazine, perphenazine, trifluoperazine**, and **thiethylperazine** are less sedating than chlorpromazine but severe dystonic reactions sometimes occur, especially in children.

Metoclopramide is an effective anti-emetic with a spectrum of activity closely resembling that of the phenothiazines but it has a peripheral action on the gut in addition to its central effect and therefore may be superior to the phenothiazines in the emesis associated with gastroduodenal, hepatic, and biliary disease. The high-dose preparation is of value in the prevention of nausea and vomiting associated with cytotoxic drug therapy. Acute dystonic reactions may occur, particularly with children and young women, but they are less frequent than with phenothiazines.

Domperidone is used for the relief of nausea and vomiting, especially when associated with cytotoxic drug therapy. It has the advantage over metoclopramide and the phenothiazines of being less likely to cause central effects such as sedation and dystonic reactions because it does not readily cross the blood-brain barrier. It may be given for the treatment of levodopa- and bromocriptine-induced vomiting in parkinsonism (section 4.9.1). Domperidone acts at the chemoreceptor trigger zone and so is unlikely to be effective in motion sickness and other vestibular disorders.

Antihistamines are active in most of these conditions, but are not usually drugs of choice.

Nabilone is a synthetic cannabinoid with anti-emetic properties, reported to be superior to prochlorperazine. It is beneficial in the relief of nausea and vomiting associated with cytotoxic drug therapy. Side-effects occur in most patients given standard doses.

Ondansetron and **granisetron** are specific ($5HT_3$) serotonin antagonists. They have a valuable role in the management of nausea and vomiting in patients receiving cytotoxics who are unable to tolerate, or whose nausea and vomiting is not controlled by, less expensive drugs.

BETAHISTINE HYDROCHLORIDE

Indications: vertigo, tinnitus, and hearing loss in Ménière's disease
Cautions: asthma; **interactions:** Appendix 1 (betahistine)
Contra-indications: phaeochromocytoma
Side-effects: nausea; rarely headache, rashes
Dose: initially 16 mg 3 times daily, preferably with food; maintenance 24–48 mg daily

PoM **Serc®** (Duphar)
Tablets, scored, betahistine hydrochloride 8 mg, net price 120-tab pack = £12.88; 16 mg (Serc®-16), 84-tab pack = £18.03. Label: 21

CHLORPROMAZINE HYDROCHLORIDE

Indications: nausea and vomiting of terminal illness (where other drugs have failed or are not available); other indications, see sections 4.2.1, 15.1.4.2
Cautions; Contra-indications; Side-effects: see section 4.2.1

Dose: by mouth, 10–25 mg every 4–6 hours
By deep intramuscular injection 25 mg initially then 25–50 mg every 3–4 hours until vomiting stops
By rectum in suppositories, chlorpromazine 100 mg every 6–8 hours

Preparations
Section 4.2.1

CINNARIZINE

Indications: vestibular disorders, such as vertigo, tinnitus, nausea, and vomiting in Ménière's disease; motion sickness; vascular disease, see section 2.6.3
Cautions; Side-effects: see under Cyclizine; also allergic skin reactions and fatigue; caution in hypotension (high doses); rarely, extrapyramidal symptoms in elderly on prolonged therapy; avoid in porphyria (see section 9.8.2)
Dose: vestibular disorders, 30 mg 3 times daily; CHILD 5–12 years half adult dose
Motion sickness, 30 mg 2 hours before travel then 15 mg every 8 hours during journey if necessary; CHILD 5–12 years half adult dose

Cinnarizine (Non-proprietary)
Tablets, cinnarizine 15 mg. Net price 20 = £1.10. Label: 2
Available from Ashbourne (Cinazière®), Norton
Stugeron® (Janssen)
Tablets, scored, cinnarizine 15 mg. Net price 20 = 98p. Label: 2
Note. A proprietary brand of cinnarizine 15 mg tablets (Marzine RF®) is on sale to the public for travel sickness
Stugeron Forte®: see section 2.6.3

CYCLIZINE

Indications: nausea, vomiting, vertigo, motion sickness, labyrinthine disorders
Cautions; Side-effects: drowsiness, occasional dry mouth and blurred vision; see also section 3.4.1 (Disadvantages of Antihistamines); cyclizine may aggravate severe heart failure and counteract the haemodynamic benefits of opioids; **interactions:** Appendix 1 (antihistamines)
DRIVING. Drowsiness may affect performance of skilled tasks (e.g. driving); effects of alcohol enhanced
Dose: by mouth, cyclizine hydrochloride 50 mg up to 3 times daily; CHILD 6–12 years 25 mg
By intramuscular or intravenous injection, cyclizine lactate 50 mg 3 times daily

Valoid® (Wellcome)
Tablets, scored, cyclizine hydrochloride 50 mg. Net price 20 = 99p. Label: 2
PoM *Injection*, cyclizine lactate 50 mg/mL. Net price 1-mL amp = 57p

DIMENHYDRINATE

Indications: nausea, vomiting, vertigo, motion sickness, labyrinthine disorders
Cautions; Side-effects: see under Cyclizine; avoid in porphyria (see section 9.8.2)

Dose: 50–100 mg 2–3 times daily; CHILD 1–6 years 12.5–25 mg, 7–12 years 25–50 mg
Motion sickness, first dose 30 minutes before journey

Dramamine® (Searle)
Tablets, scored, dimenhydrinate 50 mg. Net price 20 = 93p. Label: 2

DOMPERIDONE

Indications: see under Dose
Cautions: renal impairment; pregnancy and breast-feeding; not recommended for chronic administration; **interactions:** Appendix 1 (domperidone)
Side-effects: raised prolactin concentrations (possible galactorrhoea and gynaecomastia); acute dystonic reactions reported
Dose: by mouth, acute nausea and vomiting, (including nausea and vomiting induced by levodopa and bromocriptine), 10–20 mg every 4–8 hours, max. period of treatment 3 months; CHILD, nausea and vomiting following cytotoxic therapy or radiotherapy only, 200–400 micrograms/kg every 4–8 hours
By rectum in suppositories, 30–60 mg every 4–8 hours; CHILD, 2–12 years 30–120 mg daily according to body-weight (approximately 4 mg/kg)

PoM **Motilium®** (Sanofi Winthrop)
Tablets, f/c, domperidone 10 mg (as maleate). Net price 30-tab pack = £2.52; 100-tab pack = £8.42
Suspension, sugar-free, domperidone 5 mg/5 mL. Net price 200-mL pack = £1.85
Suppositories, domperidone 30 mg. Net price 10 = £2.72

DROPERIDOL

See section 4.2.1

GRANISETRON

Indications: nausea and vomiting induced by cytotoxic chemotherapy or radiotherapy
Cautions: pregnancy and breast-feeding
Side-effects: constipation, headache; transient increases in liver enzymes
Dose: by intravenous infusion over 5 minutes, prevention, 3 mg (up to 2 additional 3-mg infusions may be given within 24 hours); treatment, as for prevention (the two additional infusions must not be given less than 10 minutes apart); max. 9 mg in 24 hours; CHILD not yet recommended

▼ PoM **Kytril®** (SmithKline Beecham)
Infusion, granisetron (as hydrochloride) 1 mg/mL, for dilution and use as infusion, net price 3-mL amp = £36.00

HALOPERIDOL

See section 4.2.1

HYOSCINE HYDROBROMIDE
(Scopolamine hydrobromide)

Indications: motion sickness; premedication, see section 15.1.3

Cautions: elderly, urinary retention, cardiovascular disease, gastro-intestinal obstruction, hepatic or renal impairment; pregnancy and breast-feeding; **interactions:** Appendix 1 (antimuscarinics)

DRIVING. Drowsiness may affect performance of skilled tasks (e.g. driving): effects of alcohol enhanced

Contra-indications: closed-angle glaucoma

Side-effects: drowsiness, dry mouth, dizziness, blurred vision, difficulty with micturition

Dose: motion sickness, *by mouth*, 300 micrograms 30 minutes before start of journey followed by 300 micrograms every 6 hours if required; max. 3 doses in 24 hours; CHILD 4–10 years 75–150 micrograms, over 10 years 150–300 micrograms

Note. Proprietary brands of hyoscine tablets (Joyrides®, Kwells®) are on sale to the public for motion sickness)

Injection, see section 15.1.3

PoM Scopoderm TTS® (Ciba)

Patch, self-adhesive, pink, releasing hyoscine approx. 500 micrograms/72 hours when in contact with skin. Net price 2 = £2.84. Label: 2, counselling, see below

Administration: motion sickness prevention, apply 1 patch to hairless area of skin behind ear 5–6 hours before journey; replace if necessary after 72 hours, siting replacement patch behind other ear

COUNSELLING. Explain accompanying instructions to patient and in particular emphasise advice to wash hands after handling and to wash application site after removing, and to use one at a time

METHOTRIMEPRAZINE
See section 4.2.1

METOCLOPRAMIDE HYDROCHLORIDE

Indications: adults, nausea and vomiting, particularly in gastro-intestinal disorders and treatment with cytotoxics or radiotherapy; gastro-intestinal—section 1.2; migraine—section 4.7.4.1

PATIENTS UNDER 20 YEARS. Use restricted to severe intractable vomiting of known cause, vomiting of radiotherapy and cytotoxics, aid to gastro-intestinal intubation, pre-medication

Cautions: hepatic and renal impairment; elderly, young adults, and children (measure dose accurately, preferably with a pipette); may mask underlying disorders such as cerebral irritation; avoid for 3–4 days following gastro-intestinal surgery, may cause acute hypertensive response in phaeochromocytoma; pregnancy and breast-feeding; avoid in porphyria (see section 9.8.2); **interactions:** Appendix 1 (metoclopramide)

Side-effects: extrapyramidal effects (especially in children/young adults), hyperprolactinaemia, occasionally tardive dyskinesia on prolonged administration; also reported, drowsiness, restlessness, diarrhoea

Dose: by mouth, or by intramuscular injection or by intravenous injection over 1–2 minutes, 10 mg (5 mg in young adults 15–19 years under 60 kg) 3 times daily; CHILD up to 1 year (up to 10 kg) 1 mg twice daily, 1–3 years (10–14kg) 1 mg 2–3 times daily, 3–5 years (15–19 kg) 2 mg 2–3 times daily, 5–9 years (20–29 kg) 2.5 mg 3 times daily, 9–14 years (30 kg and over) 5 mg 3 times daily

Note. Daily dose of metoclopramide should not normally exceed 500 micrograms/kg, particularly for children and young adults (restricted use, see above)

For radiological examinations, as a single dose 5–10 minutes before examination, 10–20 mg (10 mg in young adults 15–19 years); CHILD under 3 years 1 mg, 3–5 years 2 mg, 5–9 years 2.5 mg, 9–14 years 5 mg

By continuous intravenous infusion (preferred method), initially (before starting chemotherapy), 2–4 mg/kg over 15–30 minutes, then 3–5 mg/kg over 8–12 hours; max. in 24 hours, 10 mg/kg

By intermittent intravenous infusion, initially (before starting chemotherapy), up to 2 mg/kg over at least 15 minutes up to 2 mg/kg over at least 15 minutes every 2 hours; max. in 24 hours, 10 mg/kg

PoM Metoclopramide (Non-proprietary)

Tablets, metoclopramide hydrochloride 10 mg, net price 20 = £1.16

Available from APS, Ashbourne (Gastroflux®), Berk (Primperan®), Cox, CP, Evans, Kerfoot, Lagap (Parmid®), Nicholas (Metramid®), Norton

Oral solution, metoclopramide hydrochloride 5 mg/5 mL, net price 100-mL pack = £1.05

Available from Berk (Primperan®, sugar-free), Lagap (Parmid® sugar-free)

Injection, metoclopramide hydrochloride 5 mg/mL, net price 2-mL amp = 24p

Available from Berk (Primperan®)

PoM Maxolon® (Beecham)

Tablets, scored, metoclopramide hydrochloride 10 mg. Net price 21-tab pack = £2.20, 84-tab pack = £8.53

Syrup, sugar-free, metoclopramide hydrochloride 5 mg/5 mL. Net price 200-mL pack = £3.48

Paediatric liquid, sugar-free, metoclopramide hydrochloride 1 mg/mL. Net price 15-mL pack with pipette = £1.37. Counselling, use of pipette

Injection, metoclopramide hydrochloride 5 mg/mL. Net price 2-mL amp = 24p

PoM Maxolon High Dose® (Beecham)

Injection, metoclopramide hydrochloride 5 mg/mL. Net price 20-mL amp = £2.43.

For dilution and use as an intravenous infusion in nausea and vomiting associated with cytotoxic chemotherapy only

Modified-release preparations

Note. All unsuitable for patients under 20 years

PoM Gastrobid Continus® (Napp)

Tablets, m/r, metoclopramide hydrochloride 15 mg. Net price 56-tab pack = £8.06. Label: 25

Dose: patients over 20 years, 1 tablet twice daily

4.6 Drugs used in nausea and vertigo

PoM Gastromax® (Farmitalia Carlo Erba)
Capsules, m/r, orange/yellow, enclosing white to light beige pellets, metoclopramide hydrochloride 30 mg. Net price 28-cap pack = £11.85. Label: 22, 25
Dose: patients over 20 years, 1 capsule daily

PoM Maxolon SR® (Beecham)
Capsules, m/r, clear, enclosing white granules, metoclopramide hydrochloride 15 mg. Net price 56-cap pack = £9.78. Label: 25
Dose: patients over 20 years, 1 capsule twice daily

Compound preparations (for migraine), section 4.7.4.1

NABILONE

Indications: nausea and vomiting caused by cytotoxic chemotherapy, unresponsive to conventional anti-emetics
Cautions: severe hepatic impairment; history of psychiatric disorder; elderly; hypertension; heart disease; **interactions:** Appendix 1 (nabilone)
DRIVING. Drowsiness may affect performance of skilled tasks (e.g. driving); effects of alcohol enhanced
Side-effects: drowsiness, vertigo, euphoria, dry mouth, ataxia, visual disturbance, concentration difficulties, sleep disturbance, dysphoria, hypotension, headache and nausea; also confusion, disorientation, hallucinations, psychosis, depression, decreased coordination, tremors, tachycardia, decreased appetite, and abdominal pain
Dose: patients over 18 years, initially 1 mg twice daily, increased if necessary to 2 mg twice daily, throughout each cycle of cytotoxic therapy and, if necessary, for 48 hours after the last dose of each cycle; max. 6 mg daily given in 3 divided doses. The first dose should be taken the night before initiation of cytotoxic treatment and the second dose 1–3 hours before the first dose of cytotoxic drug

PoM Cesamet® (Lilly)
Capsules, blue/white, nabilone 1 mg. Net price 20 = £31.76 (hosp. only). Label: 2

ONDANSETRON

Indications: see under Dose
Cautions: pregnancy and breast-feeding; moderate or severe hepatic impairment (max. 8 mg daily)
Side-effects: constipation; headache, sensation of warmth or flushing in head and over stomach; occasional alterations in liver enzymes; hypersensitivity reactions reported
Dose: moderately emetogenic chemotherapy or radiotherapy, *by mouth*, 8 mg 1–2 hours before treatment *or*, *by slow intravenous injection*, 8 mg immediately before treatment, *then* 8 mg *by mouth* every 12 hours for up to 5 days
Severely emetogenic chemotherapy, *by slow intravenous injection*, 8 mg immediately before treatment, followed by 8 mg at intervals of 2–4 hours for 2 further doses (*or* followed by 1 mg/hour *by continuous intravenous infusion* for up to 24 hours) *then* 8 mg *by mouth* every 12 hours for up to 5 days
alternatively, *by intravenous infusion* over 15 minutes, 32 mg immediately before treatment *then* 8 mg *by mouth* every 12 hours for up to 5 days
Note. Efficacy may be enhanced by addition of a single dose of dexamethasone sodium phosphate 20 mg by intravenous injection
CHILD, *by slow intravenous injection or by intravenous infusion* over 15 minutes, 5 mg/m^2 immediately before chemotherapy then, 4 mg *by mouth* every 12 hours for up to 5 days
Prevention and treatment of postoperative nausea and vomiting, *by mouth*, 8 mg 1 hour before anaesthesia, followed by 8 mg at intervals of 8 hours for 2 further doses
alternatively by slow intravenous injection, a single dose of 4 mg at induction

▼ **PoM Zofran®** (Glaxo)
Tablets, both yellow, f/c, ondansetron (as hydrochloride) 4 mg, net price 30-tab pack = £187.50; 8 mg, 10-tab pack = £90.00
Injection, ondansetron (as hydrochloride) 2 mg/mL, net price 2-mL amp = £10.50; 4-mL amp = £15.00

PERPHENAZINE

Indications: severe nausea, vomiting (see notes above); other indications, section 4.2.1
Cautions; Contra-indications; Side-effects: see section 4.2.1; extrapyramidal symptoms may occur, particularly in young adults, elderly, and debilitated; avoid in children under 14 years
Dose: 4 mg 3 times daily, adjusted according to response; max. 24 mg daily (chemotherapy-induced); ELDERLY quarter to half adult dose

Preparations: see section 4.2.1

PROCHLORPERAZINE

Indications: severe nausea, vomiting, vertigo, labyrinthine disorders (see notes above); other indications, section 4.2.1
Cautions; Contra-indications: see under Chlorpromazine Hydrochloride (section 4.2.1). Oral route only for children (avoid if less than 10 kg); elderly (see notes above)
Side-effects: see under Chlorpromazine Hydrochloride; extrapyramidal symptoms may occur, particularly in children, elderly, and debilitated
Dose: by mouth, nausea and vomiting, prochlorperazine maleate or mesylate, acute attack, 20 mg initially then 10 mg after 2 hours; prevention 5–10 mg 2–3 times daily; CHILD (over 10 kg only) 250 micrograms/kg 2–3 times daily
Labyrinthine disorders, 5 mg 3 times daily, gradually increased if necessary to 30 mg daily in divided doses, then reduced after several weeks to 5–10 mg daily
By deep intramuscular injection, nausea and vomiting, 12.5 mg when required followed if necessary after 6 hours by an oral dose, as above; CHILD not recommended

By rectum in suppositories, nausea and vomiting, 25 mg followed if necessary after 6 hours by oral dose, as above; *or* due to migraine, 5 mg 3 times daily; CHILD not recommended

PoM **Prochlorperazine** (Non-proprietary)
Tablets, prochlorperazine maleate 5 mg, net price 20 = 67p. Label: 2
Available from Ashbourne (Prozière®), Cox, Norton

PoM **Stemetil®** (Rhône-Poulenc Rorer)
Tablets, prochlorperazine maleate 5 mg (off-white), net price 84-tab pack = £2.95; 25 mg (scored), 56-tab pack = £5.19. Label: 2
Syrup, straw-coloured, prochlorperazine mesylate 5 mg/5 mL. Net price 100-mL pack = £1.66. Label: 2
Eff sachets, granules, effervescent, sugar-free, prochlorperazine mesylate 5 mg/sachet. Net price 21-sachet pack = £3.09. Label: 2, 13
Injection, prochlorperazine mesylate 12.5 mg/mL. Net price 1-mL amp = 32p; 2-mL amp = 41p
Suppositories, prochlorperazine maleate (as prochlorperazine), 5 mg, net price 10 = £4.16; 25 mg, 10 = £5.47. Label: 2

PoM **Vertigon®** (SK&F)
Spansule® (= capsules m/r), both clear/purple, enclosing yellowish-green and white pellets, prochlorperazine (as maleate), 10 mg, net price 60-cap pack = £2.24; 15 mg, 60-cap pack = £2.74. Label: 2, 25
Dose: initially 10–15 mg once or twice daily (elderly 10 mg daily). Maintenance 10–15 mg daily

Buccal preparation
PoM **Buccastem®** (R&C)
Tablets (buccal), pale yellow, prochlorperazine maleate 3 mg. Net price 4 × 15-tab pack = £6.90. Label: 2, counselling, administration, see under Dose below
Dose: 1–2 tablets twice daily; tablets are placed high between upper lip and gum and left to dissolve

PROMETHAZINE HYDROCHLORIDE

Indications: nausea, vomiting, vertigo, labyrinthine disorders, motion sickness; other indications, see sections 3.4.1, 4.1.1, 15.1.4.1
Cautions; Side-effects: see under Cyclizine but more sedating; intramuscular injection may be painful; avoid in porphyria (see section 9.8.2)
Dose: by mouth, 25–50 mg daily in single or divided doses; max. 75 mg
CHILD, motion sickness prevention, 1–5 years, 5 mg at night and following morning (1–2 years on doctors advice only); 5–10 years, 10 mg at night and following morning
By deep intramuscular injection, 25–50 mg when necessary; CHILD 5–10 years 6.25–12.5 mg
By slow intravenous injection, see section 3.4.1

Preparations
See section 3.4.1

PROMETHAZINE THEOCLATE

Indications: nausea, vertigo, labyrinthine disorders, motion sickness (acts longer than the hydrochloride)

Cautions; Side-effects: see under Promethazine Hydrochloride
Dose: 25–75 mg, max. 100 mg, daily; CHILD 5–10 years, 12.5–37.5 mg daily
Motion sickness prevention, 25 mg at bedtime on night before travelling *or* 25 mg 1–2 hours before travelling; CHILD 5–10 years, half adult dose
For severe vomiting in pregnancy, 25 mg at bedtime, increased if necessary to a max. of 100 mg daily (but see also Vomiting of Pregnancy in notes above)

Avomine® (Rhône-Poulenc Rorer)
Tablets, scored, promethazine theoclate 25 mg. Net price 10-tab pack = 93p; 28-tab pack = 93p. Label: 2

THIETHYLPERAZINE

Indications: severe nausea, vomiting, vertigo, labyrinthine disorders
Cautions; Contra-indications; Side-effects: see under Chlorpromazine Hydrochloride (section 4.2.1); young adults, elderly, and debilitated particularly susceptible to extrapyramidal effects; avoid in children under 15 years
Dose: by mouth, thiethylperazine maleate 10 mg 2–3 times daily
By intramuscular injection, thiethylperazine [base] 6.5 mg
Note: Thiethylperazine 6.5 mg ≡ thiethylperazine malate 10.86 mg ≡ thiethylperazine maleate 10.28 mg

PoM **Torecan®** (Sandoz)
Tablets, s/c, thiethylperazine *maleate* 10 mg. Net price 50 = £1.42. Label: 2
Injection, thiethylperazine 6.5 mg (as *malate*)/mL. Net price 1-mL amp = 18p

TRIFLUOPERAZINE

Indications: severe nausea and vomiting (see notes above); other indications, section 4.2.1
Cautions; Contra-indications; Side-effects: see section 4.2.1; extrapyramidal symptoms may occur, particularly in children, elderly, and debilitated
Dose: by mouth, 2–4 mg daily in divided doses *or* as a single dose of a modified-release preparation; max. 6 mg daily; CHILD 3–5 years up to 1 mg daily, 6–12 years up to 4 mg daily
By deep intramuscular injection, 1–3 mg daily in divided doses, max. 6 mg daily

Preparations
See section 4.2.1

4.7 Analgesics

4.7.1 Non-opioid analgesics
4.7.2 Opioid analgesics
4.7.3 Trigeminal neuralgia
4.7.4 Antimigraine drugs

For advice on pain relief in terminal care see Prescribing in Terminal Care, p. 12.

4.7.1 Non-opioid analgesics

The non-opioid drugs, aspirin and paracetamol, are particularly suitable for pain in musculoskeletal conditions, whereas the opioid analgesics are more suitable for severe visceral pain.

Aspirin is the analgesic of choice for headache, transient musculoskeletal pain, and dysmenorrhoea. It also has anti-inflammatory properties which may be useful, and is an antipyretic. Aspirin tablets or dispersible aspirin tablets are adequate for most purposes as they act rapidly.

Gastric irritation may be a problem; it is minimised by taking the dose after food. Numerous formulations are available which improve gastric tolerance, e.g. the buffered aspirin preparations such as aloxiprin (Palaprin Forte®) and enteric-coated aspirin. Some of these preparations have a slow onset of action and are therefore unsuitable for single-dose analgesic use though their prolonged action may be useful for night pain.

Paracetamol is similar in efficacy to aspirin, but has no demonstrable anti-inflammatory activity; it is less irritant to the stomach. Overdosage with paracetamol is particularly dangerous as it may cause hepatic damage which is sometimes not apparent for 4 to 6 days. **Benorylate** is an aspirin–paracetamol ester.

Nefopam may have a place in the relief of persistent pain unresponsive to other non-opioid analgesics. It causes little or no respiratory depression, but sympathomimetic and antimuscarinic side-effects may be troublesome.

Anti-inflammatory analgesics (see section 10.1.1) are particularly useful for the treatment of patients with chronic disease accompanied by pain and inflammation. Some of them are also used in the short-term treatment of mild to moderate pain including transient musculoskeletal pain. They are also suitable for the relief of pain in *dysmenorrhoea* and to treat pain caused by *secondary bone tumours*, many of which produce lysis of bone and release prostaglandins (see Prescribing in Terminal Care, p. 12).

Compound analgesic preparations of, for example, aspirin, paracetamol, and codeine are **not** recommended. Single-ingredient preparations should be prescribed in preference because compound preparations rarely have any advantage and complicate the treatment of overdosage. The dangers of co-proxamol (dextropropoxyphene-paracetamol) overdosage call for rapid treatment as described in Poisoning, p. 18.

It is even more desirable to **avoid** mixtures of analgesics with antihistamines or muscle relaxants; the individual components should be prescribed separately so that the dose of each can be adjusted as appropriate.

Caffeine is a weak stimulant that is often included, in small doses, in analgesic preparations. It does not contribute to the analgesic or anti-inflammatory effect of the preparation and may possibly aggravate the gastric irritation caused by aspirin. Moreover, in excessive dosage or on withdrawal caffeine may itself induce headache.

ASPIRIN

Indications: mild to moderate pain, pyrexia (see notes above); see also section 10.1.1; anti-platelet, see section 2.9

Cautions: asthma, allergic disease, impaired renal or hepatic function (avoid if severe), dehydration, pregnancy; G6PD-deficiency (see section 9.1.5); **interactions:** Appendix 1 aspirin)

Contra-indications: children under 12 years and in breast-feeding (possible link with Reye's syndrome); gastro-intestinal ulceration, haemophilia; not for treatment of gout

Side-effects: generally mild and infrequent but high incidence of gastro-intestinal irritation with slight asymptomatic blood loss, increased bleeding time, bronchospasm and skin reactions in hypersensitive patients. Prolonged administration, see section 10.1.1. Overdosage: see Emergency Treatment of Poisoning, p. 17

Dose: 300–900 mg every 4–6 hours when necessary; max. 4 g daily

Aspirin (Non-proprietary)
Tablets, aspirin 300 mg. Net price 20 = 9p. Label: 21, 32
Available from APS, Evans, Kerfoot
Dispersible tablets, aspirin 300 mg, net price 20 = 9p; 75 mg, see section 2.9. Label: 13, 21, 32
Available from APS, Cox, Evans, Kerfoot
Note. Addendum 1989 to BP 1988 directs that when soluble aspirin tablets are prescribed, dispersible aspirin tablets shall be dispensed.

Caprin® (Sinclair)
Tablets, e/c, pink, aspirin 324 mg. Net price 20 = 69p. Label: 5, 25, 32

Nu-Seals® **Aspirin** (Lilly)
Tablets, e/c, red, aspirin 300 mg, net price 100-tab pack = £5.27. Label: 5, 25, 32

Palaprin Forte® (Nicholas)
Tablets, orange, scored, aloxiprin[1] 600 mg (≡ aspirin 500 mg). To be taken dispersed in water, chewed, sucked, or swallowed whole. Net price 20 = 50p. Label: 21, 33
Dose: ½–2 tablets up to 4 times daily; max. 8 daily

1. Aloxiprin is a polymeric condensation product of aluminium oxide and aspirin

With codeine phosphate 8 mg
Co-codaprin (Non-proprietary)
Tablets, co-codaprin 8/400 (codeine phosphate 8 mg, aspirin 400 mg). Net price 20 = 34p. Label: 21, 32
Dose: 1–2 tablets every 4–6 hours when necessary; max. 8 tablets daily
Available from Cox
Dispersible tablets, co-codaprin 8/400 (codeine phosphate 8 mg, aspirin 400 mg). Net price 20 = 31p. Label: 13, 21, 32
Dose: 1–2 tablets in water every 4–6 hours; max. 8 tablets daily
Available from Cox
When co-codaprin tablets or dispersible tablets are prescribed and no strength is stated tablets, or dispersible tablets, respectively, containing codeine phosphate 8 mg and aspirin 400 mg should be dispensed.

Other compound preparations
PoM Aspav® (Roussel)
Dispersible tablets, aspirin 500 mg, papaveretum 10 mg. Net price 20 = £1.35. Label: 2, 13, 21, 32
Dose: 1–2 tablets in water every 4–6 hours if necessary; max. 8 tablets daily. Contra-indicated in women of child-bearing potential (see Appendix 4)

NHS PoM Doloxene Compound® (Lilly)
Capsules, grey/red, dextropropoxyphene napsylate 100 mg, aspirin 375 mg, caffeine 30 mg. Net price 20 = £1.34. Label: 2, 21, 32
Dose: 1 capsule 3–4 times daily; max. 4 capsules daily

NHS CD Equagesic® (Wyeth)
Tablets, pink/white/yellow, ethoheptazine citrate 75 mg, meprobamate 150 mg, aspirin 250 mg. Net price 20 = 66p. Label: 2, 21, 32
Dose: muscle pain, 1–2 tablets 3–4 times daily

NHS PoM Robaxisal Forte® (Wyeth)
Tablets, pink/white, scored, methocarbamol 400 mg, aspirin 325 mg. Net price 20 = £1.90. Label: 2, 21, 32
Dose: muscle pain, 2 tablets 4 times daily

For a list of **preparations** containing aspirin and paracetamol **on sale to the general public**, see p. 176.

PARACETAMOL
Indications: mild to moderate pain, pyrexia
Cautions: hepatic and renal impairment, alcohol dependence; **interactions**: Appendix 1 (paracetamol)
Side-effects: side-effects rare, but rashes, blood disorders, and acute pancreatitis reported; **important**: liver damage (and less frequently renal damage) following overdosage, see Emergency Treatment of Poisoning, p. 18
Dose: by mouth, 0.5–1 g every 4–6 hours to a max. of 4 g daily; CHILD 2 months 60 mg for post-immunisation pyrexia; otherwise under 3 months (on doctor's advice only), 10 mg/kg (5 mg/kg if jaundiced); 3 months–1 year 60–120 mg, 1–5 years 120–250 mg, 6–12 years 250–500 mg; these doses may be repeated every 4–6 hours when necessary (max. of 4 doses in 24 hours)
For full Joint Committee on Vaccination and Immunisation recommendation on post-immunisation pyrexia, see p. 444
Rectal route, see below

Paracetamol (Non-proprietary)
Tablets, paracetamol 500 mg. Net price 20 = 9p. Label: 29, 30
Available from APS, Cox, Evans, Kerfoot, Sterling Health (NHS Panadol®)
Soluble Tablets (= Dispersible tablets), paracetamol 500 mg. Net price 60-tab pack = £1.43. Label: 13, 29, 30
Available from Sanofi Winthrop (NHS Panadol Soluble®)
Paediatric Soluble Tablets (= Paediatric dispersible tablets), paracetamol 120 mg. Net price 24-tab pack = 62p. Label: 13, 30
Available from R&C (NHS Disprol® Junior)
Paediatric Oral Solution (= Paediatric Elixir), paracetamol 120 mg/5 mL. Net price 100 mL = 50p. Label: 30
Note. Sugar-free versions are available and can be ordered by specifying 'sugar-free' on the prescription.
Available from Berk, Evans, RP Drugs (Paldesic®), Wallace Mfg (NHS Salzone®)

Oral Suspension 120 mg/5 mL (= Paediatric Mixture), paracetamol 120 mg/5 mL. Net price 100 mL = 43p. Label: 30
Note. BP directs that when Paediatric Paracetamol Oral Suspension or Paediatric Paracetamol Mixture is prescribed Paracetamol Oral Suspension 120 mg/5 mL should be dispensed; sugar-free versions are available and can be ordered by specifying 'sugar-free' on the prescription
Available from Cupal (Cupanol® Under 6, sugar-free), R&C (Disprol®, sugar-free), Sterling Health (Panadol®, sugar-free), Wellcome (Calpol®, Calpol® sugar-free)
Oral Suspension 250 mg/5 mL (= Mixture), paracetamol 250 mg/5 mL. Net price 100 mL = £1.34. Label: 30
Available from Cupal (NHS Cupanol® Over 6, sugar-free), Wellcome (NHS Calpol® Six Plus)
Suppositories, paracetamol 125 mg. Net price 10 = £10.50. Label: 30
Dose: by rectum, CHILD 1–5 years 125–250 mg (1–2 suppositories) up to 4 times daily
Available from Novex (Alvedon®)

With codeine phosphate 8 mg
Co-codamol (Non-proprietary)
Tablets, co-codamol 8/500 (codeine phosphate 8 mg, paracetamol 500 mg). Net price 20 = 28p. Label: 29, 30
Dose: 1–2 tablets every 4–6 hours; max. 8 tablets daily; CHILD 6–12 years ½–1 tablet
Available from APS, Cox, Evans, Galen (NHS Parake®), Kerfoot, Norton, Sterling Health (NHS Panadeine®)
Effervescent or *dispersible tablets*, co-codamol 8/500 (paracetamol 500 mg, codeine phosphate 8 mg). Net price 20 = 59p. Label: 13, 29, 30
Dose: 1–2 tablets in water every 4–6 hours, max. 8 tablets daily; CHILD 6–12 years ½–1 tablet, max. 4 tablets daily
Available from Fisons (NHS Paracodol®), Sterwin
Note. The Drug Tariff allows tablets of co-codamol labelled 'dispersible' to be dispensed against an order for 'effervescent' and *vice versa*
Capsules, co-codamol 8/500 (paracetamol 500 mg, codeine phosphate 8 mg). Net price 30 = £1.68. Label: 29, 30
Dose: 1–2 capsules every 4 hours; max. 8 capsules daily
Available from Fisons (NHS Paracodol®)
When co-codamol tablets, dispersible (or effervescent) tablets, or capsules are prescribed and no strength is stated tablets, dispersible (or effervescent) tablets, or capsules, respectively, containing codeine phosphate 8 mg and paracetamol 500 mg should be dispensed.

With codeine phosphate 30 mg
PoM Solpadol® (Sanofi Winthrop)
Effervescent tablets, paracetamol 500 mg, codeine phosphate 30 mg. Contains 18.6 mmol Na$^+$/tablet; avoid in renal impairment. Net price 60-tab pack = £5.83. Label: 2, 13, 29, 30
Dose: 2 tablets in water every 4 hours; max. 8 daily

PoM Tylex® (Cilag)
Capsules, paracetamol 500 mg, codeine phosphate 30 mg. Net price 100 = £8.60. Label: 2, 29, 30
Dose: 1–2 capsules every 4 hours; max. 8 capsules daily

With dihydrocodeine tartrate 10 mg
PoM Co-dydramol (Non-proprietary)
Tablets, scored, co-dydramol 10/500 (dihydrocodeine tartrate 10 mg, paracetamol 500 mg). Net price 20 = 33p. Label: 21, 29, 30
Dose: 1–2 tablets every 4–6 hours; max. 8 tablets daily
Available from APS, Cox, Evans, Galen (NHS Galake®), Kerfoot, Napp, Norton, Sterwin

4.7 Analgesics

When co-dydramol tablets are prescribed and no strength is stated tablets containing dihydrocodeine tartrate 10 mg and paracetamol 500 mg should be dispensed.
Note. Tablets containing paracetamol 500 mg and dihydrocodeine 7.46 mg (Paramol®) are on sale to the public. The name Paramol® was formerly applied to a brand of co-dydramol tablets

With dihydrocodeine tartrate 20 or 30 mg
PoM **Remedeine**® (Napp)
Tablets, paracetamol 500 mg, dihydrocodeine tartrate 20 mg. Net price 112-tab pack = £10.98. Label: 2, 21, 29, 30
Dose: 1–2 tablets every 4–6 hours; max. 8 tablets daily
Forte tablets, paracetamol 500 mg, dihydrocodeine tartrate 30 mg. Net price 56-tab pack = £6.90. Label: 2, 21, 29, 30
Dose: 1–2 tablets every 4–6 hours; max. 8 tablets daily

Other compound preparations
PoM **Co-proxamol** (Non-proprietary)
Tablets, co-proxamol 32.5/325 (dextropropoxyphene hydrochloride 32.5 mg, paracetamol 325 mg). Net price 20 = 28p. Label: 2, 10 patient information leaflet (if available), 29, 30
Dose: 2 tablets 3–4 times daily; max. 8 tablets daily
Available from APS, Cox (NHS Cosalgesic®), Dista (NHS Distalgesic®), Evans, Kerfoot, Sterwin
When co-proxamol tablets are prescribed and no strength is stated tablets containing dextropropoxyphene hydrochloride 32.5 mg and paracetamol 325 mg should be dispensed.

NHS CD **Fortagesic**® (Sanofi Winthrop)
Tablets, pentazocine 15 mg (as hydrochloride), paracetamol 500 mg. Net price 20 = £1.40. Label: 2, 21, 29, 30
Dose: 2 tablets up to 4 times daily; CHILD 7–12 years 1 tablet every 4 hours, max. 4 tablets daily

NHS PoM **Lobak**® (Sanofi Winthrop)
Tablets, scored, chlormezanone 100 mg, paracetamol 450 mg. Net price 50 = £7.67. Label: 2, 29, 30
Dose: muscle pain, 1–2 tablets 3 times daily; max. 8 tablets daily

For a list of **preparations** containing aspirin and paracetamol **on sale to the general public**, see p. 176.

BENORYLATE
(Aspirin-paracetamol ester; 2 g benorylate is equivalent to approximately 1.15 g aspirin and 970 mg paracetamol)
Indications: mild to moderate pain; pyrexia; see also section 10.1.1
Cautions; Contra-indications; Side-effects: see under Aspirin and under Paracetamol
Note. Preparations containing aspirin are contra-indicated in children under 12 years of age owing to an association with Reye's syndrome, see notes above
Dose: 2 g twice daily, preferably after food

Preparations: see section 10.1.1

DICLOFENAC SODIUM
See section 10.1.1

DIFLUNISAL
Indications: mild to moderate pain; see also section 10.1.1
Cautions; Contra-indications; Side-effects: see section 10.1.1

Dose: 250–500 mg twice daily preferably after food

Preparations: see section 10.1.1

FENOPROFEN
Indications: mild to moderate pain, pyrexia; see also section 10.1.1
Cautions; Contra-indications; Side-effects: See section 10.1.1
Dose: 200–600 mg 3–4 times daily, after food; max. 3 g daily

PoM **Progesic**® (Lilly)
Tablets, yellow, fenoprofen 200 mg (as calcium salt). Net price 20 = £2.20. Label: 21
PoM **Fenopron**®: see section 10.1.1

FLURBIPROFEN
See section 10.1.1

IBUPROFEN
Indications: mild to moderate pain; see also section 10.1.1
Cautions; Contra-indications; Side-effects: see section 10.1.1
Dose: 1.2–1.8 g daily in divided doses, preferably after food, increased if necessary to a max. of 2.4 g daily; CHILD, fever and pain, see below

Fever and pain in children
▼ PoM **Junifen**® (Boots)
Suspension, sugar-free, ibuprofen 100 mg/5 mL, net price 150-mL pack = £2.41. Label: 21
Dose: fever and pain in children, under 1 year not recommended, 1–12 years 20 mg/kg daily in divided doses *or* 1–2 years 2.5 mL 3–4 times daily, 3–7 years 5 mL, 8–12 years 10 mL

Other preparations: see section 10.1.1

KETOPROFEN
See section 10.1.1

KETOROLAC
See section 15.1.4.2

MEFENAMIC ACID
Indications: mild to moderate pain, pyrexia in children; menorrhagia; see also section 10.1.1
Cautions; Contra-indications; Side-effects: see section 10.1.1; exclude pathological conditions before treating menorrhagia
Dose: 500 mg 3 times daily after food; CHILD over 6 months 25 mg/kg daily in divided doses for max. 7 days, except in juvenile arthritis (Still's disease)

Preparations
See section 10.1.1

NAPROXEN SODIUM
Indications: mild to moderate pain; rheumatic disease, see Naproxen, section 10.1.1
Cautions; Contra-indications; Side-effects: see section 10.1.1

Dose: 550 mg twice daily when necessary, preferably after food
Note. 275 mg naproxen sodium ≡ 250 mg naproxen but the sodium salt has a more rapid action.

PoM Synflex® (Syntex)
Tablets, orange, naproxen sodium 275 mg. Net price 20 = £2.90. Label: 21

NEFOPAM HYDROCHLORIDE
Indications: moderate pain
Cautions: hepatic or renal disease, elderly, urinary retention; **interactions:** Appendix 1 (nefopam)
Contra-indications: convulsive disorders; not indicated for myocardial infarction

Side-effects: nausea, nervousness, urinary retention, dry mouth, lightheadedness; less frequently vomiting, blurred vision, drowsiness, sweating, insomnia, tachycardia, headache; confusion and hallucinations also reported; may colour urine (pink)
Dose: by mouth, initially 60 mg (elderly, 30 mg) 3 times daily, adjusted according to response; usual range 30–90 mg 3 times daily
By intramuscular injection, 20 mg every 6 hours
Note. Nefopam hydrochloride 20 mg by injection ≡ 60 mg by mouth

PoM Acupan® (3M)
Tablets, f/c, nefopam hydrochloride 30 mg. Net price 90-tab pack = £11.73. Label: 2, 14

The following is a list of preparations on sale to the general public that contain **aspirin** or **paracetamol**, **alone** or with **other ingredients**. Other significant ingredients (such as codeine) are listed, but minor ingredients (such as caffeine) are not. For details of preparations containing ibuprofen on sale to the general public, see section 10.1.1.
Important: contact **Poisons Information Services** (p. 15) for full details of the ingredients

Actron® (aspirin, paracetamol), **Alka-Seltzer®** (aspirin), **Anadin®** (aspirin, quinine), **Anadin Extra®**, **Anadin Extra Soluble®** (both aspirin, paracetamol), **Anadin Maximum Strength®** (aspirin), **Anadin Paracetamol®** (paracetamol), **Andrews Answer®** (paracetamol), **Askit®** (aspirin, aloxiprin = polymeric product of aspirin), **Aspro®** (aspirin), **Aspro Clear®** (aspirin), **Aspro Paraclear Junior®** and **Aspro Paraclear Soluble®** (paracetamol)
Banimax® (aspirin, paracetamol), **Bayer Aspirin®** (aspirin), **Beechams Hot Lemon®**, **Hot Lemon with Honey®** or **Hot Blackcurrant®** (all paracetamol), **Beechams Powders®** (aspirin), **Beechams Powders Capsules® With Decongestant** (paracetamol, phenylephrine), **Beecham Aspirin®** and **Beechams Powders Tablets®** (aspirin), **Benylin Day and Night Cold and Flu Relief®** (*day tablets*, paracetamol, phenylpropanolamine, *night tablets*, paracetamol, diphenhydramine)
Cafadol® (paracetamol), **Calpol Extra For Adults®** (paracetamol, codeine), **Calpol Infant®** and **Calpol Six-Plus®** (both paracetamol), **Catarrh-Ex®** (paracetamol, pseudoephedrine), **Coda-med®** (paracetamol, codeine), **Codanin®** (paracetamol, codeine), **Codis 500®** (aspirin, codeine), **Cojene®** (aspirin, codeine), **Coldrex Blackcurrant Powders®**, **Hot Lemon Powders®**, and **Tablets®** (all paracetamol, phenylephrine), **Mrs. Cullen's®** (aspirin), **Cupanol Over 6®**, **Cupanol Under Six®** (both paracetamol)
Day Nurse® (paracetamol, dextromethorphan, phenylpropanolamine), **De Witt's Analgesic Pills®** (paracetamol), **Disprin®** and **Disprin Direct®** (both aspirin), **Disprin Extra®** (aspirin, paracetamol), **Disprol®**, **Disprol Junior®**, **Disprol Paediatric®** (all paracetamol), **Doan's® Backache pills** (paracetamol, sodium salicylate), **Dristan Tablets®** (aspirin, chlorpheniramine, phenylephrine), **Elkamol®** (paracetamol), **EP®** (paracetamol, codeine)
Fanalgic® (paracetamol), **Femigraine®** (aspirin, cyclizine), **Feminax®** (paracetamol, codeine, hyoscine), **Fennings Powders Adult®** and **Fennings Powders Child®** (both paracetamol), **Flurex Bedtime®** (paracetamol, diphenhydramine, pseudoephedrine), **Flurex Capsules®** and **Tablets®** (paracetamol, phenylephrine), **Fynnon® Calcium Aspirin** (aspirin)

Hedex®, **Hedex Soluble®** and **Hedex Extra®** (all paracetamol)
Junior Lemsip® (paracetamol, phenylephrine), **Laboprin DL®** (lysine acetylsalicylate), **Lem-plus Capsules®** (paracetamol, phenylephrine), **Lem-plus Powders®** (paracetamol), **Lemsip Lemon** or **Blackcurrant®**, **Lemsip Cold Relief® Capsules with Decongestant** (paracetamol, phenylephrine), **Lemsip Nightime®** (paracetamol, chlorpheniramine, dextromethorphan, phenylpropanolamine)
Medised® (paracetamol, promethazine), **Midrid®** (paracetamol, isometheptene mucate), **Migraleve®** (*pink tablets*, paracetamol, codeine, buclizine, *yellow tablets*, paracetamol, codeine), **Miradol®** (paracetamol), **Mu-Cron Tablets®** (paracetamol, phenylpropanolamine)
Night Nurse® (paracetamol, dextromethorphan, promethazine), **Nurse Sykes Powders®** (aspirin, paracetamol), **Nu Seals®** Aspirin (aspirin)
Palaprin Forte® (aloxiprin = polymeric product of aspirin), **Paldesic®** (paracetamol), **Pameton®** (paracetamol, methionine), **Panadeine®** (paracetamol, codeine), **Panadol®**, **Panadol Baby and Infant®**, **Panadol Extra®**, **Panadol Junior®** (all paracetamol), **Panaleve Junior®**, **Panaleve 6+®** (both paracetamol), **Panerel®** (paracetamol, codeine), **Paracets®** (paracetamol), **Paracodol®** (paracetamol, codeine), **Paramin®** (paracetamol), **Paramol®** (paracetamol, dihydro codeine), **Phensic®** and **Phensic Soluble®** (both aspirin), **Powerin®** (aspirin, paracetamol), **Propain®** (paracetamol, codeine, diphenhydramine)
Resolve® (paracetamol), **Rimadol®** (paracetamol), **Salzone®** (paracetamol), **Sinutab®** (paracetamol, phenylpropanolamine), **Solpadeine®** paracetamol, codeine), **SP Cold Relief Capsules®** (paracetamol, phenylphrine), **Sudafed-Co®** (paracetamol, pseudoephedrine), **Syndol®** (paracetamol, codeine, doxylamine)
Toptabs® (aspirin), **Tramil®** (paracetamol), **Triogesic®** (paracetamol, phenylpropanolamine)
Uniflu with Gregovite C® (paracetamol, codeine, diphenhydramine, phenylephrine)
Veganin® (aspirin, paracetamol, codeine), **Vicks Coldcare®** (paracetamol, dextromethorphan, phenylpropanolamine), **Vick's Medinite®** (paracetamol, dextromethorphan, doxylamine, ephedrine)

Injection, nefopam hydrochloride 20 mg/mL. Net price 1-mL amp = 74p

4.7.2 Opioid analgesics

Opioid analgesics are used to relieve moderate to severe pain particularly of visceral origin. Repeated administration may cause dependence and tolerance, but this is no deterrent in the control of pain in terminal illness, for guidelines see Prescribing in Terminal Care, p. 12.

SIDE-EFFECTS. Opioid analgesics share many side-effects though qualitative and quantitative differences exist. The most common include nausea, vomiting, constipation, and drowsiness. Larger doses produce respiratory depression and hypotension. Overdosage, see Poisoning, p. 18.

INTERACTIONS. See Appendix 1 (opioid analgesics) (**important**: special hazard with *pethidine and possibly other opioids* and MAOIs).

DRIVING. Drowsiness may affect performance of skilled tasks (e.g. driving); effects of alcohol enhanced.

CHOICE. **Morphine** remains the most valuable opioid analgesic for severe pain although it frequently causes nausea and vomiting. It is the standard against which other opioid analgesics are compared. In addition to relief of pain, morphine also confers a state of euphoria and mental detachment.

Morphine is the opioid of choice for the oral treatment of *severe pain in terminal care*. It is given regularly every 4 hours (or every 12 hours as modified-release tablets). For guidelines on dosage adjustment in terminal care, see p. 12.

Buprenorphine has both opioid agonist and antagonist properties and may precipitate withdrawal symptoms, including pain, in patients dependent on other opioids. It has abuse potential and may itself cause dependence. It has a much longer duration of action than morphine and sublingually is an effective analgesic for 6 to 8 hours. Vomiting may be a problem. Unlike most opioid analgesics its effects are only partially reversed by naloxone.

Codeine is effective for the relief of mild to moderate pain but is too constipating for long-term use.

Dextromoramide is less sedating than morphine and has a short duration of action.

Dipipanone used alone is less sedating than morphine but the only preparation available contains an anti-emetic and is therefore not suitable for regular regimens in terminal care (see p. 12).

Dextropropoxyphene given alone is a very mild analgesic somewhat less potent than codeine. Combinations of dextropropoxyphene with paracetamol (co-proxamol) or aspirin have little more analgesic effect than paracetamol or aspirin alone. An important disadvantage of co-proxamol is that overdosage (which may be combined with alcohol) is complicated by respiratory depression and acute heart failure due to the dextropropoxyphene and by hepatotoxicity due to the paracetamol. Rapid treatment is essential (see Emergency Treatment of Poisoning, p. 18).

Diamorphine (heroin) is a powerful opioid analgesic. It may cause less nausea and hypotension than morphine. In *terminal care* the greater solubility of diamorphine allows effective doses to be injected in smaller volumes and this is important in the emaciated patient.

Dihydrocodeine has an analgesic efficacy similar to that of codeine. The dose of dihydrocodeine by mouth is usually 30 mg every 4 hours; doubling the dose to 60 mg may provide some additional pain relief but this may be at the cost of more nausea and vomiting.

Meptazinol is claimed to have a low incidence of respiratory depression. It has a reported length of action of 2 to 7 hours with onset within 15 minutes, but there is an incidence of nausea and vomiting.

Methadone is less sedating than morphine and acts for longer periods. In prolonged use, methadone should not be administered more often than twice daily to avoid the risk of accumulation and opioid overdosage.

Nalbuphine has a similar efficacy to that of morphine for pain relief, but may have fewer side-effects and less abuse potential. Nausea and vomiting occur less than with other opioids but respiratory depression is similar to that with morphine.

Oxycodone is used as the pectinate in suppositories (special order, Boots) for the control of *pain in terminal care.*

Pentazocine has both agonist and antagonist properties and precipitates withdrawal symptoms, including pain in patients dependent on other opioids. By injection it is more potent than dihydrocodeine or codeine, but hallucinations and thought disturbances may occur. It is not recommended and, in particular, should be avoided after myocardial infarction as it may increase pulmonary and aortic blood pressure as well as cardiac work.

Pethidine produces a prompt but short-lasting analgesia and even in high doses it is a less potent analgesic than morphine. It is not suitable for the relief of pain in terminal care. It is used for analgesia in labour, and in the neonate is associated with less respiratory depression than other opioid analgesics (probably because its action is weaker).

Phenazocine is effective in severe pain and has less tendency to increase biliary pressure than other opioid analgesics. It can be administered sublingually if nausea and vomiting are a problem.

ADDICTS. Although caution is necessary addicts (and ex-addicts) may be treated with analgesics in the same way as other people when there is a real clinical need. Doctors are reminded that they do not require a special licence to prescribe opioid analgesics for addicts for relief of pain due to organic disease or injury.

MORPHINE SALTS

Indications: see notes above; acute pulmonary oedema; peri-operative analgesia see section 15.1.4.3

Cautions: hypotension, hypothyroidism, asthma, and decreased respiratory reserve; pregnancy and breast-feeding; may precipitate coma in hepatic impairment (but many such patients tolerate morphine well); reduce dose in renal impairment, elderly and debilitated; dependence (severe withdrawal symptoms if withdrawn abruptly); use of cough suppressants containing opioid analgesics not generally recommended in children and should be avoided altogether in those under 1 year; **interactions:** Appendix 1 (opioid analgesics)
TERMINAL CARE. In the control of pain in terminal illness these cautions should not necessarily be a deterrent to the use of opioid analgesics

Contra-indications: avoid in raised intracranial pressure or head injury (in addition to interfering with respiration, affect pupillary responses vital for neurological assessment)

Side-effects: nausea and vomiting (particularly in initial stages), constipation, and drowsiness; larger doses produce respiratory depression and hypotension; other side-effects include difficulty with micturition, ureteric or biliary spasm, dry mouth, sweating, facial flushing, vertigo, bradycardia, palpitations, postural hypotension, hypothermia, hallucinations, mood changes, dependence, miosis, urticaria and pruritus; overdosage: see Emergency Treatment of Poisoning, p. 18

Dose: acute pain, *by subcutaneous or intramuscular injection*, 10 mg every 4 hours if necessary (15 mg for heavier well-muscled patients); CHILD up to 1 month 150 micrograms/kg, 1–12 months 200 micrograms/kg, 1–5 years 2.5–5 mg, 6–12 years 5–10 mg
By slow intravenous injection, quarter to half corresponding intramuscular dose
Myocardial infarction, *by slow intravenous injection* (2 mg/minute), 10 mg followed by a further 5–10 mg if necessary; elderly or frail patients, reduce dose by half
Acute pulmonary oedema, *by slow intravenous injection* (2 mg/minute) 5–10 mg
Chronic pain, *by mouth or by subcutaneous or intramuscular injection*, 5–20 mg regularly every 4 hours; dose may be increased according to needs; oral dose should be approximately double corresponding intramuscular dose and triple to quadruple corresponding intramuscular *diamorphine* dose (see also Prescribing in Terminal Care, p. 12); *by rectum*, as suppositories, 15–30 mg regularly every 4 hours
Note. The doses stated above refer equally to morphine hydrochloride, sulphate, and tartrate; for dose of **modified-release** tablets, see next column.

Oral solutions

PoM or **CD Morphine Oral Solutions**
Oral solutions of morphine can be prescribed by writing the formula:
Morphine hydrochloride 5 mg
Chloroform water to 5 mL

Note. The proportion of morphine hydrochloride may be altered when specified by the prescriber; if above 13 mg per 5 mL the solution becomes **CD**. For sample prescription see Controlled Drugs and Drug Dependence, p. 7. It is usual to adjust the strength so that the dose volume is 5 or 10 mL.

Oramorph® (Boehringer Ingelheim)
PoM *Oral solution*, morphine sulphate 10 mg/5 mL. Net price 100-mL pack = £2.31; 250-mL pack = £5.36; 500-mL pack = £9.70. Label: 2
CD *Concentrated oral solution*, sugar-free, morphine sulphate 100 mg/5 mL. Net price 30-mL pack = £6.47; 120-mL pack = £24.15 (both with calibrated dropper). Label: 2

Tablets
CD Sevredol® (Napp)
Tablets, both f/c, scored, morphine sulphate 10 mg (blue), net price 56-tab pack = £6.47; 20 mg (pink), 56-tab pack = £12.94. Label: 2

Modified-release tablets
Note. For advice on transfer from oral solutions of morphine to modified-release tablets of morphine, see Terminal Care, p. 12

CD MST Continus® (Napp)
Tablets, all m/r, f/c, morphine sulphate 5 mg (white), net price 60-tab pack = £4.62; 10 mg (brown), 60-tab pack = £7.70; 15 mg (green) net price 60-tab pack = £13.50; 30 mg (purple), 60-tab pack = £18.49; 60 mg (orange), 60-tab pack = £36.06; 100 mg (grey), 60-tab pack = £57.10; 200 mg (green), 60-tab pack = £114.20. Label: 2, 25
Dose: severe pain uncontrolled by weaker opioids, 30 mg every 12 hours, increased to 60 mg every 12 hours when required, then further increments of 25–50% if necessary. For lower initial doses in patients who have not received other opioids, see Prescribing in Terminal Care, p. 12
CHILD severe, intractable pain in cancer, initially 200–800 micrograms/kg every 12 hours, then further increments of 30–50% if necessary
Note. Brand name prescriptions for MST Continus must also specify 'tablets' (i.e. 'MST Continus tablets').

CD SRM-Rhotard® (Farmitalia Carlo Erba)
Tablets, all m/r, f/c, morphine sulphate 10 mg (buff), net price 60-tab pack = £6.93; 30 mg (violet), 60-tab pack = £16.41; 60 mg (orange), 60-tab pack = £32.45; 100 mg (grey), 60-tab pack = £51.39. Label: 2, 25
Dose: severe pain uncontrolled by weaker opioids, 30 mg every 12 hours, increased to 60 mg every 12 hours when required, then further increments of 25–50% if necessary. For lower initial doses in patients who have not received other opioids, see Prescribing in Terminal Care, p. 12
CHILD not yet recommended
Note. Brand name prescriptions for SRM-Rhotard must also specify 'tablets' (i.e. 'SRM-Rhotard Tablets')

Injections
CD Morphine Sulphate Injection, morphine sulphate 10, 15, 20, and 30 mg/mL, net price 1- and 2-mL amp (all) = 51–86p

CD Min-I-Jet® Morphine Sulphate (IMS)
Injection, morphine sulphate 10 mg/mL, net price 2-mL disposable syringe = £5.92

CD Morphine and Atropine Injection
See section 15.1.4.3

4.7 Analgesics

Injection with anti-emetic
CAUTION. In myocardial infarction cyclizine may aggravate severe heart failure and counteract the haemodynamic benefits of opioids, see section 4.6. **Not recommended** in terminal care, see p. 12

CD Cyclimorph® (Wellcome)
Cyclimorph-10® *Injection*, morphine tartrate 10 mg, cyclizine tartrate 50 mg/mL. Net price 1-mL amp = £1.28
Dose: by subcutaneous, intramuscular, or intravenous injection, 1 mL, repeated not more often than every 4 hours, with not more than 3 doses in any 24-hour period; CHILD 1–5 years 0.25–0.5 mL as a single dose, 6–12 years 0.5–1 mL as a single dose
Cyclimorph-15® *Injection*, morphine tartrate 15 mg, cyclizine tartrate 50 mg/mL. Net price 1-mL amp = £1.33
Dose: by subcutaneous, intramuscular, or intravenous injection, 1 mL, repeated not more often than every 4 hours, with not more than 3 doses in any 24-hour period

Suppositories
CD Morphine Suppositories, morphine hydrochloride or sulphate 15 mg, net price 12 = £3.60; 30 mg, 12 = £4.80. Label: 2.
Available from Evans, Martindale
Note. Both the strength of the suppositories and the morphine salt contained in them must be specified by the prescriber

CD Sevredol® (Napp)
Suppositories, morphine sulphate 10 mg, net price 12 = £6.12; 20 mg, 12 = £7.45; 30 mg, 12 = £9.60. Label: 2

Mixed opium alkaloids
Mixed opium alkaloids do not have any advantage over morphine alone; alcoholic solutions are liable to evaporation and are **not** recommended.

CD Nepenthe (Evans)
Oral solution (= elixir), brown, anhydrous morphine 8.4 mg/mL (500 micrograms from opium tincture, 7.9 mg from morphine). Diluent syrup, life of diluted elixir 4 weeks. Net price 100-mL pack = £22.45. Label: 2
Dose: 1–2 mL, repeated not more often than every 4 hours when necessary; CHILD 6–12 years 0.5–1 mL, as a single dose
Note. This product must always be diluted when being dispensed.
CAUTION. *Nepenthe Oral Solution may become concentrated through evaporation of the solvent. It should be stored in a cool place in the original airtight container. If evaporation occurs during storage the solution should not be used because of risk of overdosage.*

ALFENTANIL
See section 15.1.4.3

BUPRENORPHINE
Indications: moderate to severe pain; peri-operative analgesia, see section 15.1.4.3
Cautions; Contra-indications; Side-effects: see under Morphine Salts, but side-effects less marked; can give rise to mild withdrawal symptoms in patients dependent on opioids; effects only partially reversed by naloxone; **interactions:** Appendix 1 (opioid analgesics)

Dose: by sublingual administration, initially 200–400 micrograms every 8 hours, increasing if necessary to 200–400 micrograms every 6–8 hours; CHILD over 6 months, 16–25 kg, 100 micrograms; 25–37.5 kg, 100–200 micrograms; 37.5–50 kg, 200–300 micrograms
By intramuscular or slow intravenous injection, 300–600 micrograms every 6–8 hours; CHILD over 6 months 3–6 micrograms/kg every 6–8 hours; max. 9 micrograms/kg

CD Temgesic® (R&C)
Tablets (sublingual), buprenorphine (as hydrochloride), 200 micrograms, net price 50 = £6.00; 400 micrograms, 50 = £12.00. Label: 2, 26
Injection, buprenorphine 300 micrograms (as hydrochloride)/mL. Net price 1-mL amp = 55p

CODEINE PHOSPHATE
Indications: mild to moderate pain
Cautions; Contra-indications; Side-effects: see under Morphine Salts but side-effects less marked; use of cough suppressants containing codeine or similar opioid analgesics not generally recommended in children and should be avoided altogether in those under 1 year; **interactions:** Appendix 1 (opioid analgesics)
Dose: by mouth, 30–60 mg every 4 hours when necessary, to a max. of 240 mg daily; CHILD 1–12 years, 3 mg/kg daily in divided doses
By intramuscular injection, 30–60 mg every 4 hours when necessary

Codeine Phosphate (Non-proprietary)
PoM *Tablets*, codeine phosphate 15 mg, net price 20 = 38p; 30 mg, 20 = 39p; 60 mg, 20 = £1.24. Label: 2
Note. As for schedule 2 controlled drugs, travellers needing to take codeine phosphate preparations abroad may require a doctor's letter explaining why they are necessary.
PoM *Syrup*, codeine phosphate 25 mg/5 mL. Net price 100 mL = 78p. Label: 2
CD *Injection*, codeine phosphate 60 mg/mL. Net price 1-mL amp = £1.35
Codeine Linctuses
See section 3.9.1

Note. Codeine is an ingredient of some compound analgesic preparations, see sections 4.7.1 and 10.1.1 (Codafen Continus®)

DEXTROMORAMIDE
Indications: severe pain
Cautions; Contra-indications; Side-effects: see under Morphine Salts, but less sedating than morphine; only short duration of action (2–3 hours); avoid in obstetric analgesia (increased risk of neonatal depression); **interactions:** Appendix 1 (opioid analgesics)
Dose: by mouth, 5 mg increasing to 20 mg, when required
By subcutaneous or intramuscular injection, 5 mg increasing to 15 mg, when required
By rectum in suppositories, 10 mg when required

CD Palfium® (Boehringer Mannheim)
Tablets, both scored, dextromoramide (as tartrate) 5 mg, net price 60-tab pack = £4.78; 10 mg (peach), 60-tab pack = £9.45. Label: 2
Injection, dextromoramide (as tartrate) 5 mg/mL, net price 1-mL amp = 20p; 10 mg/mL, 1-mL amp = 24p
Suppositories, dextromoramide 10 mg (as tartrate). Net price 10 = £2.35. Label: 2

DEXTROPROPOXYPHENE HYDROCHLORIDE

Indications: mild to moderate pain
Cautions; Contra-indications; Side effects: see under Morphine Salts but side-effects less marked; occasional hepatotoxicity; avoid in porphyria (see section 9.8.2); compound preparations special hazard in overdose, see notes above; convulsions reported in overdose
Dose: 65 mg every 6–8 hours when necessary
Note. 65 mg dextropropoxyphene hydrochloride ≡ 100 mg dextropropoxyphene napsylate

PoM **Dextropropoxyphene Capsules,** the equivalent of dextropropoxyphene hydrochloride 65 mg (as napsylate). Net price 20 = £1.19. Label: 2
Available from Lilly (NHS Doloxene®)

Note. Dextropropoxyphene is an ingredient of some compound analgesic preparations, see section 4.7.1

DIAMORPHINE HYDROCHLORIDE

Indications: see notes above; acute pulmonary oedema
Cautions; Contra-indications; Side-effects: see under Morphine Salts; **interactions:** Appendix 1 (opioid analgesics)
Dose: acute pain, *by subcutaneous or intramuscular injection*, 5 mg repeated every 4 hours if necessary (up to 10 mg for heavier well-muscled patients)
By slow intravenous injection, quarter to half corresponding intramuscular dose
Myocardial infarction, *by slow intravenous injection* (1 mg/minute), 5 mg followed by a further 2.5–5 mg if necessary; elderly or frail patients, reduce dose by half
Acute pulmonary oedema, *by slow intravenous injection* (1 mg/minute) 2.5–5 mg
Chronic pain, *by mouth or by subcutaneous or intramuscular injection*, 5–10 mg regularly every 4 hours; dose may be increased according to needs; intramuscular dose should be approximately half corresponding oral dose, and quarter to third corresponding oral *morphine* dose; see also Prescribing in Terminal Care, p. 12

CD **Diamorphine** (Non-proprietary)
Tablets, diamorphine hydrochloride 10 mg. Net price 20 = 91p. Label: 2
Injection, powder for reconstitution, diamorphine hydrochloride. Net price 5-mg amp = £1.16, 10-mg amp = £1.34, 30-mg amp = £1.60, 100-mg amp = £4.42, 500-mg amp = £20.68
Available from Evans, Napp (Diaphine®)

CD **Diamorphine Linctus**
See section 3.9.1

DIHYDROCODEINE TARTRATE

Indications: moderate to severe pain
Cautions; Contra-indications; Side-effects: see under Morphine Salts
Dose: by mouth, 30 mg every 4–6 hours when necessary, preferably after food (see also notes above); CHILD over 4 years 0.5–1 mg/kg every 4–6 hours
By deep subcutaneous or intramuscular injection, up to 50 mg every 4–6 hours

Dihydrocodeine (Non-proprietary)
PoM *Tablets*, dihydrocodeine tartrate 30 mg. Net price 20 = 62p. Label: 2, 21
PoM *Elixir*, dihydrocodeine tartrate 10 mg/5 mL. Net price 150 mL = £1.85. Label: 2, 21
CD *Injection*, dihydrocodeine tartrate 50 mg/mL. Net price 1-mL amp = 45p
Available from Napp
Note. The brand name DF118® was formerly used for dihydrocodeine tartrate preparations

PoM **DHC Continus**® (Napp)
Tablets, m/r, dihydrocodeine tartrate 60 mg (scored), net price 56-tab pack = £6.75; 90 mg, 56-tab pack = £10.63; 120 mg, 56-tab pack = £14.18. Label: 2, 25
Dose: chronic severe pain, 60–120 mg every 12 hours

Note. Dihydrocodeine is an ingredient of some compound analgesic preparations, see section 4.7.1

DIPIPANONE HYDROCHLORIDE

Indications: moderate to severe pain
Cautions; Contra-indications; Side-effects: see under Morphine Salts; **interactions:** Appendix 1 (opioid analgesics)

CD **Diconal**® (Wellcome)
Tablets, pink, scored, dipipanone hydrochloride 10 mg, cyclizine hydrochloride 30 mg. Net price 50-tab pack = £7.59. Label: 2
Dose: 1 tablet gradually increased to 3 tablets every 6 hours
CAUTION. **Not recommended** in terminal care, see p. 12

FENTANYL
See section 15.1.4.3

MEPTAZINOL

Indications: moderate to severe pain, including postoperative and obstetric pain and renal colic; peri-operative analgesia, see section 15.1.4.3
Cautions; Contra-indications; Side-effects: see under Morphine Salts
Dose: by mouth, 200 mg every 3–6 hours as required
By intramuscular injection, 75–100 mg every 2–4 hours if necessary; obstetric analgesia, 100–150 mg according to patient's weight (2 mg/kg)
By slow intravenous injection, 50–100 mg every 2–4 hours if necessary

4.7 Analgesics 181

PoM **Meptid**® (Monmouth)
Tablets, orange, f/c, meptazinol 200 mg. Net price 20 = £1.80. Label: 2
Injection, meptazinol 100 mg (as hydrochloride)/mL. Net price 1-mL amp = 79p

METHADONE HYDROCHLORIDE

Indications: severe pain, see notes above; adjunct in treatment of opioid dependence, section 4.10
Cautions; Contra-indications; Side-effects: see under Morphine Salts, but less sedating than morphine; **interactions:** Appendix 1 (opioid analgesics)
Dose: by mouth or by subcutaneous or intramuscular injection, 5–10 mg every 6–8 hours, adjusted according to response

CD **Methadone Linctus**, see section 3.9.1
CD **Methadone Mixture 1 mg/mL**, section 4.10
CD **Physeptone**® (Wellcome)
Tablets, scored, methadone hydrochloride 5 mg. Net price 50 = £3.11. Label: 2
Injection, methadone hydrochloride 10 mg/mL. Net price 1-mL amp = 86p

NALBUPHINE HYDROCHLORIDE

Indications: moderate to severe pain; peri-operative analgesia, see section 15.1.4.3
Cautions; Contra-indications; Side-effects: see under Morphine Salts; **interactions:** Appendix 1 (opioid analgesics)
Dose: by subcutaneous, intramuscular, or intravenous injection, 10–20 mg for 70-kg patient every 3–6 hours, adjusted as required; CHILD up to 300 micrograms/kg repeated once or twice as necessary
Myocardial infarction, *by slow intravenous injection*, 10–20 mg repeated after 30 minutes if necessary

PoM **Nubain**® (Du Pont)
Injection, nalbuphine hydrochloride 10 mg/mL. Net price 1-mL amp = 75p; 2-mL amp = £1.16

PAPAVERETUM

See section 15.1.4.3

PENTAZOCINE

Indications: moderate to severe pain, but see notes above
Cautions; Contra-indications; Side-effects: see under Morphine Salts; occasional hallucinations; avoid in patients dependent on opioids and in arterial or pulmonary hypertension and heart failure; avoid in porphyria (see section 9.8.2)
Dose: by mouth, pentazocine hydrochloride 50 mg every 3–4 hours preferably after food (range 25–100 mg); CHILD 6–12 years 25 mg
By subcutaneous, intramuscular, or intravenous injection, moderate pain, pentazocine 30 mg, severe pain 45–60 mg every 3–4 hours when necessary; CHILD over 1 year, *by subcutaneous or intramuscular injection*, up to 1 mg/kg, *by intravenous injection* up to 500 micrograms/kg
By rectum in suppositories, pentazocine 50 mg up to 4 times daily

CD **Pentazocine** (Non-proprietary)
Capsules, pentazocine hydrochloride 50 mg. Net price 20 = £3.51. Label: 2, 21
Tablets, pentazocine hydrochloride 25 mg. Net price 20 = £1.65. Label: 2, 21
Injection, pentazocine 30 mg (as lactate)/mL. Net price 1-mL amp = 80p; 2-mL amp = £1.54
Suppositories, pentazocine 50 mg (as lactate). Net price 20 = £9.55. Label: 2
Note. The brand name NHS Fortral® (Sanofi Winthrop) is used for all the above preparations of pentazocine

PETHIDINE HYDROCHLORIDE

Indications: moderate to severe pain, obstetric analgesia; peri-operative analgesia, see section 15.1.4.3
Cautions; Contra-indications; Side-effects: see under Morphine Salts, but less constipating than morphine; avoid in severe renal impairment; convulsions reported in overdosage; **interactions:** Appendix 1 (opioid analgesics)
Dose: by mouth, 50–150 mg every 4 hours; CHILD 0.5–2 mg/kg
By subcutaneous or intramuscular injection, 25–100 mg, repeated after 4 hours; CHILD, *by intramuscular injection*, 0.5–2 mg/kg
By slow intravenous injection, 25–50 mg, repeated after 4 hours
Obstetric analgesia, *by subcutaneous or intramuscular injection*, 50–100 mg, repeated 1–3 hours later if necessary; max. 400 mg in 24 hours

CD **Pethidine** (Roche)
Tablets, pethidine hydrochloride 50 mg, net price 20 = 39p. Label: 2
Injection, pethidine hydrochloride 50 mg/mL. Net price 1-mL amp = 11p; 2-mL amp = 14p. 10 mg/mL see section 15.1.4.3
CD **Pamergan P100**® (Martindale)
Injection, pethidine hydrochloride 50 mg, promethazine hydrochloride 25 mg/mL. Net price 2-mL amp = 45p
Dose: by intramuscular injection, for obstetric analgesia, 1–2 mL every 4 hours if necessary; severe pain, 1–2 mL every 4–6 hours if necessary; premedication, see section 15.1.4.3
Note. Although usually given intramuscularly, may be given intravenously after dilution to at least 10 mL with water for injections

PHENAZOCINE HYDROBROMIDE

Indications: severe pain
Cautions; Contra-indications; Side-effects: see under Morphine Salts, but less sedating than morphine; **interactions:** Appendix 1 (opioid analgesics)
Dose: by mouth or sublingually, 5 mg every 4–6 hours when necessary; single doses may be increased to 20 mg

Cautionary label wordings, see inside back cover　　　　　　　　　　　　　　　　Prices are **net**, see p. 1

CD Narphen® (Napp)
Tablets, scored, phenazocine hydrobromide 5 mg. Net price 100-tab pack = £25.43. Label: 2

PHENOPERIDINE
See section 15.1.4.3

4.7.3 Trigeminal neuralgia

Carbamazepine (section 4.8.1), taken during the acute stages of trigeminal neuralgia, reduces the frequency and severity of attacks if given continuously. It has no effect on other forms of headache. A dose of 100 mg once or twice a day should be given initially and the dose slowly increased until the best response is obtained; most patients require 200 mg 3–4 times daily but a few may require an increased total daily dosage of up to 1.6 g. Plasma concentrations should be monitored when high doses are given. Occasionally extreme dizziness is encountered which is a further reason for starting treatment with a small dose and increasing it slowly.

Some cases of trigeminal neuralgia respond to **phenytoin** (section 4.8.1) given alone or in conjunction with carbamazepine. A combination of phenytoin and carbamazepine is only required in very refractory cases or in those unable to tolerate high doses of carbamazepine.

4.7.4 Antimigraine drugs
4.7.4.1 Treatment of the acute migraine attack
4.7.4.2 Prophylaxis of migraine

4.7.4.1 TREATMENT OF THE ACUTE MIGRAINE ATTACK

Most migraine headaches respond to analgesics such as **aspirin** or **paracetamol** (section 4.7.1) but as peristalsis is often reduced during migraine the medication may not be sufficiently well absorbed to be effective; dispersible or effervescent preparations should therefore preferably be used.

Ergotamine is used in patients who do not respond to analgesics. It relieves migraine headache by constricting cranial arteries but visual and other prodromal symptoms are not affected and vomiting may be made worse. This can be relieved by the addition of an **anti-emetic** (see below).

The value of ergotamine is limited by difficulties in absorption and by its side-effects, particularly nausea, vomiting, abdominal pain, and muscular cramps. In some patients repeated administration may cause habituation. Rarely headache may be provoked, either by chronic overdosage or by rapid withdrawal of the drug. Doses of 6 to 8 mg per attack and 10 to 12 mg per week should **not** be exceeded. Ergotamine treatment should **not** be repeated at intervals of less than 4 days and it should **never** be prescribed prophylactically[1]; it should not be given in hemiplegic migraine.

---
1. In the management of cluster headache, a low dose of ergotamine is occasionally given on a daily basis for 1–2 weeks; ergotamine is not licensed for this purpose.

There are various ergotamine preparations designed to improve absorption and best results are obtained when the dose is given early in an attack. An aerosol form (Medihaler-Ergotamine®) is acceptable to some patients. Sublingual ergotamine (Lingraine®) probably has no advantage over oral treatment.

Dihydroergotamine is of doubtful value.

Sumatriptan is a new $5-HT_1$ agonist. It appears to be of considerable value in the treatment of an acute attack but experience is relatively limited.

Anti-emetics (section 4.6), such as **metoclopramide** by mouth or, if vomiting is likely, by intramuscular injection, or the phenothiazine and antihistamine anti-emetics, relieve the nausea associated with migraine attacks. Prochlorperazine may be given rectally if vomiting is a problem. Metoclopramide has the added advantage of promoting gastric emptying and normal peristalsis. A single dose should be given at the onset of symptoms. Oral analgesic preparations containing metoclopramide are available.

ANALGESICS
Section 4.7.1

ANALGESICS WITH ANTI-EMETICS
Migraleve® (Charwell)
Tablets, all f/c, *pink tablets*, buclizine hydrochloride 6.25 mg, paracetamol 500 mg, codeine phosphate 8 mg; *yellow tablets*, paracetamol 500 mg, codeine phosphate 8 mg. Net price 48-tab Duopack (32 pink + 16 yellow) = £4.68; 48 pink = £5.10; 48 yellow = £4.31. Label: 2, 17, 30
Dose: 2 pink tablets at onset of attack, or if it is imminent, then 2 yellow tablets every 4 hours if necessary; max. in 24 hours 2 pink and 6 yellow; CHILD 10–14 years, half adult dose

PoM **Migravess®** (Bayer)
Tablets, effervescent, scored, metoclopramide hydrochloride 5 mg, aspirin 325 mg. Net price 30-tab pack = £3.60. Label: 13, 17
Forte tablets, effervescent, scored, metoclopramide hydrochloride 5 mg, aspirin 450 mg. Net price 30-tab pack = £4.94. Label: 13, 17
Dose: tablets or Forte tablets, 2 dissolved in water at onset of attack then every 4 hours when necessary; max. 6 tablets in 24 hours; CHILD 12–15 years, half adult dose

PoM **Paramax®** (Bencard)
Tablets, scored, paracetamol 500 mg, metoclopramide hydrochloride 5 mg. Net price 42-tab pack = £3.63. Label: 17, 30
Sachets, effervescent powder, sugar-free, the contents of 1 sachet = 1 tablet; to be dissolved in ¼ tumblerful of liquid before administration. Net price 42-sachet pack = £4.79. Label: 13, 17, 30
Dose: (tablets or sachets): 2 at onset of attack then every 4 hours when necessary to max. of 6 in 24 hours (young adult 15–19 years, over 60 kg, max. of 5 in 24 hours); ADOLESCENT and YOUNG ADULT 12–19 years, 30–59 kg, 1 at onset of attack then 1 every 4 hours when necessary to max. of 3 in 24 hours

4.7 Analgesics

ERGOTAMINE TARTRATE
Indications: acute attacks of migraine and migraine variants unresponsive to analgesics
Cautions: withdraw treatment immediately if numbness or tingling of extremities develops; should not be used for migraine prophylaxis; **interactions:** Appendix 1 (ergotamine)
Contra-indications: peripheral vascular disease, coronary heart disease, obliterative vascular disease or Raynaud's syndrome, hepatic or renal impairment, sepsis, severe or inadequately controlled hypertension, hyperthyroidism, pregnancy and breast-feeding, porphyria (see section 9.8.2)
Side-effects: headache, nausea, vomiting, and abdominal pain; repeated high dosage may cause ergotism with gangrene and confusion; pleural and peritoneal fibrosis may occur with excessive use

PoM **Cafergot**® (Sandoz)
Tablets, ergotamine tartrate 1 mg, caffeine 100 mg. Net price 2 × 50-tab pack = £4.57. Label: 18, counselling, dosage
Dose: 1–2 tablets at onset; max. 4 tablets in 24 hours; not to be repeated at intervals of less than 4 days; max. 10 tablets weekly
Suppositories, ergotamine tartrate 2 mg, caffeine 100 mg. Net price 30 = £4.99. Label: 18, counselling, dosage
Dose: 1 suppository at onset; max. 2 in 24 hours; not to be repeated at intervals of less than 4 days; max. 5 suppositories weekly

PoM **Lingraine**® (Sanofi Winthrop)
Tablets (for sublingual use), green, ergotamine tartrate 2 mg. Net price 12 = £6.93. Label: 18, 26, counselling, dosage
Dose: 1 tablet at onset repeated after 30 minutes if necessary; max. 3 in 24 hours and 6 weekly

PoM **Medihaler-Ergotamine**® (3M)
Aerosol inhalation (oral), ergotamine tartrate 360 micrograms/metered inhalation. Net price 75-dose unit = £3.44. Label: 18, counselling, dosage
Dose: 360 micrograms (1 puff) repeated if necessary after 5 minutes; max. 6 inhalations in 24 hours and 15 inhalations weekly

PoM **Migril**® (Wellcome)
Tablets, scored, ergotamine tartrate 2 mg, cyclizine hydrochloride 50 mg, caffeine hydrate 100 mg. Net price 20 = £11.67. Label: 2, 18, counselling, dosage
Dose: 1 tablet at onset, followed after 30 minutes by ½–1 tablet, repeated every 30 minutes if necessary; max. 4 tablets per attack and 6 tablets weekly

DIHYDROERGOTAMINE MESYLATE
Indications: migraine attack unresponsive to analgesics
Cautions; Contra-indications; Side-effects: see under Ergotamine Tartrate, as well as numbness and tingling of extremities, precordial pain reported; also contra-indicated in shock; avoid intra-arterial injection
Dose: by subcutaneous or intramuscular injection, 1 mg repeated once after 30–60 minutes if necessary; max. 3 mg daily and 6 mg weekly

PoM **Dihydergot**® (Sandoz)
Injection, dihydroergotamine mesylate 1 mg/mL. Net price 1-mL amp = 21p

ISOMETHEPTENE MUCATE
Indications: migraine attack
Cautions: cardiovascular disease; **interactions:** Appendix 1 (sympathomimetics)
Contra-indications: glaucoma; porphyria (see section 9.8.2)
Side-effects: dizziness, circulatory disturbances

Midrid® (Shire)
Capsules, red, isometheptene mucate 65 mg, paracetamol 325 mg. Net price 20 = £2.72. Label: 17, 30
Dose: migraine, 2 capsules at onset of attack, followed by 1 capsule every hour if necessary; max. 5 capsules in 12 hours

SUMATRIPTAN
Indications: acute treatment of migraine attacks; cluster headache (subcutaneous injection only)
Cautions: not for prophylaxis; conditions which predispose to ischaemic heart disease; hepatic or renal impairment; pregnancy and breast-feeding; subcutaneous injection not yet recommended for hemiplegic migraine; **interactions:** Appendix 1 (sumatriptan)
DRIVING. Drowsiness may affect performance of skilled tasks (e.g. driving)
Contra-indications: ischaemic heart disease; previous myocardial infarction or Prinzmetal's angina; uncontrolled hypertension
CSM advice. Following reports of chest pain and tightness (coronary vasoconstriction) CSM has emphasised that sumatriptan should **not** be used in ischaemic heart disease or Prinzmetal's angina, and that use with ergotamine should be **avoided**.
Side-effects: transient pain at injection site; sensations of tingling, heat, heaviness, pressure, or tightness in any part of body; flushing, dizziness, feeling of weakness; fatigue, drowsiness, altered liver function tests, transient increase in blood pressure reported; nausea and vomiting also reported
Dose: by mouth, 100 mg as soon as possible after onset (patient not responding should not take second dose for same attack); dose may be repeated if migraine recurs; max. 300 mg in 24 hours
By subcutaneous injection using auto-injector, 6 mg as soon as possible after onset, repeated once after at least 1 hour if symptoms recur; max. 12 mg in 24 hours
ELDERLY over 65 years and CHILD not yet recommended
IMPORTANT. **Not** for intravenous injection which may cause coronary vasospasm and angina.

▼ PoM **Imigran**® (Glaxo)
Tablets, f/c, sumatriptan (as succinate) 100 mg. Net price 6-tab pack = £48.00. Label: 3, 10 patient information leaflet
Injection, sumatriptan (as succinate) 12 mg/mL (= 6 mg/0.5-mL syringe), net price, treatment pack (2 × 0.5-mL pre-filled syringes and auto-injector) = £41.14; refill pack (2 × 0.5-mL pre-filled syringes) = £39.14. Label: 3, 10 patient information leaflet

4.7.4.2 PROPHYLAXIS OF MIGRAINE

Where migraine attacks are frequent, search should be made for provocative factors such as stress or diet (chocolate, cheese, alcohol, etc.). Benzodiazepines should be avoided because of the risk of dependence. In patients with more than one attack a month, one of three main prophylactic agents may be tried: pizotifen, beta-blockers, or tricyclic antidepressants (even when the patient is not obviously depressed). Long-term treatment with any of these prophylactic drugs is undesirable; the need for continuing therapy should be reviewed at intervals of about 6 months. Oral contraceptives may precipitate or worsen migraine; patients reporting a sharp increase in frequency of migraine or focal features should be recommended alternative contraceptive measures.

Pizotifen is an antihistamine and serotonin antagonist structurally related to the tricyclic antidepressants. It affords good prophylaxis but may cause weight gain. To avoid undue drowsiness treatment may be started at 500 micrograms at night and gradually increased to 3 mg; it is rarely necessary to exceed this dose.

The **beta-blockers** propranolol, metoprolol, nadolol, and timolol (see section 2.4) are all effective. Propranolol is the most commonly used in an initial dose of 40 mg 2 to 3 times daily by mouth. Beta-blockers may also be given as a single daily dose of a long-acting preparation. The value of beta-blockers is limited by their contra-indications (see section 2.4) and by interaction with ergotamine (see Appendix 1, beta-blockers).

Tricyclic antidepressants (section 4.3.1) may usefully be prescribed in a dose, for example, of amitriptyline 10 mg at night, increasing to a maintenance dose of 50 to 75 mg at night.

There is some evidence that the **calcium-channel blockers** (see section 2.6.2), e.g. verapamil and nifedipine may be useful in migraine prophylaxis.

Cyproheptadine (see section 3.4.1), an antihistamine with serotonin-antagonist and calcium channel-blocking properties, may also be tried in refractory cases.

Clonidine (Dixarit®) is probably little better than placebo and may aggravate depression or produce insomnia. **Methysergide** has dangerous side-effects (retroperitoneal fibrosis and fibrosis of the heart valves and pleura); **important:** it should only be administered under hospital supervision.

CLONIDINE HYDROCHLORIDE

Indications: prevention of recurrent migraine (but see notes above), vascular headache, menopausal flushing; hypertension, see section 2.5.2
Cautions: depressive illness, concurrent antihypertensive therapy; avoid in porphyria (see section 9.8.2); **interactions:** Appendix 1 (clonidine)
Side-effects: dry mouth, sedation, dizziness, nausea, nocturnal restlessness; occasionally rashes
Dose: 50 micrograms twice daily, increased after 2 weeks to 75 micrograms twice daily if necessary

PoM **Dixarit**® (Boehringer Ingelheim)
Tablets, blue, s/c, clonidine hydrochloride 25 micrograms. Net price 112-tab pack = £6.13
PoM **Catapres**® (hypertension), see section 2.5.2

METHYSERGIDE

Indications: prevention of severe recurrent migraine and cluster headache in patients who are refractory to other treatment and whose lives are seriously disrupted (**important:** hospital supervision only, see notes above)
Cautions: history of peptic ulceration; avoid abrupt withdrawal of treatment; after 6 months withdraw for reassessment for at least 1 month (see also notes above)
Contra-indications: renal, hepatic, pulmonary, and cardiovascular disease, severe hypertension, collagen disease, cellulitis, urinary-tract disorders, cachectic or septic conditions, pregnancy, breast-feeding
Side-effects: nausea, vomiting, heartburn, abdominal discomfort, drowsiness, and dizziness occur frequently in initial treatment; psychic reactions, insomnia, oedema, weight gain, rashes, loss of scalp hair, cramps, arterial spasm, paraesthesias of extremities, postural hypotension, and tachycardia also occur. Retroperitoneal and other abnormal fibrotic reactions may occur on prolonged administration, requiring immediate withdrawal of treatment
Dose: 1 mg at bedtime, gradually increased to 1–2 mg 2–3 times daily with food (see notes above)
Carcinoid syndrome, usual range, 12–20 mg daily (hospital supervision)

PoM **Deseril**® (Sandoz)
Tablets, s/c, methysergide 1 mg (as maleate). Net price 50 = £4.58. Label: 2, 21

PIZOTIFEN

Indications: prevention of vascular headache including classical migraine, common migraine, and cluster headache
Cautions: urinary retention; closed-angle glaucoma, renal impairment; pregnancy and breast-feeding; **interactions:** Appendix 1 (pizotifen)
DRIVING. Drowsiness may affect performance of skilled tasks (e.g. driving); effects of alcohol enhanced
Side-effects: antimuscarinic effects, drowsiness, increased appetite and weight gain; occasionally nausea, dizziness; CNS stimulation may occur in children
Dose: 1.5 mg at night *or* 500 micrograms 3 times daily (but see also notes above), adjusted according to response within the usual range 0.5–3 mg daily; max. single dose 3 mg; max. daily dose 4.5 mg; CHILD up to 1.5 mg daily; max. single dose at night 1 mg

PoM **Sanomigran**® (Sandoz)
Tablets, both ivory-yellow, s/c, pizotifen (as hydrogen malate), 500 micrograms, net price 20 = £1.60; 1.5 mg, 28-tab pack = £7.98. Label: 2
Elixir, sugar-free, pizotifen 250 micrograms (as hydrogen malate)/5 mL. Net price 300-mL pack = £4.23. Label: 2

4.8 Antiepileptics

4.8.1 Control of epilepsy
4.8.2 Drugs used in status epilepticus
4.8.3 Febrile convulsions

4.8.1 Control of epilepsy

The object of treatment is to prevent the occurrence of seizures by maintaining an effective plasma concentration of the drug. Careful adjustment of doses is necessary, starting with low doses and increasing gradually until seizures are controlled or there are overdose effects.

The frequency of administration is determined by the plasma half-life, and should be kept as low as possible to encourage better patient compliance. Most antiepileptics, when used in average dosage, may be given twice daily. Phenobarbitone and sometimes phenytoin, which have long half-lives, may often be given as a daily dose at bedtime. However, with large doses, some antiepileptics may need to be administered 3 times daily to avoid adverse effects associated with high peak plasma concentrations. Young children metabolise antiepileptics more rapidly than adults and therefore require more frequent doses and a higher amount per kilogram body-weight.

COMBINATION THERAPY. Therapy with several antiepileptic drugs concurrently should generally be avoided. Patients are best controlled with one antiepileptic. Combinations of drugs have been used on the grounds that their therapeutic effects were additive while their individual toxicity was reduced but there is no evidence for this. In fact, toxicity may be enhanced with combination therapy. A second drug should only be added to the regimen if seizures continue despite high plasma concentrations or toxic effects. The use of more than two antiepileptics is rarely justified. Another disadvantage of multiple therapy is that drug interactions occur between the various antiepileptics (see below). Moreover, it is illogical to combine primidone and phenobarbitone as the former is largely metabolised to phenobarbitone in the liver, which is responsible for most, if not all, of its antiepileptic action.

INTERACTIONS. Owing to hepatic enzyme induction carbamazepine, phenobarbitone, phenytoin, and primidone may increase one another's metabolism; a most important example of this type of interaction between antiepileptics is reduction of the plasma-carbamazepine concentration by concurrent administration of phenytoin.

For a number of important interactions with other drugs, see **Appendix 1** and for FPA guidelines on the interaction between antiepileptics and **oral contraceptives**, see section 7.3.1

WITHDRAWAL. Abrupt withdrawal of antiepileptics, particularly the barbiturates and benzodiazepines, should be avoided, as this may precipitate severe rebound seizures. Reduction in dosage should be carried out in stages and, in the case of the barbiturates, the withdrawal process may take months. The changeover from one antiepileptic drug regimen to another should be made cautiously, withdrawing the first drug only when the new regimen has been largely established.

The decision to withdraw all antiepileptics from a seizure-free patient, and its timing, is often difficult and may depend on individual patient factors. Even in patients who have been seizure-free for several years, there is a significant risk of seizure recurrence on drug withdrawal.

DRIVING. Patients suffering from epilepsy may drive a motor vehicle (but not a heavy goods or public service vehicle) provided that they have had a seizure-free period of two years or, if subject to attacks only while asleep, have established a three-year period of asleep attacks without awake attacks. Patients affected by drowsiness should not drive or operate machinery.

PREGNANCY AND BREAST-FEEDING. During pregnancy, plasma concentrations of antiepileptics should be frequently monitored as they may fall, particularly in the later stages. There is an increased risk of teratogenicity associated with the use of anticonvulsant drugs but, generally, prescribing in pregnancy should follow the same principles as that in non-pregnant patients. **Important** see also under Prescribing in Pregnancy (Appendix 4).

Breast-feeding is acceptable with all antiepileptic drugs, taken in normal doses, with the possible exception of the barbiturates see Prescribing during Breast-feeding (Appendix 5).

PARTIAL SEIZURES WITH OR WITHOUT SECONDARY GENERALISATION

Carbamazepine and **phenytoin** are the drugs of choice for secondary generalised tonic-clonic seizures and for partial seizures themselves; controlled trials with **sodium valproate** suggest similar efficacy but more evidence is awaited. Phenobarbitone and primidone are also effective but are likely to be more sedating. Second-line drugs include clonazepam, clobazam, and acetazolamide. The new drugs **lamotrigine** and **vigabatrin** are now available where control is difficult to obtain. Partial epilepsy and secondarily generalised seizures are more difficult to control than tonic-clonic seizures occurring as part of a syndrome of primary generalised epilepsy (see below).

GENERALISED SEIZURES

TONIC-CLONIC SEIZURES (GRAND MAL). The drugs of choice for *tonic-clonic seizures* occurring as part of a syndrome of *primary generalised epilepsy* are carbamazepine, phenytoin, and sodium valproate. Phenobarbitone and primidone are also effective but may be more sedating. The new drugs **lamotrigine** and **vigabatrin** are now available where control is difficult to obtain.

ABSENCE SEIZURES (PETIT MAL). **Ethosuximide** and **sodium valproate** are the drugs of choice in simple absence seizures. Sodium valproate is also highly effective in treating the tonic-clonic seizures which may co-exist with absence seizures in primary generalised epilepsy.

MYOCLONIC SEIZURES. Myoclonic seizures (myoclonic jerks) occur in a variety of syndromes, and response to treatment varies considerably. **Sodium valproate** is the drug of choice and **clonazepam**, **ethosuximide**, and other antiepileptic drugs may be used.

ATYPICAL ABSENCE, ATONIC, AND TONIC SEIZURES. These seizure types are usually seen in childhood, in specific epileptic syndromes, or associated with cerebral damage or mental retardation. They may respond poorly to the traditional drugs. **Phenytoin**, **sodium valproate**, **clonazepam**, **ethosuximide**, and **phenobarbitone** may be tried. Other second-line antiepileptic drugs are occasionally helpful, including **acetazolamide** and **corticosteroids**.

CARBAMAZEPINE

Carbamazepine is a drug of choice for simple and complex partial seizures and for tonic-clonic seizures regardless of whether they are primary or secondary to a focal discharge. It has a wider therapeutic index than phenytoin and the relationship between dose and plasma concentration is linear, but monitoring of plasma concentrations may be helpful in determining optimum dosage. It has generally fewer side-effects than phenytoin or the barbiturates, but reversible blurring of vision, dizziness, and unsteadiness are dose-related, and may be dose-limiting. These side-effects may be reduced by altering the timing of medication. It is essential to initiate carbamazepine therapy at a low dose and build this up over one or two weeks.

CARBAMAZEPINE

Indications: all forms of epilepsy except absence seizures; trigeminal neuralgia (section 4.7.3); prophylaxis in manic-depressive illness (section 4.2.3)

Cautions: see notes above; hepatic impairment; pregnancy (**important** see notes above and Appendix 4 (neural tube screening)) and breast-feeding (see notes above); avoid sudden withdrawal; **interactions:** see p. 185 and Appendix 1 (carbamazepine)

Contra-indications: atrioventricular conduction abnormalities (unless paced); porphyria (see section 9.8.2); patients on MAOIs or within 2 weeks of MAOI therapy (theoretical grounds only)

Side-effects: gastro-intestinal disturbances, dizziness, drowsiness, headache, ataxia, confusion and agitation (elderly), visual disturbances (especially double vision and often associated with peak plasma concentrations); constipation, anorexia; generalised erythematous rash may occur in about 3% of patients; leucopenia and other blood disorders have occurred rarely; cholestatic jaundice, acute renal failure, Stevens-Johnson syndrome, toxic epidermal necrolysis, alopecia, thromboembolism, fever, proteinuria, lymph node enlargement, cardiac conduction disturbances, and hepatitis reported; hyponatraemia and oedema also reported (with higher doses)

Dose: epilepsy, initially, 100–200 mg 1–2 times daily, increased slowly to usual dose of 0.8–1.2 g daily in divided doses; in some cases 1.6 g daily may be needed; CHILD daily in divided doses, up to 1 year 100–200 mg, 1–5 years 200–400 mg, 5–10 years 400–600 mg, 10–15 years 0.6–1 g

Note. Plasma concentration for optimum response 4–12 mg/litre (20–50 micromol/litre)

PoM **Carbamazepine** (Non-proprietary)
Tablets, carbamazepine 100 mg, net price 20 = 64p; 200 mg, 20 = £1.14; 400 mg, 20 = £2.29. Label: 3

PoM **Tegretol**® (Geigy)
Tablets, all scored, carbamazepine 100 mg, net price 20 = 62p; 200 mg, 20 = £1.15; 400 mg, 56-tab pack = £6.56. Label: 3

Chewtabs, orange, carbamazepine 100 mg, net price 20 = £1.05; 200 mg, 20 = £1.96. Label: 3, 21, 24

Liquid, sugar-free, carbamazepine 100 mg/5 mL. Net price 300-mL pack = £5.72. Label: 3

PoM **Tegretol**® **Retard** (Geigy)
Tablets, modified-release, both scored, carbamazepine 200 mg (beige-orange), net price 20 = £1.50; 400 mg (brown-orange), 20 = £2.94. Label: 3, 25

Dose: epilepsy (ADULT and CHILD over 5 years), as above; trigeminal neuralgia, as section 4.7.3; total daily dose given in 2 divided doses

ETHOSUXIMIDE

Ethosuximide is the drug of choice in simple absence seizures; it may also be used in myoclonic seizures and in atypical absence, atonic, and tonic seizures.

ETHOSUXIMIDE

Indications: absence seizures

Cautions: see notes above; hepatic and renal impairment; pregnancy and breast-feeding (see notes above); avoid sudden withdrawal; avoid in porphyria (see section 9.8.2); **interactions:** Appendix 1 (ethosuximide)

Side-effects: gastro-intestinal disturbances, drowsiness, dizziness, ataxia, dyskinesia, hiccup, photophobia, headache, depression, and mild euphoria. Psychotic states, rashes, liver changes, and haematological disorders such as leucopenia and agranulocytosis occur rarely; systemic lupus erythematosus reported

Dose: initially, 500 mg daily, increased by 250 mg at intervals of 4–7 days to usual dose of 1–

4.8 Antiepileptics

1.5 g daily; occasionally up to 2 g daily may be needed; CHILD up to 6 years 250 mg daily, over 6 years 500 mg, increased gradually to a max. of 1 g daily

Note. Plasma concentration for optimum response 40–100 mg/litre (300–700 micromol/litre)

PoM **Emeside**® (LAB)
Capsules, orange, ethosuximide 250 mg. Net price 112-cap pack = £9.64
Syrup, black currant or orange, ethosuximide 250 mg/5 mL. Net price 200-mL pack = £5.22

PoM **Zarontin**® (P-D)
Capsules, orange, ethosuximide 250 mg. Net price 50 = £3.82
Syrup, red, ethosuximide 250 mg/5 mL. Net price 250-mL pack = £4.67

PHENOBARBITONE AND OTHER BARBITURATES

Phenobarbitone is an effective drug for tonic and partial seizures but may be sedative in adults and cause behavioural disturbances and hyperkinesia in children. It may be tried for atypical absence, atonic, and tonic seizures. Rebound seizures may be a problem on withdrawal. Monitoring plasma concentrations is less useful than with other drugs because tolerance occurs. **Methylphenobarbitone** is largely converted to phenobarbitone in the liver and has no advantages. **Primidone** is largely converted to phenobarbitone in the body and this is probably responsible for its antiepileptic action. A small starting dose of primidone (125 mg) is essential, and the drug should be introduced over several weeks.

PHENOBARBITONE

Indications: all forms of epilepsy except absence seizures; status epilepticus, section 4.8.2
Cautions: elderly, debilitated, children, impaired renal or hepatic function, respiratory depression (avoid if severe), pregnancy and breast-feeding (see notes above); avoid sudden withdrawal; see also notes above; avoid in porphyria (see section 9.8.2); **interactions:** see p. 185 and Appendix 1 (barbiturates and primidone)
Side-effects: drowsiness, lethargy, mental depression, ataxia and allergic skin reactions; paradoxical excitement, restlessness and confusion in the elderly and hyperkinesia in children; megaloblastic anaemia (may be treated with folic acid); overdosage: see Emergency Treatment of Poisoning, p. 19
Dose: by mouth, 60–180 mg at night; CHILD 5–8 mg/kg daily (febrile convulsions, see 4.8.3)
By intramuscular or intravenous injection, 50–200 mg, repeated after 6 hours if necessary; max. 600 mg daily; dilute injection 1 in 10 with water for injections before intravenous administration, status epilepticus, section 4.8.2

Note. For therapeutic purposes phenobarbitone and phenobarbitone sodium may be considered equivalent in effect. Plasma concentration for optimum response 15–40 mg/litre (60–180 micromol/litre)

CD [1]**Phenobarbitone Tablets,** phenobarbitone 15 mg, net price 20 = 6p; 30 mg, 20 = 7p; 60 mg, 20 = 10p; 100 mg, 20 = 18p. Label: 2
CD [1]**Phenobarbitone Sodium Tablets,** phenobarbitone sodium 30 mg, net price 20 = 13p; 60 mg, 20 = 29p. Label: 2
CD [1]**Phenobarbitone Elixir,** phenobarbitone 15 mg/5 mL in a suitable flavoured vehicle, containing alcohol 38%. Net price 100 mL = 57p. Label: 2
Note. Some hospitals supply alcohol-free formulations
CD [1]**Phenobarbitone Injection,** phenobarbitone sodium 200 mg/mL in propylene glycol 90% and water for injections 10%. Net price 1-mL amp = 63p
Note. Must be diluted before intravenous administration (see under Dose)
Available from Rhône-Poulenc Rorer (CD [1]Gardenal Sodium®), Martindale; other strengths also available from Martindale.

1. See p. 7 for prescribing requirements for phenobarbitone

METHYLPHENOBARBITONE

Indications; Cautions; Side-effects: see under Phenobarbitone
Dose: 100–600 mg daily

CD **Prominal**® (Sanofi Winthrop)
Tablets, methylphenobarbitone 30 mg, net price 20 = 72p; 60 mg, 20 = 96p; 200 mg, 20 = £2.05. Label: 2

PRIMIDONE

Indications: all forms of epilepsy except absence seizures; essential tremor (section 4.9.3)
Cautions; Side-effects: see under Phenobarbitone. Drowsiness, ataxia, nausea, visual disturbances, and rashes, particularly at first, usually reversible on continued administration; **interactions:** see p. 185 and Appendix 1 (barbiturates and primidone)
Dose: epilepsy, initially, 125 mg daily at bedtime, increased by 125 mg every 3 days to 500 mg daily in 2 divided doses then increased by 250 mg every 3 days to a max. of 1.5 g daily in divided doses; CHILD 20–30 mg/kg daily in 2 divided doses
Note. Monitor plasma concentrations of derived phenobarbitone. Optimum range as for phenobarbitone.

PoM **Mysoline**® (ICI)
Tablets, scored, primidone 250 mg. Net price 20 = 36p. Label: 2
Oral suspension, primidone 250 mg/5 mL. Net price 250-mL pack = £1.04. Label: 2

PHENYTOIN

Phenytoin is effective in tonic-clonic and partial seizures. It has a narrow therapeutic index and the relationship between dose and plasma concentration is non-linear; small dosage increases in some patients may produce large rises in plasma concentrations with acute toxic side-effects. Monitoring of plasma concentration greatly assists dosage adjustment. A few missed doses or a small change in drug absorption may result in a marked change in plasma concentration.

Phenytoin may cause coarse facies, acne, hirsutism, and gingival hyperplasia and so may be particularly undesirable in adolescent patients.

PHENYTOIN

Indications: all forms of epilepsy except absence seizures; trigeminal neuralgia (see also section 4.7.3)

Cautions: hepatic impairment (reduce dose), pregnancy and breast-feeding (see notes above); avoid sudden withdrawal; avoid in porphyria (see section 9.8.2); see also notes above; **interactions:** see p. 185 and Appendix 1 (phenytoin)

Side-effects: nausea, vomiting, mental confusion, dizziness, headache, tremor, transient nervousness, insomnia occur commonly; rarely dyskinesias, peripheral neuropathy; ataxia, slurred speech, nystagmus and blurred vision are signs of overdosage; rashes (discontinue, if mild re-introduce cautiously but discontinue immediately if recurrence), coarse facies, acne and hirsutism, fever and hepatitis; lupus erythematosus, erythema multiforme (Stevens–Johnson syndrome), toxic epidermal necrolysis, polyarteritis nodosa; lymphadenopathy; gingival hypertrophy and tenderness; rarely haematological effects, including megaloblastic anaemia (may be treated with folic acid), leucopenia, thrombocytopenia, agranulocytosis, and aplastic anaemia; plasma calcium may be lowered (rickets and osteomalacia)

Dose: by mouth, initially 3–4 mg/kg daily *or* 150–300 mg daily (as a single dose *or* in two divided doses) increased gradually as necessary (plasma monitoring, see notes above); usual dose 300–400 mg daily; max. 600 mg daily; CHILD 5–8 mg/kg daily (in 1 or 2 doses)

By intravenous injection—section 4.8.2

Note. Plasma concentration for optimum response 10–20 mg/litre (40–80 micromol/litre)

COUNSELLING. Take preferably with or after food

PoM **Phenytoin** (Non-proprietary)

Capsules, phenytoin sodium 100 mg, net price 20 = 41p. Label: 27, counselling, administration
Available from APS, Cox, Kerfoot

Tablets, coated, phenytoin sodium 50 mg, net price 20 = 22p; 100 mg, 20 = 26p. Label: 27, counselling, administration
Available from APS, Cox, Kerfoot

PoM **Epanutin**® (P-D)

Capsules, phenytoin sodium 25 mg (white/purple), net price 20 = 39p; 50 mg (white/pink), 20 = 40p; 100 mg (white/orange), 20 = 48p; 300 mg (white/green), 20 = £1.53. Label: 27, counselling, administration

Infatabs® (= tablets, chewable), yellow, scored, phenytoin 50 mg. Net price 20 = £1.10. Label: 24

Suspension, red, phenytoin 30 mg/5 mL. Net price 100 mL = 71p. Counselling, administration

Note. For an equivalent therapeutic effect, phenytoin 90 mg as phenytoin suspension 90 mg in 15 mL ≡ phenytoin sodium 100 mg as tablets or capsules. The MCA now advises that there are no clinically relevant differences in bioavailability between available phenytoin sodium tablets and capsules

VALPROATE

Sodium valproate is effective in controlling tonic-clonic seizures, particularly in primary generalised epilepsy. It is the drug of choice in myoclonic seizures, and may be tried in atypical absence, atonic, and tonic seizures. Controlled trials in partial epilepsy suggest that it has similar efficacy to that of carbamazepine and phenytoin, but more evidence is awaited. Plasma concentrations are not a useful index of efficacy, therefore routine monitoring is unhelpful. The drug has widespread metabolic effects, and may have dose-related side-effects. There has been concern over severe hepatic or pancreatic toxicity, although these effects are rare.

SODIUM VALPROATE

Indications: all forms of epilepsy

Cautions: in patients most at risk (e.g. children and those with history of liver disease) monitor liver function in first 6 months; pregnancy (**important** see notes above and Appendix 4 (neural tube screening)); breast-feeding; monitor platelet function before major surgery; may give false-positive urine tests for ketones in diabetes mellitus; avoid sudden withdrawal; see also notes above; **interactions:** see p. 185 and Appendix 1 (valproate)

Contra-indications: active liver disease; porphyria (but see section 9.8.2)

Side-effects: gastric irritation, nausea, ataxia and tremor; hyperammonaemia, increased appetite and weight gain; transient hair loss (regrowth may be curly), oedema, thrombocytopenia, and inhibition of platelet aggregation; impaired hepatic function leading rarely to fatal hepatic failure (see Cautions—withdraw treatment immediately if vomiting, anorexia, jaundice, drowsiness, or loss of seizure control occurs); amenorrhoea, rashes; rarely pancreatitis (measure plasma amylase in acute abdominal pain), leucopenia, red cell hypoplasia

Dose: by mouth, initially, 600 mg daily in divided doses, preferably after food, increasing by 200 mg/day at 3-day intervals to a max. of 2.5 g daily in divided doses, usual maintenance 1–2 g daily (20–30 mg/kg daily); CHILD up to 20 kg (about 4 years), initially 20 mg/kg daily in divided doses, may be increased gradually providing plasma concentrations monitored to 40 mg/kg daily; over 20 kg, initially 400 mg daily in divided doses increased gradually to 20–30 mg/kg daily; max. 35 mg/kg daily

4.8 Antiepileptics

By intravenous injection (over 3–5 minutes) or *by intravenous infusion*, continuation of valproate treatment when oral therapy not possible, same as current dose by oral route
Initiation of valproate therapy (when oral valproate not possible), *by intravenous injection* (over 3–5 minutes), 400–800 mg (up to 10 mg/kg) followed by *intravenous infusion* up to max. 2.5 g daily
CHILD, usually 20–30 mg/kg daily

PoM **Sodium Valproate** (Non-proprietary)
Tablets, e/c, sodium valproate 200 mg, net price 20 = £1.31; 500 mg, 20 = £3.15. Label: 5, 25
Available from Cox, Hillcross, Norton
Oral solution, sodium valproate 200 mg/5 mL. Net price 100 mL = £1.91
Available from Norton (sugar-free)

PoM **Epilim**® (Sanofi Winthrop)
Tablets (crushable), scored, sodium valproate 100 mg. Net price 20 = 80p
Tablets, both e/c, lilac, sodium valproate 200 mg, net price 20 = £1.32; 500 mg, 20 = £3.29. Label: 5, 25
Liquid, red, sugar-free, sodium valproate 200 mg/5 mL. Net price 300-mL pack = £6.04
Syrup, red, sodium valproate 200 mg/5 mL. Net price 300-mL pack = £6.04

PoM **Epilim**® **Intravenous** (Sanofi Winthrop)
Injection, powder for reconstitution, sodium valproate. Net price 400-mg vial (with 4-mL amp water for injections) = £9.00

BENZODIAZEPINES

Clonazepam is occasionally used in tonic-clonic or partial seizures, but its sedative side-effects may be prominent. **Clobazam** may be used as adjunctive therapy in the treatment of epilepsy (section 4.1.2), but the effectiveness of these and other **benzodiazepines** may wane considerably after weeks or months of continuous therapy.

CLOBAZAM
Section 4.1.2

CLONAZEPAM
Indications: all forms of epilepsy; myoclonus; status epilepticus, section 4.8.2
Cautions: see notes above; respiratory disease; hepatic and renal impairment; elderly and debilitated; pregnancy and breast-feeding (see notes above); avoid sudden withdrawal; **interactions:** see p. 185 and Appendix 1 (clonazepam)
DRIVING. Drowsiness may affect the performance of skilled tasks (e.g. driving); effects of alcohol enhanced
Contra-indications: respiratory depression; acute pulmonary insufficiency; porphyria (see section 9.8.2)
Side-effects: drowsiness, fatigue, dizziness, muscle hypotonia, coordination disturbances; hypersalivation in infants, paradoxical aggression, irritability and mental changes; rarely, blood disorders, abnormal liver-function tests; overdosage: see Emergency Treatment of Poisoning, p. 19

Dose: 1 mg (elderly, 500 micrograms), initially at night for 4 nights, increased over 2–4 weeks to a usual maintenance dose of 4–8 mg daily in divided doses; CHILD up to 1 year 250 micrograms increased as above to 0.5–1 mg, 1–5 years 250 micrograms increased to 1–3 mg, 5–12 years 500 micrograms increased to 3–6 mg

PoM **Rivotril**® (Roche)
Tablets, both scored, clonazepam 500 micrograms (beige), net price 20 = 88p; 2 mg, 20 = £1.84. Label: 2

OTHER DRUGS

Acetazolamide, a carbonic anhydrase inhibitor, is a second-line drug for both tonic-clonic and partial seizures. It is occasionally helpful in atypical absence, atonic, and tonic seizures.
Lamotrigine is a new antiepileptic for the adjunctive treatment of partial seizures and secondarily generalised tonic-clonic seizures which are not satisfactorily controlled with other antiepileptics.
Vigabatrin is a new antiepileptic for use in chronic epilepsy not satisfactorily controlled by other antiepileptics. It is useful in tonic-clonic and partial seizures but has prominent behavioural side-effects in some patients.

ACETAZOLAMIDE
Indications: see notes above
Cautions; Side-effects: see section 11.6
Dose: 0.25–1 g daily in divided doses; CHILD 125–750 mg daily

Preparations
See section 11.6

LAMOTRIGINE
Indications: adjunctive treatment of partial seizures and secondarily generalised tonic-clonic seizures not satisfactorily controlled with other antiepileptics
Cautions: closely monitor (including hepatic, renal and clotting parameters) if rash, fever, influenza-like symptoms, drowsiness, or worsening of seizure control develops, especially in first month of treatment (although causal relationship not established lamotrigine given with other antiepileptics has been associated with rapidly progressive illness with status epilepticus, multi-organ dysfunction and disseminated intravascular coagulation); avoid abrupt withdrawal (taper off over 2 weeks); pregnancy and breast-feeding; **interactions:** Appendix 1 (lamotrigine)
Contra-indications: hepatic or renal impairment
Side-effects: rashes (rarely angioedema and Stevens-Johnson syndrome); diplopia, blurred vision, dizziness, drowsiness, headache, unsteadiness, tiredness, gastro-intestinal disturbances, irritability, aggression; see also Cautions

Dose: with existing antiepileptic therapy, initially 50 mg twice daily (50 mg once daily in patients taking sodium valproate) for 14 days; usual maintenance 200–400 mg daily (100–200 mg daily in patients taking sodium valproate) in 2 divided doses
CHILD under 12 years and ELDERLY, not yet recommended

▼ PoM **Lamictal**® (Wellcome)
Tablets, both yellow, lamotrigine 50 mg, net price 56-tab pack = £32.64; 100 mg, 56-tab pack = £56.32

VIGABATRIN
Indications: epilepsy not satisfactorily controlled by other antiepileptics
Cautions: renal impairment; closely monitor neurological function; avoid sudden withdrawal; history of psychosis or behavioural problems; **interactions:** Appendix 1 (vigabatrin)
Contra-indications: pregnancy (high doses teratogenic in *animals*) and breast-feeding
Side-effects: drowsiness, fatigue, dizziness, nervousness, irritability, depression, headache; less commonly confusion, aggression, psychosis, memory disturbance, visual disturbance (e.g. diplopia); weight gain and gastro-intestinal disturbances reported; excitation and agitation in children
Dose: with current antiepileptic therapy, initially 2 g daily in single or 2 divided doses then increased or decreased according to response in steps of 0.5–1 g; usual max. 4 g daily; CHILD 3–9 years initially 1 g daily

▼ PoM **Sabril**® (Merrell)
Tablets, scored, vigabatrin 500 mg, net price 100-tab pack = £46.00. Label: 3

4.8.2 Drugs used in status epilepticus

Major status epilepticus should be *treated initially* with intravenous **diazepam** used with caution because of the risk of respiratory depression; in situations where facilities for resuscitation are not immediately available, *small doses* of diazepam can be given intravenously or the drug can be administered as a rectal solution (Stesolid®). Absorption from intramuscular injection or from suppositories is too slow for treatment of status epilepticus. When diazepam is given intravenously there may be a high risk of venous thrombophlebitis which is minimised by using an emulsion (Diazemuls®). **Clonazepam** and **lorazepam** are used; lorazepam has the advantage of a long duration of action.

To *prevent recurrence* **phenytoin sodium** may be given by slow intravenous injection, with ECG monitoring in a dose of 15 mg/kg at a rate of not more than 50 mg/minute (in adults) followed by the maintenance dosage. Intramuscular use of phenytoin is not recommended (absorption is slow and erratic) and intravenous infusion is not recommended (precipitates).

If status epilepticus *continues or returns*, **chlormethiazole** may be given by intravenous infusion. Chlormethiazole has a short half-life, and the rate of infusion can be titrated against the patient's clinical condition (see **cautions** on next page).

Paraldehyde also remains a valuable drug. Given by deep intramuscular injection or rectally it causes little respiratory depression and is therefore useful where facilities for resuscitation are poor. In some specialist centres with **intensive care facilities**, it has also been given intravenously (**must** be very well diluted, see next page).

Providing the patient has not recently received phenobarbitone or primidone, in some specialist centres with **intensive care facilities**, **phenobarbitone sodium** (section 4.8.1) is sometimes given intravenously, at a rate of 100 mg/minute, until seizures stop or until a maximum of 15 mg/kg has been given.

DIAZEPAM
Indications: status epilepticus; convulsions due to poisoning (see Emergency Treatment of Poisoning); other indications, see sections 4.1.2, 10.2.2, 15.1.4.1
Cautions; Contra-indications; Side-effects: see section 4.1.2; hypotension and apnoea may occur; when given intravenously facilities for reversing respiratory depression with mechanical ventilation must be at hand (but see also notes above)
Dose: by intravenous injection, 10–20 mg at a rate of 0.5 mL (2.5 mg) per 30 seconds, repeated if necessary after 30–60 minutes; may be followed by *intravenous infusion* to max. 3 mg/kg over 24 hours; CHILD 200–300 micrograms/kg
By rectum as rectal solution, ADULT and CHILD over 3 years 10 mg; CHILD 1–3 years and ELDERLY 5 mg; repeat after 5 minutes if necessary

PoM **Diazepam** (Non-proprietary)
Injection (solution), diazepam 5 mg/mL. See Appendix 6. Net price 2-mL amp = 25p
Available from CP

PoM **Diazemuls**® (Dumex)
Injection (emulsion), diazepam 5 mg/mL (0.5%). See Appendix 6. Net price 2-mL amp = 69p

PoM **Stesolid**® (CP)
Rectal tubes (= rectal solution), diazepam 2 mg/mL. Net price 5 × 2.5-mL (5 mg) tubes = £5.78; 4 mg/mL, 5 × 2.5-mL (10 mg) tubes = £7.37

PoM **Valium**® (Roche)
Injection (solution), diazepam 5 mg/mL. See Appendix 6. Net price 2-mL amp = 30p

Oral preparations, section 4.1.2

CLONAZEPAM
Indications: status epilepticus; other forms of epilepsy, and myoclonus, section 4.8.1
Cautions; Contra-indications; Side-effects: see section 4.8.1. Hypotension and apnoea may occur and resuscitation facilities must be available

4.8 Antiepileptics

Dose: by intravenous injection (over 30 seconds) *or by intravenous infusion*, 1 mg, repeated if necessary; CHILD all ages, 500 micrograms

PoM **Rivotril**® (Roche)
Injection, clonazepam 1 mg/mL in solvent, for dilution with 1 mL water for injections immediately before injection or as described in Appendix 6. Net price 1-mL amp (with 1 mL water for injections) = 71p

Oral preparations, section 4.8.1

CHLORMETHIAZOLE EDISYLATE
Indications: status epilepticus; other indications, see sections 4.1.1, 15.1.4.1
Cautions: see section 4.1.1 for general cautions; resuscitation facilities must be available; maintain clear airway (risk of mechanical obstruction in deep sedation); *rapid infusion* to be given only under direct medical supervision (risk of apnoea and hypotension—special care in those susceptible to cerebral or cardiac complications, e.g. the elderly); during *continuous infusion* sleep induced may lapse into deep unconsciousness and patient must be kept under close and constant observation; *prolonged infusion* may lead to accumulation and delay recovery, may also cause electrolyte imbalance (infusion does not contain electrolytes); **interactions:** Appendix 1 (chlormethiazole)
Contra-indications: acute pulmonary insufficiency
Side-effects: nasal congestion and irritation (with sneezing), conjunctival irritation, headache; localised thrombophlebitis, tachycardia and transient fall in blood pressure (apnoea and hypotension on rapid infusion); (see also section 4.1.1)
Dose: by intravenous infusion, as a 0.8% solution, initially 5–15 mL (40–120 mg)/minute up to a total of 40–100 mL (320–800 mg), then continued if necessary at a reduced rate according to response (see notes above); usual rate 0.5–1 mL (4–8 mg)/minute; CHILD initially 0.01 mL (80 micrograms)/kg/minute, then dose increased every 2–4 hours if necessary until seizures controlled or drowsiness occurs; if no seizure for 2 days dose gradually reduced every 4–6 hours (if seizures recur dose increased to previous level)
IMPORTANT. See cautions for intravenous infusion under Cautions (above)

PoM **Heminevrin**® (Astra)
Intravenous infusion 0.8%, chlormethiazole edisylate 8 mg/mL. Net price 500-mL bottle = £5.25

Oral preparations, section 4.1.1

LORAZEPAM
Indications: status epilepticus; other indications, section 4.1.2
Cautions; Contra-indications; Side-effects: see section 4.1.2; hypotension and apnoea may occur and resuscitation facilities must be available
Dose: by intravenous injection, 4 mg; CHILD 2 mg

Preparations
Section 4.1.2

PARALDEHYDE
Indications: status epilepticus
Cautions: bronchopulmonary disease, hepatic impairment; avoid intramuscular injection near sciatic nerve (causes severe causalgia); intravenous route, specialist centres only with intensive care facilities (see notes above)
Side-effects: rashes; pain and sterile abscess after intramuscular injection; rectal irritation after enema
Dose: by deep intramuscular injection, as a single dose, 5–10 mL; usual max. 20 mL daily with not more than 5 mL at any one site; CHILD up to 3 months 0.5 mL, 3–6 months 1 mL, 6–12 months 1.5 mL, 1–2 years 2 mL, 3–5 years 3–4 mL, 6–12 years 5–6 mL
By intravenous infusion, up to 4–5 mL diluted to a 4% solution with sodium chloride intravenous infusion 0.9% (specialist centres **only**, see notes above)
By rectum, 5–10 mL, administered as a 10% enema in physiological saline; CHILD as for intramuscular dose
Note. Do not use paraldehyde if it has a brownish colour or an odour of acetic acid. Avoid contact with rubber and plastics.

PoM **Paraldehyde** (Non-proprietary)
Injection, sterile paraldehyde 5-mL and 10-mL amp
Note. May temporarily be unavailable

PHENYTOIN SODIUM
Indications: status epilepticus; seizures in neurosurgery; arrhythmias, see section 2.3.2
Cautions: hypotension and heart failure; resuscitation facilities must be available; injection solutions alkaline (irritant to tissues); see also section 4.8.1; **interactions:** Appendix 1 (phenytoin)
Contra-indications: sinus bradycardia, sino-atrial block, and second- and third-degree heart block; Stokes-Adams syndrome; porphyria (see section 9.8.2)
Side-effects: intravenous injection may cause cardiovascular and CNS depression (particularly if injection too rapid) with arrhythmias, hypotension, and cardiovascular collapse; alterations in respiratory function (including respiratory arrest)
Dose: by slow intravenous injection (with blood pressure and ECG monitoring), status epilepticus, 15 mg/kg at a rate not exceeding 50 mg per minute, as a loading dose (see also

notes above). Maintenance doses of about 100 mg should be given thereafter at intervals of every 6 hours, monitored by measurement of plasma concentrations; rate and dose reduced according to weight

By intramuscular injection, not recommended (see notes above)

PoM **Epanutin Ready Mixed Parenteral**® (P-D) *Injection*, phenytoin sodium 50 mg/mL with propylene glycol 40% and alcohol 10% in water for injections. Net price 5-mL amp = £4.07

Oral preparations, section 4.8.1

4.8.3 Febrile convulsions

Brief febrile convulsions need only simple treatment such as tepid sponging or bathing, or antipyretic medication, e.g. **paracetamol** (section 4.7.1). *Prolonged febrile convulsions* (those lasting 15 minutes or longer), *recurrent convulsions*, or those occurring in a child at known risk must be treated more actively, as there is the possibility of resulting brain damage. **Diazepam** is the drug of choice given either by slow intravenous injection in a dose of 250 micrograms/kg (as Diazemuls®, section 4.8.2) or preferably rectally in solution (Stesolid®, section 4.8.2) in a dose of 500 micrograms/kg, repeated if necessary. The rectal route is preferred as satisfactory absorption is achieved within minutes and administration is much easier. Suppositories are not suitable because absorption is too slow.

Intermittent prophylaxis (i.e. the anticonvulsant administered at the onset of fever) is possible in only a small proportion of children. Again **diazepam** is the treatment of choice, orally or rectally.

The exact role of continuous prophylaxis in children at risk from prolonged or complex febrile convulsions is controversial. It is probably indicated in only a small proportion of children, including those whose first seizure occurred at under 14 months or who have pre-existing neurological abnormalities or who have had previous prolonged or focal convulsions. Thus long-term anticonvulsant prophylaxis is rarely indicated.

4.9 Drugs used in parkinsonism and related disorders

4.9.1 Dopaminergic drugs used in parkinsonism
4.9.2 Antimuscarinic drugs used in parkinsonism
4.9.3 Drugs used in essential tremor, chorea, tics, and related disorders

In idiopathic Parkinson's disease, progressive degeneration of pigment-containing cells of the substantia nigra leads to deficiency of the neurotransmitter dopamine. This, in turn, results in a neurohumoral imbalance in the basal ganglia, causing the characteristic signs and symptoms of the illness to appear. The pathogenesis of this process is still obscure and current drug therapy aims simply to correct the imbalance. Although this approach fails to prevent the progression of the disease, it greatly improves the quality and expectancy of life of most patients.

The patient should be advised at the outset of the limitations of treatment and possible side-effects. About 10 to 20% of patients are unresponsive to treatment.

ELDERLY. Antiparkinsonian drugs carry a special risk of inducing confusion in the elderly. It is particularly important to initiate treatment with low doses and to use small increments.

4.9.1 Dopaminergic drugs used in parkinsonism

Levodopa, used with a **dopa-decarboxylase inhibitor**, is the treatment of choice for patients disabled by idiopathic Parkinson's disease. It is least valuable in elderly patients and in those with long-standing disease who may not tolerate a dose large enough to overcome their deficit. It is also less valuable in patients with post-encephalitic disease who are particularly susceptible to the side-effects. Parkinsonism caused by generalised degenerative brain disease does not normally respond to levodopa. It should not be used for neuroleptic-induced parkinsonism.

Levodopa, the amino-acid precursor of dopamine, acts mainly by replenishing depleted striatal dopamine. It improves bradykinesia and rigidity more than tremor. It is generally administered in conjunction with an extracerebral dopa-decarboxylase inhibitor which prevents the peripheral degradation of levodopa to dopamine but, unlike levodopa, does not cross the blood-brain barrier. Effective brain concentrations of dopamine can thereby be achieved with lower doses of levodopa. At the same time the reduced peripheral formation of dopamine decreases peripheral side-effects such as nausea and vomiting and cardiovascular effects. There is also less delay in onset of therapeutic effect and a smoother clinical response. A disadvantage is an increased incidence of abnormal involuntary movements.

The extracerebral dopa-decarboxylase inhibitors given with levodopa are benserazide (in **co-beneldopa**) and carbidopa (in **co-careldopa**).

When co-careldopa 10/100 (10 mg of carbidopa for each 100 mg of levodopa) is used the dose of carbidopa may be insufficient to achieve full inhibition of extracerebral dopa-decarboxylase; co-careldopa 25/100 (25 mg of carbidopa for each 100 mg of levodopa) should then be used so that the daily dose of carbidopa is at least 75 mg.

Levodopa therapy should be initiated with low doses and gradually increased, by small increments, at intervals of 2 to 3 days. The final dose is usually a compromise between increased mobility and dose-limiting side-effects. Intervals between doses may be critical and should be chosen to suit the needs of the individual patient. Nausea and vomiting are rarely dose-limiting but doses should be taken after meals. Domperidone (section 4.6) may be useful in controlling vomiting. The most frequent dose-limiting side-effects of levodopa are involuntary movements and psychiatric complications. As the patient ages, the maintenance dose may need to be reduced.

During the first 6 to 18 months of levodopa therapy there may be a slow improvement in the response of the patient which is maintained for 1½ to 2 years; thereafter a slow decline may occur. Particularly troublesome is the 'on-off' effect the incidence of which increases as the treatment progresses. This is characterised by fluctuations in performance with normal performance during the 'on' period and weakness and akinesia lasting for 2 to 4 hours during the 'off' period.

'End-of-dose' deterioration may also occur where the duration of benefit after each dose becomes progressively shorter. Modified-release preparations may help with 'end-of-dose' deterioration or nocturnal immobility and rigidity.

Selegiline is a monoamine-oxidase-B inhibitor used in severe parkinsonism in conjunction with levodopa to reduce 'end-of-dose' deterioration. It has been suggested that early treatment with selegiline may also delay the need for levodopa therapy and possibly slow the rate of progression of the disease but this remains to be confirmed.

Bromocriptine acts by direct stimulation of surviving dopamine receptors. Although effective, it has no advantages over levodopa. It should be reserved for patients for whom levodopa alone is no longer adequate or who despite careful titration cannot tolerate levodopa. Its use is often limited by its side-effects and when used with levodopa, abnormal involuntary movements and confusional states are common.

Lysuride is a newly introduced drug for parkinsonism; it is similar to bromocriptine in its action.

Pergolide is another newly introduced drug; it acts mainly on dopamine D_2 receptors. Like bromocriptine and lysuride it is sometimes useful in reducing 'off' periods and in ameliorating fluctuations in the later stage of Parkinson's disease. All these dopaminergic drugs may cause serious neuropsychiatric side-effects and occasionally may cause retroperitoneal fibrosis.

Amantadine has modest antiparkinsonian effects. It improves mild bradykinetic disabilities as well as tremor and rigidity. Unfortunately only a small proportion of patients derive much benefit from this drug and tolerance to its effects occurs. However it has the advantage of being relatively free from side-effects.

LEVODOPA

Indications: parkinsonism (but not drug-induced extrapyramidal symptoms), see notes above
Cautions: pulmonary disease, peptic ulceration, cardiovascular disease, diabetes mellitus, open-angle glaucoma, skin melanoma, psychiatric illness (avoid if severe). In prolonged therapy, psychiatric, hepatic, haematological, renal, and cardiovascular surveillance is advisable. Warn patients who benefit from therapy to resume normal activities gradually; avoid abrupt withdrawal; **interactions:** Appendix 1 (levodopa)
Contra-indications: closed-angle glaucoma
Side-effects: anorexia, nausea, insomnia, agitation, postural hypotension (rarely labile hypertension), dizziness, tachycardia, arrhythmias, reddish discoloration of urine and other body fluids, rarely hypersensitivity; abnormal involuntary movements and psychiatric symptoms which include hypomania and psychosis may be dose-limiting; occasionally depression, drowsiness, and rarely headache, peripheral neuropathy reported
Dose: initially 125–500 mg daily in divided doses after meals, increased according to response (but rarely used alone, see notes above)

PoM **Brocadopa**® (Brocades)
Capsules, levodopa 125 mg, net price 20 = 71p; 250 mg, 20 = 85p; 500 mg, 20 = £1.52. Label: 14, 21

PoM **Larodopa**® (Cambridge)
Tablets, scored, levodopa 500 mg. Net price 20 = £1.34. Label: 14, 21

CO-BENELDOPA

A mixture of benserazide hydrochloride and levodopa in mass proportions corresponding to 1 part of benserazide and 4 parts of levodopa

Indications; Cautions; Contra-indications; Side-effects: see under Levodopa and notes above
Dose: expressed as levodopa, initially 50–100 mg twice daily, adjusted according to response; usual maintenance dose 400–800 mg daily in divided doses after meals

Note. When transferring patients from levodopa, 3 capsules co-beneldopa 25/100 (Madopar 125®) should be substituted for 2 g levodopa; the levodopa should be discontinued 12 hours beforehand

PoM **Madopar**® (Roche)
Capsules 62.5, blue/grey, co-beneldopa 12.5/50 (benserazide 12.5 mg (as hydrochloride), levodopa 50 mg). Net price 100-cap pack = £7.76. Label: 14, 21
Capsules 125, blue/pink, co-beneldopa 25/100 (benserazide 25 mg (as hydrochloride), levodopa 100 mg). Net price 100-cap pack = £13.51. Label: 14, 21
Capsules 250, blue/caramel, co-beneldopa 50/200 (benserazide 50 mg (as hydrochloride), levodopa 200 mg). Net price 100-cap pack = £22.46. Label: 14, 21
Dispersible tablets 62.5, scored, co-beneldopa 12.5/50 (benserazide 12.5 mg (as hydrochloride), levodopa 50 mg). Net price 100-tab pack = £8.29. Label: 14, 21, counselling, administration, see below
Dispersible tablets 125, scored, co-beneldopa 25/100 (benserazide 25 mg (as hydrochloride) levodopa 100 mg). Net price 100-tab pack = £14.70. Label: 14, 21, counselling, administration, see below
Note. The tablets may be dispersed in water or orange squash or swallowed whole

Chapter 4: Central nervous system

PoM **Madopar**® **CR** (Roche)
Capsules 125, m/r, dark green/light blue, co-beneldopa 25/100 (benserazide 25 mg (as hydrochloride), levodopa 100 mg). Net price 100-cap pack = £17.97. Label: 5, 14, 25
Dose: fluctuations in response to conventional levodopa/decarboxylase inhibitor preparations, initially 1 capsule substituted for every 100 mg of levodopa and given at same dosage frequency, subsequently increased every 2–3 days according to response; average increase of 50% needed over previous levodopa dose and titration may take up to 4 weeks; supplementary dose of conventional Madopar® may be needed with first morning dose; if response still poor to total daily dose of Madopar® CR plus Madopar® corresponding to 1.2 g levodopa, consider alternative therapy

CO-CARELDOPA

A mixture of carbidopa and levodopa; the proportions are expressed in the form *x/y* where *x* and *y* are the strengths in milligrams of carbidopa and levodopa respectively
Indications; Cautions; Contra-indications; Side-effects: see under Levodopa and notes above
Dose: expressed as levodopa, initially 100–125 mg 3–4 times daily adjusted according to response; usual maintenance dose 0.75–1.5 g daily in divided doses after food. See also under Sinemet-Plus®
Note. When transferring patients from levodopa, 3 tablets co-careldopa 25/250 (Sinemet-275®) should be substituted for 4 g levodopa; the levodopa should be discontinued 12 hours beforehand

PoM **Sinemet**® (Du Pont)
Tablets (Sinemet-110), blue, scored, co-careldopa 10/100 (carbidopa 10 mg (as monohydrate), levodopa 100 mg). Net price 20 = £1.71. Label: 14, 21
Tablets (Sinemet-275), blue, scored, co-careldopa 25/250 (carbidopa 25 mg (as monohydrate), levodopa 250 mg). Net price 20 = £3.57. Label: 14, 21

PoM **Sinemet LS**® (Du Pont)
Tablets, yellow, scored, co-careldopa 12.5/50 (carbidopa 12.5 mg (as monohydrate), levodopa 50 mg). Net price 84-tab pack = £6.87. Label: 14, 21
Note. 2 tablets Sinemet LS® ≡ 1 tablet Sinemet Plus®

PoM **Sinemet-Plus**® (Du Pont)
Tablets, yellow, scored, co-careldopa 25/100 (carbidopa 25 mg (as monohydrate), levodopa 100 mg). Net price 20 = £2.52. Label: 14, 21
Dose: initially 1 tablet 3 times daily, adjusted according to response to 8 daily in divided doses; larger doses by gradual substitution of Sinemet® for Sinemet-Plus®
Note. The daily dose of carbidopa required to achieve full inhibition of extracerebral dopa-decarboxylase is 75 mg; co-careldopa 25/100 provides an adequate dose of carbidopa when low doses of levodopa are needed

PoM **Sinemet**® **CR** (Du Pont)
Tablets, m/r, peach, co-careldopa 50/200 (carbidopa 50 mg (as monohydrate), levodopa 200 mg). Net price 56-tab pack = £21.84. Label: 14, 25
Dose: initial treatment or fluctuations in response to conventional levodopa therapy, 1 tablet twice daily; both dose and interval then adjusted according to response at intervals of not less than 3 days; if transferring from existing levodopa therapy withdraw 8 hours beforehand (12 hours for m/r levodopa preparations); 1 tablet Sinemet® CR twice daily can be substituted for a daily dose of levodopa 300–400 mg in Sinemet® conventional tablets

AMANTADINE HYDROCHLORIDE

Indications: parkinsonism (but not drug-induced extrapyramidal symptoms); antiviral, see section 5.3
Cautions: cardiovascular, hepatic, or renal disease (avoid if severe), recurrent eczema, psychosis, elderly, breast-feeding. Avoid abrupt discontinuation of treatment; **interactions:** Appendix 1 (amantadine)
DRIVING. May affect performance of skilled tasks (e.g. driving)
Contra-indications: epilepsy, gastric ulceration
Side-effects: nervousness, inability to concentrate, insomnia, dizziness, convulsions, hallucinations, gastro-intestinal disturbances, skin discoloration, dry mouth, peripheral oedema; rarely leucopenia
Dose: 100 mg daily increased if necessary to 100 mg twice daily (not later than 4 p.m.), usually in conjunction with other treatment; max. 400 mg daily (with close supervision)

PoM **Symmetrel**® (Geigy)
Capsules, brownish-red, amantadine hydrochloride 100 mg. Net price 56-cap pack = £9.46. Counselling, driving
Syrup, amantadine hydrochloride 50 mg/5 mL. Net price 150-mL pack = £3.17. Counselling, driving

BROMOCRIPTINE

Indications: parkinsonism (but not drug-induced extrapyramidal symptoms); endocrine disorders, see section 6.7.1
Cautions; Side-effects: see section 6.7.1
HYPOTENSIVE REACTIONS. Hypotensive reactions may be disturbing in some patients during the first few days of treatment and particular care should be exercised when driving or operating machinery; tolerance to bromocriptine reduced by alcohol
Dose: first week 1–1.25 mg at night, second week 2–2.5 mg at night, third week 2.5 mg twice daily, then 3 times daily increasing by 2.5 mg every 3–14 days according to response to a usual range of 10–40 mg daily; taken with food

PoM **Bromocriptine** (Non-proprietary)
Tablets, bromocriptine (as mesylate), 2.5 mg, net price 20 = £5.11. Label: 21, counselling, hypotensive reactions

PoM **Parlodel**® (Sandoz)
Tablets, both scored, bromocriptine (as mesylate), 1 mg, net price 20 = £1.86; 2.5 mg, 20 = £3.59. Label: 21, counselling, hypotensive reactions
Capsules, bromocriptine (as mesylate), 5 mg (blue/white), net price 20 = £7.04; 10 mg, 20 = £13.03. Label: 21, counselling, hypotensive reactions

LYSURIDE MALEATE
Indications: Parkinson's disease
Cautions: history of pituitary tumour; psychotic disturbance; **interactions:** Appendix 1 (lysuride)
HYPOTENSIVE REACTIONS. Hypotensive reactions may be disturbing in some patients during the first few days of treatment and particular care should be exercised when driving or operating machinery
Contra-indications: severe disturbances of peripheral circulation; coronary insufficiency, porphyria (see section 9.8.2)
Side-effects: nausea and vomiting; dizziness; headache, lethargy, malaise, drowsiness, psychotic reactions (including hallucinations); occasionally severe hypotension, rashes; rarely abdominal pain and constipation; Raynaud's phenomenon reported
Dose: initially 200 micrograms at bedtime with food increased as necessary at weekly intervals to 200 micrograms twice daily (midday and bedtime) then to 200 micrograms 3 times daily (morning, midday, and bedtime); further increases made by adding 200 micrograms each week first to the bedtime dose, then to the midday dose and finally to the morning dose; max. 5 mg daily in 3 divided doses after food

PoM **Revanil**® (Roche)
Tablets, scored, lysuride maleate 200 micrograms. Net price 100-tab pack = £24.00. Label: 21, counselling, hypotensive reactions

PERGOLIDE
Indications: adjunct to levodopa in Parkinson's disease
Cautions: arrhythmias or underlying cardiac disease, history of confusion or hallucinations, dyskinesia, pregnancy, breast-feeding; increase dose gradually and avoid abrupt withdrawal; avoid in porphyria (see section 9.8.2); **interactions:** Appendix 1 (pergolide)
HYPOTENSIVE REACTIONS. Hypotensive reactions may be disturbing in some patients during the first few days of treatment and particular care should be exercised when driving or operating machinery.
Side-effects: hallucinations, confusion, dyskinesia, somnolence, abdominal pain, nausea, dyspepsia, diplopia, rhinitis, dyspnoea, insomnia, constipation or diarrhoea, hypotension, tachycardia and arrhythmias reported
Dose: 50 micrograms daily for 2 days, increased gradually by 100–150 micrograms every third day over next 12 days, usually given in 3 divided doses; further increases of 250 micrograms every third day; usual maintenance 3 mg daily (above 5 mg daily not evaluated); during pergolide titration levodopa dose may be reduced cautiously

▼ PoM **Celance**® (Lilly)
Tablets, all scored, pergolide (as mesylate) 50 micrograms (ivory), net price 30-tab pack = £11.00; 250 micrograms (green), 20 = £8.31; 1 mg (pink), 20 = £30.00. Counselling, hypotensive reactions

SELEGILINE
Indications: Parkinson's disease or symptomatic parkinsonism (but not drug-induced extrapyramidal symptoms), either used alone (in early disease) or as an adjunct to levodopa therapy
Cautions: side-effects of levodopa may be increased, concurrent levodopa dosage may need to be reduced by 20–50%; **interactions:** Appendix 1 (selegiline)
Side-effects: hypotension, nausea and vomiting, confusion, agitation
Dose: 10 mg in the morning, or 5 mg at breakfast and midday

PoM **Eldepryl**® (Britannia)
Tablets, both scored, selegiline hydrochloride 5 mg, net price 20 = £9.30; 10 mg, 20 = £18.60

4.9.2 Antimuscarinic drugs used in parkinsonism

Antimuscarinic drugs (less correctly termed 'anticholinergics') are the other main class of drugs used in Parkinson's disease. They are less effective than levodopa in idiopathic Parkinson's disease although they often usefully supplement its action. Patients with mild symptoms, particularly where tremor predominates, may be treated initially with antimuscarinic drugs (alone or with selegiline, section 4.9.1), levodopa being added or substituted as symptoms progress. They have value in post-encephalitic parkinsonism.

Antimuscarinic drugs exert their antiparkinsonian effect by correcting the relative central cholinergic excess thought to occur in parkinsonism as a result of dopamine deficiency. In most patients their effects are only moderate, reducing tremor and rigidity to some effect but without significant action on bradykinesia. They exert a synergistic effect when used with levodopa and are also useful in reducing sialorrhoea.

The antimuscarinic drugs also reduce the symptoms of drug-induced parkinsonism as seen, for example, with antipsychotic drugs (section 4.2.1) but there is no justification for giving them simultaneously with antipsychotics unless parkinsonian side-effects occur. Tardive dyskinesia is not improved by the antimuscarinic drugs and may be made worse.

No important differences exist between the many synthetic antimuscarinic drugs available but some patients appear to tolerate one better than another. They may be taken before food if dry mouth is troublesome, or after food if gastrointestinal symptoms predominate. Those most commonly used are **orphenadrine** and **benzhexol; benztropine** and **procyclidine** are also used. Benztropine is similar to benzhexol but is excreted more slowly; changes in dose therefore need to be carried out very gradually. Both procyclidine and benztropine may be given parenterally and are effective emergency treatment for acute drug-induced dystonic reactions which may be severe.

BENZHEXOL HYDROCHLORIDE
Indications: parkinsonism; drug-induced extrapyramidal symptoms (but not tardive dyskinesia, see notes above)
Cautions: cardiovascular disease, hepatic or renal impairment; avoid abrupt discontinuation of treatment; drugs of this type liable to abuse; **interactions:** Appendix 1 (antimuscarinics)
DRIVING. May affect performance of skilled tasks (e.g. driving)
Contra-indications: untreated urinary retention, closed-angle glaucoma, gastro-intestinal obstruction
Side-effects: dry mouth, gastro-intestinal disturbances, dizziness, blurred vision; less commonly urinary retention, tachycardia, hypersensitivity, nervousness, and with high doses in susceptible patients, mental confusion, excitement, and psychiatric disturbances which may necessitate discontinuation of treatment
Dose: 1 mg daily, gradually increased; usual maintenance dose 5–15 mg daily in 3–4 divided doses

PoM **Benzhexol** (Non-proprietary)
Tablets, benzhexol hydrochloride 2 mg, net price 20 = 31p; 5 mg, 20 = 63p. Counselling, before or after food (see notes above), driving
PoM **Artane**® (Lederle)
Tablets, both scored, benzhexol hydrochloride 2 mg, net price 20 = 32p; 5 mg, 20 = 65p. Counselling, before or after food (see notes above), driving
PoM **Broflex**® (Bioglan)
Syrup, pink, benzhexol hydrochloride 5 mg/5 mL. Net price 200-mL pack = £4.34. Counselling, before or after food (see notes above), driving

BENZTROPINE MESYLATE
Indications; Cautions; Contra-indications; Side-effects: see under Benzhexol Hydrochloride, but causes sedation rather than stimulation; avoid in children under 3 years
Dose: by mouth, 0.5–1 mg daily usually at bedtime, gradually increased; max. 6 mg daily; usual maintenance dose 1–4 mg daily in single or divided doses
By intramuscular or intravenous injection, 1–2 mg, repeated if symptoms reappear

PoM **Cogentin**® (MSD)
Tablets, scored, benztropine mesylate 2 mg. Net price 20 = 29p. Label: 2
Injection, benztropine mesylate 1 mg/mL. Net price 2-mL amp = 92p

BIPERIDEN
Indications; Cautions; Contra-indications; Side-effects: see under Benzhexol Hydrochloride, but may cause drowsiness; injection may cause hypotension
Dose: by mouth, biperiden hydrochloride 1 mg twice daily, gradually increased to 2 mg 3 times daily; usual maintenance dose 3–12 mg daily in divided doses

By intramuscular or slow intravenous injection, biperiden lactate 2.5–5 mg up to 4 times daily

PoM **Akineton**® (Knoll)
Tablets, scored, biperiden hydrochloride 2 mg. Net price 100-tab pack = £4.72. Label: 2
Injection, biperiden lactate 5 mg/mL. Net price 1-mL amp = 70p

METHIXENE HYDROCHLORIDE
Indications; Cautions; Contra-indications; Side-effects: see under Benzhexol Hydrochloride
Dose: 2.5 mg 3 times daily gradually increased; usual maintenance dose 15–60 mg (elderly 15–30 mg) daily in divided doses

PoM **Tremonil**® (Sandoz)
Tablets, scored, methixene hydrochloride 5 mg. Net price 50 = £1.71. Label: 2

ORPHENADRINE HYDROCHLORIDE
Indications; Cautions; Contra-indications; Side-effects: see under Benzhexol Hydrochloride, but more euphoric; may cause insomnia; avoid in porphyria (see section 9.8.2)
Dose: by mouth, 150 mg daily in divided doses, gradually increased; max. 400 mg daily

PoM **Biorphen**® (Bioglan)
Elixir, sugar-free, orphenadrine hydrochloride 25 mg/5 mL. Net price 200-mL pack = £5.14. Counselling, driving
PoM **Disipal**® (Brocades)
Tablets, yellow, s/c, orphenadrine hydrochloride 50 mg. Net price 20 = 30p. Counselling, driving
Additives: include tartrazine

PROCYCLIDINE HYDROCHLORIDE
Indications; Cautions; Contra-indications; Side-effects: see under Benzhexol Hydrochloride
Dose: by mouth, 2.5 mg 3 times daily, gradually increased if necessary; usual max. 30 mg daily (60 mg daily in exceptional circumstances)
Acute dystonia, *by intramuscular injection*, 5–10 mg repeated if necessary after 20 minutes; max. 20 mg daily; *by intravenous injection*, 5 mg (usually effective within 5 minutes); an occasional patient may need 10 mg or more and may require up to half an hour to obtain relief

PoM **Procyclidine** (Non-proprietary)
Tablets, procyclidine hydrochloride 5 mg. Net price 20 = £1.06. Counselling, driving
PoM **Arpicolin**® (RP Drugs)
Syrup, procyclidine hydrochloride 2.5 mg/5 mL, net price 200-mL pack = £3.60; 5 mg/5 mL, 200-mL pack = £6.35. Counselling, driving
PoM **Kemadrin**® (Wellcome)
Tablets, scored, procyclidine hydrochloride 5 mg. Net price 20 = £1.17. Counselling, driving
Injection, procyclidine hydrochloride 5 mg/mL. Net price 2-mL amp = £1.49

4.9.3 Drugs used in essential tremor, chorea, tics, and related disorders

Tetrabenazine is mainly used to control movement disorders in Huntington's chorea and related disorders. It may act by depleting nerve endings of dopamine. It has useful action in only a proportion of patients and its use may be limited by the development of depression.

Haloperidol may be useful in improving motor tics and symptoms of Gilles de la Tourette syndrome and related choreas. **Pimozide** (see section 4.2.1 for CSM warning) and more recently **clonidine** (section 4.7.4.2) and **sulpiride** (section 4.2.1), are also used in Gilles de la Tourette syndrome. **Benzhexol** (section 4.9.2) at high dosage may also improve some movement disorders. It is sometimes necessary to build the dose up over many weeks, to 20 to 30 mg daily or higher. **Chlorpromazine** and **haloperidol** are used to relieve intractable hiccup (section 4.2.1).

Propranolol or another beta-adrenoceptor blocking drug (see section 2.4) may be useful in treating essential tremor or tremors associated with anxiety or thyrotoxicosis. Propranolol is given in a dosage of 40 mg 2 or 3 times daily, increased if necessary; 80 to 160 mg daily is usually required for maintenance.

Primidone in some cases provides relief from benign essential tremor; the dose is increased slowly to reduce side-effects.

HALOPERIDOL

Indications: motor tics, adjunctive treatment in choreas and Gilles de la Tourette syndrome; other indications, section 4.2.1
Cautions; Contra-indications; Side-effects: see section 4.2.1
Dose: by mouth, 0.5–1.5 mg 3 times daily adjusted according to the response; 10 mg daily or more may occasionally be necessary in Gilles de la Tourette syndrome; CHILD, Gilles de la Tourette syndrome up to 10 mg daily

Preparations: section 4.2.1

PRIMIDONE

Indications: essential tremor; epilepsy, see section 4.8.1
Cautions; Contra-indications; Side-effects: see section 4.8.1
Dose: essential tremor, initially 50 mg daily increased gradually over 2–3 weeks according to response; max. 750 mg daily

Preparations: section 4.8.1

TETRABENAZINE

Indications: movement disorders due to Huntington's chorea, senile chorea, and related neurological conditions
Cautions: pregnancy; avoid in breast-feeding; **interactions:** Appendix 1 (tetrabenazine)
DRIVING. May affect performance of skilled tasks (e.g. driving)

Side-effects: drowsiness, gastro-intestinal disturbances, depression, extrapyramidal dysfunction, hypotension
Dose: initially 12.5 mg twice daily (elderly 12.5 mg daily) gradually increased to 12.5–25 mg 3 times daily; max. 200 mg daily

PoM **Nitoman**® (Roche)
Tablets, pale yellow-buff, scored, tetrabenazine 25 mg. Net price 120-tab pack = £5.59. Label: 2

TORSION DYSTONIAS AND OTHER INVOLUNTARY MOVEMENTS

BOTULINUM A TOXIN-HAEMAGGLUTININ COMPLEX

Indications: blepharospasm and hemifacial spasm
Cautions: avoid deep or misplaced injection; pregnancy, breast-feeding
Side-effects: ptosis, diplopia; exacerbation of eyelid abnormalities, paralysis of mid-facial muscles, reduced blinking leading to keratitis and dry eyes; minor bruising and lid swelling
Dose: by subcutaneous injection, initially 120 units per affected eye, divided between 4 sites around affected eye as directed on package insert, repeated approximately every 8 weeks or as necessary (dose may be reduced to 80 or 60 units per eye)

▼ PoM **Dysport**® (Porton)
Injection, powder for reconstitution, botulinum A toxin-haemagglutinin complex, net price 500-unit vial = £170.00

4.10 Drugs used in substance dependence

ALCOHOL DEPENDENCE

Disulfiram (Antabuse®) is used as an adjunct to the treatment of alcohol dependence. It gives rise to extremely unpleasant systemic reactions after the ingestion of even small amounts of alcohol because it leads to accumulation of acetaldehyde in the body. Reactions include flushing of the face, throbbing headache, palpitations, tachycardia, nausea, vomiting, and, with large doses of alcohol, arrhythmias, hypotension, and collapse. Even the small amounts of alcohol included in many oral medicines may be sufficient to precipitate a reaction. It may be advisable for patients to carry a card warning of the danger of administration of alcohol.

Chlormethiazole (section 4.1.1) and **benzodiazepines** (section 4.1.2) are used to attenuate withdrawal symptoms but themselves have a dependence potential (section 4.1).

DISULFIRAM

Indications: adjunct in the treatment of chronic alcohol dependence (under specialist supervision)

Cautions: ensure that alcohol not consumed for at least 12 hours before initiating treatment; see also notes above; variable and occasionally severe reactions on alcohol challenge; hepatic or renal impairment, respiratory disease, diabetes mellitus, epilepsy; **interactions:** Appendix 1 (disulfiram)

ALCOHOL REACTION. Patients should be warned of unpredictable and occasionally severe nature of disulfiram-alcohol interactions. Reactions can occur in 10 minutes and last several hours (may require intensive supportive therapy). Patients should not ingest alcohol at all and should be warned of possible presence of alcohol in liquid medicines

Contra-indications: cardiac failure, coronary artery disease, psychosis and drug addiction, pregnancy

Side-effects: initially drowsiness and fatigue; nausea, vomiting, halitosis, reduced libido; rarely psychotic reactions (depression, paranoia, schizophrenia, mania), allergic dermatitis, peripheral neuritis, hepatic cell damage

Dose: 800 mg as a single dose on first day, reducing over 5 days to 100–200 mg daily; may be continued for up to 1 year

PoM **Antabuse 200**® (CP)
Tablets, scored, disulfiram 200 mg. Net price 50 = £17.50. Label: 2, counselling, alcohol reaction

---

CIGARETTE SMOKING

Nicotine chewing gum may be used as an adjunct to counselling; it is not available on the NHS.

NHS **Nicorette**® (Kabi Pharmacia)
Chewing gum, sugar-free, nicotine (as resin) 2 mg, net price pack of 30 = £2.83; pack of 105 = £7.66

NHS PoM **Nicorette Plus**® (Kabi Pharmacia)
Chewing gum, sugar-free, nicotine (as resin) 4 mg, net price pack of 105 = £10.80.
Cautions: angina, coronary artery disease; exacerbation of gastritis or peptic ulcer if swallowed
Contra-indications: pregnancy
Dose: nicotine replacement, initially one 2-mg piece to be chewed slowly for approx. 30 minutes, when urge to smoke occurs; patients needing more than 15 2-mg pieces daily may need the 4-mg strength; max. 15 pieces of 4-mg strength daily

---

OPIOID DEPENDENCE

Methadone is an opioid *agonist*. It can be substituted for opioids such as diamorphine, preventing the onset of withdrawal symptoms; it is itself addictive and should only be prescribed for those who are physically dependent on opioids. It is administered in a single daily dose usually as methadone mixture 1 mg/mL. The dose is adjusted according to the degree of dependence with the aim of gradual reduction.

Naltrexone is an opioid *antagonist*. It blocks the action of opioids such as diamorphine and precipitates withdrawal symptoms in opioid-dependent subjects. Since the euphoric action of opioid agonists is blocked by naltrexone it is given to former addicts as an aid to relapse prevention. Naltrexone should be initiated in specialist clinics only.

METHADONE HYDROCHLORIDE

Indications: adjunct in treatment of opioid dependence, see notes above; analgesia, section 4.7.2
Cautions; Contra-indications; Side-effects: section 4.7.2; overdosage: see Emergency Treatment of Poisoning, p. 18
Dose: initially 10–20 mg daily, increased by 10–20 mg daily until no signs of withdrawal or intoxication; usual dose 40–60 mg daily

CD **Methadone Mixture 1 mg/mL**
Net price 500 mL = £6.51. Label: 2
Available from Martindale, Penn (special order)

This preparation is 2½ times the strength of Methadone Linctus and is intended only for drug dependent persons for whom treatment is normally ordered on form FP10(HP)(ad) or FP10(MDA), or in Scotland on forms HBP(A) or GP10
The title includes the strength and prescriptions should be written accordingly
Syrup preserved with hydroxybenzoate esters may be incompatible with methadone hydrochloride.

NALTREXONE HYDROCHLORIDE

Indications: adjunct to prevent relapse in detoxified formerly opioid-dependent patients
Cautions: hepatic and renal impairment; liver function tests needed before and during treatment; test for opioid dependence with naloxone; avoid concomitant use of opioids but increased dose of opioid analgesic may be required for pain (monitor for opioid intoxication)
Contra-indications: patients currently dependent on opioids; acute hepatitis or liver failure
Side-effects: nausea, vomiting, abdominal pain; anxiety, nervousness, sleeping difficulty, headache, reduced energy; joint and muscle pain; less frequently, loss of appetite, diarrhoea, constipation, increased thirst; chest pain; increased sweating and lachrymation; increased energy, 'feeling down', irritability, dizziness, chills; delayed ejaculation, decreased potency; rash; occasionally, liver function abnormalities; reversible idiopathic thrombocytopenia reported
Dose: 25 mg initially then 50 mg daily; the total weekly dose may be divided and given on 3 days of the week for improved compliance (e.g. 100 mg on Monday and Wednesday, and 150 mg on Friday)

PoM **Nalorex**® (Du Pont)
Tablets, orange, scored, naltrexone hydrochloride 50 mg. Net price 50-tab pack = £79.49

5: Drugs used in the treatment of
INFECTIONS

In this chapter, drug treatment is discussed under the following headings:
- 5.1 Antibacterial drugs
- 5.2 Antifungal drugs
- 5.3 Antiviral drugs
- 5.4 Antiprotozoal drugs
- 5.5 Anthelmintics

5.1 Antibacterial drugs

- 5.1.1 Penicillins
- 5.1.2 Cephalosporins, cephamycins and other beta-lactam antibiotics
- 5.1.3 Tetracyclines
- 5.1.4 Aminoglycosides
- 5.1.5 Macrolides
- 5.1.6 Clindamycin and lincomycin
- 5.1.7 Some other antibiotics
- 5.1.8 Sulphonamides and trimethoprim
- 5.1.9 Antituberculous drugs
- 5.1.10 Antileprotic drugs
- 5.1.11 Metronidazole and tinidazole
- 5.1.12 4-Quinolones
- 5.1.13 Urinary-tract infections

CHOICE OF A SUITABLE DRUG. Before selecting an antibiotic the clinician must first consider two factors—the patient and the known or likely causative organism. Factors related to the patient which must be considered include history of allergy, renal and hepatic function, resistance to infection (i.e. whether immunocompromised), ability to tolerate drugs by mouth, severity of illness, ethnic origin, age and, if female, whether pregnant, breast-feeding or taking an oral contraceptive.

The known or likely organism and its antibiotic sensitivity, in association with the above factors, will suggest one or more antibiotics, the final choice depending on the microbiological, pharmacological, and toxicological properties.

An example of a rational approach to the selection of an antibiotic is treatment of a urinary-tract infection in a patient complaining of nausea in early pregnancy. The organism is reported as being resistant to ampicillin but sensitive to nitrofurantoin (can cause nausea), gentamicin (can only be given by injection and best avoided in pregnancy), tetracycline and co-trimoxazole (both contra-indicated in pregnancy), and cephalexin. The safest antibiotics in pregnancy are the penicillins and cephalosporins; therefore, cephalexin would be indicated for this patient.

The principles involved in selection of an antibiotic must allow for a number of variables including changing renal and hepatic function, increasing bacterial resistance, and new information on side-effects. Duration of therapy, dosage, and route of administration depend on site, type and severity of infection.

ANTIBIOTIC POLICIES. Many health authorities now place limits on the antibiotics that may be used in their hospitals, to achieve reasonable economy consistent with adequate cover, and to reduce the development of resistant organisms. An authority may indicate a range of drugs for general use, and permit treatment with other drugs only on the advice of the microbiologist or physician responsible for the control of infectious diseases.

BEFORE STARTING THERAPY. The following precepts should be considered before starting:

Viral infections should not be treated with antibiotics.

Samples should be taken for culture and sensitivity testing; **'blind'** prescribing of an antibiotic for a patient ill with unexplained pyrexia usually leads to further difficulty in establishing the diagnosis.

An up-to-date knowledge of **prevalent organisms** and their current sensitivity is of great help in choosing an antibiotic before bacteriological confirmation is available.

The **dose** of an antibiotic will vary according to a number of factors including age, weight, renal function, and severity of infection. The prescribing of the so-called 'standard' dose in serious infections may result in failure of treatment or even death of the patient therefore it is important to prescribe a dose appropriate to the condition. On the other hand, for an antibiotic with a narrow margin between the toxic and therapeutic dose (e.g. an aminoglycoside) it is also important to avoid an excessive dose and plasma concentration monitoring may be required.

The **route** of administration of an antibiotic will often depend on the severity of the infection. Life-threatening infections require intravenous therapy. Whenever possible painful intramuscular injections should be avoided in children.

Duration of therapy depends on the nature of the infection and the response to treatment. Courses should not be unduly prolonged as they are wasteful and may lead to side-effects. However, in certain infections such as tuberculosis it is necessary to continue treatment for relatively long periods. Conversely a single dose of an antibiotic may cure uncomplicated urinary-tract infections.

Suggested treatment is shown in Table 1. When the pathogen has been isolated treatment may be changed to a more appropriate antibiotic if necessary. If no bacterium is cultured the antibiotic can be continued or stopped on clinical grounds. Infections for which prophylaxis is useful are listed in Table 2.

Cautionary label wordings, see inside back cover   Prices are **net**, see p. 1

Chapter 5: Infections

Table 1. Summary of antibacterial therapy

Infection	Suggested antibacterial	Comment
1: Gastro-intestinal system		
Gastro-enteritis	Antibiotic not usually indicated	Frequently nonbacterial aetiology
Campylobacter enteritis	Erythromycin *or* ciprofloxacin	
Invasive salmonellosis	Ciprofloxacin *or* trimethoprim	Includes severe infections which may be invasive
Shigellosis	Ciprofloxacin *or* trimethoprim	Antibiotic not indicated for mild cases. Ciprofloxacin should be used for trimethoprim-resistant strains
Typhoid fever	Chloramphenicol *or* ciprofloxacin	Infections from the Indian subcontinent, the Middle-East, and South-East Asia may be chloramphenicol-resistant and ciprofloxacin may be more appropriate
Biliary-tract infection	Gentamicin *or* a cephalosporin	
Peritonitis	Gentamicin (*or* a cephalosporin) + metronidazole (*or* clindamycin)	
Peritoneal dialysis-associated peritonitis	Vancomycin[3] + gentamicin added to dialysis fluid	Discontinue either gentamicin or vancomycin when sensitivity known; treat for 5–10 days
2: Cardiovascular system		
Endocarditis caused by:		
Penicillin-sensitive streptococci (e.g. viridans streptococci)	Benzylpenicillin (*or* vancomycin if penicillin-allergic) + low-dose gentamicin (i.e. 60–80 mg twice daily)	Treat for up to 4 weeks; stop gentamicin after 2 weeks if organism fully sensitive to penicillin. Oral amoxycillin[1] may be substituted for benzylpenicillin after 2 weeks
Streptococci with reduced sensitivity to penicillin e.g. *Streptococcus faecalis*	Benzylpenicillin (*or* vancomycin[3] if penicillin-allergic) + low-dose gentamicin (i.e. 60–80 mg twice daily)	Treat for 4 weeks
Staphylococcus aureus (and *Staphylococcus epidermidis*)	Flucloxacillin[2] + *either* gentamicin *or* fusidic acid (*or* vancomycin[3] alone if penicillin-allergic)	Treat for at least 4 weeks; stop gentamicin after 2 weeks
3: Respiratory system		
Haemophilus epiglottitis	Chloramphenicol *or* cefotaxime	Give intravenously
Exacerbations of chronic bronchitis	Amoxycillin[1] *or* trimethoprim *or* tetracycline	Note that 20% of pneumococci and 15% of *Haemophilus influenzae* strains are tetracycline-resistant
Pneumonia:		
Previously healthy chest	Benzylpenicillin *or* amoxycillin[1]	Add flucloxacillin[2] if *Staphylococcus* suspected e.g. in influenza or measles; add erythromycin[4] if *Mycoplasma pneumoniae* or *Legionella* infection is suspected (severe *Legionella* infections may require addition of rifampicin)
Previously unhealthy chest	Flucloxacillin[2] + amoxycillin[1] *or* erythromycin[4] alone	Substitute erythromycin[4] (*or* rifampicin and erythromycin[4], see above) for flucloxacillin if *Legionella* infection is suspected; use erythromycin[4] if *Mycoplasma pneumoniae* infection is suspected
Hospital-acquired	A broad-spectrum cephalosporin *or* an aminoglycoside	Add erythromycin[4] if *Legionella* infection suspected
4: Central nervous system		
Meningitis caused by:		
Meningococcus	Benzylpenicillin *or* cefotaxime	Give rifampicin for 2 days before hospital discharge
Pneumococcus	Benzylpenicillin *or* cefotaxime	
Haemophilus influenzae	Chloramphenicol *or* cefotaxime	For *H. influenzae* type b give rifampicin for 4 days before hospital discharge
Listeria	Amoxycillin[1] + gentamicin	

1. Where amoxycillin is suggested ampicillin or an ester of ampicillin (see section 5.1.1.3) may be used.
2. Where flucloxacillin is suggested cloxacillin may be used.
3. Where vancomycin is suggested teicoplanin may be used.
4. Where erythromycin is suggested another macrolide (e.g. azithromycin or clarithromycin) may be used.

Table 1. Summary of antibacterial therapy (*continued*)

Infection	Suggested antibacterial	Comment
7: Urinary tract		
Acute pyelonephritis or prostatitis	Trimethoprim *or* gentamicin *or* cephalosporin *or* a 4-quinolone	Do not give trimethoprim or a 4-quinolone in pregnancy. Treat prostatitis with trimethoprim or a 4-quinolone for 4 weeks
'Lower' UTI	Trimethoprim *or* amoxycillin[1] *or* nitrofurantoin *or* oral cephalosporin	
7: Genital system		
Syphilis	Procaine penicillin (*or* tetracycline *or* erythromycin if penicillin-allergic)	Treat for 10–21 days
Gonorrhoea	Amoxycillin[1] with probenecid (*or* spectinomycin, *or* a 4-quinolone if penicillin-allergic)	Single-dose treatment in uncomplicated infection; choice depends on locality where infection acquired; contact-tracing advised; remember chlamydia
Non-gonococcal urethritis	Tetracycline *or* erythromycin	Treat for 7–21 days; contact-tracing advised
Pelvic inflammatory disease	Metronidazole + doxycycline (*or* erythromycin) *or* co-amoxiclav alone	Remember gonorrhoea; co-amoxiclav is not active against chlamydia; severely ill patients may require gentamicin (or a 'second-generation' cephalosporin) + a tetracycline
9: Blood		
Septicaemia Initial 'blind' therapy	Aminoglycoside + a penicillin *or* a cephalosporin alone *In immunocompromised*, aminoglycoside + a broad-spectrum penicillin *or* a 'third generation' cephalosporin alone	Choice depends on local resistance patterns and clinical presentation; add metronidazole if anaerobic infection suspected; add flucloxacillin[2] *or* vancomycin[3] if Gram-positive infection suspected
10: Musculoskeletal system		
Osteomyelitis and septic arthritis	Clindamycin alone *or* flucloxacillin[2] + fusidic acid. If *Haemophilus influenzae* give amoxycillin[1] *or* cefuroxime	Under 5 years of age may be *H. influenzae*. Treat acute disease for at least 6 weeks and chronic infection for at least 12 weeks
11: Eye		
Purulent conjunctivitis	Chloramphenicol *or* gentamicin eye-drops	
12: Ear, nose, and oropharynx		
Dental infections	Phenoxymethylpenicillin (*or* amoxycillin[1]) *or* erythromycin *or* metronidazole	Tetracycline for chronic destructive forms of periodontal disease
Sinusitis	Amoxycillin[1] *or* doxycycline	
Otitis externa	Flucloxacillin[2]	
Otitis media	Benzylpenicillin Phenoxymethylpenicillin	Initial i/m therapy (if possible) with benzylpenicillin, then oral therapy with phenoxymethylpenicillin
	Amoxycillin[1] if under 5 years (*or* erythromycin if penicillin-allergic)	Under 5 years of age may be *Haemophilus influenzae*
Throat infections	Benzylpenicillin Phenoxymethylpenicillin (*or* erythromycin if penicillin-allergic)	Initial i/m therapy (in severe infection) with benzylpenicillin, then oral therapy with phenoxymethylpenicillin; treat beta-haemolytic streptococcal infections for at least 10 days. Most infections are caused by viruses
13: Skin		
Impetigo	Topical fusidic acid *or* mupirocin; oral flucloxacillin[2] *or* erythromycin if widespread	Topical treatment for 7 days usually adequate; max. duration of topical treatment 14 days
Erysipelas	Phenoxymethylpenicillin	
Cellulitis	Phenoxymethylpenicillin + flucloxacillin[2] (*or* erythromycin alone if penicillin-allergic) *or* co-amoxiclav alone	Severe cellulitis may require parenteral benzylpenicillin + flucloxacillin or co-amoxiclav alone
Acne—see section 13.6		

1. Where amoxycillin is suggested ampicillin or an ester of ampicillin (see section 5.1.1.3) may be used.
2. Where flucloxacillin is suggested cloxacillin may be used.
3. Where vancomycin is suggested teicoplanin may be used.

Table 2. Summary of antibacterial prophylaxis

Infection	Antibacterial and dose
Prevention of recurrence of rheumatic fever[1]	Phenoxymethylpenicillin 250 mg twice daily *or* sulphadimidine 500 mg daily (250 mg for children)
Prevention of secondary case of meningococcal meningitis[1]	Rifampicin 600 mg every 12 hours for 2 days; CHILD 10 mg/kg (3 months–1 year, 5 mg/kg) every 12 hours for 2 days *or* ciprofloxacin 500 mg as a single dose
Prevention of secondary case of *Haemophilus influenzae* type b disease[1]	Rifampicin 600 mg once daily for 4 days (optimum regimen for adults); CHILD over 3 months 20 mg/kg once daily for 4 days (max. 600 mg daily)
Prevention of secondary case of diphtheria in non-immune patient	Erythromycin 500 mg every 6 hours for 5 days; CHILD up to 2 years 125 mg every 6 hours, 2–8 years 250 mg every 6 hours
Prevention of pneumococcal infection following splenectomy or in patients with sickle cell disease	Phenoxymethylpenicillin 500 mg every 12 hours; CHILD under 5 years 125 mg every 12 hours, 6–12 years 250 mg every 12 hours

Prevention of endocarditis in patients with heart-valve lesion, septal defect, patent ductus, or prosthetic valve
 	
Dental procedures that require antibiotic prophylaxis are:
  extractions
  scaling
  surgery involving gingival tissues.
Antibiotic prophylaxis for dental procedures may be supplemented with *chlorhexidine gel 1%* or *chlorhexidine mouthwash 0.2%*, used 5 minutes before procedure
 	
Note. Oral clindamycin now replaces oral erythromycin (which caused nausea and vomiting); if clindamycin is used, periodontal or other multistage procedures should not be repeated at intervals of less than 2 weeks
	Dental procedures *under local or no anaesthesia*, patients who have not received a penicillin more than once in the previous month, including those with a prosthetic valve (but not those who have had endocarditis), oral amoxycillin 3 g 1 hour before procedure; CHILD under 5 years quarter adult dose; 5–10 years half adult dose
	patients who are penicillin-allergic or have received a penicillin more than once in the previous month,
	oral clindamycin 600 mg 1 hour before procedure; CHILD under 5 years quarter adult dose; 5–10 years half-adult dose
	patients who have had endocarditis, amoxycillin + gentamicin, as under general anaesthesia
	
	Dental procedures *under general anaesthesia, no special risk* (including patients who have not received a penicillin more than once in the previous month),
	either i/m or i/v amoxycillin 1 g at induction, then oral amoxycillin 500 mg 6 hours later; CHILD under 5 years quarter adult dose; 5–10 years half adult dose
	or oral amoxycillin 3 g 4 hours before induction then oral amoxycillin 3 g as soon as possible after procedure; CHILD under 5 years quarter adult dose; 5–10 years half adult dose
	or oral amoxycillin 3 g + oral probenecid 1 g 4 hours before procedure;
	special risk (patients with a prosthetic valve or who have had endocarditis), i/m or i/v amoxycillin 1 g + i/m or i/v gentamicin 120 mg at induction, then oral amoxycillin 500 mg 6 hours later; CHILD under 5 years amoxycillin quarter adult dose, gentamicin 2 mg/kg; 5–10 years amoxycillin half adult dose, gentamicin 2 mg/kg
	patients who are penicillin-allergic or who have received a penicillin more than once in the previous month,
	either i/v vancomycin 1 g over at least 100 minutes then i/v gentamicin 120 mg at induction or 15 minutes before procedure; CHILD under 10 years vancomycin 20 mg/kg, gentamicin 2 mg/kg
	or i/v teicoplanin 400 mg + gentamicin 120 mg at induction or 15 minutes before procedure; CHILD under 14 years teicoplanin 6 mg/kg, gentamicin 2 mg/kg
	or i/v clindamycin 300 mg over at least 10 minutes at induction or 15 minutes before procedure then oral or i/v clindamycin 150 mg 6 hours later; CHILD under 5 years quarter adult dose; 5–10 years half adult dose
	
	Upper respiratory-tract procedures, as for dental procedures; post-operative dose may be given parenterally if swallowing is painful
	
	Genito-urinary procedures, as for *special risk* patients undergoing dental procedures under general anaesthesia except that clindamycin is not given, see above; if urine infected, prophylaxis should also cover infective organism
	
	Obstetric, gynaecological and gastro-intestinal procedures (prophylaxis required for patients with prosthetic valves or those who have had endocarditis only), as for genito-urinary procedures

Prevention of gas-gangrene in high lower-limb amputations or following major trauma	Benzylpenicillin 300–600 mg every 6 hours for 5 days *or* if penicillin-allergic give metronidazole 500 mg every 8 hours
Prevention of tuberculosis in susceptible close contacts	Isoniazid 300 mg daily for 6 months; CHILD, isoniazid 5–10 mg/kg daily *or* isoniazid 300 mg daily + rifampicin 600 mg daily (450 mg if less than 50 kg) for 3 months; CHILD isoniazid 5–10 mg/kg daily + rifampicin 10 mg/kg daily

1. For details of those who should receive chemoprophylaxis contact a consultant in communicable disease control (or a consultant in infectious diseases or the local public health laboratory). Unless there has been mouth to mouth contact, hospital workers do not generally require chemoprophylaxis.

Table 2. Summary of antibacterial prophylaxis (*continued*)

Infection	Antibacterial and adult dose
Prevention of infection in abdominal surgery	
Operations on stomach or oesophagus for carcinoma, or cholecystectomy in patients with possibly infected bile	Single dose of gentamicin *or* a cephalosporin given in 2 hours before operation
Resections of colon and rectum for carcinoma, and resections in inflammatory bowel disease	Single dose of *either* gentamicin + metronidazole *or* cefuroxime + metronidazole given in 2 hours before operation
Hysterectomy	Metronidazole as suppository *or* single i/v dose

5.1.1 Penicillins

5.1.1.1 Benzylpenicillin and phenoxymethylpenicillin
5.1.1.2 Penicillinase-resistant penicillins
5.1.1.3 Broad-spectrum penicillins
5.1.1.4 Antipseudomonal penicillins
5.1.1.5 Mecillinams

The penicillins are bactericidal and act by interfering with bacterial cell wall synthesis. They diffuse well into body tissues and fluids, but penetration into the cerebrospinal fluid is poor except when the meninges are inflamed. They are excreted in the urine in therapeutic concentrations. Probenecid blocks the renal tubular excretion of the penicillins, producing higher and more prolonged plasma concentrations (see section 10.1.4); it is not recommended in children under 2 years of age.

The most important side-effect of the penicillins is hypersensitivity, which causes rashes and, occasionally, anaphylaxis, which can be fatal. Patients who are allergic to one penicillin will be allergic to all as the hypersensitivity is related to the basic penicillin structure. A rare but serious toxic effect of the penicillins is encephalopathy due to cerebral irritation. This may result from excessively high doses but can also develop with normal doses given to patients with renal failure. The penicillins should **not** be given by intrathecal injection as they can cause encephalopathy which may be fatal.

A second problem relating to high doses of penicillin, or normal doses given to patients with renal failure, is the accumulation of electrolyte since most injectable penicillins contain either sodium or potassium.

Diarrhoea frequently occurs during oral penicillin therapy. It is most common with ampicillin and its derivatives, which can also cause pseudomembranous colitis.

5.1.1.1 BENZYLPENICILLIN AND PHENOXYMETHYLPENICILLIN

Benzylpenicillin (Penicillin G), the first of the penicillins, remains an important and useful antibiotic but is inactivated by bacterial penicillinases (beta-lactamases). It is the drug of choice for streptococcal, pneumococcal, gonococcal, and meningococcal infections and also for actinomycosis, anthrax, diphtheria, gas-gangrene, leptospirosis, syphilis, tetanus, yaws, and treatment of Lyme disease in children. Pneumococci, meningococci, and gonococci which have decreased sensitivity to penicillin have been isolated. Benzylpenicillin is inactivated by gastric acid and absorption from the gut is low; therefore it is best given by injection. Benzylpenicillin may cause convulsions after high doses by intravenous injection or in renal failure.

Procaine penicillin is a sparingly soluble salt of benzylpenicillin. It is used in intramuscular depot preparations which provide therapeutic tissue concentrations for up to 24 hours. It is the preferred choice for the treatment of syphilis; neurosyphilis requires special consideration.

Benethamine penicillin is a benzylpenicillin salt with very low solubility giving a prolonged action after intramuscular injection, though producing low plasma concentrations; it is used, with soluble and procaine penicillin, in Triplopen®.

Phenoxymethylpenicillin (Penicillin V) has a similar antibacterial spectrum to benzylpenicillin, but is less active. It is gastric acid-stable, so is suitable for oral administration. It should not be used for serious infections because absorption can be unpredictable and plasma concentrations variable. It is indicated principally for respiratory-tract infections in children, for streptococcal tonsillitis, and for continuing treatment after one or more injections of benzylpenicillin when clinical response has begun. It should not be used for meningococcal or gonococcal infections. Phenoxymethylpenicillin is used for prophylaxis against streptococcal infections following rheumatic fever.

BENZYLPENICILLIN
(Penicillin G)

Indications: tonsillitis, otitis media, erysipelas, streptococcal endocarditis, meningococcal and pneumococcal meningitis, prophylaxis in limb amputation

Cautions: history of allergy; renal impairment; **interactions:** Appendix 1 (penicillins)
Contra-indications: penicillin hypersensitivity
Side-effects: sensitivity reactions including urticaria, fever, joint pains; angioedema; anaphylactic shock in hypersensitive patients; diarrhoea after administration by mouth
Dose: by intramuscular or by slow intravenous injection or by infusion, 1.2 g daily in 4 divided doses, increased if necessary to 2.4 g daily or more (see also below); NEONATE, 30 mg/kg daily (in 2 divided doses in the first few days of life then in 3–4 divided doses); CHILD 1 month–12 years, 10–20 mg/kg daily in 4 divided doses (higher doses may be required, see also below)
Bacterial endocarditis, *by slow intravenous injection or by infusion*, 7.2 g daily in 4–6 divided doses
Meningitis, *by slow intravenous injection or by infusion*, 2.4 g every 4–6 hours; CHILD 1 month–12 years, 180–300 mg/kg daily in 4–6 divided doses
Prophylaxis in limb amputation, section 5.1, Table 2
By intrathecal injection, **not** recommended, see section 5.1.1

PoM **Crystapen**® (Glaxo)
Injection, powder for reconstitution, benzylpenicillin sodium (unbuffered). Net price 600-mg vial = 35p
Electrolytes: Na⁺ 1.68 mmol/600-mg vial

BENETHAMINE PENICILLIN
Indications: penicillin-sensitive infections; prophylaxis
Cautions; Contra-indications; Side-effects: see under Benzylpenicillin

PoM **Triplopen**® (Glaxo)
(Triple penicillin injection)
Injection, powder for reconstitution, benethamine penicillin 475 mg, procaine penicillin 250 mg, benzylpenicillin sodium 300 mg. Net price per vial = 40p
Electrolytes: Na⁺ 1.2 mmol/vial
Dose: by deep intramuscular injection, 1 vial every 2–3 days

BENZATHINE PENICILLIN
Indications: penicillin-sensitive infections
Cautions; Contra-indications; Side-effects: see under Benzylpenicillin
Dose: see below

PoM **Penidural**® (Wyeth)
Suspension, pink, benzathine penicillin 229 mg/5 mL. Net price 100 mL = £1.49. Label: 9
Dose: 10 mL 3–4 times daily; CHILD 5 mL 3–4 times daily
Paediatric drops, pink, benzathine penicillin 115 mg/mL. Net price 10 mL = £1.63. Label: 9, counselling, use of pipette
Dose: CHILD up to 5 years, 1–2 dropperfuls (approx. 77–154 mg) 3–4 times daily

PHENOXYMETHYLPENICILLIN
(Penicillin V)
Indications: tonsillitis, otitis media, erysipelas; rheumatic fever and pneumococcal infection prophylaxis
Cautions; Contra-indications; Side-effects: see under Benzylpenicillin; **interactions:** Appendix 1 (penicillins)
Dose: 250–500 mg every 6 hours, at least 30 minutes before food; CHILD, every 6 hours, up to 1 year 62.5 mg, 1–5 years 125 mg, 6–12 years 250 mg
Rheumatic fever and pneumococcal infection prophylaxis, section 5.1, Table 2

PoM **Phenoxymethylpenicillin** (Non-proprietary)
Tablets, phenoxymethylpenicillin (as potassium salt) 250 mg, net price 20 = 33p. Label: 9, 23
Available from APS (Apsin®), Berk, Boots (Stabilin V-K®), Cox, CP, Dista (Distaquaine V-K®), Evans, Kerfoot
Oral solution, phenoxymethylpenicillin (as potassium salt) for reconstitution with water, 62.5 mg/5 mL, net price 100 mL = 52p; 125 mg/5 mL, 100 mL = 47p; 250 mg/5 mL, 100 mL = 71p. Label: 9, 23
Available from APS (Apsin®), Boots (Stabilin V-K®), Cox, CP, Evans, Kerfoot

PROCAINE PENICILLIN
Indications: penicillin-sensitive infections
Cautions; Contra-indications; Side-effects: see under Benzylpenicillin; **not** for intravenous administration
Dose: see below

PoM **Bicillin**® (Brocades)
Injection, powder for reconstitution, procaine penicillin 1.8 g, benzylpenicillin sodium 360 mg. Net price 6-mL multidose vial = £1.74
Electrolytes: Na⁺ 1 mmol/vial
Dose: when reconstituted with 4.6 mL water for injections, 1 mL (procaine penicillin 300 mg, benzylpenicillin sodium 60 mg) every 12–24 hours by intramuscular injection
Primary syphilis, by intramuscular injection, 3 mL (4 mL in heavier patients) daily for 10 days (14 days for secondary or latent syphilis)
Note. Reconstitution with 4.6 mL water for injections produces 6 mL

5.1.1.2 PENICILLINASE-RESISTANT PENICILLINS

Most staphylococci are now resistant to benzylpenicillin because they produce penicillinases. **Cloxacillin** and **flucloxacillin**, however, are not inactivated by these enzymes and are thus effective in infections caused by penicillin-resistant staphylococci, which is the sole indication for their use. They are acid-stable and can, therefore, be given by mouth as well as by injection.

5.1.1 Penicillins

Flucloxacillin is better absorbed from the gut than cloxacillin and is, therefore, to be preferred for oral therapy.

Methicillin is also effective against penicillin-resistant *Staph. aureus*, but can only be given by injection because it is not acid-stable and is now seldom used.

Staph. aureus strains resistant to methicillin (methicillin-resistant *Staphylococcus aureus*, MRSA) and cloxacillin have emerged in some hospitals; some of these organisms are only sensitive to vancomycin (section 5.1.7). Other alternatives include rifampicin, teicoplanin, and ciprofloxacin.

Temocillin is a new penicillin with activity against penicillinase-producing Gram-negative bacteria (except *Pseudomonas aeruginosa*); it is not active against Gram-positive bacteria.

CLOXACILLIN

Indications: infections due to penicillinase-producing staphylococci

Cautions; Contra-indications; Side-effects: see under Benzylpenicillin (section 5.1.1.1)

Dose: by mouth, 500 mg every 6 hours, at least 30 minutes before food

By intramuscular injection, 250 mg every 4–6 hours

By slow intravenous injection or by infusion, 500 mg every 4–6 hours

Doses may be doubled in severe infections

CHILD, any route, under 2 years quarter adult dose; 2–10 years half adult dose

Note. Oral liquid preparation no longer marketed

PoM **Cloxacillin** (Non-proprietary)
Capsules, cloxacillin (as sodium salt) 250 mg, net price 20 = £3.64; 500 mg, 20 = £7.29. Label: 9, 23

PoM **Orbenin**® (Beecham)
Capsules, both orange/black, cloxacillin (as sodium salt) 250 mg, net price 20 = £3.64; 500 mg, 20 = £7.29. Label: 9, 23
Injection, powder for reconstitution, cloxacillin (as sodium salt). Net price 250-mg vial = 93p; 500-mg vial = £1.86; also available as 1-g vial
Electrolytes: Na$^+$ 0.59 mmol/250-mg vial, 1.18 mmol/500-mg vial

FLUCLOXACILLIN

Indications: infections due to penicillinase-producing staphylococci

Cautions; Contra-indications; Side-effects: see under Benzylpenicillin (section 5.1.1.1); hepatitis and cholestatic jaundice reported (may be delayed for up to 2 months after treatment); avoid in porphyria (see section 9.8.2)

Dose: by mouth, 250 mg every 6 hours, at least 30 minutes before food

By intramuscular injection, 250 mg every 6 hours

By slow intravenous injection or by infusion, 0.25–1 g every 6 hours

Doses may be doubled in severe infections

CHILD, any route, under 2 years quarter adult dose; 2–10 years half adult dose

PoM **Flucloxacillin** (Non-proprietary)
Capsules, flucloxacillin (as sodium salt) 250 mg, net price 20 = £2.70; 500 mg, 20 = £5.60. Label: 9, 23
Available from APS, Ashbourne (Fluclomix®), Berk (Ladropen®), Brocades (Stafoxil®), Cox, CP, Evans, Galen (Galfloxin®), Kerfoot

Oral solution (= elixir or syrup), flucloxacillin (as sodium salt) for reconstitution with water, 125 mg/5 mL. Net price 100 mL = £3.11. Label: 9, 23
Available from APS, Cox, CP, Norton

Oral suspension (= mixture), flucloxacillin (as magnesium salt) for reconstitution with water, 125 mg/5 mL, net price 100 mL = £3.32; 250 mg/5 mL, 100 mL = £6.64. Label: 9, 23
Available from Berk

Injection, powder for reconstitution, flucloxacillin (as sodium salt). Net price 250-mg vial = 77p; 500-mg vial = £1.53
Available from Berk

PoM **Floxapen**® (Beecham)
Capsules, both black/caramel, flucloxacillin (as sodium salt) 250 mg, net price 20-cap pack = £4.62, 28-cap pack = £6.47; 500 mg, 28-cap pack = £12.95. Label: 9, 23
Syrup, flucloxacillin 125 mg (as magnesium salt)/5 mL when reconstituted with water. Net price 100 mL = £3.32. Label: 9, 23
Syrup forte, flucloxacillin 250 mg (as magnesium salt)/5 mL when reconstituted with water. Net price 100 mL = £6.64. Label: 9, 23
Injection, powder for reconstitution, flucloxacillin (as sodium salt). Net price 250-mg vial = 93p; 500-mg vial = £1.86; 1-g vial = £3.71
Electrolytes: Na$^+$ 0.57 mmol/250-mg vial, 1.13 mmol/500-mg vial, 2.26 mmol/1-g vial

METHICILLIN SODIUM

Indications: infections due to penicillinase-producing staphylococci

Cautions; Contra-indications; Side-effects: see under Benzylpenicillin (section 5.1.1.1)

Dose: by intramuscular injection or by intravenous injection over 3–4 minutes *or by intravenous infusion*, 1 g every 4–6 hours; CHILD under 2 years quarter adult dose; 2–10 years half adult dose

PoM **Celbenin**® (Beecham)
Injection, powder for reconstitution, methicillin sodium. Net price 1-g vial = £1.88
Electrolytes: Na$^+$ 2.44 mmol/g

TEMOCILLIN

Indications: infections due to penicillinase-producing Gram-negative bacteria except pseudomonas.

Cautions; Contra-indications; Side-effects: see under Benzylpenicillin (section 5.1.1.1)

Dose: by intramuscular injection or by intravenous injection (over 3–4 minutes) *or by intravenous infusion*, 1–2 g every 12 hours

Acute uncomplicated urinary-tract infections, 1 g daily as a single dose or in divided doses

PoM **Temopen**® (Bencard)
Injection, powder for reconstitution, temocillin (as sodium salt). Net price 500-mg vial = £7.50; 1-g vial = £15.00
Electrolytes: Na⁺ 5 mmol/g

5.1.1.3 BROAD-SPECTRUM PENICILLINS

Ampicillin is active against certain Gram-positive and Gram-negative organisms but is inactivated by penicillinases including those produced by *Staphylococcus aureus* and by common Gram-negative bacilli such as *Escherichia coli*. Almost all staphylococci, 50% of *E. coli* strains and 15% of *Haemophilus influenzae* strains are now resistant. The likelihood of resistance should therefore be considered before using ampicillin for the 'blind' treatment of infections; in particular, it should not be used for hospital patients without checking sensitivity.

Ampicillin is well excreted in the bile and urine. It is principally indicated for the treatment of exacerbations of chronic bronchitis and middle ear infections, both of which are usually due to *Streptococcus pneumoniae* and *H. influenzae*, and for urinary-tract infections (section 5.1.13) and gonorrhoea.

Ampicillin can be given by mouth but less than half the dose is absorbed, and absorption is further decreased by the presence of food in the gut. Higher plasma concentrations are obtained with the ampicillin esters **bacampicillin** and **pivampicillin**; their absorption is little affected by the presence of food, and the incidence of diarrhoea is less than with ampicillin. These antibiotics should be given every 8 hours for moderate or severe infections, especially outside the renal tract.

Maculopapular rashes commonly occur with ampicillin (and amoxycillin) but are not usually related to true penicillin allergy. They almost always occur in patients with glandular fever; broad-spectrum penicillins should not therefore be used for 'blind' treatment of a sore throat. Rashes are also common in patients with chronic lymphatic leukaemia and in patients infected with the human immunodeficiency virus (HIV).

Amoxycillin is a derivative of ampicillin which differs by only one hydroxyl group and has a similar antibacterial spectrum. It is, however, better absorbed when given by mouth, producing higher plasma and tissue concentrations; unlike ampicillin, absorption is not affected by the presence of food in the stomach.

Co-amoxiclav consists of amoxycillin with the beta-lactamase inhibitor clavulanic acid. Clavulanic acid itself has no significant antibacterial activity but, by inactivating penicillinases, it makes the combination active against penicillinase-producing bacteria that are resistant to amoxycillin. These include most *Staph. aureus*, 50% of *E. coli* strains, and up to 15% of *H. influenzae* strains, as well as many *Bacteroides* and *Klebsiella* spp. **Sulbactam** is another beta-lactamase inhibitor which is available in combination with ampicillin (as Dicapen®, Unasyn®).

Combinations of ampicillin with flucloxacillin (as co-fluampicil) and ampicillin with cloxacillin (Ampiclox®) are available.

AMOXYCILLIN

Indications: see under Ampicillin; also typhoid fever and endocarditis prophylaxis
Cautions; Contra-indications; Side-effects: see under Ampicillin
Dose: by mouth, 250 mg every 8 hours, doubled in severe infections; CHILD up to 10 years, 125 mg every 8 hours, doubled in severe infections
Severe or recurrent purulent respiratory infection, 3 g every 12 hours; CHILD 2–5 years 750 mg every 12 hours, 5–10 years 1.5 g every 12 hours
Endocarditis prophylaxis, section 5.1, Table 2

Short-course oral therapy
Dental abscess, 3 g repeated after 8 hours
Urinary-tract infections, 3 g repeated after 10–12 hours
Gonorrhoea, single dose of 2–3 g with probenecid 1 g
Otitis media, CHILD 3–10 years, 750 mg twice daily for 2 days

By intramuscular injection, 500 mg every 8 hours; CHILD, 50–100 mg/kg daily in divided doses
By intravenous injection or infusion. 500 mg every 8 hours increased to 1 g every 6 hours; CHILD, 50–100 mg/kg daily in divided doses

PoM **Amoxycillin** (Non-proprietary)
Capsules, amoxycillin (as trihydrate) 250 mg, net price 20 = £2.82; 500 mg, 20 = £5.67. Label: 9
Available from APS, Ashbourne (Amix®), Berk (Almodan®), BHR (Amrit®), Cox, CP, Eastern (Amoram®), Evans, Galen (Galenamox®), Kerfoot, Lagap, Norton, Rima (Rimoxallin®)
Oral suspension, amoxycillin (as trihydrate) for reconstitution with water, 125 mg/5 mL, net price 100 mL = £1.98; 250 mg/5 mL, 100 mL = £3.24. Label: 9.
Available from APS, Ashbourne (Amix®), Berk (Almodan®), BHR (Amrit®), Cox, CP, Eastern (Amoram®), Evans, Galen (Galenamox®), Kerfoot, Lagap, Norton, Rima (Rimoxallin®)

PoM **Almodan**® (Berk)
Injection, powder for reconstitution, amoxycillin (as sodium salt), 250-mg vial, net price = 39p; 500-mg vial = 71p

PoM **Amoxil**® (Bencard)
Capsules, both maroon/gold, amoxycillin (as trihydrate), 250 mg, net price 21-cap pack = £3.67; 500 mg, 21-cap pack = £7.35. Label: 9
Dispersible tablets, sugar-free, amoxycillin 500 mg (as trihydrate). Net price 21-tab pack = £8.48. Label: 9, 13
Fiztab (= chewable tablets), sugar-free, amoxycillin (as trihydrate) 125 mg, net price 20-tab pack = £2.20; 250 mg, 20-tab pack = £4.40; 500 mg, 20-tab pack = £8.80. Label: 9, 10
patient information leaflet
Note. Dose form not suitable for children under 3 years

Syrup SF, both sugar-free, amoxycillin (as trihydrate) for reconstitution with water, 125 mg/5 mL, net price 100 mL = £2.20; 250 mg/5 mL, 100 mL = £4.40. Label: 9

Paediatric suspension, amoxycillin 125 mg (as trihydrate)/1.25 mL when reconstituted with water. Net price 20 mL = £3.30. Label: 9, counselling, use of pipette

Sachets SF, powder, sugar-free, amoxycillin 750 mg (as trihydrate)/sachet, net price 4-sachet pack = £2.86; 3 g/sachet, 2-sachet pack = £4.73; 14-sachet pack = £33.11. Label: 9, 13

Injection, powder for reconstitution, amoxycillin (as sodium salt). Net price 250-mg vial = 36p; 500-mg vial = 66p; 1-g vial = £1.31
Electrolytes: Na$^+$ 3.2 mmol/g

PoM **Flemoxin Solutab**® (Brocades)
Dispersible tablets, sugar-free, both scored, amoxycillin (as trihydrate) 375 mg, net price 10-tab pack = £2.62; 750 mg, 10-tab pack = £5.25. Label: 9, 13

Dose: 375 mg every 12 hours, doubled in severe infections; CHILD 5–10 years half usual adult dose

Severe or recurrent respiratory-tract infection, see under Dose on p. 206

AMPICILLIN

Indications: urinary-tract infections, otitis media, chronic bronchitis, invasive salmonellosis, gonorrhoea

Cautions: history of allergy; renal impairment; erythematous rashes common in glandular fever, chronic lymphatic leukaemia, and HIV infection; **interactions:** Appendix 1 (penicillins)

Contra-indications: penicillin hypersensitivity

Side-effects: nausea, diarrhoea; rashes (discontinue treatment); rarely, pseudomembranous colitis; see also under Benzylpenicillin (section 5.1.1.1)

Dose: by mouth, 0.25–1 g every 6 hours, at least 30 minutes before food

Gonorrhoea, 2–3.5 g as a single dose with probenecid 1 g

Urinary-tract infections, 500 mg every 8 hours

By intramuscular injection or intravenous injection or infusion, 500 mg every 4–6 hours; higher doses in meningitis

CHILD under 10 years, any route, half adult dose

PoM **Ampicillin** (Non-proprietary)
Capsules, ampicillin 250 mg, net price 20 = 67p; 500 mg, 20 = £1.44. Label: 9, 23
Available from APS, Berk (Vidopen®), Brocades (Amfipen®), Cox, CP, Evans, Kerfoot, Lagap, Norton, Rima (Rimacillin®)

Oral suspension, ampicillin 125 mg/5 mL when reconstituted with water, net price 100 mL = 76p; 250 mg/5 mL, 100 mL = £1.23. Label: 9, 23
Available from APS, Berk, Brocades (Amfipen®), Cox, Evans, Kerfoot, Lagap, Norton, Rima (Rimacillin®)

PoM **Penbritin**® (Beecham)
Capsules, both black/red, ampicillin (as trihydrate) 250 mg, net price 28-cap pack = £2.05; 500 mg, 28-cap pack = £4.10. Label: 9, 23

Syrup, ampicillin 125 mg (as trihydrate)/5 mL when reconstituted with water. Net price 100 mL = £1.09. Label: 9, 23

Syrup forte, ampicillin 250 mg (as trihydrate)/5 mL when reconstituted with water. Net price 100 mL = £2.17. Label: 9, 23

Paediatric suspension, ampicillin 125 mg (as trihydrate)/1.25 mL. Net price 25 mL = £2.03. Label: 9, 23, counselling, use of pipette

Injection, powder for reconstitution, ampicillin (as sodium salt). Net price 250-mg vial = 33p; 500-mg vial = 67p
Electrolytes: Na$^+$ 0.73 mmol/250-mg vial, 1.47 mmol/500-mg vial

PoM **Vidopen**® (Berk)
Injection, powder for reconstitution, ampicillin (as sodium salt). Net price 250-mg vial = 33p; 500-mg vial = 67p.

With cloxacillin

PoM **Ampiclox**® (Beecham)
Injection, ampicillin 250 mg (as sodium salt), cloxacillin 250 mg (as sodium salt). Net price per vial = £1.36
Electrolytes: Na$^+$ 1.32 mmol/vial
Dose: by intramuscular injection or intravenous injection or infusion, 1–2 vials every 4–6 hours; CHILD up to 2 years quarter adult dose, 2–10 years half adult dose

PoM **Ampiclox Neonatal**® (Beecham)
Suspension, sugar-free, ampicillin 60 mg (as trihydrate), cloxacillin 30 mg (as sodium salt)/0.6 mL when reconstituted with water. Net price 10 mL = £2.06. Label: 9, counselling, use of pipette
Dose: 0.6 mL every 4 hours

With flucloxacillin
See co-fluampicil

AMPICILLIN WITH SULBACTAM

Indications: infections due to beta-lactamase-producing organisms; prophylaxis in abdominal and obstetric procedures

Cautions; Contra-indications; Side-effects: see under Ampicillin

Dose: by intramuscular injection or by intravenous injection over 3 minutes *or by intravenous infusion,* expressed as ampicillin, 1 g every 6–8 hours, doubled for severe infections (max. 8 g daily); CHILD, expressed as ampicillin, 100 mg/kg in 3–4 divided doses (2 divided doses in neonates)

Surgical prophylaxis, expressed as ampicillin, 1–2 g at induction; may be repeated every 6–8 hours for up to 24 hours

▼ PoM **Dicapen**® (Leo)
Injection 750 mg, powder for reconstitution, ampicillin (as sodium salt) 500 mg, sulbactam (as sodium salt) 250 mg. Net price per vial = £1.23
Electrolytes: Na⁺ 2.5 mmol/vial

Injection 1.5 g, powder for reconstitution, ampicillin (as sodium salt) 1 g, sulbactam (as sodium salt) 500 mg. Net price per vial = £2.46
Electrolytes: Na⁺ 5 mmol/vial

Injection 3 g, powder for reconstitution, ampicillin (as sodium salt) 2 g, sulbactam (as sodium salt) 1 g. Net price per vial = £4.92
Electrolytes: Na⁺ 10 mmol/vial

▼ PoM **Unasyn**® (Pfizer)
Injection 750 mg, powder for reconstitution, ampicillin (as sodium salt) 500 mg, sulbactam (as sodium salt) 250 mg. Net price per vial = £1.11
Electrolytes: Na⁺ 2.5 mmol/vial

Sultamicillin (Prodrug of ampicillin–sulbactam)
▼ PoM **Unasyn**® (Pfizer)
Tablets, sultamicillin (as tosylate) 375 mg (equivalent to ampicillin 220 mg, sulbactam 147 mg). Net price 14-tab pack = £6.30. Label: 9
Dose: ADULT and CHILD over 30 kg, upper respiratory-tract, urinary-tract and other mild infections, 1 tablet twice daily
Lower respiratory-tract, skin and soft tissue infections, sinusitis, and otitis media, 2 tablets twice daily
CHILD under 30 kg, dose form not appropriate

BACAMPICILLIN HYDROCHLORIDE

Indications; Cautions; Contra-indications; Side-effects: see under Ampicillin
Dose: 400 mg 2–3 times daily, doubled in severe infections; CHILD over 5 years, 200 mg 3 times daily
Uncomplicated gonorrhoea, 1.6 g as a single dose with probenecid 1 g

PoM **Ambaxin**® (Upjohn)
Tablets, scored, bacampicillin hydrochloride 400 mg. Net price 20 = £6.34. Label: 9

CO-AMOXICLAV

A mixture of amoxycillin (as the trihydrate or as the sodium salt) and clavulanic acid (as potassium clavulanate); the proportions are expressed in the form x/y where x and y are the strengths in milligrams of amoxycillin and clavulanic acid respectively

Indications; Cautions; Contra-indications; Side-effects: see under Ampicillin and notes above; also caution in severe hepatic impairment; hepatitis, cholestatic jaundice, and erythema multiforme (including Stevens-Johnson syndrome) reported; phlebitis at injection site also reported
Dose: by mouth, expressed as amoxycillin, 250 mg every 8 hours, dose doubled in severe infections; CHILD see under preparations below (under 6 years Augmentin® '125/31 SF' suspension; 6–12 years Augmentin® '250/62 SF' suspension)

By intravenous injection or infusion, expressed as amoxycillin, 1 g every 8 hours increased to 1 g every 6 hours in more serious infections; INFANTS up to 3 months 25 mg/kg every 8 hours (every 12 hours in the perinatal period and in premature infants); CHILD 3 months–12 years, 25 mg/kg every 8 hours increased to 25 mg/kg every 6 hours in more serious infections
Surgical prophylaxis, expressed as amoxycillin, 1 g at induction; for procedures lasting longer than 1 hour dose may be repeated every 6 hours

PoM **Augmentin**® (Beecham)
Tablets, f/c, co-amoxiclav 250/125 (amoxycillin 250 mg as trihydrate, clavulanic acid 125 mg as potassium salt). Net price 21-tab pack = £7.00; 30-tab pack = £10.13. Label: 9
Dispersible tablets, sugar-free, co-amoxiclav 250/125 (amoxycillin 250 mg as trihydrate, clavulanic acid 125 mg as potassium salt). Net price 21-tab pack = £7.86. Label: 9, 13

'125/31 SF' *suspension*, sugar-free, co-amoxiclav 125/31 (amoxycillin 125 mg as trihydrate, clavulanic acid 31 mg as potassium salt)/5 mL when reconstituted with water. Net price 100 mL = £3.27. Label: 9
Dose: CHILD under 1 year 0.8 mL/kg daily in 3 divided doses; 1–6 years (10–18 kg) 5 mL every 8 hours, doubled in severe infections

'250/62 SF' *suspension*, sugar-free, co-amoxiclav 250/62 (amoxycillin 250 mg as trihydrate, clavulanic acid 62 mg as potassium salt)/5 mL when reconstituted with water. Net price 100 mL = £4.60. Label: 9
Dose: CHILD 6–12 years 5 mL every 8 hours, doubled in severe infections

Injection 600 mg, powder for preparing intravenous injections, co-amoxiclav 500/100 (amoxycillin 500 mg as sodium salt, clavulanic acid 100 mg as potassium salt). Net price per vial = £1.35
Electrolytes: Na⁺ 1.6 mmol, K⁺ 0.5 mmol/600-mg vial

Injection 1.2 g, powder for preparing intravenous injections, co-amoxiclav 1000/200 (amoxycillin 1 g as sodium salt, clavulanic acid 200 mg as potassium salt). Net price per vial = £2.70
Electrolytes: Na⁺ 3.1 mmol, K⁺ 1 mmol/1.2-g vial

CO-FLUAMPICIL

A mixture of equal parts by mass of flucloxacillin and ampicillin
Indications: mixed infections involving penicillinase-producing staphylococci
Cautions; Contra-indications; Side-effects: see under Ampicillin and Flucloxacillin
Dose: by mouth, co-fluampicil, 250/250 every 6 hours, dose doubled in severe infections; CHILD under 10 years half adult dose, dose doubled in severe infections
By intramuscular or slow intravenous injection or by intravenous infusion, co-fluampicil 250/250 every 6 hours, dose doubled in severe infections; CHILD under 2 years quarter adult dose, 2–10 years half adult dose, dose doubled in severe infections

PoM Co-fluampicil (Non-proprietary)
Capsules, co-fluampicil 250/250 (flucloxacillin 250 mg as sodium salt, ampicillin 250 mg as trihydrate). Net price 20 = £4.00. Label: 9, 23
Available from Generics (Flu-Amp®), Norton

PoM Magnapen® (Beecham)
Capsules, black/turquoise, co-fluampicil 250/250 (flucloxacillin 250 mg as sodium salt, ampicillin 250 mg as trihydrate). Net price 20-cap pack = £5.08. Label: 9, 23
Syrup, co-fluampicil 125/125 (flucloxacillin 125 mg as magnesium salt, ampicillin 125 mg as trihydrate)/5 mL when reconstituted with water. Net price 100 mL = £4.13. Label: 9, 23
Injection 500 mg, powder for reconstitution, co-fluampicil 250/250 (flucloxacillin 250 mg as sodium salt, ampicillin 250 mg as sodium salt). Net price per vial = £1.10
Electrolytes: Na⁺ 1.3 mmol/vial
Injection 1 g, powder for reconstitution, co-fluampicil 500/500 (flucloxacillin 500 mg as sodium salt, ampicillin 500 mg as sodium salt). Net price per vial = £2.20
Electrolytes: Na⁺ 2.6 mmol/vial

PIVAMPICILLIN

Indications: see under Ampicillin
Cautions; Contra-indications; Side-effects: see under Ampicillin; hepatic and renal function tests required in long-term use; avoid in porphyria (see section 9.8.2)
Dose: 500 mg every 12 hours, doubled in severe infections; CHILD up to 1 year 40–60 mg/kg daily in 2–3 divided doses; 1–5 years 350–525 mg daily; 6–10 years 525–700 mg daily; doses can be doubled in severe infections

PoM Pondocillin® (Leo)
Tablets, f/c, pivampicillin 500 mg. Net price 20 = £4.22. Label: 5, 9, 21
Suspension, sugar-free, pivampicillin 175 mg/5 mL when reconstituted with water. Net price 50 mL = £1.76; 100 mL = £2.84. Label: 5, 9, 21
Sachets, granules, off-white, pivampicillin 175 mg/sachet. Net price 10-sachet pack = £1.98. Label: 5, 9, 13, 21

With pivmecillinam

PoM Miraxid® (Fisons)
Tablets, f/c, pivampicillin 125 mg, pivmecillinam hydrochloride 100 mg. Net price 20 = £2.59. Label: 9, 21, 27, counselling, posture (see below)
Dose: 2 tablets twice daily, increased to 3 tablets twice daily for severe infections; CHILD 6–10 years 1 tablet twice daily
COUNSELLING. Swallow whole with plenty of fluid during meals while sitting or standing
Miraxid® 450 Tablets, f/c, pivampicillin 250 mg, pivmecillinam hydrochloride 200 mg. Net price 20 = £5.06. Label: 9, 21, 27, counselling, posture (see below)
Dose: 1 tablet twice daily, increased to 2 tablets twice daily for severe infections
COUNSELLING. Swallow whole with plenty of fluid during meals while sitting or standing

Paediatric suspension, pivampicillin 62.5 mg, pivmecillinam 46.2 mg/unit-dose sachet. Net price 10-sachet pack = £2.70. Label: 9, 13, 21
Dose: under 6 years 1 sachet twice daily increased to 2 sachets twice daily for severe infections, 6–10 years 2 sachets twice daily increased to 3 sachets twice daily for severe infections

PoM Pondocillin Plus® (Leo)
Tablets, f/c, pivampicillin 250 mg, pivmecillinam hydrochloride 200 mg. Net price 20 = £5.98. Label: 9, 21, 27, counselling, posture (see below)
Dose: 1 tablet twice daily, increased to 2 tablets twice daily for severe infections
COUNSELLING. Swallow whole with plenty of fluid during meals while sitting or standing

5.1.1.4 ANTIPSEUDOMONAL PENICILLINS

The carboxypenicillins, **carbenicillin** and **ticarcillin**, are principally indicated for the treatment of serious infections caused by *Pseudomonas aeruginosa* although they also have activity against certain other Gram-negative bacilli including *Proteus* spp. and *Bacteroides fragilis*. Carbenicillin has been replaced by ticarcillin which is more active against these organisms.

Timentin® (ticarcillin with clavulanic acid, section 5.1.1.3), is active against penicillinase-producing bacteria resistant to ticarcillin.

The ureidopenicillins, **azlocillin** and **piperacillin**, have a broad spectrum and are both more active than ticarcillin against *Ps. aeruginosa*.

For pseudomonas septicaemias (especially in neutropenia or endocarditis) these antipseudomonal penicillins should be given with an aminoglycoside (e.g. gentamicin or netilmicin, section 5.1.4) as there is a synergistic effect. Penicillins and aminoglycosides must not, however, be mixed in the same syringe or infusion.

Owing to the sodium content of many of these antibiotics, high doses may lead to hypernatraemia.

AZLOCILLIN

Indications: infections due to *Pseudomonas aeruginosa*, see notes above
Cautions; Contra-indications; Side-effects: see under Benzylpenicillin (section 5.1.1.1); **interactions**: Appendix 1 (penicillins)
Dose: by intravenous injection, 2 g every 8 hours Serious infections, by intravenous infusion, 5 g every 8 hours; PREMATURE INFANT 50 mg/kg every 12 hours; NEONATE 100 mg/kg every 12 hours; INFANT 7 days–1 year 100 mg/kg every 8 hours; CHILD 1–14 years 75 mg/kg every 8 hours

PoM Securopen® (Bayer)
Injection, powder for reconstitution, azlocillin (as sodium salt). Net price 500-mg vial = £1.62; 1-g vial = £3.21; 2-g vial = £5.02
Electrolytes: Na⁺ 1.08 mmol/500-mg vial, 2.17 mmol/1-g vial, 4.33 mmol/2-g vial

Infusion, powder for reconstitution, azlocillin (as sodium salt). Net price 5-g vial = £11·80 (also available with 50 mL water for injections, transfer needle, and infusion bag)
Electrolytes: Na$^+$ 10.84 mmol/5-g vial

CARBENICILLIN

Indications: infections due to *Pseudomonas aeruginosa* and *Proteus* spp., see notes above
Cautions; Contra-indications: see under Benzylpenicillin (section 5.1.1.1)
Side-effects: see under Benzylpenicillin (section 5.1.1.1); also hypokalaemia, alteration in platelet function
Dose: *by slow intravenous injection or rapid infusion*, severe systemic infections, 5 g every 4–6 hours; CHILD 250–400 mg/kg daily in divided doses
By intramuscular injection, urinary-tract infections, 2 g every 6 hours; CHILD 50–100 mg/kg daily in divided doses

PoM **Pyopen**® (Beecham)
Injection, powder for reconstitution, carbenicillin (as sodium salt). Net price 1-g vial = £1.54; 5-g vial = £7.50
Electrolytes: Na$^+$ 5.4 mmol/1-g vial, 27.1 mmol/5-g vial

PIPERACILLIN

Indications: infections due to *Pseudomonas aeruginosa*, see notes above
Cautions; Contra-indications; Side-effects: see under Benzylpenicillin (section 5.1.1.1)
Dose: *by intramuscular or by slow intravenous injection or by intravenous infusion*, 100–150 mg/kg daily (in divided doses), increased to 200–300 mg/kg daily in severe infections, and to at least 16 g daily in life-threatening infections; single doses over 2 g intravenous route only

PoM **Pipril**® (Lederle)
Injection, powder for reconstitution, piperacillin (as sodium salt). Net price 1-g vial = £3.07; 2-g vial = £6.08; 4-g vial = £12.01
Infusion, powder for reconstitution, piperacillin 4 g (as sodium salt), with 50-mL bottle water for injections and transfer needle. Net price complete unit = £12.80
Electrolytes: Na$^+$ 1.94 mmol/g

TICARCILLIN

Indications: infections due to *Pseudomonas* and *Proteus* spp, see notes above.
Cautions; Contra-indications; Side-effects: see under Benzylpenicillin (section 5.1.1.1)
Dose: *by slow intravenous injection* over 3–4 minutes *or by intravenous infusion*, 15–20 g daily in divided doses; CHILD 200–300 mg/kg daily in divided doses
Urinary-tract infections, *by intramuscular or slow intravenous injection*, 3–4 g daily in divided doses; CHILD 50–100 mg/kg daily in divided doses

PoM **Ticar**® (Beecham)
Injection, powder for reconstitution, ticarcillin (as sodium salt). Net price 1-g vial = £1.68; 5-g vial = £6.84
Infusion, powder for reconstitution, ticarcillin 5 g (as sodium salt) in infusion bottle, with transfer needle and diluent. Net price complete unit = £8.03
Electrolytes: Na$^+$ 5.3 mmol/1-g vial, 26.7 mmol/5-g vial

With clavulanic acid
PoM **Timentin**® (Beecham)
Injection 1.6 g, powder for reconstitution, ticarcillin 1.5 g (as sodium salt), clavulanic acid 100 mg (as potassium salt). Net price per vial = £3.04
Injection 3.2 g, powder for reconstitution, ticarcillin 3 g (as sodium salt), clavulanic acid 200 mg (as potassium salt). Net price per vial = £6.08
Electrolytes: Na$^+$ 16 mmol, K$^+$ 1 mmol/3.2-g vial
Dose: *by intravenous infusion*, 3.2 g every 6–8 hours increased to every 4 hours in more severe infections; CHILD 80 mg/kg every 6–8 hours (every 12 hours in neonates)

5.1.1.5 MECILLINAMS

Mecillinam and **pivmecillinam** have significant activity against many Gram-negative bacteria including salmonellae, but excluding *Ps. aeruginosa*. Pivmecillinam is given by mouth and subsequently hydrolysed to mecillinam, which is the active drug and must itself be given by injection.

MECILLINAM

Indications: severe infections due to Gram-negative enteric bacteria
Cautions; Contra-indications; Side-effects: see under Benzylpenicillin (section 5.1.1.1); liver and renal function tests on long-term use
Dose: *by intramuscular or by slow intravenous injection or by intravenous infusion*, 5–15 mg/kg every 6–8 hours

PoM **Selexidin**® (Leo)
Injection, powder for reconstitution, mecillinam. Net price 400-mg vial = £1.22

PIVMECILLINAM

Indications: see under Dose below
Cautions; Contra-indications; Side-effects: see under Benzylpenicillin (section 5.1.1.1); also liver and renal function tests required in long-term use
Dose: acute uncomplicated cystitis, 400 mg initially, then 200 mg every 8 hours for 3 days (10-tab pack)
Chronic or recurrent bacteriuria, 400 mg every 6–8 hours
Salmonellosis, 1.2–2.4 g daily for 14 days (14–28 days for carriers)
COUNSELLING. Tablets should be swallowed whole with plenty of fluid during meals while sitting or standing

5.1.2 Cephalosporins, cephamycins, and other beta-lactams

PoM Selexid® (Leo)
Tablets, f/c, pivmecillinam hydrochloride 200 mg. Net price 20 = £4.48. Label: 9, 21, 27, counselling, posture (see Dose above)
Suspension, granules, pivmecillinam 100 mg/single-dose sachet. Net price 20 sachets = £4.03. Label: 9, 13, 21

With pivampicillin
See under Pivampicillin (section 5.1.1.3)

5.1.2 Cephalosporins, cephamycins, and other beta-lactam antibiotics

Antibiotics discussed in this section include the **cephalosporins**, such as cefotaxime, ceftazidime, cefuroxime, cephalexin and cephradine, the **cephamycin**, cefoxitin, the **monobactam**, aztreonam, and the **carbapenem** imipenem (a thienamycin derivative).

CEPHALOSPORINS AND CEPHAMYCINS

The cephalosporins are broad-spectrum antibiotics but in spite of the number of cephalosporins currently available there are few absolute indications for their use. All have a similar antibacterial spectrum although individual agents have differing activity against certain organisms. The pharmacology of the cephalosporins is similar to that of the penicillins, excretion being principally renal and blocked by probenecid.

The principal side-effect of the cephalosporins is hypersensitivity and about 10% of penicillin-sensitive patients will also be allergic to the cephalosporins. Haemorrhage due to interference with blood clotting factors has been associated with several cephalosporins.

Cephradine and **cefazolin** have generally been replaced by the newer cephalosporins mentioned below.

Cefuroxime and **cephamandole** are 'second generation' cephalosporins and are less susceptible than the earlier cephalosporins to inactivation by penicillinases. They are, therefore, active against certain bacteria which are resistant to the other drugs and have greater activity against *H. influenzae* and *Neisseria gonorrhoeae*.

Cefotaxime, **ceftazidime**, **ceftizoxime**, and **cefodizime** are 'third generation' cephalosporins with greater activity than the 'second generation' cephalosporins against certain Gram-negative bacteria. However, they are less active than cefuroxime and cephamandole against Gram-positive bacteria, most notably *Staphylococcus aureus*. Their broad antibacterial spectrum may encourage superinfection with resistant bacteria or fungi.

Cefsulodin and **ceftazidime** have good activity against pseudomonas. Ceftazidime is also active against other Gram-negative bacteria. Cefsulodin has a very much narrower spectrum and should be used only for pseudomonal infections.

Cefoxitin, a cephamycin antibiotic, is active against bowel flora including *Bacteroides fragilis* and because of this it has been recommended for abdominal sepsis such as peritonitis.

ORALLY ACTIVE CEPHALOSPORINS. The orally active 'first generation' cephalosporins, **cephalexin**, **cephradine**, and **cefadroxil** and the 'second generation' cephalosporin, **cefaclor** have a similar antimicrobial spectrum. They are useful for urinary-tract infections which do not respond to other drugs or which occur in pregnancy. Cefaclor has good activity against *Haemophilus influenzae*, but is associated with protracted skin reactions especially in children. Cefadroxil has a longer duration of action than the other cephalosporins but poor activity against *H. influenzae*. **Cefuroxime axetil**, an ester of the 'second generation' cephalosporin cefuroxime, has the same antibacterial spectrum as the parent compound; gastro-intestinal side-effects are quite common.

Cefixime has a longer duration of action than the other cephalosporins that are active by mouth. It is presently only indicated for acute infections.

CEFACLOR

Indications: infections due to sensitive Gram-positive and Gram-negative bacteria, but see notes above
Cautions: penicillin sensitivity; renal impairment; false positive urinary glucose (if tested for reducing substances) and false positive Coombs' test; **interactions:** Appendix 1 (cephalosporins)
Contra-indications: cephalosporin hypersensitivity; porphyria (see section 9.8.2)
Side-effects: diarrhoea and rarely pseudomembranous colitis (CSM has warned both more likely with higher doses), nausea and vomiting; allergic reactions including rashes, pruritus, urticaria, serum sickness-like reactions with rashes, fever and arthralgia, and anaphylaxis; erythema multiforme, toxic epidermal necrolysis reported; eosinophilia and rarely thrombocytopenia or neutropenia; disturbances in liver enzymes, transient hepatitis and cholestatic jaundice; other side-effects reported include reversible interstitial nephritis, hyperactivity, nervousness, sleep disturbances, confusion, hypertonia, and dizziness.
Dose: 250 mg every 8 hours, doubled for severe infections; max. 4 g daily; CHILD over 1 month, 20 mg/kg daily in 3 divided doses, doubled for severe infections, max. 1 g daily; *or* 1 month–1 year, 62.5 mg every 8 hours; 1–5 years, 125 mg; over 5 years, 250 mg; doses doubled for severe infections

PoM Distaclor® (Dista)
Capsules, cefaclor 250 mg (violet/white), net price 21-cap pack = £10.83; 500 mg (violet/grey), 20 = £20.63. Label: 9
Suspension, both pink, cefaclor for reconstitution with water, 125 mg/5 mL, net price 100 mL = £5.16; 250 mg/5 mL, 100 mL = £10.32. Label: 9

CEFADROXIL

Indications: see under Cefaclor; see also notes above

Cautions; Contra-indications; Side-effects: see under Cefaclor

Dose: patients over 40 kg, 0.5–1 g twice daily; skin, soft tissue, and simple urinary-tract infections, 1 g daily; CHILD under 1 year, 25 mg/kg daily in divided doses; 1–6 years, 250 mg twice daily; over 6 years, 500 mg twice daily

PoM Baxan® (Bristol-Myers)
Capsules, cefadroxil 500 mg (as monohydrate). Net price 20 = £6.63. Label: 9
Suspension, cefadroxil (as monohydrate) for reconstitution with water, 125 mg/5 mL, net price 60 mL = £1.75; 250 mg/5 mL, 60 mL = £3.48; 500 mg/5 mL, 60 mL = £5.21. Label: 9

CEFIXIME

Indications: see under Cefaclor and notes above

Cautions; Contra-indications; Side-effects: see under Cefaclor

Dose: 200–400 mg daily as a single dose or in 2 divided doses; CHILD 8 mg/kg daily as a single dose or in 2 divided doses *or* 6 months–1 year 75 mg; 1–4 years 100 mg; 5–10 years 200 mg; 11–12 years 300 mg

▼ **PoM Suprax®** (Lederle)
Tablets, f/c, scored, cefixime 200 mg. Net price 20 = £27.39. Label: 9
Paediatric oral suspension, cefixime 100 mg/5 mL when reconstituted with water. Net price 37.5 mL (with double-ended spoon for measuring 3.75 mL or 5 mL since dilution not recommended) = £6.53; 75 mL = £11.72. Label: 9

CEFODIZIME

Indications: see under Dose

Cautions; Contra-indications; Side-effects: see under Cefaclor

Dose: by intramuscular or intravenous injection or by intravenous infusion, lower respiratory-tract infection (including pneumonia and bronchopneumonia), 1 g every 12 hours
Upper and lower urinary-tract infections (including acute and chronic pyelonephritis and cystitis), 1 g every 12 hours *or* 2 g daily (as a single dose); single doses over 1 g intravenous route only

▼ **PoM Timecef®** (Roussel)
Injection, powder for reconstitution, cefodizime (as sodium salt), net price 1-g vial = £11.32
Electrolytes: Na$^+$ 3.18 mmol/g

CEFOTAXIME

Indications: see under Cefaclor; surgical prophylaxis; see also notes above

Cautions; Contra-indications; Side-effects: see under Cefaclor

Dose: by intramuscular or intravenous injection, moderate to serious infection, 1 g every 8 hours; life-threatening infection, 2 g every 8 hours; exceptionally, for life-threatening infections due to organisms less sensitive to cefotaxime, up to 12 g daily
Urinary-tract and mild to moderate infections, 1 g every 12 hours
Gonorrhoea 1 g as a single dose
In severe renal impairment, doses to be halved after initial dose of 1 g. NEONATE, 50 mg/kg daily in 2–4 divided doses; in severe infections 150–200 mg/kg daily. CHILD, 100–150 mg/kg daily in 2–4 divided doses; in severe infections, up to 200 mg/kg daily
By intravenous infusion, 1–2 g over 20–60 minutes

PoM Claforan® (Roussel)
Injection, powder for reconstitution, cefotaxime (as sodium salt). Net price 500-mg vial = £2.48; 1-g vial = £4.95; 2-g vial = £9.90
Electrolytes: Na$^+$ 2.09 mmol/g

CEFOXITIN

Indications: see under Cefaclor; surgical prophylaxis; more active against Gram-negative bacteria

Cautions; Contra-indications; Side-effects: see under Cefaclor

Dose: by intramuscular or by slow intravenous injection or by infusion, 1–2 g every 6–8 hours, increased in severe infections; max. 12 g daily; CHILD up to 1 week 20–40 mg/kg every 12 hours; 1–4 weeks 20–40 mg/kg every 8 hours; over 1 month 20–40 mg/kg every 6–8 hours

PoM Mefoxin® (MSD)
Injection, powder for reconstitution, cefoxitin (as sodium salt). Net price 1-g vial = £4.92; 2-g vial = £9.84
Electrolytes: Na$^+$ 2.3 mmol/g

CEFSULODIN SODIUM

Indications: infections due to sensitive strains of *Ps. aeruginosa*; surgical prophylaxis

Cautions; Contra-indications; Side-effects: see under Cefaclor

Dose: by intramuscular injection, or by slow intravenous injection, or by intravenous infusion, 1–4 g daily in 2–4 divided doses increased in severe infections to 6 g daily or more; CHILD 20–50 mg/kg daily

PoM Monaspor® (Ciba)
Injection, powder for reconstitution, cefsulodin sodium. Net price 500-mg vial = £5.65; 1-g vial = £11.30
Electrolytes: Na$^+$ 1.8 mmol/g

CEFTAZIDIME
Indications: see under Cefaclor; see also notes above
Cautions; Contra-indications; Side-effects: see under Cefaclor
Dose: by intramuscular injection or intravenous injection or infusion, 1 g every 8 hours *or* 2 g every 12 hours; 2 g every 8–12 hours in severe infections; single doses over 1 g intravenous route only; elderly usual max. 3 g daily; CHILD, up to 2 months 25–60 mg/kg daily in 2 divided doses, over 2 months 30–100 mg/kg daily in 2–3 divided doses; up to 150 mg/kg daily if immunocompromised or meningitis; intravenous route recommended for children
Urinary-tract and less serious infections, 0.5–1 g every 12 hours
Pseudomonal lung infection in cystic fibrosis, ADULT with normal renal function 100–150 mg/kg daily in 3 divided doses; CHILD up to 150 mg/kg daily; intravenous route recommended for children

PoM **Fortum**® (Glaxo)
Injection, powder for reconstitution, ceftazidime (as pentahydrate), with sodium carbonate. Net price 250-mg vial = £2.48; 500-mg vial = £4.95; 1-g vial = £9.90; 2-g vial (for injection and for infusion) = £19.80
Electrolytes: Na⁺ 2.3 mmol/g

CEFTIZOXIME
Indications: see under Cefaclor; see also notes above
Cautions; Contra-indications; Side-effects: see under Cefaclor
Dose: by deep intramuscular or slow intravenous injection or by intravenous infusion, 1–2 g every 8–12 hours increased in severe infections up to 8 g daily, in 3 divided doses; CHILD over 3 months 30–60 mg/kg daily in 2–4 divided doses, increased to 100–150 mg/kg daily for severe infections
Gonorrhoea, *by intramuscular injection*, 1 g as a single dose
Urinary-tract infections, *by deep intramuscular or slow intravenous injection or by infusion*, 0.5–1 g every 12 hours

PoM **Cefizox**® (Wellcome)
Injection, powder for reconstitution, ceftizoxime (as sodium salt). Net price 500-mg vial = £2.76; 1-g vial = £5.50; 2-g vial = £11.00
Electrolytes: Na⁺ 2.6 mmol/g

CEFUROXIME
Indications: see under Cefaclor; surgical prophylaxis; more active against *H. influenzae* and *N. gonorrhoeae*
Cautions; Contra-indications; Side-effects: see under Cefaclor

Dose: by mouth (as cefuroxime axetil), 250 mg twice daily in most infections including mild to moderate lower respiratory-tract infections (e.g. bronchitis); doubled for more severe lower respiratory-tract infections or if pneumonia suspected
Urinary-tract infection, 125 mg twice daily, doubled in pyelonephritis
Gonorrhoea, 1 g as a single dose
CHILD over 3 months, 125 mg twice daily, if necessary doubled in child over 2 years with otitis media
By intramuscular injection or intravenous injection or infusion, 750 mg every 6–8 hours; 1.5 g every 6–8 hours in severe infections; single doses over 750 mg intravenous route only
CHILD usual dose 60 mg/kg daily (range 30–100 mg/kg daily) in 3–4 divided doses (2–3 divided doses in neonates)
Gonorrhoea, 1.5 g as a single dose by intramuscular injection (divided between 2 sites)
Surgical prophylaxis, 1.5 g by intravenous injection at induction; may be supplemented with 750 mg intramuscularly 8 and 16 hours later (abdominal, pelvic, and orthopaedic operations) *or* followed by 750 mg intramuscularly every 8 hours for further 24–48 hours (cardiac, pulmonary, oesophageal, and vascular operations)
Meningitis, 3 g intravenously every 8 hours; CHILD, 200–240 mg/kg daily (in 3–4 divided doses) reduced to 100 mg/kg daily after 3 days or on clinical improvement; NEONATE, 100 mg/kg daily reduced to 50 mg/kg daily

PoM **Zinacef**® (Glaxo)
Injection, powder for reconstitution, cefuroxime (as sodium salt). Net price 250-mg vial = 88p; 750-mg vial = £2.64; 1.5-g vial (for injection and for infusion) = £5.29
Electrolytes: Na⁺ 1.8 mmol/750-mg vial

PoM **Zinnat**® (Glaxo)
Tablets, both f/c, cefuroxime 125 mg (as cefuroxime axetil), net price 14-tab pack = £6.30; 250 mg, 14-tab pack = £12.60. Label: 9, 21, 25
Suspension, cefuroxime (as cefuroxime axetil) 125 mg/5 mL when reconstituted with water. Net price 70 mL = £7.20. Label: 9, 21
Sachets, cefuroxime (as cefuroxime axetil) 125 mg/sachet, net price 14-sachet pack = £7.20. Label: 9, 13, 21

CEPHALEXIN
Indications: see under Cefaclor
Cautions; Contra-indications; Side-effects: see under Cefaclor
Dose: 250 mg every 6 hours *or* 500 mg every 8–12 hours increased to 1–1.5 g every 6–8 hours for severe infections; CHILD, 25 mg/kg daily in divided doses, doubled for severe infections, max. 100 mg/kg daily; *or* under 1 year, 125 mg every 12 hours; 1–5 years, 125 mg every 8 hours; 6–12 years, 250 mg every 8 hours

Chapter 5: Infections

PoM Cephalexin (Non-proprietary)
Capsules, cephalexin 250 mg, net price 20 = £2.44; 500 mg, 20 = £4.80. Label: 9
Tablets, cephalexin 250 mg, net price 20 = £2.44; 500 mg, 20 = £4.80. Label: 9
Oral suspension, cephalexin for reconstitution with water, 125 mg/5 mL, net price 100 mL = £1.27; 250 mg/5 mL, 100 mL = £2.55. Label: 9

PoM Ceporex® (Glaxo)
Capsules, both caramel/grey, cephalexin 250 mg, net price 20 = £3.00, 28-cap pack = £4.47; 500 mg, 20 = £5.88, 28-cap pack = £8.72. Label: 9
Tablets, all pink, f/c, cephalexin 250 mg, net price 20 = £3.00, 28-tab pack = £4.47; 500 mg, 20 = £5.88, 28-tab pack = £8.72; 1 g (scored), 14-tab pack = £8.72. Label: 9
Paediatric drops, orange, cephalexin 125 mg/1.25 mL when reconstituted with water. Net price 10 mL = £1.52. Label: 9, counselling, use of pipette
Suspension, both yellow, cephalexin 125 mg/5 mL, net price 100 mL = £1.59; 250 mg/5 mL, 100 mL = £3.19. Label: 9
Syrup, all orange, cephalexin for reconstitution with water, 125 mg/5 mL, net price 100 mL = £1.59; 250 mg/5 mL, 100 mL = £3.19; 500 mg/5 mL, 100 mL = £6.19. Label: 9

PoM Keflex® (Lilly)
Capsules, cephalexin 250 mg (green/white), net price 28-cap pack = £3.57; 500 mg (pale green/dark green), 28-cap pack = £6.97. Label: 9
Tablets, both peach, cephalexin 250 mg, net price 28-tab pack = £3.57; 500 mg (scored), 28-tab pack = £6.97. Label: 9
Suspension, cephalexin for reconstitution with water, 125 mg/5 mL (pink), net price 100 mL = £1.27; 250 mg/5 mL (orange), 100 mL = £2.55. Label: 9

CEPHAMANDOLE

Indications: see under Cefaclor; surgical prophylaxis
Cautions; Contra-indications; Side-effects: see under Cefaclor
Dose: by deep intramuscular injection or intravenous injection over 3–5 minutes *or by intravenous infusion*, 0.5–2 g every 4–8 hours; CHILD over 1 month, 50–100 mg/kg daily in 3–6 divided doses increased to 150 mg/kg daily for severe infections
Surgical prophylaxis, *by intramuscular or intravenous injection*, 1–2 g 30–60 minutes before surgery followed by 1–2 g every 6 hours for 24–48 hours (up to 72 hours for implantation of prostheses)

PoM Kefadol® (Dista)
Injection, powder for reconstitution, cephamandole (as nafate) with sodium carbonate. Net price 1-g vial = £3.91
Electrolytes: Na$^+$ 1.19 mmol/1-g vial

CEPHAZOLIN

Indications: see under Cefaclor; surgical prophylaxis
Cautions; Contra-indications; Side-effects: see under Cefaclor
Dose: by intramuscular injection or intravenous injection or infusion, 0.5–1 g every 6–12 hours; CHILD, 25–50 mg/kg daily (in divided doses), increased to 100 mg/kg daily in severe infections

PoM Kefzol® (Lilly)
Injection, powder for reconstitution, cephazolin (as sodium salt). Net price 500-mg vial = £2.45; 1-g vial = £4.63
Electrolytes: Na$^+$ 2.1 mmol/g

CEPHRADINE

Indications: see under Cefaclor; surgical prophylaxis
Cautions; Contra-indications; Side-effects: see under Cefaclor
Dose: by mouth, 250–500 mg every 6 hours *or* 0.5–1 g every 12 hours; CHILD, 25–50 mg/kg daily in divided doses
By intramuscular injection or intravenous injection or infusion, 0.5–1 g every 6 hours, increased to 8 g daily in severe infections; CHILD 50–100 mg/kg daily in 4 divided doses

PoM Velosef® (Squibb)
Capsules, cephradine 250 mg (orange/blue), net price 20-cap pack = £3.55; 500 mg, 20-cap pack = £7.00. Label: 9
Syrup, cephradine 250 mg/5 mL when reconstituted with water. Net price 100 mL = £4.22. Label: 9
Injection, powder for reconstitution, cephradine. Net price 500-mg vial = 99p; 1-g vial = £1.95

OTHER BETA-LACTAM ANTIBIOTICS

Aztreonam is a monocyclic beta-lactam ('monobactam') antibiotic with an antibacterial spectrum limited to Gram-negative aerobic bacteria including *Pseudomonas aeruginosa*, *Neisseria meningitidis*, and *Haemophilus influenzae*; it should not be used alone for 'blind' treatment since it is not active against Gram-positive organisms. Aztreonam is also effective against *Neisseria gonorrhoeae* (but not against concurrent chlamydial infection). Side-effects are similar to those of the other beta-lactams although aztreonam may be less likely to cause hypersensitivity in penicillin-sensitive patients.

Imipenem, a carbapenem, is the first thienamycin beta-lactam antibiotic; it has a broad spectrum of activity which includes many aerobic and anaerobic Gram-positive and Gram-negative bacteria. Imipenem is partially inactivated in the kidney by enzymatic activity and is therefore administered in combination with **cilastatin**, a specific enzyme inhibitor, which blocks its renal metabolism. Side-effects are similar to those of other beta-lactam antibiotics; neurotoxicity has been observed at very high dosage or in renal failure.

AZTREONAM

Indications: Gram-negative infections including *Pseudomonas aeruginosa*, *Haemophilus influenzae*, and *Neisseria meningitidis*
Cautions: hypersensitivity to beta-lactam antibiotics; hepatic impairment; reduce dose in renal impairment; **interactions:** Appendix 1 (aztreonam)
Contra-indications: aztreonam hypersensitivity; pregnancy and breast-feeding
Side-effects: nausea, vomiting, diarrhoea, abdominal cramps; mouth ulcers, altered taste; jaundice and hepatitis; blood disorders (including thrombocytopenia and neutropenia); urticaria and rashes
Dose: by intramuscular injection or intravenous injection or infusion: 1 g every 8 hours *or* 2 g every 12 hours; 2 g every 6–8 hours for severe infections (including systemic *Pseudomonas aeruginosa* and lung infections in cystic fibrosis); single doses over 1 g intravenous route only
CHILD over 1 week, *by intravenous injection or infusion*, 30 mg/kg every 6–8 hours increased in severe infections for child of 2 years or older to 50 mg/kg every 6–8 hours; max. 8 g daily
Urinary-tract infections, 0.5–1 g every 8–12 hours
Gonorrhoea/cystitis, *by intramuscular injection*, 1 g as a single dose

PoM **Azactam**® (Squibb)
Injection, powder for reconstitution, aztreonam. Net price 500-mg vial = £4.48; 1-g vial = £8.95; 2-g vial and 2-g bottle (for preparing infusion) (both) = £17.90

IMIPENEM WITH CILASTATIN

Indications: aerobic and anaerobic Gram-positive and Gram-negative infections
Cautions: hypersensitivity to penicillins, cephalosporins and other beta-lactam antibiotics; renal impairment; CNS disorders (e.g. epilepsy); pregnancy
Contra-indications: hypersensitivity to imipenem or cilastatin; breast-feeding
Side-effects: nausea, vomiting, diarrhoea (pseudomembranous colitis reported), taste disturbances; blood disorders, positive Coombs test; allergic reactions (with rash, pruritus, urticaria, fever, anaphylactic reactions, rarely toxic epidermal necrolysis); myoclonic activity, convulsions, confusion and mental disturbances reported; slight increases in liver enzymes and bilirubin reported; increases in serum creatinine and blood urea; local reactions: erythema, pain and induration, and thrombophlebitis
Dose: by deep intramuscular injection, mild to moderate infections, in terms of imipenem, 500–750 mg every 12 hours; gonococcal urethritis or cervicitis, 500 mg as a single dose
By intravenous infusion, in terms of imipenem, 1–2 g daily in 3–4 divided doses; less sensitive organisms, up to 50 mg/kg daily (to max. 4 g daily); CHILD 3 months and older, 60 mg/kg (up to max. of 2 g) daily in 4 divided doses

PoM **Primaxin**® (MSD)
Intramuscular injection, powder for reconstitution, imipenem (as monohydrate) 500 mg with cilastatin (as sodium salt) 500 mg. Net price 15-mL vial = £15.00
Electrolytes: Na⁺ 1.47 mmol/vial
Intravenous infusion, powder for reconstitution, imipenem (as monohydrate) 250 mg with cilastatin (as sodium salt) 250 mg. Net price 60-mL vial = £9.00
Electrolytes: Na⁺ 0.86 mmol/vial
Intravenous infusion, powder for reconstitution, imipenem (as monohydrate) 500 mg with cilastatin (as sodium salt) 500 mg. Net price 120-mL vial = £15.00
Electrolytes: Na⁺ 1.72 mmol/vial

5.1.3 Tetracyclines

The tetracyclines are broad-spectrum antibiotics whose value has decreased owing to increasing bacterial resistance. They remain, however, the treatment of choice for infections caused by chlamydia (trachoma, psittacosis, salpingitis, urethritis, and lymphogranuloma venereum), rickettsia (including Q-fever), mycoplasma (respiratory and genital infections), brucella (doxycycline with rifampicin), and the spirochaete, *Borrelia burgdorferi* (Lyme disease). They are also used in acne, in destructive (refractory) periodontal disease, in exacerbations of chronic bronchitis (because of their activity against *Haemophilus influenzae*), and for leptospirosis in penicillin hypersensitivity (as an alternative to erythromycin).

Microbiologically, there is little to choose between the various tetracyclines, the only exception being **minocycline** which has a broader spectrum, is active against *Neisseria meningitidis* and has been used for meningococcal prophylaxis; however it may cause dizziness and vertigo.

The tetracyclines are deposited in growing bone and teeth (being bound to calcium) causing staining and occasionally dental hypoplasia, and should **not** be given to children under 12 years or to pregnant women. With the exception of **doxycycline** and **minocycline** the tetracyclines may exacerbate renal failure and should **not** be given to patients with kidney disease. Absorption of tetracyclines is decreased by milk (except doxycycline and minocycline), antacids, and calcium, iron, and magnesium salts.

TETRACYCLINE

Indications: exacerbations of chronic bronchitis; brucellosis (see also notes above), chlamydia, mycoplasma, and rickettsia; pleural effusions due to malignancy or cirrhosis; acne vulgaris (see section 13.6)

Cautions: breast-feeding; hepatic impairment (avoid intravenous administration); renal impairment (avoid if severe); rarely causes photosensitivity; **interactions:** Appendix 1 (tetracyclines)

Contra-indications: severe renal impairment, pregnancy (see also Appendix 4), children under 12 years of age, systemic lupus erythematosus

Side-effects: nausea, vomiting, diarrhoea; erythema (discontinue treatment); headache and visual disturbances may indicate benign intracranial hypertension; pseudomembranous colitis reported

Dose: by mouth, 250 mg every 6 hours, increased in severe infections to 500 mg every 6–8 hours
Acne, see section 13.6
Primary, secondary, or latent syphilis, 500 mg every 6 hours for 15 days
Non-gonococcal urethritis, 500 mg every 6 hours for 7–14 days (21 days if failure or relapse following the first course)
By intramuscular injection, 100 mg every 8–12 hours, or every 4–6 hours in severe infections
By intravenous infusion, 500 mg every 12 hours; max. 2 g daily
Pleural effusions, see under Achromycin® intravenous infusion

COUNSELLING. Tablets or capsules should be swallowed whole with plenty of fluid while sitting or standing

PoM **Tetracycline Tablets,** coated, tetracycline hydrochloride 250 mg. Net price 20 = 30p. Label: 7, 9, 23, counselling, posture, see above

PoM **Achromycin®** (Lederle)
Capsules, orange, tetracycline hydrochloride 250 mg. Net price 20 = 95p. Label: 7, 9, 23, counselling, posture, see above
Tablets, orange, f/c, tetracycline hydrochloride 250 mg. Net price 20 = 67p. Label: 7, 9, 23, counselling, posture, see above
Intramuscular injection, powder for reconstitution, tetracycline hydrochloride 100 mg, procaine hydrochloride 40 mg. Net price per vial = £1.09
Intravenous infusion, powder for reconstitution, tetracycline hydrochloride. Net price 250-mg vial = £1.27; 500-mg vial = £2.43
Dose: infections, see above
Recurrent pleural effusions, by intrapleural instillation, 500 mg in 30–50 mL sodium chloride intravenous infusion 0.9%

PoM **Sustamycin®** (Boehringer Mannheim)
Capsules, m/r, light blue/dark blue, tetracycline hydrochloride 250 mg. Net price 20 = £2.12. Label: 7, 9, 23, 25
Dose: 2 capsules initially, then 1 every 12 hours

PoM **Tetrabid-Organon®** (Organon)
Capsules, m/r, purple/yellow, tetracycline hydrochloride 250 mg. Net price 20 = £1.73. Label: 7, 9, 23, 25
Dose: 2 capsules initially, then 1 every 12 hours; acne, 1 daily

PoM **Tetrachel®** (Berk)
Capsules, orange, tetracycline hydrochloride 250 mg. Net price 20 = 30p. Label: 7, 9, 23, counselling, posture, see above
Tablets, orange, f/c, tetracycline hydrochloride 250 mg. Net price 20 = 30p. Label: 7, 9, 23, counselling, posture, see above

Compound preparations

PoM **Deteclo®** (Lederle)
Tablets, blue, f/c, tetracycline hydrochloride 115.4 mg, chlortetracycline hydrochloride 115.4 mg, demeclocycline hydrochloride 69.2 mg. Net price 20 = £2.54. Label: 7, 9, 11, 23, counselling, posture, see above
Dose: 1 tablet every 12 hours; 3–4 tablets daily in more severe infections

PoM **Mysteclin®** (Squibb)
Tablets, orange, s/c, tetracycline hydrochloride 250 mg, nystatin 250 000 units. Net price 20 = £1.34. Label: 7, 9, 23, counselling, posture, see above

CHLORTETRACYCLINE HYDROCHLORIDE

Indications; Cautions; Contra-indications; Side-effects: see under Tetracycline
Dose: 250–500 mg every 6 hours

PoM **Aureomycin®** (Lederle)
Capsules, yellow, chlortetracycline hydrochloride 250 mg. Net price 20 = £2.36. Label: 7, 9, 23

DEMECLOCYCLINE HYDROCHLORIDE

Indications: see under Tetracycline; also inappropriate secretion of antidiuretic hormone, section 6.5.2
Cautions; Contra-indications; Side-effects: see under Tetracycline, but photosensitivity is more common
Dose: 150 mg every 6 hours *or* 300 mg every 12 hours

PoM **Ledermycin®** (Lederle)
Capsules, red, demeclocycline hydrochloride 150 mg. Net price 20 = £4.24. Label: 7, 9, 11, 23

DOXYCYCLINE

Indications: see under Tetracycline; brucellosis (with rifampicin); also chronic prostatitis and sinusitis
Cautions; Contra-indications; Side-effects: see under Tetracycline, but may be used in renal impairment; avoid in porphyria (see section 9.8.2)

Dose: 200 mg on first day, then 100 mg daily; severe infections (including chronic urinary-tract infections), 200 mg daily
Acne, 50 mg daily for 6–12 weeks or longer
COUNSELLING. Capsules should be swallowed whole with plenty of fluid during meals while sitting or standing

PoM **Doxycycline** (Non-proprietary)
Capsules, doxycycline 100 mg (as hydrochloride). Net price 20 = £9.32. Label: 6, 9, 27, counselling, posture, see above
Available from APS, Ashbourne (Demix®), Hillcross, Kerfoot, Lagap (Doxylar®), Norton

PoM **Nordox**® (Panpharma)
Capsules, green, doxycycline 100 mg (as hydrochloride). Net price 10-cap pack = £4.66. Label: 6, 9, 27, counselling, posture, see above

PoM **Vibramycin**® (Invicta)
Capsules, doxycycline (as hydrochloride) 50 mg (green/ivory), net price 28-cap pack = £7.74; 100 mg (green), 8-cap pack = £4.18. Label: 6, 9, 27, counselling, posture, see above

PoM **Vibramycin-D**® (Invicta)
Dispersible tablets, off-white, doxycycline 100 mg. Net price 8-tab pack = £4.91. Label: 6, 9, 13

LYMECYCLINE
Indications; Cautions; Contra-indications; Side-effects: see under Tetracycline
Dose: 408 mg every 12 hours

PoM **Tetralysal 300**® (Farmitalia Carlo Erba)
Capsules, lymecycline 408 mg (≡ tetracycline 300 mg). Net price 20-cap pack = £3.04. Label: 6, 9

MINOCYCLINE
Indications: see under Tetracycline; also meningococcal carrier state
Cautions; Contra-indications: see under Tetracycline, but may be used in renal impairment
Side-effects: see under Tetracycline; also dizziness and vertigo (more common in women); severe exfoliative rashes and liver damage reported
Dose: 100 mg twice daily
Acne, 50 mg twice daily for minimum course of 6 weeks (*caution*: higher doses associated with hyperpigmentation of acne lesions)

PoM **Minocycline** (Non-proprietary)
Tablets, minocycline (as hydrochloride) 50 mg, net price 84-tab pack = £27.68; 100 mg, 20-tab pack = £13.17. Label: 6, 9
Available from Ashbourne (Blemix®)

PoM **Minocin**® (Lederle)
Tablets, both f/c, minocycline (as hydrochloride) 50 mg (beige), net price 84-tab pack = £27.68; 100 mg (orange), 20-tab pack = £13.17. Label: 6, 9

PoM **Minocin MR**® (Lederle)
Capsules, m/r, yellow/brown (enclosing yellow and orange pellets), minocycline hydrochloride 100 mg. Net price 49-cap pack = £27.68. Label: 6, 25
Dose: acne, 1 capsule daily

OXYTETRACYCLINE
Indications; Cautions; Contra-indications; Side-effects: see under Tetracycline; avoid in porphyria (see section 9.8.2)
Dose: 250–500 mg every 6 hours

PoM **Oxytetracycline** (Non-proprietary)
Tablets, coated, oxytetracycline dihydrate 250 mg, net price 20 = 24p. Label: 7, 9, 23
Available from APS, Ashbourne (Oxytetramix®), Berk (Berkmycen®, contain tartrazine), Cox, CP, DDSA (Oxymycin®), Evans, Kerfoot, Norton

PoM **Imperacin**® (ICI)
Tablets, yellow, f/c, oxytetracycline dihydrate 250 mg. Net price 20 = 49p. Label: 7, 9, 23
Additives: include tartrazine

PoM **Terramycin**® (Pfizer)
Capsules, yellow, oxytetracycline 250 mg (as hydrochloride). Net price 28-cap pack = 96p. Label: 7, 9, 23
Tablets, yellow, s/c, oxytetracycline 250 mg (as dihydrate). Net price 28-tab pack = 96p. Label: 7, 9, 23

5.1.4 Aminoglycosides

These include amikacin, gentamicin, kanamycin, neomycin, netilmicin, streptomycin, and tobramycin. All are bactericidal and active against some Gram-positive and many Gram-negative organisms. Amikacin, gentamicin, and tobramycin are also active against *Pseudomonas aeruginosa*; streptomycin is active against *Mycobacterium tuberculosis* and is now almost entirely reserved for tuberculosis (section 5.1.9).

The aminoglycosides are not absorbed from the gut (although there is a risk of absorption in inflammatory bowel disease and liver failure) and must therefore be given by injection for systemic infections.

Excretion is principally via the kidney and accumulation occurs in renal impairment.

Most side-effects of this group of antibiotics are dose-related therefore care must be taken with dosage and whenever possible treatment should not exceed 7 days. The important side-effects are ototoxicity, and to a lesser degree nephrotoxicity; they occur most commonly in the elderly and in patients with renal failure.

If there is impairment of renal function (or high pre-dose plasma concentrations) the interval between doses must be increased; if the renal impairment is severe the dose itself should be reduced as well.

Aminoglycosides may impair neuromuscular transmission and should not be given to patients with myasthenia gravis; large doses given during surgery have been responsible for a transient myasthenic syndrome in patients with normal neuromuscular function.

Aminoglycosides should not be given with potentially ototoxic diuretics (e.g. frusemide and ethacrynic acid); if concurrent use is unavoidable administration of the aminoglycoside and of the diuretic should be separated by as long a period as practicable.

Neomycin is too toxic for parenteral administration and can only be used for infections of the skin or mucous membranes or to reduce the bacterial population of the colon prior to bowel surgery or in hepatic failure. Oral administration may lead to malabsorption. Small amounts of neomycin may be absorbed from the gut in patients with hepatic failure and, as these patients may also be uraemic, cumulation may occur with resultant ototoxicity.

PREGNANCY. Where possible, the aminoglycosides should be avoided in pregnancy as they cross the placenta and can cause fetal eighth nerve damage.

PLASMA CONCENTRATIONS. Plasma concentration monitoring avoids both excessive and subtherapeutic concentrations, thus preventing toxicity and, at the same time, ensuring efficacy.

If possible plasma concentrations of aminoglycosides should be measured in all patients and **must** be determined in infants *or* if high doses are being given, *or* if there is renal impairment, *or* if treatment lasts longer than 7 days.

Note. Plasma concentrations should be measured approximately one hour after intravenous or intramuscular injection, and also just before the next dose.

Gentamicin is the most important of the aminoglycosides and is widely used for the treatment of serious infections. It is the aminoglycoside of choice in the UK. It has a broad spectrum but is inactive against anaerobes and has poor activity against haemolytic streptococci and pneumococci. When used for the 'blind' therapy of undiagnosed serious infections it is usually given in conjunction with a penicillin and/or metronidazole.

The daily dose is up to 5 mg/kg given in divided doses every 8 hours (if renal function is normal); whenever possible treatment should not exceed 7 days. Higher doses are occasionally indicated for serious infections, especially in the neonate or the compromised host. A lower dose of 80 mg twice daily (60 mg for lighter or elderly patients) in association with benzylpenicillin is sufficient for endocarditis due to oral streptococci (often termed *Streptococcus viridans*) and gut streptococci.

Amikacin is a derivative of kanamycin and has one important advantage over gentamicin in that it is stable to 8 of the 9 classified aminoglycoside-inactivating enzymes whereas gentamicin is inactivated by 5. It is principally indicated for the treatment of serious infections caused by Gram-negative bacilli resistant to gentamicin.

Kanamycin has been superseded by other aminoglycosides.

Netilmicin has similar activity to gentamicin, but may cause less ototoxicity in those needing treatment for longer than 10 days. Netilmicin is active against a number of gentamicin-resistant Gram-negative bacilli but is less active against *Ps. aeruginosa* than gentamicin or tobramycin.

Tobramycin is similar to gentamicin. It is slightly more active against *Ps. aeruginosa* but shows less activity against certain other Gram-negative bacteria.

GENTAMICIN

Indications: septicaemia and neonatal sepsis; meningitis and other CNS infections; biliary tract infection, acute pyelonephritis or prostatitis, endocarditis caused by *Strep. viridans* or *strep. faecalis* (with a penicillin)

Cautions: renal impairment, infants and elderly (adjust dose and monitor renal, auditory and vestibular function together with plasma gentamicin concentrations); avoid prolonged use; **interactions:** Appendix 1 (aminoglycosides)

Contra-indications: pregnancy, myasthenia gravis

Side-effects: vestibular damage, reversible nephrotoxicity; rarely, hypomagnesaemia on prolonged therapy, pseudomembranous colitis; see also notes above

Dose: by intramuscular or by slow intravenous injection over at least 3 minutes *or by intravenous infusion*, 2–5 mg/kg daily (in divided doses every 8 hours). In renal impairment the interval between successive doses should be increased to 12 hours when the creatinine clearance is 30–70 mL/minute, 24 hours for 10–30 mL/minute, 48 hours for 5–10 mL/minute, and after twice-weekly dialysis for less than 5 mL/minute

CHILD up to 2 weeks, 3 mg/kg every 12 hours; 2 weeks–12 years, 2 mg/kg every 8 hours

By intrathecal injection, 1 mg daily (increased if necessary to 5 mg daily), with 2–4 mg/kg daily *by intramuscular injection* (in divided doses every 8 hours)

Endocarditis prophylaxis, section 5.1, table 2

Note. One-hour ('peak') concentration should not exceed 10 mg/litre; pre-dose ('trough') concentration should be less than 2 mg/litre

PoM **Gentamicin** (Non-proprietary)

Injection (without preservative), gentamicin (as sulphate), net price 10 mg/mL, 1-mL amp = 50p, 2-mL vial = £1.08; 40 mg/mL, 1-mL amp = £1.26, 2-mL amp = £1.72, 2-mL vial = £1.77

Available from David Bull

5.1.4 Aminoglycosides 219

PoM **Cidomycin**® (Roussel)
Injection, gentamicin 40 mg (as sulphate)/mL. Net price 2-mL amp or vial = £1.59
Paediatric injection, gentamicin 10 mg (as sulphate)/mL. Net price 2-mL vial = 67p
Intrathecal injection, gentamicin 5 mg (as sulphate)/mL. Net price 1-mL amp = 79p

PoM **Genticin**® (Nicholas)
Injection, gentamicin 40 mg (as sulphate)/mL. Net price 2-mL amp or vial = £1.58

PoM **Isotonic Gentamicin Injection** (Baxter)
Intravenous infusion, gentamicin 800 micrograms (as sulphate)/mL in sodium chloride intravenous infusion 0.9%. Net price 100-mL (80-mg) Viaflex® bag = £1.65
Electrolytes: Na$^+$ 15.4 mmol/100-mL bag

AMIKACIN

Indications: serious Gram-negative infections resistant to gentamicin
Cautions; Contra-indications; Side-effects: see under Gentamicin
Dose: by intramuscular or by slow intravenous injection or by infusion, 15 mg/kg daily in 2 divided doses
Note. One-hour ('peak') concentration should not exceed 30 mg/litre; pre-dose ('trough') concentration should be less than 10 mg/litre

PoM **Amikin**® (Bristol-Myers)
Injection, amikacin 250 mg (as sulphate)/mL. Net price 2-mL vial = £10.14
Paediatric injection, amikacin 50 mg (as sulphate)/mL. Net price 2-mL vial = £2.36

KANAMYCIN

Indications: superseded by other aminoglycosides (see notes above)
Cautions; Contra-indications; Side-effects: see under Gentamicin
Dose: by intramuscular injection, 250 mg every 6 hours *or* 500 mg every 12 hours
By intravenous infusion, 15–30 mg/kg daily in divided doses every 8–12 hours
Note. One-hour ('peak') concentration should not exceed 30 mg/litre; pre-dose ('trough') concentration should be less than 10 mg/litre

PoM **Kannasyn**® (Sanofi·Winthrop)
Powder (for preparing injections), kanamycin (as acid sulphate). Net price 1-g vial = £22.16

NEOMYCIN SULPHATE

Indications: bowel sterilisation prior to surgery, see also notes above
Cautions; Contra-indications; Side-effects: see under Gentamicin but too toxic for systemic use, see notes above; avoid in renal impairment
Dose: by mouth, bowel sterilisation, 1 g every 4 hours

PoM **Neomycin Elixir**, neomycin sulphate 100 mg/5 mL. Net price 100 mL = 66p
PoM **Mycifradin**® (Upjohn)
Tablets, neomycin sulphate 500 mg. Net price 20 = £3.60

PoM **Nivemycin**® (Boots)
Tablets, neomycin sulphate 500 mg. Net price 20 = £2.06
Elixir, neomycin sulphate 100 mg/5 mL. Net price 100 mL = 66p

NETILMICIN

Indications: serious Gram-negative infections resistant to gentamicin
Cautions; Contra-indications; Side-effects: see under Gentamicin
Dose: by intramuscular injection or by intravenous injection over 3–5 minutes or by intravenous infusion, 4–6 mg/kg daily, as a single daily dose or in divided doses every 8 or 12 hours; in severe infections, up to 7.5 mg/kg daily in divided doses every 8 hours (reduced as soon as clinically indicated, usually within 48 hours) NEONATE up to 1 week, 3 mg/kg every 12 hours; INFANT over 1 week, 2.5–3 mg/kg every 8 hours; CHILD 2–2.5 mg/kg every 8 hours
Urinary-tract infection, 150 mg as a single daily dose for 5 days
Gonorrhoea, 300 mg as a single dose
Note. For divided daily dose regimens, one-hour ('peak') concentration should not exceed 12 mg/litre; pre-dose ('trough') concentration should be less than 2 mg/litre

PoM **Netillin**® (Schering-Plough)
Injection, netilmicin (as sulphate) 10 mg/mL, net price 1.5-mL (15-mg) amp = £1.49; 50 mg/mL, 1-mL (50-mg) amp = £2.21; 100 mg/mL, 1-mL (100-mg) amp = £2.88; 1.5-mL (150-mg) amp = £4.11, 2-mL (200-mg) amp = £5.33

TOBRAMYCIN

Indications: see under Gentamicin and notes above
Cautions; Contra-indications; Side-effects: see under Gentamicin
Dose: by intramuscular injection or by slow intravenous injection or by intravenous infusion, 3 mg/kg daily in divided doses every 8 hours; in severe infections up to 5 mg/kg daily in divided doses every 6–8 hours (reduced to 3 mg/kg as soon as clinically indicated); NEONATE 2 mg/kg every 12 hours; CHILD over 1 week 2–2.5 mg/kg every 8 hours
Urinary-tract infection, *by intramuscular injection*, 2–3 mg/kg daily as a single dose
Note. One-hour ('peak') concentration should not exceed 10 mg/litre; pre-dose ('trough') concentration should be less than 2 mg/litre

PoM **Nebcin**® (Lilly)
Injection, tobramycin (as sulphate) 10 mg/mL, net price 2-mL (20-mg) vial = £1.08; 40 mg/mL, 1-mL (40-mg) vial = £1.46, 2-mL (80-mg) vial = £2.63

5.1.5 Macrolides

Erythromycin has an antibacterial spectrum that is similar but not identical to that of penicillin; it is thus an alternative in penicillin-allergic patients.

Indications for erythromycin include respiratory infections in children, whooping-cough, legionnaires' disease, and campylobacter enteritis. It has activity against gut anaerobes and has been used with neomycin for prophylaxis before bowel surgery. It is active against many penicillin-resistant staphylococci but some are now also resistant to erythromycin. Erythromycin is also active against chlamydia and mycoplasmas.

Erythromycin causes nausea, vomiting, and diarrhoea in some patients; in mild to moderate infections this can be avoided by giving a lower dose (250 mg 4 times daily) but if a more serious infection, such as Legionella pneumonia, is suspected higher doses are needed.

Azithromycin is a new macrolide with slightly less activity than erythromycin against Gram-positive bacteria but enhanced activity against some Gram-negative organisms. Plasma concentrations are very low but tissue concentrations are much higher. It has a long plasma half-life and once daily dosage is recommended.

Clarithromycin is an erythromycin derivative with slightly greater activity than the parent compound. Tissue concentrations are higher than with erythromycin. It is given twice daily.

Azithromycin and clarithromycin cause fewer gastro-intestinal side-effects than erythromycin.

Spiramycin is also a macrolide (see section 5.4.7).

ERYTHROMYCIN

Indications: alternative to penicillin in hypersensitive patients; sinusitis, diphtheria and whooping cough prophylaxis; legionnaires' disease; chronic prostatitis; acne vulgaris (see section 13.6)

Cautions: hepatic and renal impairment; pregnancy and breast-feeding; **interactions:** Appendix 1 (erythromycin)

Contra-indications: porphyria (see section 9.8.2); estolate contra-indicated in liver disease

Side-effects: nausea, vomiting, abdominal discomfort, diarrhoea after large doses; reversible hearing loss also reported after large doses; if given for more than 14 days may occasionally cause cholestatic jaundice

Dose: by mouth, ADULT and CHILD over 8 years, 250–500 mg every 6 hours *or* 0.5–1 g every 12 hours (see notes above); up to 4 g daily in severe infections; CHILD up to 2 years 125 mg every 6 hours, 2–8 years 250 mg every 6 hours, doses doubled for severe infections

Acne, see section 13.6

Early syphilis, 500 mg 4 times daily for 14 days

By intravenous infusion, ADULT and CHILD severe infections, 50 mg/kg daily by continuous infusion *or* in divided doses every 6 hours; mild infections (oral treatment not possible), 25 mg/kg daily

PoM **Erythromycin** (Non-proprietary)
Tablets, e/c, erythromycin 250 mg, net price 20 = 86p; 500 mg, 20 = £2.03. Label: 5, 9, 25
Available from APS, Ashbourne (Rommix®), Berk (Erycen®), Cox, CP, Evans, Kerfoot, Norton
Mixture, erythromycin (as ethyl succinate) 125 mg/5 mL, net price 100 mL = £1.47; 250 mg/5 mL, 100 mL = £2.17; 500 mg/5 mL, 100 mL = £3.59. Label: 9
Available from APS, Ashbourne (Rommix®), Berk, Cox, CP, Evans, Kerfoot, Norton, RP Drugs (Arpimycin®)

PoM **Erythromycin Lactobionate** (Non-proprietary)
Intravenous infusion, powder for reconstitution, erythromycin (as lactobionate). Net price 1-g vial = £9.60
Available from David Bull

PoM **Erymax®** (P-D)
Capsules, opaque orange/clear orange, enclosing orange and white e/c pellets, erythromycin 250 mg. Net price 30-cap pack = £6.25. Label: 5, 9, 25
Dose: 1 every 6 hours *or* 2 every 12 hours; acne, 1 twice daily then 1 daily after 1 month

PoM **Erythrocin®** (Abbott)
Tablets, both f/c, erythromycin (as stearate), 250 mg, net price 20 = £2.13; 500 mg, 20 = £4.48. Label: 9
Intravenous infusion, powder for reconstitution, erythromycin (as lactobionate). Net price l-g vial = £8.63

PoM **Erythromid®** (Abbott)
Tablets, orange, e/c, f/c, erythromycin 250 mg. Net price 20 = 86p. Label: 5, 9, 25

PoM **Erythromid DS®** (Abbott)
Tablets, e/c, f/c, erythromycin 500 mg. Net price 20 = £1.94. Label: 5, 9, 25

PoM **Erythroped®** (Abbott)
Suspension PI, erythromycin 125 mg (as ethyl succinate)/5 mL when reconstituted with water. Net price 140 mL = £2.13. Label: 9
Suspension PI SF, sugar-free, erythromycin 125 mg (as ethyl succinate)/5 mL when reconstituted with water. Net price 140 mL = £2.20. Label: 9
Granules PI, erythromycin (as ethyl succinate) 125 mg/sachet. Net price 28-sachet pack = £2.99. Label: 9, 13
Suspension, erythromycin 250 mg (as ethyl succinate)/5 mL when reconstituted with water. Net price 140 mL = £4.04. Label: 9
Suspension SF, sugar-free, erythromycin 250 mg (as ethyl succinate)/5 mL when reconstituted with water. Net price 140 mL = £4.28. Label: 9
Granules, erythromycin (as ethyl succinate) 250 mg/sachet. Net price 28-sachet pack = £5.05. Label: 9, 13
Suspension forte, erythromycin 500 mg (as ethyl succinate)/5 mL when reconstituted with water. Net price 140 mL = £7.16. Label: 9
Granules forte, erythromycin (as ethyl succinate) 500 mg/sachet. Net price 28-sachet pack = £8.17. Label: 9, 13

5.1.6 Clindamycin

PoM **Erythroped A**® (Abbott)
Tablets, yellow, f/c, erythromycin 500 mg (as ethyl succinate). Net price 28-tab pack = £6.47. Label: 9
Granules, erythromycin 1 g (as ethyl succinate)/sachet. Net price 14-sachet pack = £7.50. Label: 9, 13

PoM **Ilosone**® (Dista)
Capsules, ivory/red, erythromycin 250 mg (as estolate). Net price 20 = £4.15. Label: 9
Tablets, pink, erythromycin 500 mg (as estolate). Net price 12-tab pack = £4.96. Label: 9
Suspension, orange, erythromycin 125 mg (as estolate)/5 mL. Net price 100 mL = £2.51. Label: 9
Suspension forte, orange, erythromycin 250 mg (as estolate)/5 mL. Net price 100 mL = £4.89. Label: 9

AZITHROMYCIN

Indications: respiratory-tract infections; otitis media; skin and soft-tissue infections; uncomplicated genital chlamydial infections
Cautions; Side-effects: see under Erythromycin; caution in renal impairment, pregnancy and breast-feeding; mild neutropenia reported; **interactions:** Appendix 1 (azithromycin)
Contra-indications: hepatic impairment
Dose: 500 mg once daily for 3 days *or* 500 mg once daily on first day then 250 mg daily for 4 days; CHILD 10 mg/kg on first day then 5 mg/kg once daily for 4 days; *or* body-weight 15–25 kg, 200 mg on first day then 100 mg once daily for 4 days; body-weight 26–35 kg, 300 mg on first day then 150 mg once daily; body-weight 36–45 kg, 400 mg on first day then 200 mg once daily
Genital chlamydial infections, 1 g as a single dose

▼ PoM **Zithromax**® (Richborough)
Capsules, azithromycin (as dihydrate) 250 mg. Net price 4-cap pack = £9.99, 6-cap. pack = £14.99. Label: 5, 9, 23
Oral suspension, azithromycin (as dihydrate) 200 mg/5 mL when reconstituted with water. Net price 15-mL pack = £7.05, 22.5-mL pack = £10.35, 30-mL pack = £13.80. Label: 5, 9, 23

CLARITHROMYCIN

Indications: respiratory-tract infections, mild to moderate skin and soft tissue infections
Cautions; Side-effects: see under Erythromycin; reduce dose in renal impairment; headache reported rarely
Dose: 250 mg every 12 hours for 7 days, increased in severe infections to 500 mg every 12 hours for up to 14 days; CHILD under 12 years not yet recommended

▼ PoM **Klaricid**® (Abbott)
Tablets, yellow, f/c, clarithromycin 250 mg. Net price 14-tab pack = £10.98. Label: 9

5.1.6 Clindamycin

Clindamycin has only a limited use because of serious side-effects. Its most serious toxic effect is pseudomembranous colitis (see section 1.5) which may be fatal and is most common in middle-aged and elderly women, especially following operation. Although it can occur with most antibiotics it is more frequently seen with clindamycin. Patients should therefore discontinue treatment immediately if diarrhoea develops.

Clindamycin is active against Gram-positive cocci, including penicillin-resistant staphylococci and also against many anaerobes, especially *Bacteroides fragilis*. It is well concentrated in bone and excreted in bile and urine.

Clindamycin is recommended for staphylococcal joint and bone infections such as osteomyelitis, and intra-abdominal sepsis. Clindamycin is also used for endocarditis prophylaxis (section 5.1, Table 2).

CLINDAMYCIN

Indications: staphylococcal bone and joint infections, peritonitis; endocarditis prophylaxis, section 5.1, Table 2
Cautions: discontinue immediately if diarrhoea or colitis develops; hepatic or renal impairment; monitor liver function and blood counts on prolonged therapy and in neonates and infants; pregnancy; **interactions:** Appendix 1 (clindamycin)
Contra-indications: diarrhoeal states
Side-effects: diarrhoea (discontinue treatment), abdominal discomfort, nausea, vomiting, pseudomembranous colitis; rash; jaundice and altered liver function tests; neutropenia, eosinophilia, agranulocytosis and thrombocytopenia reported; pain, induration, and abscess after intramuscular injection; thrombophlebitis after intravenous injection
Dose: by mouth, 150–300 mg every 6 hours; up to 450 mg every 6 hours in severe infections; CHILD, 3–6 mg/kg every 6 hours
COUNSELLING. Patients should discontinue immediately and contact doctor if diarrhoea develops; capsules should be swallowed with a glass of water.
By deep intramuscular injection or by intravenous infusion, 0.6–2.7 g daily in 2–4 divided doses; life-threatening infection, up to 4.8 g daily; single doses above 600 mg by intravenous infusion only; single doses by intravenous infusion not to exceed 1.2 g
CHILD over 1 month, 15–40 mg/kg daily in 3–4 divided doses; severe infections, at least 300 mg daily regardless of weight
Endocarditis prophylaxis, section 5.1, Table 2

PoM **Dalacin C**® (Upjohn)
Capsules, clindamycin (as hydrochloride) 75 mg (lavender), net price 20 = £4.92; 150 mg, (lavender/maroon), 20 = £9.07. Label: 9, 27, counselling, see above (diarrhoea)

Paediatric suspension, pink, clindamycin 75 mg (as palmitate hydrochloride)/5 mL when reconstituted with purified water (freshly boiled and cooled). Net price 100 mL = £6.62. Label: 9, 27, counselling, see above (diarrhoea)
Injection, clindamycin 150 mg (as phosphate)/mL. Net price 2-mL amp = £5.17; 4-mL amp = £10.29

5.1.7 Some other antibiotics

Antibacterials discussed in this section include chloramphenicol, fusidic acid, spectinomycin, glycopeptide antibiotics (vancomycin and teicoplanin), and the polymyxins (colistin and polymyxin B).

Chloramphenicol is a potent, potentially toxic, broad-spectrum antibiotic which should be reserved for the treatment of life-threatening infections, particularly those caused by *Haemophilus influenzae*, and also for typhoid fever.

Its toxicity renders it unsuitable for systemic use except in the circumstances indicated above.

Eye-drops of chloramphenicol (see section 11.3.1) are useful for bacterial conjunctivitis.

CHLORAMPHENICOL

Indications: see notes above
Cautions: avoid repeated courses and prolonged treatment; reduce doses in hepatic or renal impairment; blood counts required before and periodically during treatment; may cause 'grey syndrome' in neonates (monitor plasma concentrations); **interactions:** Appendix 1 (chloramphenicol)
Contra-indications: pregnancy (see also Appendix 4), breast-feeding, porphyria (see section 9.8.2)
Side-effects: blood disorders including irreversible aplastic anaemia (aplastic anaemia attributed to chloramphenicol has terminated in leukaemia), peripheral neuritis, optic neuritis, erythema multiforme, nausea, vomiting, diarrhoea, nocturnal haemoglobinuria reported)
Dose: by mouth or by intravenous injection or infusion, 50 mg/kg daily in 4 divided doses (exceptionally, can be doubled for severe infections such as septicaemia and meningitis, providing high doses reduced as soon as clinically indicated); CHILD, haemophilus epiglottitis and pyogenic meningitis, 50–100 mg/kg daily in divided doses (high dosages decreased as soon as clinically indicated); INFANTS under 2 weeks 25 mg/kg daily (in 4 divided doses), 2 weeks–1 year 50 mg/kg daily (in 4 divided doses)
Note. Plasma concentration monitoring required in neonates and preferred in those under 4 years of age; recommended peak plasma concentration 15–25 mg/litre; pre-dose ('trough') concentration should not exceed 15 mg/litre

PoM **Chloromycetin®** (P-D)
Capsules, white/grey, chloramphenicol 250 mg. Net price 20 = £1.64
Suspension, chloramphenicol 125 mg (as palmitate)/5 mL. Net price 100 mL = £3.85
Injection, powder for reconstitution, chloramphenicol (as sodium succinate). Net price 300 mg vial = £5.16; 1.2-g vial = £5.03
Electrolytes: Na⁺ 0.94 mmol/300-mg vial, 3.75 mmol/1.2-g vial

PoM **Kemicetine®** (Farmitalia Carlo Erba)
Injection, powder for reconstitution, chloramphenicol (as sodium succinate). Net price 1-g vial = 99p
Electrolytes: Na⁺ 3.14 mmol/g

Fusidic acid and its salts are narrow-spectrum antibiotics. The only indication for their use is in infections caused by penicillin-resistant staphylococci, especially osteomyelitis, as they are well concentrated in bone; a second antistaphylococcal antibiotic is usually required to prevent emergence of resistance.

SODIUM FUSIDATE

Indications: see notes above
Cautions: liver-function tests required
Side-effects: nausea, vomiting, rashes, reversible jaundice, especially after high dosage or rapid infusion (withdraw therapy if persistent)
Dose: see under Preparations, below

PoM **Fucidin®** (Leo)
Tablets, f/c, sodium fusidate 250 mg. Net price 20 = £13.89. Label: 9
Dose: 500 mg every 8 hours, doubled for severe infections
Suspension, orange, fusidic acid 250 mg (≡ sodium fusidate 175 mg)/5 mL. Do not dilute. Net price 50 mL = £7.77. Label: 9, 21
Dose: as fusidic acid, ADULT 750 mg every 8 hours; CHILD up to 1 year 50 mg/kg daily (in 3 divided doses), 1–5 years 250 mg every 8 hours, 5–12 years 500 mg every 8 hours
Note. Fusidic acid is incompletely absorbed and doses recommended for suspension are proportionately higher than those for sodium fusidate tablets

Intravenous infusion, powder for reconstitution, diethanolamine fusidate 580 mg (≡ sodium fusidate 500 mg), with buffer. Net price per vial (with diluent) = £4.65
Electrolytes: Na⁺ 14 mmol/vial when reconstituted with buffer
Dose: as diethanolamine fusidate, by intravenous infusion, ADULT over 50 kg, 580 mg 3 times daily; ADULT under 50 kg and CHILD, 6–7 mg/kg 3 times daily

Spectinomycin is active against Gram-negative organisms, including *N. gonorrhoeae*. Its only indication is the treatment of gonorrhoea caused by penicillin-resistant organisms or in a penicillin-allergic patient.

SPECTINOMYCIN

Indications: see notes above
Cautions: pregnancy and breast-feeding; **interactions:** Appendix 1 (spectinomycin)
Side-effects: nausea, dizziness, urticaria, fever
Dose: by deep intramuscular injection, 2 g; up to 4 g in difficult-to-treat cases and in geographical areas of resistance; CHILD over 2 years, if no alternative treatment, 40 mg/kg

PoM **Trobicin**® (Upjohn)
Injection, powder for reconstitution, spectinomycin (as hydrochloride). Net price 2-g vial (with diluent) = £8.16

VANCOMYCIN AND TEICOPLANIN

The glycopeptide antibiotics vancomycin and teicoplanin have bactericidal activity against aerobic and anaerobic Gram-positive bacteria.

Vancomycin is the drug of choice for antibiotic-associated pseudomembranous colitis, for which it is given by mouth; a dose of 125 mg every 6 hours for 7 to 10 days is considered to be adequate; it is not absorbed by mouth. It has a limited use by the intravenous route in the prophylaxis and treatment of endocarditis and other serious infections caused by Gram-positive cocci including multi-resistant staphylococci. It has a relatively long duration of action and can therefore be given every 12 hours; plasma concentrations should be monitored (especially in patients with renal impairment in whom the dose may need marked reduction). It is ototoxic and nephrotoxic.

Teicoplanin is very similar to vancomycin but has a significantly longer duration of action allowing once daily administration. Unlike vancomycin, teicoplanin can be given by intramuscular as well as by intravenous injection.

VANCOMYCIN

Indications: see notes above
Cautions: extravasation at injection site may cause necrosis and thrombophlebitis; blood counts and hearing, liver, and kidney function tests required; reduce dose in elderly; **interactions:** Appendix 1 (vancomycin)
Contra-indications: if possible avoid parenteral administration in patients with renal impairment or a history of deafness
Side-effects: after parenteral administration nausea, chills, fever, urticaria, rashes, 'red man' syndrome (on rapid intravenous injection), eosinophilia, tinnitus (discontinue use), renal impairment
Dose: by mouth, 125 mg every 6 hours for 7–10 days, see notes above; CHILD, half adult dose
By intravenous infusion, 500 mg over at least 60 minutes every 6 hours *or* 1 g over at least 100 minutes every 12 hours; NEONATE up to 1 week, 15 mg/kg initially then 10 mg/kg every 12 hours; INFANT 1–4 weeks, 15 mg/kg initially then 10 mg/kg every 8 hours; CHILD over 1 month, 10 mg/kg every 6 hours

Note. Plasma concentration monitoring required; peak plasma concentration should not exceed 30 mg/litre; pre-dose ('trough') concentration should not exceed 10 mg/litre

Endocarditis prophylaxis, section 5.1, table 2

PoM **Vancocin**® (Lilly)
Matrigel capsules, vancomycin (as hydrochloride) 125 mg (blue/peach), net price 20-cap pack = £63.08; 250 mg (blue/grey), 20-cap pack = £126.16
Injection, powder for reconstitution, vancomycin (as hydrochloride). Net price 500-mg vial = £10.69

TEICOPLANIN

Indications: potentially serious Gram-positive infections including endocarditis, dialysis-associated peritonitis, and serious infections due to *Staphylococcus aureus*
Cautions: blood counts and liver and kidney function tests required; reduce dose in renal impairment (and monitor renal and auditory function on prolonged administration or if other nephrotoxic drugs given); reduce dose in elderly
Side-effects: nausea, vomiting, diarrhoea; rash, fever, bronchospasm, anaphylactic reactions; dizziness, headache; blood disorders including eosinophilia, leucopenia, and thrombocytopenia; disturbances in liver enzymes, transient increase of serum creatinine; tinnitus, mild hearing loss, and vestibular disorders also reported; local reactions include erythema, pain, and thrombophlebitis
Dose: by intravenous injection or infusion, 400 mg initially, subsequently 200 mg daily; severe infections, 400 mg every 12 hours for 3 doses initially, subsequently 400 mg daily; the subsequent doses can alternatively be given *by intramuscular injection*
CHILD *by intravenous injection or infusion*, initially 6 mg/kg every 12 hours for 3 doses, subsequently 3 mg/kg daily (severe infections, 6 mg/kg daily)
Endocarditis prophylaxis, section 5.1, Table 2

PoM **Targocid**® (Merrell)
Injection, powder for reconstitution, teicoplanin, net price 200-mg vial (with diluent) = £26.72; 400-mg vial (with diluent) = £53.44
Electrolytes: Na$^+$ <0.5 mmol/200- and 400-mg vial

POLYMYXINS

The polymyxin antibiotics, colistin and polymyxin B, are active against Gram-negative organisms, including *Pseudomonas aeruginosa*. They are **not** absorbed by mouth and thus need to be given by injection to obtain a systemic effect; however, they are toxic and have few, if any, indications for systemic use.

Colistin is used in bowel sterilisation regimens in neutropenic patients; it is **not** recommended for gastro-intestinal infections.

Both colistin and polymyxin B are included in some preparations for topical application.

COLISTIN

Indications: see notes above

Cautions: reduce dose in renal impairment; **interactions:** Appendix 1 (polymyxins)

Contra-indications: myasthenia gravis; porphyria (see section 9.8.2)

Side-effects: perioral and peripheral paraesthesia, vertigo, muscle weakness, apnoea, nephrotoxicity

Dose: by mouth, bowel sterilisation, 1.5–3 million units every 8 hours

By intramuscular injection or intravenous injection or infusion, 2 million units every 8 hours (but see notes above)

PoM Colomycin® (Pharmax)

Tablets, scored, colistin sulphate 1.5 million units. Net price 50 = £63.60

Syrup, pink, colistin sulphate 250 000 units/5 mL when reconstituted with water. Net price 80 mL = £3.79

Injection, powder for reconstitution, colistin sulphomethate sodium. Net price 500 000-unit vial = £1.25; 1 million-unit vial = £1.83

Electrolytes, (before reconstitution) Na$^+$ < 0.5 mmol/ 500 000- and 1 million-unit vial

POLYMYXIN B SULPHATE

Indications; Cautions; Contra-indications; Side-effects: see under Colistin

Dose: by slow intravenous infusion, 15 000– 25 000 units/kg daily in divided doses

PoM Aerosporin® (Wellcome)

Injection, powder for reconstitution, polymyxin B sulphate. Net price 500 000-unit vial = £13.81

5.1.8 Sulphonamides and trimethoprim

The importance of the sulphonamides as chemotherapeutic agents has decreased as a result of increasing bacterial resistance and their replacement by antibiotics which are generally more active and less toxic.

The principal indication for sulphonamides used alone is urinary-tract infections caused by sensitive organisms.

Sulphamethoxazole and trimethoprim have been used in combination (as co-trimoxazole) because of their synergistic activity. Increasing bacterial resistance to sulphonamides and the high incidence of sulphonamide-related side-effects have however diminished the value of co-trimoxazole.

Indications for **co-trimoxazole** include urinary-tract infections, prostatitis, exacerbations of chronic bronchitis, and invasive salmonella infections, but trimethoprim alone is now preferred. High doses of co-trimoxazole are used for *Pneumocystis carinii* infections. Co-trimoxazole is no longer recommended for gonorrhoea.

Trimethoprim can be used alone for the treatment of urinary- and respiratory-tract infections and for prostatitis and invasive salmonella infections. Side-effects are less than with co-trimoxazole especially in older patients; therefore it should be used in place of co-trimoxazole for most infections (except pneumocystis).

Side-effects of the sulphonamides include rashes, which are common, the Stevens-Johnson syndrome (erythema multiforme), renal failure (especially with the less soluble preparations), and blood dyscrasias, notably marrow depression and agranulocytosis.

Side-effects of co-trimoxazole are similar to those of the sulphonamides but a particular watch should be kept for haematological effects and special care should be taken in patients who may be folate deficient such as the elderly and chronic sick. There have been recent reports of deaths in patients over the age of 65 years being treated with co-trimoxazole and almost certainly associated with the sulphonamide component. For this reason co-trimoxazole should be used with care in the elderly and preferably only if there is no acceptable alternative. The effect on the fetus is unknown and the drugs should not be used in pregnancy.

The **longer-acting sulphonamide**, sulfametopyrazine which is highly bound to plasma proteins, has the advantage of requiring less frequent administration, but toxic effects due to accumulation are more likely to occur.

For *topical preparations* of sulphonamides used in the treatment of burns see section 13.10.1.1.

CO-TRIMOXAZOLE

A mixture of trimethoprim and sulphamethoxazole in the proportions of 1 part to 5 parts

Indications: invasive salmonellosis, typhoid fever, bone and joint infections due to *Haemophilus influenzae*, urinary-tract infections, sinusitis, exacerbations of chronic bronchitis, gonorrhoea in penicillin-allergic patients

Cautions: blood counts in prolonged treatment, maintain adequate fluid intake, renal impairment, breast-feeding; photosensitivity; elderly patients (**important:** see notes above); **interactions:** Appendix 1 (co-trimoxazole)

Contra-indications: pregnancy, infants under 6 weeks (risk of kernicterus), renal or hepatic failure, jaundice, blood disorders; porphyria (see section 9.8.2)

Side-effects: nausea, vomiting, glossitis, rashes, erythema multiforme (includes Stevens-Johnson syndrome), epidermal necrolysis, eosinophilia, agranulocytosis, granulocytopenia,

5.1.8 Sulphonamides and trimethoprim

purpura, leucopenia; megaloblastic anaemia due to trimethoprim

Dose: *by mouth*, 960 mg every 12 hours, increased to 1.44 g in severe infections; 480 mg every 12 hours if treated for more than 14 days; CHILD, every 12 hours, 6 weeks to 5 months, 120 mg; 6 months to 5 years, 240 mg; 6–12 years, 480 mg

Prophylaxis of recurrent urinary-tract infection, 480 mg at night; CHILD 6–12 mg/kg at night

Gonorrhoea, 1.92 g every 12 hours for 2 days, or 2.4 g followed by a further dose of 2.4 g after 8 hours but see notes above

High-dose therapy for *Pneumocystis carinii* infections, 120 mg/kg daily in divided doses for 14 days

By intramuscular injection or intravenous infusion, 960 mg every 12 hours

Note. 480 mg of co-trimoxazole consists of sulphamethoxazole 400 mg and trimethoprim 80 mg

PoM Co-trimoxazole (Non-proprietary)
Tablets, co-trimoxazole 480 mg, net price 20 = £1.00; 960 mg, 20 = £3.23. Label: 9
Available from APS, Ashbourne (Comixco®), Cox (480 mg), CP, DDSA (Fectrim®, Fectrim® Forte), Evans (480 mg), Kerfoot (960 mg), Lagap (Laratrim® 960 mg), Norton
Dispersible tablets, co-trimoxazole 480 mg. Net price 20 = 97p. Label: 9, 13
Available from APS, Ashbourne (Comixco® Disp), Kerfoot, Norton (Comox®)
Paediatric oral suspension, co-trimoxazole 240 mg/5 mL. Net price 100 mL = £2.09. Label: 9
Available from APS, Ashbourne (Comixco®), CP, Lagap (Laratrim®), Norton, RP Drugs (Chemotrim®)
Oral suspension, co-trimoxazole 480 mg/5 mL. Net price 100 mL = £3·00. Label: 9
Available from APS, CP, Evans, Lagap (Laratrim®)
Strong sterile solution, co-trimoxazole 96 mg/mL. For dilution and use as an intravenous infusion. Net price 5-mL amp = £1.51, 10-mL amp = £2.83, 20-mL vial = £5.37
Available from David Bull

PoM Bactrim® (Roche)
Drapsules® (= tablets), orange, f/c, co-trimoxazole 480 mg. Net price 20 = £2.49. Label: 9
Tablets (dispersible), yellow, scored, co-trimoxazole 480 mg. Net price 20 = £2.49. Label: 9, 13
Double-strength tablets, scored, co-trimoxazole 960 mg. Net price 20 = £3.54. Label: 9
Adult suspension, yellow, co-trimoxazole 480 mg/5 mL. Net price 100 mL = £3.00. Label: 9
Paediatric syrup, sugar-free, yellow, co-trimoxazole 240 mg/5 mL. Net price 100 mL = £2.09. Label: 9

PoM Septrin® (Wellcome)
Tablets, co-trimoxazole 480 mg. Net price 20 = £3.03. Label: 9
Dispersible tablets, orange, sugar-free, co-trimoxazole 480 mg. Net price 20 = £3.22. Label: 9, 13
Forte tablets, scored, co-trimoxazole 960 mg. Net price 20 = £5.05. Label: 9

Adult suspension, co-trimoxazole 480 mg/5 mL. Net price 100 mL = £4.74. Label: 9
Paediatric suspension, sugar-free, co-trimoxazole 240 mg/5 mL. Net price 100 mL = £2.63. Label: 9
Intramuscular injection, co-trimoxazole 320 mg/mL. Net price 3-mL amp = £2.71
Intravenous infusion, co-trimoxazole 96 mg/mL. To be diluted before use. Net price 5-mL amp = £1.59

SULFAMETOPYRAZINE

Indications: urinary-tract infections, chronic bronchitis
Cautions; Contra-indications; Side-effects: see under Co-trimoxazole
Dose: 2 g once weekly

PoM Kelfizine W® (Farmitalia Carlo Erba)
Tablets, sulfametopyrazine 2 g. Tablets to be taken in water. Net price 1 = £1.25. Label: 9, 13

SULPHADIAZINE

Indications: meningococcal meningitis
Cautions; Contra-indications; Side-effects: see under Co-trimoxazole; avoid in severe renal impairment
Dose: *by deep intramuscular injection or intravenous infusion*, 2 g initially then 1 g every 6 hours for 2 days, followed by oral treatment for a further 5 days

PoM Sulphadiazine (Non-proprietary)
Tablets, sulphadiazine 500 mg. Net price 20 = £1.34. Label: 9, 27
Available from CP
Injection, sulphadiazine 250 mg (as sodium salt)/mL. Net price 4-mL amp = 94p
Available from Rhône-Poulenc Rorer

SULPHADIMIDINE

Indications: urinary-tract infections; meningococcal meningitis
Cautions; Contra-indications; Side-effects: see under Co-trimoxazole
Dose: *by mouth*, 2 g initially, then 0.5–1 g every 6–8 hours

PoM Sulphadimidine (Non-proprietary)
Tablets, sulphadimidine 500 mg. Net price 20 = £2.00. Label: 9, 27
Available from CP

TRIMETHOPRIM

Indications: urinary-tract infections, acute and chronic bronchitis
Cautions: renal impairment, breast-feeding, predisposition to folate deficiency, blood counts required on long-term therapy; **interactions:** Appendix 1 (trimethoprim)

Contra-indications: severe renal impairment, pregnancy, neonates; porphyria (see section 9.8.2)

Side-effects: gastro-intestinal disturbances including nausea and vomiting, pruritus, rashes, depression of haemopoiesis

Dose: *by mouth*, acute infections, 200 mg every 12 hours; urinary-tract infections, 300 mg daily *or* 200 mg twice daily; CHILD, twice daily, 2–5 months 25 mg, 6 months–5 years 50 mg, 6–12 years 100 mg

Chronic infections and prophylaxis, 100 mg at night; CHILD 1–2 mg/kg at night

By slow intravenous injection or infusion, 150–250 mg every 12 hours; CHILD under 12 years, 6–9 mg/kg daily in 2–3 divided doses

PoM **Trimethoprim** (Non-proprietary)
Tablets, trimethoprim 100 mg, net price 20 = 64p; 200 mg, 20 = 94p. Label: 9
Available from APS, Berk (Trimopen®), Cox, CP, Evans, Kerfoot, Lagap (Trimogal®), Norton

PoM **Ipral®** (Squibb)
Tablets, trimethoprim 100 mg, net price 20 = 80p; 200 mg, 20 = £1.71. Label: 9

PoM **Monotrim®** (Duphar)
Tablets, both scored, trimethoprim 100 mg, net price 20 = 82p; 200 mg, 20 = £1.44. Label: 9
Suspension, sugar-free, trimethoprim 50 mg/5 mL. Net price 100 mL = £1.77. Label: 9
Injection, trimethoprim 20 mg (as lactate)/mL. Net price 5-mL amp = 68p

PoM **Trimopan®** (Berk)
Suspension, sugar-free, trimethoprim 50 mg/5 mL. Net price 100 mL = £1.37. Label: 9

5.1.9 Antituberculous drugs

Tuberculosis is treated in two phases—an *initial phase* using at least three drugs and a *continuation phase* using two drugs. Treatment requires specialised knowledge, particularly where the disease involves resistant organisms or non-respiratory organs.

The regimens given below are recommended by the Joint Tuberculosis Committee of the British Thoracic Society for the treatment of tuberculosis in the UK; variations occur in other countries.

INITIAL PHASE. The concurrent use of at least three drugs during the initial phase is designed to reduce the population of viable bacteria as rapidly as possible and to prevent the emergence of drug-resistant bacteria. Treatment of choice for the initial phase is the daily use of isoniazid, rifampicin, and pyrazinamide; ethambutol is added if drug resistance is thought likely. Streptomycin is now rarely used in the UK but it may be added if the organism is resistant to isoniazid. The initial phase drugs should be continued for 2 months.

CONTINUATION PHASE. After the initial phase, treatment is continued for a further 4 months with isoniazid and rifampicin; longer treatment may be necessary for bone and joint infections, for meningitis, or for resistant organisms.

Recommended dosage for standard unsupervised 6-month regimen

Isoniazid (for 6 months)	ADULT 300 mg daily; CHILD 10 mg/kg (max. 300 mg) daily
Rifampicin (for 6 months)	ADULT under 50 kg 450 mg daily, 50 kg and over 600 mg daily; CHILD 10 mg/kg daily
Pyrazinamide (for first 2 months only)	ADULT under 50 kg 1.5 g, 50 kg and over 2 g daily; CHILD 35 mg/kg daily

Note. Ethambutol and streptomycin are included in treatment regimens if resistance is suspected; see notes below for doses

PREGNANCY AND BREAST-FEEDING. The standard regimen (above) may be used during pregnancy and breast-feeding; pyridoxine supplements are advisable. Streptomycin should not be given in pregnancy

CHILDREN. As for adults, children are given isoniazid, rifampicin, and pyrazinamide for the first 2 months followed by isoniazid and rifampicin during the next 4 months. If pyrazinamide is omitted from the initial phase, then treatment with isoniazid and rifampicin should be given for 9 months. Ethambutol should be **avoided** in young children because of the difficulty in testing eyesight and in obtaining reports of visual symptoms (see below).

NON-COMPLIANT PATIENTS. Treatment needs to be fully supervised in patients who cannot be relied upon to comply with the treatment regimen. These patients are given isoniazid, rifampicin, and pyrazinamide 3 times a week under supervision for the first 2 months followed by isoniazid and rifampicin three times a week for a further 4 months.

Recommended dosage for intermittent supervised treatment

Isoniazid (for 6 months)	ADULT and CHILD 15 mg/kg 3 times a week
Rifampicin (for 6 months)	ADULT 600–900 mg 3 times a week; CHILD 15 mg/kg 3 times a week
Pyrazinamide (for first 2 months only)	ADULT under 50 kg 2 g 3 times a week, 50 kg and over 2.5 g; CHILD 50 mg/kg 3 times a week
	or
	ADULT under 50 kg 3 g twice a week, 50 kg and over 3.5 g; CHILD 75 mg/kg twice a week

Note. Ethambutol and streptomycin are included in treatment regimens if resistance is suspected; see notes below for doses

IMMUNOCOMPROMISED PATIENTS. Immunocompromised patients may develop tuberculosis owing to reactivation of previously latent disease or to new infection. Multi-resistant *Mycobacterium tuberculosis* may be present or the infection may be caused by other mycobacteria e.g. *M. avium* complex. Culture should always be carried out and

5.1.9 Antituberculous drugs

the type of organism and its sensitivity confirmed. A minimum duration of treatment of 9 months is currently recommended.

> Major causes of treatment failure are incorrect prescribing by the physician and inadequate compliance by the patient. Avoid both excessive and inadequate dosage. Treatment should be supervised by a specialist physician.

Isoniazid is cheap and highly effective. Like rifampicin it should always be included in any antituberculous regimen unless there is a specific contra-indication. Its only common side-effect is peripheral neuropathy which is more likely to occur where there are pre-existing risk factors such as diabetes and alcoholism and in chronic renal failure and malnutrition. In these circumstances pyridoxine 10 mg daily should be given prophylactically from the start of treatment. Other side-effects such as hepatitis and psychosis are rare.

Rifampicin is a key component of any antituberculous regimen. Like isoniazid it should always be included unless there is a specific contra-indication.

During the first two months of rifampicin administration transient disturbance of liver function with elevated serum transaminases is common but generally does not require interruption of treatment. Occasionally more serious liver toxicity requires a change of treatment particularly in those with pre-existing liver disease.

On intermittent treatment six toxicity syndromes have been recognised—influenzal, abdominal, and respiratory symptoms, shock, renal failure, and thrombocytopenic purpura—and can occur in 20 to 30% of patients.

Rifampicin induces hepatic enzymes which accelerate the metabolism of several drugs including oestrogens, corticosteroids, phenytoin, sulphonylureas, and anticoagulants. The effectiveness of oral contraceptives is reduced and alternative family planning advice should be offered.

Pyrazinamide is a bactericidal drug only active against intracellular dividing forms of *Mycobacterium tuberculosis*; it exerts its main effect only in the first two or three months. It is particularly useful in tuberculous meningitis because of good meningeal penetration. It is not active against *M. bovis*.

Ethambutol is included in a treatment regimen if resistance is suspected; it can be omitted if the risk of resistance is low. For unsupervised treatment ethambutol is given in a dose of 25 mg/kg daily in the initial phase followed by 15 mg/kg daily in the continuation phase (*or* 15 mg/kg daily throughout); in fully supervised intermittent treatment ethambutol is given in a dose of 30 mg/kg 3 times a week *or* 45 mg/kg twice a week.

Side-effects of ethambutol are largely confined to visual disturbances in the form of loss of acuity, colour blindness, and restriction of visual fields.

These toxic effects are more common where excessive dosage is used or the patient's renal function is impaired, in which case the drug should be **avoided**. The earliest features of ocular toxicity are subjective and patients should be advised to discontinue therapy immediately if they develop deterioration in vision and promptly seek further advice. Early discontinuation of the drug is almost always followed by recovery of eyesight. Patients who cannot understand warnings about visual side-effects should, if possible, be given an alternative drug. In particular, ethambutol should be **avoided** in children until they are at least 6 years old and capable of reporting symptomatic visual changes accurately.

Ophthalmic examination should be performed prior to treatment and at intervals during treatment.

Streptomycin is now rarely used in the UK except for resistant organisms. It is given intramuscularly in a standard dose of 1 g daily, reduced to 500–750 mg in patients under 50 kg or those over 40 years of age. For fully supervised intermittent treatment streptomycin is given in a dose of 1 g 3 times a week, reduced to 750 mg 3 times a week in patients under 50 kg. Children are given streptomycin in a dose of 15–20 mg/kg daily or for fully supervised intermittent treatment, 15–20 mg/kg 3 times a week. Plasma drug concentrations should be measured, particularly in patients with impaired renal function in whom streptomycin must be used with great care. Side-effects increase after a cumulative dose of 100 g, which should only be exceeded in exceptional circumstances.

Second-line drugs available for infections caused by resistant organisms, or when first-line drugs cause unacceptable side-effects, include capreomycin, cycloserine, and prothionamide (no longer on UK market).

CAPREOMYCIN

Indications: in combination with other drugs, tuberculosis resistant to first-line drugs

Cautions: renal, hepatic, or auditory impairment; monitor renal, hepatic, auditory, and vestibular function and electrolytes; pregnancy (teratogenic in *animals*) and breast-feeding; **interactions:** Appendix 1 (capreomycin)

Side-effects: hypersensitivity reactions including urticaria and rashes; leucocytosis or leucopenia, rarely thrombocytopenia; changes in liver function tests; nephrotoxicity, electrolyte disturbances; hearing loss with tinnitus and vertigo; neuromuscular block after large doses, pain and induration at injection site

Dose: by deep intramuscular injection, 1 g daily (not more than 20 mg/kg) for 2–4 months, then 1 g 2–3 times each week

PoM **Capastat**® (Dista)
Injection, powder for reconstitution, capreomycin sulphate 1 million units (≡ capreomycin approx. 1 g). Net price per vial = £2.28

CYCLOSERINE

Indications: in combination with other drugs, tuberculosis resistant to first-line drugs

Cautions: discontinue (or reduce dose) if allergic dermatitis or symptoms of CNS toxicity; reduce dose in renal impairment (avoid if severe); monitor haematological, renal, and hepatic function; pregnancy and breast-feeding; **interactions:** Appendix 1 (cycloserine)

Contra-indications: severe renal impairment, epilepsy, depression, severe anxiety, psychotic states, alcohol dependence, porphyria (see section 9.8.2)

Side-effects: mainly neurological, including headache, dizziness, vertigo, drowsiness, tremor, convulsions; psychosis, depression; rashes; megaloblastic anaemia; changes in liver function tests

Dose: initially 250 mg every 12 hours for 2 weeks increased according to blood concentration and response to max. 500 mg every 12 hours; CHILD initially 10 mg/kg daily adjusted according to blood concentration and response

Note. Blood concentration monitoring required especially in renal impairment or if dose exceeds 500 mg daily or if signs of toxicity; blood concentration should not exceed 30 mg/litre

PoM Cycloserine (Lilly)
Capsules, red/grey cycloserine 250 mg, net price 20 = £11.35. Label: 2, 8

ETHAMBUTOL HYDROCHLORIDE

Indications: tuberculosis, in combination with other drugs

Cautions: reduce dose in renal impairment; elderly; pregnancy; warn patients to report visual changes—see notes above

Contra-indications: young children (see notes), optic neuritis, poor vision

Side-effects: optic neuritis, red/green colour blindness, peripheral neuritis

Dose: ADULT and CHILD over 6 years, see notes above

PoM Myambutol® (Lederle)
Tablets, ethambutol hydrochloride 100 mg (yellow), net price 20 = £1.45; 400 mg (grey), 20 = £5.23. Label: 8

PoM Mynah® (Lederle)
Mynah 250 tablets, yellow, ethambutol hydrochloride 250 mg, isoniazid 100 mg. Net price 84-tab pack = £16.45. Label: 8, 23
Mynah 300 tablets, orange, ethambutol hydrochloride 300 mg, isoniazid 100 mg. Net price 84-tab pack = £19.66. Label: 8, 23

ISONIAZID

Indications: tuberculosis, in combination with other drugs; prophylaxis—section 5.1, Table 2

Cautions: impaired liver and kidney function, epilepsy, history of psychosis, alcoholism, breast-feeding; **interactions:** Appendix 1 (isoniazid)

Contra-indications: drug-induced liver disease, porphyria (see section 9.8.2)

Side-effects: nausea, vomiting, hypersensitivity reactions including rashes, peripheral neuritis with high doses (pyridoxine prophylaxis, see notes above), convulsions, psychotic episodes, agranulocytosis; hepatitis (especially over age of 35); systemic lupus erythematosus-like syndrome reported

Dose: *by mouth or by intramuscular or intravenous injection*, see notes above

PoM Isoniazid Tablets, isoniazid 50 mg, net price 20 = 32p; 100 mg, 20 = 35p. Label: 8, 22

PoM Isoniazid Elixir (BPC)
Elixir, isoniazid 50 mg, citric acid monohydrate 12.5 mg, sodium citrate 60 mg, concentrated anise water 0.05 mL, compound tartrazine solution 0.05 mL, glycerol 1 mL, double-strength chloroform water 2 mL, water to 5 mL. Label: 8, 22
Isoniazid oral solution (isoniazid 50 mg/5 mL) available from Penn, RP Drugs (both special order)

PoM Rimifon® (Cambridge)
Injection, isoniazid 25 mg/mL. Net price 2-mL amp = 9p

PYRAZINAMIDE

Indications: tuberculosis in combination with other drugs

Cautions: impaired renal function, diabetes, gout; **interactions:** Appendix 1 (pyrazinamide)

Contra-indications: liver damage, porphyria (see section 9.8.2)

Side-effects: hepatotoxicity including fever, anorexia, hepatomegaly, jaundice, liver failure; nausea, vomiting, arthralgia, sideroblastic anaemia, urticaria

Dose: see notes above

PoM Zinamide® (MSD)
Tablets, scored, pyrazinamide 500 mg. Net price 20 = £1.44. Label: 8

RIFAMPICIN

Indications: see under Dose

Cautions: reduce dose in hepatic impairment (see Appendix 2; liver function tests and blood counts in hepatic disorders and on prolonged therapy); pregnancy (see Appendix 4); advise patients on oral contraceptives to use additional means; discolours soft contact lenses; see also notes above; **interactions:** Appendix 1 (rifampicin)

Note. If treatment interrupted re-introduce with low dosage and increase gradually; discontinue permanently if serious side-effects develop

Contra-indications: jaundice, porphyria (see section 9.8.2)

Side-effects: gastro-intestinal symptoms including anorexia, nausea, vomiting, diarrhoea (pseudomembranous colitis reported); those occurring mainly on intermittent therapy include influenzal syndrome (with chills, fever, dizziness, bone pain), respiratory symptoms (including shortness of breath), collapse and shock, haemolytic anaemia, acute renal failure, and thrombocytopenic purpura; alterations of liver function, jaundice; flushing, urticaria, and rashes; other side-effects reported include oedema, muscular weakness and myopathy, leucopenia, eosinophilia, menstrual disturbances; urine, saliva, and other body secretions coloured orange-red

Dose: brucellosis, legionnaires' disease and serious staphylococcal infections, in combination with other drugs, *by mouth or by intravenous infusion*, 0.6–1.2 g daily in 2–4 divided doses

Tuberculosis, in combination with other drugs, see notes above

Leprosy, section 5.1.10

Prophylaxis of meningococcal meningitis and *Haemophilus influenzae* (type b) infection, section 5.1, Table 2

PoM **Rifampicin** (Non-proprietary)
Capsules, rifampicin 150 mg, net price 20 = £3.44; 300 mg, 20 = £6.88. Label: 8, 14, 22, counselling, see lenses above
Available from Generics

PoM **Rifadin**® (Merrell)
Capsules, rifampicin 150 mg (blue/red), net price 20 = £3.82; 300 mg (red), 20 = £7.64. Label: 8, 14, 22, counselling, see lenses above
Syrup, red, rifampicin 100 mg/5 mL. Do not dilute. Net price 120 mL = £3.71. Label: 8, 14, 22, counselling, see lenses above
Intravenous infusion, powder for reconstitution, rifampicin. Net price 600-mg vial (with solvent) = £8.00
Electrolytes: Na⁺ <0.5 mmol/vial

PoM **Rimactane**® (Ciba)
Capsules, rifampicin 150 mg (red), net price 56-tab pack = £9.63; 300 mg (red/brown), 56-tab pack = £19.26. Label: 8, 14, 22, counselling, see lenses above
Syrup, red, rifampicin 100 mg/5 mL. Do not dilute. Net price 100 mL = £2.78. Label: 8, 14, 22, counselling, see lenses above
Intravenous infusion, powder for reconstitution, rifampicin. Net price 300-mg vial (with diluent) = £7.28
Electrolytes: Na⁺ < 0.5 mmol/vial
Note. Owing to risk of contact sensitisation care must be taken to avoid contact during preparation and infusion

Combined preparations
PoM **Rifater**® (Merrell)
Tablets, pink-beige, s/c, rifampicin 120 mg, isoniazid 50 mg, pyrazinamide 300 mg. Net price 20 = £4.40. Label: 8, 14, 22, counselling, see lenses above
Dose: initial treatment of pulmonary tuberculosis, patients up to 40 kg 3 tablets daily preferably before breakfast, 40–49 kg 4 tablets daily, 50–64 kg 5 tablets daily, 65 kg or more, 6 tablets daily; not suitable for use in children

PoM **Rifinah 150**® (Merrell)
Tablets, pink, rifampicin 150 mg, isoniazid 100 mg. Net price 84-tab pack = £16.59. Label: 8, 14, 22, counselling, see lenses above
Dose: ADULT under 50 kg, 3 tablets daily, preferably before breakfast

PoM **Rifinah 300**® (Merrell)
Tablets, orange, rifampicin 300 mg, isoniazid 150 mg. Net price 56-tab pack = £21.93. Label: 8, 14, 22, counselling, see lenses above
Dose: ADULT 50 kg and over, 2 tablets daily, preferably before breakfast

PoM **Rimactazid 150**® (Ciba)
Tablets, pink, s/c, rifampicin 150 mg, isoniazid 100 mg. Net price 84-tab pack = £14.93. Label: 8, 14, 22, counselling, see lenses above
Additives: include gluten
Dose: ADULT under 50 kg, 3 tablets daily, preferably before breakfast

PoM **Rimactazid 300**® (Ciba)
Tablets, orange, s/c, rifampicin 300 mg, isoniazid 150 mg. Net price 56-tab pack = £19.74. Label: 8, 14, 22, counselling, see lenses above
Additives: include gluten
Dose: ADULT 50 kg and over, 2 tablets daily, preferably before breakfast

STREPTOMYCIN

Indications: tuberculosis, in combination with other drugs
Cautions; Contra-indications; Side-effects: see under Aminoglycosides, section 5.1.4; also hypersensitivity reactions, paraesthesia of mouth
Dose: by deep intramuscular injection, see notes above

PoM **Streptomycin Sulphate** (Evans)
Injection, powder for reconstitution, streptomycin (as sulphate). Net price 1-g vial = £5.62

5.1.10 Antileprotic drugs

Advice from a member of the Panel of Leprosy Opinion is essential for the treatment of leprosy (Hansen's disease). Details of the Panel can be obtained from the Department of Health telephone 071-972 3272.

For over twenty years the mainstay of leprosy treatment was dapsone monotherapy but resistance to dapsone became an increasing concern. The World Health Organization has made recommendations to overcome this problem of dapsone resistance and to prevent the emergence of resistance to other antileprotic drugs. These recommendations are based on the same principles as for the chemotherapy of tuberculosis. Drugs recommended are **dapsone, rifampicin,** and **clofazimine;** ethionamide or prothionamide (which are not marketed in the UK) are no longer recommended unless absolutely necessary.

A three-drug regimen is recommended for *multibacillary leprosy* (lepromatous, borderline-lepromatous, and borderline leprosy) and a two-drug regimen for those suffering from *paucibacillary leprosy* (borderline-tuberculoid, tuberculoid, and indeterminate). These regimens, which are widely applicable throughout the world (with minor local variations), are as follows:

Multibacillary leprosy (3-drug regimen)
Rifampicin   600 mg once-monthly, supervised (450 mg for those weighing less than 35 kg)
Dapsone   100 mg daily, self-administered
Clofazimine   300 mg once-monthly, supervised, *and* 50 mg daily, self-administered

Note. Substitution of clofazimine with ethionamide or prothionamide is no longer recommended unless absolutely necessary; administration (in a dose of 250–375 mg daily) should be under medical supervision, with periodic checks for hepatotoxicity

Treatment should be given for at least 2 years and be continued, wherever possible, up to smear negativity. It should be continued unchanged during both type I (reversal) or type II (erythema nodosum leprosum) reactions which, if severe, should receive their own specific treatment (e.g. prednisolone or increased clofazimine dosage).

Paucibacillary leprosy (2-drug regimen)
Rifampicin   600 mg once-monthly, supervised (450 mg for those weighing less than 35 kg)
Dapsone   100 mg daily, self-administered

Treatment should be given for 6 months. If treatment is interrupted the regimen should be recommenced where it was left off to complete the full course.

Neither the multibacillary nor the paucibacillary antileprosy regimen is sufficient to treat tuberculosis, therefore patients who also have tuberculosis should be given appropriate antituberculous drugs in addition to the antileprosy regimen.

DAPSONE

Indications: leprosy, dermatitis herpetiformis
Cautions: cardiac or pulmonary disease; anaemia (treat severe anaemia before starting); G6PD-deficiency (including breast-feeding of affected children, see section 9.1.5); pregnancy; avoid in porphyria (see section 9.8.2); **interactions:** Appendix 1 (dapsone)
Side-effects: (dose-related and uncommon at doses used for leprosy), neuropathy, allergic dermatitis, anorexia, nausea, vomiting, headache, insomnia, tachycardia, anaemia, hepatitis, agranulocytosis
Dose: leprosy, 1–2 mg/kg daily, see notes above
Dermatitis herpetiformis, see specialist literature

PoM **Dapsone Tablets,** dapsone 50 mg, net price 20 = 55p; 100 mg, 20 = 74p. Label: 8

CLOFAZIMINE

Indications: leprosy
Cautions: hepatic and renal impairment—function tests required

Side-effects: nausea, giddiness, headache, and diarrhoea with high doses, skin and urine coloured (red), lesions discoloured (blue-black)
Dose: leprosy, see notes above
Lepromatous lepra reactions, dosage increased to 300 mg daily for max. of 3 months

PoM **Lamprene®** (Geigy)
Capsules, brown, clofazimine 100 mg. Net price 20 = £1.65. Label: 8, 14, 21

RIFAMPICIN
Section 5.1.9

5.1.11 Metronidazole and tinidazole

Metronidazole is an antimicrobial drug with high activity against anaerobic bacteria and protozoa; indications include trichomonal vaginitis (section 5.4.3), bacterial vaginosis (notably *Gardnerella vaginalis* infections), and *Entamoeba histolytica* and *Giardia lamblia* infections (section 5.4.2). It is also used for surgical and gynaecological sepsis in which its activity against colonic anaerobes, especially *Bacteroides fragilis*, is important. Metronidazole is also effective in the treatment of pseudomembranous colitis (in a dose of 400 mg by mouth three times daily). Topical metronidazole (see section 13.10.1.2) reduces the odour produced by anaerobic bacteria in fungating tumours; it is also used in he management of rosacea.

Tinidazole is similar to metronidazole but has a longer duration of action.

METRONIDAZOLE

Indications: anaerobic infections, see under Dose below; protozoal infections, section 5.4.2
Cautions: disulfiram-like reaction with alcohol, hepatic impairment; pregnancy and breast-feeding (manufacturer advises avoidance of high-dose regimens); **interactions:** Appendix 1 (metronidazole)
Side-effects: nausea, vomiting, unpleasant taste, and gastro-intestinal disturbances; rashes, urticaria and angioedema; rarely drowsiness, headache, dizziness, ataxia, and darkening of urine; on prolonged or intensive therapy peripheral neuropathy, transient epileptiform seizures, and leucopenia
Dose: anaerobic infections (usually treated for 7 days), *by mouth*, 800 mg initially then 400 mg every 8 hours; *by rectum*, 1 g every 8 hours for 3 days, then 1 g every 12 hours; *by intravenous infusion*, 500 mg every 8 hours; CHILD, any route, 7.5 mg/kg every 8 hours
Leg ulcers and pressure sores, *by mouth*, 400 mg every 8 hours for 7 days
Bacterial vaginosis, *by mouth*, 400 mg twice daily for 7 days *or* 2 g as a single dose
Acute ulcerative gingivitis, *by mouth*, 200 mg every 8 hours for 3 days; CHILD 1–3 years 50 mg every 8 hours for 3 days; 3–7 years 100 mg every 12 hours; 7–10 years 100 mg every 8 hours

Acute dental infections, *by mouth*, 200 mg every 8 hours for 3–7 days

Surgical prophylaxis, *by mouth*, 400 mg every 8 hours started 24 hours before surgery, then continued postoperatively *by intravenous infusion* or *by rectum* (see below) until oral administration can be resumed; CHILD 7.5 mg/kg every 8 hours

By rectum, 1 g every 8 hours; CHILD 125–250 mg every 8 hours

By intravenous infusion, 500 mg shortly before surgery then every 8 hours until oral administration can be started; CHILD, 7.5 mg/kg every 8 hours

PoM **Metronidazole** (Non-proprietary)
Tablets, metronidazole 200 mg, net price 20 = 70p; 400 mg, 20 = £1.45. Label: 4, 9, 21, 25, 27
Available from APS, Cox, CP, DDSA (Vaginyl®), Evans, Kerfoot, Lagap (Metrolyl®), Lederle (Zadstat®), Norton
Intravenous infusion, metronidazole 5 mg/mL. Net price 20-mL amp = £1.80
Available from David Bull

PoM **Flagyl**® (Rhône-Poulenc Rorer)
Tablets, both f/c, ivory, metronidazole 200 mg, net price 21-tab pack = £2.19; 400 mg, 14-tab pack = £3.11. Label: 4, 9, 21, 25, 27
Intravenous infusion, metronidazole 5 mg/mL. Net price 20-mL amp = £2.06; 100-mL Viaflex® bag = £3.50
Electrolytes: Na$^+$ 13.6 mmol/100-mL bottle or bag
Suppositories, metronidazole 500 mg, net price 10 = £6.77; 1 g, 10 = £10.28. Label: 4, 9

PoM **Flagyl S**® (Rhône-Poulenc Rorer)
Suspension, metronidazole 200 mg (as benzoate)/5 mL. Net price 100 mL = £4.53. Label: 4, 9, 23

PoM **Metrogel**®: see section 13.10.1.2
PoM **Metrotop**®: see section 13.10.1.2

PoM **Metrolyl**® (Lagap)
Intravenous infusion, metronidazole 5 mg/mL. Net price 100-mL Steriflex® bag = £4.05
Electrolytes: Na$^+$ 14.53 mmol/100-mL bag
Suppositories, metronidazole 500 mg, net price 10 = £4.25; 1 g, 10 = £6.80. Label: 4, 9

PoM **Zadstat**® (Lederle)
Suppositories, metronidazole 500 mg, net price 10 = £4.25; 1 g, 10 = £6.80. Label: 4, 9

With antifungal

PoM **Flagyl Compak**® (Rhône-Poulenc Rorer)
Treatment pack, tablets, off-white, f/c, metronidazole 400 mg, with pessaries, yellow, nystatin 100 000 units. Net price 14 tablets and 14 pessaries (with applicator) = £4.24
Dose: for mixed trichomonal and candidal infections, 1 tablet twice daily for 7 days and 1 pessary inserted twice daily for 7 days *or* 1 pessary at night for 14 nights

TINIDAZOLE

Indications: anaerobic infections, see under Dose below; protozoal infections, section 5.4.2
Cautions; Side-effects: see under Metronidazole; pregnancy (manufacturer advises avoidance in first trimester)

Dose: anaerobic infections *by mouth*, 2 g initially, followed by 1 g daily *or* 500 mg twice daily, usually for 5–6 days
Bacterial vaginosis and acute ulcerative gingivitis, a single 2-g dose
Abdominal surgery prophylaxis, a single 2-g dose approximately 12 hours before surgery

PoM **Fasigyn**® (Pfizer)
Tablets, f/c, tinidazole 500 mg. Net price 20-tab pack = £11.50. Label: 4, 9, 21, 25

5.1.12 4-Quinolones

Antibacterials discussed in this section include acrosoxacin, ciprofloxacin, enoxacin, ofloxacin, and the urinary antiseptics cinoxacin, nalidixic acid, and norfloxacin.

Acrosoxacin is used only in the treatment of gonorrhoea in patients allergic to penicillins or who have strains resistant to penicillins and other antibiotics.

Nalidixic acid and **cinoxacin** are effective in uncomplicated urinary-tract infections; **norfloxacin** has also been introduced for the treatment of urinary-tract infections.

Ciprofloxacin is active against both Gram-positive and Gram-negative bacteria. It is particularly active against Gram-negative bacteria, including salmonella, shigella, campylobacter, neisseria, and pseudomonas. Ciprofloxacin only has moderate activity against Gram-positive bacteria such as *Streptococcus pneumoniae* and *Strep. faecalis*; it is not the drug of first choice for pneumococcal pneumonia. It is active against chlamydia and some mycobacteria. Most anaerobic organisms are not susceptible. Uses for ciprofloxacin include infections of the respiratory (but not for pneumococcal pneumonia, see above) and urinary tracts, and of the gastro-intestinal system, and gonorrhoea and septicaemia caused by sensitive organisms.

Enoxacin is used for urinary-tract infections, skin and soft-tissue infections, gonorrhoea, and shigellosis.

Ofloxacin is used for urinary-tract infections, lower respiratory-tract infections, gonorrhoea, and non-gonococcal urethritis and cervicitis.

Temafloxacin has been withdrawn owing to reports of serious adverse effects (including hypoglycaemia, hepatic dysfunction, haemolytic anaemia, renal dysfunction and anaphylaxis).

CAUTIONS. 4-Quinolones should be used with caution in patients with epilepsy or a history of epilepsy, in hepatic or renal impairment, in pregnancy, during breast-feeding, and in children or adolescents (arthropathy has developed in weight-bearing joints in young *animals*). The CSM has warned that 4-quinolones may induce **convulsions** in patients with or without a history of convulsions; taking NSAIDs at the same time may also induce them. Other **interactions**: Appendix 1 (4-quinolones).

SIDE-EFFECTS. Common side-effects of the 4-quinolones include nausea, vomiting, abdominal pain, diarrhoea (rarely pseudomembranous colitis), headache, dizziness, sleep disorders, rash, pruritus, anaphylaxis, photosensitivity, increase in blood urea and creatinine, transient disturbances in liver enzymes and bilirubin, arthralgia and myalgia, blood disorders (including eosinophilia, leucopenia, thrombocytopenia, and altered prothrombin concentration). Less frequent side-effects include anorexia, restlessness, hallucinations, confusion, and disturbances in vision, taste and smell.

CIPROFLOXACIN

Indications: Gram-negative and Gram-positive infections, see notes above
Cautions; Side-effects: see notes above; avoid excessive alkalinity of urine and ensure adequate fluid intake (risk of crystalluria); not recommended in children or growing adolescents; G6PD deficiency (see section 9.1.5); anaphylaxis reported, particularly in AIDS patients, also reported dyspepsia, tremor, convulsions, jaundice and hepatitis with necrosis, renal failure, nephritis, vasculitis, Stevens-Johnson syndrome and tachycardia
DRIVING. May impair performance of skilled tasks (e.g. driving); effects of alcohol enhanced
Dose: by mouth, respiratory-tract infections, 250–750 mg twice daily
Urinary-tract infections, 250–500 mg twice daily
Gonorrhoea, 250 mg as a single dose
Most other infections, 500–750 mg twice daily
Prophylaxis of meningococcal meningitis, section 5.1, Table 2
By intravenous infusion (over 30–60 minutes), 200 mg twice daily
Urinary-tract infections, 100 mg twice daily
Gonorrhoea, 100 mg as a single dose
CHILD not recommended (see above) but where benefit outweighs risk, *by mouth*, 7.5–15 mg/kg daily in 2 divided doses *or by intravenous infusion*, 5–10 mg/kg daily in 2 divided doses

PoM **Ciproxin®** (Baypharm)
Tablets, f/c, scored, ciprofloxacin (as hydrochloride) 250 mg. Net price 20 = £15.00. Label: 5, 9, 25, counselling, driving
Intravenous infusion, ciprofloxacin 2 mg (as lactate)/mL. Net price 50-mL bottle = £12.00; 100-mL bottle = £24.00
Electrolytes: Na⁺ 15.4 mmol/100-mL bottle

ACROSOXACIN

(Rosoxacin)
Indications: gonorrhoea
Cautions; Side-effects: see notes above; avoid frequent repeat doses in patients under 18 years
DRIVING. May impair performance of skilled tasks (e.g, driving)
Dose: 300 mg as a single dose on an empty stomach

PoM **Eradacin®** (Sanofi Winthrop)
Capsules, red/yellow, acrosoxacin 150 mg. Net price 20-cap pack = £29.04. Label: 2, 23

CINOXACIN

Indications: urinary-tract infections
Cautions; Side-effects: see notes above; avoid in severe renal impairment; also reported, peripheral and oral oedema, tinnitus, perineal burning
Dose: 500 mg every 12 hours; prophylaxis, 500 mg at night

PoM **Cinobac®** (Lilly)
Capsules, green/orange, cinoxacin 500 mg. Net price 14-cap pack = £6.88. Label: 9

ENOXACIN

Indications: urinary-tract and skin infections, gonorrhoea, shigellosis
Cautions; Side-effects: see notes above; also reported, dyspepsia, dry mouth and throat, stomatitis, palpitation and tachycardia, oedema, fatigue, tremor, convulsions, tinnitus
Dose: urinary-tract infections, 200 mg twice daily for 3 days; complicated infections, 400 mg (elderly 200 mg) twice daily for 7–14 days
Skin infections, 400 mg (elderly 200 mg) twice daily for 7–14 days
Chancroid, 400 mg (elderly 200 mg) every 12 hours for 3 doses
Gonorrhoea, 400 mg as a single dose
Shigellosis, 400 mg (elderly 200 mg) twice daily for 5 days

PoM **Comprecin®** (P-D)
Tablets, f/c, blue, enoxacin 200 mg. Net price 6-tab pack = £2.50. Label: 9

NALIDIXIC ACID

Indications: urinary-tract infections
Cautions; Side-effects: see notes above; avoid in porphyria (see section 9.8.2) and if history of convulsive disorders, avoid strong sunlight, false positive urinary glucose (if tested for reducing substances); caution in G6PD deficiency (see section 9.1.5); also reported toxic psychosis and convulsions, weakness, increased intracranial pressure, paraesthesia, cranial nerve palsy, cholestasis, metabolic acidosis
Dose: 1 g every 6 hours for 7 days, reduced in chronic infections to 500 mg every 6 hours; CHILD over 3 months max. 50 mg/kg daily in divided doses; reduced in prolonged therapy to 30 mg/kg daily

PoM **Nalidixic Acid** (Non-proprietary)
Tablets, nalidixic acid 500 mg. Net price 56-tab pack = £10.80. Label: 9, 11
Available from Norton

PoM **Mictral**® (Sanofi Winthrop)
Granules, effervescent, nalidixic acid 660 mg, sodium citrate (as sodium citrate and citric acid) 4.1 g/sachet (Na⁺ 41 mmol/sachet). Net price 9-sachet pack = £5.11. Label: 9, 11, 13
Dose: 1 sachet in water 3 times daily for 3 days

PoM **Negram**® (Sanofi Winthrop)
Tablets, beige, nalidixic acid 500 mg. Net price 56-tab pack = £11.96. Label: 9, 11
Suspension, pink, sugar-free, nalidixic acid 300 mg/5 mL. Diluent syrup, life of diluted suspension 14 days. Net price 150 mL = £11.98. Label: 9, 11

PoM **Uriben**® (RP Drugs)
Suspension, pink, nalidixic acid 300 mg/5 mL. Net price 200 mL = £14.00; 500 mL = £30.00. Label: 9, 11

NORFLOXACIN

Indications: see under Dose
Cautions; Side-effects: see notes above; avoid in prepubital children and growing adolescents; also reported, anorexia, depression, anxiety, tinnitus, toxic epidermal necrolysis, Stevens-Johnson syndrome
Dose: urinary-tract infections, 400 mg twice daily for 7–10 days (for 3 days in uncomplicated lower urinary-tract infections)
Chronic relapsing urinary-tract infections, 400 mg twice daily for 12 weeks; may be reduced to 400 mg once daily if adequate suppression within first 4 weeks

▼ PoM **Utinor**® (MSD)
Tablets, norfloxacin 400 mg. Net price 6-tab pack = £2.88, 14-tab pack = £6.72. Label: 5, 9

OFLOXACIN

Indications: see under Dose
Cautions; Side-effects: see notes above; caution in history of psychiatric illness and in G6PD deficiency; avoid strong sunlight; avoid in epilepsy or history of epilepsy and in children and adolescents; also reported, loss of appetite, anxiety, unsteady gait and tremor, paraesthesia, neuropathy, psychotic reactions (discontinue treatment); tachycardia, anaemia and agranulocytosis; on intravenous infusion, hypotension and local reactions (including thrombophlebitis)
DRIVING. May affect performance of skilled tasks (e.g. driving)
Dose: by mouth, urinary-tract infections, 200–400 mg daily preferably in the morning, increased if necessary in upper urinary-tract infections to 400 mg twice daily
Lower respiratory-tract infections, 400 mg daily preferably in the morning, increased if necessary to 400 mg twice daily
Uncomplicated gonorrhoea, 400 mg as a single dose
Non-gonococcal urethritis and cervicitis, 400 mg daily in single or divided doses
By intravenous infusion (over at least 30 minutes), complicated urinary-tract infection, 200 mg daily

Lower respiratory-tract infection, 200 mg twice daily
Septicaemia, 200 mg twice daily
Severe or complicated infections, dose may be increased to 400 mg twice daily

PoM **Tarivid**® (Hoechst, Roussel)
Tablets, scored, yellow-white, ofloxacin 200 mg, net price 10-tab pack = £7.38, 20-tab pack = £14.75. Label: 5, 9, 11, counselling, driving
▼ *Intravenous infusion*, ofloxacin (as hydrochloride) 2 mg/mL, net price 50-mL bottle = £15.80; 100-mL bottle = £22.57

5.1.13 Urinary-tract infections

Urinary-tract infection is more common in women than in men; when it occurs in men there is frequently an underlying abnormality of the renal tract. Recurrent episodes of infection are an indication for radiological investigation especially in children in whom untreated pyelonephritis may lead to permanent kidney damage.

Escherichia coli is the most common cause of urinary-tract infection. Less common causes include Proteus and Klebsiella spp. *Pseudomonas aeruginosa* infections are almost invariably associated with functional or anatomical abnormalities of the renal tract. *Staphylococcus epidermidis* and *Enterococcus faecalis* infection may complicate catheterisation or instrumentation. Whenever possible a specimen of urine should be collected for culture and sensitivity testing before starting antibiotic therapy.

Uncomplicated lower urinary-tract infections often respond to ampicillin, nalidixic acid, nitrofurantoin, or trimethoprim given for 5–7 days; those caused by fully sensitive bacteria respond to two 3-g doses of amoxycillin (section 5.1.1.3). Bacterial resistance, however, especially to ampicillin (to which approximately 50% of *E. coli* are now resistant), has increased the importance of urine culture prior to therapy. Alternatives for resistant organisms include co-amoxiclav (amoxycillin with clavulanic acid), an oral cephalosporin, and ciprofloxacin. Hexamine should **not** be used as it is only bacteriostatic, requires acid urine, and frequently causes side-effects.

Long-term low dose therapy may be required in selected patients to prevent *recurrence of infection*; indications include frequent relapses and significant kidney damage. Trimethoprim and nitrofurantoin have been recommended for long-term therapy.

Acute pyelonephritis can be associated with septicaemia and is best treated initially by injection of a broad-spectrum antibiotic such as cefuroxime or gentamicin especially if the patient is vomiting or severely ill.

Prostatitis can be difficult to cure and requires treatment for several weeks with an antibiotic which penetrates prostatic tissue such as trimethoprim, erythromycin, or ciprofloxacin.

Where infection is localised and associated with an indwelling *catheter* a bladder instillation is often effective (see section 7.4.4).

Patients with *heart-valve lesions* undergoing instrumentation of the urinary tract should be given a parenteral antibiotic to prevent bacteraemia and endocarditis (section 5.1, Table 2).

Urinary-tract infection in *pregnancy* may be asymptomatic and requires prompt treatment to prevent progression to acute pyelonephritis. Penicillins and cephalosporins can be given in pregnancy but trimethoprim, sulphonamides, 4-quinolones, and tetracyclines should be avoided.

In *renal failure* antibiotics normally excreted by the kidney accumulate with resultant toxicity unless the dose is reduced. This applies especially to the aminoglycosides which should be used with great caution; tetracyclines, hexamine, and nitrofurantoin should be avoided altogether.

NITROFURANTOIN

Indications: urinary-tract infections

Cautions: monitor lung and liver function on long-term therapy, especially in the elderly; susceptibility to peripheral neuropathy; false positive urinary glucose (if tested for reducing substances); urine may be coloured yellow or brown; **interactions:** Appendix 1 (nitrofurantoin)

Contra-indications: impaired renal function, infants less than 1 month old, G6PD deficiency (including late pregnancy, and breast-feeding of affected infants, see section 9.1.5), porphyria (see section 9.8.2)

Side-effects: anorexia, nausea, vomiting, and diarrhoea; acute and chronic pulmonary reactions; peripheral neuropathy; also reported, angioedema, urticaria, rash and pruritus; rarely, cholestatic jaundice, hepatitis, exfoliative dermatitis, erythema multiforme, pancreatitis, arthralgia, blood disorders (including agranulocytosis, thrombocytopenia, and aplastic anaemia), and transient alopecia

Dose: 50–100 mg every 6 hours with food; CHILD 3 mg/kg daily in 4 divided doses

Prophylaxis (but see Cautions), 50–100 mg at night; CHILD 1 mg/kg at night

PoM **Nitrofurantoin** (Non-proprietary)
Tablets, nitrofurantoin 50 mg and 100 mg. Label: 9, 14, 21
Available from Biorex

PoM **Furadantin**® (Norwich Eaton)
Tablets, all yellow, scored, nitrofurantoin 50 mg, net price 20 = £1.96; 100 mg, 20 = £3.29. Label: 9, 14, 21
Suspension, yellow, sugar-free, nitrofurantoin 25 mg/5 mL. Net price 300 mL = £4.50. Label: 9, 14, 21

PoM **Macrodantin**® (Norwich Eaton)
Capsules, nitrofurantoin 50 mg (yellow/white), net price 28-cap pack = £3.05; 100 mg (yellow), 20 = £3.49. Label: 9, 14, 21

HEXAMINE HIPPURATE
(Methenamine hippurate)

Indications: prophylaxis and long-term treatment of recurrent urinary-tract infections

Cautions: pregnancy; **interactions:** Appendix 1 (hexamine)

Contra-indications: severe renal impairment, dehydration, metabolic acidosis

Side-effects: gastro-intestinal disturbances, bladder irritation, rash

Dose: 1 g every 12 hours (may be increased in patients with catheters to 1 g every 8 hours); CHILD 6–12 years 500 mg every 12 hours

Hiprex® (3M)
Tablets, scored, hexamine hippurate 1 g. Net price 60-tab pack = £5.75. Label: 9

5.2 Antifungal drugs

Fungal infections are frequently associated with a defect in host resistance which should, if possible, be corrected otherwise drug therapy may fail. Similarly, treatment of dermatophyte infection may be unsuccessful until the animal source has been removed or controlled.

For local treatment of fungal infections see also sections 7.2.2 (genital), 7.4.4 (bladder), 11.3.2 (eye), 12.1.1 (ear), 12.3.3 (oropharynx), and 13.10.2 (skin).

POLYENE ANTIFUNGALS. The polyene antifungals include amphotericin and nystatin.

Amphotericin is not absorbed from the gut and is the only polyene antibiotic which can be given parenterally. It is used for the treatment of systemic fungal infections and is active against most fungi and yeasts. It is highly protein bound and penetrates poorly into body fluids and tissues. When given parenterally amphotericin is toxic and side-effects are common.

A formulation of amphotericin encapsulated in liposomes is now available and is apparently significantly less toxic than the parent compound. It is therefore being recommended for systemic mycoses when amphotericin alone is contra-indicated because of toxicity, especially nephrotoxicity.

Nystatin is not absorbed when given by mouth and is too toxic for parenteral use. It is active against a number of yeasts and fungi but is principally used for *Candida albicans* infections of skin and mucous membranes. It is also used in the treatment of intestinal candidiasis.

IMIDAZOLE ANTIFUNGALS. The imidazole antifungals include clotrimazole, econazole, isoconazole, ketoconazole, miconazole, sulconazole, and tioconazole; they are active against a wide range of fungi and yeasts. Their main indications are vaginal candidiasis and dermatophyte infections. Clotrimazole, econazole, isoconazole, sulconazole, and tioconazole are used for local treatment.

5.2 Antifungal drugs

Miconazole is used for local treatment and can be given by mouth for oral and intestinal infection; it can also be given parenterally for systemic infections including aspergillosis, candidiasis, and cryptococcosis but the injection contains polyethoxylated castor oil which may give rise to hypersensitivity reactions.

Ketoconazole is significantly better absorbed after oral administration than the other imidazoles, but has been associated with fatal hepatotoxicity. The CSM has advised that prescribers should weigh the potential benefits of ketoconazole treatment against the liver damage risk and should carefully monitor patients both clinically and biochemically. It should **not** be given for superficial fungal infections.

TRIAZOLE ANTIFUNGALS. The triazole antifungals include fluconazole and itraconazole which are absorbed by mouth.

Fluconazole is an oral triazole antifungal indicated for local and systemic candidiasis and cryptococcal infections.

Itraconazole is indicated for oropharyngeal and vulvovaginal candidiasis, pityriasis versicolor, and tinea corporis and pedis; it is metabolised in the liver and should not be given to patients with a history of liver disease.

OTHER ANTIFUNGALS. **Flucytosine** is a synthetic antifungal drug which is only active against yeasts and has been used for the treatment of systemic candidiasis, cryptococcosis, and torulopsosis. It is well absorbed from the gut and distributed widely in the body. Side-effects are uncommon but bone-marrow depression can occur and weekly blood counts are necessary during prolonged therapy. Synergy has been demonstrated with amphotericin. Resistance to flucytosine is not uncommon and can develop during therapy; sensitivity testing is, therefore, essential before and during treatment.

Griseofulvin is selectively concentrated in keratin and is the drug of choice for widespread or intractable dermatophyte infections. It is well absorbed from the gut but is inactive when applied topically. It is more effective in skin than in nail infections and treatment must be continued for several weeks or even months. Side-effects are uncommon.

Terbinafine, an allylamine antifungal, has recently been introduced for ringworm infections where oral treatment is considered appropriate.

AMPHOTERICIN

Indications: See under Dose
Cautions: when given parenterally, toxicity common (close supervision necessary); hepatic and renal-function tests, blood counts, and plasma electrolyte monitoring required; other nephrotoxic drugs, corticosteroids (avoid except to control reactions), antineoplastics; frequent change of injection site (irritant); **interactions:** Appendix 1 (amphotericin)

Side-effects: when given parenterally, anorexia, nausea and vomiting, diarrhoea, epigastric pain; febrile reactions, headache, muscle and joint pain; anaemia; disturbances in renal function (including hypokalaemia and hypomagnesaemia) and renal toxicity; also cardiovascular toxicity (including arrhythmias), blood disorders, neurological disorders (including hearing loss, diplopia, convulsions, peripheral neuropathy), abnormal liver function (discontinue treatment), rash, anaphylactoid reactions
Dose: by mouth, intestinal candidiasis, 100–200 mg every 6 hours
By intravenous infusion, see under Preparations, below

PoM Fungilin® (Squibb)
Tablets, yellow, scored, amphotericin 100 mg. Net price 56-tab pack = £8.32. Label: 9
Lozenges—see section 12.3.2
Suspension, yellow, sugar-free, amphotericin 100 mg/mL. Net price 12 mL = £2.31. Label: 9, counselling, use of pipette

PoM Fungizone® (Squibb)
Intravenous infusion, powder for reconstitution, amphotericin (as sodium deoxycholate complex). Net price 50-mg vial = £3.70
Electrolytes: Na⁺ <0.5 mmol/vial
Dose: by intravenous infusion, systemic fungal infections, 250 micrograms/kg daily, gradually increased if tolerated to 1 mg/kg daily; max. (severe infection) 1.5 mg/kg daily or on alternate days
Note. Prolonged treatment usually necessary; if interrupted for longer than 7 days recommence at 250 micrograms/kg daily and increase gradually

Liposomal amphotericin
▼ PoM AmBisome® (Vestar)
Intravenous infusion, powder for reconstitution, amphotericin 50 mg encapsulated in liposomes. Net price 50-mg vial = £119.00
Electrolytes: Na⁺ <0.5 mmol/vial
Dose: systemic mycoses where toxicity (particularly nephrotoxicity) precludes use of conventional amphotericin, by intravenous infusion, initially 1 mg/kg daily as a single dose increased gradually if necessary to 3 mg/kg daily as a single dose

FLUCONAZOLE

Indications: see under Dose
Cautions: renal impairment; pregnancy (toxicity at high doses in *animal* studies) and breast-feeding; children (use only if imperative and if no alternative treatment; not recommended under 1 year); raised liver enzymes **interactions:** Appendix 1 (fluconazole)
Side-effects: nausea, abdominal discomfort, diarrhoea, and flatulence; occasionally abnormalities of liver enzymes; rarely rash (discontinue treatment)

Dose: acute or recurrent vaginal candidiasis, *by mouth*, a single dose of 150 mg

Mucosal candidiasis (except vaginal), *by mouth*, 50 mg daily (100 mg daily in unusually difficult infections) given for 7–14 days in oropharyngeal candidiasis (max. 14 days except in severely immunocompromised patients); for 14 days in atrophic oral candidiasis associated with dentures; for 14–30 days in other mucosal infections (e.g. oesophagitis, candiduria)

Systemic candidiasis and cryptococcal infections (including meningitis), *by mouth or intravenous infusion*, 400 mg initially then 200 mg daily, increased if necessary to 400 mg daily; treatment continued according to response (at least 6–8 weeks for cryptococcal meningitis)

Prevention of relapse of cryptococcal meningitis in AIDS patients after completion of primary therapy, at least 100 mg daily

Prevention of fungal infections in immunocompromised patients following cytotoxic chemotherapy or radiotherapy, 50 mg daily; 100 mg daily if risk of severe recurrent infections

CHILD over 1 year (see Cautions), *by mouth or by intravenous infusion*, superficial candidal infections, 1–2 mg/kg daily; systemic candidiasis and cryptococcal infections, 3–6 mg/kg daily

PoM **Diflucan**® (Pfizer)
Capsules, fluconazole 50 mg (blue/white), net price 7-cap pack = £16.61; 150 mg (blue), single-capsule pack = £7.12; 200 mg (purple/white), 7-cap pack = £66.42. Label: 50 and 200 mg, 9

Oral suspension, fluconazole for reconstitution with water, 50 mg/5 ml, net price 35 mL = £16.61; 200 mg/5 ml, 35 mL = £66.42. Label: 9

Intravenous infusion, fluconazole 2 mg/mL in sodium chloride intravenous infusion 0.9%, net price 25-mL bottle = £7.32; 100-mL bottle = £29.28
Electrolytes: Na⁺ 15 mmol/100-mL bottle

FLUCYTOSINE

Indications: systemic yeast infections

Cautions: hepatic impairment, renal impairment (reduce dose and monitor plasma concentrations), blood disorders, liver-function tests and blood counts required; pregnancy, breast-feeding

Side-effects: nausea, vomiting, diarrhoea, rashes, thrombocytopenia, leucopenia

Dose: *by mouth or intravenous infusion*, 200 mg/kg daily in 4 divided doses; extremely sensitive organisms, 100–150 mg/kg daily may be sufficient

Note. Plasma concentration for optimum response 25–50 mg/litre (200–400 micromol/litre)

PoM **Alcobon**® (Roche)
Tablets, scored, flucytosine 500 mg. Net price 20 = £9.43 (hosp. only)

Intravenous infusion, flucytosine 10 mg/mL. Net price 250-mL infusion bottle and giving set = £16.56 (hosp. only)
Electrolytes: Na⁺ 34.44 mmol/250-mL bottle

GRISEOFULVIN

Indications: dermatophyte infections of the skin, scalp, hair and nails, where topical therapy has failed or is inappropriate

Cautions: rarely aggravation or precipitation of systemic lupus erythematosus; breast feeding; **interactions:** Appendix 1 (griseofulvin) DRIVING. May impair performance of skilled tasks (e.g. driving); effects of alcohol enhanced

Contra-indications: liver failure, porphyria (see section 9.8.2); pregnancy

Side-effects: headache, nausea, vomiting, rashes, photosensitivity; dizziness, fatigue, agranulocytopenia and leucopenia reported; lupus erythematosus, erythema multiforme, toxic epidermal necrolysis, peripheral neuropathy, confusion and impaired co-ordination also reported

Dose: 500 mg daily, in divided doses or as a single dose, in severe infection dose may be doubled, reducing when response occurs; CHILD, 10 mg/kg daily in divided doses or as a single dose

PoM **Fulcin**® (ICI)
Tablets, griseofulvin 125 mg (scored), net price 20 = 63p; 500 mg (f/c), 20 = £2.35. Label: 9, 21, counselling, driving

Oral suspension, brown, griseofulvin 125 mg/5 mL. Net price 100 mL = £1.13. Label: 9, 21, counselling, driving

PoM **Grisovin**® (Glaxo)
Tablets, both f/c, griseofulvin 125 mg, net price 20 = 47p; 500 mg, 20 = £1.75. Label: 9, 21, counselling, driving

ITRACONAZOLE

Indications: oropharyngeal and vulvovaginal candidiasis; pityriasis versicolor and other dermatophyte infections

Cautions: avoid if history of liver disease; pregnancy (toxicity in *animal* studies) and breast-feeding; **interactions:** Appendix 1 (itraconazole)

Side-effects: nausea, abdominal pain, dyspepsia, headache

Dose: oropharyngeal candidiasis, 100 mg daily (200 mg daily in AIDS or neutropenia) for 15 days

Vulvovaginal candidiasis, 200 mg twice daily for 1 day

Pityriasis versicolor, 200 mg daily for 7 days

Tinea corporis and tinea cruris, 100 mg daily for 15 days

Tinea pedis and tinea manuum, 100 mg daily for 30 days

Max. period of treatment, 30 days
CHILD not yet recommended

PoM **Sporanox**® (Janssen)
Capsules, blue/pink, enclosing coated beads, itraconazole 100 mg. Net price 4-cap pack = £5.99; 15-cap pack = £22.46. Label: 5, 9, 21, 25

KETOCONAZOLE

Indications: systemic mycoses, serious chronic resistant mucocutaneous candidiasis, serious resistant gastro-intestinal mycoses, chronic resistant vaginal candidiasis, resistant dermatophyte infections of skin or finger nails (not toe nails); prophylaxis of mycoses in immunosuppressed patients

Cautions: **important:** monitor liver function clinically and biochemically—for treatment lasting longer than 14 days perform liver function tests before starting, 14 days after starting, then at monthly intervals (for details see data sheet); pregnancy (teratogenicity in *animal* studies), packs carry a warning to avoid in pregnancy; avoid in porphyria (see section 9.8.2); **interactions:** Appendix 1 (ketoconazole)

Contra-indications: hepatic impairment

Side-effects: nausea, vomiting, abdominal pain; headache; rashes, urticaria, pruritus; rarely thrombocytopenia, gynaecomastia; fatal liver damage—for CSM advice see notes above, risk of developing hepatitis greater if given for longer than 14 days

Dose: 200 mg once daily with food, usually for 14 days; if response inadequate after 14 days continue until at least 1 week after symptoms have cleared and cultures become negative; max. 400 mg daily.

CHILD, 3 mg/kg daily

Chronic resistant vaginal candidiasis, 400 mg daily with food for 5 days

PoM **Nizoral**® (Janssen)
Tablets, scored, ketoconazole 200 mg. Net price 30-tab pack = £15.69. Label: 5, 9, 21
Suspension, pink, ketoconazole 100 mg/5 mL. Net price 100 mL with pipette = £7.16. Label: 5, 9, 21, counselling, use of pipette

MICONAZOLE

Indications: see under Dose

Cautions: change infusion site to avoid phlebitis; pregnancy; avoid in porphyria (see section 9.8.2); **interactions:** Appendix 1 (miconazole)

Side-effects: nausea and vomiting, pruritus, rashes

Dose: by mouth as tablets, oral and intestinal fungal infections, 250 mg every 6 hours for 10 days or up to 2 days after symptoms clear; as oral gel, see under Daktarin® oral gel

By intravenous infusion, systemic fungal infections, initially, 600 mg every 8 hours; CHILD, max. 15 mg/kg every 8 hours up to 40 mg/kg/day

Daktarin® (Janssen)
PoM *Tablets,* scored, miconazole 250 mg. Net price 20 = £14.89. Label: 9, 21
Note. Can be sucked for oral treatment
PoM ¹*Oral gel,* sugar-free, miconazole 25 mg/mL. Net price 80 g = £5.00. Label: 9, counselling advised, hold in mouth, after food
Dose: oral and intestinal fungal infections, 5–10 mL in the mouth after food 4 times daily;

retain near lesions before swallowing; CHILD under 2 years, 2.5 mL twice daily, 2–6 years, 5 mL twice daily, over 6 years, 5 mL 4 times daily
Localised lesions, smear affected area with clean finger; a 15-g tube (net price £1.70) also available
1. 15-g tube can be sold to public

PoM *Intravenous solution,* miconazole 10 mg/mL. For dilution and use as an infusion. Net price 20-mL amp = £1.47 (hosp. only)
Note. Contains polyethoxylated castor oil which has been associated with anaphylaxis

NYSTATIN

Indications: candidiasis

Side-effects: nausea, vomiting, diarrhoea at high doses

Dose: by mouth, intestinal candidiasis 500 000 units every 6 hours, doubled in severe infections; CHILD 100 000 units 4 times daily

For use as a mouthwash in oral candidiasis, see section 12.3.2

PoM **Nystatin** (Non-proprietary)
Oral suspension, nystatin 100 000 units/mL. Net price 30 mL with pipette = £2.50. Label: 9, counselling, use of pipette

PoM **Nystan**® (Squibb)
Tablets, brown, s/c, nystatin 500 000 units. Net price 56-tab pack = £4.70. Label: 9
Pastilles—see section 12.3.2
Suspension, yellow, nystatin 100 000 units/mL. Net price 30 mL with pipette = £2.50. Label: 9, counselling, use of pipette
Suspension, gluten-, lactose-, and sugar-free, nystatin 100 000 units/mL when reconstituted with water. Net price 24 mL with pipette = £1.67. Label: 9, counselling, use of pipette

PoM **Nystatin-Dome**® (Lagap)
Suspension, yellow, nystatin 100 000 units/mL. Net price 30 mL with 1-mL spoon = £2.50. Label: 9, counselling, use of 1-mL spoon

TERBINAFINE

Indications: dermatophyte infections of the nails, ringworm infections (including tinea pedis, cruris, and corporis) where oral therapy appropriate (due to site, severity or extent)

Cautions: hepatic and renal impairment; pregnancy, breast-feeding; **interactions:** Appendix 1 (terbinafine)

Side-effects: abdominal discomfort, loss of appetite, nausea, diarrhoea; rash, urticaria

Dose: 250 mg daily usually for 2–6 weeks in tinea pedis, 2–4 weeks in tinea cruris, 4 weeks in tinea corporis, 6 weeks–3 months or longer in nail infections; CHILD not yet recommended

▼ PoM **Lamisil**® (Sandoz)
Tablets, off-white, scored, terbinafine 250 mg (as hydrochloride), net price 14-tab pack = £23.75, 28-tab pack = £45.80. Label: 9

5.3 Antiviral drugs

The specific therapy of virus infections is generally unsatisfactory and treatment is, therefore, primarily symptomatic. Fortunately, the majority of infections resolve spontaneously.

HERPES SIMPLEX AND VARICELLA–ZOSTER

Acyclovir is active against herpes viruses but does not eradicate them. It is effective only if started at the onset of infection. Uses of acyclovir include the systemic treatment of varicella–zoster and the systemic and topical treatment of herpes simplex infections of the skin and mucous membranes (including initial and recurrent genital herpes); it is also used topically in the eye. It can be life-saving in herpes simplex and varicella–zoster infections in the immunocompromised, and is also used in the immunocompromised for prevention of recurrence and prophylaxis. See also section 11.3.3 (eye) and section 13.10.3 (skin, including herpes labialis).

Idoxuridine is also only effective if started at the onset of infection; it is too toxic for systemic use. It has been used topically in the treatment of herpes simplex lesions of the skin and external genitalia with variable results; it has also been used topically in the treatment of zoster, but evidence of its value is dubious. See also section 11.3.3 (eye) and section 13.10.3 (skin, including herpes labialis).

Inosine pranobex has been used by mouth for herpes simplex infections; its effectiveness has not been established. **Amantadine** has also been used by mouth but, again, its effectiveness has not been established; it has also been used for the prophylaxis of influenza A infections.

ACYCLOVIR

Indications: herpes simplex and varicella–zoster
Cautions: maintain adequate hydration; reduce dose in renal impairment; pregnancy; **interactions:** Appendix 1 (acyclovir)
Side-effects: rashes; gastro-intestinal disturbances; rises in bilirubin and liver-related enzymes, increases in blood urea and creatinine, decreases in haematological indices, headache, neurological reactions, fatigue; on intravenous infusion, severe local inflammation (sometimes leading to ulceration), also confusion, hallucinations, agitation, tremors, somnolence, psychosis, convulsions and coma
Dose: by mouth,
Herpes simplex, treatment, 200 mg (400 mg in the immunocompromised) 5 times daily, usually for 5 days; CHILD under 2 years, half adult dose, over 2 years, adult dose
Herpes simplex, prevention of recurrence, 200 mg 4 times daily *or* 400 mg twice daily possibly reduced to 200 mg 2 or 3 times daily and interrupted every 6–12 months
Herpes simplex, prophylaxis in the immunocompromised, 200–400 mg 4 times daily; CHILD under 2 years, half adult dose, over 2 years, adult dose
Herpes zoster, 800 mg 5 times daily for 7 days

By intravenous infusion over 1 hour, herpes simplex or recurrent varicella-zoster 5 mg/kg every 8 hours; doubled in primary and recurrent varicella-zoster in the immunocompromised, and in simplex encephalitis; CHILD up to 3 months 10 mg/kg every 8 hours; 3 months–12 years, 250 mg/m^2 every 8 hours, dose doubled in the immunocompromised and in simplex encephalitis
By topical application, herpes simplex (*cream* or *eye ointment* as appropriate) every 4 hours (5 times daily), see sections 13.10.3 and 11.3.3
Note. Cream should not be used on mucous membranes

PoM **Zovirax**® (Wellcome)
Tablets, acyclovir 200 mg (blue), net price 25-tab pack = £28.89; 400 mg (pink), 56-tab pack = £105.95; 800 mg (blue, scored), 35-tab pack = £113.00. Label: 9
Suspension, off-white, sugar-free, acyclovir 200 mg/5 mL. Net price 125 mL = £28.89. Label: 9
Intravenous infusion, powder for reconstitution, acyclovir (as sodium salt). Net price 250-mg vial = £10.91; 500-mg vial = £20.22
Electrolytes: Na$^+$ 1.1 mmol/250-mg vial
Cream, see section 13.10.3
Eye ointment, see section 11.3.3

AMANTADINE HYDROCHLORIDE

Indications: see under Dose; parkinsonism, see section 4.9.1
Cautions; Contra-indications; Side-effects: see section 4.9.1
Dose: herpes zoster, 100 g twice daily for 14 days, if necessary extended for a further 14 days for post-herpetic neuralgia
Influenza A$_2$, treatment, 100 twice daily for 5–7 days; prophylaxis 100 g twice daily for as long as required (usually 7–10 days); CHILD 10–15 years, 100 g daily

Preparations
See section 4.9.1

IDOXURIDINE

See sections 11.3.3 (eye) and 13.10.3 (skin including herpes labialis)

INOSINE PRANOBEX

Indications: see under Dose
Cautions: avoid in renal impairment; history of gout or hyperuricaemia
Side-effects: reversible increases in serum and urinary uric acid
Dose: mucocutaneous herpes simplex, 1 g 4 times daily for 7–14 days
Adjunctive treatment of genital warts, 1 g 3 times daily for 14–28 days

PoM **Imunovir**® (Leo)
Tablets, inosine pranobex 500 mg. Net price 100 = £37.24. Label: 9

HUMAN IMMUNODEFICIENCY VIRUS

Zidovudine inhibits the human immunodeficiency virus (HIV) but does not eradicate it from the body; it is not therefore a cure for AIDS but may delay progression of the disease. It is now also being recommended for asymptomatic HIV antibody positive individuals.

Zidovudine is toxic and expensive and should only be prescribed by those experienced in its use.

ZIDOVUDINE
(Azidothymidine, AZT)

Indications: management of advanced human immunodeficiency virus (HIV) disease such as acquired immunodeficiency syndrome (AIDS) or AIDS-related complex; early symptomatic or asymptomatic HIV infection with markers indicating risk of disease progression

Cautions: haematological toxicity (blood tests at least every 2 weeks for first 3 months then at least once a month, early disease with good bone marrow reserves may require less frequent tests e.g. every 1–3 months); adjust dose according to data sheet if anaemia or myelosuppression; renal and hepatic impairment; elderly; pregnancy; avoid in breast-feeding; **interactions:** Appendix 1 (zidovudine)

Contra-indications: abnormally low neutrophil counts or haemoglobin values (see data sheet)

Side-effects: anaemia (often requiring transfusion), neutropenia, and leucopenia (all more frequent with high dose and advanced disease); also include, nausea and vomiting, anorexia, abdominal pain, headache, rash, fever, myalgia, paraesthesia, insomnia, malaise, and asthenia

Dose: by mouth, symptomatic disease, 200 mg every 4 hours (total 1.2 g daily) for 70-kg patient; for advanced disease with poorer tolerance dose may be reduced to maintenance of 100 mg every 4 hours (total 600 mg daily); daily dosage can be given in 4–5 divided doses
Asymptomatic disease, initially 500 mg daily increased if disease progresses to 1.5 g daily CHILD over 3 months initially 180 mg/m^2 every 6 hours

By intravenous infusion, patients temporarily unable to take oral zidovudine, 2.5 mg/kg every 4 hours; not to be given for more than 2 weeks

PoM **Retrovir**® (Wellcome)
Capsules, white/blue band, zidovudine 100 mg, net price 100 = £119.00; 250 mg (blue/white), 40-cap pack = £119.00
Syrup, zidovudine 50 mg/5 mL. Net price 200-mL pack with 10-mL oral syringe = £23.80
▼*Injection,* zidovudine 20 mg/mL. For dilution and use as an intravenous infusion. Net price 10 mL vial = £11.94

CYTOMEGALOVIRUS (CMV)

Ganciclovir is related to acyclovir but with enhanced activity against cytomegalovirus; it is much more toxic than acyclovir and indicated only for life- or sight-threatening *cytomegalovirus infections in immunocompromised* patients. It can cause leucopenia and thrombocytopenia and is also a potential carcinogen. It should therefore only be prescribed when the potential benefit outweighs the risks of adverse reactions. Ganciclovir causes profound myelosuppression when given with zidovudine; the two should not normally be given together particularly during initial ganciclovir therapy.

Foscarnet is also active against cytomegalovirus and is indicated for cytomegalovirus retinitis in patients with AIDS in whom ganciclovir is contraindicated or is inappropriate. It is not recommended for the treatment of CMV infections other than retinitis or for use in non-AIDS patients. Foscarnet is a toxic drug which can cause impairment of renal function in up to 50% of patients.

GANCICLOVIR

Indications: life-threatening or sight-threatening cytomegalovirus infections in immunocompromised patients only (consult data sheet)

Cautions: haematological toxicity (blood counts required every 1–2 days for first 14 days—see data sheet); renal impairment; concomitant administration of drugs that inhibit replication of rapidly dividing cells (e.g. pentamidine, co-trimoxazole); history of exposure to irradiation or to drugs toxic to bone marrow (avoid concomitant zidovudine during induction); increased risk of seizures with imipenem; potential carcinogen; ensure adequate hydration after administration; vesicant—infuse only into veins with adequate blood flow; **not** for neonatal or congenital cytomegalovirus; **interactions:** Appendix 1 (ganciclovir)

Contra-indications: pregnancy (includes effective contraception during treatment and barrier contraception for men for 90 days after treatment); breast-feeding (until 72 hours after last dose); hypersensitivity to ganciclovir or acyclovir; abnormally low neutrophil counts (see data sheet)

Side-effects: most frequent, neutropenia and thrombocytopenia; anaemia and eosinophilia; fever, rash, abnormal liver function tests; raised blood urea nitrogen or serum creatinine; also sepsis, facial oedema, sore throat, epistaxis, malaise; other side-effects reported have included all body systems, including cardiovascular, CNS and special senses, gastro-intestinal, metabolic, musculoskeletal, respiratory, dermatological, urogenital (see data sheet); local reactions at injection site

Dose: by intravenous infusion over 1 hour, initially 5 mg/kg every 12 hours for 14–21 days; maintenance (for patients at risk of relapse of retinitis) 6 mg/kg daily on 5 days per week *or* 5 mg/kg daily every day
In renal impairment, consult data sheet for dosage reduction

PoM Cymevene® (Syntex)
Intravenous infusion, powder for reconstitution, ganciclovir (as sodium salt). Net price 500-mg vial = £32.42

Electrolytes: Na⁺ 2 mmol/500-mg vial
CAUTION IN HANDLING. Wear polythene gloves and safety glasses when reconstituting; if solution contacts skin or mucosa immediately wash with soap and water

FOSCARNET SODIUM
Indications: cytomegalovirus retinitis in patients with AIDS in whom ganciclovir is inappropriate
Cautions: renal impairment (avoid if severe), hypocalcaemia, monitor serum creatinine and serum calcium concentrations every second day; ensure adequate hydration
Contra-indications: pregnancy, breast-feeding
Side-effects: nausea, vomiting, headache, fatigue, rash; impairment of renal function including acute renal failure, symptomatic hypocalcaemia; decreased haemoglobin concentration; rarely hypoglycaemia, convulsions; thrombophlebitis if given undiluted by peripheral vein
Dose: by intravenous infusion, 20 mg/kg over 30 minutes then 21–200 mg/kg daily according to renal function for 2–3 weeks

▼ PoM Foscavir® (Astra)
Intravenous infusion, foscarnet sodium hexahydrate 24 mg/mL. Net price 500-mL bottle = £53.58

RESPIRATORY SYNCYTIAL VIRUS

Tribavirin inhibits a wide range of DNA and RNA viruses. It is given by inhalation for the treatment of severe bronchiolitis caused by the respiratory syncytial virus in infants, especially when they have other serious diseases. It is also effective in lassa fever.

TRIBAVIRIN
(Ribavirin)
Indications: severe respiratory syncytial virus bronchiolitis in infants and children
Cautions: maintain standard supportive respiratory and fluid management therapy; monitor equipment for precipitation
Contra-indications: pregnancy
Side-effects: reticulocytosis; also worsening respiration, bacterial pneumonia, and pneumothorax reported
Dose: by aerosol inhalation or nebulisation (via small particle aerosol generator) of solution containing 20 mg/mL for 12–18 hours for at least 3 days; max. 7 days

PoM Virazid® (Britannia)
Inhalation, tribavirin 6 g for reconstitution with 300 mL water for injections. Net price 3 × 6-g vials = £585.00

5.4 Antiprotozoal drugs
5.4.1 Antimalarials
5.4.2 Amoebicides
5.4.3 Trichomonacides
5.4.4 Antigiardial drugs
5.4.5 Leishmaniacides
5.4.6 Trypanocides
5.4.7 Drugs for toxoplasmosis
5.4.8 Drugs for pneumocystis pneumonia

Advice on specific problems available from:

Birmingham	021-766 6611
Glasgow	041-946 7120
Liverpool	051-708 9393
London	071-387 4411 (treatment)
	071-637 9899 (travel prophylaxis)
	071-636 8636 (travel prophylaxis)
	071-636 7921 (recorded advice)
	071-927 2212 (recorded advice)
	071-927 2435 (recorded advice)
Oxford	(0865) 225214

5.4.1 Antimalarials

Recommendations on the prophylaxis and treatment of malaria reflect guidelines agreed by UK malaria specialists.

The centres listed above should be consulted for advice on special problems.

TREATMENT OF MALARIA

If the infective species is **not known** or if the infection is **mixed** initial treatment should be with quinine, mefloquine, or halofantrine as for *falciparum malaria* (next column).

---

1. For chloroquine-sensitive strains of falciparum malaria chloroquine is effective *by mouth* in the dosage schedule outlined under benign malarias but it should **not** be used unless there is an **unambiguous exposure history** in one of the few remaining areas of chloroquine sensitivity.
   If the patient with a *chloroquine-sensitive infection* is seriously ill, chloroquine is given by *continuous intravenous infusion*. The dosage (for adults and children) is chloroquine 10 mg/kg (of base) infused over 8 hours, followed by three 8-hour infusions of 5 mg/kg (of base) each. *Oral therapy* is started as soon as possible to complete the course; the total cumulative dose for the course should be 25 mg/kg of base.
2. Valid for quinine hydrochloride, dihydrochloride, and sulphate; not valid for quinine bisulphate which contains a correspondingly smaller amount of quinine.
3. In intensive care units the loading dose can alternatively be given as quinine salt[2] 7 mg/kg infused over 30 minutes followed immediately by 10 mg/kg over 4 hours then (after 8 hours) maintenance dose as described.
4. **Important:** the loading dose of 20 mg/kg should **not** be used if the patient has received quinine (or quinidine) or mefloquine or possibly halofantrine during the previous 24 hours
5. Maintenance dose should be reduced to 5–7 mg/kg of salt if parenteral treatment is required for more than 48 hours.

FALCIPARUM MALARIA (TREATMENT)

Falciparum malaria (malignant malaria) is caused by *Plasmodium falciparum*. In most parts of the world *P. falciparum* is now resistant to chloroquine which should not therefore be given for treatment[1].

Quinine, mefloquine, or **halofantrine** can be given *by mouth* if the patient can swallow tablets and there are no serious manifestations (e.g. impaired consciousness); quinine should be given *by intravenous infusion* (see below) if the patient is seriously ill or unable to take tablets.

The adult dosage regimen for **quinine** *by mouth* is:

600 mg (of quinine salt[2]) every 8 hours for 7 days *and* (if quinine resistance known or suspected) *either followed by* **Fansidar**® 3 tablets as a single dose
or (if Fansidar®-resistant) *followed by* **tetracycline** 250 mg every 6 hours for 7 days when renal function has returned to normal.

Alternatively **mefloquine** or **halofantrine** may be given instead of quinine.

The adult dosage regimen for **mefloquine** *by mouth* is:

20 mg/kg (of mefloquine base) as a single dose (up to maximum 1.5 g) *or preferably* as 2 divided doses 6–8 hours apart.

The adult dosage regimen for **halofantrine** *by mouth* is:

1.5 g of halofantrine hydrochloride divided into three doses of 500 mg given at intervals of 6 hours; this course should be repeated after an interval of 1 week.

It is not necessary to give Fansidar® or tetracycline after mefloquine or halofantrine treatment.

If the patient is seriously ill, **quinine** should be given *by intravenous infusion*. The adult dosage regimen for quinine *by infusion* is:

loading dose[3] of 20 mg/kg[4] (up to maximum 1.4 g) of quinine salt[2] infused over 4 hours *then after 8–12 hours* maintenance dose of 10 mg/kg[5] (up to maximum 700 mg) of quinine salt[2] infused over 4 hours every 8–12 hours (until patient can swallow tablets to complete the 7-day course) *either followed by* Fansidar® *or* (when renal function has returned to normal) tetracycline as above.

CHILDREN.
Oral. Quinine is well tolerated by children although the salts are bitter. The dosage regimen for quinine *by mouth* for children is:

10 mg/kg (of quinine salt[2]) every 8 hours for 7 days *then* (if quinine resistance known or suspected)
Fansidar® as a single dose: up to 4 years ½ tablet, 5–6 years 1 tablet, 7–9 years 1½ tablets, 10–14 years 2 tablets.

Alternatively mefloquine or halofantrine may be given instead of quinine; it is not necessary to give Fansidar® after mefloquine or halofantrine treatment. The dosage regimen for mefloquine *by mouth* for children is calculated on a mg/kg basis as for adults (see above). The dosage regimen for halofantrine *by mouth* for children over 37 kg is the same as for adults (see above); the dosage regimen for halofantrine for smaller children is reduced as follows:

weight under 23 kg, no suitable dose form;
weight 23–31 kg, 3 doses of 250 mg at intervals of 6 hours;
weight 32–37 kg, 3 doses of 375 mg at intervals of 6 hours.

This course of halofantrine should be repeated after an interval of 1 week.

Parenteral. The dosage regimen for quinine *by intravenous infusion* for children is calculated on a mg/kg basis as for adults (see above).

BENIGN MALARIAS (TREATMENT)

Benign malaria is usually caused by *Plasmodium vivax* and less commonly by *P. ovale* and *P. malariae*. **Chloroquine**[6] is the drug of choice for the treatment of benign malarias.

The adult dosage regimen for **chloroquine** *by mouth* is:

initial dose of 600 mg (of base) *then*
a single dose of 300 mg after 6 to 8 hours *then*
a single dose of 300 mg daily for 2 days
(approximate total cumulative dose of 25 mg/kg of base)

Chloroquine alone is adequate for *P. malariae* infections but in the case of *P. vivax* and *P. ovale*, a *radical cure* (to destroy parasites in the liver and thus prevent relapses) is required. This is achieved with **primaquine**[7] in an adult dosage of 15 mg daily for 14 to 21 days given after the chloroquine; a 21-day course is recommended for Chesson-type strains of *P. vivax* from south-east Asia and western Pacific.

CHILDREN. The dosage regimen of chloroquine for benign malaria in children is:

initial dose of 10 mg/kg (of base) *then*
a single dose of 5 mg/kg after 6–8 hours *then*
a single dose of 5 mg/kg daily for 2 days

For a *radical cure* children are then given primaquine[7] in a dose of 250 micrograms/kg daily.

1–5. See previous page.
6. Halofantrine and mefloquine are also active in benign malarias but are not required since chloroquine is usually effective.
7. Before starting primaquine the blood should be tested for glucose-6-phosphate dehydrogenase (G6PD) activity as the drug can cause haemolysis in patients who are deficient in the enzyme. If the patient is G6PD deficient primaquine, in a dose for adults of 30 mg once a week (children 500–750 micrograms/kg once a week) for 8 weeks, has been found useful and without undue harmful effects.

PROPHYLAXIS AGAINST MALARIA

The recommendations on prophylaxis reflect guidelines agreed by UK malaria specialists; the advice is aimed at residents of the UK who travel to endemic areas for short stays. The choice of drug takes account of:
- risk of exposure to malaria;
- extent of drug resistance;
- efficacy of the recommended drugs;
- side-effects of the drugs;
- patient-related criteria (e.g. age, pregnancy, renal or hepatic impairment).

NETS AND REPELLENTS. The most important point to remember is that **prophylaxis is relative and not absolute**, and that breakthrough can occur with any of the drugs recommended anywhere in the world. Personal protection against being bitten, e.g. use of mosquito nets, repellents etc. is **very important**.

LENGTH OF PROPHYLAXIS. Prophylaxis should be started one week before travel into an endemic area (or if not possible at earliest opportunity up to 1 or 2 days before travel); it should be continued for at least 4 weeks after leaving. Administration of mefloquine should be restricted to a period of 3 months (including the dose 1 week beforehand and 4 weeks after).

CHILDREN. The following prophylactic doses are based on guidelines agreed by UK malaria experts and may differ from advice in data sheets. If in doubt telephone centres listed on p. 240.

Age	Weight (kg)	Chloroquine Proguanil	Maloprim®
0–5 weeks		$\frac{1}{8}$	—
6 weeks– 11 months		$\frac{1}{4}$	—
1–5 years	10–19	$\frac{1}{2}$	$\frac{1}{4}$
6–11 years	20–39	$\frac{3}{4}$	$\frac{1}{2}$
12 years	40	adult dose	adult dose

Fraction of adult dose

Note. Weight is a better guide than age for children over 6 months old. Specialist advice should be obtained for use of Maloprim® in children under 1 year of age.

Prophylaxis is required in **breast-fed infants**; although antimalarials are excreted in milk, the amounts are too variable to give reliable protection.

PREGNANCY. Chloroquine and proguanil may be given in usual doses in areas where *P. falciparum* strains are sensitive; in the case of proguanil, folate supplements should be given. Maloprim® is contra-indicated in the first trimester; folate supplements should be given if Maloprim® is prescribed in the second and third trimester. The centres listed on p. 240 should be consulted for advice on prophylaxis in resistant areas.

SPECIFIC RECOMMENDATIONS. Specific recommendations by geographical regions are given below.

North Africa and the Middle East
(risk: generally low; transmission confined to rural areas and may be seasonal)

> chloroquine 300 mg (as base) once weekly
>
> *or*
>
> proguanil hydrochloride 200 mg once daily

Above recommendations apply to some areas of Turkey (south coast and border with Syria) and also to Mauritius. No chemoprophylaxis needed for Algeria, Libya, Morocco, Tunisia, or tourist areas of Egypt; *both* chloroquine *and* proguanil needed for Afghanistan, Iran, and Oman.

Sub-Saharan Africa
(includes East, Central and West Africa, north-east corner of South Africa (including Kruger National Park) and also Madagascar) (risk: very high)

> *both*
> chloroquine 300 mg (as base) once weekly
> *and*
> proguanil hydrochloride 200 mg once daily

Mefloquine alone is an option for short-term travellers (administration restricted to 3 months) to Cameroon, Kenya, Malawi, Tanzania, Uganda, Zaire, and Zambia; see Mefloquine p. 244 for details of regimen.

South Asia
(Bangladesh, Bhutan, India, Nepal, Pakistan, and Sri Lanka) (risk: variable)

> *both*
> chloroquine 300 mg (as base) once weekly
> *and*
> proguanil hydrochloride 200 mg once daily

South-East Asia
(risk: varies from very low to substantial)

> *both*
> chloroquine 300 mg (as base) once weekly
> *and*
> proguanil hydrochloride 200 mg once daily

Mefloquine alone is an option for short-term travellers (administration restricted to 3 months); see Mefloquine p. 244 for details of regimen.

No chemoprophylaxis needed for tourist areas and cities of Brunei, China, Hong Kong, peninsular west Malaysia, Philippines, Sarawak, Singapore, and Thailand (all very low risk).

5.4 Antiprotozoal drugs

Oceania (Papua New Guinea, Solomon Islands, Vanuatu) (risk: very high)

> both
> Maloprim® 1 tablet once weekly
> and
> chloroquine 300 mg (as base) once weekly

Mefloquine alone is an option for short-term travellers (administration restricted to 3 months); see Mefloquine (p. 244) for details of regimen.

Latin America
(risk: variable to high)

Variable risk areas:

> chloroquine 300 mg (as base) once weekly

or

> proguanil hydrochloride 200 mg once daily

Used for variable risk areas which include Argentina (a few areas), Belize, rural Costa Rica, Dominican Republic, El Salvador, Guatemala, Haiti, Honduras, rural Mexico, Nicaragua, rural Paraguay, and Peru (below 1500 m)

Variable to high risk areas:

> both
> chloroquine 300 mg (as base) once weekly
> and
> proguanil hydrochloride 200 mg once daily

Used for variable to high risk areas which include Bolivia (below 2500 m), rural Brazil, Colombia, Equador, French Guiana, Guyana, Panama, Suriname, and rural Venezuela.
Mefloquine alone is an option for short-term travellers (administration restricted to 3 months) to the Amazonas region of Brazil; see Mefloquine (p. 244) for details of regimen.

> TREATMENT COURSES. Adults travelling to areas of chloroquine-resistance who are unlikely to have easy access to medical care should carry a treatment course. Self-medication should be **avoided** if medical help is accessible; prophylaxis should be continued during and after the attack. In view of the continuing emergence of resistant strains and of the different regimens required for different areas expert advice should be sought on the best treatment course for an individual patient.

CHLOROQUINE

Indications: chemoprophylaxis and treatment of malaria; rheumatoid arthritis and lupus erythematosus—see section 10.1.3

Cautions: hepatic and renal impairment, pregnancy (but for malaria benefit outweighs risk, see Appendix 4, Antimalarials), may exacerbate psoriasis, neurological disorders (especially history of epilepsy), severe gastro-intestinal disorders, G6PD deficiency (see section 9.1.5); elderly; ophthalmic examination and long-term therapy, see p. 368; avoid concurrent therapy with hepatotoxic drugs—other **interactions**: Appendix 1 (chloroquine)

Side-effects: gastro-intestinal disturbances, headache, visual disturbances, irreversible retinal damage, corneal opacities, depigmentation or loss of hair, skin reactions; rarely blood disorders (thrombocytopenia, agranulocytosis, and aplastic anaemia), psychosis

Dose: see notes above

PoM* **Avloclor**® (ICI)
Tablets, scored, chloroquine phosphate 250 mg (≡chloroquine base 155 mg). Net price 20-tab pack = 70p. Label: 5
* Can be sold to the public provided it is licensed and labelled for the prophylaxis of malaria

Nivaquine® (Rhône-Poulenc Rorer)
PoM* *Tablets*, f/c, yellow, chloroquine sulphate 200 mg (≡chloroquine base 150 mg). Net price 28-tab pack = £1.04. Label: 5
* Can be sold to the public provided it is licensed and labelled for the prophylaxis of malaria

PoM* *Syrup*, golden, chloroquine sulphate 68 mg/5 mL (≡chloroquine base 50 mg/5 mL). Net price 100 mL = £2.18. Label: 5
* Can be sold to the public provided it is licensed and labelled for the prophylaxis of malaria

PoM *Injection*, chloroquine sulphate 54.5 mg/mL (≡chloroquine base 40 mg/mL). Net price 5-mL amp = 52p

HALOFANTRINE HYDROCHLORIDE

Indications: treatment of uncomplicated chloroquine-resistant falciparum malaria, see notes above

Cautions: discontinue breast-feeding during treatment; not indicated for cerebral or complicated malaria

Contra-indications: pregnancy

Side-effects: diarrhoea, abdominal pain, nausea, vomiting; transient elevation of serum transaminases; pruritus also reported

Dose: see notes above

▼ PoM **Halfan**® (SK&F)
Tablets, scored, halofantrine hydrochloride 250 mg. Net price 12-tab pack = £13.96

MEFLOQUINE

Indications: chemoprophylaxis and treatment of chloroquine-resistant falciparum malaria, see notes above

Cautionary label wordings, see inside back cover

Cautions: exclude pregnancy before starting chemoprophylaxis (**important teratogenic risk**) avoid for chemoprophylaxis in severe hepatic and in renal impairment; avoid frequent or prolonged administration (accumulation occurs due to long half-life); not recommended in young children (under 15 kg); **interactions:** Appendix 1 (mefloquine)
COUNSELLING. May affect performance of skilled tasks
Contra-indications: chemoprophylaxis in pregnancy (teratogenic in *animals*, **avoid** pregnancy **during** and for **3 months after**), breast-feeding, and history of psychiatric disturbances or convulsions
Side-effects: nausea, vomiting, diarrhoea, abdominal pain, anorexia; dizziness and loss of balance; rarely bradycardia, headache, neuropsychiatric disturbances (discontinue treatment), weakness, paraesthesia, rash, pruritus, and disturbances in liver function tests; erythema multiforme (and Stevens-Johnson syndrome) reported
Dose: short-term chemoprophylaxis (administration restricted to 3 months), 250 mg each week starting 1 week before departure and continued for 4 weeks after leaving malarious area; CHILD 15–19 kg (2–5 years) quarter adult dose, 20–30 kg (6–8 years) half adult dose, 31–45 kg (9–11 years) three-quarters adult dose
Longer chemoprophylaxis (more than total of 3 months), not recommended
Treatment, see notes above

▼ PoM **Lariam**® (Roche)
Tablets, scored, mefloquine 250 mg (as hydrochloride). Net price 8-tab pack = £14.53. Label: 21, 25, 27

PRIMAQUINE

Indications: eradication of *Plasmodium vivax* and *P. ovale* malaria
Cautions: G6PD deficiency (see notes above); systemic diseases associated with granulocytopenia (e.g. rheumatoid arthritis, lupus erythematosus); pregnancy and breast-feeding; **interactions:** Appendix 1 (primaquine)
Side-effects: nausea, vomiting, abdominal pain; less commonly methaemoglobinaemia, haemolytic anaemia especially in G6PD deficiency
Dose: see notes above

Primaquine (ICI)
Tablets, brown, s/c, primaquine 7.5 mg (as phosphate). Net price 20 = 12p

PROGUANIL HYDROCHLORIDE

Indications: chemoprophylaxis of malaria
Cautions: severe renal impairment; pregnancy (folate supplements needed); **interactions:** Appendix 1 (proguanil)
Side-effects: mild gastric intolerance; occasionally mouth ulcers and stomatitis; skin reaction and hair loss reported
Dose: see notes above

Paludrine® (ICI)
Tablets, scored, proguanil hydrochloride 100 mg. Net price 20 = 87p. Label: 21

PYRIMETHAMINE

Indications: malaria (but used only in combination with dapsone or sulphadoxine); toxoplasmosis (section 5.4.7)
Cautions: hepatic or renal impairment, folate supplements in pregnancy, blood counts required with prolonged treatment; **interactions:** Appendix 1 (pyrimethamine)
Side-effects: depression of haematopoiesis with high doses, rashes, insomnia

Daraprim® (Wellcome)
Tablets, scored, pyrimethamine 25 mg. Net price 30-tab pack = £2.22
Dose: not recommended alone

With sulfadoxine
ADDITIONAL CAUTIONS: Severe adverse reactions on long-term use therefore not for prophylaxis; pregnancy (see also Appendix 4) and breast-feeding (see also Appendix 5); **interactions:** Appendix 1
PoM **Fansidar**® (Roche)
Tablets, scored, pyrimethamine 25 mg, sulfadoxine 500 mg. Net price 10-tab pack = £2.52
Dose: treatment, see notes above
Chemoprophylaxis, not recommended by UK experts.

With dapsone
ADDITIONAL CAUTIONS: G6PD deficiency (see section 9.1.5); pregnancy (see also Appendix 4) and breast-feeding (see also Appendix 5); **interactions:** Appendix 1
PoM **Maloprim**® (Wellcome)
Tablets, scored, pyrimethamine 12.5 mg, dapsone 100 mg. Net price 30-tab pack = £2.76
Dose: limited use, see Chemoprophylaxis

QUININE

Indications: falciparum malaria; nocturnal leg cramps, see section 10.2.2
Cautions: atrial fibrillation, conduction defects, heart block, pregnancy; G6PD deficiency (see section 9.1.5); **interactions:** Appendix 1 (quinine)
Contra-indications: haemoglobinuria, optic neuritis
Side-effects: cinchonism, including tinnitus, headache, nausea, abdominal pain, rashes, visual disturbances (including temporary blindness), confusion; hypersensitivity reactions including angioedema, blood disorders (including thrombocytopenia and intravascular coagulation), and acute renal failure; hypoglycaemia (especially after parenteral administration)
Dose: see notes above
Note. Quinine (anhydrous base) 100 mg ≡ quinine bisulphate 169 mg ≡ quinine dihydrochloride 122 mg ≡ quinine hydrochloride 122 mg ≡ quinine sulphate 121 mg. Quinine bisulphate 300-mg tablets are available but provide smaller amounts of quinine than the dihydrochloride, hydrochloride, or sulphate

5.4 Antiprotozoal drugs

PoM **Quinine Dihydrochloride Tablets**, quinine dihydrochloride 300 mg. Net price 20 = £2.34

PoM **Quinine Hydrochloride Tablets**, quinine hydrochloride 300 mg. Net price 20 = £1.84

PoM **Quinine Sulphate Tablets**, coated, quinine sulphate 200 mg, net price 20 = 74p; 300 mg, 20 = 72p

PoM **Quinine Dihydrochloride Injection**, quinine dihydrochloride 300 mg/mL. For dilution and use as an infusion. 1- and 2-mL amps

Injection available from Martindale and Penn (both special order) or from specialist centres (see p. 240)

Note. Intravenous injection of quinine is so hazardous that it has been superseded by infusion

5.4.2 Amoebicides

Metronidazole is the drug of choice for *acute invasive amoebic dysentery* for it is very effective against vegetative amoebae in ulcers at a dosage of 800 mg three times daily for 5 days; it is also effective against amoebae which may have migrated to the liver. It is given either for 10 days, or for 5 days followed by a 10-day course of diloxanide furoate. **Tinidazole** is also effective.

Diloxanide furoate is the drug of choice in *chronic intestinal amoebiasis* in which only cysts and not vegetative forms of *Entamoeba histolytica* are present in the faeces; metronidazole and tinidazole are relatively ineffective. Diloxanide furoate is relatively free from toxic effects in therapeutic doses and the usual course is of 10 days, given alone for chronic infections or following 5 days of metronidazole in acute dysenteric infections.

For *amoebic abscesses* of the liver **metronidazole** is effective in doses of 400 mg 3 times daily for 5–10 days; the course may be repeated after 2 weeks if necessary. Aspiration of the abscess is indicated where it is suspected that it may rupture or where there is no improvement after 72 hours of metronidazole; the aspiration may need to be repeated. Aspiration aids penetration of metronidazole and, for abscesses with more than 100 mL of pus, if carried out in conjunction with drug therapy, may reduce the period of disability.

If metronidazole or tinidazole are not available emetine may be used but its side-effects are much more marked. Diloxanide is not effective against hepatic amoebiasis, but a 10-day course should be given at the completion of metronidazole or tinidazole treatment to destroy any amoebae in the gut.

DILOXANIDE FUROATE

Indications: chronic amoebiasis—see notes

Side-effects: flatulence, vomiting, urticaria, pruritus

Dose: 500 mg every 8 hours for 10 days; CHILD 20 mg/kg daily in 3 divided doses.

See also notes above

PoM **Furamide**® (Boots)

Tablets, scored, diloxanide furoate 500 mg. Label: 9

Available only on direct order from Boots

PoM **Entamizole**® (Boots)

Tablets, off-white, diloxanide furoate 250 mg, metronidazole 200 mg. Label: 4, 9, 21, 25

Available only on direct order from Boots

Dose: amoebiasis, 2 tablets 3 times daily for 5 days; CHILD 5–12 years ½–1 tablet, according to age, for 5 days

Treatment may be extended to 10 days in refractory cases; not suitable for prolonged (e.g. prophylactic) use

METRONIDAZOLE

Indications: see under Dose below; anaerobic infections, section 5.1.11

Cautions; Side-effects: section 5.1.11

Dose: by mouth, invasive intestinal amoebiasis, 800 mg every 8 hours for 5 days; CHILD 1–3 years 200 mg every 8 hours; 3–7 years 200 mg every 6 hours; 7–10 years 400 mg every 8 hours

Extra-intestinal amoebiasis (including liver abscess) and symptomless amoebic cyst passers, 400–800 mg every 8 hours for 5–10 days; CHILD 1–3 years 100–200 mg every 8 hours; 3–7 years 100–200 mg every 6 hours; 7–10 years 200–400 mg every 8 hours

Urogenital trichomoniasis, 200 mg every 8 hours for 7 days *or* 400 mg every 12 hours for 7 days, *or* 800 mg in the morning and 1.2 g at night for 2 days, *or* 2 g as a single dose; CHILD 1–3 years 50 mg every 8 hours for 7 days; 3–7 years 100 mg every 12 hours; 7–10 years 100 mg every 8 hours

Giardiasis, 2 g daily for 3 days; CHILD 1–3 years 500 mg daily; 3–7 years 600–800 mg daily; 7–10 years 1 g daily

Preparations

Section 5.1.11

TINIDAZOLE

Indications: see under Dose below; anaerobic infections, section 5.1.11

Cautions; Side-effects: section 5.1.11

Dose: intestinal amoebiasis, 2 g daily for 2–3 days; CHILD 50–60 mg/kg daily for 3 days

Amoebic involvement of liver, 1.5–2 g daily for 3–5 days; CHILD 50–60 mg/kg daily for 5 days

Urogenital trichomoniasis and giardiasis, single 2-g dose (repeated once if necessary); CHILD single dose of 50–75 mg/kg

Preparations

Section 5.1.11

5.4.3 Trichomonacides

Metronidazole (section 5.4.2) is the treatment of choice for *Trichomonas vaginalis* infection.

If metronidazole is ineffective, **nimorazole** may be tried; it is usually given as a single 2-g dose, with food. A further 2-g dose may be given if there is no clinical improvement.

Alcohol should be avoided during treatment with both metronidazole and nimorazole.

NIMORAZOLE

Indications: trichomoniasis; acute ulcerative gingivitis, see section 12.3.2
Contra-indications: active CNS disease, severe renal failure
Side-effects: nausea, vomiting, rashes, vertigo, drowsiness, ataxia (discontinue treatment), intolerance to alcohol
Dose: see notes above

Naxogin 500® (Farmitalia Carlo Erba)
Tablets, scored, nimorazole 500 mg. Net price 8-tab pack = £1.74. Label: 4, 21

5.4.4 Antigiardial drugs

Metronidazole (section 5.4.2) is the treatment of choice for *Giardia lamblia* infections, given by mouth in a dosage of 2 g daily for 3 days or 400 mg every 8 hours for 5 days.

Alternative treatments are **tinidazole** (section 5.4.2) 2 g as a single dose or **mepacrine hydrochloride** 100 mg every 8 hours for 5–7 days.

MEPACRINE HYDROCHLORIDE

Indications: giardiasis
Cautions: hepatic impairment, elderly, history of psychosis; avoid in psoriasis; **interactions:** Appendix 1 (mepacrine)
Side-effects: gastro-intestinal disturbances; dizziness, headache; with large doses nausea, vomiting and occasionally transient acute toxic psychosis and CNS stimulation; on prolonged treatment yellow discoloration of skin and urine, chronic dermatoses (including severe exfoliative dermatitis), hepatitis, aplastic anaemia; also reported blue/black discoloration of palate and nails and corneal deposits with visual disturbances
Dose: 100 mg every 8 hours for 5–7 days; CHILD 2 mg/kg every 8 hours

Mepacrine Hydrochloride
Tablets, mepacrine hydrochloride 100 mg. Net price 20 = 28p. Label: 4, 9, 14, 21
Available from Boots (special order)

5.4.5 Leishmaniacides

Cutaneous leishmaniasis frequently heals spontaneously but if skin lesions are extensive or unsightly, treatment is indicated, as it is in visceral leishmaniasis (kala-azar).

Sodium stibogluconate, an organic pentavalent antimony compound, is the treatment of choice for visceral leishmaniasis. The dose is 20 mg/kg daily (max. 850 mg) for at least 20 days by intramuscular or intravenous injection; the dosage varies with different geographical regions and expert advice should be obtained. Skin lesions are treated for 10 days.

Pentamidine isethionate (section 5.4.8) has been used in antimony-resistant visceral leishmaniasis, but although the initial response is often good, the relapse rate is high; it is associated with serious side-effects.

SODIUM STIBOGLUCONATE

Indications: leishmaniasis
Cautions: intravenous injections must be given slowly and stopped if coughing or substernal pain develops; intramuscular injection painful
Contra-indications: pneumonia, myocarditis, nephritis, hepatitis
Side-effects: anorexia, vomiting, coughing, substernal pain
Dose: see notes above

PoM **Pentostam**® (Wellcome)
Injection, sodium stibogluconate equivalent to pentavalent antimony 100 mg/mL. Net price 100-mL bottle = £68.01

5.4.6 Trypanocides

The prophylaxis and treatment of trypanosomiasis is difficult and differs according to the strain of organism. Expert advice should therefore be obtained.

5.4.7 Drugs for toxoplasmosis

Most infections caused by *Toxoplasma gondii* are self-limiting, and treatment is not necessary. Exceptions are patients with eye involvement (toxoplasma choroidoretinitis), and those who are immunosuppressed. The treatment of choice is a combination of pyrimethamine and sulphadiazine, given for several weeks (expert advice **essential**). Pyrimethamine is a folate antagonist, and adverse reactions to this combination are relatively common (folinic acid supplements and weekly blood counts needed).

If toxoplasmosis is acquired in pregnancy, transplacental infection may lead to severe disease in the fetus. The pyrimethamine and sulphadiazine combination is best avoided in pregnancy but there are encouraging reports with spiramycin (not on UK market).

5.4.8 Drugs for Pneumocystis pneumonia

Pneumonia caused by *Pneumocystis carinii* occurs in immunosuppressed or severely debilitated patients. It is the commonest cause of pneumonia in AIDS. **Co-trimoxazole** (section 5.1.8) in high dosage is the drug of choice for the treatment of pneumocystis pneumonia. **Pentamidine isethionate** is an alternative to co-trimoxazole and is particularly indicated for patients with a history of adverse reactions to, or who have not responded to, co-trimoxazole. Pentamidine isethionate is a potentially toxic drug that can cause severe hypotension during or immediately after administration; it should only be administered by those experienced in its use. Pentamidine isethionate is given by intravenous infusion but can also be administered by inhalation which reduces side-effects (although systemic absorption may still occur); intermittent prophylactic inhalation may prevent relapse.

PENTAMIDINE ISETHIONATE

Indications: see under Dose (should only be given by specialists)

Cautions: risk of severe hypotension following administration (establish baseline blood pressure and administer with patient lying down; monitor blood pressure closely during administration, and at regular intervals, until treatment concluded); hepatic and renal impairment; hypertension or hypotension; hyperglycaemia or hypoglycaemia; leucopenia, thrombocytopenia, or anaemia; carry out laboratory monitoring for all functions according to data sheet

Side-effects: severe reactions, sometimes fatal, due to hypotension, hypoglycaemia, pancreatitis, and arrhythmias; also leucopenia, thrombocytopenia, acute renal failure, hypocalcaemia; also reported: azotaemia, abnormal liver-function tests, leucopenia, anaemia, hyperkalaemia, nausea and vomiting, dizziness, syncope, flushing, hyperglycaemia, rash, and taste disturbances; bronchoconstriction reported on inhalation; discomfort, pain, induration, abscess formation, and muscle necrosis at injection site

Dose: Pneumocystis carinii pneumonia, *by intravenous infusion*, 4 mg/kg daily for at least 14 days (reduced according to data sheet in renal impairment)

By inhalation of nebulised solution (using suitable equipment—see data sheet) 600 mg pentamidine isethionate daily for 3 weeks; secondary prevention, 300 mg every 4 weeks *or* 150 mg every 2 weeks

Visceral leishmaniasis (Kala-azar), *by deep intramuscular injection*, 3–4 mg/kg on alternate days to max. total of 10 injections; course may be repeated if necessary

Cutaneous leishmaniasis, *by deep intramuscular injection*, 3–4 mg/kg once or twice weekly until condition resolves (but see also section 5.4.5)

Trypanosomiasis, *by deep intramuscular injection or intravenous infusion*, 4 mg/kg daily on alternate days to total of 7–10 injections

Note. Direct bolus intravenous injection should be avoided whenever possible and **never** given rapidly; intramuscular injections should be deep and preferably given into the buttock

PoM **Pentacarinat**® (Rhône-Poulenc Rorer)
Injection, powder for reconstitution, pentamidine isethionate. Net price 300-mg vial = £15.98
Nebuliser solution, pentamidine isethionate. Net price 300-mg bottle = £16.87

5.5 Anthelmintics

5.5.1 Drugs for threadworms
5.5.2 Ascaricides
5.5.3 Taenicides
5.5.4 Drugs for hookworms
5.5.5 Schistosomicides
5.5.6 Filaricides
5.5.7 Drugs for guinea worms
5.5.8 Drugs for strongyloidiasis

Advice on prophylaxis and treatment of helminth infections is available from:

Birmingham	021-766 6611
Glasgow	041-946 7120
Liverpool	051-708 9393
London	071-387 4411 (treatment)

5.5.1 Drugs for threadworms
(pinworms, *Enterobius vermicularis*)

Anthelmintics are effective in threadworm infections, but their use needs to be combined with hygienic measures to break the cycle of autoinfection. All members of the family require treatment.

Adult threadworms do not live for longer than 6 weeks and for development of fresh worms, ova must be swallowed and exposed to the action of digestive juices in the upper intestinal tract. Direct multiplication of worms does not take place in the large bowel. Adult female worms lay ova on the peri-anal skin which causes pruritus; scratching the area then leads to ova being transmitted on fingers to the mouth, often via food eaten with unwashed hands. Washing hands and scrubbing nails before each meal and after each visit to the toilet is essential. A bath taken immediately after rising will remove ova laid during the night.

Mebendazole is the drug of choice for patients of all ages over 2 years. It is given as a single dose; as reinfection is very common, a second dose may be given after 2–3 weeks.

Piperazine salts are preferably given daily for 7 days (followed by a second course if necessary 7 days later); single-dose preparations are also available.

Pyrantel is equally effective. It is given as a single dose; cure-rates are improved if one or two further doses are given at intervals of 2 weeks.

MEBENDAZOLE

Indications: threadworm, roundworm, whipworm, and hookworm infections

Cautions: pregnancy (toxicity in *rats*)

Note. The package insert in the Vermox® pack includes the statement that it is not suitable for women known to be pregnant or children under 2 years

Side-effects: rarely abdominal pain, diarrhoea

Dose: threadworms, ADULT and CHILD over 2 years, 100 mg as a single dose; if reinfection occurs second dose may be needed after 2–3 weeks; CHILD under 2 years, not yet recommended

Roundworms—section 5.5.2

[1]PoM **Vermox**® (Janssen)
Tablets, pink, scored, chewable, mebendazole 100 mg. Net price 6-tab pack = £1.57
Suspension mebendazole 100 mg/5 mL. Net price 30 mL = £1.82

1. Can be sold to the public if supplied for the oral treatment of enterobiasis in a container or package containing only a single dose of not more than 100 mg of mebendazole; a proprietary brand (Ovex®) is also on sale to the public.

PIPERAZINE

Indications: threadworm and roundworm infections

Cautions: renal impairment (avoid if severe), liver disease, neurological disease; epilepsy, pregnancy (see also Appendix 4 (packs on sale to the general public carry a warning to avoid in epilepsy and pregnancy); **interactions:** Appendix 1 (piperazine)

Side-effects: nausea, vomiting, colic, diarrhoea, allergic reactions including urticaria, bronchospasm, and rare reports of Stevens-Johnson syndrome and angioedema; rarely dizziness, muscular incoordination ('worm wobble'); drowsiness, confusion and clonic contractions in patients with neurological or renal abnormalities

Dose: see under Preparations, below

Piperazine Citrate (Non-proprietary)
Elixir, piperazine hydrate 750 mg/5 mL (as citrate)
Available from Cupal (Expelix®)
Dose: threadworms, 15 mL once daily for 7 days; CHILD 2–3 years 5 mL once daily for 7 days, 4–6 years 7.5 mL once daily for 7 days, 7–12 years 10 mL once daily for 7 days; repeat course after 1 week if necessary
Roundworms, 30 mL as a single dose; CHILD 1–3 years 10 mL as a single dose, 4–5 years 15 mL as a single dose, 6–8 years 20 mL as a single dose, 9–12 years 25 mL as a single dose; repeat dose after 2 weeks

Pripsen® (R&C)
Oral powder, cream, piperazine phosphate 4 g and sennosides 15.3 mg/sachet. Net price two-dose sachet pack = £1.31. Label: 13
Dose: threadworms, stirred into a small glass of milk or water and drunk immediately, ADULT and CHILD over 6 years, 1 sachet, repeat after 14 days; INFANT 3 months–1 year, one-third sachet (2.5 mL powder); CHILD 1–6 years, two-thirds sachet (5 mL powder), repeat after 14 days
Roundworms, first dose as for threadworms; repeat at monthly intervals for up to 3 months if reinfection risk

5.5.2 Ascaricides
(common roundworm infections)

Levamisole (not on UK market) is very effective against ascaris and is generally considered to be the drug of choice. It is very well tolerated; mild nausea or vomiting has been reported in about 1% of treated patients; it is given as a single dose of 120–150 mg in adults.

Mebendazole (section 5.5.1) is also active against *Ascaris lumbricoides*; the usual dose is 100 mg twice daily for 3 days. **Pyrantel** is also an effective broad-spectrum anthelmintic and a single dose of 10 mg/kg (max. 1 g) is usually sufficient to eradicate ascaris; it may occasionally produce mild nausea but experience shows it to be a very safe drug. **Piperazine** may also be given in a single adult dose equivalent to 4–4.5 g of piperazine hydrate see Piperazine, above.

PYRANTEL

Indications: roundworm, threadworm, and hookworm infections

Cautions: liver disease; **interactions:** Appendix 1 (pyrantel)

Side-effects: see notes above

Dose: ADULT and CHILD over 6 months, *Ascaris lumbricoides* alone, a single dose of 5 mg/kg; mixed infections involving *Ascaris lumbricoides*, single dose of 10 mg/kg
Hookworm—section 5.5.4
Threadworm—section 5.5.1

PoM **Combantrin®** (Pfizer)
Tablets, orange, pyrantel 125 mg (as embonate). Net price 6-tab pack = 64p

5.5.3 Taenicides
(tapeworms)

Niclosamide (Yomesan®, *Bayer*, not on UK market) is the most widely used drug for tapeworm infections and side-effects are limited to occasional gastro-intestinal upset, light-headedness, and pruritus; it is not effective against larval worms. Fears of developing cysticercosis in *Taenia solium* infections have proved unfounded. All the same, it is wise to anticipate this possibility by using an anti-emetic on wakening.

Praziquantel (not on UK market) is effective as niclosamide and is given as a single dose of 10–20 mg/kg after a light breakfast.

5.5.4 Drugs for hookworms
(ancylostomiasis, necatoriasis)

Hookworms live in the upper small intestine and draw blood from the point of their attachment to their host. An iron-deficiency anaemia may thereby be produced and, if present, effective treatment of the infection requires not only expulsion of the worms but treatment of the anaemia.

Mebendazole (section 5.5.1) has a useful broad-spectrum activity, and is effective against hookworms; the usual dose is 100 mg twice daily for 3 days.

Pyrantel (section 5.5.2) is also very effective against hookworms; its side-effects are limited to occasional nausea and vomiting. The usual dose is 10 mg/kg (max. 1 g) given as a single dose. **Bephenium** is still widely used and its side-effects are limited to occasional nausea and vomiting. A single dose of 2.5 g is given and repeated after 1–2 days. It is unpleasant to take and activity against *Necator americanus* is unreliable.

BEPHENIUM

Indications: roundworm and hookworm infections

Side-effects: nausea, vomiting, diarrhoea, headache, vertigo

Dose: see notes above

Alcopar® (Wellcome)
Granules, yellow/green, bephenium 2.5 g (as hydroxynaphthoate)/sachet. Net price per sachet = 84p. Label: 13

5.5.5 Schistosomicides
(bilharziasis)

Adult *Schistosoma haematobium* worms live in the genito-urinary veins and adult *S. mansoni* in those of the colon and mesentery. *S. japonicum* is more widely distributed in veins of the alimentary tract and portal system.

Praziquantel (Biltricide®, not on UK market) is effective against all human schistosomes. The dose is 40 mg/kg as a single oral dose (60 mg/kg in 3 divided doses on one day for *S. japonicum* infections). No serious toxic effects have been reported. Of all the available schistosomicides, it has the most attractive combination of effectiveness, broad-spectrum activity, and low toxicity.

Oxamniquine (Vansil®, *Pfizer*) is effective against *S. mansoni* infections only. It is a quinoline compound given by mouth; the dosage ranges from 15 mg/kg as a single dose to a total of 60 mg/kg over 2 to 3 days according to the geographical region. It can occasionally cause convulsions.

Metriphonate (Bilarcil®, not on UK market) is an organophosphorus compound which is only effective against *S. haematobium* infections. It is given by mouth in 3 doses of 7.5 mg/kg at intervals of 2 weeks. As it reduces plasma-cholinesterase concentrations it should be used with caution in patients likely to be frequently exposed to organophosphorus insecticides.

Hycanthone, lucanthone, niridazole, and stibocaptate have now been superseded.

5.5.6 Filaricides

Diethylcarbamazine (Hetrazan®, *Lederle*) is effective against microfilariae and adults of *Loa loa*, *Wuchereria bancrofti*, and *Brugia Malayi*. To minimise reactions treatment is commenced with a dose of 1 mg/kg and increased gradually over 3 days to 6 mg/kg daily in divided doses; this dosage is maintained for 21 days and usually gives a radical cure for these infections. Close medical supervision is necessary particularly in the early phase of treatment.

In heavy infections there may be a febrile reaction, and in heavy *Loa loa* infection there is a small risk of encephalopathy. In such cases treatment must be given under careful in-patient supervision and stopped at the first sign of cerebral involvement (and specialist advice sought).

Diethylcarbamazine can cause such serious reactions in onchocerciasis, that it should no longer be used for this infection. Suramin has also been used for onchocerciasis but is now obsolete because of its toxicity.

Ivermectin (Mectizan®, *MSD*, not on UK market) is very effective in *onchocerciasis* and it is now the drug of choice. A single dose of 150 micrograms/kg by mouth produces a prolonged reduction in microfilarial levels. Retreatment at intervals of 6 to 12 months depending on symptoms must be given until the adult worms die out. Reactions are usually slight and most commonly take the form of temporary aggravation of itching and rash.

5.5.7 Drugs for guinea worms
(dracontiasis)

Guinea worms, *Dracunculus medinensis*, may be killed and their removal from the tissues facilitated by a course of **niridazole** (Ambilhar®, not on UK market). Use of niridazole does not obviate the concomitant need for sterile dressing of the ulcer caused by a guinea worm and for its extraction, wherever possible, under sterile conditions. In India, mebendazole has been reported as effective at a dosage of 200 mg twice daily for 7 days. **Metronidazole** has also been reported to be effective in a dose of 400 mg three times daily for 5 days.

5.5.8 Drugs for strongyloidiasis

Adult *Strongyloides stercoralis* live in the gut and produce larvae which penetrate the gut wall and invade the tissues, setting up a cycle of auto-infection. **Thiabendazole** is the drug of choice, at a dosage of 25 mg/kg every 12 hours for 3 days. **Albendazole** (Zentel®, *SmithKline Beecham*, not on UK market) is an alternative with fewer side-effects; it is given in a dose of 400 mg daily for 3 days, repeated after 3 weeks if necessary.

THIABENDAZOLE

Indications: strongyloidiasis, cutaneous and visceral larva migrans, dracontiasis, symptoms of trichinosis; secondary treatment for threadworm when mixed with above infestations; adjunct in hookworm, whipworm, or roundworm
Cautions: hepatic or renal impairment, discontinue if hypersensitivity reactions occur; **interactions**: Appendix 1 (thiabendazole)
DRIVING. May impair performance of skilled tasks (e.g. driving)
Contra-indications: pregnancy (teratogenesis in *animal* studies)
Side-effects: anorexia, nausea, vomiting, dizziness, diarrhoea, headache, pruritus, drowsiness; hypersensitivity reactions including fever, chills, angioedema, rashes, erythema multiforme; rarely tinnitus, collapse, parenchymal liver damage
Dose: see notes above

PoM **Mintezol®** (MSD)
Tablets, orange, chewable, thiabendazole 500 mg. Net price 6-tab pack = 62p. Label: 3, 21, 24

6: Drugs used in the treatment of disorders of the
ENDOCRINE SYSTEM

In this chapter, drug treatment is discussed under the following headings:
6.1 Drugs used in diabetes
6.2 Thyroid and antithyroid drugs
6.3 Corticosteroids
6.4 Sex hormones
6.5 Hypothalamic and pituitary hormones
6.6 Drugs affecting bone metabolism
6.7 Other endocrine drugs

6.1 Drugs used in diabetes

6.1.1 Insulin
6.1.2 Oral antidiabetic drugs
6.1.3 Diabetic ketoacidosis
6.1.4 Treatment of hypoglycaemia
6.1.5 Treatment of diabetic neuropathy
6.1.6 Diagnostic and monitoring agents for diabetes mellitus

6.1.1 Insulin

6.1.1.1 Short-acting insulin
6.1.1.2 Intermediate- and long-acting insulins
6.1.1.3 Hypodermic equipment

Insulin plays a key role in the body's regulation of carbohydrate, fat, and protein metabolism. Diabetes mellitus is due to a deficiency in insulin synthesis and secretion. Patients are generally described as insulin-dependent diabetics (type 1) or non-insulin-dependent diabetics (type 2), although many of the latter need insulin to maintain satisfactory control.

Insulin is a polypeptide hormone of complex structure. It is extracted mainly from pork pancreas and purified by crystallisation; it can also be made biosynthetically by recombinant DNA technology using *Escherichia coli* or semisynthetically by enzymatic modification of porcine material (see under Human Insulins, below). All insulin preparations are to a greater or lesser extent immunogenic in man but immunological resistance to insulin action is uncommon.

Insulin is inactivated by gastro-intestinal enzymes, and must therefore be given by injection; the subcutaneous route is ideal for most circumstances. It is usually injected into the upper arms, thighs, buttocks, or abdomen; there may be increased absorption from a limb site if the limb is used in strenuous exercise. Insulin is usually administered using a syringe and needle but portable injection devices (section 6.1.1.3) which hold insulin in cartridge form and meter the required dose are rapidly growing in popularity.

Insulin can also be given by continuous subcutaneous infusion using soluble insulin in an infusion pump. This technique now has an established though limited place in the treatment of diabetes, and provides for continuous basal insulin infusion with preprandial boosts. Its chief benefit is the considerable improvement in quality of life enjoyed by some patients, and, at times, the elimination of troublesome hypoglycaemia. It is unsuitable for emotionally or psychiatrically disturbed patients, and thus does not provide a general solution for 'brittle' diabetics. There are many disadvantages to this technique. Patients using it must be well-motivated, reliable, and able to monitor their own blood glucose, and must have access to expert advice both day and night.

Minor allergic reactions at the sites of injections during the first few weeks of treatment are uncommon, usually transient and require no treatment. Fat hypertrophy sometimes develops at sites of insulin injection and can to some extent be avoided by rotation of injection sites.

CHOICE OF TREATMENT. About 25% of diabetics require insulin treatment; apart from those presenting in ketoacidosis, insulin is needed by most of those with a rapid onset of symptoms, weight loss, weakness, and sometimes vomiting, often associated with ketonuria. The majority of those who are obese can be managed by restriction of carbohydrate or energy intake alone or with the subsequent administration of oral hypoglycaemic drugs. Most children require insulin from the outset.

MANAGEMENT OF DIABETIC PATIENTS. The aim of treatment is to achieve the best possible control of plasma glucose without making the patient obsessional, and avoiding disabling hypoglycaemia; close co-operation is needed between the patient and the medical team. Mixtures of available insulin preparations may be required and these combinations have to be worked out for the individual patient. Insulin requirements may be affected by variations in lifestyle, infection, and corticosteroids, and sometimes by a very small amount when the oral contraceptive pill is taken. In pregnancy insulin requirements should be assessed frequently by an experienced diabetic physician.

The energy and carbohydrate intake must be adequate to allow normal growth and development but obesity must be avoided. The carbohydrate intake must be regulated and should be distributed throughout the day. Fine control of plasma glucose can be achieved by moving portions of carbohydrate from one meal to another without altering the total intake.

Insulin doses are determined on an individual basis, by gradually increasing the dose but avoiding troublesome hypoglycaemic reactions.

There are 3 main types of insulin preparations:
1. those of **short** duration which have a relatively rapid onset of action, namely soluble forms of insulin;
2. those with an **intermediate** action, e.g. Isophane Insulin Injection and Insulin Zinc Suspension; and
3. those whose action is slower in onset and lasts for **long** periods, e.g. Human Ultratard®.

The *duration of action* of different insulin preparations varies considerably from one patient to another, and needs to be assessed for every individual; those indicated below are only approximations. The type of insulin used and its dose and frequency of administration depend on the particular needs of the patient. Most patients are best started on insulins of intermediate action twice daily and a short-acting insulin can later be added to cover any hyperglycaemia which may follow breakfast or evening meal.

Some recommended insulin regimens

Insulin	Regimen
1. Short-acting insulin mixed with Intermediate-acting insulin	twice daily (before meals)
2. Short-acting insulin mixed with Intermediate-acting insulin	before breakfast
Short-acting insulin	before evening meal
Intermediate-acting insulin	bedtime
3. Short-acting insulin	three times daily (before breakfast, midday and evening meal)
Intermediate-acting insulin	bedtime
4. Short-acting insulin mixed with Intermediate-acting insulin	before breakfast (sufficient in some cases)

HUMAN INSULINS. There are differences in the amino-acid sequence in animal and human insulins; most available insulins are either porcine in origin or of human sequence prepared by modification of porcine material (emp) or biosynthetically (crb, prb, or pyr). Preparations of human sequence insulin should theoretically be less immunogenic, but in trials no real advantage has been shown.

HYPOGLYCAEMIA. This is a potential hazard when the type of insulin is changed, especially when converting from beef to human insulin. The conversion from beef to human sequence insulin should always be undertaken with specialist advice; it is usual to reduce the total dose by about 10%, with careful monitoring for the first few days. When changing from porcine to human sequence insulin, a dose change is not usually needed, but careful monitoring is advised. Loss of warning of hypoglycaemia is a common problem among insulin-treated diabetics and can be a serious hazard, especially for drivers. The cause is not known, but very tight control of diabetes appears to lower the blood glucose concentration needed to trigger hypoglycaemic symptoms. Beta-blockers can also blunt hypoglycaemic awareness (and can delay recovery).

Some patients have reported loss of warning of hypoglycaemia after transfer to human insulin. Patients should be warned of this possibility and if they believe that human insulin is responsible for their loss of warning it is reasonable to transfer them back to porcine insulin. When prescribing insulin great care should be taken to specify whether a human or an animal preparation is required. Indications for changing from animal to human preparations must be very carefully considered in the light of these reported problems.

DRIVING. Car drivers need to be particularly careful to avoid hypoglycaemia (see above) and should be warned of the problems. They should normally check their blood glucose concentration before driving and, on long journeys, at intervals of approximately two hours. If hypoglycaemia occurs a car driver should switch off the ignition until recovery is complete, which may take up to 15 minutes or longer. Driving is not permitted when hypoglycaemic awareness has been lost.

UNITS. The word 'unit' should **not** be abbreviated.

6.1.1.1 SHORT-ACTING INSULIN

Soluble Insulin is a short-acting form of insulin. For maintenance regimens it is usual to inject it 15 to 30 minutes before meals.

Soluble insulin is the only appropriate form of insulin for use in diabetic emergencies and at the time of surgical operations. It has the great advantage that it can be given intravenously and intramuscularly, as well as subcutaneously.

When injected subcutaneously, soluble insulin has a rapid onset of action (after 30 to 60 minutes), a peak action between 2 and 4 hours, and a duration of action of up to 8 hours. Human sequence preparations tend to have a more rapid onset and a shorter overall duration.

When injected intravenously, soluble insulin has a very short half-life of only about 5 minutes and its effect disappears within 30 minutes.

SOLUBLE INSULIN
(Insulin Injection; Neutral Insulin)
A sterile solution of insulin (i.e. bovine or porcine) or of human insulin; pH 6.6–8.0

Indications: diabetes mellitus; diabetic ketoacidosis (section 6.1.3)

Cautions: see notes above; reduce dose in renal impairment; **interactions:** Appendix 1 (antidiabetics)

Side-effects: see notes above; local reactions and fat hypertrophy at injection site; overdose causes hypoglycaemia

Dose: by subcutaneous, intramuscular, or intravenous injection or intravenous infusion, according to patient's requirements
COUNSELLING. Show bottle to patient and confirm that patient is expecting the version dispensed

Highly purified animal
Hypurin Neutral® (CP)
Injection, soluble insulin (bovine, highly purified) 100 units/mL. Net price 10-mL vial = £8.95
Velosulin® (Novo Nordisk Wellcome)
Injection, soluble insulin (porcine, highly purified) 100 units/mL. Net price 10-mL vial = £7.85

Human sequence
Human Actrapid® (Novo Nordisk)
Injection, soluble insulin (human, pyr) 100 units/mL. Net price 10-mL vial = £8.45
Human Actrapid Penfill® (Novo Nordisk)
Injection, soluble insulin (human, pyr) 100 units/mL. Net price 5 × 1.5-mL cartridge (for NHS NovoPen® devices) = £7.69
Human Velosulin® (Novo Nordisk Wellcome)
Injection, soluble insulin (human, emp) 100 units/mL. Net price 10-mL vial = £8.45
Humulin S® (Lilly)
Injection, soluble insulin (human, prb) 100 units/mL. Net price 10-mL vial = £9.49, cartridge (for NHS B-D pen®), 5 × 1.5-mL = £8.01
Pur-In® Neutral (CP)
Injection, soluble insulin (human, emp) 100 units/mL. Net price 10-mL vial = £8.45, 5 × 3-mL cartridge (for NHS Pur-In Pen® device) = £15.38

Mixed preparations, see Biphasic Insulin and Biphasic Isophane Insulin (section 6.1.1.2)

6.1.1.2 INTERMEDIATE- AND LONG-ACTING INSULINS

When given by subcutaneous injection intermediate- and long-acting insulins have an onset of action of approximately 1–2 hours, a maximal effect at 4–12 hours, and a duration of 16–35 hours. Some are given twice daily in conjunction with short-acting (soluble) insulin, and others are given once daily, particularly in elderly patients. They can be mixed with soluble insulin in the syringe, essentially retaining the properties of the two components, although there may be some blunting of the initial effect of the soluble insulin component (especially on mixing with protamine zinc insulin, see below).

Isophane Insulin is a suspension of insulin with protamine which is of particular value for initiation of twice-daily insulin regimens. Patients usually mix isophane with soluble insulin but ready-mixed preparations may be appropriate (**Biphasic Isophane Insulin**).

Biphasic Insulin is another ready-mixed insulin suitable for twice-daily injection.

Insulin Zinc Suspension (Amorphous) has an intermediate duration of action and **Insulin Zinc Suspension (Crystalline)** a more prolonged duration of action. These preparations may be used independently or in **Insulin Zinc Suspension** (30% amorphous, 70% crystalline).

Protamine Zinc Insulin is usually given once-daily in conjunction with short-acting (soluble) insulin. It has the drawback of binding with the soluble insulin when mixed in the same syringe, and is now rarely used.

INSULIN ZINC SUSPENSION
(Insulin Zinc Suspension (Mixed); I.Z.S.)
A sterile neutral suspension of bovine and/or porcine insulin or of human insulin in the form of a complex obtained by the addition of a suitable zinc salt; consists of rhombohedral crystals (10–40 microns) and of particles of no uniform shape (not exceeding 2 microns)

Indications: diabetes mellitus (long acting)
Cautions; Side-effects: see under Soluble Insulin (section 6.1.1.1)
Dose: by subcutaneous injection, according to patient's requirements
COUNSELLING. Show bottle to patient and confirm that patient is expecting the version dispensed

Highly purified animal
Hypurin Lente® (CP)
Injection, insulin zinc suspension (bovine, highly purified) 100 units/mL. Net price 10-mL vial = £8.95
Lentard MC® (Novo Nordisk)
Injection, insulin zinc suspension (bovine and porcine, highly purified) 100 units/mL. Net price 10-mL vial = £6.89

Human sequence
Human Monotard® (Novo Nordisk)
Injection, insulin zinc suspension (human, pyr) 100 units/mL. Net price 10-mL vial = £8.45
Humulin Lente® (Lilly)
Injection, insulin zinc suspension (human, prb) 100 units/mL. Net price 10-mL vial = £9.49

INSULIN ZINC SUSPENSION (AMORPHOUS)
(Amorph. I.Z.S.)
A sterile neutral suspension of bovine or porcine insulin in the form of a complex obtained by the addition of a suitable zinc salt; consists of particles of no uniform shape (not exceeding 2 microns)

Indications: diabetes mellitus (intermediate acting)
Cautions; Side-effects: see under Soluble Insulin (section 6.1.1.1)
Dose: by subcutaneous injection, according to patient's requirements
COUNSELLING. Show bottle to patient and confirm that patient is expecting the version dispensed

Semitard MC® (Novo Nordisk)
Injection, insulin zinc suspension (amorphous) (porcine, highly purified) 100 units/mL. Net price 10-mL vial = £7.49

INSULIN ZINC SUSPENSION (CRYSTALLINE)
(Cryst. I.Z.S.)
A sterile neutral suspension of bovine insulin or of human insulin in the form of a complex obtained by the addition of a suitable zinc salt; consists of rhombohedral crystals (10–40 microns)

Indications: diabetes mellitus (duration of action, see below)
Cautions; Side-effects: see under Soluble Insulin (section 6.1.1.1)
Dose: by subcutaneous injection, according to patient's requirements
COUNSELLING. Show bottle to patient and confirm that patient is expecting the version dispensed

Human sequence
Human Ultratard® (Novo Nordisk) (long acting)
Injection, insulin zinc suspension, crystalline (human, pyr) 100 units/mL. Net price 10-mL vial = £8.45
Humulin Zn® (Lilly) (intermediate acting)
Injection, insulin zinc suspension, crystalline (human, prb) 100 units/mL. Net price 10-mL vial = £9.49

ISOPHANE INSULIN
(Isophane Insulin Injection; Isophane Protamine Insulin Injection; Isophane Insulin (NPH))
A sterile suspension of bovine or porcine insulin or of human insulin in the form of a complex obtained by the addition of protamine sulphate or another suitable protamine

Indications: diabetes mellitus (intermediate acting)
Cautions; Side-effects: see under Soluble Insulin (section 6.1.1.1); protamine may cause allergic reactions
Dose: by subcutaneous injection, according to patient's requirements
COUNSELLING. Show bottle to patient and confirm that patient is expecting the version dispensed

Highly purified animal
Hypurin Isophane® (CP)
Injection, isophane insulin (bovine, highly purified) 100 units/mL. Net price 10-mL vial = £8.95
Insulatard® (Novo Nordisk Wellcome)
Injection, isophane insulin (porcine, highly purified) 100 units/mL. Net price 10-mL vial = £7.85

Human sequence
Human Insulatard® (Novo Nordisk Wellcome)
Injection, isophane insulin (human, emp) 100 units/mL. Net price 10-mL vial = £8.45
Human Protaphane® (Novo Nordisk)
Injection, isophane insulin (human, pyr) 100 units/mL. Net price 10-mL vial = £8.45
Human Protaphane Penfill® (Novo Nordisk)
Injection, isophane insulin (human, pyr) 100 units/mL. Net price 5 × 1.5-mL cartridge (for NHS Novopen® devices) = £8.10

Humulin I® (Lilly)
Injection, isophane insulin (human, prb) 100 units/mL. Net price 10-mL vial = £9.49, cartridge (for NHS B-D pen®), 5 × 1.5 mL = £8.01
Pur-In® Isophane (CP)
Injection, isophane insulin (human, emp) 100 units/mL. Net price 10-mL vial = £8.45, 5 × 3-mL cartridge (for NHS Pur-In Pen® device) = £16.20

Mixed preparations, see Biphasic Isophane Insulin (below)

PROTAMINE ZINC INSULIN
(Protamine Zinc Insulin Injection)
A sterile suspension of insulin in the form of a complex obtained by the addition of a suitable protamine and zinc chloride; this preparation was included in BP 1980 but is not included in BP 1988

Indications: diabetes mellitus (long acting)
Cautions; Side-effects: see under Soluble Insulin (section 6.1.1.1); protamine may cause allergic reactions; see also notes above
Dose: by subcutaneous injection, according to patient's requirements
COUNSELLING. Show bottle to patient and confirm that patient is expecting the version dispensed

Hypurin Protamine Zinc® (CP)
Injection, protamine zinc insulin (bovine, highly purified) 100 units/mL. Net price 10-mL vial = £9.60

BIPHASIC INSULINS

BIPHASIC INSULIN
(Biphasic Insulin Injection)
A sterile suspension of crystals containing bovine insulin in a solution of porcine insulin

Indications: diabetes mellitus (intermediate acting)
Cautions; Side-effects: see under Soluble Insulin (section 6.1.1.1)
Dose: by subcutaneous injection, according to patient's requirements
COUNSELLING. Show bottle to patient and confirm that patient is expecting the version dispensed

Rapitard MC® (Novo Nordisk)
Injection, biphasic insulin (highly purified) 100 units/mL. Net price 10-mL vial = £6.89

BIPHASIC ISOPHANE INSULIN
(Biphasic Isophane Insulin Injection)
A sterile buffered suspension of porcine insulin complexed with protamine sulphate (or another suitable protamine) in a solution of porcine insulin *or* a sterile buffered suspension of human insulin complexed with protamine sulphate (or another suitable protamine) in a solution of human insulin

Indications: diabetes mellitus (intermediate acting)

Cautions; Side-effects: see under Soluble Insulin (section 6.1.1.1); protamine may cause allergic reactions

Dose: *by subcutaneous injection*, according to the patient's requirements

COUNSELLING. Show bottle to patient and confirm that patient is expecting the version dispensed

Highly purified animal
Initard 50/50® (Novo Nordisk Wellcome)
Injection, biphasic isophane insulin (porcine, highly purified), 50% soluble, 50% isophane. 100 units/mL. Net price 10-mL vial = £7.85

Mixtard 30/70® (Novo Nordisk Wellcome)
Injection, biphasic isophane insulin (porcine, highly purified), 30% soluble, 70% isophane, 100 units/mL. Net price 10-mL vial = £7.85

Human sequence
Human Actraphane 30/70® (Novo Nordisk)
Injection, biphasic isophane insulin (human, pyr), 30% soluble, 70% isophane, 100 units/mL. Net price 10-mL vial = £8.45

Human Initard 50/50® (Novo Nordisk Wellcome)
Injection, biphasic isophane insulin (human, emp), 50% soluble, 50% isophane, 100 units/mL. Net price 10-mL vial = £8.45

Human Mixtard 30/70® (Novo Nordisk Wellcome)
Injection, biphasic isophane insulin (human, emp), 30% soluble, 70% isophane, 100 units/mL. Net price 10-mL vial = £8.45

Humulin M1® (Lilly)
Injection, biphasic isophane insulin (human, prb), 10% soluble, 90% isophane, 100 units/mL. Net price 10-mL vial = £9.49, 5 × 1.5-mL cartridge (for NHS B-D pen®) = £8.01

Humulin M2® (Lilly)
Injection, biphasic isophane insulin (human, prb), 20% soluble, 80% isophane, 100 units/mL. Net price 10-mL vial = £9.49, 5 × 1.5-mL cartridge (for NHS B-D pen®) = £8.01

Humulin M3® (Lilly)
Injection, biphasic isophane insulin (human, prb), 30% soluble, 70% isophane, 100 units/mL. Net price 10-mL vial = £9.49, 5 × 1.5-mL cartridge (for NHS B-D pen®) = £8.01

Humulin M4® (Lilly)
Injection, biphasic isophane insulin (human, prb), 40% soluble, 60% isophane, 100 units/mL. Net price 10-mL vial = £9.49, 5 × 1.5-mL cartridge (for NHS B-D pen®) = £8.01

PenMix 10/90 Penfill® (Novo Nordisk)
Injection, biphasic isophane insulin (human, pyr), 10% soluble, 90% isophane, 100 units/mL. Net price 5 × 1.5-mL cartridge (for NHS Novopen® devices) = £8.10

PenMix 20/80 Penfill® (Novo Nordisk)
Injection, biphasic isophane insulin (human, pyr), 20% soluble, 80% isophane, 100 units/mL. Net price 5 × 1.5-mL cartridge (for NHS Novopen® devices) = £8.10

PenMix 30/70 Penfill® (Novo Nordisk)
Injection, biphasic isophane insulin (human, pyr), 30% soluble, 70% isophane, 100 units/mL. Net price 5 × 1.5-mL cartridge (for NHS Novopen® devices) = £8.10

PenMix 40/60 Penfill® (Novo Nordisk)
Injection, biphasic isophane insulin (human, pyr), 40% soluble, 60% isophane, 100 units/mL. Net price 5 × 1.5-mL cartridge (for NHS Novopen® devices) = £8.10

PenMix 50/50 Penfill® (Novo Nordisk)
Injection, biphasic isophane insulin (human, pyr), 50% soluble, 50% isophane, 100 units/mL. Net price 5 × 1.5-mL cartridge (for NHS Novopen® devices) = £8.10

Pur-In® Mix 15/85 (CP)
Injection, biphasic isophane insulin (human, emp), 15% soluble, 85% isophane, 100 units/mL. Net price 10-mL vial = £8.45, 5 × 3-mL cartridge (for NHS Pur-In Pen® device) = £16.20

Pur-In® Mix 25/75 (CP)
Injection, biphasic isophane insulin (human, emp), 25% soluble, 75% isophane, 100 units/mL. Net price 10-mL vial = £8.45, 5 × 3-mL cartridge (for NHS Pur-In Pen® device) = £16.20

Pur-In® Mix 50/50 (CP)
Injection, biphasic isophane insulin (human, emp), 50% soluble, 50% isophane, 100 units/mL. Net price 10-mL vial = £8.45, 5 × 3-mL cartridge (for NHS Pur-In Pen® device) = £16.20

6.1.1.3 HYPODERMIC EQUIPMENT

Patients should be advised on the safe disposal of lancets, single-use syringes, and needles. Suitable arrangements for the safe disposal of contaminated waste must be made before these products are prescribed for patients who are carriers of infectious diseases.

Injection devices
NHS **Autopen®** (Owen Mumford)
Injection device, for use with Lilly and Novo Nordisk 1.5-mL insulin cartridges; allows adjustment of dosage in multiples of one unit, max. 16 units (single unit version); two units, max. 32 units (two unit version). Net price (both) = £13.96

NHS **B-D Pen®** (Becton Dickinson)
Injection device, for use with Lilly 1.5-mL insulin cartridges; allows adjustment of dosage in multiples of one unit, max. 30 units. Available only from clinics.

NHS **NovoPen II®** (Novo Nordisk)
Injection device, for use with Penfill® insulin cartridges; allows adjustment of dosage in multiples of two units, max. 36 units. Available only from clinics

NHS **Penject®** (Hypoguard)
Injection device, for use with B-D U100 1-mL syringe; allows adjustment of dosage in multiples of two units. Net price = £18.40

NHS **Pur-In Pen®** (CP)
Injection devices, for use with Pur-In® insulin cartridges; allows adjustment of dosage in multiples of one unit (Pur-In Pen® 1), two units (Pur-In Pen® 2), and four units (Pur-In Pen® 4); max. 40 units. Available only from clinics

6.1 Drugs used in diabetes

Lancets
Lancets may be used on their own or in an automatic "finger pricking" device such as NHS Autoclix® (BM Diagnostics) or NHS Glucolet® (Bayer Diagnostics). Various devices take different lancets, Monolet® and Unilet G® are compatible with most devices. Available from Bayer Diagnostics (Ames®), Becton Dickinson (B-D Microfine®), Sherwoods (Monolet®, Monolet® Extra), Owen Mumford (Unilet G®, Unilet®)

Needles
Hypodermic Needle, Sterile single use (Drug Tariff). For use with re-usable glass syringe, sizes 0.5 mm (25G), 0.45 mm (26G), 0.4 mm (27G). Net price 100-needle pack = £2.20

Needle Clipping Device (Drug Tariff). Consisting of a clipper to remove needle from its hub and container from which cut-off needles cannot be retrieved; designed to hold 1200 needles, not suitable for use with lancets. Net price = £1.04
Available from Becton Dickinson (B-D Safe-clip®)

Subcutaneous infusion pumps
NHS **MS36**® (Graseby Medical)
Infusion pump, for use with any brand of U100 soluble insulin. Net price = £782.00

Syringes
Clickcount® (Hypoguard). Calibrated glass with Luer taper conical fitting, supplied with dosage chart and strong box for blind patients for whom the Pre-Set syringe is unsuitable. Net price 1 mL = £14.50

Hypodermic Syringe (Drug Tariff). Calibrated glass with Luer taper conical fitting, for use with U100 insulin. Net price 0.5 mL and 1 mL = £9.72
Available from Rand Rocket

Pre-Set U100 Insulin Syringe (Drug Tariff). Calibrated glass with Luer taper conical fitting, supplied with dosage chart and strong box, for blind patients. Net price 1 mL = £15.81
Available from Rand Rocket

U100 Insulin Syringe with Needle (Drug Tariff). Disposable with fixed or separate needle for single use, colour coded orange, sizes 0.5 mm (25G), 0.45 mm (26G), 0.4 mm (27G), 0.36 mm (28G). Net price 0.5 mL and 1 mL (with needle) = 10p
Available from Becton Dickinson (Lo-Dose®, Plastipak®), Rand Rocket (Clinipak®)

6.1.2 Oral antidiabetic drugs
6.1.2.1 Sulphonylureas
6.1.2.2 Biguanides
6.1.2.3 Guar gum

Oral antidiabetic drugs are used for non-insulin-dependent (type 2) diabetes; they should not be prescribed until patients have been shown not to respond adequately to at least one month's restriction of energy and carbohydrate intake. They should be used to augment the effect of diet, and not to replace it.

6.1.2.1 SULPHONYLUREAS

The sulphonylureas act mainly by augmenting insulin secretion and consequently are effective only when some residual pancreatic beta-cell activity is present; during long-term administration they also have an extrapancreatic action. All may lead to hypoglycaemia 4 hours or more after food but this is usually an indication of overdose, and is relatively uncommon.

There are several sulphonylureas but there is no evidence for any difference in their effectiveness. Only **chlorpropamide** has appreciably more side-effects, mainly because of its very prolonged duration of action and the consequent hazard of hypoglycaemia, but also as a result of the common and unpleasant chlorpropamide-alcohol flush phenomenon. Selection of an individual sulphonylurea depends otherwise on the age of the patient and renal function (see below), or more generally just on personal preference.

Elderly patients are particularly prone to the dangers of hypoglycaemia when long-acting sulphonylureas are used; **chlorpropamide**, and also preferably **glibenclamide**, should be avoided in these patients and replaced by others, such as **gliclazide** or **tolbutamide**.

CAUTIONS AND CONTRA-INDICATIONS. These drugs tend to encourage weight gain and should only be prescribed if poor control and symptoms persist despite adequate attempts at dieting. They should not be used during breast-feeding, and caution is needed in the elderly and those with hepatic and renal insufficiency because of the hazard of hypoglycaemia. The short-acting tolbutamide may be used in renal impairment, as may gliquidone and gliclazide which are principally metabolised and inactivated in the liver. Sulphonylureas should be avoided in porphyria (see section 9.8.2).

Insulin therapy should be instituted temporarily during intercurrent illness (such as myocardial infarction, coma, infection, and trauma) and during surgery since control of diabetes with the sulphonylureas is often inadequate in such circumstances. Insulin therapy is also usually substituted during pregnancy. Sulphonylureas are contra-indicated in the presence of ketoacidosis.

SIDE-EFFECTS. These are generally mild and infrequent and include gastro-intestinal disturbances and headache.

Chlorpropamide may cause facial flushing after drinking alcohol; this effect is not normally witnessed with other sulphonylureas. Chlorpropamide may also enhance the effect of antidiuretic hormone and very rarely may cause hyponatraemia.

Sensitivity reactions (usually in first 6–8 weeks of therapy) include transient rashes which rarely progress to erythema multiforme and exfoliative dermatitis, fever, and jaundice; photosensitivity has also rarely been reported with chlorpropamide. Blood disorders are rare too but include thrombocytopenia, agranulocytosis, and aplastic anaemia. All these phenomena are very rare.

Cautionary label wordings, see inside back cover

CHLORPROPAMIDE

Indications: diabetes mellitus (for use in diabetes insipidus, see section 6.5.2)
Cautions; Contra-indications; Side-effects: see notes above; **interactions:** Appendix 1 (antidiabetics)
Dose: initially 250 mg daily (elderly patients 100–125 mg but avoid—see notes above), adjusted according to response; max. 500 mg daily; taken with breakfast

PoM **Chlorpropamide** (Non-proprietary)
Tablets, chlorpropamide 100 mg, net price 20 = 18p; 250 mg, 20 = 27p. Label: 4
Available from APS, Cox, CP

PoM **Diabinese**® (Pfizer)
Tablets, scored, chlorpropamide 100 mg, net price 28-tab pack = 56p; 250 mg, 28-tab pack = £1.23. Label: 4

GLIBENCLAMIDE

Indications: diabetes mellitus
Cautions; Contra-indications; Side-effects: see notes above; **interactions:** Appendix 1 (antidiabetics)
Dose: initially 5 mg daily (elderly patients 2.5 mg (but see also notes above)), adjusted according to response; max. 15 mg daily; taken with breakfast

PoM **Glibenclamide** (Non-proprietary)
Tablets, glibenclamide 2.5 mg, net price 20 = 67p; 5 mg, 20 = 78p
Available from APS (Libanil®), Ashbourne (Diabetamide®), Berk (Calabren®), Cox, CP, Evans, Generics, Kerfoot, Lagap (Malix®)

PoM **Daonil**® (Hoechst)
Tablets, scored, glibenclamide 5 mg. Net price 28-tab pack = £2.70

PoM **Semi-Daonil**® (Hoechst)
Tablets, scored, glibenclamide 2.5 mg. Net price 28-tab pack = £1.62

PoM **Euglucon**® (Roussel)
Tablets, glibenclamide 2.5 mg, net price 28-tab pack = £1.62; 5 mg (scored), 28-tab pack = £2.70

GLICLAZIDE

Indications: diabetes mellitus
Cautions; Contra-indications; Side-effects: see notes above; **interactions:** Appendix 1 (antidiabetics)
Dose: initially, 40–80 mg daily, adjusted according to response; up to 160 mg as a single dose, with breakfast; higher doses divided; max. 320 mg daily

PoM **Diamicron**® (Servier)
Tablets, scored, gliclazide 80 mg. Net price 60 = £6.48

GLIPIZIDE

Indications: diabetes mellitus
Cautions; Contra-indications; Side-effects: see notes above; **interactions:** Appendix 1 (antidiabetics)
Dose: initially 2.5–5 mg daily, adjusted according to response; max. 40 mg daily; up to 15 mg may be given as a single dose before breakfast; higher doses divided

PoM **Glibenese**® (Pfizer)
Tablets, scored, glipizide 5 mg. Net price 56-tab pack = £3.30

PoM **Minodiab**® (Farmitalia Carlo Erba)
Tablets, glipizide 2.5 mg, net price 60 = £3.39; 5 mg (scored), 60 = £4.74

GLIQUIDONE

Indications: diabetes mellitus
Cautions; Contra-indications; Side-effects: see notes above; **interactions:** Appendix 1 (antidiabetics)
Dose: initially 15 mg daily before breakfast, adjusted to 45–60 mg daily in 2 or 3 divided doses; max. single dose 60 mg, max. daily dose 180 mg

PoM **Glurenorm**® (Sanofi Winthrop)
Tablets, scored, gliquidone 30 mg. Net price 100 = £16.35

TOLAZAMIDE

Indications: diabetes mellitus
Cautions; Contra-indications; Side-effects: see notes above; **interactions:** Appendix 1 (antidiabetics)
Dose: initially 100–250 mg daily with breakfast adjusted according to response; max. 1 g daily; higher doses divided

PoM **Tolanase**® (Upjohn)
Tablets, both scored, tolazamide 100 mg, net price 20 = £1.13; 250 mg, 20 = £2.46

TOLBUTAMIDE

Indications: diabetes mellitus
Cautions; Contra-indications; Side-effects: see notes above; **interactions:** Appendix 1 (antidiabetics)
Dose: 0.5–1.5 g (max. 2 g) daily in divided doses (see notes above)

PoM **Tolbutamide** (Non-proprietary)
Tablets, tolbutamide 500 mg. Net price 20 = 29p
Available from APS, Cox, CP, Evans, Kerfoot

PoM **Rastinon**® (Hoechst)
Tablets, scored, tolbutamide 500 mg. Net price 20 = 68p

6.1.2.2 BIGUANIDES

Metformin, the only available biguanide, has a different mode of action from the sulphonylureas, and is not interchangeable with them. It exerts its effect mainly by decreasing gluconeogenesis and by increasing peripheral utilisation of glucose; since it only acts in the presence of endogenous insulin it is only effective in diabetics with some residual functioning pancreatic islet cells. Metformin is used in the treatment of non-insulin-dependent diabetics when strict dieting and sulphonylurea treatment have failed to control diabetes, especially in overweight patients, in whom it may, if necessary, be used first. It can be used alone or with a sulphonylurea. It does not exert a hypoglycaemic action in non-diabetic subjects unless given in overdose. Gastro-intestinal side-effects are initially common, and may persist in some patients, particularly when very high doses such as 3 g daily are given.

Metformin is not free from the hazard of lactic acidosis but this occurs almost exclusively in renal failure patients, in whom it should not be used.

METFORMIN HYDROCHLORIDE
Indications: diabetes mellitus (see notes above)
Cautions: see notes above; **interactions:** Appendix 1 (antidiabetics)
Contra-indications: hepatic or renal impairment (withdraw if renal impairment suspected), predisposition to lactic acidosis, heart failure, severe infection or trauma, dehydration, alcohol dependence; pregnancy, breast-feeding
Side-effects: anorexia, nausea, vomiting, diarrhoea (usually transient), lactic acidosis (withdraw treatment), decreased vitamin-B_{12} absorption
Dose: 500 mg every 8 hours *or* 850 mg every 12 hours with or after food; max. 3 g daily in divided doses though most physicians limit this to 2 g daily (see notes above)

PoM **Metformin** (Non-proprietary)
Tablets, coated, metformin hydrochloride 500 mg, net price 21-tab pack = 50p, 84-tab pack = £2.02; 850 mg, 20 = 81p. Label: 21
Available from APS, Berk, Cox, CP, Evans, Kerfoot, Lagap (Orabet®), Norton

PoM **Glucophage®** (Lipha)
Tablets, f/c, metformin hydrochloride 500 mg, net price 84 = £2.11; 850 mg, 56 = £2.34. Label: 21

6.1.2.3 GUAR GUM

Guar gum, if taken in adequate quantities, results in some reduction of postprandial plasma-glucose concentrations in diabetes mellitus, probably by retarding carbohydrate absorption. It is also used to relieve symptoms of the dumping syndrome.

Flatulence limits its use.

GUAR GUM
Indications: see notes above
Cautions: maintain adequate fluid intake; **interactions:** Appendix 1 (guar gum)
COUNSELLING. Preparations that swell in contact with liquid should always be carefully swallowed with water and should not be taken imediately before going to bed.
Contra-indications: gastro-intestinal obstruction
Side-effects: flatulence, abdominal distension, intestinal obstruction

Guarem® (Rybar)
Granules, ivory, sugar-free, guar gum 5 g/sachet. Net price 100 sachets = £16.45. Label: 13, counselling, food (see below), administration (see above)
Dose: 5 g stirred into 200 mL fluid 3 times daily immediately before main meals (or sprinkled on food and eaten accompanied by 200 mL fluid)

Guarina® (Norgine)
Granules, dispersible, guar gum 5 g/sachet. Net price 60 sachets = £8.95. Label: 13, counselling, food (see below), administration (see above)
Dose: 5 g stirred into 150 mL fluid immediately before main meals up to 3 times daily (or sprinkled on food and eaten accompanied by 150 mL of fluid)

6.1.3 Diabetic ketoacidosis

Soluble insulin, the only form of insulin that may be given intravenously, is used in the management of diabetic ketoacidotic and hyperosmolar non-ketotic coma. It is preferable to use the type of soluble insulin that the patient has been using previously. It is necessary to achieve and to maintain an adequate plasma-insulin concentration until the metabolic disturbance is brought under control.

Insulin is best given by *intravenous infusion*, using an infusion pump, and diluted to 1 unit/mL (care in mixing, see Appendix 6). Adequate plasma concentrations can usually be maintained with infusion rates of 6 units/hour for adults and 0.1 units/kg/hour for children. Blood glucose is expected to decrease by about 5 mmol/hour; if the response is inadequate the infusion rate can be doubled or quadrupled. When the plasma glucose has fallen to 10 mmol/litre the infusion rate can be reduced to 1 to 2 units/hour for adults (about 0.02 units/kg/hour for children) and continued until the patient is ready to take food by mouth. The insulin infusion should not be stopped before subcutaneous insulin has been started.

No matter how large, a bolus intravenous injection of insulin can only provide an adequate plasma concentration for a short time, therefore if facilities for intravenous infusion are not available the insulin is given by *intramuscular injection*. An initial loading dose of 20 units intramuscularly is followed by 6 units intramuscularly every hour until the plasma glucose concentration has fallen to 10 mmol/litre; intramuscular injections are then given every 2 hours. Although absorption of insulin is usually rapid after intramuscular injection, it may be impaired in the presence of hypotension and poor tissue perfusion; moreover depots of insulin may build up during treatment therefore late hypoglycaemia should be watched for and treated appropriately.

Intravenous replacement of fluid and electrolytes with **sodium chloride** intravenous infusion is an essential part of the management of ketoacidosis; **potassium chloride** is included in the infusion as appropriate to prevent the hypokalaemia induced by the insulin. **Sodium bicarbonate** infusion (1.26% or 2.74%) is only used in cases of extreme acidosis and shock since the acid-base disturbance is normally corrected by the insulin. **Glucose** solution (10%) is infused once the blood glucose has decreased below 10 mmol/litre but insulin infusion must continue.

For the role of glucose, see section 9.2.2.

6.1.4 Treatment of hypoglycaemia

Initially, glucose or 3 or 4 lumps of sugar should be taken with a little water. If necessary, this may be repeated in 10 to 15 minutes.

If hypoglycaemia causes unconsciousness, up to 50 mL of **50% glucose intravenous infusion** should be given intravenously (see section 9.2.2).

Glucagon can be given as an alternative to parenteral glucose in hypoglycaemia. It is a polypeptide hormone produced by the alpha cells of the islets of Langerhans. Its action is to increase plasma glucose concentration by mobilising glycogen stored in the liver. It has the advantage that it can be injected by any route (intramuscular, subcutaneous, or intravenous) in a dose of 1 mg (1 unit) in circumstances when an intravenous injection of glucose would be difficult or impossible to administer. It may be issued to close relatives of insulin-treated patients for emergency use in hypoglycaemic attacks. It is often advisable to prescribe on an 'if necessary' basis to all hospitalised insulin-treated patients, so that it may be given rapidly by the nurses during an hypoglycaemic emergency. If not effective in 20 minutes intravenous glucose should be given.

GLUCAGON

Indications: acute hypoglycaemia
Cautions: see notes above. Ineffective in chronic hypoglycaemia, starvation, and adrenal insufficiency
Contra-indications: insulinoma, phaeochromocytoma, glucagonoma
Side-effects: nausea, vomiting, rarely hypersensitivity reactions
Dose: by subcutaneous, intramuscular, or intravenous injection, adults and children 0.5–1 unit repeated after 20 minutes if necessary
Note. 1 unit of glucagon = 1 mg of glucagon or glucagon hydrochloride

PoM **Glucagon Injection,** powder for reconstitution, glucagon (as hydrochloride, with lactose). Net price 1-unit vial (Lilly) = £5.16; (Novo Nordisk) = £4.62; 10-unit vial (Novo Nordisk) = £27.06 (all with diluent)

CHRONIC HYPOGLYCAEMIA

Diazoxide, administered by mouth, is useful in the management of patients with chronic hypoglycaemia from excess endogenous insulin secretion, either from an islet cell tumour or islet cell hyperplasia. It has no place in the management of acute hypoglycaemia.

DIAZOXIDE

Indications: chronic intractable hypoglycaemia (for use in hypertensive crisis see section 2.5.1)
Cautions: ischaemic heart disease, pregnancy, labour, impaired renal function; haematological examinations and blood pressure monitoring required during prolonged treatment; growth, bone, and developmental checks in children; **interactions:** Appendix 1 (diazoxide)
Side-effects: anorexia, nausea, vomiting, hyperuricaemia, hypotension, oedema, tachycardia, arrhythmias, extrapyramidal effects; hypertrichosis on prolonged treatment
Dose: by mouth, adults and children, initially 5 mg/kg daily in 2–3 divided doses

PoM **Eudemine**® (A&H)
Tablets—discontinued
Note. Diazoxide powder is available on named patient basis for extemporaneous preparation of oral suspension.

6.1.5 Treatment of diabetic neuropathy

Optimal diabetic control is beneficial for the management of *painful neuropathy*. Most patients should be treated with insulin, and relief may probably be accelerated by continuous insulin infusion. **Non-opioid analgesics** such as aspirin and paracetamol (see section 4.7.1) are indicated. Relief may also be obtained with the **tricyclic antidepressants**, amitriptyline, imipramine, and nortriptyline (see section 4.3.1) with or without a low dose of a **phenothiazine** (see section 4.2). **Carbamazepine** (see section 4.8.1) or mexiletine may be useful; lignocaine has also been used but needs further evaluation.

In *autonomic neuropathy* diabetic diarrhoea can often be aborted by two or three doses of **tetracycline** 250 mg (see section 5.1.3). Otherwise **codeine phosphate** (see section 1.4.2) is the best drug, but all other antidiarrhoeal preparations can be tried. **Anti-emetics** or **cisapride** may control vomiting in gastroparesis. In the rare cases where they do not, erythromycin (especially when given intravenously) has been shown to be of benefit but further studies are needed.

In *neuropathic postural hypotension* an increased salt intake and the use of the **mineralocorticoid** fludrocortisone 100 to 400 micrograms daily (see section 6.3.1) help by increasing plasma volume but uncomfortable oedema is a common side-effect. Fludrocortisone can also be combined with **flurbiprofen** (see section 10.1.1) and **ephedrine hydrochloride** (see section 3.1.1.2).

Gustatory sweating can be treated with **antimuscarinics** (see section 1.2), poldine methylsulphate is the best but propantheline bromide may also be used; side-effects are common. In some patients with *neuropathic oedema*, **ephedrine hydrochloride** 30 to 60 mg three times daily offers impressive relief.

6.1.6 Diagnostic and monitoring agents for diabetes mellitus

BLOOD GLUCOSE MONITORING

Blood glucose monitoring gives a direct measure of the glucose concentration at the time of the test and can detect hypoglycaemia as well as hyperglycaemia. It is a method of assessing diabetic control, especially where tight control is essential e.g. in pregnancy. Patients should be properly trained in the use of blood glucose monitoring systems and to take appropriate action on the results obtained. Inadequate understanding of the normal fluctuations in blood glucose may lead to confusion and inappropriate action.

Blood glucose concentration evaluation may be carried out visually (using a colour comparison chart) or by means of a meter. Meters give a more precise reading and are useful for patients with poor eyesight or who are colour blind.

Note: In the U.K. blood glucose concentration is expressed in mmol/litre and the British Diabetic Association advises its members that these units should be used for self blood glucose monitoring. In other European countries units of mg/100 mL (or mg/dL) are commonly used.

It is advisable to check that the meter is pre-set in the correct units.

Test strips
BM-Test 1–44® (BM Diagnostics)
Reagent strips, for blood glucose monitoring, visual range (1–44 mmol/litre) meter range (0.5–27.7 mmol/litre), suitable for use with Reflolux® S. Net price 50-strip pack = £12.95
Dextrostix® (Bayer Diagnostics)
Reagent strips, for blood glucose monitoring, visual range (1.4–14 mmol/litre). Net price 50-strip pack = £12.36
ExacTech® (MediSense)
Biosensor strips, for blood glucose monitoring, range (2.2–25mmol/litre), for use with ExacTech® meter only. Net price 50-strip pack = £12.43
Glucostix® (Bayer Diagnostics)
Reagent strips, for blood glucose monitoring, visual range (1–44 mmol/litre), meter range (2–22 mmol/litre), suitable for use with Glucometer® II with memory, Glucometer® GX. Net price 50-strip pack = £12.36

Hypoguard® GA (Hypoguard)
Reagent strips, for blood glucose monitoring, visual range (1–22 mmol/litre), meter range (0–22 mmol/litre), suitable for use with Hypocount® GA. Net price 50-strip pack = £11.18
Hypoguard® Supreme (Hypoguard)
Reagent strips, for blood glucose monitoring, visual range (1–22 mmol/litre), meter range (2–22 mmol/litre), suitable for use with Hypocount® Supreme meter. Net price 50-strip pack = £12.00

Meters
NHS **ExacTech®** (MediSense)
Meter (Sensor) for blood glucose monitoring for use with ExacTech® test strips. ExacTech Companion = £39.00, ExacTech Companion starter pack = £49.00, ExacTech Pen = £39.00, ExacTech Pen starter pack = £49.00
NHS **Glucometer®** (Bayer Diagnostics)
Meters for blood glucose monitoring for use with Glucostix® test strips. Glucometer II with memory = £49.00, Glucometer GX = £39.00
NHS **Hypocount®** (Hypoguard)
Meters for blood glucose monitoring, Hypo-Count GA (for use with Hypoguard GA® test strips) = £55.00, Hypocount® Supreme (for use with Hypoguard® Supreme test strips) = £49.00
NHS **Reflolux® S** (BM Diagnostics)
Meter for blood glucose monitoring (for use with BM-Test 1–44® test strips) = £29.00

URINALYSIS

Glucose
Qualitative and semiquantitative tests range from reagent strips specific to glucose in urine to reagent tablets which detect all reducing sugars in urine. They vary in the time taken to perform the test and colour changes. Training of patients in the performance of the test and correct evaluation of results is essential.

Clinistix® (Bayer Diagnostics)
Reagent strips, for detection of glucose in urine. Net price 50-strip pack = £2.42
Clinitest® (Bayer Diagnostics)
Reagent tablets, for detection of glucose and other reducing substances in urine. Pocket set (test tube, dropper and 36 tablets), net price = £2.96, 36-tab pack = £1.49, 6-test tube pack = £1.74, 6-dropper pack = £1.74, NHS test tube rack set (6 tubes and 2 droppers) = £4.38
Diabur Test 5000® (BM Diagnostics)
Reagent strips, for detection of glucose in urine. Net price 50-strip pack = £2.11
Diastix® (Bayer Diagnostics)
Reagent strips, for detection of glucose in urine. Net price 50-strip pack = £2.06

Ketones
Acetest® (Bayer Diagnostics)
Reagent tablets, for detection of ketones in urine. Net price 100-tab pack = £2.64
Ketostix® (Bayer Diagnostics)
Reagent strips, for detection of ketones in urine. Net price 50-strip pack = £2.06
Ketur Test® (BM Diagnostics)
Reagent strips, for detection of ketones in urine. Net price 50-strip pack = £2.02

Protein
Albustix® (Bayer Diagnostics)
Reagent strips, for detection of protein in urine. Net price 50-strip pack = £2.84

Albym Test® (BM Diagnostics)
Reagent strips, for detection of protein in urine. Net price 50-strip pack = £2.72

NHS **Micral-Test®** (BM Diagnostics)
Reagent strips, for detection of albumin in urine, visual range (0–100 mg/litre). Net price 30-strip pack = £30.00. Used in clinics

GLUCOSE TOLERANCE TEST

The **glucose** tolerance test is used in the diagnosis of diabetes mellitus. In the UK this generally involves giving 75 g of glucose BP (= dextrose monohydrate) by mouth to the fasting patient, and measuring plasma concentrations at intervals. At an international level, however, confusion has arisen because in different pharmacopoeias the title 'glucose' can mean the anhydrous form or the monohydrate. Sources at the World Health Organisation have therefore suggested that the form of dextrose should be standardised as anhydrous, and that the standard amount should be 75 g. The equivalent value (and titles) in the UK are:

Anhydrous glucose BP (anhydrous dextrose) 75 g = Glucose BP (dextrose monohydrate) 82.5 g

6.2 Thyroid and antithyroid drugs

6.2.1 Thyroid hormones
6.2.2 Antithyroid drugs

6.2.1 Thyroid hormones

Thyroid hormones are used in hypothyroidism (myxoedema), and also in diffuse non-toxic goitre, Hashimoto's thyroiditis (lymphadenoid goitre), and thyroid carcinoma. Neonatal hypothyroidism requires prompt treatment for normal development.

Thyroxine sodium is the treatment of choice for *maintenance* therapy. The initial dose should not exceed 100 micrograms daily, preferably before breakfast, or 25 to 50 micrograms in elderly patients or those with cardiac disease, increased by 25 to 50 micrograms at intervals of at least 4 weeks. The usual maintenance dose to relieve hypothyroidism is 100 to 200 micrograms daily which can be administered as a single dose.

In infants a daily dose of 10 micrograms/kg up to a maximum of 50 micrograms daily should be given; subsequent therapy should reach 100 micrograms daily by 5 years and adult doses by 12 years, guided by clinical response, growth assessment, and measurements of plasma thyroxine and thyroid-stimulating hormone.

Liothyronine sodium has a similar action to thyroxine but is more rapidly metabolised; 20 micrograms is equivalent to 100 micrograms of thyroxine. Its effects develop after a few hours and disappear within 24 to 48 hours of discontinuing treatment. It may be used in *severe hypothyroid states* when a rapid response is desired.

Liothyronine by intravenous injection is the treatment of choice in *hypothyroid coma*. Adjunctive therapy includes intravenous fluids, hydrocortisone, and antibiotics; assisted ventilation is often required.

Dried **thyroid** should **not** be used as its effects are unpredictable.

THYROXINE SODIUM

Indications: hypothyroidism
Cautions: cardiovascular disorders, prolonged myxoedema, adrenal insufficiency; **interactions:** Appendix 1 (thyroxine)
Side-effects: arrhythmias, anginal pain, tachycardia, cramps in skeletal muscles, headache, restlessness, excitability, flushing, sweating, diarrhoea, excessive weight loss
Dose: see notes above

PoM **Thyroxine** (Non-proprietary)
Tablets, thyroxine sodium 25 micrograms, net price 20 = 9p; 50 micrograms, 20 = 4p; 100 micrograms, 20 = 5p
Various strengths available from APS, Cox, CP, Evans (including Eltroxin®), Kerfoot

LIOTHYRONINE SODIUM

(L-Tri-iodothyronine sodium)
Indications: see notes above
Cautions; Contra-indications; Side-effects: see under Thyroxine Sodium; has a more rapid effect
Dose: by mouth, initially 10–20 micrograms daily in 2–3 divided doses gradually increased to 20 micrograms 3 times daily; elderly patients should receive smaller initial doses, gradually increased; CHILD, adult dose reduced in proportion to body-weight
By slow intravenous injection, hypothyroid coma, 5-20 micrograms repeated every 12 hours or more frequently (every 4 hours if necessary); alternatively 50 micrograms initially then 25 micrograms every 8 hours reducing to 25 micrograms twice daily

PoM **Tertroxin®** (Evans)
Tablets, scored, liothyronine sodium 20 micrograms. Net price 100-tab pack = 90p
PoM **Triiodothyronine** (Evans)
Injection, powder for reconstitution, liothyronine sodium (with dextran). Net price 20-microgram amp = £3.60

6.2.2 Antithyroid drugs

Antithyroid drugs are used to prepare patients for thyroidectomy. They are also used for prolonged periods in the hope of inducing life-long remission. In the UK carbimazole is the most commonly used drug. Propylthiouracil may be used in patients who suffer sensitivity reactions to carbimazole; sensitivity is not necessarily displayed to both drugs. Both drugs act primarily by interfering with the synthesis of thyroid hormones.

6.2 Thyroid and antithyroid drugs

> **CSM warning (neutropenia and agranulocytosis)**
> Doctors are reminded of the importance of recognising bone marrow suppression induced by carbimazole and the need to stop treatment promptly.
> 1. Patient should be asked to report symptoms and signs suggestive of infection, especially sore throat.
> 2. A white blood cell count should be performed if there is any clinical evidence of infection.
> 3. Carbimazole should be stopped promptly if there is clinical or laboratory evidence of neutropenia.

Carbimazole is given in a daily dose of 30 to 60 mg and maintained at this dose until the patient becomes euthyroid, usually after 4 to 8 weeks; the dose may then be progressively reduced to a maintenance of between 5 and 15 mg daily; therapy is usually given for 18 months. Children may be given 15 mg daily, adjusted according to response. Rashes are common, and propylthiouracil may then be substituted. Pruritus and rashes can also be treated with antihistamines without discontinuing therapy, however patients should be advised to report any sore throat immediately because of the rare complication of agranulocytosis see CSM warning, above.

Propylthiouracil is given in a daily dose of 300–600 mg and maintained on this dose until the patient becomes euthyroid; the dose may then be progressively reduced to a maintenance of between 50 and 150 mg daily.

Although antithyroid drugs have a short half-life they need only be given once daily because of their prolonged effect on the thyroid. Overtreatment with the rapid development of hypothyroidism is not uncommon and should be avoided particularly during pregnancy since it can cause fetal goitre.

A combination of carbimazole, 20 to 60 mg daily with thyroxine, 50 to 150 micrograms daily, may be used in a *blocking-replacement regimen*; therapy is again usually given for 18 months. The blocking-replacement regimen is not suitable during pregnancy.

Unless operation or use of radioactive iodine is planned, treatment should be for at least a year.

Before partial thyroidectomy **iodine** may be given for 10 to 14 days in addition to carbimazole or propylthiouracil to assist control and reduce vascularity of the thyroid. Iodine should not be used for long-term treatment since its antithyroid action tends to diminish.

Radioactive sodium iodide (^{131}I) solution is used increasingly for the treatment of thyrotoxicosis at all ages, particularly where medical therapy or compliance is a problem, in patients with cardiac disease, and in patients who relapse after thyroidectomy.

Propranolol is useful for rapid relief of thyrotoxic symptoms and may be used in conjunction with antithyroid drugs or as an adjunct to radioactive iodine. Beta-blockers are also useful in neonatal thyrotoxicosis and in supra-ventricular arrhythmias due to hyperthyroidism. Propranolol may be used in conjunction with iodine to prepare mildly thyrotoxic patients for surgery but it is still preferable to make the patient euthyroid with carbimazole before surgery. Laboratory tests of thyroid function are not altered by beta-blockers. Most experience in treating thyrotoxicosis has been gained with propranolol but **nadolol** and **sotalol** are also used. For doses and preparations of beta-blockers see section 2.4.

Thyrotoxic crisis ('thyroid storm') requires emergency treatment with intravenous administration of fluids, propranolol (5 mg) and hydrocortisone (100 mg every 6 hours, as sodium succinate), as well as oral iodine solution and carbimazole or propylthiouracil which may need to be administered by nasogastric tube.

PREGNANCY AND BREAST-FEEDING. Radioactive iodine therapy is contra-indicated during pregnancy. Propylthiouracil and carbimazole can be given. Both drugs cross the placenta and in high doses may cause fetal goitre and hypothyroidism. Rarely, carbimazole has been associated with aplasia cutis of the neonate.

Carbimazole and propylthiouracil transfer to breast milk but this does not preclude breast-feeding as long as neonatal development is closely monitored.

CARBIMAZOLE

Indications: hyperthyroidism
Cautions: large goitre; pregnancy, breast-feeding (see notes)
Side-effects: nausea, headache, rashes and pruritus, arthralgia; rarely alopecia, agranulocytosis **(see CSM warning above)**, jaundice
Dose: see notes above

PoM **Neo-Mercazole**® (Nicholas)
Tablets, both pink, carbimazole 5 mg, net price 100-tab pack = £2.49; 20 mg, 100-tab pack = £9.22

IODINE AND IODIDE

Indications: thyrotoxicosis (pre-operative)
Cautions: pregnancy, children; not for long-term treatment
Contra-indications: breast-feeding
Side-effects: hypersensitivity reactions including coryza-like symptoms, headache, lachrymation, conjunctivitis, pain in salivary glands, laryngitis, bronchitis, rashes; on prolonged treatment depression, insomnia, impotence; goitre in infants of mothers taking iodides

Aqueous Iodine Oral Solution (Lugol's Solution), iodine 5%, potassium iodide 10% in purified water, freshly boiled and cooled, total iodine 130 mg/mL. Net price 100 mL = £1.47. Label: 27
Dose: 0.1–0.3 mL 3 times daily well diluted with milk or water

PROPYLTHIOURACIL
Indications: hyperthyroidism
Cautions; Side-effects: see under Carbimazole; also rarely tendency to haemorrhage; reduce dose in renal impairment; systemic lupus erythematosus reported
Dose: see notes above

PoM **Propylthiouracil**® (Non-proprietary)
Tablets, propylthiouracil 50 mg. Net price 20 = £1.94
Available from CP, Evans

6.3 Corticosteroids

6.3.1 Replacement therapy
6.3.2 Comparisons of corticosteroids
6.3.3 Disadvantages of corticosteroids
6.3.4 Clinical management

6.3.1 Replacement therapy

The adrenal cortex normally secretes hydrocortisone (cortisol) which has glucocorticoid activity and weak mineralocorticoid activity. It also secretes the mineralocorticoid aldosterone.

In deficiency states, physiological replacement is best achieved with a combination of **hydrocortisone**[1] and the mineralocorticoid **fludrocortisone**; hydrocortisone alone does not usually provide sufficient mineralocorticoid activity for complete replacement.

In *Addison's disease* or following adrenalectomy, **hydrocortisone** 20 to 30 mg daily by mouth is usually required. This is given in 2 doses, the larger in the morning and the smaller in the evening, mimicking the normal diurnal rhythm of cortisol secretion. The optimum daily dose is determined on the basis of clinical response. Glucocorticoid therapy is supplemented by fludrocortisone 50 to 300 micrograms daily.

In *acute adrenocortical insufficiency*, **hydrocortisone** is given intravenously (preferably as sodium succinate) in doses of 100 mg every 6 to 8 hours in sodium chloride intravenous infusion 0.9%.

In *hypopituitarism* glucocorticoids should be given as in adrenocortical insufficiency, but since the production of aldosterone is also regulated by the renin-angiotensin system a mineralocorticoid is not usually required. Additional replacement therapy with thyroxine (section 6.2.1) and sex hormones (section 6.4) should be given as indicated by the pattern of hormone deficiency.

Corticosteroid cover for *adrenalectomy*, for *hypophysectomy* or for operations on patients on long-term treatment with corticosteroids is determined logically from the knowledge that in a normal person major stress will not lead to the secretion of more than 300 mg of cortisol in 24 hours; once the stress is over, cortisol production rapidly returns to its usual level of approximately 20 mg per 24 hours. A simple way of mimicking this is to administer hydrocortisone. On the day of operation hydrocortisone 100 mg (usually as the succinate) is given by intramuscular or intravenous injection with the premedication, and repeated every 8 hours. In the absence of complications, the dose can be halved every 24 hours until a normal maintenance dose of 20 to 30 mg per 24 hours is reached on the 5th postoperative day.

CORTISONE ACETATE
Section 6.3.4

FLUDROCORTISONE ACETATE
Indications: mineralocorticoid replacement in adrenocortical insufficiency
Cautions; Contra-indications; Side-effects: section 6.3.3
Dose: adrenocortical insufficiency, 50–300 micrograms daily; CHILD 5 micrograms/kg daily

PoM **Florinef**® (Squibb)
Tablets, pink, scored, fludrocortisone acetate 100 micrograms. Net price 20 = 96p. Label: 10 steroid card

HYDROCORTISONE
Section 6.3.4

6.3.2 Comparisons of corticosteroids

Betamethasone, dexamethasone, hydrocortisone, prednisolone, and prednisone are used for their anti-inflammatory effect; the following table shows equivalent anti-inflammatory doses.

Equivalent Anti-inflammatory Doses of Glucocorticoids

Drug	Equivalent anti-inflammatory dose (mg)
Betamethasone	0.75
Cortisone acetate	25
Dexamethasone	0.75
Hydrocortisone	20
Methylprednisolone	4
Prednisolone	5
Prednisone	5
Triamcinolone	4

Note. This table takes no account of mineralocorticoid effects (see text below), nor does it take account of variations in duration of action.

In comparing the relative potencies of corticosteroids in terms of their anti-inflammatory (glucocorticoid) effects it should be borne in mind that high anti-inflammatory (glucocorticoid) activity in itself is of no advantage unless it occurs

---

1. Cortisone has generally been superseded by hydrocortisone; management with the more potent synthetic glucocorticoids such as prednisolone (with fludrocortisone) though practicable, offers no advantage. They tend to have less mineralocorticoid activity than hydrocortisone and their greater glucocorticoid activity is only of advantage in the treatment of inflammatory and neoplastic disease.

in conjunction with relatively low mineralocorticoid activity so that the mineralocorticoid effect on water and electrolytes is not also increased.

The mineralocorticoid activity of **fludrocortisone** is so high that its anti-inflammatory activity is of no clinical relevance.

The mineralocorticoid effects of **cortisone** and **hydrocortisone** are too high for them to be used on a long-term basis for inflammatory disease suppression since fluid retention would be too great, but they are suitable for adrenal replacement therapy (section 6.3.1); hydrocortisone is preferred because cortisone is only active after conversion in the liver to hydrocortisone. Hydrocortisone is also used by intravenous injection for the emergency management of some conditions (section 6.3.4). The relatively moderate anti-inflammatory potency of hydrocortisone makes it a first-choice topical corticosteroid for the management of inflammatory skin conditions because side-effects (both topical and caused by absorption) are less marked (see section 13.4); cortisone is not active topically.

Prednisolone has predominantly glucocorticoid activity and is the corticosteroid most commonly used by mouth for long-term administration. **Prednisone** has a similar level of glucocorticoid activity but is only active after conversion in the liver to prednisolone; it is therefore not recommended.

Betamethasone and **dexamethasone** have very high glucocorticoid activity in conjunction with insignificant mineralocorticoid activity. This makes them particularly suitable for high-dose therapy in conditions where water retention would be a disadvantage (see *cerebral oedema*, section 6.3.4).

They also have a long duration of action and this, coupled with their lack of mineralocorticoid action makes them particularly suitable for conditions which require suppression of corticotrophin secretion (see *congenital adrenal hyperplasia*, section 6.3.4). Some esters of betamethasone and of **beclomethasone** exert a considerably more marked topical effect (e.g. on the skin or the lungs) than when given by mouth; use is made of this to obtain topical effects without corresponding systemic activity (e.g. for skin applications and asthma inhalations).

Stimulation of the adrenal cortex by **tetracosactrin** has been used as an alternative to corticosteroids to control certain diseases; there is no close relationship between the dose producing satisfactory clinical improvement and the equivalent dose of oral corticosteroid producing the same degree of improvement.

6.3.3 Disadvantages of corticosteroids

Overdosage or prolonged use may exaggerate some of the normal physiological actions of corticosteroids.

Mineralocorticoid effects include *hypertension, sodium and water retention and potassium loss*.

They are most marked with fludrocortisone, but are significant with cortisone, hydrocortisone, corticotrophin, and tetracosactrin. Mineralocorticoid actions are negligible with the high potency glucocorticoids, betamethasone and dexamethasone, and occur only slightly with methylprednisolone, prednisolone, prednisone, and triamcinolone.

Glucocorticoid effects include *diabetes* and *osteoporosis* which is a danger, particularly in the elderly, as it may result in osteoporotic fractures for example of the hip or vertebrae; in addition administration of high doses is associated with *avascular necrosis* of the femoral head. *Mental disturbances* may occur; a serious paranoid state or depression with risk of suicide may be induced, particularly in patients with a history of mental disorder. *Euphoria* is frequently observed. *Muscle wasting* (proximal myopathy) may also occur.

Corticosteroid therapy is weakly linked with *peptic ulceration*; the use of soluble or enteric-coated preparations to reduce the risk is speculative only. Modification of tissue reactions may result in spread of *infection*; suppression of clinical signs may allow septicaemia or tuberculosis to reach an advanced stage before being recognised.

High doses of corticosteroids may cause *Cushing's syndrome*, with moon face, striae, and acne; it is usually reversible on withdrawal of treatment, but this must always be gradually tapered to avoid symptoms of acute adrenal insufficiency (see Adrenal Suppression).

In children, administration of corticosteroids may result in *suppression of growth*. Corticosteroids given in high dosage during *pregnancy* may affect adrenal development in the child (but see also Appendix 4).

For details of the adverse effects of topical and of systemic corticosteroid therapy on the *skin*, see sections 13.4 and 13.5.

For details of the adverse effects of topical and of systemic corticosteroid therapy on the *eye*, see section 11.4.

ADRENAL SUPPRESSION. Administration of corticosteroids suppresses the secretion of corticotrophin and may lead to adrenal atrophy; withdrawal of treatment must therefore be gradual to avoid symptoms of *acute adrenal insufficiency*. When long-term treatment is to be discontinued, the dose should be reduced gradually over a period of several weeks or months depending on the dosage and duration of the therapy. Too rapid a reduction of corticosteroid dosage can lead to *acute adrenal insufficiency, hypotension,* and *death*. A number of minor withdrawal symptoms may also result such as *rhinitis, conjunctivitis, loss of weight, arthralgia,* and *painful itchy skin nodules*.

Adrenal atrophy can persist for years after stopping prolonged corticosteroid therapy, therefore any illness or surgical emergency may require temporary reintroduction of corticosteroid therapy to compensate for lack of sufficient adrenocortical response. Anaesthetists **must** therefore know whether a patient is taking or has been taking corticosteroids to avoid a precipitous fall in blood pressure during anaesthesia or in the immediate postoperative period. Patients should therefore carry cards giving details of their dosage and possible complications. These 'steroid cards' can be obtained from local Family Practitioner Committees or

>DHSS Printing and Stationery Unit,
>Room 110, North Fylde Central Office,
>Norcross, Blackpool FY5 3TA

In Scotland 'steroid cards' are available from Health Boards. In Northern Ireland they may be obtained from Central Services Agency, 27 Adelaide St, Belfast BT2 8FH.

Pharmacists may also obtain 'steroid cards' from the Royal Pharmaceutical Society of Great Britain.

Interactions: see Appendix 1 (corticosteroids).

6.3.4 Clinical management

Corticosteroids should not be used unless the benefits justify the hazards; the lowest dose that will produce an acceptable response should be used (see also under Administration, below). Dosage varies widely in different diseases and in different patients.

If the use of a corticosteroid can save or prolong life, as in *exfoliative dermatitis*, *pemphigus*, *acute leukaemia* or *acute transplant rejection*, high doses may need to be given, as the complications of therapy are likely to be less serious than the effects of the disease itself.

When long-term corticosteroid therapy is used in relatively benign chronic diseases such as *rheumatoid arthritis* the danger of treatment may become greater than the disabilities produced by the disease. To minimise side-effects the maintenance dose should be kept as low as possible (see also section 10.1.2.1).

When potentially less harmful measures are ineffective corticosteroids are used topically for the treatment of *inflammatory conditions of the skin* (see section 13.4). Corticosteroids should be avoided or used only under specialist supervision in *psoriasis* (see section 13.5).

Corticosteroids are used both topically (by rectum) and systemically (by mouth or intravenously) in the management of *ulcerative colitis* and *Crohn's disease* (see sections 1.5 and 1.7.2).

Use can be made of the mineralocorticoid activity of fludrocortisone to treat *postural hypotension* in autonomic neuropathy (see section 6.1.5).

Very high doses of corticosteroids have been given by intravenous injection in *septic shock*. However a recent study (using methylprednisolone sodium succinate) did not demonstrate efficacy and, moreover, suggested a higher mortality in some subsets of patients given the high-dose corticosteroid therapy.

Dexamethasone and betamethasone have little if any mineralocorticoid action and their long duration of action makes them particularly suitable for suppressing corticotrophin secretion in *congenital adrenal hyperplasia* where the dose should be tailored to the individual on clinical grounds and by measurement of adrenal androgens and 17-hydroxyprogesterone. In common with all glucocorticoids their suppressive action on the hypothalamic-pituitary-adrenal axis is greatest and most prolonged when they are given at night. In most normal subjects a single dose of 1 mg of dexamethasone at night, depending on weight, is sufficient to inhibit corticotrophin secretion for 24 hours. This is the basis of the 'overnight dexamethasone suppression test' for diagnosing Cushing's syndrome.

Betamethasone and dexamethasone are also appropriate for conditions where water retention would be a disadvantage, as for example in treating traumatic *cerebral oedema* with doses of 12 to 20 mg daily.

In acute hypersensitivity reactions such as *angioedema* of the upper respiratory tract and *anaphylactic shock*, corticosteroids are indicated as an adjunct to emergency treatment with adrenaline (see section 3.4.3). In such cases hydrocortisone (as sodium succinate) by intravenous injection in a dose of 100 to 300 mg may be required.

Corticosteroids are preferably used by inhalation in the management of *asthma* (see section 3.2) but systemic therapy in association with bronchodilators is required for the emergency treatment of severe acute asthma (see section 3.1.1).

Corticosteroids may also be useful in conditions such as *rheumatic fever*, *chronic active hepatitis*, and *sarcoidosis*; they may also lead to remissions of acquired *haemolytic anaemia*, and some cases of the *nephrotic syndrome* (particularly in children) and *thrombocytopenic purpura*.

Corticosteroids can improve the prognosis of serious conditions such as *systemic lupus erythematosus*, *temporal arteritis*, and *polyarteritis nodosa*; the effects of the disease process may be suppressed and symptoms relieved, but the underlying condition is not cured, although it may ultimately burn itself out. It is usual to begin therapy in these conditions at fairly high dose, such as 40 to 60 mg prednisolone daily, and then to reduce the dose to the lowest commensurate with disease control.

For other reference to the use of corticosteroids see section 11.4 (eye), 12.1.1 (otitis externa), 12.2.1 (allergic rhinitis), and 12.3.1 (aphthous ulcers).

ADMINISTRATION. Whenever possible *local treatment* with creams, intra-articular injections, inhalations, eye-drops, or enemas should be used in preference to *systemic treatment*. The suppressive action of a corticosteroid on cortisol secretion is least when it is given in the morning, therefore in an attempt to reduce pituitary-adrenal suppression a corticosteroid (usually prednisolone) should normally be taken as a single dose in the morning. In an attempt to reduce pituitary-adrenal suppression further, the total dose for two

6.3 Corticosteroids

days can sometimes be taken as a single dose on alternate days; alternate-day administration has not been very successful in the management of asthma (see section 3.2) but it can be suitable for rheumatoid arthritis (see section 10.1.2). Pituitary-adrenal suppression can also be reduced by means of intermittent therapy with short courses. In some conditions it may be possible to reduce the dose of corticosteroid by adding a small dose of an immunosuppressive drug (see section 8.2.1).

CHILDREN. In children the indications for corticosteroids are the same as for adults but risks are greater. The implications of starting these drugs are serious, and they should be used only when specifically indicated, in a minimal dosage, and for the shortest possible time. Prolonged or continuous treatment is rarely justified.

PREDNISOLONE
Indications: suppression of inflammatory and allergic disorders; see also notes above
Cautions; Contra-indications; Side-effects: section 6.3.3
Dose: by mouth, initially, up to 10–20 mg daily (severe disease, up to 60 mg daily), preferably taken in the morning after breakfast; can often be reduced within a few days but may need to be continued for several weeks or months Maintenance, usual range, 2.5–15 mg daily, but higher doses may be needed; cushingoid side-effects increasingly likely with doses above 7.5 mg daily
See also section 3.2 (asthma), section 8.2.2 (immunosuppression), and section 10.1.2 (rheumatic diseases)
By intramuscular injection, prednisolone acetate, 25–100 mg once or twice weekly (for preparation see section 10.1.2.2)

PoM **Prednisolone** (Non-proprietary)
Tablets, prednisolone 1 mg, net price 20 = 7p; 5 mg, 20 = 15p. Label: 10 steroid card, 21
Available from APS, Cox, CP, Evans, Kerfoot
Tablets, both e/c, prednisolone 2.5 mg (brown), net price 20 = 22p; 5 mg (red), 20 = 41p. Label: 5, 10 steroid card, 25
Available from APS, Biorex, Cox, Kerfoot (2.5 mg)

PoM **Deltacortril Enteric**® (Pfizer)
Tablets, both e/c, prednisolone 2.5 mg (brown), net price 56-tab pack = 62p; 5 mg (red), 56-tab pack = £1.18. Label: 5, 10 steroid card, 25

PoM **Deltastab**® (Boots)
Tablets, scored, prednisolone 1 mg, net price 20 = 6p; 5 mg, 20 = 14p. Label: 10 steroid card, 21
Injection, see section 10.1.2.2

PoM **Precortisyl**® (Roussel)
Tablets, prednisolone 1 mg, net price 20 = 7p; 5 mg (scored), 20 = 15p. Label: 10 steroid card, 21

PoM **Precortisyl Forte**® (Roussel)
Tablets, scored, prednisolone 25 mg. Net price 20 = £1.56. Label: 10 steroid card, 21

I am a patient on—

STEROID TREATMENT

which must not be stopped abruptly

and in the case of intercurrrent illness may have to be increased

full details are available from the hospital or general practitioners shown overleaf →

STC1

INSTRUCTIONS

1 DO NOT STOP taking the steroid drug except on medical advice. Always have a supply in reserve.

2 In case of feverish illness, accident, operation (emergency or otherwise), diarrhoea or vomiting the steroid treatment MUST be continued. Your doctor may wish you to have a LARGER DOSE or an INJECTION at such times.

3 If the tablets cause indigestion consult your doctor AT ONCE.

4 Always carry this card while receiving steroid treatment and show it to any doctor, dentist, nurse or midwife or anyone else who is giving you treatment.

5 After your treatment has finished you must still tell any doctor, dentist, nurse or midwife or anyone else who is giving you treatment that you have had steroid treatment.

Cautionary label wordings, see inside back cover

PoM Prednesol® (Glaxo)
Tablets, pink, scored, soluble, prednisolone 5 mg (as sodium phosphate). Net price 20 = £1.15. Label: 10 steroid card, 13, 21

PoM Sintisone® (Farmitalia Carlo Erba)
Tablets, scored, prednisolone steaglate 6.65 mg (≡ prednisolone 5 mg). Net price 20 = £1.29. Label: 10 steroid card, 21

BETAMETHASONE

Indications: suppression of inflammatory and allergic disorders; congenital adrenal hyperplasia; cerebral oedema; see also notes above
Cautions; Contra-indications; Side-effects: section 6.3.3
Dose: by mouth, usual range 0.5–5 mg daily. See also Administration (above)
By intramuscular injection or slow intravenous injection or infusion, 4–20 mg, repeated up to 4 times in 24 hours; CHILD, *by slow intravenous injection*, up to 1 year 1 mg, 1–5 years 2 mg, 6–12 years 4 mg

PoM Betnelan® (Evans)
Tablets, scored, betamethasone 500 micrograms. Net price 100-tab pack = £3.63. Label: 10 steroid card, 21

PoM Betnesol® (Evans)
Tablets, pink, scored, soluble, betamethasone 500 micrograms (as sodium phosphate). Net price 100-tab pack = £3.20. Label: 10 steroid card, 13, 21
Injection, betamethasone 4 mg (as sodium phosphate)/mL. Net price 1-mL amp = 65p. Label: 10 steroid card

CORTISONE ACETATE

Indications: section 6.3.1
Cautions; Contra-indications; Side-effects: section 6.3.3
Dose: by mouth, replacement therapy, 25–37.5 mg daily in divided doses

PoM Cortistab® (Boots)
Tablets, both scored, cortisone acetate 5 mg, net price 20 = 15p; 25 mg, 20 = 62p. Label: 10 steroid card, 21

PoM Cortisyl® (Roussel)
Tablets, scored, cortisone acetate 25 mg. Net price 20 = £1.19. Label: 10 steroid card, 21

DEXAMETHASONE

Indications: suppression of inflammatory and allergic disorders; shock; diagnosis of Cushing's disease, congenital adrenal hyperplasia; cerebral oedema; see also notes above
Cautions; Contra-indications; Side-effects: section 6.3.3; perineal irritation may follow intravenous administration of the phosphate ester
Dose: by mouth, usual range 0.5–9 mg daily. See also Administration (above)
See also section 8.1 (chemotherapy emesis)

By intramuscular injection or slow intravenous injection or infusion (as dexamethasone phosphate), initially 0.5–20 mg; CHILD 200–500 micrograms/kg daily
Cerebral oedema (as dexamethasone phosphate), *by intravenous injection*, 10 mg initially, then 4 mg *by intramuscular injection* every 6 hours as required for 2–10 days

PoM Dexamethasone (Organon)
Tablets, dexamethasone 500 micrograms, net price 20 = 64p; 2 mg, 20 = £1.73. Label: 10 steroid card, 21
Injection, dexamethasone sodium phosphate 5 mg/mL (≡ dexamethasone 4 mg/mL, dexamethasone phosphate 4.8 mg/mL). Net price 1-mL amp = 83p; 2-mL vial = £1.27. Label: 10 steroid card

PoM Decadron® (MSD)
Tablets, scored, dexamethasone 500 micrograms. Net price 20 = 91p. Label: 10 steroid card, 21
Injection, dexamethasone phosphate 4 mg/mL (≡ dexamethasone 3.33 mg/mL, dexamethasone sodium phosphate 4.17 mg/mL). Net price 2-mL vial = £1.76. Label: 10 steroid card

PoM Decadron Shock-Pak® (MSD)
Injection, dexamethasone 20 mg/mL (≡ dexamethasone sodium phosphate 25 mg/mL). Net price 5-mL vial = £15.13. Label: 10 steroid card
Dose: shock, *by intravenous injection or infusion*, 2–6 mg/kg, repeated if necessary after 2–6 hours (but see section 6.3.2)

FLUDROCORTISONE
See section 6.3.1

HYDROCORTISONE

Indications: adrenocortical insufficiency (section 6.3.1); suppression of inflammatory and allergic disorders; shock; see also notes above
Cautions; Contra-indications; Side-effects: section 6.3.3; perineal irritation may follow intravenous administration of the phosphate ester
Dose: by mouth, replacement therapy, 20–30 mg daily in divided doses—see section 6.3.1
By intramuscular injection or slow intravenous injection or infusion, 100–500 mg, 3–4 times in 24 hours or as required; CHILD *by slow intravenous injection* up to 1 year 25 mg, 1–5 years 50 mg, 6–12 years 100 mg
Anaphylactic shock—see notes above and section 3.4.3

Oral preparations

PoM Hydrocortistab® (Boots)
Tablets, scored, hydrocortisone 20 mg. Net price 20 = 62p. Label: 10 steroid card, 21

PoM Hydrocortone® (MSD)
Tablets, scored, hydrocortisone 10 mg, net price 20 = 46p; 20 mg, 20 = 71p. Label: 10 steroid card, 21

Parenteral preparations

PoM Efcortelan Soluble® (Glaxo)
Injection, powder for reconstitution, hydrocortisone (as sodium succinate). Net price 100-mg vial (with 2-mL amp water for injections) = 67p. Label: 10 steroid card

PoM Efcortesol® (Glaxo)
Injection, hydrocortisone 100 mg (as sodium phosphate)/mL. Net price 1-mL amp = 75p; 5-mL amp = £3.40. Label: 10 steroid card

PoM Solu-Cortef® (Upjohn)
Injection, powder for reconstitution, hydrocortisone (as sodium succinate). Net price 100-mg vial (with 2-mL amp water for injections) = £1.02; without water for injections = 96p. Label: 10 steroid card

METHYLPREDNISOLONE

Indications: suppression of inflammatory and allergic disorders; cerebral oedema; see also notes above

Cautions; Contra-indications; Side-effects: section 6.3.3; rapid intravenous administration of large doses has been associated with cardiovascular collapse

Dose: by mouth, usual range 2–40 mg daily. See also Administration (above)

By intramuscular injection or slow intravenous injection or infusion, initially 10–500 mg; graft rejection, up to 1 g daily *by intravenous infusion* for up to 3 days

Oral preparations

PoM Medrone® (Upjohn)
Tablets, scored, methylprednisolone 2 mg (pink), net price 30-tab pack = £2.69; 4 mg, 30-tab pack = £5.16; 16 mg, 14-tab pack = £6.68; 100 mg (blue), 20-tab pack = £40.27. Label: 10 steroid card, 21

Parenteral preparations

PoM Methylprednisolone Sodium Succinate (Non-proprietary)
Injection, powder for reconstitution, methylprednisolone (as sodium succinate) (all with solvent). Net price 125-mg vial = £3.56; 500-mg vial = £10.59; 1-g vial = £19.09
Available from Evans

PoM Solu-Medrone® (Upjohn)
Injection, powder for reconstitution, methylprednisolone (as sodium succinate) (all with solvent). Net price 40-mg vial = £1.32; 125-mg vial = £3.96; 500-mg vial = £11.77; 1-g vial = £21.21; 2-g vial = £40.27. Label: 10 steroid card

Intramuscular depot

PoM Depo-Medrone® (Upjohn)
Injection (aqueous suspension), methylprednisolone acetate 40 mg/mL. Net price 1-mL vial = £2.59; 2-mL vial = £4.65; 3-mL vial = £6.75. Label: 10 steroid card
Dose: by deep intramuscular injection, 40–120 mg, repeated every 2–3 weeks if required

Cautionary label wordings, see inside back cover

PREDNISONE

Indications: suppression of inflammatory and allergic disorders; see also notes above

Cautions; Contra-indications; Side-effects: section 6.3.3. Avoid in liver disease

Dose: see Prednisolone

PoM Prednisone (Non-proprietary)
Tablets, prednisone 5 mg, net price 20 = 15p. Label: 10 steroid card, 21

PoM Decortisyl® (Roussel)
Tablets, scored, prednisone 5 mg. Net price 20 = 15p. Label: 10 steroid card, 21

TRIAMCINOLONE

Indications: suppression of inflammatory and allergic disorders; see also notes above

Cautions; Contra-indications; Side-effects: section 6.3.3. Triamcinolone in high dosage has a greater tendency to cause proximal myopathy and should be avoided in chronic therapy

Dose: by mouth, 2–24 mg daily. See also Administration (above)

By deep intramuscular injection, into gluteal muscle, 40 mg of acetonide for depot effect, repeated at intervals according to the patient's response; max. single dose 100 mg

PoM Kenalog® (Squibb)
Injection (aqueous suspension), triamcinolone acetonide 40 mg/mL. Net price 1-mL vial (intramuscular/intra-articular) = £1.70; 1-mL syringe (intramuscular only) = £2.11; 2-mL syringe (intramuscular only) = £3.66. Label: 10 steroid card

PoM Ledercort® (Lederle)
Tablets, triamcinolone 2 mg (blue), net price 20 = £1.94; 4 mg, 20 = £3.87. Label: 10 steroid card, 21

6.4 Sex hormones

Sex hormones are described under the following section headings:
- **6.4.1** Female sex hormones
- **6.4.2** Male sex hormones and antagonists
- **6.4.3** Anabolic steroids

6.4.1 Female sex hormones
6.4.1.1 Oestrogens and HRT
6.4.1.2 Progestogens

6.4.1.1 OESTROGENS AND HRT

Oestrogens are necessary for the development of female secondary sexual characteristics; they also stimulate myometrial hypertrophy with endometrial hyperplasia.

Oestrogen therapy is given cyclically or continuously for a number of gynaecological conditions. If long-term therapy is required a progestogen should be added cyclically to prevent cystic hyperplasia of the endometrium and possible transformation to cancer. This cyclical addition of a progestogen is not necessary if the patient has had a hysterectomy.

Prices are **net**, see p. 1

PRIMARY AMENORRHOEA. After assessment by a specialist an oestrogen such as ethinyloestradiol 10 micrograms on alternate days (increasing to max. of 50 micrograms daily) is administered continuously together with cyclical progestogen, or a low-dose combined oral contraceptive is given (see section 7.3.1).

HORMONE REPLACEMENT THERAPY (HRT). Menopausal *vasomotor symptoms* and menopausal *vaginitis* are alleviated by administration of small doses of oestrogen. There is also good evidence that small doses of oestrogen given for several years starting in the perimenopausal period will diminish postmenopausal *osteoporosis* and reduce the incidence of *stroke and myocardial infarction*. There is an increased risk of *endometrial cancer* (countered by cyclical progestogen, see below) and, after some years of use, possibly a slightly increased risk of *breast cancer*.

Hormone replacement therapy (HRT) is indicated for menopausal women whose lives are inconvenienced by *vaginal atrophy* or *vasomotor instability*. Vaginal atrophy may respond to a short course of oestrogen cream given for a few weeks and repeated if necessary. Oral therapy is needed for vasomotor symptoms and should be given for at least a year; in a woman with a uterus cyclical progestogen should be added to reduce the risk of endometrial cancer (see above). Hormone replacement therapy is also indicated for women with *early natural or surgical menopause (before age 45)*, since they are at high risk of osteoporosis; in a woman with a uterus cyclical progestogen should again be added to reduce the risk of endometrial cancer (see above); hormone replacement therapy should be given to the age of at least 50 and possibly for a further 10 years.

Long-term hormone replacement therapy in general is almost certainly favourable in risk benefit terms for menopausal women *without a uterus* because they do not require cyclical progestogen therapy; it should probably be continued for about 10 years. The picture is less clear for menopausal women *with a uterus* because the need for cyclical administration of progestogen may blunt the protective effect of low-dose oestrogen against myocardial infarction and stroke; any effect of the progestogen (favourable or otherwise) on breast cancer is not yet known. Nevertheless, risk factors for osteoporosis should be borne in mind and, if there are several, consideration given to hormone replacement therapy. Risk factors include *recent corticosteroid therapy or any disease predisposing to osteoporosis, thinness, lack of exercise, alcoholism or smoking, and fracture of a hip or forearm before the age of 65; women of Afro-Caribbean origin appear to be less susceptible than those who are white or Asian*.

Choice. The choice of oestrogen for hormone replacement therapy is not straightforward and depends on an overall balance of indication, risk, and convenience. Vaginitis in a woman with a uterus can only be treated for a few weeks with an oestrogen, without addition of cyclical progestogen; this constraint includes topical cream (see section 7.2.1) since a significant amount is absorbed through the vaginal mucosa. Oestrogen therapy alone is suitable for long-term continuous therapy in a woman without a uterus. A woman with a uterus requires a regimen of oestrogen with cyclical progestogen for the last 10 to 13 days of the cycle. All oral preparations of oestrogen are subject to first-pass metabolism in the liver and intestine, therefore subcutaneous or transdermal administration reflects more closely endogenous hormone activity. In the case of subcutaneous implants, problems have been encountered with the recurrence of vasomotor symptoms at supraphysiological plasma concentrations; moreover, there is evidence of prolonged endometrial stimulation after discontinuation (calling for continued cyclical progestogen).

Providing calcium intake is adequate calcium supplements do not confer additional benefit on hormone replacement therapy (see section 9.5.1).

SUPPRESSION OF LACTATION. Oestrogens are no longer used to suppress lactation because of their association with thrombo-embolism. **Bromocriptine** (section 6.7.1) is used where necessary.

HEREDITARY HAEMORRHAGIC TELANGIECTASIA. Ethinyloestradiol 0.5 mg to 1 mg daily is used under **specialist supervision** in the management of hereditary haemorrhagic telangiectasia.

NEOPLASIA. Stilboestrol is used mainly in neoplastic conditions (see section 8.3.1)

ETHINYLOESTRADIOL

Indications: see notes above; breast cancer, see section 8.3.1

Cautions: prolonged exposure to unopposed oestrogens may increase risk of development of endometrial cancer (see notes above); breastfeeding, diabetes, epilepsy, asthma, hypertension, migraine, cardiac or renal disease, history of jaundice, contact lenses (may irritate); may interfere with results of thyroid-function tests and cortisol estimations by increasing concentrations of hormone-binding protein; **interactions:** Appendix 1 (oestrogens)

SURGERY. For a warning on oestrogens and elective surgery, see Combined Oral Contraceptives, section 7.3.1

Contra-indications: pregnancy; oestrogen-dependent cancer, active thrombophlebitis or thromboembolic disorders (higher doses also contra-indicated if history, see Combined Oral Contraceptives, section 7.3.1), hepatic impairment, Dubin-Johnson and Rotor syndromes, endometriosis, porphyria (see section 9.8.2), sickle-cell anaemia (but see also Oral Contraceptives, section 7.3.1), undiagnosed vaginal bleeding, history of herpes gestationis; deterioration of otosclerosis

Side-effects: nausea and vomiting, weight gain, breast enlargement and tenderness, withdrawal bleeding, sodium retention with oedema and hypertension (minimal for HRT), changes in liver function, jaundice, thrombosis (but for

HRT see notes above), rashes and chloasma, depression, headache, endometrial carcinoma in postmenopausal women

Dose: menopausal symptoms 10–20 micrograms daily continuously *or* for 21 days, repeated after 7 days, with progestogen from day 17 to day 26 of cycle if uterus intact

PoM **Ethinyloestradiol** (Non-proprietary)
Tablets, ethinyloestradiol 10 micrograms, net price 20 = 49p; 20 micrograms, 20 = 62p; 50 micrograms, 20 = £1.14; 1 mg, 20 = £2.55
Available from Evans (10 and 50 micrograms, 1 mg)

MESTRANOL

Indications: see notes above and under preparations
Cautions; Contra-indications; Side-effects: see under Ethinyloestradiol
Dose: see below

With progestogen
Note. Unsuitable for use as or with an oral contraceptive

PoM **Syntex Menophase®** (Syntex)
Tablets, 5 pink, mestranol 12.5 micrograms; 8 orange, mestranol 25 micrograms; 2 yellow, mestranol 50 micrograms; 3 green, mestranol 25 micrograms and norethisterone 1 mg; 6 blue, mestranol 30 micrograms and norethisterone 1.5 mg; 4 lavender, mestranol 20 micrograms and norethisterone 750 micrograms. Net price per pack = £3.33
Dose: menopausal symptoms (including osteoporosis prophylaxis), if uterus intact 1 tablet daily, starting with a pink tablet on Sunday, then in sequence (without interruption)

OESTRADIOL

Indications: see notes above and under preparations
Cautions; Contra-indications; Side-effects: see under Ethinyloestradiol; transdermal delivery systems may cause erythema and itching
Dose: see below

Oestrogen-only
PoM **Oestradiol Implants** (Organon)
Implant, oestradiol 25 mg, net price each = £6.60; 50 mg, each = £13.20; 100 mg, each = £25.30
Dose: by implantation, oestrogen replacement, including osteoporosis prophylaxis (with cyclical progestogen on 10–13 days of each cycle if uterus intact, see notes above), 25–100 mg as required (usually every 4–8 months)

PoM **Climaval®** (Sandoz)
Tablets, oestradiol valerate 1 mg (grey-blue), net price 3 × 28-tab pack = £7.20; 2 mg (blue), 3 × 28-tab pack = £7.20
Dose: menopausal symptoms (if patient has had a hysterectomy), 1–2 mg daily (for up to 24 months)

PoM **Estraderm TTS®** (Ciba)
TTS 25 patch, self-adhesive, releasing oestradiol approx. 25 micrograms/24 hours when in contact with skin. Net price 8-patch pack = £6.75. Label: 10 patient information leaflet, counselling, see below

TTS 50 patch, self-adhesive, releasing oestradiol approx. 50 micrograms/24 hours when in contact with skin. Net price 8-patch pack = £7.45. Label: 10 patient information leaflet, counselling, see below

TTS 100 patch, self-adhesive, releasing oestradiol approx. 100 micrograms/24 hours when in contact with skin. Net price 8-patch pack = £8.20. Label: 10 patient information leaflet, counselling, see below

Dose: menopausal symptoms (including osteoporosis prophylaxis in case of Estraderm TTS 50 only), 1 patch to be applied twice weekly on continuous basis; give progestogen on 12 days a month (unless patient has had hysterectomy); therapy should be initiated with TTS 50 for first month, subsequently adjusted to lowest effective dose; max. one TTS 100 daily
COUNSELLING. Patch should be removed after 3–4 days and replaced with fresh patch on slightly different site; recommended sites: clean, dry, unbroken areas of skin on trunk below waistline; not to be applied on or near breasts

PoM **Hormonin®** (Shire)
Tablets, pink, oestradiol 600 micrograms, oestriol 270 micrograms, oestrone 1.4 mg. Net price 20 = £1.34
Dose: menopausal symptoms (including osteoporosis prophylaxis), with progestogen for 12–13 days per cycle if uterus intact, 1–2 tablets daily
Note. Hormonin® tablets can be given continuously or cyclically (21 days out of 28)

PoM **Progynova®** (Schering Health Care)
Tablets, both s/c, oestradiol valerate 1 mg (beige), net price 21-tab pack = £1.98; 2 mg (blue), 21-tab pack = £1.98
Dose: menopausal symptoms (short-term), 1 mg daily for 21 days, interval of at least 7 days before next course; increased to 2 mg daily if required

With progestogen
Note. Unsuitable for use as or with an oral contraceptive

PoM **Cyclo-Progynova®** (Schering Health Care)
1-mg Tablets, all s/c, 11 beige, oestradiol valerate 1 mg; 10 brown, oestradiol valerate 1 mg and norgestrel 500 micrograms (≡ levonorgestrel 250 micrograms). Net price per pack = £3.50
Dose: menopausal symptoms (including osteoporosis prophylaxis), if uterus intact, 1 beige tablet daily for 11 days, starting on 5th day of menstruation (or at any time if cycles have ceased or are infrequent), then 1 brown tablet daily for 10 days, followed by a 7-day interval
2-mg Tablets, all s/c, 11 white, oestradiol valerate 2 mg; 10 brown, oestradiol valerate 2 mg and norgestrel 500 micrograms (≡ levonorgestrel 250 micrograms). Net price per pack = £3.50
Dose: see above, but starting with 1 white tablet daily (instead of 1 beige tablet) if symptoms not fully controlled with lower strength

Chapter 6: Endocrine system

▼ PoM **Estracombi**® (Ciba)
Combination pack of 4-self adhesive patches of *Estraderm TTS*® *50* (releasing oestradiol approx. 50 micrograms/24 hours when in contact with skin) and 4 patches of *Estragest TTS*® (releasing oestradiol approx. 50 micrograms/24 hours and norethisterone acetate 250 micrograms/24 hours when in contact with skin). Net price per pack = £9.95. Label: 10 patient information leaflet, counselling, see below
Dose: menopausal symptoms (including osteoporosis prophylaxis) if uterus intact, starting within 5 days of onset of menstruation (or any time if cycles have ceased or are infrequent), 1 *Estraderm TTS*® *50* patch to be applied twice weekly for 2 weeks followed by 1 *Estragest TTS*® patch twice weekly for 2 weeks; subsequent courses are repeated without interval
COUNSELLING. Patch should be removed after 3–4 days and replace with fresh patch on slightly different site; recommended sites: clean, dry, unbroken areas of skin on trunk below waistline; not to be applied on or near breasts

PoM **Estrapak 50**® (Ciba)
Calendar pack, 8 self-adhesive patches, releasing oestradiol approx. 50 micrograms/24 hours when in contact with skin, and 12 tablets, red, norethisterone acetate 1 mg. Net price per pack = £8.45. Label: 10 patient information leaflet, counselling, see below
Dose: menopausal symptoms (including osteoporosis prophylaxis) if uterus intact, starting within 5 days of onset of menstruation (or at any time if cycles have ceased or are infrequent), apply 1 patch twice weekly on continuous basis, and take 1 tablet daily on days 15–26 of each 28-day treatment cycle
COUNSELLING. Patch should be removed after 3–4 days and replaced with fresh patch on slightly different site; recommended sites: clean, dry, unbroken areas of skin on trunk below waistline; not to be applied on or near breasts

PoM **Nuvelle**® (Schering Health Care)
Tablets, all s/c, 16 white, oestradiol valerate 2 mg; 12 pink, oestradiol valerate 2 mg and levonorgestrel 75 micrograms. Net price 3 × 28-tab pack = £13.77
Dose: climacteric symptoms of menopause, 1 white tablet daily for 16 days, starting on 5th day of menstruation (or any time if cycles have ceased or are infrequent) then 1 pink tablet daily for 12 days; subsequent courses are repeated without interval

PoM **Trisequens**® (Novo Nordisk)
Trisequens® *tablets,* 12 blue, oestradiol 2 mg, oestriol 1 mg; 10 white, oestradiol 2 mg, oestriol 1 mg, norethisterone acetate 1 mg; 6 red, oestradiol 1 mg, oestriol 500 micrograms. Net price 28-tab pack = £3.74; 3 × 28-tab pack = £11.22
Dose: menopausal symptoms (including osteoporosis prophylaxis), if uterus intact, 1 blue tablet daily, starting on 5th day of menstruation (or at any time if cycles have ceased or are infrequent), then 1 tablet daily in sequence (without interruption)

Trisequens Forte® *tablets,* 12 yellow, oestradiol 4 mg, oestriol 2 mg; 10 white, oestradiol 4 mg, oestriol 2 mg, norethisterone acetate 1 mg; 6 red, oestradiol 1 mg, oestriol 500 micrograms. Net price 28-tab pack = £3.74; 3 × 28-tab pack = £11.22
Dose: menopausal symptoms (but not osteoporosis prophylaxis), see under Trisequens®, starting with 1 yellow tablet daily (instead of 1 blue tablet) if symptoms not fully controlled with lower strength

OESTRIOL

Indications: see notes above and under preparations
Cautions; Contra-indications; Side-effects: see under Ethinyloestradiol
Dose: see below

PoM **Ovestin**® (Organon)
Tablets, oestriol 250 micrograms. Net price 20 = 60p. Label: 25
Dose: genito-urinary symptoms associated with oestrogen-deficiency states, 0.5–3 mg daily, as single dose, for up to 1 month, then 0.5–1 mg daily until restoration of epithelial integrity (short-term use)
Infertility associated with poor cervical penetration, 0.25–1 mg daily, as single dose, on days 6–15 of cycle (with regular monitoring)
Ingredient of Hormonin® and (with progestogen) of Trisequens®, see Oestradiol

OESTROGENS, CONJUGATED

Indications: see notes above and under preparations
Cautions; Contra-indications; Side-effects: see under Ethinyloestradiol
Dose: see below

PoM **Premarin**® (Wyeth)
Tablets, all s/c, conjugated oestrogens 625 micrograms (maroon), net price 21-tab pack = £1.38; 1.25 mg (yellow), 21-tab pack = £2.27; 2.5 mg (purple), 20 = £2.30
Dose: menopausal symptoms including osteoporosis prophylaxis, (with progestogen for 10–12 days per cycle if uterus intact), 0.625–1.25 mg daily

With progestogen
Note. Unsuitable for use as or with an oral contraceptive
PoM **Prempak-C**® (Wyeth)
0.625 Calendar pack, all s/c, 28 maroon tablets, conjugated oestrogens 625 micrograms; 12 light brown tablets, norgestrel 150 micrograms (≡levonorgestrel 75 micrograms). Net price per pack = £4.06
Dose: menopausal symptoms (including osteoporosis prophylaxis), if uterus intact, 1 maroon tablet daily on continuous basis, starting on 1st day of menstruation (or at any time if cycles have ceased or are infrequent), and 1 brown tablet daily on days 17–28 of each 28-day treatment cycle; subsequent courses are repeated without interval

1.25 Calendar pack, all s/c, 28 yellow tablets, conjugated oestrogens 1.25 mg; 12 light brown tablets, norgestrel 150 micrograms (≡levonorgestrel 75 micrograms). Net price per pack = £4.06
Dose: see above, but taking 1 yellow tablet daily on continuous basis (instead of 1 maroon tablet) if symptoms not fully controlled with lower strength

PIPERAZINE OESTRONE SULPHATE
(Estropipate)
Indications: see notes above and under preparations
Cautions; Contra-indications; Side-effects: see under Ethinyloestradiol
Dose: see below

PoM **Harmogen**® (Abbott)
Tablets, peach, scored, piperazine oestrone sulphate 1.5 mg. Net price 20 = £1.65
Dose: menopausal symptoms, 1.5–4.5 mg daily in single or divided doses for 21–28 days, repeated after 5–7 days if necessary; if given for longer reduced to lowest dose (and given with progestogen for 12 days per month if uterus intact)

TIBOLONE

Tibolone combines oestrogenic and progestogenic activity with weak androgenic activity. It has recently been introduced for the treatment of vasomotor symptoms of the menopause. It is given continuously, without cyclical progestogen.

TIBOLONE
Indications: see under Dose
Cautions: renal impairment, epilepsy, migraine, diabetes mellitus, hypercholesterolaemia; withdraw if signs of thrombo-embolic disease, abnormal liver function tests or cholestatic jaundice; induce withdrawal bleeding with a progestogen if transferring from another form of HRT; **interactions:** Appendix 1 (tibolone)
Contra-indications: hormone-dependent tumours, history of cardiovascular or cerebrovascular disease (e.g. thrombophlebitis, thrombo-embolism), uninvestigated vaginal bleeding, severe liver disease, pregnancy, breast-feeding
Side-effects: weight changes, ankle oedema, dizziness, seborrhoeic dermatitis, vaginal bleeding, headache, gastro-intestinal disturbances, increased facial hair
Dose: vasomotor symptoms following natural or surgical menopause, 2.5 mg daily
Note. Unsuitable for use in the premenopause and as or with an oral contraceptive; also unsuitable for use within 12 months of the last menstrual period (may cause irregular bleeding)

▼ PoM **Livial**® (Organon)
Tablets, tibolone 2.5 mg. Net price 28-tab pack = £13.20

6.4 Sex hormones 271

6.4.1.2 PROGESTOGENS

Progestogens modify some of the effects of, and act mainly on tissues sensitised by, oestrogens; their effects are inhibited by oestrogen excess. There are two main groups of progestogen, the naturally occurring hormone *progesterone* and its analogues (allyloestrenol, dydrogesterone, hydroxyprogesterone, and medroxyprogesterone) and the *testosterone* analogues e.g. norethisterone. Progesterone and its analogues are less androgenic than the testosterone derivatives and neither progesterone nor dydrogesterone causes virilisation. Other synthetic derivatives are variably metabolised into testosterone and oestrogen; thus side-effects vary with the preparation and the dose.

Progestogens are used in many menstrual disorders, including *severe dysmenorrhoea*, and *menorrhagia*. **Norethisterone** and **dydrogesterone** may be given alone on a cyclical basis during part of the menstrual cycle or in conjunction with an oestrogen. Where contraception is also required in younger women, however, the best choice is a combined oral contraceptive (see section 7.3.1).

Where *endometriosis* requires drug treatment, it may respond to a progestogen, e.g. norethisterone, administered on a continuous basis. Alternatively, danazol (section 6.7.3) may be given.

Progestogens have been widely advocated for the alleviation of *premenstrual symptoms* but no convincing physiological basis for such treatment has been shown.

The progestogens desogestrel, ethynodiol, levonorgestrel, and norethisterone are used in combined oral and in progestogen-only *contraceptives* (see sections 7.3.1 and 7.3.2). Levonorgestrel is the active isomer and has twice the potency of racemic norgestrel.

Progestogens are also used in conjunction with oestrogens in *hormone replacement therapy* in menopausal women with an intact uterus (see section 6.4.1.1). See section 8.3.2 for use in *neoplastic disease*.

Progestogens have been used in *habitual abortion* but there is no evidence of benefit. If they are used for this purpose they should be of the true progesterone-derivative type, e.g. **hydroxyprogesterone hexanoate** to avoid any masculinisation of a female fetus.

PROGESTERONE
Indications: see under Dose and notes above
Cautions: diabetes, breast-feeding, hypertension; hepatic, cardiac, or renal disease; **interactions:** Appendix 1 (progestogens)
Contra-indications: undiagnosed vaginal bleeding, missed or incomplete abortion, past severe arterial disease or current high risk (e.g. family history, together with cholesterol above 6.5 mmol/litre), mammary carcinoma; porphyria (see section 9.8.2)

Cautionary label wordings, see inside back cover

Prices are **net**, see p. 1

Side-effects: acne, urticaria, oedema, weight gain, gastro-intestinal disturbances, changes in libido, breast discomfort, premenstrual symptoms, irregular menstrual cycles; rarely jaundice. Injection may be painful
Dose: by vagina or rectum, premenstrual syndrome, 200 mg daily to 400 mg twice daily starting at day 12–14 and continued until onset of menstruation (but not recommended, see notes above); rectally if barrier methods of contraception are used, or if vaginal infection
By deep intramuscular injection into buttock, embryo transfer, consult manufacturer's literature

PoM **Cyclogest**® (Hoechst)
Suppositories, progesterone 200 mg, net price 15 = £5.40; 400 mg, 15 = £7.83

PoM **Gestone**® (Paines & Byrne)
Injection, progesterone 25 mg/mL, 1-mL amp = 34p; 50 mg/mL, 1-mL amp = 44p, 2-mL amp = 58p

ALLYLOESTRENOL

Indications: habitual abortion, but see notes above
Cautions; Contra-indications; Side-effects: see under Progesterone and notes above
Dose: habitual abortion, 5–10 mg daily for at least 16 weeks (but see notes above)

PoM **Gestanin**® (Organon)
Tablets, allyloestrenol 5 mg. Net price 20 = £1.99

DESOGESTREL

Ingredient of combined oral contraceptives (section 7.3.1)

DYDROGESTERONE

Indications: see under Dose and notes above
Cautions; Contra-indications; Side-effects: see under Progesterone and notes above; breakthrough bleeding may occur (increase dose)
Dose: endometriosis, 10 mg 2–3 times daily from 5th to 25th day of cycle or continuously
Infertility, irregular cycles, 10 mg twice daily from 11th to 25th day for at least 6 cycles
Habitual abortion, 10 mg twice daily from day 11 to day 25 of cycle until conception, then continuously until 20th week of pregnancy and gradually reduced (but see notes above)
Dysfunctional uterine bleeding, 10 mg twice daily (together with an oestrogen) for 5–7 days to arrest bleeding; 10 mg twice daily (together with an oestrogen) from 11th to 25th day of cycle to prevent bleeding
Dysmenorrhoea, 10 mg twice daily from 5th to 25th day of cycle
Amenorrhoea, 10 mg twice daily from 11th to 25th day of cycle with oestrogen therapy from 1st to 25th day of cycle
Premenstrual syndrome, 10 mg twice daily from 12th to 26th day of cycle increased if necessary (but not recommended, see notes above)

Hormone replacement therapy, with continuous oestrogen therapy, 10 mg twice daily, for the first 12–14 days of each calendar month; with cyclical oestrogen, 10 mg twice daily for the last 12–14 days of each treatment cycle

PoM **Duphaston**® (Duphar)
Tablets, scored, dydrogesterone 10 mg. Net price 60-tab pack = £10.05

ETHYNODIOL DIACETATE

Ingredient of combined and progestogen-only oral contraceptives (sections 7.3.1 and 7.3.2)

GESTODENE

Ingredient of combined oral contraceptives (section 7.3.1)

HYDROXYPROGESTERONE HEXANOATE

Indications: habitual abortion but see notes above
Cautions; Contra-indications; Side-effects: see under Progesterone and notes above
Dose: by intramuscular injection, 250–500 mg weekly during first half of pregnancy

PoM **Proluton* Depot**® (Schering Health Care)
Injection (oily), hydroxyprogesterone hexanoate 250 mg/mL. Net price 1-mL amp = £2.35; 2-mL amp = £3.69
*formerly Primolut Depot®

LEVONORGESTREL

Ingredient of combined and progestogen-only oral contraceptives (sections 7.3.1 and 7.3.2)

MEDROXYPROGESTERONE ACETATE

Indications: see under Dose; for use as a contraceptive, see section 7.3.2; for use in malignant disease, see section 8.3.2
Cautions; Contra-indications; Side-effects: see under Progesterone and notes above; disturbances of normal menstrual cycle and irregular bleeding may occur; contra-indicated in pregnancy
Dose: by mouth, 2.5–10 mg daily for 5–10 days beginning on 16th–21st day of cycle, repeated for 2 cycles in dysfunctional uterine bleeding and 3 cycles in secondary amenorrhoea
Mild to moderate endometriosis, 10 mg 3 times daily for 90 consecutive days, beginning on 1st day of cycle
By deep intramuscular injection, endometriosis, 50 mg weekly or 100 mg every 2 weeks

PoM **Depo-Provera**® **50mg/mL** (Upjohn)
Injection (aqueous suspension), medroxyprogesterone acetate 50 mg/mL. Net price 3-mL vial = £4.17; 5-mL vial = £6.85

PoM **Provera**® (Upjohn)
Tablets, both scored, medroxyprogesterone acetate 5 mg, net price 20-tab pack = £2.58, 100-tab pack = £12.87; 10 mg, 50-tab pack = £12.87

NORETHISTERONE

Indications: see under Dose; for use as a contraceptive see sections 7.3.1 and 7.3.2
Cautions; Contra-indications; Side-effects: see under Progesterone but more virilising and greater incidence of liver disturbances and jaundice; avoid in pregnancy; exacerbation of epilepsy and migraine
Dose: endometriosis 10 mg daily starting on 5th day of cycle (increased if spotting occurs to 25 mg daily in divided doses to prevent breakthrough bleeding)
Menorrhagia, 5 mg 3 times daily for 10 days to arrest bleeding; to prevent bleeding 5 mg twice daily from 19th to 26th day
Dysmenorrhoea, 5 mg 3 times daily from 5th to 24th day for 3–4 cycles
Premenstrual syndrome, 5 mg 2–3 times daily from 19th to 26th day for several cycles (but not recommended, see notes above)
Postponement of menstruation, 5 mg 3 times daily starting 3 days before anticipated onset

PoM **Menzol**® (Schwarz)
Tablets, scored, norethisterone 5 mg. Net price 3 × 24-tab (8-day) 'Planapak' = £7.70; 3 × 60-tab (20-day) 'Planapak' = £19.35
PoM **Primolut N**® (Schering Health Care)
Tablets, norethisterone 5 mg. Net price 20 = £1.63
PoM **Utovlan**® (Syntex)
Tablets, scored, norethisterone 5 mg. Net price 20 = £1.54

NORGESTIMATE

Ingredient of combined oral contraceptive (section 7.3.1)

NORGESTREL

Ingredient of combined and progestogen-only oral contraceptives (section 7.3.1) and of combined preparations for menopausal symptoms (section 6.4.1.1)

6.4.2 Male sex hormones and antagonists

Androgens cause masculinisation; they may be used as replacement therapy in castrated adults and in those who are hypogonadal due to either pituitary or testicular disease. In the normal male they depress spermatogenesis and inhibit pituitary gonadotrophin secretion. Androgens also have an anabolic action which led to the development of anabolic steroids (section 6.4.3).

Androgens are useless as a treatment of impotence and impaired spermatogenesis unless there is associated hypogonadism; they should not be given until the hypogonadism has been properly investigated. Treatment should be under expert supervision.

When given to patients with hypopituitarism they can lead to normal sexual development and potency but not to fertility. If fertility is desired, the usual treatment is with gonadotrophins or pulsatile gonadotrophin-releasing hormone (section 6.5.1) which will stimulate spermatogenesis as well as androgen production.

Caution should be used when androgens or chorionic gonadotrophin are used in treating boys with delayed puberty since the fusion of epiphyses is hastened and may result in short stature.

Androgens are still quite useful in occasional women with disseminated cancer of the breast despite their masculinising effects.

Intramuscular depot preparations of **testosterone esters** are preferred for replacement therapy. Testosterone enanthate or propionate or alternatively Sustanon®, which consists of a mixture of testosterone esters and has a longer duration of action, may be used. Satisfactory replacement therapy can sometimes be obtained with 1 mL of Sustanon 250®, given by intramuscular injection once a month, although more frequent dose intervals are often necessary. Implants of testosterone have been superseded for hypogonadism but are still occasionally used. Menopausal women are also sometimes given implants of testosterone (in a dose of 50–100 mg every 4–8 months) as an adjunct to hormone replacement therapy.

Of the orally active preparations, **testosterone undecanoate** and **mesterolone** are available. Methyltestosterone and other 17α-alkyl derivatives of testosterone are no longer on the UK market because they sometimes cause dose-related cholestatic jaundice.

TESTOSTERONE AND ESTERS

Indications: see under preparations
Cautions: cardiac, renal, or hepatic impairment (see Appendix 2), elderly, ischaemic heart disease, hypertension, epilepsy, migraine, skeletal metastases (risk of hypercalcaemia), pre-pubital boys (see notes above)
Contra-indications: breast cancer in men, prostatic cancer, hypercalcaemia, pregnancy, breast-feeding, nephrosis
Side-effects: sodium retention with oedema, hypercalcaemia, increased bone growth, priapism, precocious sexual development and premature closure of epiphyses in pre-pubertal males, virilism in women, and suppression of spermatogenesis in men

Oral
PoM **Restandol**® (Organon)
Capsules, red-brown, testosterone undecanoate 40 mg in oily solution. Net price 60 = £15.78. Label: 21, 25
Dose: androgen deficiency, 120–160 mg daily for 2–3 weeks; maintenance 40–120 mg daily

Intramuscular
PoM **Primoteston Depot**® (Schering Health Care)
Injection (oily), testosterone enanthate 250 mg/mL. Net price 1-mL amp = £4.13
Dose: by slow intramuscular injection, hypogonadism, initially 250 mg every 2–3 weeks; maintenance 250 mg every 3–6 weeks
Breast cancer, 250 mg every 2–3 weeks

PoM **Sustanon 100**® (Organon)
Injection (oily), testosterone propionate 20 mg, testosterone phenylpropionate 40 mg, and testosterone isocaproate 40 mg/mL. Net price 1-mL amp = £1.11
Dose: by deep intramuscular injection, androgen deficiency, 1 mL every 2 weeks

PoM **Sustanon 250**® (Organon)
Injection (oily), testosterone propionate 30 mg, testosterone phenylpropionate 60 mg, testosterone isocaproate 60 mg, and testosterone decanoate 100 mg/mL. Net price 1-mL amp = £2.61
Dose: by deep intramuscular injection, androgen deficiency, 1 mL usually every 3 weeks

PoM **Virormone**® (Paines & Byrne)
Injection, testosterone propionate 50 mg/mL. Net price 2-mL amp = 46p
Dose: by intramuscular injection, androgen deficiency, 50 mg 2–3 times weekly
Delayed puberty, 50 mg weekly
Breast cancer, 100 mg 2–3 times weekly

Implant
PoM **Testosterone** (Organon)
Implant, testosterone 100 mg, net price = £5.61; 200 mg = £10.45
Dose: by implantation, male hypogonadism, 600 mg every 6 months
Menopausal women, see notes above

MESTEROLONE

Indications: see under Dose
Cautions; Contra-indications; Side-effects: see under Testosterone Esters; spermatogenesis unimpaired
Dose: androgen deficiency, 25 mg 3–4 times daily for several months, reduced to 50–75 mg daily in divided doses for maintenance

PoM **Pro-Viron**® (Schering Health Care)
Tablets, scored, mesterolone 25 mg. Net price 50 = £7.91

ANTI-ANDROGENS

Cyproterone acetate is an anti-androgen used in the treatment of severe hypersexuality and sexual deviation in the male; it inhibits spermatogenesis and produces reversible infertility. Abnormal sperm forms are produced. Cyproterone acetate is also used in the treatment of acne and hirsutism in women (see section 13.6) and in prostatic cancer (see section 8.3.4). As hepatic tumours have been produced in *animal* studies, careful consideration should be given to the risk/benefit ratio before treatment.

CYPROTERONE ACETATE

Indications: see notes above; prostate cancer, see section 8.3.4

Cautions: impaired ability to drive and operate machinery; ineffective for male hypersexuality in chronic alcoholism (relevance to prostate cancer not known); blood counts and monitor hepatic function, adrenocortical function and blood glucose regularly; diabetes mellitus, adrenocortical insufficiency
Contra-indications: (do not apply in prostate cancer) hepatic disease, malignant or wasting disease, severe depression, history of thromboembolic disorders; youths under 18 years (may arrest bone maturation and testicular development)
Side-effects: fatigue and lassitude, weight changes, changes in hair pattern, gynaecomastia (rarely leading to galactorrhoea and benign breast nodules); rarely osteoporosis; inhibition of spermatogenesis (see notes above); liver abnormalities reported in *animals*
Dose: male hypersexuality, 50 mg twice daily after food

PoM **Androcur**® (Schering Health Care)
Tablets, scored, cyproterone acetate 50 mg. Net price 56-tab pack = £32.23. Label: 2, 21

6.4.3 Anabolic steroids

All the anabolic steroids have some androgenic activity but they cause less virilisation than androgens in women. Their protein-building property led to the hope that they might be widely useful in medicine but this hope has not been realised. They have, for example, been given for osteoporosis in women and in cases of wasting. Their use as body builders or tonics is quite unjustified; they are abused by some athletes.

Anabolic steroids are used in the treatment of some *aplastic anaemias* (see section 9.1.3) and to reduce the itching of *chronic biliary obstruction* (see Prescribing in Terminal Care).

NANDROLONE

Indications: osteoporosis in postmenopausal women; aplastic anaemia, see section 9.1.3
Cautions: cardiac and renal impairment, hepatic impairment (see Appendix 2), hypertension, diabetes mellitus, epilepsy, migraine; monitor skeletal maturation in young patients; skeletal metastases (risk of hypercalcaemia); interactions: Appendix 1 (anabolic steroids)
Contra-indications: severe hepatic impairment, prostate cancer, male breast cancer, pregnancy, porphyria (see section 9.8.2)
Side-effects: acne, sodium retention with oedema, virilisation with high doses including voice changes (sometimes irreversible), amenorrhoea, inhibition of spermatogenesis, premature epiphyseal closure; abnormal liver-function tests reported with high doses; liver tumours reported occasionally on prolonged treatment with anabolic steroids
Dose: see next page

PoM **Deca-Durabolin**® (Organon)
Injection (oily), nandrolone decanoate 25 mg/mL, net price 1-mL amp = £1.75, 1-mL syringe = £1.88; 50 mg/mL, 1-mL amp = £3.37, 1-mL syringe = £3.57
Dose: by deep intramuscular injection, 50 mg every 3 weeks

PoM **Deca-Durabolin 100**®, see section 9.1.3

PoM **Durabolin**® (Organon)
Injection (oily), nandrolone phenylpropionate 25 mg/mL, net price 1-mL amp = 86p; 50 mg/mL, 1-mL syringe = £1.70
Dose: by deep intramuscular injection, 50 mg weekly

STANOZOLOL

Indications: see under Dose
Cautions; Contra-indications; Side-effects: see under Nandrolone. Headache, dyspepsia, euphoria, depression, cramp, and occasionally hair loss, also reported; cholestatic jaundice occasionally reported
Dose: by mouth, vascular manifestations of Behcet's disease, 10 mg daily
Hereditary angioedema, 2.5–10 mg daily to control attacks, reduced for maintenance (2.5 mg 3 times weekly may be sufficient); CHILD 1–6 years initially 2.5 mg daily, 6–12 years initially 2.5–5 mg daily, reduced for maintenance
Note: In hereditary angioedema restricted to well-established cases who have experienced serious attacks (and not for premenopausal women except in life-threatening situations)

PoM **Stromba**® (Sanofi Winthrop)
Tablets, scored, stanozolol 5 mg. Net price 56-tab pack = £24.48

6.5 Hypothalamic and pituitary hormones and anti-oestrogens

Hypothalamic and pituitary hormones are described under the following section headings:
6.5.1 Hypothalamic and anterior pituitary hormones and anti-oestrogens
6.5.2 Posterior pituitary hormones and antagonists

Use of preparations in these sections requires detailed prior investigation of the patient and *should be reserved for specialist centres.*

6.5.1 Hypothalamic and anterior pituitary hormones and anti-oestrogens

ANTI-OESTROGENS

The anti-oestrogens **clomiphene**, **cyclofenil**, and **tamoxifen** are used in the treatment of female infertility due to secondary amenorrhoea (e.g. polycystic ovarian disease). They induce gonadotrophin release by occupying oestrogen receptors in the hypothalamus, thereby interfering with feedback mechanisms; chorionic gonadotrophin is sometimes used as an adjunct. Care is taken to avoid hyperstimulation and multiple pregnancies.

CLOMIPHENE CITRATE

Indications: anovulatory infertility—see notes above
Cautions: see notes above; polycystic ovary syndrome (cysts may enlarge during treatment), incidence of multiple births increased
Contra-indications: hepatic disease, ovarian cysts, endometrial carcinoma, pregnancy, abnormal uterine bleeding
Side-effects: visual disturbances (withdraw), ovarian hyperstimulation (withdraw), hot flushes, abdominal discomfort, occasionally nausea, vomiting, depression, insomnia, breast tenderness, weight gain, rashes, dizziness, hair loss
Dose: 50 mg daily for 5 days (starting on 2nd to 5th day of menstrual cycle or at any time if cycles have ceased); in absence of ovulation second course of 100 mg daily for 5 days may be given; most patients who are going to respond will do so to first course; 3 courses should constitute adequate therapeutic trial; long-term cyclical therapy not recommended

PoM **Clomid**® (Merrell)
Tablets, yellow, scored, clomiphene citrate 50 mg. Net price 20 = £6.73

PoM **Serophene**® (Serono)
Tablets, scored, clomiphene citrate 50 mg. Net price 20 = £6.73

CYCLOFENIL

Indications: anovulatory infertility—see notes above
Contra-indications: see under Clomiphene Citrate
Side-effects: hot flushes, abdominal discomfort, nausea; rarely cholestatic jaundice
Dose: 200 mg twice daily for 10 days starting on 3rd day of natural or induced bleeding, repeated for at least 3 cycles

PoM **Rehibin**® (Serono)
Tablets, scored, cyclofenil 100 mg. Net price 20 = £3.70

TAMOXIFEN
See section 8.3.4

ANTERIOR PITUITARY HORMONES

CORTICOTROPHINS
Tetracosactrin an analogue of corticotrophin (ACTH) is used to test adrenocortical function; corticotrophin itself is no longer commercially available in the UK. Failure of the plasma cortisol concentration to rise after intramuscular administration indicates adrenocortical insufficiency.

Both corticotrophin and tetracosactrin were formerly used as alternatives to corticosteroids in conditions such as Crohn's disease or rheumatoid arthritis; their value was limited by the variable and unpredictable therapeutic response and by the waning of their effect with time.

TETRACOSACTRIN

Indications: see notes above

Cautions; Contra-indications; Side-effects: see section 6.3.3 and Corticotrophin; important risk of anaphylaxis (medical supervision; see data sheet)

PoM **Synacthen**® (Ciba)
Injection, tetracosactrin 250 micrograms (as acetate)/mL. Net price 1-mL amp = 93p
Dose: diagnostic, *by intramuscular or intravenous injection*, 250 micrograms as a single dose

PoM **Synacthen Depot**® (Ciba)
Injection (aqueous suspension), tetracosactrin 1 mg (as acetate)/mL, with zinc phosphate complex; also contains benzyl alcohol. Net price 1-mL amp = £1.05; 2-mL vial = £1.92
Dose: by intramuscular injection, initially 1 mg daily (or every 12 hours in acute cases); subsequently reduced to 1 mg every 2–3 days, then 1 mg weekly (or 500 micrograms every 2–3 days)

GONADOTROPHINS

Follicle-stimulating hormone (FSH) is used in the treatment of infertile women with proven hypopituitarism or who have not responded to clomiphene; it is used in conjunction with luteinising hormone (LH). Follicle-stimulating hormone is contained in **menotrophin** (which also contains luteinising hormone) and **urofollitrophin**; luteinising hormone is contained in **chorionic gonadotrophin**. Treatment requires careful monitoring to avoid the ovarian hyperstimulation syndrome and multiple pregnancy.

The gonadotrophins are also occasionally used in the treatment of oligospermia associated with hypopituitarism. There is no justification for their use in primary gonadal failure.

Chorionic gonadotrophin has also been used in delayed puberty in the male to stimulate endogenous testosterone production, but has little advantage over testosterone (section 6.4.2).

CHORIONIC GONADOTROPHIN

(Human Chorionic Gonadotrophin; HCG)
A preparation of a glycoprotein fraction secreted by the placenta and obtained from the urine of pregnant women having the action of the pituitary luteinising hormone

Indications: see notes above

Cautions: see notes above; cardiac or renal impairment, asthma, epilepsy, migraine

Side-effects: oedema (particularly in males—reduce dose), headache, tiredness, mood changes, gynaecomastia, local reactions; sexual precocity with high doses; may aggravate ovarian hyperstimulation

Dose: by intramuscular injection, according to patient's requirements

PoM **Gonadotraphon LH**® (Paines & Byrne)
Injection, powder for reconstitution, chorionic gonadotrophin. Net price 500-unit amp = 98p; 1000-unit amp = £1.25; 5000-unit amp = £3.71 (all with solvent)

PoM **Pregnyl**® (Organon)
Injection, powder for reconstitution, chorionic gonadotrophin. Net price 500-unit amp = 69p; 1500-unit amp = £2.07; 5000-unit amp = £3.08 (all with solvent)

PoM **Profasi**® (Serono)
Injection, powder for reconstitution, chorionic gonadotrophin. Net price 500-unit amp = 69p; 1000-unit amp = 95p; 2000-unit amp = £1.75; 5000-unit amp = £3.08 (all with solvent)

MENOTROPHIN

Indications: see notes above

Cautions: ovarian cysts, adrenal or thyroid disorders, hyperprolactinoma or pituitary tumour

Side-effects: ovarian hyperstimulation, multiple pregnancy; local reactions

Dose: by deep intramuscular injection, according to patient's response

PoM **Humegon**® (Organon)
Injection, powder for reconstitution, human menopausal gonadotrophins as follicle-stimulating hormone 75 units, luteinising hormone 75 units. Net price per amp = £8.80; follicle-stimulating hormone 150 units, luteinising hormone 150 units, 1 amp = £16.00 (both with solvent)

PoM **Pergonal**® (Serono)
Injection, powder for reconstitution, menotrophin as follicle-stimulating hormone 75 units, luteinising hormone 75 units. Net price per amp (with solvent) = £9.79

UROFOLLITROPHIN

Extract of the urine of postmenopausal women containing follicle-stimulating hormone

Indications: see notes above

Cautions; Side-effects: see under Menotrophin

Dose: by deep intramuscular injection, according to patient's response

PoM **Metrodin**® (Serono)
Injection, powder for reconstitution, urofollitrophin as follicle-stimulating hormone 75 units. Net price per amp (with solvent) = £9.79

GROWTH HORMONE

Growth hormone is used in the treatment of short stature due to growth hormone deficiency (including short stature in Turner syndrome); only the human type is effective as growth hormone is species specific. Growth hormone of human origin

6.5 Hypothalamic and pituitary hormones and anti-oestrogens

(HGH; somatotrophin) has been replaced by a growth hormone of human sequence, **somatropin**, produced using recombinant DNA technology.

SOMATROPIN
(Biosynthetic Human Growth Hormone)
Indications: see notes above
Cautions: only patients with open epiphyses; relative deficiencies of other pituitary hormones (notably hypothyroidism); diabetes mellitus (adjustment of antidiabetic therapy may be necessary); avoid in pregnancy (theoretical risk)
Side-effects: antibody formation; local reactions (rotate subcutaneous injection sites to prevent lipo-atrophy); in Turner syndrome temporary exacerbation of lymphoedema reported
Dose: 0.5–0.7 units/kg (Turner syndrome, 1 unit/kg) weekly divided into 6 or 7 doses for *subcutaneous injection* (alternatively divided into 2 or 3 doses for *intramuscular injection*, but more painful)

PoM **Genotropin**® (Kabi Pharmacia)
Injection, powder for reconstitution, somatropin (rbe), net price 4-unit vial (with diluent) = £30.50; 12-unit vial (with diluent) = £91.50
KabiPen injection, two-compartment cartridge containing powder for reconstitution, somatropin (rbe) and diluent. Net price 16-unit pack = £122.00. For use with NHS KabiPen® device (available free from clinics)
KabiQuick injection, two-compartment single-dose syringe containing powder for reconstitution, somatropin (rbe) and diluent. Net price 2-unit syringe = £16.00, 3-unit syringe = £24.00, 4-unit syringe = £32.00
KabiVial injection, two-compartment cartridge containing powder for reconstitution, somatropin (rbe) and diluent. Net price 4-unit vial = £30.50, 16-unit vial = £122.00

PoM **Humatrope**® (Lilly)
Injection, powder for reconstitution, somatropin (rbe) and diluent, net price 4-unit vial = £30.50; 16-unit vial = £122.00

PoM **Norditropin**® (Novo Nordisk)
Injection, powder for reconstitution, somatropin (epr), net price 12-unit vial (with diluent) = £91.50
PenSet 12 injection, powder for reconstitution, somatropin (epr), net price 12-unit vial (with diluent in cartridge and needle) = £96.08. For use with NHS Nordiject® 12 device (available free from clinics)
PenSet 24 injection, powder for reconstitution, somatropin (epr), net price 24-unit vial (with diluent in cartridge and needle) = £192.15. For use with NHS Nordiject® 24 device (available free from clinics)

PoM **Saizen**® (Serono)
Injection, powder for reconstitution, somatropin (rmc), net price 4-unit vial (with diluent) = £30.50; 10-unit vial (with diluent) = £76.25

HYPOTHALAMIC HORMONES

Gonadorelin (gonadotrophin-releasing hormone, LH-RH) when injected intravenously in normal subjects leads to a rapid rise in plasma concentrations of both luteinising hormone (LH) and follicle-stimulating hormone (FSH). It has not proved to be very helpful, however, in distinguishing hypothalamic from pituitary lesions. Gonadorelin is also used for treatment of infertility, particularly in the female. Gonadorelin **analogues** are indicated in breast and prostate cancer (see section 8.3.4), and in endometriosis (see section 6.7.2).

Thyrotrophin-releasing hormone (TRH, **protirelin**) may be of value in difficult cases of hyperthyroidism but has been superseded largely by immunoassays. Failure of plasma thyrotrophin (TSH) concentration to rise after intravenous injection indicates excess circulating thyroid hormones. Impaired or absent responses also occur in some euthyroid patients with single adenoma, multinodular goitre, or endocrine exophthalmos; patients with hypopituitarism show a reduced or delayed rise.

GONADORELIN
(LH-RH)
Indications: see preparations below
Side-effects: rarely, nausea, headache, abdominal pain, increased menstrual bleeding; rarely, hypersensitivity reaction on repeated administration of large doses; irritation at injection site
Dose: see below

PoM **Fertiral**® (Hoechst)
Injection, gonadorelin 500 micrograms/mL. Net price 2-mL amp = £34.30
For amenorrhoea and infertility due to abnormal release of LH–RH (endogenous gonadorelin), *by pulsatile subcutaneous infusion*, initially 10–20 micrograms over 1 minute, repeated every 90 minutes for max. of 6 months; pulsatile intravenous infusion (in association with heparin) may be required

PoM **HRF**® (Monmouth)
Injection, powder for reconstitution, gonadorelin. Net price 100-microgram vial = £8.12; 500-microgram vial = £17.73 (both with diluent)
For assessment of pituitary function (adults), *by subcutaneous or intravenous injection*, 100 micrograms

PoM **Relefact LH-RH**® (Hoechst)
Injection, gonadorelin 100 micrograms/mL. Net price 1-mL amp = £9.68
For assessment of pituitary function, *by intravenous injection*, 100 micrograms

PoM **Relefact LH-RH/TRH**® (Hoechst)
Injection, gonadorelin 100 micrograms, protirelin 200 micrograms/mL. Net price 1-mL amp = £11.18
For assessment of anterior pituitary reserve by intravenous injection, 1 mL

PROTIRELIN

Indications: assessment of thyroid function and thyroid stimulating hormone reserve

Cautions: severe hypopituitarism, myocardial ischaemia, bronchial asthma and obstructive airways disease, pregnancy

Side-effects: after rapid intravenous administration desire to micturate, flushing, dizziness, nausea, strange taste; transient increase in pulse rate and blood pressure; rarely bronchospasm

Dose: by intravenous injection, 200 micrograms; CHILD 1 microgram/kg

PoM **TRH-Roche**® (Cambridge)
Injection, protirelin 100 micrograms/mL. Net price 2-mL amp = £1.50 (hosp. only)

6.5.2 Posterior pituitary hormones and antagonists

POSTERIOR PITUITARY HORMONES

DIABETES INSIPIDUS. **Vasopressin** (antidiuretic hormone, ADH) is used in the treatment of *pituitary* ('cranial') *diabetes insipidus* as its analogues **lypressin** or **desmopressin**. Dosage is tailored to produce a slight diuresis every 24 hours to avoid water intoxication. Treatment may be required for a limited period only in diabetes insipidus following trauma or pituitary surgery.

Desmopressin has a longer duration of action than vasopressin or lypressin; unlike vasopressin and lypressin it has no vasoconstrictor effect. It is given intranasally for maintenance therapy, and by injection in the postoperative period or in unconscious patients. Desmopressin is also used in the differential diagnosis of diabetes insipidus. Following a dose of 2 micrograms intramuscularly or 20 micrograms intranasally, restoration of the ability to concentrate urine after water deprivation confirms a diagnosis of cranial diabetes insipidus. Failure to respond occurs in nephrogenic diabetes insipidus.

In *nephrogenic* and *partial pituitary diabetes insipidus* benefit may be gained from the paradoxical antidiuretic effect of thiazides (see section 2.2.1) e.g. chlorthalidone 100 mg twice daily reduced to maintenance dose of 50 mg daily.

Chlorpropamide (section 6.1.2.1) is also useful in partial pituitary diabetes insipidus, and probably acts by sensitising the renal tubules to the action of remaining endogenous vasopressin; it is given in doses of up to 350 mg daily in adults and 200 mg daily in children, care being taken to avoid hypoglycaemia. Carbamazepine (see section 4.8.1) is also sometimes useful (in a dose of 200 mg once or twice daily); its mode of action may be similar to that of chlorpropamide.

OTHER USES. Desmopressin injection is also used to boost factor VIII concentrations in mild to moderate haemophilia.

Vasopressin infusion is used to control variceal bleeding in portal hypertension, prior to more definitive treatment and with variable results. Terlipressin, a new derivative of vasopressin, is used similarly.

Oxytocin, another posterior pituitary hormone, is indicated in obstetrics (see section 7.1.1).

VASOPRESSIN

Indications: pituitary diabetes insipidus; bleeding from oesophageal varices

Cautions: heart failure, asthma, epilepsy, migraine or other conditions which might be aggravated by water retention; renal impairment (see also contra-indications); pregnancy

Contra-indications: vascular disease (especially disease of coronary arteries) unless extreme caution, chronic nephritis (until reasonable blood nitrogen concentrations attained)

Side-effects: pallor, nausea, belching, abdominal cramps, desire to defaecate, hypersensitivity reactions, constriction of coronary arteries (may cause anginal attacks and myocardial ischaemia)

Dose: by subcutaneous or intramuscular injection, diabetes insipidus, 5–20 units every four hours

By intravenous infusion, initial control of variceal bleeding, 20 units over 15 minutes

Synthetic vasopressin
PoM **Pitressin**® (P-D)
Injection, argipressin (synthetic vasopressin) 20 units/mL. Net price 1-mL amp = £5.00 (hosp. only)

DESMOPRESSIN

Indications: see under Dose

Cautions: see under Vasopressin; less pressor activity, but still need for considerable caution in renal impairment, cardiovascular disease and hypertension (not indicated for nocturnal enuresis or nocturia in these circumstances); also need for considerable caution in cystic fibrosis

Dose: intranasally

Diabetes insipidus, diagnosis, ADULT and CHILD, 20 micrograms

Diabetes insipidus, treatment, ADULT, 10–40 micrograms daily (in one or two divided doses); CHILD, 5–20 micrograms; infants may require lower doses

Primary nocturnal enuresis, ADULT and CHILD (over 7 years), 20–40 micrograms at bedtime (**important:** see also cautions); withdraw for at least one week for reassessment after 3 months

Nocturia associated with multiple sclerosis, ADULT (under 65 years), 10–20 micrograms at bedtime (**important:** see also cautions)

Renal function testing, ADULT, 40 micrograms; CHILD (1–15 years), 20 micrograms; CHILD (under 1 year), 10 micrograms (avoid fluid overload)

6.6 Drugs affecting bone metabolism

6.6.1 Calcitonin
6.6.2 Bisphosphonates

See also plicamycin (section 8.1.2), calcium (section 9.5.1.1), phosphorus (section 9.5.2), vitamin D (section 9.6.4), and oestrogens in postmenopausal osteoporosis (section 6.4.1.1).

6.6.1 Calcitonin

Calcitonin is involved with parathyroid hormone in the regulation of bone turnover and hence in the maintenance of calcium balance and homoeostasis. It is used to lower the plasma-calcium concentration in some patients with hypercalcaemia (notably when associated with malignant disease). In the treatment of severe Paget's disease of bone it is used mainly for relief of pain but it is also effective in relieving some of the neurological complications, for example deafness. The prolonged use of **porcine calcitonin** can lead to the production of neutralising antibodies. **Salcatonin** (synthetic salmon calcitonin) is less immunogenic and thus more suitable for long-term therapy. When changing treatment in Paget's disease, calcitonin (pork) 80 units is equivalent to salcatonin 50 units.

CALCITONIN (PORK)

Indications: Paget's disease of bone; hypercalcaemia
Cautions: see notes above; may contain trace of thyroid; skin test if history of allergy; pregnancy and breast-feeding (avoid—inhibits lactation in *animals*)
Side-effects: nausea, vomiting, flushing, tingling of hands, unpleasant taste, inflammatory reactions at injection site
Dose: hypercalcaemia, *by subcutaneous or intramuscular injection*, initially 4 units/kg daily adjusted according to clinical and biochemical response (higher doses more conveniently given as salcatonin, see below)
Paget's disease of bone, *by subcutaneous or intramuscular injection*, dose range 80 units 3 times weekly to 160 units daily in single or divided doses; in patients with bone pain or nerve compression syndromes, 80–160 units daily for 3–6 months

PoM **Calcitare**® (Rhône-Poulenc Rorer)
Injection, powder for reconstitution, porcine calcitonin. Net price 160-unit vial (with gelatin diluent) = £11.36

SALCATONIN

Indications: see under Dose
Cautions; Side-effects: see under Calcitonin (pork) and notes above
Dose: hypercalcaemia, *by subcutaneous or intramuscular injection*, range from 5–10 units/kg daily *to* 400 units every 6–8 hours adjusted according to clinical and biochemical response

---

By injection
Diabetes insipidus, diagnosis (*subcutaneous or intramuscular*), ADULT and CHILD, 2 micrograms
Diabetes insipidus, treatment (*subcutaneous, intramuscular or intravenous*), ADULT, 1–4 micrograms daily; CHILD 400 nanograms
Renal function testing (*subcutaneous or intramuscular*), ADULT and CHILD, 2 micrograms (avoid fluid overload)
Mild to moderate haemophilia and von Willebrands disease, post lumbar puncture headache, fibrinolytic response testing, consult data sheet

PoM **DDAVP**® (Ferring)
Intranasal solution, desmopressin 100 micrograms/mL. Net price 2.5-mL dropper bottle and catheter = £9.50
Injection, desmopressin 4 micrograms/mL. Net price 1-mL amp = £1.07

PoM **Desmospray**® (Ferring)
Nasal spray, desmopressin 10 micrograms/metered spray. Net price 5-mL unit = £19.92

LYPRESSIN

Indications: pituitary diabetes insipidus
Cautions; Contra-indications; Side-effects: see under Vasopressin; less hypersensitivity; also nasal congestion with ulceration of mucosa
Dose: intranasally, 2.5–10 units 3–7 times daily

PoM **Syntopressin**® (Sandoz)
Nasal spray, lypressin 50 units/mL, 2.5 units/squeeze. Net price 5-mL bottle = £3.49

TERLIPRESSIN

Indications: bleeding from oesophageal varices
Cautions; Contra-indications; Side-effects: see under Vasopressin, but effects are milder
Dose: by intravenous injection, 2 mg followed by 1 or 2 mg every 4 to 6 hours until bleeding is controlled, for up to 72 hours

PoM **Glypressin**® (Ferring)
Injection, terlipressin, powder for reconstitution. Net price 1-mg vial with 5 mL diluent = £19.00 (hosp. only)

ANTIDIURETIC HORMONE ANTAGONISTS

Demeclocycline (see section 5.1.3) may be used in the treatment of hyponatraemia resulting from inappropriate secretion of antidiuretic hormone. It is thought to act by directly blocking the renal tubular effect of antidiuretic hormone. Initially 0.9 to 1.2 g is given daily in divided doses, reduced to 600–900 mg daily for maintenance.

(no additional benefit with over 8 units/kg every 6 hours); *by slow intravenous infusion* (Miacalcic® only), 5–10 units/kg over at least 6 hours
Paget's disease of bone, *by subcutaneous or intramuscular injection*, dose range 50 units 3 times weekly to 100 units daily, in single or divided doses; in patients with bone pain or nerve compression syndromes, 50–100 units daily for 3–6 months

Bone pain in neoplastic disease, *by subcutaneous or intramuscular injection*, 200 units every 6 hours *or* 400 units every 12 hours for 48 hours; may be repeated at discretion of physician

Postmenopausal osteoporosis, *by subcutaneous or intramuscular injection*, 100 units daily with dietary calcium and vitamin D supplements (see sections 9.5.1.1 and 9.6.4)

PoM **Calsynar**® (Rhône-Poulenc Rorer)
Injection, salcatonin 100 units/mL in saline/acetate, net price 1-mL amp = £8.12; 200 units/mL in saline/acetate, 2-mL vial = £29.20
For subcutaneous or intramuscular injection only

PoM **Miacalcic**® (Sandoz)
Injection, salcatonin 50 units/mL, net price 1-mL amp = £3.65; 100 units/mL, 1-mL amp = £7.31; 200 units/mL, 2-mL vial = £26.28
For subcutaneous or intramuscular injection and for dilution and use as an intravenous infusion

6.6.2 Bisphosphonates

Disodium etidronate is used mainly in the treatment of *Paget's disease* of bone. It is adsorbed onto hydroxyapatite crystals, so slowing both their rate of growth and dissolution, and reduces the increased rate of bone turnover associated with the disease. Disodium etidronate is also highly effective in the treatment of *hypercalcaemia of malignancy*; more recently **disodium pamidronate** and **sodium clodronate** have been introduced for this purpose as well.

Disodium etidronate is now available with calcium carbonate for *established vertebral osteoporosis*.

DISODIUM ETIDRONATE

Indications: see under Dose
Cautions: reduce dose in mild renal impairment (avoid if moderate to severe); **interactions:** Appendix 1 (bisphosphonates)
Contra-indications: moderate to severe renal impairment; pregnancy and breast-feeding; avoid oral administration in severe inflammatory conditions of gastro-intestinal tract; not indicated for osteoporosis in presence of hypercalcaemia or hypercalciuria
Side-effects: nausea, diarrhoea; asymptomatic hypocalcaemia; increased bone pain in Paget's disease and increased risk of fractures with high doses (discontinue if fractures occur); rarely skin reactions (including angioedema); abdominal pain and constipation reported; transient taste loss also reported

Dose: Paget's disease of bone, *by mouth*, 5 mg/kg as a single daily dose for up to 6 months; doses above 10 mg/kg daily for up to 3 months may be used with caution but doses above 20 mg/kg daily are not recommended
Hypercalcaemia of malignancy, *by intravenous infusion*, 7.5 mg/kg daily for 3 days; repeat once if necessary after at least 7 days; *by mouth*, on day after last intravenous dose, 20 mg/kg as a single daily dose for 30 days; max. recommended treatment period 90 days
Established vertebral osteoporosis, see under *Didronel PMO*®

COUNSELLING. Avoid food for at least 2 hours before and after oral treatment, particularly calcium-containing products

PoM **Didronel**® (Norwich Eaton)
Tablets, disodium etidronate 200 mg. Net price 60-tab pack = £37.62. Counselling, food and calcium (see above)

PoM **Didronel IV**® (Norwich Eaton)
Injection, disodium etidronate 50 mg/mL. For dilution and use as an infusion. Net price 6-mL amp = £16.43

With calcium carbonate
For cautions and side-effects of calcium carbonate see section 9.5.1.1

PoM **Didronel PMO**® (Norwich Eaton)
Tablets, 14 white, disodium etidronate 400 mg; 76 pink, effervescent, calcium carbonate 1.25 g (Cacit®). Net price per pack = £40.20. Label: 10 patient information leaflet, C, food and calcium (see above)
Dose: established vertebral osteoporosis (90-day cycles) 1 etidronate daily for 14 days, then 1 calcium daily for 76 days; recommended duration of therapy, 3 years

DISODIUM PAMIDRONATE

Note. Disodium pamidronate was formerly called aminohydroxypropylidenediphosphonate disodium (APD)
Indications: hypercalcaemia of malignancy
Cautions: renal impairment (divide daily dose if severe); possibility of convulsions due to electrolyte disturbances; **interactions:** Appendix 1 (bisphosphonates)
Contra-indications: pregnancy and breast-feeding
Side-effects: nausea, diarrhoea; asymptomatic hypocalcaemia; transient rise in body temperature; occasional lymphocytopenia and hypomagnesaemia
Dose: by slow intravenous infusion, according to plasma calcium concentration 15–60 mg in single infusion or in divided doses over 2–4 days; max. 90 mg per treatment course (see Appendix 6)

PoM **Aredia**® (Ciba)
Intravenous solution, disodium pamidronate (anhydrous) 3 mg/mL. For dilution and use as infusion. Net price 5-mL amp = £24.16

SODIUM CLODRONATE
Indications: hypercalcaemia of malignancy
Cautions: monitor renal and hepatic function and white cell count; **interactions:** Appendix 1 (bisphosphonates)
Contra-indications: moderate to severe renal impairment; pregnancy and breast-feeding, avoid oral administration in severe inflammatory conditions of gastro-intestinal tract
Side-effects: nausea, diarrhoea; asymptomatic hypocalcaemia; rarely skin reactions
Dose: by mouth, 1.6 g daily in single or 2 divided doses increased if necessary to a max. of 3.2 g daily; max. recommended treatment period 6 months
   COUNSELLING. Avoid food for 1–2 hours before and after treatment, particularly calcium-containing products e.g. milk
By slow intravenous infusion, 300 mg daily for max. 7–10 days

▼ PoM **Bonefos**® (Boehringer Ingelheim)
Capsules, yellow, sodium clodronate 400 mg. Net price 112-cap pack = £194.00. Counselling, food and calcium
Concentrate (= intravenous solution), sodium clodronate 60 mg/mL, for dilution and use as infusion. Net price 5-mL amp = £14.80

▼ PoM **Loron**® (Boehringer Mannheim)
Capsules, sodium clodronate 400 mg. Net price 120-cap pack = £207.85. Label: 10 patient information leaflet, counselling, food and calcium
Intravenous solution, sodium clodronate 30 mg/mL, for dilution and use as infusion. Net price 10-mL amp = £14.80

6.7 Other endocrine drugs

This section includes:
6.7.1 Bromocriptine
6.7.2 Danazol, gestrinone, and gonadorelin analogues
6.7.3 Metyrapone and trilostane

6.7.1 Bromocriptine

Bromocriptine is a stimulant of dopamine receptors in the brain; it also inhibits release of prolactin by the pituitary. Bromocriptine is used for the suppression of lactation when simpler measures fail, for the treatment of galactorrhoea and cyclical benign breast disease, and for the treatment of prolactinomas (when it reduces both plasma prolactin concentration and tumour size). Bromocriptine also inhibits the release of growth hormone and is sometimes used in the treatment of acromegaly, the success rate is much lower than with prolactinomas.

For the use of bromocriptine in parkinsonism, see section 4.9.1.

BROMOCRIPTINE
Indications: see notes above
Cautions: monitor for pituitary enlargement, particularly during pregnancy, annual gynaecological assessment (post-menopausal, every 6 months), monitor for peptic ulceration in acromegalic patients; contraceptive advice if appropriate (oral contraceptives may increase prolactin concentrations); at high dosage caution in patients with history of psychotic disorders or with severe cardiovascular disease and monitor for retroperitoneal fibrosis; avoid in porphyria (see section 9.8.2); **interactions:** Appendix 1 (bromocriptine)
HYPOTENSIVE REACTIONS. Hypotensive reactions may be disturbing in some patients during the first few days of treatment and particular care should be exercised when driving or operating machinery; tolerance to bromocriptine reduced by alcohol
Side-effects: nausea, vomiting, constipation, headache, dizziness, postural hypotension, drowsiness, reversible pallor of fingers and toes particularly in patients with Raynaud's syndrome; *high doses*, confusion, psychomotor excitation, hallucinations, dyskinesia, dry mouth, leg cramps, pleural effusions (may necessitate withdrawal of treatment), retroperitoneal fibrosis reported (monitoring required)
Dose: prevention/suppression of lactation for medical reasons, 2.5 mg on 1st day (prevention) or daily for 2–3 days (suppression); then 2.5 mg twice daily for 14 days
Hypogonadism/galactorrhoea, infertility, initially 1–1.25 mg at bedtime, increased gradually; usual dose 7.5 mg daily in divided doses, increased if necessary to a max. of 30 mg daily. Usual dose in infertility without hyperprolactinaemia, 2.5 mg twice daily
Cyclical benign breast disease and cyclical menstrual disorders (particularly breast pain), 1–1.25 mg at bedtime, increased gradually; usual dose 2.5 mg twice daily
Acromegaly, initially 1–1.25 mg at bedtime, increase gradually to 5 mg every 6 hours
Prolactinoma, initially 1–1.25 mg at bedtime; increased gradually to 5 mg every 6 hours (occasional patients may require up to 30 mg daily)
Doses should be taken with food

PoM **Bromocriptine** (Non-proprietary)
Tablets, bromocriptine (as mesylate), 2.5 mg, net price 20 = £5.11. Label: 21, counselling, hypotensive reactions
Available from APS, Berk, Cox, Kerfoot, Norton

PoM **Parlodel**® (Sandoz)
Tablets, both scored, bromocriptine (as mesylate) 1 mg, net price 20 = £1.86; 2.5 mg, 20 = £3.59. Label: 21, counselling, see above
Capsules, bromocriptine (as mesylate) 5 mg (blue/white), net price 20 = £7.04; 10 mg, 20 = £13.03. Label: 21, counselling, hypotensive reactions

6.7.2 Danazol, gestrinone and gonadorelin analogues

Danazol inhibits pituitary gonadotrophins; it combines androgenic activity with antioestrogenic and antiprogestogenic activity. It is used in the treatment of *endometriosis* and has also been used for *menorrhagia* and other *menstrual disorders*, *mammary dysplasia*, and *gynaecomastia* where other measures proved unsatisfactory. It may also be effective in the long-term management of *hereditary angioedema*.

Gestrinone has general actions similar to those of danazol and has recently been introduced for the treatment of endometriosis.

DANAZOL

Indications: see notes above and under Dose

Cautions: cardiac, hepatic, or renal impairment (avoid if severe), elderly, polycythaemia, epilepsy, diabetes mellitus, hypertension, migraine, lipoprotein disorder, history of thrombosis; withdraw if virilisation (may be irreversible on continued use); non-hormonal contraceptive methods should be used, if appropriate; **interactions:** Appendix 1 (danazol)

Contra-indications: pregnancy, ensure that patients with amenorrhoea are not pregnant; breast-feeding; severe hepatic, renal or cardiac impairment; thrombo-embolic disease; uninvestigated vaginal bleeding; androgen-dependent tumours; porphyria (see section 9.8.2)

Side-effects: nausea, dizziness, rashes, backache, nervousness, headache, weight gain; menstrual disturbances, flushing and reduction in breast size; skeletal muscle spasm, hair loss; androgenic effects including acne, oily skin, oedema, hirsutism, voice changes and rarely clitoral hypertrophy (see also Cautions); insulin resistance; leucopenia and thrombocytopenia reported; benign intracranial hypertension and visual disturbances also reported; rarely cholestatic jaundice

Dose: usual range 200–800 mg daily in up to 4 divided doses; in women all doses should start during menstruation, preferably on the first day
Endometriosis, initially 400 mg daily in up to 4 divided doses, adjusted according to response, usually for 6 months
Menorrhagia, 200 mg daily, usually for 3 months
Severe cyclical mastalgia, 200–300 mg daily usually for 3–6 months
Benign breast cysts, 300 mg daily usually for 3–6 months
Gynaecomastia, 400 mg daily in divided doses for 6 months (adolescents 200 mg daily, increased to 400 mg daily if no response after 2 months)
For pre-operative thinning of endometrium, 400–800 mg daily for 3–6 weeks
CHILD, precocious puberty, no longer recommended

PoM **Danazol** (Non-proprietary)
Capsules, danazol 100 mg, net price 20 = £6.10; 200 mg, 20 = £12.08
Available from APS, Generics

PoM **Danol**® (Sanofi Winthrop)
Capsules, danazol 100 mg (grey/white), net price 100-cap pack = £30.50; 200 mg (pink/white), 56-cap pack = £33.83.

GESTRINONE

Indications: endometriosis

Cautions; Contra-indications; Side-effects: see under Danazol; **Interactions:** Appendix 1 (gestrinone)

Dose: 2.5 mg twice weekly starting on first day of cycle with second dose 3 days later, repeated on same two days preferably at same time each week; duration of treatment usually 6 months
MISSED DOSES. one missed dose — 2.5 mg as soon as possible and maintain original sequence; two or more missed doses — discontinue, re-start on first day of new cycle (following negative pregnancy test)

▼ PoM **Dimetriose**® (Roussel)
Capsules, gestrinone 2.5 mg, net price 8-cap pack = £75.00

GONADORELIN ANALOGUES

Gonadorelin analogues, after an initial stimulation phase, down-regulate pituitary gonadotrophin secretion, leading to inhibition of ovarian steroid secretion and are thus effective in the treatment of endometriosis.

BUSERELIN

Indications: endometriosis; prostate cancer, see section 8.3.4

Cautions; Contra-indications; Side-effects: see under Nafarelin

Dose: 300 micrograms (one spray in each nostril) three times daily starting on first or second day of menstrual cycle; max. duration of treatment 6 months
COUNSELLING. Avoid use of nasal decongestants before and for at least 30 minutes after treatment.

▼ PoM **Suprecur**® (Hoechst)
Nasal spray, buserelin 150 micrograms (as acetate)/metered spray. Net price 2 × 100-dose pack (with metered dose pumps) = £81.00.
Counselling, see above

GOSERELIN

Indications: endometriosis; breast cancer and prostate cancer, see section 8.3.4

Cautions; Contra-indications; Side-effects: see under Nafarelin; also irritation at injection site

Dose: by subcutaneous injection into anterior abdominal wall, 3.6 mg every 28 days (local anaesthetic if required); max. duration of treatment 6 months

Preparations
See section 8.3.4

LEUPRORELIN ACETATE
Indications: endometriosis; prostate cancer, see section 8.3.4
Cautions; Contra-indications; Side-effects: see under Nafarelin; also irritation at injection site, rotate injection site periodically
Dose: by subcutaneous or by intramuscular injection, 3.75 mg every 4 weeks, starting during the first 5 days of menstrual cycle; max. duration of treatment 6 months

Preparations
See section 8.3.4

NAFARELIN
Indications: endometriosis
Cautions: ovarian cysts; non-hormonal method of contraception should be used throughout treatment
Contra-indications: pregnancy, breast-feeding; undiagnosed vaginal bleeding
Side-effects: hot flushes, vaginal dryness, change in libido, headache, emotional lability, myalgia, decreased breast size, irritation of nasal mucosa, rarely sensitivity reactions such as shortness of breath, chest pain, urticaria, rash, pruritus; ovarian cysts (may require withdrawal); decrease in trabecular bone density (repeat courses not recommended)
Dose: 200 micrograms twice daily as one spray in one nostril in the morning and one spray in the other nostril in the evening starting between second and fourth day of menstrual cycle; max. duration of treatment 6 months
COUNSELLING. Avoid use of nasal decongestants before and for at least 30 minutes after treatment

▼ PoM **Synarel**® (Syntex)
Nasal spray, nafarelin 200 micrograms (as acetate)/metered spray. Net price 60-dose unit = £101.35. Label: 10 patient information leaflet, Counselling, see above

BREAST PAIN (MASTALGIA)

Once any serious underlying cause has been ruled out, most women will respond to reassurance and reduction in dietary fat; withdrawal of an oral contraceptive or of hormone replacement therapy may help resolve the pain.

Women whose symptoms persist for longer than 6 months may require drug treatment. Danazol is the most effective but may be unacceptable owing to its unpleasant side-effects (which occur in about one-third of patients). Bromocriptine (section 6.7.1) like danazol is associated with unpleasant side-effects. Gamolenic acid (section 13.5) can be useful and, with its lack of antioestrogenic side-effects, may be preferred particularly in younger women who wish to continue taking an oral contraceptive; whereas bromocriptine and danazol act within 2 months, gamolenic acid may require 4 months to take effect.

Symptoms recur in about 50% of women within 2 years of withdrawal of therapy but may be less severe.

6.7.3 Metyrapone and trilostane

Metyrapone is a competitive inhibitor of 11β-hydroxylation in the adrenal cortex; the resulting inhibition of cortisol production leads to an increase in ACTH production which, in turn, leads to increased synthesis and release of cortisol precursors. It may be used as a test of anterior pituitary function.

Although most types of *Cushing's syndrome* are treated surgically, that which occasionally accompanies carcinoma of the bronchus is not usually amenable to surgery. Metyrapone has been found helpful in controlling the symptoms of the disease; it is also used in other forms of Cushing's syndrome to prepare the patient for surgery. The dosages used are either low, and tailored to cortisol production, or high, in which case corticosteroid replacement therapy is also needed.

Trilostane inhibits the synthesis of mineralocorticoids and glucocorticoids by the adrenal cortex, and may be useful in Cushing's syndrome and primary hyperaldosteronism. It appears to be less effective than metyrapone for Cushing's syndrome.

METYRAPONE
Cautions: gross hypopituitarism (risk of precipitating acute adrenal failure); many drugs interfere with estimation of steroids
Contra-indications: pregnancy, breast-feeding
Side-effects: occasional nausea, vomiting, dizziness, headache, hypotension
Dose: in the assessment of pituitary function 750 mg every 4 hours for 6 doses; CHILD 15 mg/kg (minimum 250 mg) every 4 hours for 6 doses
Management of Cushing's syndrome, range 0.25–6 g daily, tailored to cortisol production; see also section 6.3.1
Resistant oedema due to increased aldosterone secretion in cirrhosis, nephrosis, and congestive heart failure, 2.5–4.5 g daily in divided doses (with a glucocorticoid)
Note. Metyrapone should only be used under specialist advice; corticosteroid replacement therapy needed with high doses

PoM **Metopirone**® (Ciba)
Capsules, metyrapone 250 mg. Net price 20 = £4.18. Label: 21

TRILOSTANE
Indications: see notes above
Cautions: impaired liver and kidney function, monitor circulating corticosteroids and blood-electrolyte concentrations; non-hormonal contraceptive methods should be used, if appropriate; **interactions:** Appendix 1 (trilostane)
Contra-indications: pregnancy
Side-effects: rarely flushing, nausea, rhinorrhoea with high doses
Dose: 60 mg 4 times daily for at least 3 days, then adjusted according to patient's response; usual dose range 120–480 mg daily in divided doses
Note. Trilostane should only be used under specialist advice; corticosteroid replacement therapy may be needed in severe illness or surgery

PoM **Modrenal**® (Farillon)
Capsules, pink/black, trilostane 60 mg. Net price 20 = £7.92

7: Drugs used in
OBSTETRICS, GYNAECOLOGY, and URINARY-TRACT DISORDERS

In this chapter, drugs and appliances are discussed under the following headings:
7.1 Drugs used in obstetrics
7.2 Treatment of vaginal and vulval conditions
7.3 Contraceptives
7.4 Drugs for genito-urinary disorders
7.5 Appliances for urinary disorders

For hormonal therapy of gynaecological disorders see sections 6.4.1 and 6.5.1.

7.1 Drugs used in obstetrics

7.1.1 Prostaglandins and oxytocics
7.1.2 Mifepristone
7.1.3 Myometrial relaxants

Note. Because of the complexity of dosage regimens in obstetrics, in all cases detailed specialist literature should be consulted.

7.1.1 Prostaglandins and oxytocics

Prostaglandins and oxytocics are used to induce abortion or induce or augment labour and to minimise blood loss from the placental site. They include oxytocin, ergometrine, and the prostaglandins. All induce uterine contractions with varying degrees of pain according to the strength of contractions induced.

INDUCTION OF ABORTION. **Dinoprostone**, given by the *extra-amniotic* route is the preferred prostaglandin for the induction of late therapeutic abortion. Extra-amniotic **dinoprostone** is also of value as an adjunct in 'priming' the cervix prior to suction termination but is less commonly used nowadays.

Gemeprost is a prostaglandin available in the form of pessaries to ripen and soften the cervix before induction of abortion, particularly in primigravida.

INDUCTION AND AUGMENTATION OF LABOUR. **Oxytocin** (*Syntocinon®*) is administered by slow intravenous infusion, preferably using an infusion pump, to induce or augment labour, often in conjunction with amniotomy. Uterine activity must be monitored carefully and hyperstimulation avoided. Large doses of oxytocin may result in excessive fluid retention.

Dinoprostone is available as vaginal tablets and vaginal gels for the induction of labour at term. The intravenous and oral routes are rarely used.

PREVENTION AND TREATMENT OF HAEMORRHAGE. Bleeding due to *incomplete abortion* can be controlled with **ergometrine** and **oxytocin** (*Syntometrine®*) given intravenously or intramuscularly, the dose being adjusted according to the patient's condition and blood loss. This is commonly used prior to surgical evacuation of the uterus, particularly when surgery is delayed. Oxytocin and ergometrine combined are more effective in early pregnancy than either drug alone.

For the routine management of the *third stage of labour* ergometrine 500 micrograms with oxytocin 5 units (Syntometrine® 1 mL) is given by intramuscular injection with or after delivery of the shoulders. Intravenous injection is recommended for the prevention of postpartum haemorrhage in *high-risk cases*, giving either ergometrine 125–250 micrograms alone *or* oxytocin 5–10 units, after delivery of the shoulders (repeated if necessary); alternatively intravenous infusion of oxytocin 10–20 units/500 mL can be given after delivery of the shoulders, particularly when the uterus is *atonic*. If these measures are ineffective the use of **carboprost** is considered.

CARBOPROST

Indications: postpartum haemorrhage due to uterine atony in patients unresponsive to ergometrine and oxytocin

Cautions: history of glaucoma or raised intraocular pressure, asthma, hypertension, hypotension, anaemia, jaundice, diabetes, history of epilepsy, uterine scars; excessive dosage may cause uterine rupture

Contra-indications: acute pelvic inflammatory disease, cardiac, renal, pulmonary, or hepatic disease

Side-effects: nausea, vomiting and diarrhoea, hyperthermia and flushing, bronchospasm; less frequent effects include raised blood pressure, dyspnoea, and pulmonary oedema; chills, headache, diaphoresis, dizziness, and erythema and pain at injection site also reported

Dose: by deep intramuscular injection, 250 micrograms repeated if necessary at intervals of 1½ hours (in severe cases the interval may be reduced but should not be less than 15 minutes); total dose should not exceed 12 mg (48 doses)

▼ PoM **Hemabate**® (Upjohn)
Injection, carboprost as trometamol salt (tromethamine salt) 250 micrograms/mL, net price 1-mL amp = £16.50 (hosp. only)

DINOPROSTONE
Indications: see notes above
Cautions: asthma, glaucoma and raised intra-ocular pressure; excessive dosage may cause uterine rupture; continuous administration for more than 2 days not recommended; see also notes above
Contra-indications: hypertonic uterine inertia, mechanical obstruction of delivery, placenta praevia, predisposition to uterine rupture, severe toxaemia, untreated pelvic infection, fetal distress, grand multiparas and multiple pregnancy, prior history of difficult or traumatic delivery; avoid extra-amniotic route in cervicitis or vaginitis
Side-effects: nausea, vomiting, diarrhoea, flushing, shivering, headache, dizziness, temporary pyrexia and raised white blood cell count, uterine hypertonus, unduly severe uterine contractions; all dose-related and more common after intravenous administration; also local tissue reaction and erythema after intravenous administration
Dose: see under Preparations, below
IMPORTANT. Do not confuse dose of **Prostin E2**® vaginal **gel** with that of **Prostin E2**® vaginal **tablets**—not bioequivalent. In addition, do not confuse **Prostin E2**® vaginal gel with **Prepidil**® cervical gel—different site of administration and different indication—see under Preparations, below.

PoM **Prepidil**® (Upjohn)
Cervical gel, dinoprostone 200 micrograms/mL in disposable syringe. Net price 2.5-mL syringe (500 micrograms) = £14.72
Dose: by cervix, pre-induction cervical softening and dilation, inserted into cervical canal (just below level of internal cervical os), 500 micrograms [single dose gel]

PoM **Prostin E2**® (Upjohn)
Tablets, dinoprostone 500 micrograms. Net price 10-tab pack = £14.93 (hosp. only)
Dose: by mouth, induction of labour, 500 micrograms, followed by 0.5–1 mg (max. 1.5 mg) at hourly intervals
Intravenous solution, for dilution and use as an infusion, dinoprostone 1 mg/mL, net price 0.75-mL amp = £7.43; 10 mg/mL, 0.5-mL amp = £14.93 (both hosp. only; rarely used, see data sheet for dose and indications)
Extra-amniotic solution, dinoprostone 10 mg/mL. Net price 0.5-mL amp (with diluent) = £16.05 (hosp. only; less commonly used nowadays, see data sheet for dose and indications)
Vaginal gel, dinoprostone 400 micrograms/mL, net price 2.5 mL (1 mg) = £14.52; 800 micrograms/mL, 2.5 mL (2 mg) = £16.00
Dose: by vagina, induction of labour, inserted high into posterior fornix (avoid administration into cervical canal), 1 mg (unfavourable primigravida 2 mg), followed after 6 hours by 1–2 mg if required; max. [gel] 3 mg (unfavourable primigravida 4 mg)
Vaginal tablets, dinoprostone 3 mg. Net price 8-vaginal tab pack = £65.04
Dose: by vagina, induction of labour, inserted high into posterior fornix, 3 mg, followed after 6–8 hours by 3 mg if labour is not established; max. 6 mg [vaginal tablets]
Note. Prostin E2 Vaginal Gel and Vaginal Tablets are **not** bioequivalent

DINOPROST
Indications: see notes above
Cautions; Contra-indications; Side-effects: see under Dinoprostone and notes above

PoM **Prostin F2 alpha**® (Upjohn)
Intra-amniotic injection, dinoprost 5 mg (as trometamol salt)/mL. Net price 4-mL amp = £19.71 (hosp. only; rarely used, see data sheet for dose and indications)

ERGOMETRINE MALEATE
Indications: see notes above
Cautions: toxaemia, cardiac disease, hypertension, sepsis, multiple pregnancy; porphyria (see section 9.8.2)
Contra-indications: 1st and 2nd stages of labour, vascular disease, impaired pulmonary, hepatic, and renal function
Side-effects: nausea, vomiting, transient hypertension, vasoconstriction
Dose: by intramuscular injection, 200–500 micrograms (onset about 5–7 minutes, duration about 45 minutes)
By intravenous injection for emergency control of haemorrhage, 100–500 micrograms (onset about 1 minute)
See also notes above

PoM **Ergometrine Injection,** ergometrine maleate 500 micrograms/mL. Net price 1-mL amp = 29p

With oxytocin, see Syntometrine®, p. 286

GEMEPROST
Indications: see under Dose
Cautions: obstructive airways disease, cardiovascular insufficiency, raised intra-ocular pressure, cervicitis or vaginitis
Side-effects: vaginal bleeding and uterine pain; nausea, vomiting, or diarrhoea; headache, muscle weakness, dizziness, flushing, chills, backache, dyspnoea, chest pain, palpitations and mild pyrexia; uterine rupture reported (most commonly in multiparas or if history of uterine surgery)
Dose: by vagina in pessaries, softening and dilation of the cervix to facilitate transcervical operative procedures in first trimester, inserted into posterior fornix, 1 mg 3 hours before surgery
Second trimester abortion, inserted into posterior fornix, 1 mg every 3 hours for max. of 5 administrations; second course may begin 24 hours after start of treatment
Second trimester intra-uterine death, inserted into posterior fornix, 1 mg every 3 hours for max. of 5 administrations only; monitor for coagulopathy

PoM **Cervagem**® (Farillon)
Pessaries, gemeprost 1 mg. Net price 1 pessary = £20.96

OXYTOCIN
Indications: see under Dose and notes above
Cautions: hypertension, pressor drugs (may precipitate severe hypertension), multiple pregnancy, high parity, previous Caesarean section
Contra-indications: hypertonic uterine action, mechanical obstruction to delivery, failed trial labour, severe toxaemia, predisposition to amniotic fluid embolism, fetal distress, and placenta praevia
Side-effects: high doses cause violent uterine contractions leading to rupture and fetal asphyxiation, arrhythmias, maternal hypertension and subarachnoid haemorrhage, water intoxication
Dose: *by slow intravenous infusion*, induction of labour and augmentation of labour in hypotonic uterine inertia, as a solution containing 1 unit per litre, 1–3 milliunits per minute, adjusted according to response
Missed abortion, as a solution containing 10–20 units/500 mL given at a rate of 10–30 drops/minute, increased in strength by 10–20 units/500 mL every hour to a max. strength of 100 units/500 mL

PoM **Syntocinon**® (Sandoz)
Injection, oxytocin 1 unit/mL, net price 2-mL amp = 18p; 5 units/mL, 1-mL amp = 20p; 10 units/mL, 1-mL amp = 23p, 5-mL amp = 84p

With ergometrine
PoM **Syntometrine**® (Sandoz)
Injection, ergometrine maleate 500 micrograms, oxytocin 5 units/mL. Net price 1-mL amp = 19p
Dose: by intramuscular injection, 1 mL; by intravenous injection, 0.5–1 mL

7.1.1.1 DUCTUS ARTERIOSUS

MAINTENANCE OF PATENCY
Alprostadil (prostaglandin E₁) is used to maintain patency of the ductus arteriosus in neonates with congenital heart defects, prior to corrective surgery in centres where intensive care is immediately available.

ALPROSTADIL
Indications: congenital heart defects in neonates prior to corrective surgery
Cautions: see notes above; history of haemorrhage, avoid in hyaline membrane disease, monitor arterial pressure
Side-effects: apnoea (particularly in infants under 2 kg), flushing, bradycardia, hypotension, tachycardia, cardiac arrest, oedema, diarrhoea, fever, convulsions, disseminated intravascular coagulation, hypokalaemia; cortical proliferation of long bones, weakening of the wall of the ductus arteriosus and pulmonary artery may follow prolonged use
Dose: *by intravenous infusion,* initially 50–100 nanograms/kg/minute, then decreased to lowest effective dose

PoM **Prostin VR**® (Upjohn)
Intravenous solution, alprostadil 500 micrograms/mL in alcohol. For dilution and use as an infusion. Net price 1-mL amp = £56.96 (hosp. only)

CLOSURE OF DUCTUS ARTERIOSUS
Prostaglandin E₁ has the role of dilating the ductus arteriosus; indomethacin is believed to close it by inhibiting prostaglandin synthesis.

INDOMETHACIN
Indications: patent ductus arteriosus in premature infants (under specialist supervision)
Cautions: may mask symptoms of infection; may reduce renal function by 50% or more and precipitate renal insufficiency especially in infants with heart failure, sepsis, or hepatic impairment, or who are receiving nephrotoxic drugs; if urine volume reduced, discontinue until output returns to normal; may induce hyponatraemia; monitor renal function and electrolytes
Contra-indications: untreated infection, bleeding, congenital heart disease where patency of ductus arteriosus necessary for satisfactory pulmonary or systemic blood flow; thrombocytopenia, coagulation defects, necrotising enterocolitis, renal impairment
Side-effects: include haemorrhagic, renal, gastrointestinal, metabolic, and coagulation disorders; fluid retention, and exacerbation of infection
Dose: *by intravenous injection,* over 5–10 seconds, 3 doses at intervals of 12–24 hours, age less than 48 hours, 200 micrograms/kg then 100 micrograms/kg then 100 micrograms/kg; age 2–7 days, 200 micrograms/kg then 200 micrograms/kg then 200 micrograms/kg; age over 7 days, 200 micrograms/kg then 250 micrograms/kg then 250 micrograms/kg; solution prepared with 1–2 mL sodium chloride 0.9% or water for injections (not glucose and no preservatives)
If ductus arteriosus reopens a second course of 3 injections may be given

PoM **Indocid PDA**® (Morson)
Injection, powder for reconstitution, indomethacin (as sodium trihydrate). Net price 3 × 1-mg vials = £22.50 (hosp. only)

7.1.2 Mifepristone

MIFEPRISTONE
Indications: medical alternative to surgical termination of intra-uterine pregnancy of up to 63 days gestation (based on first day of last menstrual period and/or ultrasound scan)
Cautions: asthma, chronic obstructive airways disease; cardiovascular disease or risk factors; prosthetic heart valves or history of infective endocarditis (prophylaxis recommended, see section 5.1 table 2); not recommended in hepatic or renal impairment; avoid aspirin and NSAIDs for at least 8–12 days after mifepristone administration
Contra-indications: pregnancy of 64 days gestation and over, suspected ectopic pregnancy; chronic adrenal failure, long-term corticosteroid therapy, haemorrhagic disorders and anticoagulant therapy; women over 35 years, moderate or heavy smokers (smoking and alcohol must be avoided after taking and for at least 2 days after the gemeprost pessary); porphyria (see section 9.8.2)

Side-effects: vaginal bleeding (may be severe), malaise, faintness, nausea, vomiting, rashes; uterine pain after gemeprost (may be severe and require parenteral opioids); uterine and urinary-tract infections reported

Dose: by mouth, 600 mg in a single dose in presence of doctor and observed for at least 2 hours after administration; followed 36–48 hours later (unless abortion already complete) by gemeprost 1 mg *by vagina* as pessaries, observed for at least 6 hours after insertion with follow-up visit 8–12 days later (if treatment fails essential that pregnancy be terminated by another method)

Note. Careful monitoring essential for 6 hours after administration of gemeprost pessary (risk of profound hypotension)

▼ PoM **Mifegyne**® (Roussel)
Tablets, yellow, mifepristone 200 mg. Net price 3-tab pack = £42.90 (supplied to NHS hospitals and premises approved under Abortion Act 1967). Label: 10 patient information leaflet

7.1.3 Myometrial relaxants

Beta$_2$-adrenoceptor stimulants (sympathomimetics) relax uterine muscle and are used in selected cases in an attempt to inhibit *premature labour.*

They should not be used unless a clear benefit is likely. Tachycardia is the commonest side-effect and may be extreme if atropine is also administered.

ISOXSUPRINE HYDROCHLORIDE

Indications: uncomplicated premature labour
Cautions: may cause hypotension in the newborn; see notes above
Contra-indications: recent arterial haemorrhage, heart disease, premature detachment of placenta, severe anaemia, infection
Side-effects: hypotension, tachycardia, flushing, nausea, vomiting
Dose: by intravenous infusion, initially 200–300 micrograms/minute gradually increased to 500 micrograms/minute until labour is arrested; subsequently *by intramuscular injection,* 10 mg every 3 hours for 24 hours, then every 4–6 hours for 48 hours

PoM **Duvadilan**® (Duphar)
Injection, isoxsuprine hydrochloride 5 mg/mL. Net price 2-mL amp = 35p

RITODRINE HYDROCHLORIDE

Indications: uncomplicated premature labour; fetal asphyxia due to hypertonic uterine action
Cautions: diabetes mellitus (monitor blood sugar during intravenous treatment), cardiac disorders, thyrotoxicosis, treatment with corticosteroids, anaesthetics, potassium-depleting diuretics (depresses potassium plasma concentrations); monitor blood pressure and pulse; **interactions:** Appendix 1 (sympathomimetics, beta$_2$)

Contra-indications: haemorrhage, hypertension, pre-eclampsia, cord compression, infection
Side-effects: nausea, vomiting, flushing, sweating, tremor; hypokalaemia, tachycardia and hypotension with high doses
Dose: by intravenous infusion, premature labour, initially 50 micrograms/minute, gradually increased to 150–350 micrograms/minute and continued for 12–48 hours after contractions have ceased; or *by intramuscular injection,* 10 mg every 3–8 hours continued for 12–48 hours after contractions have ceased; then *by mouth,* 10 mg 30 minutes before termination of intravenous infusion, repeated every 2 hours for 24 hours, followed by 10–20 mg every 4–6 hours, max. 120 mg daily

Fetal asphyxia due to hypertonic uterine action, *by intravenous infusion,* 50 micrograms/minute increased as necessary to a max. of 350 micrograms/minute, while preparations are made for delivery

PoM **Yutopar**® (Duphar)
Tablets, buff, scored, ritodrine hydrochloride 10 mg. Net price 90-tab pack = £19.80
Injection, ritodrine hydrochloride 10 mg/mL. Net price 5-mL amp = £2.15

SALBUTAMOL

Indications: uncomplicated premature labour
Cautions; Contra-indications; Side-effects: see under Ritodrine Hydrochloride
Dose: by intravenous infusion, 10 micrograms/minute gradually increased to max. of 45 micrograms/minute until contractions have ceased, then gradually reduced; or *by intravenous or intramuscular injection,* 100–250 micrograms repeated according to patient's response; subsequently *by mouth* 4 mg every 6–8 hours

Preparations: see section 3.1.1.1

TERBUTALINE SULPHATE

Indications: uncomplicated premature labour
Cautions; Contra-indications; Side-effects: see under Ritodrine Hydrochloride
Dose: by intravenous infusion, 10 micrograms/minute (as a 0.0005% solution) for 1 hour, gradually increased to a max. of 25 micrograms/minute until contractions have ceased, then reduced; subsequently *by subcutaneous injection,* 250 micrograms every 6 hours for 3 days, and *by mouth,* 5 mg every 8 hours until 37th week of pregnancy

Preparations: see section 3.1.1.1

7.2 Treatment of vaginal and vulval conditions

7.2.1 Topical hormones
7.2.2 Anti-infective drugs

Symptoms are primarily referable to the vulva, but infections almost invariably involve the vagina which should also be treated. Applications to the vulva alone are likely to give only symptomatic relief without cure.

Aqueous medicated douches may disturb normal vaginal acidity and bacterial flora.

Topical anaesthetic agents give only symptomatic relief and may cause sensitivity reactions. They are indicated only in cases of pruritus where specific local causes have been excluded.

Systemic drugs are required in the treatment of infections such as gonorrhoea and syphilis (see section 5.1).

7.2.1 Topical hormones

Application of cream containing an oestrogen may be used on a short-term basis to improve the quality of the vaginal epithelium in menopausal atrophic vaginitis. For further comment see section 6.4.1.1.

Topical oestrogens are also used prior to vaginal surgery in postmenopausal women for prolapse when there is epithelial atrophy.

> Topical oestrogens should be used in the minimum effective amount and treatment discontinued as soon as possible to minimise absorption of the oestrogen.

OESTROGENS, TOPICAL

Indications: see notes above
Cautions; Contra-indications; Side-effects: see Ethinyloestradiol (section 6.4.1.1); contra-indicated in pregnancy and lactation; discontinue treatment and examine patients periodically to assess need for further treatment

PoM Ortho® Dienoestrol (Cilag)
Cream, dienoestrol 0.01%. Net price 78 g with applicator = £2.61
Condoms: damages latex condoms and diaphragms
Insert 1–2 applicatorfuls daily for 1–2 weeks, then gradually reduced to 1 applicatorful 1–3 times weekly if necessary; attempts to reduce or discontinue should be made at 3–6 month intervals with re-examination

PoM Ortho-Gynest® (Cilag)
Intravaginal cream, oestriol 0.01%. Net price 78 g with applicator = £5.40
Condoms: damages latex condoms and diaphragms
Insert 1 applicatorful daily, preferably in evening; reduced to 1 applicatorful twice a week; attempts to reduce or discontinue should be made at 3–6 month intervals with re-examination
Pessaries, oestriol 500 micrograms. Net price 15 pessaries = £5.29
Condoms: damages latex condoms and diaphragms
Insert 1 pessary daily, preferably in the evening, until improvement occurs; maintenance 1 pessary twice a week; attempts to reduce or discontinue should be made at 3–6 month intervals with re-examination

PoM Ovestin® (Organon)
Intravaginal cream, oestriol 0.1%. Net price 15 g with applicator = £4.74
Condoms: effect on latex condoms and diaphragms not yet known
Insert 1 applicator-dose daily for 2–3 weeks, then reduce to twice a week (discontinue every 2–3 months for 4 weeks to assess need for further treatment); post-menopausal surgery, 1 applicator-dose daily for 2 weeks, resuming 2 weeks after surgery

PoM Premarin® (Wyeth)
Vaginal cream, conjugated oestrogens 625 micrograms/g. Net price 42.5 g with calibrated applicator = £2.19
Condoms: effect on latex condoms and diaphragms not yet known
Insert 1–2 g daily, starting on 5th day of cycle, for 3 weeks, followed by 1-week interval; if therapy long term, oral progestogen for 10–12 days at end of each cycle essential

PoM Tampovagan® Stilboestrol and Lactic Acid (Norgine)
Pessaries, stilboestrol 500 micrograms, lactic acid 5%. Net price 10 pessaries = £8.28
Condoms: no evidence of damage to latex condoms and diaphragms
Insert 2 pessaries at night for 1–2 weeks then reduce (short-term only, see notes above)

PoM Vagifem® (Novo Nordisk)
Vaginal tablets, f/c, m/r, oestradiol 25 micrograms in disposable applicators. Net price 15-applicator pack = £14.99
Condoms: no evidence of damage to latex condoms and diaphragms
Insert 1 tablet daily for 2 weeks then reduce to 1 tablet twice weekly; discontinue after 3 months to assess need for further treatment

7.2.2 Anti-infective drugs

Effective specific treatments are available for the common vaginal infections.

FUNGAL INFECTIONS

Candidal vulvitis can be treated locally with cream but is almost invariably associated with vaginal infection which should be treated as well. *Vaginal candidiasis* is treated primarily with antifungal pessaries or cream inserted high into the vagina (including the time of menstruation).

Nystatin is a well established treatment. One or two pessaries are inserted for 14 to 28 nights; they may be supplemented with cream for vulvitis and to treat other superficial sites of infection.

Imidazole drugs (clotrimazole, econazole, isoconazole, and miconazole) appear to be equally effective in shorter courses of 3 to 14 days according to the preparation used; single dose preparations are also available, which is an advantage when compliance is a problem. Vaginal applications may be supplemented with cream for vulvitis and to treat other superficial sites of infection.

Recurrence is common if the full course of treatment is not completed and is also particularly likely if there are predisposing factors such as antibiotic therapy, oral contraceptive use, pregnancy, or diabetes mellitus. Possible reservoirs of infection may also lead to recontamination and should be treated. These include other skin sites such as the digits, nail beds, and umbilicus as well as the gut and the bladder. The partner may also be the source of re-infection and should be treated with cream at the same time.

Oral treatment with fluconazole or itraconazole may be necessary in resistant or recurrent infection (see section 5.2); oral ketoconazole has been associated with fatal hepatotoxicity (see section 5.2 for CSM warning).

7.2 Treatment of vaginal and vulval conditions

Preparations for vaginal and vulval candidiasis

Canesten® (Baypharm)
Cream (topical), clotrimazole 1%. Net price 20 g = £1.82; 50 g = £4.26
Condoms: effect on latex condoms and diaphragms not yet known
Apply to anogenital area 2–3 times daily
PoM[1] *Vaginal cream*, clotrimazole 2%. Net price 35 g (with 5-g applicators) = £5.22
Condoms: effect on latex condoms and diaphragms not yet known
Insert 5 g twice daily for 3 days or once nightly for 6 nights
Vaginal cream (10% VC®), clotrimazole 10%. Net price 5-g applicator pack = £3.43
Condoms: effect on latex condoms and diaphragms not yet known
Insert 5 g at night as a single dose
PoM[1] *Vaginal tablets*, clotrimazole 100 mg, net price 6 = £2.64; 200 mg, 3 = £2.58
Insert 200 mg for 3 nights *or* 100 mg for 6 nights
PoM[1] *Vaginal tablets (Canesten 1®)*, clotrimazole 500 mg. Net price 1 with applicator = £2.58
Insert 1 at night as a single dose
PoM[1] *Duopak*, clotrimazole 100-mg vaginal tablets and cream (topical) 1%. Net price 6 tabs and 20 g cream = £4.35
Condoms: effect on latex condoms and diaphragms not yet known

Ecostatin® (Squibb)
Cream (topical), econazole nitrate 1%. Net price 15 g = £1.49; 30 g = £2.75
Condoms: damages latex condoms and diaphragms
Apply to anogenital area twice daily
PoM[1] *Pessaries*, econazole nitrate 150 mg. Net price 3 with applicator = £3.96
Condoms: damages latex condoms and diaphragms
Insert 1 pessary for 3 nights
PoM[1] *Pessary (Ecostatin 1®)*, econazole nitrate 150 mg, formulated for single-dose therapy. Net price 1 pessary with applicator = £4.40
Condoms: damages latex condoms and diaphragms
Insert 1 pessary at night as a single dose
PoM[1] *Twinpack*, econazole nitrate 150-mg pessaries and cream 1%. Net price 3 pessaries and 15 g cream = £4.98
Condoms: damages latex condoms and diaphragms

PoM[1] Gyno-Daktarin® (Janssen)
Intravaginal cream, miconazole nitrate 2%. Net price 78 g with applicators = £4.95
Condoms: damages latex condoms and diaphragms
Insert 5-g applicatorful twice daily for 7 days; *topical*, apply to anogenital area twice daily
Pessaries, miconazole nitrate 100 mg. Net price 14 = £4.04
Condoms: damages latex condoms and diaphragms
Insert 1 pessary twice daily for 7 days
Tampons, coated with miconazole nitrate 100 mg. Net price 10 = £3.83
Condoms: damages latex condoms and diaphragms
Insert 1 tampon night and morning for 5 days
Combipack, miconazole nitrate 100-mg pessaries and cream (topical) 2%. Net price 14 pessaries and 15 g cream = £5.94
Condoms: damages latex condoms and diaphragms
Ovule (Gyno-Daktarin 1®), miconazole nitrate 1.2 g in a fatty basis. Net price 1 = £3.95
Condoms: damages latex condoms and diaphragms
Insert 1 ovule at night as a single dose
Note. On sale to public as *Femeron*

PoM[1] Gyno-Pevaryl® (Cilag)
Cream, econazole nitrate 1%. Net price 15 g = £1.74; 30 g = £3.45
Condoms: no evidence of damage to latex condoms and diaphragms
Apply to anogenital area 2–3 times daily for 14 days
Pessaries, econazole nitrate 150 mg. Net price 3 pessaries = £3.17
Condoms: damages latex condoms and diaphragms
Insert 1 pessary for 3 nights
Pessary (Gyno-Pevaryl 1®), econazole nitrate 150 mg, formulated for single-dose therapy. Net price 1 pessary with applicator = £4.40
Condoms: damages latex condoms and diaphragms
Insert 1 pessary at night as a single dose
Combipack, econazole nitrate 150-mg pessaries, econazole nitrate 1% cream (to be applied to anogenital area). Net price 3 pessaries and 15 g cream = £4.98
Condoms: damages latex condoms and diaphragms
CP pack (Gyno-Pevaryl 1®), econazole nitrate 150-mg pessary, econazole nitrate 1% cream (to be applied to anogenital area). Net price 1 pessary and 15 g cream = £5.84
Condoms: damages latex condoms and diaphragms

PoM Nizoral® (Janssen)
Cream (topical), ketoconazole 2%. Net price 30 g = £3.81
Apply to anogenital area once or twice daily

PoM Nystan® (Squibb)
Gel (topical), nystatin 100 000 units/g. Net price 30 g = £2.66
Condoms: no evidence of damage to latex condoms and diaphragms
Apply to anogenital area 2–4 times daily
Vaginal cream, nystatin 100 000 units/4-g application. Net price 60 g with applicator = £3.26
Condoms: damages latex condoms and diaphragms
Insert 1–2 applicatorfuls at night for at least 14 nights
Pessaries, yellow, nystatin 100 000 units. Net price 28-pessary pack = £1.96
Condoms: no evidence of damage to latex condoms and diaphragms
Insert 1–2 pessaries at night for at least 14 nights

Pevaryl® (Cilag)
Cream, econazole nitrate 1%. Net price 30 g = £2.65
Condoms: effect on latex condoms and diaphragms not yet known
Apply to anogenital area 2–3 times daily

PoM[1] Travogyn® (Schering Health Care)
Vaginal tablets (=pessaries), isoconazole nitrate 300 mg. Net price 2 = £3.90
Condoms: effect on latex condoms and diaphragms not yet known
Insert 2 pessaries as a single dose at night

---

1. Can be sold to the public for the treatment of *vaginal candidiasis*. Until packs labelled '**P**' are available, those labelled '**PoM**' can be sold providing the pharmacist deletes **PoM** from the pack and substitutes a capital **P** and provides *each purchaser* with a copy of the **patient information leaflet** supplied by the Royal Pharmaceutical Society of Great Britain.

OTHER INFECTIONS

Vaginal preparations intended to restore normal acidity (Aci-Jel®) may prevent recurrence of vaginal infections and permit the re-establishment of the normal vaginal flora.

Trichomonal infections commonly involve the lower urinary tract as well as the genital system and need systemic treatment with metronidazole, nimorazole, or tinidazole (see sections 5.4.2 and 5.4.3).

Bacterial infections with Gram-negative organisms are particularly common in association with gynaecological operations and trauma. Metronidazole is effective against certain Gram-negative organisms, especially *Bacteroides* spp. and may be used prophylactically in gynaecological surgery.

Antibacterial creams such as Sultrin® are used in the treatment of mixed bacterial infections but are of unproven value; they are ineffective against *Candida* spp. and *Trichomonas vaginalis*.

Acyclovir may be used in the treatment of genital infection due to *herpes simplex virus*, the HSV type 2 being a major cause of genital ulceration. It has a beneficial effect on virus shedding and healing, generally giving relief from pain and other symptoms. See section 5.3 for systemic preparations, and section 13.10.3 for cream.

Preparations for other vaginal infections

Aci-Jel® (Cilag)
Vaginal jelly, acetic acid 0.92% in a buffered (pH 4) basis. Net price 85 g with applicator = £3.37
Condoms: no evidence of damage to latex condoms and diaphragms

Non-specific infections, insert 1 applicatorful twice daily to restore vaginal acidity

Betadine® (Napp)
Caution: avoid in pregnancy (and if planned) in and breast-feeding; renal impairment (see appendix 3)
Side-effects: rarely sensitivity; may interfere with thyroid function

Vaginal Cleansing Kit, solution, povidone-iodine 10%. Net price 250 mL = £2.78
Condoms: no evidence of damage to latex condoms and diaphragms

To be diluted and used once daily, preferably in the morning; may be used with Betadine® pessaries or vaginal gel

Pessaries, brown, povidone-iodine 200 mg. Net price 28 pessaries with applicator = £5.11
Condoms: no evidence of damage to latex condoms and diaphragms

Vaginal gel, brown, povidone-iodine 10%. Net price 80 g with applicator = £2.33
Condoms: no evidence of damage to latex condoms and diaphragms

Vaginal infections or pre-operatively, insert 1 moistened pessary night and morning for up to 14 days *or* use morning pessary with 5-g gel at night *or* morning douche with pessary (or 5-g gel) at night

PoM **Sultrin®** (Cilag)
Indications: bacterial vaginitis and cervicitis
Contra-indications: pregnancy
Side-effects: sensitivity

Cream, sulphathiazole 3.42%, sulphacetamide 2.86%, sulphabenzamide 3.7%. Net price 78 g with applicator = £3.48
Condoms: damages latex condoms and diaphragms

Vaginal tablets, sulphathiazole 172.5 mg, sulphacetamide 143.75 mg, sulphabenzamide 184 mg. Net price 20 with applicator = £2.94
Condoms: effect on latex condoms and diaphragms not yet known

Insert 1 pessary or applicatorful of cream twice daily for 10 days, then once daily if necessary

7.3 Contraceptives

The criteria by which contraceptive methods should be judged are effectiveness, acceptability, and freedom from side-effects.

Hormonal contraception is the most effective method of fertility control, short of sterilisation, but has unwanted major and minor side-effects, especially for certain groups of women.

Intra-uterine devices have a high use-effectiveness but may produce undesirable side-effects, especially menorrhagia, or be otherwise unsuitable in a significant proportion of women; their use is generally inadvisable in nulliparous women because of the increased risk of pelvic sepsis and infertility.

Barrier methods alone (condoms, diaphragms, and caps) are less effective but can be very reliable for well-motivated couples if used in conjunction with a **spermicide**. Occasionally sensitivity reactions occur.

7.3.1 Combined oral contraceptives

Oral contraceptives containing an oestrogen and a progestogen are the most effective preparations for general use. The oestrogen content ranges from 20 to 50 micrograms and generally a preparation with the lowest oestrogen and progestogen content which gives good cycle control and minimal side-effects in the individual patient is chosen.

DOSAGE. The dosage regimen for *combined oral contraceptives* is usually 1 tablet daily for 21 days, followed by a 7-day interval during which withdrawal bleeding occurs. Additional contraceptive precautions are unnecessary in the first cycle if the tablets are started on the first day of the menses as is now usually recommended. If the first course is started on the 5th day of the cycle ovulation may not be inhibited during that cycle and additional contraceptive precautions should therefore be taken during the first 7 days[1] or when changing from a high to a low oestrogen preparation.

The tablet should be taken at approximately the same time each day. If it is delayed by longer than 12 hours, contraceptive protection may be lost.

1. Formerly 14 days but family planning organisations now consider 7 days to be enough.

CAUTIONS. Combined oral contraceptives carry a small risk of thrombo-embolic and cardiovascular complications. This increases with age, obesity, and cigarette smoking, and with predisposing conditions such as diabetes, hypertension, and familial hyperlipidaemia.

Hypertension may develop as the result of therapy but when it is due to contraceptive usage reversion to normotension occurs on cessation of treatment.

Critical factors which limit effectiveness are vomiting, severe diarrhoea, and some drug interactions (see below).

INTERACTIONS. The effectiveness of both *combined* and *progestogen-only* oral contraceptives may be considerably reduced by interaction with drugs that induce hepatic enzyme activity (e.g. **carbamazepine, griseofulvin, phenytoin, phenobarbitone, primidone**, and, above all, **rifampicin**).

FPA advice relating to a *short-term course of an enzyme-inducing drug* is that additional contraceptive precautions should be taken whilst taking the enzyme-inducing drug and for at least 7 days after stopping it; if these 7 days run beyond the end of a packet the new packet should be started immediately without a break (in the case of ED tablets the inactive ones should be omitted). **Important**: it should be noted that **rifampicin** is such a potent enzyme-inducing drug that even if a course lasts for less than 7 days the additional contraceptive precautions should be continued for at least 4 weeks after stopping it.

FPA advice relating to a *long-term course of an enzyme-inducing drug* in a woman unable to use an alternative method of contraception is to take an oral contraceptive containing ethinyloestradiol 50 micrograms or more; 'tricycling' with standard ('monophasic') tablets (i.e. taking 3 packets without a break followed by a short tablet-free interval of 4 days) is useful. **Important**: it should be noted that **rifampicin** is such a potent enzyme-inducing drug that an alternative method of contraception (such as an IUD) is **always** recommended. Since the excretory function of the liver does not return to normal for several weeks after stopping an enzyme-inducing drug, FPA advice relating to *withdrawal* is that extra contraceptive measures are required for 4 to 8 weeks after stopping.

In the case of *combined* oral contraceptives some **broad-spectrum antibiotics** (e.g. ampicillin) may interfere with oestrogen absorption. FPA advice is that additional contraceptive precautions should be taken whilst taking a *short course of a broad-spectrum antibiotic* and for 7 days after stopping. If these 7 days run beyond the end of a packet the next packet should be started immediately without a break (in the case of ED tablets the inactive ones should be omitted). If the course *exceeds 2 weeks*, resistance to this interference develops, and additional precautions become unnecessary.

SURGERY. Oestrogen-containing oral contraceptives should be discontinued (and adequate alternative contraceptive arrangements made) 4 weeks before major elective surgery and all surgery to the legs; they should normally be recommenced at the first menses occurring at least 2 weeks after the procedure. When discontinuation is not possible, e.g. after trauma or if, by oversight, a patient admitted for an elective procedure is still on an oestrogen-containing oral contraceptive, some consideration should be given to subcutaneous heparin prophylaxis. These recommendations do not apply to minor surgery with short duration of anaesthesia, e.g. laparoscopic sterilisation or tooth extraction, or to women taking oestrogen-free hormonal contraceptives.

For hormone replacement therapy the evidence of an increased risk is questionable, which suggests that it need not normally be stopped before major elective surgery (particularly as heparin prophylaxis is usual in this age group). For reference to supraphysiological concentrations of oestradiol implants see section 6.4.1.

MISSED PILL. It is important to bear in mind that the critical time for loss of protection is when a pill is forgotten at the *beginning* or *end* of a cycle. The following advice is now recommended by family planning organisations:

'If you forget a pill, take it as soon as you remember, and the next one at your normal time. If you are 12 or more hours late with any pill (especially the first or last in the packet) the pill may not work. As soon as you remember, continue normal pill taking. However, you will not be protected for the next seven days and must either not have sex or use another method such as the sheath. If these seven days run beyond the end of your packet, start the next packet at once when you have finished the present one, i.e. do not have a gap between packets. This will mean you may not have a period until the end of two packets but this does you no harm. Nor does it matter if you see some bleeding on tablet-taking days. If you are using everyday (ED) pills—miss out the seven inactive pills. If you are not sure which these are, ask your doctor.'

CHILDBIRTH. Following childbirth oral contraception can be started at any time after 3 to 4 weeks postpartum (not earlier because of the increased risk of thrombosis in relation to the combined pill, and of breakthrough bleeding in relation to the progestogen-only pill). If they are started later than 4 weeks postpartum extra contraceptive precautions should be taken for first 7 days. Lactation may be affected by combined oral contraceptives as described in Appendix 5.

ORAL CONTRACEPTIVES (Combined)

Indications: contraception; menstrual symptoms, see section 6.4.1.2

Cautions: see notes above; diabetes, hypertension, cardiac or renal disease, migraine, epilepsy, depression, asthma, immobilisation, contact lenses (may irritate), varicose veins; cigarette-smokers, (particularly those over 35 years) obesity, breast-feeding, sickle-cell anaemia (safety not established); **interactions:** Appendix 1 (contraceptives, oral)

Contra-indications: pregnancy; thrombosis and history of any thrombo-embolic disease, after evacuation of hydatidiform mole (until return to normal of urine and plasma gonadotrophin values); recurrent jaundice, acute and chronic liver disease, porphyria (see section 9.8.2), Dubin-Johnson and Rotor syndromes, hyperlipidaemia, mammary, endometrial or hepatic carcinoma, severe or focal migraine, undiagnosed vaginal bleeding, history of pruritus of pregnancy or herpes gestationis, deterioration of otosclerosis

Side-effects: nausea, vomiting, headache, breast tenderness, changes in body weight, thrombosis (more common in blood groups A, B, and AB than O), changes in libido, depression, chloasma, hypertension, impairment of liver function, hepatic tumours, reduced menstrual loss, 'spotting' in early cycles, amenorrhoea; rarely photosensitivity

Dose: see notes above

Ethinyloestradiol 20 micrograms

Mercilon® has been reported to give much better cycle control than Loestrin 20®. It is one of the options for any woman proposing to take an oral contraceptive, and is particularly appropriate for obese patients and for older women (provided oral contraceptive use otherwise suitable).

PoM **Loestrin 20**® (P-D)
Tablets, blue-grey, f/c, norethisterone acetate 1 mg, ethinyloestradiol 20 micrograms. Net price 3 × 21-tab pack = £2.58

PoM **Mercilon**® (Organon)
Tablets, desogestrel 150 micrograms, ethinyloestradiol 20 micrograms. Net price 3 × 21-tab pack = £7.20

Ethinyloestradiol 30 micrograms

Standard strength from which the initial choice is usually selected. Highly effective if the pill-free interval is not lengthened by dose omissions. Of these, Conova 30®, Eugynon 30®, and Ovran 30® are not good first choices since the others have less of the apparently unfavourable effects on plasma lipids.

PoM **Conova 30**® (Gold Cross)
Tablets, f/c, ethynodiol diacetate 2 mg, ethinyloestradiol 30 micrograms. Net price 21-tab pack = 80p

PoM **Eugynon 30**® (Schering Health Care)
Tablets, s/c, levonorgestrel 250 micrograms, ethinyloestradiol 30 micrograms. Net price 21-tab pack = 69p

PoM **Femodene**® (Schering Health Care)
Tablets, s/c, gestodene 75 micrograms, ethinyloestradiol 30 micrograms. Net price 3 × 21-tab pack = £5.70

PoM **Femodene ED**® (Schering Health Care)
As for Femodene and in addition 7 white placebo tablets. Net price 3 × 28-tab pack = £5.70

PoM **Loestrin 30**® (P-D)
Tablets, green, f/c, norethisterone acetate 1.5 mg, ethinyloestradiol 30 micrograms. Net price 3 × 21-tab pack = £3.78

PoM **Marvelon**® (Organon)
Tablets, desogestrel 150 micrograms, ethinyloestradiol 30 micrograms. Net price 3 × 21-tab pack = £4.44

PoM **Microgynon 30**® (Schering Health Care)
Tablets, beige, s/c, levonorgestrel 150 micrograms, ethinyloestradiol 30 micrograms. Net price 21-tab pack = 60p

PoM **Minulet**® (Wyeth)
Tablets, s/c, gestodene 75 micrograms, ethinyloestradiol 30 micrograms. Net price 3 × 21-tab pack = £5.70

PoM **Ovran 30**® (Wyeth)
Tablets, levonorgestrel 250 micrograms, ethinyloestradiol 30 micrograms. Net price 21-tab pack = 57p

PoM **Ovranette**® (Wyeth)
Tablets, levonorgestrel 150 micrograms, ethinyloestradiol 30 micrograms. Net price 21-tab pack = 62p

---

Ethinyloestradiol 35 micrograms

In common with the 30-microgram strength (above), standard strength from which the initial choice is usually selected. Highly effective if the pill-free interval is not lengthened by dose omissions.

PoM **Brevinor**® (Syntex)
Tablets, norethisterone 500 micrograms, ethinyloestradiol 35 micrograms. Net price 3 × 21-tab pack = £1.72

PoM **Cilest**® (Cilag)
Tablets, blue, norgestimate 250 micrograms, ethinyloestradiol 35 micrograms. Net price 3 × 21-tab pack = £5.70

PoM **Neocon 1/35**® (Ortho)
Tablets, peach, norethisterone 1 mg, ethinyloestradiol 35 micrograms. Net price 3 × 21-tab pack = £2.27

PoM **Norimin**® (Syntex)
Tablets, yellow, norethisterone 1 mg, ethinyloestradiol 35 micrograms. Net price 3 × 21-tab pack = £1.95

PoM **Ovysmen**® (Ortho)
Tablets, norethisterone 500 micrograms, ethinyloestradiol 35 micrograms. Net price 3 × 21-tab pack = £1.70

Ethinyloestradiol 50 micrograms

Increased security but possibility of increased side-effects. Used mainly in circumstances of reduced bioavailability (e.g. during long-term use of enzyme-inducing antiepileptics—see FPA advice under Interactions on p. 291).

PoM **Ovran**® (Wyeth)
Tablets, levonorgestrel 250 micrograms, ethinyloestradiol 50 micrograms. Net price 21-tab pack = 37p

7.3 Contraceptives

Mestranol 50 micrograms

In common with the ethinyloestradiol 50-microgram strength (above), increased security but possibility of increased side-effects. Used mainly in circumstances of reduced bioavailability (e.g. during long-term use of enzyme-inducing antiepileptics—see FPA advice under Interactions on p. 291).

PoM **Norinyl-1**® (Syntex)
Tablets, norethisterone 1 mg, mestranol 50 micrograms. Net price 3 × 21-tab pack = £1.88

PoM **Ortho-Novin 1/50**® (Ortho)
Tablets, norethisterone 1 mg, mestranol 50 micrograms. Net price 3 × 21-tab pack = £2.35

Phased formulations

A little more complex for the user to take, but provide better cycle control (with low metabolic effect) than equivalent fixed-dose levonorgestrel or norethisterone formulations.

PoM **BiNovum**® (Ortho)
Tablets, 7 white, norethisterone 500 micrograms, ethinyloestradiol 35 micrograms; 14 peach, norethisterone 1 mg, ethinyloestradiol 35 micrograms. Net price 3 × 21-tab pack = £2.24
Dose: 1 tablet daily for 21 days, starting with a white tablet on 1st day of cycle, and repeated after a 7-day interval

PoM **Logynon**® (Schering Health Care)
Tablets, all s/c, 6 light brown, levonorgestrel 50 micrograms, ethinyloestradiol 30 micrograms; 5 white, levonorgestrel 75 micrograms, ethinyloestradiol 40 micrograms; 10 ochre, levonorgestrel 125 micrograms, ethinyloestradiol 30 micrograms. Net price 21-tab pack = 95p
Dose: 1 tablet daily for 21 days, starting with tablet marked 1 on 1st day of cycle, and repeated after a 7-day interval

PoM **Logynon ED**® (Schering Health Care)
As for Logynon and in addition 7 white placebo tablets. Net price 28-tab pack = 95p
Dose: 1 tablet daily starting in red sector on 1st day of cycle continuing in sequence without interruption

PoM **Synphase**® (Syntex)
Tablets, 7 white, norethisterone 500 micrograms, ethinyloestradiol 35 micrograms; 9 yellow, norethisterone 1 mg, ethinyloestradiol 35 micrograms; 5 white, norethisterone 500 micrograms, ethinyloestradiol 35 micrograms. Net price 21-tab pack = £1.11
Dose: 1 tablet daily for 21 days, starting with tablet marked 1 on the 5th day of the cycle, and repeated after a 7-day interval

PoM **Triadene**® (Schering Health Care)
Tablets, all s/c, 6 beige, gestodene 50 micrograms, ethinyloestradiol 30 micrograms; 5 dark brown, gestodene 70 micrograms, ethinyloestradiol 40 micrograms; 10 white, gestodene 100 micrograms, ethinyloestradiol 30 micrograms. Net price 3 × 21-tab pack = £7.95
Dose: 1 tablet daily for 21 days, starting with tablet marked 'start' on 1st day of cycle, and repeated after 7-day interval

PoM **Tri-Minulet**® (Wyeth)
Tablets, s/c, 6 beige, gestodene 50 micrograms, ethinyloestradiol 30 micrograms; 5 dark brown, gestodene 70 micrograms, ethinyloestradiol 40 micrograms; 10 white, gestodene 100 micrograms, ethinyloestradiol 30 micrograms. Net price 3 × 21-tab pack = £7.95
Dose: 1 tablet daily for 21 days, starting with tablet marked 1 on the 1st day of the cycle, and repeated after a 7-day interval

PoM **Trinordiol**® (Wyeth)
Tablets, all s/c, 6 light brown, levonorgestrel 50 micrograms, ethinyloestradiol 30 micrograms; 5 white, levonorgestrel 75 micrograms, ethinyloestradiol 40 micrograms; 10 ochre, levonorgestrel 125 micrograms, ethinyloestradiol 30 micrograms. Net price 3 × 21-tab pack = £3.28
Dose: 1 tablet daily for 21 days, starting with tablet marked 1 on 1st day of cycle, and repeated after a 7-day interval

PoM **TriNovum**® (Ortho)
Tablets, 7 white, norethisterone 500 micrograms, ethinyloestradiol 35 micrograms; 7 light peach, norethisterone 750 micrograms, ethinyloestradiol 35 micrograms; 7 peach, norethisterone 1 mg, ethinyloestradiol 35 micrograms. Net price 3 × 21-tab pack = £2.83
Dose: 1 tablet daily for 21 days, starting with a white tablet on 1st day of cycle, and repeated after a 7-day interval

PoM **TriNovum ED**® (Ortho)
As for TriNovum and in addition 7 green placebo tablets. Net price 3 × 28-tab pack = £2.97
Dose: 1 tablet daily starting in the white sector on 1st day of cycle continuing in sequence without interruption

Emergency contraception

Combined oral contraceptives may also be given for occasional emergency use after unprotected intercourse. Two tablets of a preparation containing levonorgestrel 250 micrograms and ethinyloestradiol 50 micrograms ([1]Schering PC4®) are taken within 72 hours, and a further 2 tablets 12 hours later. The patient should be counselled on administration and should always consult her doctor approximately 3 weeks after using this treatment.

PoM **Schering PC4**® (Schering Health Care)
Tablets, s/c, levonorgestrel 250 micrograms, ethinyloestradiol 50 micrograms. Net price 4-tab pack = £1.40. For post-coital contraception as an occasional emergency measure; should not be administered if menstrual bleeding overdue or if unprotected intercourse occurred more than 72 hours previously
Dose: 2 tablets as soon as possible after coitus (up to 72 hours) then 2 tablets after 12 hours

1. **Ovran**® (see p. 292) also contains levonorgestrel 250 micrograms and ethinyloestradiol 50 micrograms but is not licensed or packed for post-coital contraception.

7.3.2 Progestogen-only contraceptives

When oestrogens are contra-indicated, progestogen-only preparations may offer a suitable alternative but the oral preparations have a higher failure rate than combined preparations. They are suitable for older patients who may be at risk from oestrogen, heavy smokers, and those in whom oestrogens cause severe side-effects. Menstrual irregularities (oligomenorrhoea, menorrhagia) are more common but patients tend to revert to a more regular cyclical menstrual pattern on long treatment. Oral preparations are started on the 1st day of the cycle and taken every day at the same time without a break. Additional contraceptive precautions are unnecessary when initiating treatment with progestogen-only contraceptives. When changing from a combined oral contraceptive to a progestogen-only preparation treatment should start on the day following completion of the combined oral contraceptive course so that there is no break in tablet taking.

The tablet should be taken at the same time each day. If it is delayed by longer than 3 hours, contraceptive protection may be lost.

MISSED PILL. The following advice is now recommended by family planning organisations:

'If you forget a pill, take it as soon as you remember and carry on with the next pill at the right time. If the pill was more than three hours overdue you are not protected. Continue normal pill-taking but you must also use another method, such as the sheath, for the next 7 days[1]. If you have vomiting or very severe diarrhoea the pill may not work. Continue to take it, but you may not be protected from the first day of vomiting or diarrhoea. Use another method, such as the sheath, for any intercourse during the stomach upset and for the next 7 days[1].'

Medroxyprogesterone acetate (Depo-Provera®) is a long-acting progestogen given by intramuscular injection; it is as effective as the combined oral preparations but should never be given without *full counselling backed by the manufacturer's approved leaflet*. It is useful for short-term interim contraception, for example, before vasectomy becomes effective. It may also be used as a long-term contraceptive for women who are unable to use any other method, after counselling on the long and short-term effects. Transient infertility and irregular cycles may occur after discontinuation of treatment. Heavy bleeding has been reported in patients given medroxyprogesterone acetate in the immediate puerperium (the first dose is best delayed until 6 to 7 weeks postpartum). **Norethisterone enanthate** (Noristerat®) is a long-acting progestogen given as an oily injection which provides contraception for 8 weeks.

Progestogen-only preparations can be administered in the early puerperium without adverse effects (except increased bleeding); lactation is not affected.

---

1. Family planning organisations formerly recommended 48 hours

PROGESTOGEN-ONLY CONTRACEPTIVES

Indications: contraception

Cautions: diabetes, hypertension, heart disease, past ectopic pregnancy (oral preparations only), functional ovarian cysts, malabsorption syndromes; migraine which is severe or focal or has begun for first time on a combined oral contraceptive; active liver disease, recurrent cholestatic jaundice, and history of jaundice in pregnancy; **interactions:** see p. 291 and Appendix 1 (contraceptives, oral)

Contra-indications: pregnancy, undiagnosed vaginal bleeding, past severe arterial disease or current high risk (e.g. family history, together with cholesterol above 6.5 mmol/litre); liver adenoma; after evacuation of hydatidiform mole (until return to normal of urine and plasma gonadotrophin values); carcinoma of the breast and other sex hormone dependent cancers; porphyria (see section 9.8.2)

Side-effects: menstrual irregularities (see also notes above); nausea and vomiting, headache, breast discomfort, depression, skin disorders, weight changes. For other critical factors affecting contraceptive efficacy such as vomiting, diarrhoea, enzyme induction, and for comment on progestogen-only contraceptives and surgical operations, see under Combined Oral Contraceptives (section 7.3.1)

Dose: by mouth, 1 tablet daily at the same time, preferably early in the evening, starting on 1st day of cycle then continuously

PoM **Femulen**® (Gold Cross)
Tablets, ethynodiol diacetate 500 micrograms. Net price 28-tab pack = 94p

PoM **Micronor**® (Ortho)
Tablets, norethisterone 350 micrograms. Net price 3 × 28-tab pack = £1.89

PoM **Microval**® (Wyeth)
Tablets, levonorgestrel 30 micrograms. Net price 35-tab pack = £1.00

PoM **Neogest**® (Schering Health Care)
Tablets, brown, s/c, norgestrel 75 micrograms (= levonorgestrel 37.5 micrograms). Net price 35-tab pack = 78p

PoM **Norgeston**® (Schering Health Care)
Tablets, s/c, levonorgestrel 30 micrograms. Net price 35-tab pack = 78p

PoM **Noriday**® (Syntex)
Tablets, norethisterone 350 micrograms. Net price 3 × 28-tab pack = £1.79

Parenteral preparations

PoM **Depo-Provera**® (Upjohn)
Injection (aqueous suspension), medroxyprogesterone acetate 150 mg/mL, net price 1-mL vial = £4.17

Note. The 150 mg/mL strength of Depo-Provera is also available in a 3.3-mL vial for use in cancer (see section 8.3.2), and a 50 mg/mL strength is available in 1-, 3-, and 5-mL vials for endometriosis.

Dose: by deep intramuscular injection, 150 mg in first 5 days of cycle or first 6 weeks after parturition (delay until 6 weeks after parturition if breast-feeding); for long-term contraception, repeated every 3 months

PoM **Noristerat**® (Schering Health Care)
Injection (oily), norethisterone enanthate 200 mg/mL. Net price 1-mL amp = £3.00
Dose: by deep intramuscular injection into gluteal muscle, short-term contraception, 200 mg in first 5 days of cycle or immediately after parturition (duration 8 weeks); may be repeated once after 8 weeks (withhold breast-feeding for neonates with severe or persistent jaundice requiring medical treatment)

7.3.3 Spermicidal contraceptives

Spermicidal contraceptives are useful additional safeguards but do **not** give adequate protection if used alone; they are suitable for use with barrier methods. They have two components: a spermicide and a vehicle which itself may have some inhibiting effect on sperm activity.

CSM Advice. Oil-based vaginal and rectal preparations are likely to damage condoms and contraceptive diaphragms made from latex rubber, and may render them less effective as a barrier method of contraception and as a protection from sexually transmitted diseases (including AIDS).

Condoms: no evidence of harm to latex condoms and diaphragms with the products listed below

C-Film® (FP)
Film, nonoxinol '9' 67 mg in a water-soluble basis. Net price 10 films = £1.34
Delfen® (Ortho)
Foam, nonoxinol '9' 12.5%, pressurised aerosol unit in a water-miscible basis. Net price 20 g (with applicator) = £4.65
Double Check® (FP)
Pessaries, nonoxinol '9' 6% in a water-soluble basis. Net price 10 pessaries = £1.08
Note. A pack including 10 condoms, called Two's Company®, costs £2.42 but is not prescribable on NHS
Duracreme® (LRC)
Cream, nonoxinol '9' 2% in a water-soluble basis. Net price 100-g tube = £2.60; applicator = 75p
Duragel® (LRC)
Gel, nonoxinol '9' 2% in a water-soluble basis. Net price 100-g tube = £2.60; applicator = 75p
Gynol II® (Ortho)
Jelly, nonoxinol '9' 2% in a water-soluble basis. Net price 81 g = £2.61; applicator = 75p
Ortho-Creme® (Ortho)
Cream, nonoxinol '9' 2% in a water-miscible basis. Net price 70 g = £2.44; applicator = 75p
Orthoforms® (Ortho)
Pessaries, nonoxinol '9' 5% in a water-soluble basis. Net price 15 pessaries = £2.40
Ortho-Gynol® (Ortho)
Jelly, *p*-di-isobutylphenoxypolyethoxyethanol 1% in a water-soluble basis. Net price 81 g = £2.44; applicator = 75p
Staycept® (Syntex)
Jelly, octoxinol 1% in a water-soluble basis. Net price 80 g = £1.98
Pessaries, nonoxinol '9' 6% in a water-soluble basis. Net price 10 pessaries = £1.43

7.3.4 Contraceptive devices

INTRA-UTERINE DEVICES

The intra-uterine device (IUD) is suitable for older parous women but should be a last-resort contraceptive for young nulliparous women because of the increased risk of pelvic inflammatory disease and infertility. Inert intra-uterine devices are no longer on the UK market but may still be worn by some women.

Smaller devices have now been introduced in order to minimise side-effects; these consist of a plastic carrier wound with copper wire; some also have a central core of silver with the aim of preventing fragmentation of the copper. Family planning organisations now recommend that the replacement time for these devices should be 5 years; any copper intrauterine device licensed currently in the UK, which is fitted in a woman over the age of 40, may remain in the uterus until menopause.

The timing and technique of fitting an intra-uterine device play a critical part in its subsequent performance and call for proper training and experience. Devices should not be fitted during the heavy days of the period; they are best fitted after the end of menstruation and before the calculated time of implantation.

An intra-uterine device should not be removed in mid-cycle unless an additional contraceptive was used for the previous 7 days. If removal is essential (e.g. to treat severe pelvic infection) post-coital contraception should be considered.

If an intra-uterine device fails and the woman wishes to continue to full-term the device should be removed in the first trimester if possible.

INTRA-UTERINE CONTRACEPTIVE DEVICES

Indications: see notes above
Cautions: anaemia, heavy menses, history of pelvic inflammatory disease, diabetes, valvular heart disease (antibiotic cover needed), epilepsy, increased risk of expulsion if inserted before uterine involution; gynaecological examination before insertion, 3 months after, and yearly; remove if pregnancy occurs; anticoagulant therapy (avoid if possible); if pregnancy occurs, increased likelihood that it may be tubal
Contra-indications: pregnancy, severe anaemia, very heavy menses, history of ectopic pregnancy or tubal surgery, distorted or small uterine cavity, genital malignancy, pelvic inflammatory disease, immunosuppressive therapy, *copper devices:* copper allergy, Wilson's disease, medical diathermy
Side-effects: uterine or cervical perforation, displacement, pelvic infection, heavy menses, dysmenorrhoea, allergy; *on insertion:* some pain and bleeding (helped by giving an NSAID, such as ibuprofen half-an-hour before insertion); occasionally, epileptic seizure, vasovagal attack

PoM Multiload® Cu250 (Organon)
Intra-uterine device, copper wire, surface area approx. 250 mm^2 wound on vertical stem of plastic carrier, 3.6 cm length, with 2 down-curving flexible arms, monofilament thread attached to base of vertical stem; preloaded in inserter. Net price, each = £6.75
For uterine length over 7 cm; replacement every 3 years (but see notes above)

PoM Multiload® Cu250 Short (Organon)
Intra-uterine device, as above, with vertical stem length 2.5 cm. Net price, each = £6.75
For uterine length 5–7 cm; replacement every 3 years (but see notes above)

PoM Multiload® Cu375 (Organon)
Intra-uterine device, as above, with copper surface area approx. 375 mm^2. Net price, each = £8.75
For uterine length over 7 cm; replacement every 5 years (see notes above)

PoM Novagard® (Kabi Pharmacia)
Intra-uterine device, copper wire with silver core, surface area approx. 200 mm^2 wound on vertical stem of T-shaped plastic carrier, impregnated with barium sulphate for radio-opacity, monofilament thread attached to base of vertical stem; partially preloaded in inserter. Dimensions: transverse arms, vertical stem, both 3.2 cm. Net price, each = £9.90
For uterine length over 5.5 cm; replacement every 5 years (see notes above)

PoM Nova-T® (Schering Health Care)
Intra-uterine device, copper wire with silver core, surface area approx. 200 mm^2 wound on vertical stem of T-shaped plastic carrier, impregnated with barium sulphate for radio-opacity, threads attached to base of vertical stem. Net price, each = £9.90
For uterine length over 6.5 cm; replacement every 5 years (see notes above)

PoM Ortho Gyne-T® (Ortho)
Intra-uterine device, copper wire, surface area 200 mm^2, wound on vertical stem of T-shaped plastic carrier, impregnated with barium sulphate for radio-opacity, tail plastic thread attached to base of vertical stem. Net price each = £8.99
For uterine length over 6.5 cm; replacement every 3 years (but see notes above)

PoM Ortho Gyne-T® 380 Slimline (Ortho)
Intra-uterine device, as above, with copper wire surface area 320 mm^2 and copper collar surface 30 mm^2 on distal portion of each arm. Net price = £9.40
For uterine length over 6.5 cm; replacement every 4 years (but see notes above)

OTHER CONTRACEPTIVE DEVICES

Contraceptive caps
Type A contraceptive pessary. Translucent rubber, sizes 1 to 5 (55–75 mm rising in steps of 5 mm), net price = £5.14
Available from Lamberts (Dumas Vault Cap®)

Type B contraceptive pessary. Opaque rubber, sizes 22 to 31 mm (rising in steps of 3 mm), net price = £6.10
Available from Lamberts (Prentif Cavity Rim Cervical Cap®)

Type C contraceptive pessary. Translucent rubber, sizes 1 to 3 (45, 48 and 51 mm), net price = £5.14
Available from Lamberts (Vimule Cap®)

Contraceptive diaphragms
Type A Diaphragm with flat metal spring. Transparent rubber with flat metal spring, sizes 55–95 mm (rising in steps of 5 mm), net price = £5.49
Available from Cilag (Ortho-White®), LRC (Durex Flat Spring®)

Type B Diaphragm with coiled metal rim. Opaque rubber with coiled metal rim, sizes 55–95 mm (rising in steps of 5 mm), net price = £5.53
Available from Cilag (Ortho®)

NHS Arcing Spring Diaphragm. Opaque rubber with arcing spring, sizes 60–95 mm (rising in steps of 5 mm)
Available from Cilag (All-Flex®, net price = £6.35), LRC (Durex Arcing Spring®, net price = £6.29)

Fertility thermometer
Fertility (Ovulation) Thermometer (Zeal)
Mercury in glass thermometer, range 35 to 39°C (graduated in 0.1°C). Net price = £1.40
For monitoring ovulation for the rhythm method of contraception

7.4 Drugs for genito-urinary disorders

7.4.1 Drugs for urinary retention
7.4.2 Drugs for urinary frequency, enuresis, and incontinence
7.4.3 Drugs used in urological pain
7.4.4 Bladder instillations and urological surgery
7.4.5 Drugs for impotence

For drugs used in the treatment of urinary-tract infections see section 5.1.13.

7.4.1 Drugs for urinary retention

Acute retention is painful and is treated by catheterisation.

Chronic retention is painless and often long-standing. Catheterisation is unnecessary unless there is deterioration of renal function. After the cause has initially been established and treated, drugs may be required to increase detrusor muscle tone.

PARASYMPATHOMIMETICS

Parasympathomimetics produce the effects of parasympathetic nerve stimulation; they possess the muscarinic rather than the nicotinic effects of acetylcholine and improve voiding efficiency by increasing detrusor muscle contraction. In the absence of obstruction to the bladder outlet they have a limited role in the relief of urinary retention. Generalised parasympathomimetic side-effects such as sweating, bradycardia, and intestinal colic may occur, particularly in the elderly.

Carbachol and **bethanechol** are choline esters that have been used in postoperative urinary retention. Bethanechol has a more selective action on the bladder than carbachol but the use of both has now been superseded by catheterisation.

Distigmine inhibits the breakdown of acetylcholine. It may help patients with an upper motor neurone neurogenic bladder.

BETHANECHOL CHLORIDE

Indications: urinary retention (but see notes above)
Contra-indications: intestinal or urinary obstruction or where increased muscular activity of urinary or gastro-intestinal tract harmful; asthma, bradycardia, hyperthyroidism, recent myocardial infarction, epilepsy, hypotension, parkinsonism, vagotonia, peptic ulceration, pregnancy; **interactions**: Appendix 1 (cholinergics)
Side-effects: parasympathomimetic effects such as nausea, vomiting, sweating, blurred vision, bradycardia, and intestinal colic
Dose: 10–25 mg 3–4 times daily half an hour before food

PoM **Myotonine**® (Glenwood)
Tablets, both scored, bethanechol chloride 10 mg, net price 20 = 90p; 25 mg, 20 = £1.15. Label: 22

CARBACHOL

Indications: urinary retention, but see notes above
Contra-indications; Side-effects: see under Bethanechol Chloride but side-effects more acute
Dose: by mouth, 2 mg 3 times daily half an hour before food
By subcutaneous injection (acute symptoms, postoperative urinary retention) 250 micrograms, repeated twice if necessary at 30-minute intervals
Note: Inadvertent intravenous administration of carbachol is **extremely hazardous** and calls for emergency treatment with atropine.

PoM **Carbachol** (Non-proprietary)
Tablets, carbachol 2 mg. Net price 20 = £1.06. Label: 22
Injection, carbachol 250 micrograms/mL.

DISTIGMINE BROMIDE

Indications: urinary retention due to upper motor lesions; myasthenia gravis, see section 10.2.1
Cautions: asthma, bradycardia, hyperthyroidism, recent myocardial infarction, epilepsy, hypotension, parkinsonism, vagotonia, peptic ulceration, pregnancy; **interactions:** Appendix 1 (cholinergics)
Contra-indications: intestinal or urinary obstruction or where increased muscular activity of urinary or gastro-intestinal tract harmful
Side-effects: see under Bethanechol Chloride, but action slower therefore side-effects less acute; see also Neostigmine (section 10.2.1)
Dose: by mouth, 5 mg daily or on alternate days, half an hour before breakfast
By intramuscular injection, 500 micrograms 12 hours after surgery to prevent urinary retention; may be repeated every 24 hours

PoM **Ubretid**® (Rhône-Poulenc Rorer)
Tablets, scored, distigmine bromide 5 mg. Net price 30-tab pack = £19.50. Label: 22
Injection, distigmine bromide 500 micrograms/mL. Net price 1-mL amp = 82p

ALPHA-BLOCKERS

The selective alpha-blockers **indoramin** and **prazosin** (see section 2.5.4) relax smooth muscle in benign prostatic hyperplasia producing an increase in urinary flow-rate and an improvement in obstructive symptoms. Both have a low incidence of side-effects, although sedation, dizziness, and hypotension may occur; since they are antihypertensives, caution is needed if a patient is receiving antihypertensive treatment (see **Interactions**, Appendix 1, alpha-blockers). Hospital supervision is preferable.

7.4.2 Drugs for urinary frequency, enuresis, and incontinence

URINARY INCONTINENCE

Antimuscarinic drugs such as **oxybutynin** and **flavoxate** are used to treat *urinary frequency*; they increase bladder capacity by diminishing unstable detrusor contractions. All these drugs may cause dry mouth and blurred vision and may precipitate glaucoma. Oxybutynin has a high level of side-effects which limits its use; the dosage needs to be carefully assessed, particularly in the elderly. Flavoxate has less marked side-effects but is also less effective. Propantheline was formerly widely used in urinary incontinence but had a low response rate with a high incidence of side-effects; it is now primarily indicated in adult enuresis. The tricyclic antidepressants imipramine, amitriptyline, and nortriptyline (see section 4.3.1) are sometimes effective in the management of the unstable bladder because of their antimuscarinic properties.

FLAVOXATE HYDROCHLORIDE

Indications: urinary frequency and incontinence; dysuria, urgency; bladder spasms due to catheterisation
Cautions; Contra-indications: see under Oxybutynin Hydrochloride (antimuscarinic effect considerably less marked)
Side-effects: antimuscarinic side-effects (see Atropine Sulphate, section 1.2); see also notes above
Dose: 200 mg 3 times daily

PoM **Urispas**® (Syntex)
Tablets, s/c, flavoxate hydrochloride 100 mg. Net price 100-tab pack = £5.45

OXYBUTYNIN HYDROCHLORIDE

Indications: urinary frequency and incontinence, neurogenic bladder instability and nocturnal enuresis
Cautions: frail elderly; hepatic or renal impairment; hyperthyroidism; cardiac disease where increase in rate undesirable; prostatic hypertrophy; hiatus hernia with reflux oesophagitis; pregnancy and breast-feeding; **interactions:** Appendix 1 (antimuscarinics)
Contra-indications: intestinal obstruction or atony, severe ulcerative colitis or toxic megacolon; significant bladder outflow obstruction; glaucoma
Side-effects: antimuscarinic side-effects (see under Atropine Sulphate, section 1.2); see also notes above

Dose: 5 mg 2–3 times daily increased if necessary to max. 5 mg 4 times daily
ELDERLY 2.5–3 mg twice daily initially, increased to 5 mg twice daily according to response and tolerance
CHILD over 5 years, neurogenic bladder instability, 5 mg twice daily increased if necessary to max. 5 mg 3 times daily; nocturnal enuresis (preferably over 7 years, see notes below), 5 mg 2–3 times daily (last dose before bedtime)

▼ PoM **Cystrin**® (Farmitalia Carlo Erba)
Tablets, oxybutynin hydrochloride 3 mg, net price 100-tab pack = £17.20; 5 mg (scored), 100-tab pack = £28.67. Label: 3

▼ PoM **Ditropan**® (S&N Pharm.)
Tablets, both blue, scored, oxybutynin hydrochloride 2.5 mg, net price 84-tab pack = £12.04; 5 mg, 84-tab pack = £24.08. Label: 3

PROPANTHELINE BROMIDE
Indications: adult enuresis, see notes above
Cautions; Contra-indications: see under Oxybutynin Hydrochloride
Side-effects: antimuscarinic side-effects (see Atropine Sulphate, section 1.2); see also notes above
Dose: 15–30 mg 2–3 times daily one hour before meals

Preparations
See section 1.2

NOCTURNAL ENURESIS

Nocturnal enuresis is a normal occurrence in young children but persists in as many as 5% by 10 years of age. In the absence of urinary-tract infection simple measures such as bladder training or the use of an alarm system may be successful. Drug therapy is not appropriate for children under 7 years of age and should be reserved for when alternative measures have failed. The possible side-effects and potential toxicity of these agents if taken in overdose should be borne in mind when they are prescribed.

The most widely used treatment is with tricyclics such as **amitriptyline**, **imipramine**, and less often **nortriptyline** (see section 4.3.1). They are effective, but behaviour disturbances may occur and relapse is common after withdrawal. Treatment should not normally exceed 3 months unless a full physical examination (including ECG) is given.

Desmopressin, an analogue of vasopressin, is also used for nocturnal enuresis (see section 6.5.2).

The sympathomimetic drug **ephedrine** may also be useful.

EPHEDRINE HYDROCHLORIDE
Indications: nocturnal enuresis
Cautions; Contra-indications; Side-effects: see under Ephedrine Hydrochloride (section 3.1.1.2)
Dose: CHILD 7–8 years 30 mg, 9–12 years 45 mg, 13–15 years 60 mg at bedtime

Preparations
See section 3.1.1.2

7.4.3 Drugs used in urological pain

The acute pain of *ureteric colic* may be relieved with **pethidine**; **diclofenac** is also effective and compares favourably with pethidine.

Lignocaine gel is a useful topical application in *urethral pain* or to relieve the discomfort of catheterisation (see section 15.2).

ALKALINISATION OF URINE

Alkalinisation of urine may be undertaken with **sodium bicarbonate**, or alternatively with potassium citrate. The alkalinising action may relieve the discomfort of *cystitis* caused by lower urinary tract infections. Sodium bicarbonate, in particular, is also used as a urinary alkalinising agent in some metabolic and renal disorders (see section 9.2.2).

POTASSIUM CITRATE
Indications: relief of discomfort in mild urinary-tract infections; alkalinisation of urine
Cautions: renal impairment, cardiac disease; elderly; *interactions:* Appendix 1 (potassium salts)
Side-effects: hyperkalaemia on prolonged high dosage, mild diuresis
Dose: see under preparations

Potassium Citrate Mixture (BP)
(Potassium Citrate Oral Solution)
Oral solution, potassium citrate 30%, citric acid monohydrate 5% in a suitable vehicle with a lemon flavour. Extemporaneous preparations should be recently prepared according to the following formula: potassium citrate 3 g, citric acid monohydrate 500 mg, syrup 2.5 mL, quillaia tincture 0.1 mL, lemon spirit 0.05 mL, double-strength chloroform water 3 mL, water to 10 mL. Contains about 28 mmol K^+/10 mL. Label: 27
Dose: 10 mL 3 times daily well diluted with water
Note. Concentrates for preparation of Potassium Citrate Mixture BP are available from Evans, Hillcross

Effercitrate® (Typharm)
Tablets, effervescent, the equivalent of potassium citrate 1.5 g (13.9 mmol K^+), citric acid 250 mg (1 tablet ≡ 5 mL potassium citrate mixture). Net price 12 = £1.60. Label: 13
Dose: ADULT and CHILD over 6 years, 2 tablets dissolved in a tumblerful of water up to 3 times daily; CHILD 1–6 years 1 tablet

SODIUM BICARBONATE

Indications: relief of discomfort in mild urinary-tract infections; alkalinisation of urine
Cautions; Side-effects: see section 1.1.2; also caution in elderly
Dose: 3 g in water every 2 hours until urinary pH exceeds 7; maintenance of alkaline urine 5–10 g daily

Sodium Bicarbonate Powder. Net price 50 g = 5p. Label: 13

ACIDIFICATION OF URINE

Acidification of urine has been undertaken with **ascorbic acid** but it is not always reliable.

For pH-modifying solutions for the maintenance of indwelling urinary catheters, see section 7.4.4.

ASCORBIC ACID
Indications: acidification of urine but see notes above
Dose: by mouth, 4 g daily in divided doses

Preparations
See section 9.6.3

OTHER PREPARATIONS FOR URINARY DISORDERS

A terpene mixture (Rowatinex®) is claimed to be of benefit in *urolithiasis* for the expulsion of calculi.

Rowatinex® (Monmouth)
Capsules, yellow, e/c, anethol 4 mg, borneol 10 mg, camphene 15 mg, cineole 3 mg, fenchone 4 mg, pinene 31 mg. Net price 50 = £7.54. Label: 25
Dose: 1 capsule 3–4 times daily

7.4.4 Bladder instillations and urological surgery

INFECTED BLADDERS. Various solutions are available as irrigations or washouts.

Initial treatment is with **sterile sodium chloride solution 0.9%** (physiological saline).

Aqueous **chlorhexidine** (see section 13.11.2) is effective against a wide range of common urinary-tract pathogens but not against most *Pseudomonas* spp. Solutions containing 1 in 5000 (0.02%) are used but they may irritate the mucosa and cause burning and haematuria (in which case they should be discontinued); solutions containing 1 in 10000 (0.01%) are usually preferred postoperatively.

Bladder irrigations of **amphotericin** 100 micrograms/mL (see section 5.2) may be of value in mycotic infections.

DISSOLUTION OF BLOOD CLOTS. Clot retention is usually treated by irrigation with sterile **sodium chloride solution 0.9%** but sterile **sodium citrate** solution for bladder irrigation (3%) may also be helpful. **Streptokinase-streptodornase** (Varidase Topical®, see section 13.11.7) is an alternative.

LOCALLY ACTING CYTOTOXIC DRUGS. **Doxorubicin** (see section 8.1.2) is used to treat recurrent superficial bladder tumours, carcinoma-in-situ, and some papillary tumours. An instillation (50 mg in 50 mL of sterile sodium chloride solution 0.9%) is retained in the bladder for one hour and treatment repeated monthly. Although systemic side-effects are few, it may cause frequency, urgency, dysuria, and occasionally reduction in bladder capacity.

Mitomycin (see section 8.1.2) is used for recurrent bladder tumours. A solution containing 20 to 40 mg in 40 mL of sterile water is instilled weekly for 4 weeks then monthly for at least 11 months.

Thiotepa (see section 8.1.1) is used for bladder tumours of low to medium grade malignancy. A solution containing 30–60 mg in 60 mL of sterile water is retained in the bladder for 2 hours. It is given weekly for 4 weeks. The concentration should be reduced if there is evidence of bone-marrow suppression.

INTERSTITIAL CYSTITIS. Dimethyl sulphoxide may be used for symptomatic relief in patients with interstitial cystitis (Hunner's ulcer). 50 mL of a 50% solution (Rimso-50®) is instilled into the bladder, retained for 15 minutes, and voided by the patient. Treatment is repeated at intervals of 2 weeks. Bladder spasm and hypersensitivity reactions may occur and long-term use requires ophthalmic, renal, and hepatic assessment at 6-monthly intervals.

CHLORHEXIDINE
Indications: bladder washouts, see notes above and section 13.11.2

DIMETHYL SULPHOXIDE
Indications: bladder washouts, see notes above

PoM **Rimso-50®** (Britannia)
Bladder instillation, sterile, dimethyl sulphoxide 50%, in aqueous solution. Net price 50 mL = £19.80

SODIUM CHLORIDE
Indications: bladder washouts, see notes above

Available from Baxter, Kendall

SODIUM CITRATE
Indications: bladder washouts, see notes above

Sterile Sodium Citrate Solution for Bladder Irrigation, sodium citrate 3%, dilute hydrochloric acid 0.2%, in purified water, freshly boiled and cooled, and sterilised

UROLOGICAL SURGERY

Endoscopic surgery within the urinary tract requires an isotonic irrigant as there is a high risk of fluid absorption; if this occurs in excess, hypervolaemia, haemolysis, and renal failure may result. **Glycine irrigation solution 1.5%** is the irrigant of choice for transurethral resection of the prostate gland and bladder tumours; **sterile sodium chloride solution 0.9%** (physiological saline) is used for percutaneous renal surgery.

GLYCINE

Indications: bladder irrigation during urological surgery; see notes above
Cautions; Side-effects: see notes above

Glycine Irrigation Solution (Non-proprietary)
Irrigation solution, glycine 1.5% in water for injections
Available from Baxter, Kendall

MAINTENANCE OF INDWELLING URINARY CATHETERS

The deposition which occurs in catheterised patients is usually chiefly composed of phosphate and to minimise this the catheter (if latex) should be changed at least as often as every 6 weeks. If the catheter is to be left for longer periods a silicone catheter should be used. If bladder washouts are required at frequent intervals this usually indicates that the catheter needs to be changed.

CATHETER PATENCY SOLUTIONS

Chlorhexidine 0.02%. Available from CliniMed (Uro-Tainer Chlorhexidine®, 100-mL sachet = £1.98), Galen (Uriflex C®, 100-mL sachet = £1.75)

Mandelic acid 1%. Available from CliniMed (Uro-Tainer Mandelic Acid®, 100-mL sachet = £1.98)

Sodium chloride 0.9%. Available from CliniMed (Uro-Tainer Sodium Chloride®, 100-mL sachet = £1.89, Uro-Tainer M®, with integral drug additive port, 50- and 100-mL sachets = £2.23), Galen (Uriflex S®, 100-mL sachet = £1.65, Uriflex SP® with integral drug additive port, 100-mL sachet = £1.96)

Solution G, citric acid 3.23%, magnesium oxide 0.38%, sodium bicarbonate 0.7%, disodium edetate 0.01%. Available from CliniMed (Uro-Tainer Suby G®, 100-mL sachet = £1.98), Galen (Uriflex G®, 100-mL sachet = £1.75)

Solution R, citric acid 6%, gluconolactone 0.6%, magnesium carbonate 2.8%, disodium edetate 0.01%. Available from CliniMed (Uro-Tainer Solution R®, 100-mL sachet = £1.98), Galen (Uriflex R®, 100-mL sachet = £1.75)

7.4.5 Drugs for impotence

Reasons for failure to produce a satisfactory erection include psychogenic, vascular, neurogenic, and endocrine abnormalities. Intracavernosal injection of vasoactive drugs under careful medical supervision is used for both diagnostic and therapeutic purposes.

The most effective treatment for impotence has been shown to be direct injection of the smooth muscle relaxant **papaverine** into the corpus cavernosum. The usual dose of papaverine by intracavernosal injection is 7.5 mg initially increased according to response to a range of 30–60 mg.

Patients with neurological or psychogenic impotence are more sensitive to the effect of papaverine than those with vascular abnormalities.
Phentolamine (0.25–1.25 mg) can be added if the response is inadequate.

Persistence of the erection for longer than 4 hours is an emergency requiring aspiration of the corpora; if aspiration fails, 1 mg of metaraminol can be diluted to 5 mL with sodium choride injection 0.9% and given by careful slow injection into the corpora.

Other side-effects include vasovagal attacks and syncope; caution is needed in patients with cardiovascular disease and ischaemic attacks.

Local side-effects include haematoma and burning pain at the site of injection and fibrotic changes in the corpora cavernosa (which may lead to Peyronie-like erectile distortion).

Note. Papaverine is available from Boots, Martindale, and Penn (all special order)

7.5 Appliances for urinary disorders

Urostomy pouches are included here but associated products (e.g. skin protectives and adhesives) are in section 1.8

UROSTOMY POUCHES

Body's Care range
Rubber bags (Body's Care)
Black butyl, one-piece pouch, odourless. Net price 1 day pouch (tap outlet) = £25.84; 1 night pouch (tap outlet) = £27.12
White rubber, one-piece pouch. Net price 1 day pouch (tap outlet) = £12.92; 1 night pouch (tap outlet) = £14.89

Bullen range
Lenbul (Bullen)
Day bag (= pouch), one-piece pouch. Net price 1 pouch with tap outlet = £13.42; 1 pouch with large opening (for 4-inch flange with tap outlet) = £13.93; 1 pouch with metal strip = £15.02
Night bag (= pouch). Net price 1 pouch with tap outlet = £15.34; 1 pouch with large opening = £15.92
One-piece flange and bag (= pouch) with tap outlet. Net price 1 (1- or 2-inch hole) = £28.19
Baby's bag (= pouch) and flange with tap outlet. Net price 1 (1¼- or 2-inch hole, with or without night tube) = £39.19
Child's rubber cap and bag (= pouch) with non-reflux valve. Net price 1 small, 1 small with metal strip, or 1 large = £26.56; 1 large with metal strip = £28.56
Urostomy sets. Net price 1 LOP-U appliance (wire ring retainer with 1.5-inch elastic belt for small flange, 10 one-piece flanges and lightweight bags with 1-inch hole, 30 3.5 × 3.5-inch double-sided adhesive plasters) = £37.20; 1 OPR-U appliance (waterproof canvas retaining shield waistband, 2 one-piece flanges and bags with 1- or 2-inch hole and tap outlet, 30 3.5 × 3.5-inch double-sided adhesive plasters) = £77.59; 1 SR-U appliance (plastic retainer ring shield with 1-inch elastic belt for medium flange, 1 Lenbul® 1.5-inch diameter flange, 1 Lenbul® day and 1 night bag with tap outlet, 30 3.5 × 3.5-inch double-sided adhesive plasters) = £58.27

7.5 Appliances for urinary disorders

Coloplast range
Stoma Urine (Coloplast)
Maxi, one-piece pouch with zinc oxide adhesive. Net price 30 pouches (13-mm hole) = £67.20
Midi, one-piece pouch with zinc oxide adhesive. Net price 30 pouches (13-mm hole) = £67.20
URO 2002® (Coloplast)
Two-piece pouch. Net price 20 small pouches (100 mL, to fit 40 mm base plate) = £48.60; 20 large pouches (375 mL, to fit 40 or 60 mm base plate) = £48.60
Base plate. Net price 5 plates (40 mm, to fit 10–35 mm stoma) or 5 plates (60 mm, to fit 10–55 mm stoma) = £12.80
Night drainage system. Net price 10 pouches (1.65 litre), 1 tube, and 2 connectors = £12.50; hospital pack, 10 pouches (1.65 litre), 5 tubes, and 10 connectors = £17.60

ConvaTec range
Surgicare System® **2** (ConvaTec)
Two-piece pouch, with non-reflux valve, clear. Net price 10 (small or standard) pouches (32, 38, 45, or 57 mm flange) = £19.99; 10 standard pouches (70 mm flange) = £21.65, (100 mm flange) = £32.60
Surgicare System® **2 Combihesive**(ConvaTec)
Two-piece pouch with Accuseal® tap, and textured backing, clear. Net price 10 standard pouches (32, 38, 45, or 57 mm flange) = £20.49

DePuy range
Raymed® (DePuy)
Butyl night bag (= pouch), one-piece pouch. Net price 1 pouch with screwcap outlet = £24.95; 1 pouch with tap outlet = £25.80

Drew range
Urostomy bags (Drew)
Urostomy bag (= pouch), one-piece pouch. Net price 50 pouches (D1/2, OSTO 06) = £73.41
Rubber bags (Drew)
Rubber bag (= pouch), one-piece pouch. Net price 1 pouch screwcap outlet (OSTO 16) = £12.57; 1 pouch (OSTO 17) tap outlet = £13.19
Ureterostomy appliance (Drew)
Ureterostomy appliance. Net price 1 appliance, 1–1.25 inch (D1/2, OSTO 05) = £37.24

Hollister range
Classic (Hollister)
Karaya 5® seal and regular adhesive with attachment for optional belt, one-piece pouch, clear. Net price 20 pouches (series 741, 23-cm pouch: 19, 25, 32, 38, 44, or 51 mm holes; series 746, 40-cm pouch and series 748, 30-cm pouch: 25, 32, 38, 44, or 51 mm holes) including 1 standard drain tube = £56.84
Regular adhesive with attachment for optional belt, one-piece pouch, clear. Net price 20 pouches (series 740, 23-cm pouch: 19, 25, 32, 38, 44, or 51 mm holes; series 745, 40-cm pouch and series 747, 30-cm pouch: 25, 32, 38, 44, or 51 mm holes) including 1 standard drain tube = £43.24
Regular adhesive only (beltless), one-piece pouch, clear. Net price 20 pouches (series 744, 23-cm pouch: 19, 25, 32, 38, 44, or 51 mm holes), including 1 standard drain tube = £43.24
First Choice® (Hollister)
Urostomy pouch with synthetic skin barrier and Microporous II adhesive (series 146). Net price 10 pouches (13–64 mm starter hole, 19, 25, 32, 38, 44, or 51 mm holes) = £40.00
Guardian® (Hollister)
Guardian, two-piece pouch with wide-bore tap and non-reflux valve (series 470). Net price 10 pouches (25-cm for max. 25, 38, or 51 mm stomas), including 1 drain tube adaptor = £21.04

Lo-profile® (Hollister)
Karaya 5® seal and Microporous II adhesive with gasket for optional belt, one-piece pouch, with non-reflux valve, clear (series 143). Net price 10 pouches (25-cm pouch: 19, 25, 32, 38, 44, or 51 mm gasket), including 1 Lo-profile drain tube = £47.93
Microporous II adhesive only (beltless) one-piece pouch with non-reflux valve (series 142). Net price 10 pouches (25-cm pouch: 19, 25, 32, 38, 44, or 51 mm holes), including 1 Lo-profile drain tube = £36.40

Rüsch range
Rubber bags (Rüsch)
Black rubber (Birkbeck®), one-piece pouch with tap outlet. Net price 1 day pouch (19 mm hole) = £27.17; 1 night pouch (19 mm hole) = £29.64
Pink rubber, one-piece pouch with tap outlet. Net price 1 day pouch (19 mm hole) = £27.17; 1 night pouch (19 mm hole) = £29.64
White rubber, one-piece pouch with tap outlet. Net price 1 day pouch (19, 25, or 28 mm holes) = £14.76; 1 night pouch (19, 25, or 28 mm holes) = £15.16
White rubber (Glasgow), one-piece pouch. Net price 1 pouch (small or large tap) = £18.03
White rubber transverse, one-piece pouch. net price 1 left or right pouch (small, medium, or large) = £18.03

Salts range
Koenig Rutzen (Salts)
All rubber white rubber tap bag (= pouch), one-piece pouch with tap outlet. Net price 1 small or medium pouch (both 25, 32, or 38 mm holes) or 1 large pouch (25, 32, 38, 44, or 51 mm holes) = £14.24
All rubber black butyl bag (= pouch), one-piece pouch with tap outlet and non-reflux valve. Net price 1 medium or large pouch (both 19, 25, 32, or 38 mm holes) = £33.89; special size holes also available to order
All rubber MB black butyl bag (= pouch), one-piece pouch with tap outlet, bridge, and non-reflux valve. Net price 1 small, medium, or large pouch (all 19, 25, 32, or 38 mm holes) = £39.63; special size holes also available to order
Black butyl, reinforced bag (= pouch), one-piece pouch with tap outlet and non-reflux valve. Net price 1 medium or large pouch (both 19, 25, 32, or 38 mm holes) = £41.53; special size holes also available to order
MB black butyl, reinforced bag (= pouch), one-piece pouch with tap outlet and non-reflux valve. Net price 1 medium or large pouch (both 19, 25, 32, or 38 mm holes) = £47.58; special size holes also available to order
Rubber bags (Salts)
Black rubber bag (= pouch) (for use with flange), two-piece pouch with tap outlet. Net price 1 small, medium, or large pouch = £18.73; special size holes also available to order
White rubber bag (= pouch) for use with flange, two-piece pouch with tap outlet. Net price 1 small, medium, or large pouch = £7.33
Light White (Salts)
Urostomy pouch with Realistic® washer, one-piece pouch, white. Net price 20 large pouches (all 25, 32, or 38 mm holes) = £95.53
Urostomy pouch with Realistic® washer, one-piece pouch, clear. Net price 20 large or small pouches (all 25, 32, or 38 mm holes) = £95.53
Urostomy pouch, one-piece pouch, white. Net price 20 large pouches (25, 32, or 38 mm holes) = £71.79
Urostomy pouch, one-piece pouch, clear. Net price 20 large or small pouches (25, 32, or 38 mm holes) = £71.79
Urostomy pouch, one-piece pouch with adhesive, white. Net price 20 large pouches (25, 32, or 38 mm holes) = £75.81
Urostomy pouch, one-piece pouch with adhesive, clear. Net price 20 large or small pouches (both 25, 32, or 38 mm holes) = £75.81

Cautionary label wordings, see inside back cover

Prices are **net**, see p. 1

Simplicity 1® (Salts)
Paediatric Uri-bag, one-piece pouch, 13 mm starter hole. Net price 15 pouches = £36.33

Simcare range
Carshalton (Simcare)
Bag (= pouch), one-piece pouch. Net price 10 oval or triangular pouches (both 25, 32, or 38 mm) with acrylic plaster = £16.46
Set, one-piece pouch. Net price 20 oval or triangular pouches with plasters, bodyplate, clamp, connector, and medium belt (both 25, 32, or 38 mm holes) = £56.00
Chiron Non-disposable (Simcare)
Butyl rubber bag (= pouch), one-piece pouch with stopcock outlet, odourless, black. Net price 1 day bag (22 mm) = £29.46
Latex rubber bag (= pouch), one-piece pouch with stopcock outlet. Net price (both 38 mm) 1 day bag = £20.40; 1 night bag = £23.14
Rubber child-size bag (= pouch), one-piece pouch with stopcock outlet, white. Net price 1 = £17.12
Rubber day bag (= pouch), one-piece pouch, white with stopcock outlet. Net price 1 (38 mm) = £20.40
Rubber night bag (= pouch), one-piece, white. Net price 1 (38, 44, or 51 mm) = £23.14
Chiron (Simcare)
Ileal bladder appliance, set comprises 1 web and elastic belt 25 mm wide, 1 wire pressure frame, 1 St Mark's pattern rubber flange (without diaphragm), 2 rubber day pouches with stopcock outlet, 30 double-sided plasters. Net price = £65.73
Mitcham (Simcare)
Maxi, one-piece pouch. Net price 10 pouches with adhesive flange (25, 32, or 38 mm) = £33.54, 10 pouches with nonadhesive flange (25, 32, or 38 mm) = £27.39
Mini, one-piece pouch. Net price 10 pouches with adhesive flange (19, 25, or 32 mm) = £33.54, 10 pouches with nonadhesive flange (25 mm or 32 mm) = £27.39
Standard, one-piece pouch. Net price 10 pouches with adhesive flange (19, 25, 32 or 38 mm) = £33.54, 10 pouches with nonadhesive flange (19, 25, 32, or 38 mm) = £27.39, 1 pouch with nonadhesive flange and foam pads (25, 32, or 38 mm) = £4.78
Rediflow (Simcare)
Adhesive set, may be worn with belt. Net price 20 pouches (19, 25, 32, 38, 44, or 51 mm) = £49.29

Ward range
Ward
Ureterostomy bag (= pouch) with tap outlet. Net price 1 night pouch = £16.32; 1 day pouch (19, 35, or 54 mm hole) = £15.28

DRAINABLE DRIBBLING APPLIANCES

Re-usable for at least 1 month (with exception of Alexa®)

Body's Care range
Bag (Body's Care)
Dribbling bag with loops and tapes. Net price 1 = £13.78
Urinal (Body's Care)
Drip male urinal with tap. Net price 1 = £36.88; 1 replacement belt = £9.11

Bullen range
Bags (Bullen)
Net price 10 Dribblet® bags = £20.09; 10 Dribblet® sheath bags = £45.09

DePuy range
Aquadry® (DePuy)
Male incontinence pouch. Net price 1 (with short or long tube) = £6.15
Drip type urinal. Net price 1 = £46.25

Henleys range
Alexa® dribbler bag (Henleys)
Plain bag, with draw strings. Net price 100 bags = £4.22; 100 bags with non-reflux valve = £16.25

Rüsch range
Peoplecare® (Rüsch)
Male drip urinal. Net price 1 = £41.39

Ward range
Bags (Ward)
Male dribbling bag with diaphragm and belt. Net price 1 = £22.71
Plastic dribbling bag. Net price 1 = £11.30

INCONTINENCE BELTS

Average life 6 months

Body's Care range
Waist belt for kipper bags (Body's Care)
Net price 1 = £4.55; 1 (with webbing band) = £4.55

Rüsch range
Peoplecare® (Rüsch)
Waist and support strap for kipper bag. Net price 1 = £5.84
Rubber belt. Net price 1 = £3.21

Simcare range
Belts (Simcare)
Rubber belt. Net price 1 = £4.62
Elastic support. Net price 1 (small, medium, or large) = £9.89
Web belt (small, medium, or large) = £9.58

Ward range
Belts (Ward)
Waist belt for black kipper bag. Net price 1 = £4.16
Rubber belt for PP (pubic pressure) urinal. Net price 1 = £3.60

Willis range
Belts (Willis)
Waist band 2-inch white web with looped strap to support bag. Net price 1 (38 or 46 inch) = £4.09; 1 (larger than 46 inch) = £4.38

INCONTINENCE SHEATHS

Unless otherwise indicated the incontinence sheaths (also known as penile sheaths or external catheters) listed below are of the soft, flexible, latex type. Each sheath may be left in place for 1 to 3 days between changes

Bard range
Reliasheath® (Bard)
Incontinence sheath with adhesive strip. Net price 30 sheaths (20, 25, 30, 35, or 40 mm) = £31.21
Uriplan® (Bard)
Incontinence sheath. Net price 30 sheaths (20, 25, 30, 35, or 40 mm) = £20.90
Uro sheath® (washable; may be used many times). Net price 1 (25, 35, or 40 mm) = £4.36

Camp range
Posey® (Camp)
Incontinence sheath. Net price 10 sheaths (incontinence sheath A) = £4.65; 10 sheaths ('Fastflow' incontinence sheath, 25, 30, or 35 mm) = £5.80

7.5 Appliances for urinary disorders

Coloplast range
Conveen® (Coloplast)
Incontinence sheath, with anti-kink design and Uriliner® adhesive strip. Net price 30 sheaths (20, 25, 30, 35, or 40 mm) = £37.50
Conveen self-sealing Urisheath® (Coloplast)
Incontinence sheath. Net price 30 sheaths (25, 30, or 35 mm) = £36.90

DePuy range
Aquadry® (DePuy)
Incontinence sheath. Net price 10 sheaths (small, medium, large, or extra-large) = £8.78; 10 sheaths with bulbous end (small, medium, or large) = £25.32
Aquadry Freedom® (DePuy)
Freedom® incontinence sheath, self-adhesive. Net price 30 sheaths (small, medium, or large) = £37.00
Freedom Plus® incontinence sheath, self-adhesive. Net price 30 sheaths (small, medium, or large) = £37.00

EMS Medical range
Sheaths (EMS Medical)
Incontinence sheath. Net price 100 sheaths (25, 30, or 35 mm) = £42.00; 30 sheaths (with liner; 25, 30, or 35 mm) = £28.30

Fry Surgical range
Uridom® (Fry Surgical)
Incontinence sheath, with adhesive strip. Net price 30 sheaths = £26.10

Hospital Management and Supplies range
Macrodom® (Hospital Management and Supplies)
Incontinence sheath, including adhesive strip. Net price 30 sheaths (with 2-inch tube) = £18.25; 25 sheaths (with 5-inch tube) = £19.17
Macrodom Plus® (Hospital Management and Supplies)
Incontinence sheath, including adhesive strip. Net price 30 sheaths (small, medium, or large) = £23.00

Incare range
Male incontinence sheath (Incare)
Incontinence sheath, self adhesive. Net price 15 sheaths (22, 26, 30, or 34 mm) = £20.70

Mediplus range
Medimates® (Mediplus)
Incontinence sheath with single-sided adhesive strip. Net price 30 sheaths (straight, 20, 25, 30, 35, or 40 mm; bulb, 25, 30, or 35 mm) = £28.30
Incontinence sheath with double-sided adhesive strip. Net price 30 sheaths (straight, 20, 25, 30, 35, or 40 mm; bulb, 25, 30, or 35 mm) = £30.20

North West Medical range
Uridrop® (North West Medical)
Incontinence sheath. Net price 30 sheaths (paediatric = 42 or 55 mm; sizes 1, 2, 3, or 4 = 70, 80, 100, or 107 mm) = £11.20
Incontinence sheath, with Uristrip® adhesive strip. Net price 30 sheaths (paediatric = 42 or 55 mm; sizes 1, 2, 3, or 4 = 70, 80, 100, or 107 mm) = £22.40

Payne range
Incontiaid® (Payne)
Incontinence sheath. Net price 10 sheaths, with adhesive strip (sizes 20, 25, 30, 35 or 40 mm) = £11.50; 1 sheath, without adhesive strip (sizes 20, 25, 30, 35 or 40 mm) = 75p; 10 adhesive strips = £3.75

Rüsch range
Dryaid® (Rüsch)
Incontinence sheath. Net price 20 sheaths (with adhesive strip; small, medium, or extra-large) = £25.20; 20 sheaths (without adhesive strip; small, medium, large, or extra-large) = £14.60
Portasheath® (Rüsch)
Incontinence sheath. Net price 25 sheaths (25, 30, or 35 mm) = £20.50
Secure external catheter kit, with adhesive strip. Net price 10 sheaths (25, 30, or 35 mm) = £8.40

Salts range
Heritage Cohesive/Sheath Pack® (Salts)
Incontinence sheath, with adhesive. Net price 30 sheaths (17, 22, 25, 32, or 34 mm) = £29.78
Male continence sheath (Salts)
Incontinence sheath. Net price 10 sheaths (17, 22, 25, 32, or 34 mm) = £6.72

Seton range
Incontinence sheath (Seton)
Incontinence sheath. Net price 30 sheaths (small, medium, large, or extra-large) = £27.80; 30 sheaths with self-adhesive liner (small, medium, large, or extra-large) = £33.12

Sherwood range
Texas Catheter® (Sherwood)
Incontinence sheath, with adhesive strip. Net price 12 sheaths = £8.28
Uri Drain® (Sherwood)
Incontinence sheath, with double-sided adhesive strap (25, 30, or 35 mm). Net price 10 = £7.65

Simcare range
Continence sheath (Simcare)
Incontinence sheath. Net price 1 sheath (small, medium, large, or extra-large) = £1.19
Uro Flo® (Simcare)
Incontinence sheath, straight, including adhesive liner. Net price 30 sheaths (small, medium, or large) = £34.81
Uro Flo Mk2® (Simcare)
Incontinence sheath, bulbous, with adhesive liner. Net price 30 sheaths (small, medium, or large) = £34.81
Male incontinence sheath (Simcare)
Incontinence sheath. Net price 100 sheaths = £57.67

Simpla range
Bubble U® (Simpla)
Incontinence sheath, with adhesive foam strip. Net price 30 sheaths (small, medium, large, or extra-large) = £24.30
Incontinence sheath, with self-adhesive Uriseal® liner. Net price 30 sheaths (small, medium, large, or extra-large) = £34.95

S&N range
Regard® (S&N)
Incontinence sheath, with liners. Net price 30 sheaths (small, medium, large, or extra-large) = £31.50

Vygon range
Peniflow® (Vygon)
Incontinence sheath. Net price 40 sheaths = £44.38

FIXING STRIPS AND ADHESIVES

Bio Diagnostics
Urifix® tape. Net price 5 m = £4.90
Camp
Posey® sheath holder. Net price 12 (adult) = £12.00; 12 (paediatric) = £10.20

Chapter 7: Obstetrics, gynaecology, and urinary-tract disorders

ConvaTec
Urihesive® strips. Net price 15 = £5.50
DePuy
Aquadry® medical adhesive (brush-on). Net price 1 = £3.25 Aquadry® penile liners. Net price 20 = £7.50
Dow Corning
Adhesive B (Silicone adhesive aerosol). Net price 207 g = £8.97
355 medical adhesive (brush-on silicone adhesive). Net price 1 = £2.72
EMS Medical
Urifix® tape. Net price 5 m = £5.30
North West Medical
Uristrip® adhesive strip. Net price 30 = £11.20
Payne
Incontiaid® sheath holder. Net price 1 = 85p
Rüsch
Dryaid® strip. Net price 20 strips = £10.60
Salts
Heritage® sheath collar pack. Net price 30 = £3.42
NHS Cohesive® strips for use with sheaths. Net price 10 = £4.50

LEG BAGS

Most plastic bags suitable for use for 5–7 days; rubber bags re-usable for 4–6 months

Bard range
Uriplan® (Bard)
  Leg bag, plastic, shaped, with tap outlet and elastic Velcro straps. Net price 10 bags (350 mL, direct inlet) = £21.63; 10 bags (350 mL, 12 inch inlet tube) = £21.32; 10 bags (500 mL, direct inlet) = £21.84; 10 bags (500 mL, 4 or 12 inch inlet tube) = £21.93; 10 bags (750 mL, direct inlet, or 4, 12, or 15 inch inlet tube) = £22.05
Seton Urisac® (Bard)
  Leg bag, plastic. Net price 10 bags (350 mL, short tube) = £10.61; 10 bags (350 mL, long tube) = £10.92; 10 bags (500 mL, short tube) = £11.54; 10 bags (500 mL, long tube) = £11.86; 10 bags (750 mL, short tube) = £12.17; 10 bags (750 mL, long tube) = £12.69

Body's Care range
Leg bags (Body's Care)
  Kipper bag, black, white, or clear. Net price 1 bag = £20.90
  Leg drainage bag, plastic, with tap outlet. Net price 10 bags (350 or 500 mL) = £17.90; 10 bags (750 mL) = £18.70

Coloplast range
Conveen® (Coloplast)
  Standard leg bag, plastic. Net price, with 1 set Velcro bands, 10 bags (500 mL, 10 or 40 cm tube) = £17.40
  Contour leg bag, plastic, shaped, sterile with sample port. Net price, with 1 set Velcro bands, 10 bags (600 mL, 5 or 30 cm tube; 800 mL, 45 cm tube) = £21.80; 10 non-sterile bags (600 mL, 45-cm adjustable tube) = £21.80

ConvaTec range
Accuseal® (ConvaTec)
  Leg bag, plastic. Net price 10 bags (500 mL) = £15.81
DePuy range
Aquadry® (DePuy)
  Catheter drainage bag, plastic. Net price 10 bags (small) = £20.65; 10 bags (large) = £21.20
  Leg bag, plastic. Net price 10 bags (350, 500, or 750 mL, short or long tube) = £19.95

EMS Medical range
Leg drainage bags (EMS)
  Leg bag, plastic. Net price 10 bags (500 mL, short or long tube) = £12.85

Incare range
Urinary leg bag (Incare)
  Leg bag, plastic. Net price 10 bags (540 mL, 37 cm tube) = £21.94; 10 bags (540 mL, direct inlet) = £21.41

Payne range
Incontiaid® (Payne)
  Leg bag, plastic. Net price 1 bag = £2.20
Single-chambered Bags (Payne)
  Leg bag, single-chambered. Net price 1 bag (rubber, with box outlet tap) = £41.94; 1 rubber bag (for night use) = £45.80; 1 bag (for female use) = £34.03; 1 bag (rubber, kipper-style) = £34.03; 1 bag (rubber, Ross type) = £38.84

Pharma-Plast range
Careline® (Pharma-Plast)
  Leg bag, plastic, with tap outlet and overnight connection tube. Net price, with 1 pair Velcro straps, 10 bags (350 mL, short or long tube) = £19.00; 10 bags (500 mL, short or long tube) = £19.50; 10 bags (750 mL, short or long tube) = £20.00

Rüsch range
Leg bag (Rüsch)
  Leg bag, plastic. Net price 10 bags (short tube, 350 or 500 mL) = £13.00; 10 bags (long tube, 350 or 500 mL) = £13.90; 10 bags (750 mL) = £9.30
Kipper bags (Rüsch)
  Leg bag. Net price 1 bag (clear/white plastic or all black plastic or rubber, with strap and buckle) = £24.40; 1 bag (clear/white plastic, without strap and buckle) = £20.00

Salts range
Heritage® (Salts)
  Leg bag, plastic. Net price 10 bags (500 mL, short tube) = £12.40; 10 bags (500 mL, long tube) = £12.62; 10 bags (750 mL, short tube) = £13.82; 10 bags (750 mL, long tube) = £14.15; 5 leg bag packs = £8.85

Sherwood range
Argyle® (Sherwood)
  Leg bag, plastic. Net price (350, 500 or 750 mL, short or long tube) = £20.50

Simcare range
NHS **Meredith®** (Simcare)
  Top outlet bag. Net price 25 bags (2 litres) = £42.89
PVC drainage bag (Simcare)
  Leg bag, plastic. Net price 1 bag (small or large) = £3.26
Rubber bags (Simcare)
  Leg bag, rubber, with leg strap. Net price = £30.20
Uro-Flo® (Simcare)
  Standard leg bag, plastic. Net price 10 bags (350, 500 or 750 mL, 5 or 30 cm tube) = £12.73
  Xtend® leg bag, plastic, sterile. Net price 10 bags (500 mL, 6–20 cm or 22–36 cm tube) = £22.58

Simpla range
Trident® (Simpla)
  Leg bag, plastic. Net price 10 bags (350 mL, short tube) = £21.70; 10 bags (500 mL, short or long tube) = £21.93; 10 bags (750 mL, short, long, or adjustable long tube) = £22.04

7.5 Appliances for urinary disorders

S&N range
Regard® (S&N)
Leg bag, plastic. Net price 10 bags (350 mL, short tube) = £21.70; 10 bags (500 mL, short tube or adjustable long tube) = £21.93; 10 bags (750 mL, adjustable long tube) = £22.04

Universal range
Unicorn® (Universal)
Leg bag, plastic. Net price 10 bags (350 mL, short tube) = £17.60; 10 bags (500 mL, short or long tube) = £17.80; 10 bags (750 mL, short or long tube) = £18.00

Wallace range
Leg bags (Wallace)
Leg bag, with valve outlet, natural latex straps, and plastic tube. Net price 10 bags (350 mL, short tube) = £21.02; 10 bags (350 mL, long tube) = £21.61; 10 bags (500 mL, short tube) = £21.48; 10 bags (500 mL, long tube) = £22.03; 10 bags (750 mL, short tube) = £21.80; 10 bags (750 mL, long tube) = £21.92
Leg bag, with twist tap, elastic straps, and plastic tube. Net price 10 bags (750 mL, short tube) = £21.84; 10 bags (750 mL, long tube, 30 cm) = £21.96
Tri-form® leg bag, plastic. Net price 10 bags (500 mL, short tube) = £21.45; 10 bags (500 mL, medium tube) = £21.70; 10 bags (500 mL, long tube) = £21.99

Ward range
Kipper bag (Ward)
Leg bag, kipper type, rubber. Net price 1 bag (black, clear, or white) = £18.95
Leg drainage bag (Ward)
Leg bag, plastic. Net price 10 bags (350 mL) = £9.43; 10 bags (500 mL) = £9.45; 10 bags (750 mL) = £9.99
Comfort® (Ward)
Leg bag, plastic. Net price 10 bags (350 mL) = £9.19; 10 bags (500 mL) = £9.45; 10 bags (750 mL) = £9.94

Willis range
Leg bags (Willis)
Rubber bag, for catheter drainage, short neck leg strap. Net price 1 bag = £24.18; 1 bag with web belt and support strap) = £28.29
Rubber bag, female, for catheter drainage, with conical mount. Net price 1 bag = £22.95; 1 bag (with web belt and support strap) = £27.06
Rubber bag, single-chambered, with olive mount. Net price 1 bag = £24.30; 1 bag (with web belt and support strap) = £28.29

NIGHT DRAINAGE BAGS

Suitable for night-time use for collection of urine from indwelling catheters or from incontinence sheaths; bag hangers normally supplied through community nursing service.
Drainage bags have life of 5–7 nights

Bard
Uriplan® drainage bag. Net price 10 bags = £9.77
Body's Care
2 litre drainage bag with tap outlet. Net price 1 bag = £1.22
Coloplast
Conveen® 1.5 litre drainage bag with 90 cm tube. Net price 10 bags = £11.00
ConvaTec
Surgicare System® 2 drainage bag. Net price 5 bags (Accuseal®) = £7.10; 5 bags (night) = £7.10
DePuy
Urine drainage bag. Net price 1 bag = £1.15
Aqua® range 2 litre urine drainage bag. Net price 10 bags (Aqua® 2, non-drainable) = £1.90; 10 bags (Aqua® 4) = £8.60

EMS Medical
2 litre urine drainage bag. Net price 10 bags = £9.80
Hospital Management and Supplies
Macpak® range. Net price 10 bags (Macpak® 1, non-drainable) = £1.47; 5 bags (Macpak® 3, drainable) = £3.86; 10 bags (Macpak® 5, non-drainable) = £1.46
Pharma-Plast
Careline® range, 2 litre urine drainage bag with 90 cm inlet tube. Net price 10 bags (Careline® E1, non-drainable) = £1.66; 10 bags (Careline® E2, non-drainable, with non-reflux valve) = £1.76; 5 bags (Careline® E4, with non-reflux valve and tap outlet) = £4.34
Rand Rocket
Urine drainage bag (non-drainable, short or long tube). Net price 25 bags = £3.75
Rüsch
Drainage bags, 2 litre. Net price 10 bags (C) = £10.00; 10 bags with non-reflux valve and plug (CV) = £11.10; 10 bags with non-reflux valve and tap (CVT) = £11.50; 10 bags with non-reflux valve and wide bore tap (DVT) = £10.60
Salts
2 litre H2 urine drainage bag. Net price 10 bags with non-reflux valve and tap = £10.15
Sherwood
Argyle® 2 litre urinary drainage bag. Net price 10 bags = £9.20
Simcare
Uro-flo® night drainage bag. Net price 10 bags (female or male) = £12.41
Simpla
Urine drainage bag. Net price 10 bags (S1, non-drainable) = £1.98; 10 bags (S2, non-drainable with non-reflux valve) = £2.11; 10 bags (night, short tube) = £9.86; 10 bags (S4, long tube) = £10.48
S&N
Regard® overnight drainage bag. Net price 10 bags = £9.11
Wallace
Community INBEDS night bag. Net price 10 bags = £11.97
Ward
2 litre drainage bag with push/pull outlet. Net price 10 bags = £9.94

SUSPENSORY SYSTEMS

Drainage bag with support; bags may be used for 5–7 days

Bard
Urisac® Portabag® with belt. Net price 10 bags (plastic) = £10.25; 1 belt = £6.00
EMS Medical
Drainage bag with Shepheard Sporran belt. Net price 10 bags (plastic) = £12.85; 1 belt = £6.70
Rüsch
Portabag® with Portabelt®. Net price 10 bags (plastic) = £14.90; 1 belt = £8.32
Wallace
Holster bag with leg bag holster. Net price 10 bags (400 mL, plastic) = £16.86; 1 holster (24–30, 30–36, or 36–44 inch) = £7.85

TUBING AND ACCESSORIES

Bard
General purpose tubing. Net price 96 inch = £1.82
Urinary drainage economy tube. Net price 48 inch = £1.16
Adaptor for Uro sheath® (penile sheath to leg bag) 8 inch. Net price 1 = 92p

Uriplan® leg bag straps (washable). Net price 5 pairs = £10.63
Latex leg bag straps. Net price 10 pairs = £2.18
Seton range foam/Velcro leg bag straps. Net price 10 pairs = £4.14
Urisac® tapes. Net price 10 pairs = £4.58
Body's Care
Velcro leg straps. Net price 1 pair = £1.48
Leg bag connecting tube. Net price 1 = £1.16; 1 (with mount) = £1.96
Coloplast
Velcro bands (washable). Net price 10 pairs = £30.70
ConvaTec
Accuseal® leg bag extension tube. Net price 10 tubes = £5.84
Accuseal® catheter adaptor. Net price 10 = £4.78
DePuy
Leg bag connecting tube. Net price 10 = £6.55
Aquadry® leg straps. Net price 5 pairs = £8.75
EMS Medical
Velcro leg straps. Net price 10 = £5.00
Incare
Leg bag straps. Net price 1 pair (14 inch, calf or 23 inch, thigh) = £2.39
MMG
G-Strap. Net price 'adult' or 'short', 5 = £10.00; 'abdomen', 5 = £11.00
Payne
Rubber extension tube, 6 inch. Net price = £2.89
Rubber leg strap. Net price 1 = £1.02
Velcro leg strap. Net price 1 = 80p
Portex
Tapered adaptor (catheter to leg bag). Net price 1 = £5.20; 1 (stepped) = £7.30
Rüsch
Connecting tubes, net price 1 tube for kipper bag = £2.43; 14 inch connecting tube for drip urinal = £2.42; 1 connecting tube for all urinals with female connector = £3.51
Salts
Heritage® leg bag extension tube. Net price 2 tubes = £1.77
Sherwood
Argyle® foam and Velcro strap, washable. Net price 1 (75 cm, leg) = £1.69; 1 (150 cm, abdomen) = £3.17
Argyle Suregrip® general purpose tube, internal diameter 7 mm, length 2.7 m. Net price 50 tubes = £34.50
Argyle Penrose® tubing, internal diameter 6, 8, 10, 13, 16, 19, or 25 mm and length 44 cm. Net price 50 = £29.50
Simcare
Stopcock for Chiron plastic urinal bags (in place of screw-cap). Net price 1 = £3.85
Rubber extension tube (with mounts). Net price = £3.85
Rubber tubing (length, 1.5 m). Net price 1 = £9.00
Plastic connector with tube. Net price 1 = £2.58
Female connector for Mitcham bag. Net price = £1.78
Leg straps. Net price 5 pairs = £11.24
Night bag connector. Net price 1 = £1.09
Spare 'O' rings for pubic pressure urinal. Net price 5 = £1.02
Uro-Flo® elastic Velcro leg straps. Net price 5 pairs = £3.66
Paul (Penrose) tubing. Net price 10 (6, 13, 19, or 25 mm) = £11.04; 10 (32, 38, 44, or 51 mm) = £11.04
Simpla
Leg bag straps. Net price 20 pairs (foam) = £11.29; 5 pairs (elasticated, washable) = £11.13
Wallace
Leg bag extension tube. Net price 10 (30 cm) = £23.46; 10 (60 cm) = £25.80
Silgrip® leg straps. Net price 5 pairs (elasticated or Side-Fix thigh-fitting) = £11.10; 5 pairs (Side-Fix calf-fitting) = £10.55

URINAL SYSTEMS

Patients generally have two urinal systems (one to wash and one to wear). Each appliance should last for 6 months

Bard
Uriplan Mcguire® urinal and adaptor. Net price (waist sizes 66–81 cm, 81–96 cm, or 96–112 cm) = £51.03
Male day and night urinal. Net price 1 (14 oz) = £38.10; 1 (20 oz) = £33.74
Mobile paraplegic day and night urinal. Net price 1 = £41.63
Uriplan Mcguire® adaptor and tubing. Net price = £6.89
Bell and Croyden
Fridjohn male urinal. Net price 1 = £40.61
Male urinal, day and night use. Net price 1 (with long or short bag) = £37.35
Body's Care
Male day and night urinal with tap, covered bag, with band and suspensory, and leg strap with air vent. Net price 1 = £43.30
Male night urinal with tap, covered bag, with band and suspensory. Net price 1 = £52.68
Male day and night urinal with tap, long tube, covered bag, with band and suspensory with air vent. Net price 1 = £51.19
Male day and night urinal with tap, double bag, air vent, inflating rim, with band understraps. Net price 1 = £54.21
Male day and night urinal with tap, covered bag, diaphragm top, and air vent. Net price 1 = £46.85
Male day and night urinal with tap, improved pattern, inflating rim, short air vent, with band and understrap. Net price 1 = £51.41; 1 (with extension tube) = £54.27; 1 (with long bag) = £52.15
Male day and night urinal with tap, air vent, diaphragm top, with band and understrap. Net price 1 (with long bag) = £49.87; 1 (with short bag) = £46.21; 1 (with extension tube) = £49.71
Male day and night urinal with tap, air vent, with band and suspensory. Net price 1 (long bag) = £44.41
Male day urinal with tap, to contain penis and scrotum. Net price 1 (short bag, with band and understrap) = £41.87; 1 (with inner sheath and air vent) = £43.51
Male jockey appliance with tap. Net price 1 = £46.32
Spares
 Replacement belt. Net price 1 = £9.11
 Outer receiver. Net price 1 = £10.60
 Inner sheath. Net price 5 = £10.92
 Plastic bags. Net price 5 = £11.98
 Rubber bag. Net price 1 = £19.45
 Ring. Net price 1 = 79p
Stoke Mandeville male urinal with tap (specify sheath size). Net price 1 = £49.18; 1 (with double bag) = £59.04; 1 replacement sheath (specify size) = £4.87
Male pubic pressure urinal with tap (specify sheath size). Net price 1 (with rubber bag) = £52.59; 1 (with 5 plastic bags) = £49.50
Spares
 Flange with sheaths. Net price 1 = £24.59
 Cone. Net price (curved, small, medium, or large; straight, small, medium, large, or extra-large) = £9.75
 Plastic bag. Net price 1 (small or large) = £11.98
 Rubber bag. Net price 1 = £19.08
 Rubber belt. Net price 1 = £3.50
Progress® long life plastic urinal. Net price 1 (inner sheath or scrotal) = £20.78
Fridjohn urinal. Net price 1 = £62.11
YB wet urinal. Net price 1 = £50.40
Essex appliance. Net price 1 = £42.08
One-piece belt. Net price 1 (rubber or plastic bag coverlet) = £42.20

7.5 Appliances for urinary disorders

Bullen
Child urinal. Net price 1 (with transverse bag) = £64.58; 1 (with medium-size long bag) = £62.41
Male urinal. Net price 1 (with large-size long bag) = £68.59

DePuy
Aquadry® urinal. Net price 1 (paediatric; scrotal support: adult or adolescent; pubic pressure: adult, adolescent or paediatric understrap; rubber understrap: adult or adolescent) = £47.90; 1 (long-term) = £46.75
Spares
Bag (except for drip type and long-term). Net price 5 (250 or 325 mL) = £10.85
Flange (child: 0.5, 0.675, 0.75, 0.875, 1, 1.125, or 1.25 inch; adult: 1, 1.125, 1.25, 1.375, 1.5, 1.675, or 1.75 inch). Net price 1 = £23.60
Cones. Net price 1 (small, medium, or large, curved or straight) = £9.90
Rubber belt. Net price 1 (adult or child) = £2.75

Ellis
Hallam modular urinal. Net price 1 = £28.75; 1 spare bag = £1.53; 1 spare belt = £3.41

LRC
Dry sheaths. Net price 144 = £14.00

Payne
Male incontinence appliance with rubber belt. Net price 1 (MK1 with combined rubber flange and understraps) = £53.23; 1 (MK2 with rubber flange and fabric facepiece) = £57.24; 1 (MK3 with combined rubber flange, understraps, and coned top) = £47.24; (MK9, with rubber flange and fabric facepiece) = £59.65
Lightweight male incontinence appliance. Net price 1 (MK4 with fabric facepiece and separate long flanged plastic bag with foam pad) = £33.75; 1 (MK5, with fabric facepiece, separate flange, and long flanged plastic bag with rubber belt) = £47.40; 1 (MK6 with combined flange and understraps, and long flanged plastic bag with rubber belt) = £41.57; 1 (MK10, with fabric facepiece, separate flange, and long flanged plastic bag with rubber belt) = £49.81
Spares
Rubber flange. Net price 1 (with feathered diaphragm, MK2, MK5, MK9, MK10) = £15.41; 1 (MK1, MK6) = £23.86; 1 (with feathered diaphragm and combined reinforced top, MK3) = £27.07
Material facepiece. Net price 1 facepiece with belt and loop (MK2, MK4, MK5) = £17.87; 1 facepiece with support belt, loop and scrotal = £20.28
Flange support with wide belt and scrotal support (MK9, MK10). Net price 1 = £20.28
Reinforced cone top (MK1, MK2, MK9). Net price 1 = £10.38
Bag (MK1, MK2, MK3, MK9). Net price 1 plastic bag = £2.62; 1 rubber bag = £15.68
Bag, long flange plastic. Net price 1 MK4 bag = £4.01; 1 MK5, MK6, MK10 bag = £3.53
Belt (MK1, MK3, MK6). Net price 1 (elastic) = £7.12; 1 (web) = £4.98; 1 (rubber) = £3.37
Night connector (MK1, MK2, MK3, MK9). Net price 1 = £3.37
Payne's urine director. Net price 1 = £19.05
Stoke Mandeville condom urinal complete. Net price 1 = £43.92
Spares
Kipper bag. Net price 1 = £24.72
Belt. Net price 1 (38, 46, or 60 inch) = £5.24
Rubber tube and connector. Net price 1 = £1.93; rubber tubing (GU or SM) = £3.96 per metre; nylon connector (latex: 8 mm or 10 mm; red: 8 mm or 10 mm) 1 = £1.12
Dry incontinence sheath. Net price 144 = £14.00
Pubic pressure urinal complete with bag. Net price 1 (rubber or plastic bag) = £53.23
Spares
Pubic pressure flange with sheath (1-inch flange with 0.5, 0.625, 0.75, or 0.875 inch sheath; 1.25-inch flange with 0.875 or 1 inch sheath; 1.5-inch flange with 1.125 or 1.25 inch sheath; 1.75-inch flange with 1.375, 1.5, or 1.625 inch sheath). Net price 1 = £23.86
Coned top. Net price 1 (straight or curved: small, medium, or large; straight: extra-large) = £10.38
Replacements
Rubber bag with vent tube (MK1, MK2, MK3, MK9). Net price 1 = £18.83
Reinforced cone top with vent tube (MK1, MK2, MK3, MK9). Net price 1 = £13.64
Latex tubing, 8 or 10 mm bore. Net price per metre = £3.96
Condom set. Net price 1 = £45.80; 1 (with 40 oz bag) = £56.82
Urinal replacement parts
Nylon stud (GU or SM). Net price 1 = £1.12; 1 (with latex tube) = £1.93
Waist belt for single-chambered bag. Net price 1 (38, 46, or 60 inch) = £5.24

Rüsch
Thames urinal with bag and connecting tube. Net price 1 (standard or long bag) = £68.33
Severn urinal with bag and connecting tube. Net price 1 (standard, long, or 5 plastic bags) = £68.33; 5 Severn spare sheaths = £26.79
Mersey urinal with bag and connecting tube. Net price 1 (standard, long, or 5 plastic bags) = £68.33
Wye, male, MkII, light-weight urinal. Net price 1 (with separate connecting tube and on/off valve) = £22.08; 1 (with long night extension tube) = £25.79; 1 (with short or long bag) = £36.78
Arizona male urinal. Net price 1 = £68.33
'55' male urinal for paraplegic patients. Net price 1 = £67.31; 6 spare sheaths = £31.45
Stoke Mandeville pattern male urinal with double chamber rubber collection bag. Net price 1 (20, 24, 25, 28, 32, 35, 38, 42, 45, 48, 51, 54, 57, 60, or 63 mm sheath) = £68.33; 1 spare sheath = £6.31
Sahara one-piece top pubic pressure urinal with bag. Net price 1 paediatric (with small rubber collection bag or 5 small plastic collection bags) = £65.14; 1 standard or large (with standard or long rubber collection bag or 5 medium plastic collection bags, and connecting tube) = £65.14
Peoplecare® pubic pressure male urinal. Net price 1 paediatric (flange 25 mm and sheath 13, 16, 19, or 22 mm; or flange 29 mm and sheath 22 or 25 mm; or flange 32 mm and sheath 19, 22, or 25 mm) = £21.16; 1 adult (flange 38 mm and sheath 19, 22, 25, 29, or 32 mm; or flange 44 mm and sheath 35, 38, or 41 mm) = £21.16
Spares:
Pubic pressure bag, standard. Net price 1 (medium) = £10.92; 1 (large) = £13.53; 1 (curved top, small, medium, or large) = £8.24; 1 (straight top, small, medium, large, or extra-large) = £8.24
Transverse rubber bag with tap. Net price 1 = £22.35
Pubic pressure flange for transverse rubber bag with tap. Net price 1 (double-based) = £21.16; 1 (adult, rubber) = £24.39
Kipper inco set with 1 black rubber kipper bag, 10 penile sheaths, waist and support strap, and connecting tube. Net price 1 = £36.61

Salts
Male pubic pressure urinal with rubber bag or 4 plastic bags. Net price 1 = £43.56
Spares
Pubic pressure flange with sheath (1-inch flange with 0.5, 0.625, 0.75, or 0.875 inch sheath; 1.25-inch flange with 0.75, 0.875, or 1 inch sheath; 1.5-inch flange with 0.75, 0.875, 1, 1.125 inch sheath; 1.75-inch flange with 1.375, 1.5, or 1.625 inch sheath). Net price 1 = £20.91
Cone. Net price 1 (small, medium, or large: straight or curved; extra-large: straight) = £9.31

Pubic pressure flange belt. Net price 1 = £18.37
Bags. Net price 4 (plastic, child or adult) = £10.23; 1 (rubber, child, adult, or transverse) = £10.23
Belt. Net price = £3.11

Simcare

Male pubic pressure urinal, child, with integral flange. Net price 1 (rubber bag, straight cone, medium) = £50.93; 1 (plastic bag, curved cone, small or medium) = £49.79

Spares

Pubic pressure flange with integral sheath for child. Net price 1 (25-mm flange with 13, 16, 19, or 22 mm sheath; 29-mm flange with 22 or 25 mm sheath; 32-mm flange with 22 or 25 mm sheath) = £28.03

Cone. Net price 1 (small, medium, or large, straight or curved; extra-large, straight) = £11.86

Pubic pressure flange, double-based. Net price 1 (child, 32 mm; adult, 38 or 44 mm) = £25.07

Chailey male urinal. Net price 1 (child, plastic bag) = £52.41; 1 (adolescent or adult, rubber bag) = £46·99; 1 (adolescent or adult, plastic bag) = £59.52

Spares

Curved top with integral sheath and straps. Net price 1 (child: 22-mm sheath; adult: 22, 25, 29, 32, 35, 38, or 44 mm sheath) = £31.36

Belt, rubber. Net price 1 (61 or 91 cm) = £4.62

Bags, plastic (also suitable for pubic pressure and Chiron® urinals). Net price 1 (wide neck, adult, or child) = £3.09

Bags, rubber (also suitable for pubic pressure and Chiron® urinals). Net price 1 child size = £14.91; 1 adult size = £20.45

Male pubic pressure urinal, adult, with integral flange. Net price 1 (rubber bag, various sizes) = £59.01; 1 (plastic bag, various sizes) = £54.98

Replacement pubic pressure flange. Net price 1 = £28.03

Male pubic pressure urinal, adult, with double-based flange. Net price 1 (rubber bag, various sizes) = £59.01; 1 (plastic bag, various sizes) = £54.98

Replacement sheath. Net price 10 = £1.08

Bag, rubber, for pubic pressure urinals. Net price 1 (adult, with vent tube) = £24.46; 1 (adult, double) = £26.19

Stoke Mandeville urinal. Net price 1 (sheath type) = £53.76; 1 (double rubber bag) = £69.88

Spares

Bag. Net price 1 = £26.19; 1 (with top) = £49.62

Sheath. Net price 1 = £7.33; 10 (for sheath type) = £3.22

Net suspensory. Net price 1 = £15.50

Chiron male rubber urinal with webbing belt. Net price 1 = £48.39

Male one-piece urinal. Net price = £46.07

Surrey model lightweight urinal. Net price = (MKI or MKII) = £43.77

Spares

Bag. Net price 10 = £27.39

Foam pad. Net price 5 (76 mm/32 mm) = £5.39

Chiron urinal. Net price 1 (male, plastic, rubber sheaths) = £25.04; 1 (geriatric, film-type sheaths) = £36.36; 1 (rubber sheaths) = £36.36

Spares

Sheath. Net price 1 (rubber) = £4.62; 10 (non-allergenic film type) = 86p

Net suspensory. Net price 1 = £10.87

Male urinal for bed use. Net price 1 = £40.84

Pubic flange, large opening. Net price 1 = £18.77

Transverse rubber bag and stopcock. Net price 1 (child) = £27.65

Steeper

Paraplegic male urinal for day and night use with porthole swan-neck top, adjustable elastic belt with linen front 4 buttonholes, and understraps suitable for sitting patients. Net price 1 = £54.36

Male rubber urinal for day use, porthole top, straight neck and inner sheath, adjustable elastic belt with linen front, 4 buttonholes, and understraps. Net price 1 = £40.15; 1 (with swan-neck) = £43.41

Male urinal, rabbit eared, with inner sheath complete with waistband. Net price 1 = £38.50

Elastic waistband, adjustable with linen front, 4 buttonholes, and tape understraps for porthole type urinals. Net price 1 = £6.82

Adjustable waistband. Net price 1 = £3.77

Scrotal pouch for rabbit eared urinal. Net price 1 = £4.25

Male dribbling bag (rubber), curved with porthole diaphragm and adjustable webbing belt. Net price 1 = £19.61

Pubic pressure urinal with double-based flange, disposable film sheaths, and 4 plastic bags. Net price 1 = £35.86

Ward

Jockey male urinal. Net price 1 = £59.44

Varsity male urinal. Net price 1 = £45.88

Male urinal. Net price 1 (day use, covered bag, complete with belt suspensory and thigh strap) = £37.95; 1 (day and night, covered bag, air vent, belt suspensory) = £39.29; 1 (day and night, short bag and belt) = £40.67; 1 (day and night, short covered bag and belt) = £44.07; (day and night, double chamber bag) = £45.81; 1 (day and night, long bag and belt) = £40.67

Paraplegic male urinal. Net price 1 = £55.57

Stoke Mandeville Pattern. Net price 1 = £53.39; 1 (removable rubber sheath, double chamber rubber bag, thigh strap and belt) = £47.95

Spare sheath. Net price 1 = £4.96

Male pubic pressure urinal. Net price 1 (rubber bag) = £49.75; 1 (plastic bag) = £44.08

Spares

Pubic pressure flange. Net price 1 = £22.82

Pubic pressure cone; Net price 1 = £9.02

Bags. Net price 1 (rubber) = £12.36; 1 (plastic) = £2.48

Male urinal. Net price 1 (day, covered bag complete with belt) = £36.12; 1 (day and night or night, covered bag complete with belt, suspensory, and thigh strap) = £47.73; 1 (day and night, long tube, air vent, rubber bag, complete with belt and thigh strap) = £43.32

Male urinal. Net price 1 (night, covered bag complete with belt, suspensory, and thigh strap) = £47.73

Male dribbling bag and tapes. Net price 1 = £17.63

Male urinal. Net price 1 (day and night, short covered bag or short bag and belt) = £40.67

Male urinal. Net price 1 (sheath and disc type with long rubber belt or sheath and suspensory with short or long covered bag) = £44.33

Male urinal. Net price 1 (conical top with short or long rubber bag) = £25.30

Night urinal. Net price 1 (with long tube) = £21.38

Stoke Mandeville sheath-type urinal, with 30 rubber film sheaths, rubber bag, and thigh strap and belt. Net price 1 = £42.46

St Peters pattern suprapubic bag. Net price 1 = £26.15

Willis

Male urinal, day and night, air tube to bag, inner sheath and diaphragm to receiver, web belt and cotton suspensory bag. Net price 1 = £44.68; 1 (bag covered with Coutil®, elastic leg strap) = £46.50; 1 (long narrow Coutil®-covered bag, web belt and cotton suspensory bag) = £46.50

Male urinal, receiver to contain penis and scrotum, web waist band, and tape understraps. Net price 1 (day, night, or small build) = £42.66

Male urinal, long rubber bag with 2 leg straps, loops and straps, flanged receiver, air tube, diaphragm and short conical inner sheath, web band and cotton suspensory bag. Net price 1 (day and night) = £44.14

7.5 Appliances for urinary disorders

Male urinal, short rubber bag, detachable bag and night tube, web belt and cotton suspensory bag. Net price 1 (day and night) = £35.57

Spares for above urinals
 White web waist band. Net price 1 (29, 36, or 44–48 inch) = £4.00
 Suspension bag. Net price 1 (small, medium, or large) = £4.49

URETHRAL CATHETERS

Urethal catheter sizes are designated by the Charrière (Ch) gauge system; when the size is not stated by the prescriber the Drug Tariff recommends that size 14 or 16 be supplied. For the Foley catheter, if the balloon size is not stated, the 10 mL size should be supplied for adults, 5 mL for paediatric use (balloon sizes are defined as the amount of fluid required to fully inflate the volume of lumen).

Foley catheters for short-/medium-term use in adults
Bard
 Uriplan®, teflon-coated latex, male or female. Net price, male (12-26 Ch: 10-mL balloon; 16-28 Ch: 30-mL balloon), 1 catheter = £1.90; female (Ch 12-26: 10-mL balloon), 1 catheter = £2.85; pre-filled with sterile water (Ch 12-26: 10-mL balloon), 1 catheter = £2.16
Rüsch
 Soft Simplastic®, PVC, male or female. Net price, male (12-26 Ch: 10-mL balloon; 16-26 Ch: 30-mL balloon), 1 catheter = £4.10; female (12-22 Ch: 10-mL balloon; 16-22 Ch: 30-mL balloon), 1 catheter = £4.10
 100 plus®, teflon-coated latex, male or female. Net price male (12-26 Ch: 10-mL balloon; 16-26 Ch: 30-mL balloon), 1 catheter = £1.84; female (12-22 Ch: 10-mL balloon; 16-32 Ch: 30-mL balloon), 1 catheter = £2.36
Simcare
 Eschmann Folatex®, latex, male or female. Net price, male (12-30 Ch: 10- or 30-mL balloon), 1 catheter = £1.72; female (12-30 Ch: 10- or 30-mL balloon), 1 catheter = £3.03

Foley catheters for short-/medium-term use in children
All 8-10 Ch: 5-mL balloon
Bard
 Uriplan®, teflon-coated latex. Net price 1 catheter = £5.24
Rüsch
 100 plus®, teflon-coated latex. Net price 1 catheter = £3.94
Simcare
 Eschmann Folatex®, latex. Net price 1 catheter = £3.15

Foley catheters for long-term use in adults
Bard
 Biocath®, hydrogel-coated, male or female. Net price, male (12-26 Ch: 10- or 30-mL balloon), 1 catheter = £5.93; female (12-26 Ch: 10-mL balloon), 1 catheter = £5.93; pre-filled with sterile water, male or female (12-26 Ch: 10-mL balloon), 1 catheter = £6.18
 Uriplan®, silicone elastomer-coated latex, male or female. Net price, male (12-26 Ch: 10-mL balloon; 16-28 Ch: 30-mL balloon), 1 catheter = £6.57; female (16-26 Ch: 30-mL balloon), 1 catheter = £6.57; pre-filled with sterile water, male or female (12-26 Ch: 10-mL balloon), 1 catheter = £7.21
 Uriplan®, all silicone. Net price (12-24 Ch: 10-mL balloon; 16-24 Ch: 30-mL balloon), 1 catheter = £6.78
Dow Corning
 Silastic®, silicone-coated. Net price (12-24 Ch: 10-mL balloon; 16-28 Ch: 30-mL balloon), 1 catheter = £6.73

Rüsch
 Silikon 100®, male or female. Net price, male (12-26 Ch: 10-mL balloon; 18-20 Ch: 20-mL balloon; 22-26 Ch: 30-mL balloon), 1 catheter = £5.84; female (12-22 Ch: 10-mL balloon; 18-20 Ch: 20-mL balloon; 22 Ch: 30-mL balloon), 1 catheter = £5.84
 Ultrasil®, silicone elastomer-coated latex, male. Net price (12-26 Ch: 10-mL balloon; 16-26 Ch: 30-mL balloon), 1 catheter = £5.05
Sherwood
 Argyle®, all silicone, male or female. Net price, male (12-26 Ch: 10-mL balloon; 16 Ch: 20-mL balloon; 18-26 Ch: 30-mL balloon), 1 catheter = £5.60; female (12-18 Ch: 10-mL balloon), 1 catheter = £5.60
Simcare
 Eschmann Folatex-S®, all silicone, male or female. Net price, male (12-26 Ch: 10-mL balloon; 18 Ch: 20-mL balloon; 20-26 Ch: 30-mL balloon), 1 catheter = £6.79; female (12-26 Ch: 10-mL balloon; 18 Ch: 20-mL balloon; 20-26 Ch: 30-mL balloon), 1 catheter = £6.20
Simpla
 All silicone, male or female. Net price, male (12-26 Ch: 10-mL balloon; 16-18 Ch: 20-mL balloon; 20-26 Ch: 30-mL balloon), 1 catheter = £6.80; female (12-18 Ch: 10-mL balloon; 20-26 Ch: 30-mL balloon), 1 catheter = £6.75

Foley catheters for long-term use in children
All 8-10 Ch: 5-mL balloon
Bard
 Biocath®, hydrogel-coated. Net price 1 catheter = £5.93
Rüsch
 Silikon 100®. Net price 1 catheter = £5.84
Sherwood
 Argyle®, all silicone. Net price 1 catheter = £6.29
Simpla
 All silicone. Net price 1 catheter = £6.97

Nelaton catheters ('ordinary' cylindrical catheter)
Astra Meditec
 Lofric®, PVC, single use, male, female, or paediatric. Net price, male (8-24 Ch); female (8-18 Ch); paediatric (6-10 Ch), 5-catheter pack (all) = £6.10
Bard
 Reliacath®, teflon-coated latex, 14 Ch. Net price 5-catheter pack = £5.94
 Reliacath®, plastic, male, female, or paediatric. Net price, male or female (12-18 Ch), 5-catheter pack = £5.44; paediatric (8-10 Ch), 5-catheter pack = £5.44
EMS
 PVC, male or female, 8-14 Ch. Net price, male, 1 catheter = 95p, 5-catheter pack = £3.95; female, 1 catheter = 98p, 5-catheter pack = £4.25
 PVC, paediatric/female, 6 Ch. Net price 1 catheter = 98p, 5-catheter pack = £4.25
Pennine
 Male, female, or paediatric. Net price, male (12-18 Ch), 10-catheter pack = £3.08; female (12-14 Ch), 10-catheter pack = £2.80; paediatric (6-10 Ch), 10-catheter pack = £2.80
Portex
 PVC, male or female, 8-14 Ch. Net price, male, 5-catheter pack = £6.26; female, 5-catheter pack = £5.98
Rüsch
 Riplex Jacques®, PVC, male or female 8-18 Ch. Net price, male, 1 catheter = £1.41, 5-catheter pack = £6.06; female, 1 catheter = £1.26, 5-catheter pack = £5.51
 Jacques®, soft red rubber, Ch 8-18. Net price 1 catheter = £1.26, 5-catheter pack = £5.25
Simcare
 PVC, male or female, 8-14 Ch. Net price, male, 5-catheter pack = £6.33; female, 5-catheter pack = £6.09

8: Drugs used in the treatment of
MALIGNANT DISEASE and for IMMUNOSUPPRESSION

In this chapter, drug treatment is discussed under the following headings:
- 8.1 Cytotoxic drugs
- 8.2 Drugs affecting the immune response
- 8.3 Sex hormones and hormone antagonists in malignant disease

Malignant disease may be treated by surgery, radiotherapy, and/or chemotherapy. Certain tumours are highly sensitive to chemotherapy but many are not, and inappropriate drug administration in these circumstances can only increase morbidity or mortality.

of the drug names, or proprietary names, identify the regimen used. Drug combinations are frequently more toxic than single drugs but may have the advantage in certain tumours of enhanced response and increased survival. However for some tumours, single-agent chemotherapy remains the treatment of choice.

> Most cytotoxic drugs are teratogenic, and all may cause life-threatening toxicity; administration should, where possible, be confined to those experienced in their use.
>
> Because of the complexity of dosage regimens in the treatment of malignant disease, dose statements have been omitted from some of the drug entries in this chapter. *In all cases detailed specialist literature should be consulted.*
>
> Prescriptions should **not** be repeated except on the instructions of a specialist.

8.1 Cytotoxic drugs

- 8.1.1 Alkylating drugs
- 8.1.2 Cytotoxic antibiotics
- 8.1.3 Antimetabolites
- 8.1.4 Vinca alkaloids and etoposide
- 8.1.5 Other antineoplastic drugs

Great care is needed when prescribing these drugs as damage to normal tissue, which may be irreversible, is an almost invariable consequence of their use. These drugs should rarely, if ever, be used empirically in a patient with cancer, and administration should always be regarded as a clinical trial with clear objectives in mind.

> **CRM guidelines on cytotoxic drug handling:**
> 1. Trained personnel should reconstitute cytotoxics;
> 2. Reconstitution should be carried out in designated areas;
> 3. Protective clothing (including gloves) should be worn;
> 4. The eyes should be protected and means of first aid should be specified;
> 5. Pregnant staff should not handle cytotoxics;
> 6. Adequate care should be taken in the disposal of waste material, including syringes, containers, and absorbent material.

In a minority of cancers, chemotherapy may result in cure, or marked prolongation of survival. Here short-term drug-related toxicity, which may be severe, is acceptable. However, for the majority of patients, modest survival prolongation or palliation of symptoms will be the aim, and an attempt should be made to use relatively non-toxic treatments, or to consider the use of other effective modalities, e.g. radiotherapy.

Cytotoxics may be used either singly, or in combination. In the latter case, the initial letters

Cytotoxic drugs fall naturally into a number of classes, each with characteristic antitumour activity, sites of action, and toxicity. A knowledge of sites of metabolism and excretion is important, as impaired drug handling as a result of disease is not uncommon and may result in enhanced toxic effects. A number of side-effects are characteristic of particular agents or groups of drugs, e.g. neurotoxicity of vinca alkaloids, and details will be provided in the appropriate sections. Most toxic effects are, however, common to many of these drugs and will be briefly outlined here.

EXTRAVASATION OF INTRAVENOUS DRUGS. A number of drugs will cause severe local tissue necrosis if leakage into the extravascular compartment occurs. Recommended modes of administration must be adhered to. Infusion of vesicant drugs should be stopped immediately if local pain is experienced. Where doubt exists as to whether significant leakage has occurred, the infusion should be discontinued and the cannula resited in another vein. There are no proven antidotes for extravasation, but general recommendations include elevation of the limb and application of ice packs three or four times daily until pain and swelling settle; if ulceration occurs plastic surgery may be required.

HYPERCALCAEMIA. Hypercalcaemia is a common complication of malignant disease. Treatment of the underlying malignancy may resolve it, but drugs which specifically lower serum calcium are often also required (see section 9.5.1.2).

HYPERURICAEMIA. Hyperuricaemia, which can result in uric acid crystal formation in the urinary tract with associated renal dysfunction is a complication of the treatment of non-Hodgkin's lymphoma and leukemia. Allopurinol (see section 10.1.4) should be started 24 hours before treating such tumours, and should be continued for 7 to 10 days; patients should be adequately hydrated. The dose of mercaptopurine or azathioprine should be reduced if allopurinol needs to be given concomitantly (see Appendix 1).

NAUSEA AND VOMITING. Nausea and vomiting is a source of considerable distress to many patients receiving chemotherapy. It should be anticipated and, where possible, prevented with anti-emetic treatment tailored to the chemotherapy regimen and the response of the patient.

If first-line anti-emetics are ineffective treatment should be escalated as below. Hospital admission may be necessary.

Group 1: severe emesis unlikely
Drugs in this group include alkylating drugs by mouth, intravenous fluorouracil, vinca alkaloids, and methotrexate.

Phenothiazines (e.g. prochlorperazine) or domperidone, given by mouth, when necessary, will often suffice. Premedication with these drugs is often useful before intravenous chemotherapy, treatment being continued for up to 24 hours afterwards. Both prochlorperazine and domperidone are also available as suppositories which is useful for patients who develop vomiting despite oral therapy.

Group 2: moderate emesis
Drugs in this group include intravenous cyclophosphamide and doxorubicin; premedication is essential for all drugs in this group. Most patients can be treated on an out-patient basis therefore, if possible, the anti-emetics should be given by mouth.

Anti-emetics in group 1 are given when necessary but it is usually preferable to give in addition dexamethasone 10 mg by mouth before and 6 hours after chemotherapy, and/or lorazepam 1 to 2 mg by mouth given similarly. Lorazepam has the advantage of causing drowsiness and amnesia, but patients cannot drive after it. Nabilone is also suitable, but may cause dysphoria. Ondansetron may also have a valuable role.

Patients in group 1 with an unsatisfactory response can be transferred to drugs in this group.

Group 3: severe emesis
Drugs in this group include mustine, dacarbazine, and cisplatin. They commonly cause severe emesis, particularly if used in combination.

A simple well-tolerated anti-emetic regimen is dexamethasone 10 mg by mouth with lorazepam 1 to 2 mg by mouth, given before and 6 hours after chemotherapy. Out-patients should be warned not to drive. Dexamethasone and lorazepam can also be given intravenously to inpatients; the dose of lorazepam is titrated according to the patient's level of consciousness (drowsiness should be obtained with 2 to 4 mg). This regimen should be avoided in patients with chronic chest disease and care is necessary in the elderly.

Alternatively, or in addition, high-dose metoclopramide can be given by intravenous infusion but it may cause dystonic reactions in younger patients (see section 4.6).

The specific ($5HT_3$) serotonin antagonists, granisetron and ondansetron, control the nausea and vomiting that occurs within 24 hours of chemotherapy but are relatively ineffective in delayed emesis (as occurs with cisplatin). There is evidence that addition of dexamethasone (e.g. 10 mg by mouth or intravenously) will enhance their efficacy. Administration of repeated doses of these specific serotonin antagonists has not been shown to be more effective than administration of a single dose.

Patients in group 2 with an unsatisfactory response can be transferred to drugs in this group.

BONE-MARROW SUPPRESSION. All cytotoxic drugs except vincristine and bleomycin cause marrow depression. This commonly occurs 7 to 10 days after administration, but is delayed for certain drugs, such as carmustine, lomustine, and melphalan. Peripheral blood counts must be checked prior to each treatment, and doses should be reduced or therapy delayed if marrow recovery has not occurred. Fever occurring in a neutropenic patient (neutrophil count less than 0.8×10^9/litre) is an indication for immediate parenteral broad-spectrum antibiotic therapy (see section 5.1, Table 1), once appropriate bacteriological investigations have taken place.

ALOPECIA. Reversible hair loss is a common complication, although it varies in degree between drugs and individual patients. No pharmacological methods of preventing this are available.

REPRODUCTIVE FUNCTION. Most cytotoxic drugs are teratogenic and should not be administered during pregnancy, especially during the first trimester (but for transplant therapy, see below).

Contraceptive advice should be offered where appropriate before cytotoxic therapy begins. Regimens that do not contain an alkylating drug may have less effect on fertility, but those with an alkylating drug will render almost all males permanently sterile early in a treatment course (there is no effect on potency). Pre-treatment counselling and consideration of sperm storage may be appropriate. Females are less severely affected, though the span of reproductive life may be shortened by the onset of a premature menopause. No increase in fetal abnormalities or abortion-rate has been recorded in patients who remain fertile after cytotoxic chemotherapy.

Transplant therapy. Female transplanted patients immunosuppressed with azathioprine should not discontinue it on becoming pregnant; although spontaneous abortion may be more common, congenital fetal abnormalities are not increased in successful pregnancies. There is less experience of cyclosporin in pregnancy; although compatible with normal pregnancy, retardation of fetal growth has been reported. Any risk to the offspring of azathioprine-treated men is small.

8.1.1 Alkylating drugs

Extensive experience is available with these drugs, which are among the most widely used in cancer chemotherapy. They act by damaging DNA, thus interfering with cell replication. In addition to the side-effects common to many cytotoxic drugs (section 8.1), there are two problems associated with prolonged usage. Firstly, gametogenesis is often severely affected (see above). Secondly, prolonged use of these drugs, particularly when combined with extensive irradiation, is associated with a marked increase in the incidence of acute non-lymphocytic leukaemia.

Cyclophosphamide is widely used in the treatment of chronic lymphocytic leukaemia, the lymphomas, and solid tumours. It may be given orally or intravenously and is inactive until metabolised by the liver. A urinary metabolite of cyclophosphamide, acrolein, may cause haemorrhagic cystitis; this is a serious complication and if it occurs cyclophosphamide is not normally used again. An increased fluid intake, for example 3 to 4 litres per day after intravenous injection, will help avoid this complication. When high-dose therapy is used mesna will also help prevent this complication.

Ifosfamide is related to cyclophosphamide; like cyclophosphamide it is given with mesna to reduce urothelial toxicity.

Chlorambucil is commonly used to treat chronic lymphocytic leukaemia, the indolent non-Hodgkin's lymphomas, Hodgkin's disease, and ovarian cancer. Side-effects, apart from marrow suppression, are uncommon, although rashes may occur.

Melphalan is used to treat myeloma and occasionally solid tumours and lymphomas. Marrow toxicity is delayed and it is usually given at intervals of 4–6 weeks.

Busulphan is used almost exclusively to treat chronic myeloid leukaemia. Frequent blood counts are necessary as excessive myelosuppression may result in irreversible bone-marrow aplasia. Hyperpigmentation of the skin is a common side-effect and, rarely, progressive pulmonary fibrosis may occur.

Lomustine (CCNU) is a lipid-soluble nitrosourea and may be given orally. It is mainly used to treat Hodgkin's disease and certain solid tumours. Marrow toxicity is delayed, and the drug is therefore given at intervals of 4 to 6 weeks. Permanent marrow damage may occur with prolonged use. Nausea and vomiting are common and moderately severe.

Carmustine is given intravenously. It has similar activity and toxicities to lomustine and is most commonly given to patients with myeloma, lymphoma, and brain tumours. Cumulative renal damage and delayed pulmonary fibrosis may occur.

Mustine is now much less commonly used. It is a very toxic drug which causes severe vomiting. The freshly prepared injection must be given into a fast-running intravenous infusion. Local extravasation causes severe tissue necrosis.

Estramustine is a stable combination of an oestrogen and mustine, designed to deliver mustine to the oestrogen receptor site of a tumour, for example prostate cancer. It has both a local cytotoxic effect and (by reducing testosterone concentrations) a hormonal effect.

Treosulfan is used to treat ovarian cancer.

Thiotepa is usually used as an intracavitary drug for the treatment of malignant effusions or bladder cancer. It is also occasionally used to treat breast cancer, but requires parenteral administration.

Mitobronitol is occasionally used to treat chronic myeloid leukaemia; it is available on a named-patient basis only (as *Myelobromol*®, Sinclair).

BUSULPHAN

Indications: chronic myeloid leukaemia
Cautions; Side-effects: see section 8.1 and notes above; avoid in porphyria (see section 9.8.2)
Dose: induction of remission, 60 micrograms/kg to max. 4 mg daily; maintenance, 0.5–2 mg daily

PoM **Myleran**® (Wellcome)
Tablets, busulphan 500 micrograms, net price 25 = £3.53; 2 mg, 25 = £5.32

CARMUSTINE

Indications: see notes above
Cautions; Side-effects: see section 8.1 and notes above; irritant to tissues

PoM **BiCNU**® (Bristol-Myers)
Injection, powder for reconstitution, carmustine. Net price 100-mg vial (with diluent) = £12.50

CHLORAMBUCIL

Indications: see notes above (for use as an immunosuppressant see section 8.2.1)
Cautions; Side-effects: see section 8.1 and notes above; caution in renal impairment; avoid in porphyria (see section 9.8.2)
Dose: used alone, usually 100–200 micrograms/kg daily for 4–8 weeks

PoM **Leukeran**® (Wellcome)
Tablets, both yellow, chlorambucil 2 mg, net price 25 = £8.55; 5 mg, 25 = £13.04

CYCLOPHOSPHAMIDE

Indications: see notes above
Cautions; Side-effects: see section 8.1 and notes above; reduce dose in renal impairment; avoid in porphyria (see section 9.8.2); **interactions:** Appendix 1 (cyclophosphamide)

PoM **Cyclophosphamide** (Farmitalia Carlo Erba)
Tablets, pink, s/c, cyclophosphamide (anhydrous) 50 mg. Net price 20 = £1.91. Label: 27
Injection, powder for reconstitution, cyclophosphamide. Net price 107-mg vial = 95p; 214-mg vial = £1.35; 535-mg vial = £2.36; 1.07-g vial = £4.12

8.1 Cytotoxic drugs

PoM **Endoxana**® (ASTA Medica)
Tablets, s/c, cyclophosphamide 50 mg, net price 100-tab pack = £9.13. Label: 27
Injection, powder for reconstitution, cyclophosphamide. Net price 107-mg vial = 79p; 214-mg vial = £1.13; 535-mg vial = £1.97; 1.069-g vial = £3.44

ESTRAMUSTINE PHOSPHATE
Indications: prostate cancer
Cautions: see section 8.1
Contra-indications: peptic ulceration, severe liver or cardiac disease
Side-effects: see section 8.1; also gynaecomastia, altered liver function, cardiovascular disorders (angina and rare reports of myocardial infarction)
Dose: 0.14–1.4 g daily in divided doses (usual range 0.56–1.12 g daily)

PoM **Estracyt**® (Kabi Pharmacia)
Capsules, estramustine phosphate 140 mg (as disodium salt). Net price 20 = £27.17. Label: 21, counselling, should not be taken with dairy products

IFOSFAMIDE
Indications: see notes above
Cautions; Side-effects: see section 8.1 and notes under Cyclophosphamide; reduce dose in renal impairment; **interactions:** Appendix 1 (ifosfamide)

PoM **Mitoxana**® (ASTA Medica)
Injection, powder for reconstitution, ifosfamide. Net price 500-mg vial = £6.74; 1-g vial = £11.76; 2-g vial = £21.65 (hosp. only)

LOMUSTINE
Indications: see notes above
Cautions; Side-effects: see section 8.1 and notes above
Dose: used alone, 120–130 mg/m² body-surface every 6–8 weeks

PoM **CCNU**® (Lundbeck)
Capsules, lomustine 10 mg (blue/white), net price 20 = £9.42; 40 mg (blue), 20 = £23.69

MELPHALAN
Indications: myelomatosis; see also notes above
Cautions; Side-effects: see section 8.1 and notes above; reduce dose in renal impairment
Dose: by mouth, 150–300 micrograms/kg daily for 4–6 days, repeated after 4–8 weeks

PoM **Alkeran**® (Wellcome)
Tablets, melphalan 2 mg, net price 25 = £11.73; 5 mg, 25 = £20.75
Injection, powder for reconstitution, melphalan. Net price 100-mg vial (with solvent and diluent) = £51.38

Cautionary label wordings, see inside back cover

MUSTINE HYDROCHLORIDE
Indications: Hodgkin's disease—see notes above
Cautions; Side-effects: see section 8.1 and notes above; irritant to tissues (also caution in handling—vesicant and a nasal irritant)

PoM **Mustine Hydrochloride** (Boots)
Injection, powder for reconstitution, mustine hydrochloride. Net price 10-mg vial = £1.48

THIOTEPA
Indications: see notes above and section 7.4.4
Cautions; Side-effects: see section 8.1; **interactions:** Appendix 1 (thiotepa)

PoM **Thiotepa** (Lederle)
Injection, powder for reconstitution, thiotepa, net price 15-mg vial = £4.85

TREOSULFAN
Indications: see notes above
Cautions; Side-effects: see section 8.1
Dose: by mouth, courses of 1–2 g daily in 4 divided doses to provide total dose of 21–28 g over initial 8 weeks

PoM **Treosulfan** (Leo)
Capsules, treosulfan 250 mg. Net price 20 = £9.04. Label: 25
Injection, powder for reconstitution, treosulfan. Net price 5 g in infusion bottle with transfer needle = £20.63

UROTHELIAL TOXICITY

Urothelial toxicity, commonly manifest by haemorrhagic cystitis, is a problem peculiar to the use of cyclophosphamide or ifosfamide and is caused by a metabolite (acrolein). **Mesna** reacts specifically with this metabolite in the urinary tract, preventing toxicity. Mesna is given simultaneously with cyclophosphamide or ifosfamide, and further doses are given orally or intravenously 4 and 8 hours after treatment.

MESNA
Indications: see notes above
Side-effects: above max. therapeutic doses, gastro-intestinal disturbances, fatigue, headache, limb pains, depression, irritability, lack of energy, rash

PoM **Uromitexan**® (ASTA Medica)
Injection, mesna 100 mg/mL. Net price 4-mL amp = £1.36; 10-mL amp = £2.95

Note. For oral administration contents of ampoule are taken in fruit juice

8.1.2 Cytotoxic antibiotics

Drugs within this group are widely used. Many cytotoxic antibiotics act as radiomimetics and simultaneous use of radiotherapy should be **avoided** as it may result in markedly enhanced normal tissue toxicity.

Doxorubicin is one of the most successful and widely used antitumour drugs, and is used to treat the acute leukaemias, lymphomas, and a variety of solid tumours. It is given by fast running infusion, commonly at 21-day intervals. Local extravasation will cause severe tissue necrosis. Common toxic effects include nausea and vomiting, myelosuppression, alopecia, and mucositis. This drug is largely excreted by the biliary tract, and an elevated bilirubin concentration is an indication for reducing the dose. Supraventricular tachycardia related to drug administration is an uncommon complication. Higher cumulative doses are associated with development of a cardiomyopathy. It is customary to limit total cumulative doses to 450–550 mg/m^2 body-surface area as symptomatic and potentially fatal heart failure is increasingly common above this level. Patients with pre-existing cardiac disease, the elderly, and those who have received myocardial irradiation should be treated cautiously. Cardiac monitoring, for example by sequential radionuclide ejection fraction measurement, may assist in safely limiting total dosage. Evidence is available to suggest that weekly low dose administration may be associated with less cardiac damage.

Epirubicin is structurally related to doxorubicin and clinical trials suggest that it is as effective in the treatment of breast cancer. A maximum cumulative dose of 0.9–1 g/m^2 is recommended to help avoid cardiotoxicity.

Aclarubicin and **idarubicin** are newly introduced anthracyclines with general properties similar to those of doxorubicin.

Mitozantrone is structurally related to doxorubicin and preliminary work suggests that it has equal activity in breast cancer; it is well tolerated apart from myelosuppression and dose-related cardiotoxicity; cardiac examinations are recommended after a cumulative dose of 160 mg/m^2 if this complication is to be avoided.

Bleomycin is used to treat the lymphomas, certain solid tumours and, by the intracavitary route, malignant effusions. It is unusual in that it causes little marrow suppression. Dermatological toxicity is common; increased pigmentation particularly affecting the flexures and subcutaneous sclerotic plaques may occur. Mucositis is also relatively common and an association with Raynaud's phenomenon is reported. Hypersensitivity reactions manifest by chills and fevers commonly occur a few hours after drug administration and may be prevented by simultaneous administration of a corticosteroid, for example hydrocortisone intravenously. The principal problem associated with the use of bleomycin is progressive pulmonary fibrosis. This is dose related, occurring more commonly at cumulative doses greater than 300 units and in the elderly. Basal lung crepitations or suspicious chest X-ray changes are an indication to stop therapy with this drug. Patients who have received extensive treatment with bleomycin (e.g. cumulative dose more than 100 units) may be at risk of developing respiratory failure if a general anaesthetic is given with high inspired oxygen concentrations. Anaesthetists should be warned of this.

Dactinomycin is principally used to treat paediatric cancers. Its side-effects are similar to those of doxorubicin, except that cardiac toxicity is not a problem.

Plicamycin (mithramycin) is no longer used as a cytotoxic, but has found a useful (though diminishing) role in low dose in the emergency therapy of hypercalcaemia due to malignant disease (for general management of hypercalcaemia, see section 9.5.1.2).

Mitomycin is used to treat upper gastro-intestinal and breast cancers. It causes delayed marrow toxicity and is usually administered at 6-weekly intervals. Prolonged use may result in permanent marrow damage. It is a relatively toxic drug and may cause lung fibrosis and renal damage.

ACLARUBICIN

Indications: acute non-lymphocytic leukaemia in patients who have relapsed or are resistant or refractory to first-line chemotherapy

Cautions; Side-effects: see section 8.1 and notes above; caution in hepatic and renal impairment; irritant to tissues

▼ PoM **Aclacin**® (Lundbeck)
Injection, powder for reconstitution, aclarubicin 20 mg (as hydrochloride). Net price 20-mg vial = £29.20

BLEOMYCIN

Indications: squamous cell carcinoma; see also notes above

Cautions; Side-effects: see section 8.1 and notes above; reduce dose in renal impairment; also caution in handling—irritant to skin

PoM **Bleomycin**® (Lundbeck)
Injection, powder for reconstitution, bleomycin (as sulphate). Net price 15-unit amp = £15.97
Note. Ampoules previously labelled as containing '15 mg' of bleomycin contained 15 units. The ampoules are now labelled only as units.

DACTINOMYCIN

(Actinomycin D)
Indications: see notes above
Cautions; Side-effects: see section 8.1 and notes above; irritant to tissues

PoM **Cosmegen Lyovac**® (MSD)
Injection, powder for reconstitution, dactinomycin, net price 500-microgram vial = £1.50

DOXORUBICIN HYDROCHLORIDE

Indications: see notes above and section 7.4.4
Cautions; Side-effects: see section 8.1 and notes above; reduce dose in hepatic impairment; also caution in handling—irritant to skin and tissues

PoM **Doxorubicin Rapid Dissolution** (Farmitalia Carlo Erba)
Injection, powder for reconstitution, doxorubicin hydrochloride, net price 10-mg vial = £17.66; 50-mg vial = £88.30
Note. This preparation has replaced Adriamycin®

PoM **Doxorubicin Solution for Injection** (Farmitalia Carlo Erba)
Injection, doxorubicin hydrochloride 2 mg/mL, net price 5-ml vial = £19.43; 25-mL vial = £97.15

EPIRUBICIN HYDROCHLORIDE
Indications: see notes above
Cautions; Side-effects: see section 8.1 and notes above; reduce dose in hepatic impairment; irritant to tissues

PoM **Pharmorubicin® Rapid Dissolution** (Farmitalia Carlo Erba)
Injection, powder for reconstitution, epirubicin hydrochloride. Net price 10-mg vial = £17.66; 20-mg vial = £35.32; 50-mg vial = £88.30

PoM **Pharmorubicin® Solution for Injection** (Farmitalia Carlo Erba)
Injection, epirubicin hydrochloride 2 mg/mL, net price 5-mL vial = £19.43; 25-mL vial = £97.15

IDARUBICIN HYDROCHLORIDE
Indications: acute leukaemias—see notes above
Cautions; Side-effects: see section 8.1 and notes above; caution in hepatic and renal impairment; also caution in handling—irritant to skin and tissues

PoM **Zavedos®** (Farmitalia Carlo Erba)
Injection, powder for reconstitution, idarubicin hydrochloride, net price 5-mg vial = £63.30; 10-mg vial = £126.60

MITOMYCIN
Indications: see notes above
Cautions; Side-effects: see section 8.1 and notes above; irritant to tissues

PoM **Mitomycin C Kyowa®** (Martindale)
Injection, powder for reconstitution, mitomycin. Net price 2-mg vial = £6.02; 10-mg vial = £19.81; 20-mg vial = £37.78 (hosp. only)

MITOZANTRONE
Indications: see notes above
Cautions; Side-effects: see section 8.1 and notes above; intrathecal administration not recommended

PoM **Novantrone®** (Lederle)
Intravenous infusion, mitozantrone 2 mg (as hydrochloride)/mL, net price 10-mL vial = £150.43; 12.5-mL vial = £188.05; 15-mL vial = £225.60

PLICAMYCIN
(Mithramycin)
Indications: refractory hypercalcaemia associated with malignancy—see notes above
Cautions; Side-effects: see section 8.1 and notes above; caution in hepatic or renal impairment (see Appendixes 2 and 3); irritant to tissues
Dose: by intravenous infusion, 25 micrograms/kg daily for 3–4 days, repeated if necessary at intervals of 7 days or longer; maintenance, 25 micrograms/kg 1–3 times each week

PoM **Mithracin®** (Pfizer)
Injection, powder for reconstitution, plicamycin, net price 2.5-mg vial = £7.51 (hosp. only)

8.1.3 Antimetabolites

Antimetabolites are incorporated into new nuclear material or combine irreversibly with vital cellular enzymes, preventing normal cellular division.

Methotrexate inhibits the enzyme dihydrofolate reductase, essential for the synthesis of purines and pyrimidines. It may be given orally, intravenously, intramuscularly, or intrathecally. High-dose methotrexate cannot generally be recommended except in clinical trials.

Methotrexate is used as maintenance therapy for childhood acute lymphoblastic leukaemia. Other uses include choriocarcinoma, non-Hodgkin lymphomas, and a number of solid tumours. Intrathecal methotrexate is used in the CNS prophylaxis of childhood acute lymphoblastic leukaemia, and as a therapy for established meningeal cancer or lymphoma.

Methotrexate causes myelosuppression, mucositis, and rarely pneumonitis. It is **contra-indicated** if significant renal impairment is present, as the kidney is its route of excretion. It should also be **avoided** if a significant pleural effusion or ascites is present as it tends to accumulate at these sites, and its subsequent return to the circulation will be associated with myelosuppression. For similar reasons blood counts should be carefully monitored when intrathecal methotrexate is given.

Oral or parenteral folinic acid (see below) will help prevent, and speed recovery from, methotrexate mucositis or myelosuppression.

Cytarabine acts by interfering with pyrimidine synthesis. It may be given subcutaneously, intravenously, or intrathecally. Its predominant use is in the induction of remission and maintenance therapy of acute myeloblastic leukaemia. It is a potent myelosuppressant and requires careful haematological monitoring.

Fluorouracil may be given orally but is usually given intravenously. It is used to treat a number of solid tumours, including colon and breast cancer. It may also be used topically for certain malignant skin lesions. Toxicity is unusual, but may include myelosuppression, mucositis, and rarely a cerebellar syndrome.

Mercaptopurine is used almost exclusively as maintenance therapy for the acute leukaemias.

The dose should be reduced if the patient is receiving concurrent allopurinol as this drug interferes with the metabolism of mercaptopurine.

Thioguanine is used orally to induce remission and for maintenance in acute myeloid leukaemia.

Azathioprine, a derivative of the antimetabolite mercaptopurine, is commonly used as an immunosuppressant (section 8.2.1).

CYTARABINE

Indications: acute leukaemias
Cautions; Side-effects: see section 8.1 and notes above

PoM **Cytarabine** (Non-proprietary)
Injection, powder for reconstitution, cytarabine. Net price 100-mg vial = £2.89; 500-mg vial = £15.45; 1-g vial = £31.50
Available from David Bull
PoM **Alexan**® (Pfizer)
Injection, cytarabine 20 mg/mL. Net price 2-mL amp = £1.06; 5-mL amp = £2.65
PoM **Alexan**® **100** (Pfizer)
Injection, cytarabine 100 mg/mL. Net price 1-mL amp = £2.65; 10-mL amp = £26.46. For intravenous infusion only
PoM **Cytosar**® (Upjohn)
Injection, powder for reconstitution, cytarabine. Net price 100-mg vial = £3.17; 500-mg vial = £15.45. For intravenous injection or infusion and subcutaneous injection only

FLUOROURACIL

Indications: see notes above
Cautions; Side-effects: see section 8.1; also caution in handling—irritant; **interactions:** Appendix 1 (fluorouracil)
Dose: by mouth, maintenance 15 mg/kg weekly; max. in one day 1 g

PoM **Fluorouracil** (Non-proprietary)
Injection, fluorouracil 25 mg/mL (as sodium salt). Net price 10-mL vial = £1.91; 20-mL vial = £3.67; 100-mL vial = £17.78
Available from David Bull
PoM **Fluoro-uracil** (Roche)
Capsules, blue/orange, fluorouracil 250 mg. Net price 30-cap pack = £35.38. Label: 21
Injection, fluorouracil 25 mg/mL (as sodium salt). Net price 10-mL amp = £1.42
Note. The injection solution can also be given by mouth in fruit juice
PoM **Efudix**® (Roche)
Cream, fluorouracil 5%. Net price 20 g = £3.75

MERCAPTOPURINE

Indications: acute leukaemias
Cautions; Side-effects: see section 8.1 and notes above; reduce dose in renal impairment; avoid in porphyria (see section 9.8.2); **interactions:** Appendix 1 (mercaptopurine)
Dose: initially 2.5 mg/kg daily

PoM **Puri-Nethol**® (Wellcome)
Tablets, fawn, scored, mercaptopurine 50 mg. Net price 25 = £19.22

METHOTREXATE

Indications: see notes above
Cautions; Side-effects: see section 8.1 and notes above; reduce dose in renal impairment; dose-related toxicity in hepatic impairment (avoid in non-malignant conditions, e.g. psoriasis); avoid in porphyria (see section 9.8.2); **interactions:** Appendix 1 (methotrexate)
Dose: by mouth, leukaemia in children (maintenance), 15 mg/m^2 weekly in combination with other drugs; psoriasis, 10–25 mg weekly

PoM **Methotrexate** (Lederle)
Tablets, yellow, scored, methotrexate 2.5 mg, net price 20 = £2.17
Injection, methotrexate 25 mg (as sodium salt)/mL. Net price 1-mL vial = £1.94; 2-mL vial = £2.69; 4-mL vial = £5.14; 8-mL vial = £10.28; 20-mL vial = £25.71; 40-mL vial = £45.71; 200-mL vial = £205.71
Injection, powder for reconstitution, methotrexate (as sodium salt). Net price 500-mg vial = £32.00
PoM **Maxtrex**® (Farmitalia Carlo Erba)
Tablets, both yellow, scored, methotrexate 2.5 mg, net price 20 = £2.14; 10 mg, 20 = £9.70

THIOGUANINE

Indications: acute leukaemias
Cautions; Side-effects: see section 8.1 and notes above; reduce dose in renal impairment
Dose: initially 2–2.5 mg/kg daily

PoM **Lanvis**® (Wellcome)
Tablets, yellow, scored, thioguanine 40 mg. Net price 25-tab pack = £46.48

FOLINIC ACID RESCUE

Folinic acid (leucovorin) is used to counteract the folate-antagonist action of methotrexate and thus speed recovery from methotrexate-induced mucositis or myelosuppression. It does not counteract the antibacterial activity of folate antagonists such as trimethoprim.

Folinic acid also interacts with fluorouracil; when the two are used together in metastatic colonic cancer a favourable effect has been demonstrated on response-rate and probably also on survival.

FOLINIC ACID

Indications: see notes above
Cautions: avoid simultaneous administration of methotrexate; as for Folic Acid (section 9.1.2) **not** indicated for pernicious anaemia or other megaloblastic anaemias where vitamin B$_{12}$ deficient
Side-effects: rarely, pyrexia after parenteral adminstration
Dose: as an antidote to methotrexate (started 8–24 hours after the beginning of methotrexate

8.1 Cytotoxic drugs 317

infusion), in general up to 120 mg in divided doses over 12–24 hours *by intramuscular or intravenous injection or infusion*, followed by 12–15 mg *intramuscularly or* 15 mg *by mouth* every 6 hours for the next 48 hours
Suspected methotrexate overdosage, immediate administration of an equal or higher dose of folinic acid

PoM **Calcium Folinate** (Non-proprietary)
Tablets, scored, folinic acid (as calcium salt) 15 mg. Net price 10-tab pack = £42.28

PoM **Calcium Leucovorin** (Lederle)
Tablets, scored, folinic acid 15 mg (as calcium salt). Net price 10-tab pack = £42.28
Injection, folinic acid 3 mg (as calcium salt)/mL. Net price 1-mL amp = £1.09
Injection, powder for reconstitution, folinic acid (as calcium salt). Net price 15-mg vial = £4.57; 30-mg vial = £8.57; 350-mg vial (Lederfolin®) = £99.98

PoM **Refolinon®** (Farmitalia Carlo Erba)
Tablets, yellow, scored, folinic acid 15 mg (as calcium salt). Net price 30 = £105.00
Injection, folinic acid 3 mg (as calcium salt)/mL. Net price 10-mL amp = £6.70

8.1.4 Vinca alkaloids and etoposide

These interfere with microtubule assembly, causing metaphase arrest. All have similar activity but vary in the predominant site of toxicity.

The vinca alkaloids are used to treat the acute leukaemias, lymphomas, and some solid tumours (e.g. breast and lung cancer). They commonly cause peripheral and autonomic neuropathy. This side-effect is most obvious with vincristine, and is manifest by peripheral paraesthesia, loss of deep tendon reflexes, and abdominal bloating and constipation. If these symptoms are severe, doses should be reduced. Significant new motor weakness is a **contra-indication** to further use of these drugs. Recovery of the nervous system is generally slow but complete. Intrathecal administration of **all** vinca alkaloids is **contra-indicated** (usually fatal).

Vincristine causes virtually no myelosuppression. Its use may be associated with alopecia; hyponatraemia, as a result of inappropriate ADH secretion, has been described.

Vinblastine is a more myelosuppressive drug than vincristine, but causes less neurotoxicity.

Vindesine is the most recent addition to the vinca alkaloid group. It has a similar range of clinical activity, and side-effects intermediate between those of the above two drugs.

Etoposide may be given orally or intravenously, the dose when used orally being double that when given intravenously. There is limited clinical evidence to suggest that administration in divided doses over 3–5 days may be beneficial; courses may not be repeated more frequently than at intervals of 21 days. It has useful activity in small cell carcinoma of the bronchus, the lymphomas, and testicular teratoma. Toxic effects include alopecia, myelosuppression, nausea, and vomiting.

ETOPOSIDE
Indications: see notes above
Cautions; Contra-indications; Side-effects: see section 8.1 and notes above; irritant to tissues

PoM **Vepesid®** (Bristol-Myers)
Capsules, etoposide 50 mg, net price 20 = £113.95; 100 mg, 10-tab pack = £99.57
Injection, etoposide 20 mg/mL. To be diluted. Net price 5-mL vial = £14.58
Caution: may dissolve certain types of filter

VINBLASTINE SULPHATE
Indications: see notes above
Cautions; Contra-indications; Side-effects: see section 8.1 and notes above; caution in handling—avoid contact with eyes; irritant to tissues
Note. IMPORTANT. Intrathecal injection **contra-indicated**

PoM **Vinblastine** (Non-proprietary)
Injection, vinblastine sulphate 1 mg/mL. Net price 10-mL vial = £11.00
Available from David Bull
Injection, powder for reconstitution, vinblastine sulphate. Net price 10-mg vial (with diluent) = £11.25
Available from David Bull, Lederle

PoM **Velbe®** (Lilly)
Injection, powder for reconstitution, vinblastine sulphate. Net price 10-mg amp (with diluent) = £10.29

VINCRISTINE SULPHATE
Indications: see notes above
Cautions; Contra-indications; Side-effects: see section 8.1 and notes above; caution in handling—avoid contact with eyes; irritant to tissues
Note. IMPORTANT. Intrathecal injection **contra-indicated**

PoM **Vincristine** (Non-proprietary)
Injection, vincristine sulphate 1 mg/mL. Net price 1-mL vial = £9.80; 2-mL vial = £19.00; 5-mL vial = £39.60; 1-mL syringe = £10·49; 2-mL syringe = £19.00
Available from David Bull
Injection, powder for reconstitution, vincristine sulphate, net price, 1-mg vial = £3.42; 2-mg vial = £6.86; 5-mg vial = £17.14 (all with diluent)
Available from David Bull, Lederle

PoM **Oncovin®** (Lilly)
Injection, vincristine sulphate 1 mg/mL, net price 1-mL vial = £10.31; 2-mL vial = £20.40

VINDESINE SULPHATE
Indications: see notes above
Cautions; Contra-indications; Side-effects: see section 8.1 and notes above; caution in handling—avoid contact with eyes; irritant to tissues
Note. IMPORTANT. Intrathecal injection **contra-indicated**

PoM **Eldisine®** (Lilly)
Injection, powder for reconstitution, vindesine sulphate, net price 5-mg vial (with diluent) = £51.77 (hosp. only)

8.1.5 Other antineoplastic drugs

Amsacrine has an action and toxic effects similar to those of doxorubicin (section 8.1.2). It is used as second-line treatment in refractory acute myeloid leukaemia. Side-effects include myelosuppression and mucositis; electrolytes should be monitored as fatal arrhythmias have occurred in association with hypokalaemia.

AMSACRINE
Indications: see notes above
Cautions; Side-effects: see section 8.1 and notes above; reduce dose in renal or hepatic impairment; also caution in handling—irritant to skin and tissues

PoM **Amsidine**® (P-D)
Concentrate for intravenous infusion, amsacrine 5 mg (as lactate)/mL, when reconstituted by mixing two solutions. Net price 1.5-mL amp with 13.5-mL vial = £32.60 (hosp. only)
Note. Use glass apparatus for reconstitution

Carboplatin is a derivative of cisplatin which has probably equivalent activity in ovarian cancer. It is also active in small cell lung cancer and is under trial in a variety of other malignancies. Carboplatin is better tolerated than cisplatin; nausea and vomiting are reduced in severity and nephrotoxicity, neurotoxicity, and ototoxicity are much less of a problem than with cisplatin. It is, however, more myelosuppressive than cisplatin.

CARBOPLATIN
Indications: see notes above
Cautions; Side-effects: see section 8.1 and notes above; reduce dose in renal impairment

PoM **Paraplatin**® (Bristol-Myers)
Injection, carboplatin 10 mg/mL. Net price 5-mL vial = £22.86; 15-mL vial = £68.57; 45-mL vial = £205.71

Cisplatin has an alkylating action. It has useful antitumour activity in certain solid tumours including ovarian cancer and testicular teratoma. It is, however, a toxic drug. Common problems include severe nausea and vomiting, nephrotoxicity (pretreatment hydration mandatory and renal function should be closely monitored), myelotoxicity, ototoxicity (high tone hearing loss and tinnitus), peripheral neuropathy, and hypomagnesaemia. These toxic effects commonly necessitate dose reduction or drug withdrawal. It is preferable that treatment with this drug be supervised by specialists familiar with its use.

CISPLATIN
Indications: see notes above
Cautions; Side-effects: see section 8.1 and notes above; reduce dose in renal impairment; **interactions:** Appendix 1 (cisplatin)

PoM **Cisplatin** (Non-proprietary)
Injection, cisplatin 1 mg/mL. Net price 10-mL vial = £2.90; 50-mL vial = £14.00; 100-mL vial = £27.00
Injection, powder for reconstitution, cisplatin 10-mg vial, net price = £2.50; 50-mg vial = £12.10; 150-mg vial = £68.57; 450-mg vial = £205.71
Various strengths available from David Bull, Farmitalia Carlo Erba, Lederle

Crisantaspase is the enzyme asparaginase produced by *Erwinia chrysanthemi*. It is used (usually intramuscularly) almost exclusively in acute lymphoblastic leukaemia. Facilities for the management of anaphylaxis should be available. Side-effects also include nausea, vomiting, CNS depression, and liver function and blood lipid changes; careful monitoring is therefore necessary and the urine is tested for glucose to exclude hyperglycaemia.

CRISANTASPASE
Indications; Cautions; Side-effects: see notes above

PoM **Erwinase**® (Porton)
Injection, powder for reconstitution, crisantaspase. Net price 20 × 10000-unit vial = £650.00

Dacarbazine is not commonly used on account of its toxicity. It has been used to treat melanoma and, in combination therapy, the soft tissue sarcomas. It is also a component of a commonly used second-line combination for Hodgkin's disease (ABVD—doxorubicin [Adriamycin®], bleomycin, vinblastine, and dacarbazine). The predominant side-effects are myelosuppression and intense nausea and vomiting.

DACARBAZINE
Indications: see notes above
Cautions; Side-effects: see section 8.1; also caution in handling—irritant to skin and tissues

PoM **DTIC-Dome**® (Bayer)
Injection, powder for reconstitution, dacarbazine. Net price 100-mg vial = £4.83; 200-mg vial = £7.40

Hydroxyurea is an orally active drug used mainly in the treatment of chronic myeloid leukaemia. Myelosuppression, nausea, and skin reactions are the most common toxic effects.

HYDROXYUREA
Indications: see notes above
Cautions; Side-effects: see section 8.1 and notes above
Dose: 20–30 mg/kg daily *or* 80 mg/kg every third day

PoM **Hydrea**® (Squibb)
Capsules, pink/green, hydroxyurea 500 mg. Net price 20 = £2.39

Procarbazine is most often used in Hodgkin's disease, for example in MOPP (mustine, vincristine [Oncovin®], procarbazine, and prednisolone) chemotherapy. It is given orally. Toxic effects include nausea, myelosuppression, and a hypersensitivity rash preventing further use of this drug. It is a mild monoamine-oxidase inhibitor but dietary restriction is not considered necessary. Alcohol ingestion may cause a disulfiram-like reaction.

PROCARBAZINE
Indications: see notes above
Cautions; Side-effects: see section 8.1 and notes above; reduce dose in renal impairment; **interactions:** Appendix 1 (procarbazine)
Dose: initially 50 mg daily, increased by 50 mg daily to 250–300 mg daily in divided doses; maintenance (on remission) 50–150 mg daily to cumulative total of at least 6 g

PoM **Natulan**® (Cambridge)
Capsules, ivory, procarbazine 50 mg (as hydrochloride). Net price 50-cap pack = £3.44. Label: 4

Razoxane has limited activity in the leukaemias, and is little used.

RAZOXANE
Indications: see notes above
Cautions; Side-effects: see section 8.1
Dose: acute leukaemias, 150–500 mg/m² daily for 3–5 days

PoM **Razoxin**® (ICI)
Tablets, scored, razoxane 125 mg. Net price 30-tab pack = £27.56

8.2 Drugs affecting the immune response

8.2.1 Cytotoxic immunosuppressants
8.2.2 Corticosteroids and other immunosuppressants
8.2.3 Immunostimulants
8.2.4 Interferons
8.2.5 Aldesleukin

8.2.1 Cytotoxic immunosuppressants

These drugs are used to suppress rejection in organ transplant recipients and are also used to treat a variety of auto-immune and collagen diseases (see section 10.1.3). They are non-specific in their action and careful monitoring of peripheral blood counts is required, with dose adjustments for marrow toxicity. Patients receiving these drugs will be prone to atypical infections.

Azathioprine is widely used for transplant recipients and is also used to treat a number of auto-immune conditions, usually when corticosteroid therapy alone has provided inadequate control. This drug is metabolised to mercaptopurine, and doses should be reduced when concurrent therapy with allopurinol is given. The predominant toxic effect is myelosuppression, although hepatic toxicity is also well recognised.

Cyclophosphamide and chlorambucil (section 8.1.1) are less commonly prescribed as immunosuppressants.

AZATHIOPRINE
Indications: see notes above
Cautions; Side-effects: see section 8.1 and notes above; also rashes; reduce dose in severe hepatic or renal impairment; **interactions:** Appendix 1 (azathioprine)
Dose: by mouth, 2–2.5 mg/kg daily. Chronic active hepatitis, 1–1.5 mg/kg daily Suppression of transplant rejection, loading dose, up to 5 mg/kg; maintenance 1–4 mg/kg daily
By intravenous injection, suppression of transplant rejection, loading dose, up to 5 mg/kg; maintenance dose (if oral route not possible), 1–2.5 mg/kg daily

PoM **Azathioprine** (Non-proprietary)
Tablets, azathioprine 50 mg. Net price 20 = £5.71
Available from APS, Ashbourne (Immunoprin®), Berk (Berkaprine®), Cox, CP, Evans, Kerfoot, Penn (Azamune®)

PoM **Imuran**® (Wellcome)
Tablets, both f/c, azathioprine 25 mg (orange), net price 100-tab pack = £39.35; 50 mg (yellow), 100-tab pack = £65.61
Injection, powder for reconstitution, azathioprine (as sodium salt). Net price 50-mg vial = £16.54

8.2.2 Corticosteroids and other immunosuppressants

Prednisolone is widely used in oncology. It has a marked antitumour effect in acute lymphoblastic leukaemia, Hodgkin's disease, and the non-Hodgkin lymphomas. It is also active in hormone-sensitive breast cancer and may cause useful disease regression. Finally, it has a role in the palliation of symptomatic end-stage malignant disease when it may produce a sense of well-being.

The corticosteroids are also powerful immunosuppressants. They are used to prevent organ transplant rejection, and in high dose to treat rejection episodes. For notes on corticosteroids see section 6.3.

Cyclosporin is a fungal metabolite and potent immunosuppressant which is virtually non-myelotoxic but markedly nephrotoxic. It has found particular use in the field of organ and tissue transplantation, for prevention of graft rejection following bone marrow, kidney, liver, pancreas, heart, and heart-lung transplantation, and for prophylaxis of graft-versus-host disease.

Antilymphocyte immunoglobulin, obtained from immunised horses, has mainly been used

CYCLOSPORIN

Indications: see notes above, and under Dose
Cautions: monitor liver and kidney function; other immunosuppressants; over-suppression may increase susceptibility to infection and lymphoma; avoid during pregnancy, breast-feeding; avoid in porphyria (see section 9.8.2); **interactions:** Appendix 1 (cyclosporin)
Side-effects: hepatic and renal impairment; tremor, gastro-intestinal disturbances, hypertrichosis; gum hyperplasia; hyperkalaemia; *occasionally* facial oedema, hypertension, fluid retention, and convulsions; serum creatinine, urea, bilirubin, and liver enzymes may be increased; burning sensation in hands and feet during first week of oral administration
Dose: organ transplantation, used alone, 10–15 mg/kg as a single dose *by mouth* 4–12 hours before transplantation followed by 10–15 mg/kg daily for 1–2 weeks post-operatively then reduced to 2–6 mg/kg daily for maintenance (dose may be adjusted by monitoring blood concentrations and renal function); maintenance dose lower and reached sooner with concomitant immunosuppressant therapy (e.g. corticosteroids); if necessary one-third oral dose can be given *by intravenous infusion* over 2–6 hours
Bone-marrow transplantation, prevention and treatment of graft-versus-host disease, 3–5 mg/kg daily *by intravenous infusion* over 2–6 hours from day before transplantation to 2 weeks post-operatively (or 12.5–15 mg/kg daily *by mouth*) then 12.5 mg/kg daily *by mouth* for 3–6 months then tailed off
Severe psoriasis where conventional therapy ineffective or inappropriate (*by mouth only*), consult data sheet for additional precautions and dose
COUNSELLING. Total daily dose may be taken as a single dose or in 2 divided doses. To mask taste, mix with cold milk, chocolate drink, or fruit juice immediately before taking. Do not use plastic cup. Keep medicine measure away from other liquids

PoM **Sandimmun**® (Sandoz)
Capsules, cyclosporin 25 mg (pale pink), net price 30-cap pack = £21.07; 50 mg (yellow), 30-cap pack = £41.25; 100 mg (dusky pink), 30-cap pack = £78.29
Oral solution, oily, yellow, sugar-free, cyclosporin 100 mg/mL. Net price 50 mL = £117.31. Counselling, administration
Concentrate for intravenous infusion (oily), cyclosporin 50 mg/mL. To be diluted before use. Net price 1-mL amp = £1.82; 5-mL amp = £8.60
Note. Contains polyethoxylated castor oil which has been associated with anaphylaxis

PREDNISOLONE
See section 6.3.4

8.2.3 Immunostimulants

A suspension of inactivated *Corynebacterium parvum* organisms may be used by the intracavitary route to treat malignant effusions.

CORYNEBACTERIUM PARVUM VACCINE

Indications: see notes above
Cautions: avoid within 10 days of thoracotomy
Side-effects: pyrexia common; abdominal pain, nausea and vomiting
Dose: *by intrapleural or intraperitoneal injection*, 7–14 mg

PoM **Coparvax**® (Wellcome)
Injection, powder for reconstitution, *Corynebacterium parvum* (inactivated). Net price 7-mg vial = £63.09

8.2.4 Interferons

The interferons (alfa, beta, and gamma) are naturally occurring proteins with complex effects on immunity and cell function. Recently alfa interferon (formerly called lymphoblastoid interferon) has shown some antitumour effect in certain lymphomas and solid tumours. Side-effects are dose-related, but commonly include influenza-like symptoms, lethargy, and depression. Myelosuppression may also occur, particularly affecting granulocyte counts. Finally, cardiovascular problems (hypotension, hypertension, and arrhythmias), and hepatotoxicity have been reported. Avoid in pregnancy unless compelling reasons for use (see Appendix 4); **interactions:** Appendix 1 (interferons).

PoM **Intron A**® (Schering-Plough)
Injection, powder for reconstitution, interferon alfa-2b (rbe). Net price 3-million unit vial = £16.96; 5-million unit vial = £28.26; 10-million unit vial = £56.52 (all with water for injection); 30-million unit vial = £169.56
For use in AIDS-related Kaposi's sarcoma, hairy cell leukaemia, chronic myelogenous leukaemia, condyloma acuminata, chronic active hepatitis B, and maintenance of remission in multiple myeloma

PoM **Roferon-A**® (Roche)
Injection, powder for reconstitution, interferon alfa-2a (rbe). Net price 3 million-unit vial = £16.96; 4.5 million-unit vial = £25.44; 9 million-unit vial = £50.88; 18 million-unit vial = £101.77 (all with syringe, needles, and water for injection)
For use in AIDS-related Kaposi's sarcoma, hairy cell leukaemia, chronic myelogenous leukaemia, recurrent or metastatic renal cell carcinoma, and chronic active hepatitis B

PoM **Wellferon**® (Wellcome)
Injection, interferon alfa-N1 (lns) 3 million units/mL, net price 1-mL vial = £19.93; 10 million units/mL, net price 1-mL vial = £64.55
For use in hairy cell leukaemia and chronic active hepatitis B

8.2.5 Aldesleukin

Aldesleukin (recombinant interleukin-2) is licensed for use by intravenous infusion in metastatic renal cell carcinoma. This is a very toxic drug which, although responsible for tumour shrinkage in a small proportion of patients, has not been shown to increase survival. Toxicity is universal and often severe. A common acute problem is the development of a capillary leak syndrome causing pulmonary oedema and hypotension. Bone marrow, hepatic, renal, thyroid, and CNS toxicity is also common. It is for use in **specialist units only**.

▼ PoM **Proleukin**® (EuroCetus)
Injection, powder for reconstitution, aldesleukin. Net price 18-million unit vial = £125.00
For metastatic renal cell carcinoma, **excluding** patients in whom all three of the following prognostic factors are present: performance status of Eastern Co-operative Oncology Group of 1 or greater, more than one organ with metastatic disease sites, and a period of less than 24 months between initial diagnosis of primary tumour and date of evaluation of treatment.

8.3 Sex hormones and hormone antagonists in malignant disease

8.3.1 Oestrogens
8.3.2 Progestogens
8.3.3 Androgens
8.3.4 Hormone antagonists

Hormonal manipulation has an important role in the treatment of metastatic breast, prostate, and endometrial cancer, and a more marginal role in the treatment of hypernephroma. These treatments are not curative, but may provide excellent palliation of symptoms in selected patients, sometimes for a period of years. Tumour response, and treatment toxicity should be carefully monitored and treatment changed if progression occurs or side-effects exceed benefit.

8.3.1 Oestrogens

Stilboestrol may be used in low dosage to treat symptomatic metastases from prostate cancer. It is less commonly used in postmenopausal women with breast cancer. Toxicity is common and dose-related side-effects include nausea, fluid retention, and venous and arterial thrombosis. Impotence and gynaecomastia always occur in men, and withdrawal bleeding may be a problem in women. Hypercalcaemia and bone pain may also occur in breast cancer.

Fosfestrol is also used for prostate cancer; it is activated by the enzyme acid phosphatase to produce stilboestrol. Side-effects are as for stilboestrol; in addition, perineal pain may complicate intravenous use.

Ethinyloestradiol is the most potent oestrogen available; unlike other oestrogens it is only slowly metabolised in the liver. It is used in breast cancer.

Polyestradiol is a long-acting oestrogen.

STILBOESTROL

Indications: see notes above
Cautions; Side-effects: cardiovascular disease (sodium retention with oedema, thromboembolism), hepatic impairment (jaundice), feminising effects in men; see also notes above
Dose: breast cancer, 10–20 mg daily
Prostate cancer, 1–3 mg daily

PoM **Stilboestrol Tablets**, stilboestrol 1 mg, net price 56 = £7.76; 5 mg, 28 = £6.61

ETHINYLOESTRADIOL

Indications: see notes above; other indications, see section 6.4.1.1
Cautions; Side-effects: see under Stilboestrol and notes above
Dose: breast cancer, 1–3 mg daily

Preparations
See section 6.4.1.1

FOSFESTROL TETRASODIUM

Indications: prostate cancer
Cautions; Contra-indications; Side-effects: see under Stilboestrol and notes above; nausea and vomiting; after intravenous injection, perineal irritation and pain in bony metastases
Dose: by slow intravenous injection, 552–1104 mg daily for at least 5 days; maintenance 276 mg 1–4 times weekly
By mouth, maintenance 100–200 mg 3 times daily, reducing to 100–300 mg daily in divided doses

PoM **Honvan**® (ASTA Medica)
Tablets, fosfestrol tetrasodium 100 mg. Net price 20 = £1.87
Injection, fosfestrol tetrasodium 55.2 mg/mL. Net price 5-mL amp = 92p

POLYESTRADIOL PHOSPHATE

Indications: prostate cancer
Cautions; Side-effects: see under Stilboestrol and notes above
Dose: by deep intramuscular injection, 80–160 mg every 4 weeks; maintenance 40–80 mg

PoM **Estradurin**® (Kabi Pharmacia)
Injection, powder for reconstitution, polyestradiol phosphate (with mepivacaine and nicotinamide). Net price 40-mg vial = £2.18; 80-mg vial = £3.51 (both with diluent)

8.3.2 Progestogens

Progestogens are used largely as second- or third-line therapy in breast cancer. They are also used to treat endometrial cancer and hypernephroma, but are little used for prostate cancer. **Medroxyprogesterone** or **megestrol** are usually chosen and can be given orally; high-dose or parenteral treatment cannot be recommended. Side-effects are mild but may include nausea, fluid retention, and weight gain.

GESTRONOL HEXANOATE

Indications: see notes above; benign prostatic hypertrophy

Cautions; Contra-indications; Side-effects: see under Progesterone (section 6.4.1.2) and notes above

Dose: endometrial cancer, *by intramuscular injection*, 200–400 mg every 5–7 days
Benign prostatic hypertrophy, *by intramuscular injection*, 200 mg every week, increased to 300–400 mg every week if necessary

PoM **Depostat**® (Schering Health Care)
Injection (oily), gestronol hexanoate 100 mg/mL. Net price 2-mL amp = £4.28

MEDROXYPROGESTERONE ACETATE

Indications: see notes above; other indications, see section 6.4.1.2

Cautions; Contra-indications; Side-effects: see under Progesterone (section 6.4.1.2) and notes above; glucocorticoid effects at high dose may lead to a cushingoid syndrome

Dose: by mouth, endometrial, prostate, and renal cancer, 100–500 mg daily; breast cancer, various doses in range 0.4–1.5 g daily
By deep intramuscular injection into the gluteal muscle, various doses in range 1 g daily down to 250 mg weekly

PoM **Depo-Provera**® (Upjohn)
Injection, medroxyprogesterone acetate 150 mg/mL. Net price 3.3-mL (500-mg) vial = £12.49

PoM **Farlutal**® (Farmitalia Carlo Erba)
Tablets, both scored, medroxyprogesterone acetate 100 mg, net price 20 = £8.32; 250 mg, 50 = £52.03
Tablets, scored, medroxyprogesterone acetate 500 mg. Net price 56 = £116.54. Label: 27
Injection, medroxyprogesterone acetate 200 mg/mL. Net price 2.5-mL vial = £14.24; 5-mL vial = £23.73

PoM **Provera**® (Upjohn)
Tablets, medroxyprogesterone acetate 100 mg (scored), net price 20 = £8.32; 200 mg (scored), 20 = £16.47; 400 mg, 30 = £48.89
Tablets, medroxyprogesterone acetate 5 mg and 10 mg, see section 6.4.1.2

MEGESTROL ACETATE

Indications: see notes above

Cautions; Contra-indications; Side-effects: see under Progesterone (section 6.4.1.2) and notes above

Dose: breast cancer, 160 mg daily in single or divided doses; endometrial cancer, 40–320 mg daily in divided doses

PoM **Megace**® (Bristol-Myers)
Tablets, both scored, megestrol acetate 40 mg, net price 20 = £5.08; 160 mg (off-white), 30-tab pack = £29.30

NORETHISTERONE

Indications: see notes above; other indications, see section 6.4.1.2

Cautions; Contra-indications; Side-effects: see section 6.4.1.2 and notes above

Dose: breast cancer, 40 mg daily, increased to 60 mg daily if required

Preparations
See section 6.4.1.2

NORETHISTERONE ACETATE

Indications: see notes above

Cautions; Contra-indications; Side-effects: see under Norethisterone (section 6.4.1.2) and notes above

Dose: breast cancer, 10 mg 3 times daily, increased to 60 mg daily if required

PoM **SH 420**® (Schering Health Care)
Tablets, scored, norethisterone acetate 10 mg. Net price 20 = £4.95

8.3.3 Androgens

The androgens are given parenterally and are predominantly used as second- or third-line therapy for metastatic breast cancer.

TESTOSTERONE ESTERS

Indications: see notes above; other indications, see section 6.4.2

Cautions; Contra-indications; Side-effects: see under Testosterone and Esters (section 6.4.2)

Dose: see under Preparations

PoM **Primoteston Depot**® : see section 6.4.2
PoM **Virormone**® : see section 6.4.2

8.3.4 Hormone antagonists

SEX HORMONE DEPENDENT TUMOURS

BREAST CANCER. **Tamoxifen** is an oestrogen receptor antagonist and at a dose of 20 mg daily is the hormonal treatment of choice for breast cancer in postmenopausal women with metastatic disease; it is also increasingly commonly used as a first-line treatment for premenopausal women in whom it is equivalent in effect to oophorectomy. Overall, approximately 30% of patients with metastatic breast cancer respond to hormonal manipulation. This figure is increased to 60% in patients with oestrogen receptor positive tumours; receptor negative tumours respond in less than 10%.

Adjuvant hormonal treatment with tamoxifen is also the treatment of choice in postmenopausal patients with high-risk breast cancer after treatment of the primary. Such treatment has consistently prolonged the period between diagnosis and the development of metastases; a modest increase in survival has been reported in some studies.

Side-effects are unusual with tamoxifen but patients with bony metastases may experience an exacerbation of pain, sometimes associated with hypercalcaemia. This reaction commonly precedes tumour response. Amenorrhoea commonly develops in premenopausal women.

Patients with non-threatening metastases unresponsive to tamoxifen may still respond to a secondary hormonal treatment. Certainly patients who initially respond to tamoxifen should receive second-line hormone treatment. No clear guidelines are available; for premenopausal patients oophorectomy or a progestogen (section 8.3.2) may be used; for postmenopausal patients a progestogen or aminoglutethimide (see below) may be used. Patients who respond can be given further hormones on relapse; refractory patients are better treated with chemotherapy or palliative therapy.

Aminoglutethimide has largely replaced adrenalectomy in postmenopausal women with breast cancer; it acts predominantly by inhibiting the conversion of androgens to oestrogens in the peripheral tissues. Corticosteroid replacement therapy is necessary (see section 6.3.1). Early toxicity is common and may include drowsiness, drug fever, and a morbilliform eruption; these side-effects generally settle spontaneously. The dose of aminoglutethimide is usually increased to 500 mg daily over 2 to 4 weeks. Hepatic enzyme induction occurs, and may require modification of the doses of other drugs (e.g. oral anticoagulants).

Goserelin, a gonadotrophin-releasing hormone (GnRH) analogue is now also indicated for management of advanced breast cancer.

PROSTATE CANCER. Metastatic cancer of the prostate is commonly responsive to hormonal treatment designed to deprive the cancer of androgen. Treatment is probably best reserved for symptomatic metastatic disease. The standard treatment is bilateral subcapsular orchidectomy, which commonly results in responses lasting 12–18 months. Alternatively, a gonadotrophin-releasing hormone (GnRH) analogue such as **buserelin**, **goserelin**, or **leuprorelin** may be given. These are as effective as orchidectomy or **stilboestrol** (section 8.3.1) but are expensive and require parenteral administration, at least initially. They cause initial stimulation of luteinising hormone release by the pituitary, which in turn causes testosterone secretion by the testis; this is followed by inhibition of luteinising hormone release with achievement of an anorchic state. During the first 1 to 2 weeks of treatment a number of patients develop a tumour 'flare' which may cause spinal cord compression or increased bone pain. When such problems are anticipated, alternative treatments (e.g. orchidectomy) or the additional use of an anti-androgen such as cyproterone acetate or flutamide (see below) are recommended; anti-androgen treatment should be started 3 days before the GnRH analogue and continued for at least 3 weeks. Other side-effects of GnRH analogues are similar to those of orchidectomy.

Cyproterone acetate is an anti-androgen which has been used as first-line therapy; it has a number of theoretical advantages, but is expensive. **Flutamide** is also an anti-androgen; it is being studied alone and in combination for prostate cancer and may have a role in preventing and treating the 'flare' which can occur in patients treated with gonadotrophin-releasing hormone analogues.

Alternatives after orchidectomy include cyproterone acetate or prednisolone. Such second-line treatment may palliate symptoms, but rarely results in appreciable disease regression.

AMINOGLUTETHIMIDE

Indications: see notes above and under Dose
Cautions: see notes above; avoid in porphyria (see section 9.8.2); **interactions:** Appendix 1 (aminoglutethimide)
Side-effects: see notes above; dizziness, somnolence, lethargy; unsteadiness at higher doses; less frequently nausea, vomiting, diarrhoea; rash (sometimes with fever) reported; allergic alveolitis and blood disorders (regular blood counts) also reported; altered thyroid function
Dose: breast or prostate cancer, 250 mg daily, increased once a week to max. 250 mg 4 times daily (lower doses may be adequate, see notes above); given with a glucocorticoid (and sometimes with a mineralocorticoid as well)
Cushing's syndrome due to malignant disease, 250 mg daily, increased gradually to 1 g daily in divided doses (occasionally 1.5–2 g daily); glucocorticoid given only if necessary

PoM **Orimeten**® (Ciba)
Tablets, scored, aminoglutethimide 250 mg. Net price 56-tab pack = £18.38

BUSERELIN

Indications: prostate cancer; endometriosis, see section 6.7.2
Cautions: during first month monitor patients at risk of ureteric obstruction or spinal cord compression, see notes above
Side-effects: initial increase in bone pain (due to transient increases in plasma testosterone); hot flushes, decreased libido, infrequent gynaecomastia, urticaria
Dose: by subcutaneous injection, 500 micrograms every 8 hours for 7 days, then *intranasally*, 1 spray into each nostril 6 times daily
COUNSELLING. Avoid use of nasal decongestants before and for at least 30 minutes after treatment.

PoM **Suprefact**® (Hoechst)
Injection, buserelin 1 mg (as acetate)/mL. Net price treatment pack of 2 × 5.5-mL vial = £30.37
Nasal spray, buserelin 100 micrograms (as acetate)/metered spray. Net price treatment pack of 4 × 10-g bottle with spray pump = £99.92. Counselling, see above

CYPROTERONE ACETATE

Indications: prostate cancer, see notes above; other indications, see section 6.4.2

Cautions: hepatic disease; risk of recurrence of thrombo-embolic disease; severe depression; see also section 6.4.2

Contra-indications: none in prostate cancer; for contra-indications relating to other indications see section 6.4.2

Side-effects: see section 6.4.2

Dose: prostate cancer, 300 mg daily in 2–3 divided doses after food

PoM **Cyprostat**® (Schering Health Care)
Tablets, scored, cyproterone acetate 50 mg. Net price 84-tab pack = £48.35 (hosp. only); 168-tab pack = £96.70. Label: 3, 21

FLUTAMIDE

Indications: prostate cancer, see notes above

Cautions: cardiac disease (sodium retention with oedema); monitor hepatic function; **interactions:** Appendix 1 (flutamide)

Side-effects: gynaecomastia (sometimes with galactorrhoea); nausea, vomiting, diarrhoea, increased appetite, insomnia, tiredness; other side-effects reported include decreased libido, inhibition of spermatogenesis, gastric and chest pain, headache, dizziness, cholestatic jaundice, oedema, blurred vision, thirst, rashes, pruritus, haemolytic anaemia, systemic lupus erythematosus-like syndrome, and lymphoedema

Dose: 250 mg 3 times daily (see also notes above)

PoM **Drogenil** (Schering-Plough)
Tablets, yellow, scored, flutamide 250 mg, net price 84-tab pack = £110.00

GOSERELIN

Indications: breast cancer; prostate cancer; endometriosis, see section 6.7.2

Cautions; Side-effects: see under Buserelin; also rashes (reversible without stopping therapy); bruising at injection site

Dose: see below

PoM **Zoladex**® (ICI)
Implant, goserelin 3.6 mg (as acetate) in syringe applicator. Net price each = £125.40
Dose: by *subcutaneous injection* into anterior abdominal wall, 3.6 mg every 28 days (local anaesthetic if desired)

LEUPRORELIN ACETATE

Indications: prostate cancer; endometriosis, see section 6.7.2

Cautions; Side-effects: see under Buserelin; also, infrequently, peripheral oedema, fatigue, nausea, irritation at injection site; rotate injection site periodically

Dose: by *subcutaneous* or by *intramuscular injection*, 3.75 mg every 4 weeks (see also notes above)

▼ PoM **Prostap SR**® (Lederle)
Injection (microcapsule powder for aqueous suspension), leuprorelin acetate, net price 3.75-mg vial with 2-mL vehicle-filled syringe = £125.40

TAMOXIFEN

Indications: breast cancer, see notes above

Cautions: **interactions:** Appendix 1 (tamoxifen)

Contra-indications: pregnancy; porphyria (see section 9.8.2)

Side-effects: hot flushes, vaginal bleeding (but suppression of menstruation in some pre-menopausal women), gastro-intestinal disturbances, dizziness; rarely fluid retention, visual disturbances (retinopathy reported); see also notes above

Dose: breast cancer, 20–40 mg daily as a single dose or in 2 divided doses

Anovulatory infertility, 20 mg daily on second to fifth days of cycle inclusive; if necessary increased to 40 mg daily then 80 mg daily for subsequent courses; if cycles irregular, start initial course on any day, with subsequent course starting 45 days later *or* on second day of cycle if menstruation occurs

PoM **Tamoxifen** (Non-proprietary)
Tablets, tamoxifen (as citrate) 10 mg, net price 30-tab pack = £6.64; 20 mg, 30-tab pack = £9.69; 40 mg, 30-tab pack = £22.00
Various strengths available from APS, Ashbourne (Oestrifen®), Berk (Emblon®), Cox, CP, Evans, Farmitalia Carlo Erba, Kerfoot, Lederle (Noltam®), Tillotts (Tamofen®)

PoM **Nolvadex**® (ICI)
Tablets, tamoxifen (as citrate) 10 mg, net price 30-tab pack = £6.20; 20 mg (Nolvadex-D®), 30-tab pack = £9.35; 40 mg (scored, Nolvadex-Forte®), 30-tab pack = £22.20

GASTRO-ENTEROPANCREATIC TUMOURS

Octreotide is a long-acting analogue of the hypothalamic release-inhibiting hormone somatostatin; it is indicated for the relief of symptoms associated with gastro-enteropancreatic endocrine tumours and for the short-term treatment of acromegaly before intervention.

OCTREOTIDE

Indications: see under Dose

Cautions: occasional sudden escape from symptomatic control with rapid recurrence of severe symptoms; in insulinoma may increase depth and duration of hypoglycaemia (close observation initially and with dose changes; marked fluctuations may be reduced by increasing administration frequency); in diabetes mellitus may reduce insulin or oral antidiabetic requirements; monitor thyroid function on long-term therapy; ultrasonic examination of gall bladder before and at intervals of 6–12 months during treatment; avoid abrupt withdrawal (see side-effects below); **interactions:** Appendix 1 (octreotide)

Contra-indications: pregnancy (unless compelling reasons) and breast-feeding

Side-effects: gastro-intestinal disturbances including anorexia, nausea, vomiting, abdominal pain and bloating, flatulence, diarrhoea, and steatorrhoea; symptoms may be reduced by injecting between meals or at bedtime; impairment of postprandial glucose tolerance (rarely persistent hyperglycaemia on chronic administration); hepatic disturbance reported; gall stone formation reported after long-term treatment (abrupt withdrawal may result in biliary hypercontractility with associated biliary colic and pancreatitis); pain and irritation at injection site (rotate sites)

Dose: symptoms associated with carcinoid tumours with features of carcinoid syndrome, VIPomas, glucagonomas, *by subcutaneous injection*, initially 50 micrograms once or twice daily, gradually increased according to response to 200 micrograms 3 times daily (higher doses required exceptionally); maintenance doses variable; in carcinoid tumours discontinue after 1 week if no effect; if rapid response required, initial dose *by intravenous injection* (with ECG monitoring and after dilution to a concentration of 10–50% with sodium chloride 0.9% injection)

Acromegaly, *by subcutaneous injection*, 100–200 micrograms 3 times daily

PoM **Sandostatin**® (Sandoz)

Injection, octreotide (as acetate) 50 micrograms/mL, net price 1-mL amp = £2.98; 100 micrograms/mL, 1-mL amp = £5.60; 200 micrograms/mL, 5-mL vial = £55,78; 500 micrograms/mL, 1-mL amp = £27.13

9: Drugs affecting
NUTRITION and BLOOD

In this chapter drugs and preparations are discussed under the following headings:
- **9.1** Anaemias and some other blood disorders
- **9.2** Electrolyte and water replacement
- **9.3** Intravenous nutrition
- **9.4** Oral nutrition
- **9.5** Minerals
- **9.6** Vitamins
- **9.7** Bitters and tonics
- **9.8** Metabolic disorders

9.1 Anaemias and some other blood disorders

- **9.1.1** Iron-deficiency anaemias
- **9.1.2** Megaloblastic anaemias
- **9.1.3** Hypoplastic and haemolytic anaemias
- **9.1.4** Autoimmune thrombocytopenic purpura
- **9.1.5** G6PD deficiency
- **9.1.6** Drugs used in neutropenia

Before initiating treatment for anaemia it is essential to determine which type is present. Iron salts may be harmful and result in iron overload if given alone to patients with anaemias other than those due to iron deficiency.

9.1.1 Iron-deficiency anaemias

9.1.1.1 Oral iron
9.1.1.2 Parenteral iron

Treatment is only justified in the presence of a demonstrable iron-deficiency state.

Prophylaxis is justifiable in pregnancy, menorrhagia, after subtotal or total gastrectomy, and in the management of low birth-weight infants such as premature babies, twins, and in infants delivered by caesarean section.

9.1.1.1 ORAL IRON

Iron salts should be given by mouth unless there are good reasons for using another route.

Ferrous salts show only marginal differences between one another in efficiency of absorption of iron, but ferric salts are much less well absorbed. Haemoglobin regeneration rate is little affected by the type of salt used provided sufficient iron is given, and in most patients the time factor is not critical. Choice of preparation is thus usually decided by incidence of side-effects and cost.

The oral dose of elemental iron should be 100 to 200 mg daily; it is customary to give this as dried **ferrous sulphate**, 200 mg three times daily. If side-effects arise, dosage can be reduced or a change made to an alternative iron salt. It should be remembered, however, that an apparent improvement in tolerance on changing to another salt may be due to its lower content of elemental iron. The incidence of side-effects due to ferrous sulphate is no greater than with other iron salts when compared on the basis of equivalent amounts of elemental iron.

Iron content of different iron salts

Iron salt	Amount	Content of ferrous iron
Ferrous fumarate	200 mg	65 mg
Ferrous gluconate	300 mg	35 mg
Ferrous glycine sulphate	225 mg	40 mg
Ferrous succinate	100 mg	35 mg
Ferrous sulphate	300 mg	60 mg
Ferrous sulphate, dried	200 mg	60 mg[1]

1. Good quality dried ferrous sulphate 200 mg may now contain approximately 65 mg ferrous iron

THERAPEUTIC RESPONSE. The haemoglobin concentration should rise by about 100–200 mg per 100 mL (1–2 g per litre) per day. After the haemoglobin has risen to normal, treatment should be continued for a further three months in an attempt to replenish the iron stores. Epithelial tissue changes such as atrophic glossitis and koilonychia are usually improved although the response is often slow.

COMPOUND PREPARATIONS. Some oral preparations contain ascorbic acid to aid absorption, or the iron is in the form of a chelate, which can be shown experimentally to produce a modest increase in absorption of iron. However, the therapeutic advantage is minimal and cost may be increased.

There is neither theoretical nor clinical justification for the inclusion of other therapeutically active ingredients, such as the B group of vitamins (except folic acid for pregnant women, see Iron and Folic Acid below).

MODIFIED-RELEASE CAPSULES AND TABLETS. These are designed to release iron gradually as the capsule or tablet passes along the gut so that a smaller amount of iron is present in the lumen at any one time. It is claimed that each dose unit contains enough iron for 24 hours, thus permitting once daily dosage.

These preparations are likely to carry the iron past the first part of the duodenum into an area of the gut where conditions for iron absorption are poor. The low incidence of side-effects may well be because of the small amounts of iron available under these conditions and so the preparations have no therapeutic advantage and should not be used.

SIDE-EFFECTS. Because iron salts are astringent, gastro-intestinal irritation may occur. Nausea and epigastric pain are dose-related but the relationship between dose and altered bowel habit (constipation or diarrhoea) is less clear. Oral iron, particularly modified-release preparations may

9.1 Anaemias and some other blood disorders

exacerbate diarrhoea in patients with inflammatory bowel disease; care is also needed in patients with intestinal strictures and diverticulae.

Iron preparations taken orally may have a constipating effect particularly in older patients, occasionally leading to faecal impaction.

FERROUS SULPHATE

Indications: iron-deficiency anaemia
Cautions: interactions: Appendix 1 (iron)
Side-effects: see notes above
Dose: ferrous iron, therapeutic, 120–180 mg daily in divided doses; prophylactic, 60 mg daily; CHILD, therapeutic, daily in divided doses, up to 1 year 36 mg, 1–5 years 72 mg, 6–12 years 120 mg
See also under Preparations
COUNSELLING. Although iron preparations are best absorbed on an empty stomach they may be taken after food to reduce gastro-intestinal side-effects; they may discolour stools

Ferrous Sulphate (Non-proprietary)
Tablets, coated, dried ferrous sulphate 200 mg (60 mg[1] iron), net price 20 = 9p
Dose: prophylactic, 1 tablet daily; therapeutic, 1 tablet 2–3 times daily
1. Good quality dried ferrous sulphate 200 mg may now contain approximately 65 mg iron

Ferrous Sulphate Oral Solution, Paediatric, BP
(Paediatric Ferrous Sulphate Mixture)
Mixture, ferrous sulphate 1.2% and a suitable antoxidant in a suitable vehicle with an orange flavour. Extemporaneous preparations should be recently prepared according to the following formula: ferrous sulphate 60 mg, ascorbic acid 10 mg, orange syrup 0.5 mL, double-strength chloroform water 2.5 mL, water to 5 mL
Dose: therapeutic, CHILD up to 1 year, 5 mL 3 times daily; 1–5 years, 10 mL 3 times daily; 6–12 years, 15 mL 3 times daily *or* 25 mL twice daily. To be taken well diluted with water

Modified-release preparations
Feospan® (SK&F)
Spansule® (= capsules m/r), clear/red, enclosing green and red pellets, dried ferrous sulphate 150 mg (47 mg iron). Net price 30-cap pack = 90p. Label: 25
Dose: 1–2 capsules daily; CHILD over 1 year 1 capsule daily; can be opened and sprinkled on food
Ferrograd® (Abbott)
Filmtabs® (= tablets f/c), m/r, red, dried ferrous sulphate 325 mg (105 mg iron). Net price 5 × 30-tab pack = £4.12. Label: 25
Dose: 1 tablet daily before food
Slow-Fe® (Ciba)
Tablets, m/r, dried ferrous sulphate 160 mg (50 mg iron). Net price 28-tab pack = 43p. Label: 25
Dose: prophylactic, 1 tablet daily; therapeutic, 2 tablets daily; CHILD over 6 years, 1 tablet daily

FERROUS FUMARATE

Indications; Cautions; Side-effects: see under Ferrous Sulphate
Dose: see under preparations below

Fersaday® (Evans)
Tablets, orange, f/c, ferrous fumarate 304 mg (100 mg iron). Net price 28-tab pack = 45p
Dose: prophylactic, 1 tablet daily; therapeutic, 1 tablet twice daily

Fersamal® (Evans)
Tablets, brown, ferrous fumarate 200 mg (65 mg iron). Net price 20 = 14p
Dose: 1–2 tablets 3 times daily
Syrup, brown, ferrous fumarate 140 mg (45 mg iron)/5 mL. Net price 200 mL = £1.47
Dose: 10–20 mL twice daily; PREMATURE INFANT 0.6–2.4 mL/kg daily; CHILD up to 6 years 2.5–5 mL twice daily
Galfer® (Galen)
Capsules, red/green, ferrous fumarate 290 mg (100 mg iron). Net price 20 = 52p
Dose: 1 capsule 1–2 times daily before food
Syrup, brown, ferrous fumarate 140 mg (45 mg iron)/5 mL. Net price 100 mL = £2.54
Dose: 10 mL 1–2 times daily before food; CHILD (full-term infant and young child) 2.5–5 mL 1–2 times daily

Modified-release preparations
Ferrocap® (Consolidated)
Capsules, m/r, green/orange, enclosing brown and white granules, ferrous fumarate 330 mg (110 mg iron). Net price 30-cap pack = 99p. Label: 25
Dose: 1 capsule daily

FERROUS GLUCONATE

Indications; Cautions; Side-effects: see under Ferrous Sulphate
Dose: see under preparations below

Ferrous Gluconate (Non-proprietary)
Tablets, red, coated, ferrous gluconate 300 mg (35 mg iron). Net price 20 = 12p
Dose: prophylactic, 2 tablets daily before food; therapeutic, 4–6 tablets daily in divided doses before food; CHILD 6–12 years, prophylactic, 1–3 tablets daily
Fergon® (Sanofi Winthrop)
Tablets, red, s/c, ferrous gluconate 300 mg (35 mg iron). Net price 20 = 44p
Dose: see above

FERROUS GLYCINE SULPHATE

Indications; Cautions; Side-effects: see under Ferrous Sulphate
Dose: see under preparations below

Plesmet® (Napp)
Syrup, ferrous glycine sulphate equivalent to 25 mg iron/5 mL. Net price 100 mL = 74p
Dose: 5–10 mL 3 times daily; CHILD 2–5 mL 2–3 times daily, according to age

Modified-release preparations
Ferrocontin Continus® (ASTA Medica)
Tablets, m/r, red, f/c, ferrous glycine sulphate equivalent to 100 mg iron. Net price 30-tab pack = 99p. Label: 25
Dose: 1 tablet daily

FERROUS SUCCINATE

Indications; Cautions; Side-effects: see under Ferrous Sulphate
Dose: see under preparations below

Ferromyn® (Wellcome)
Elixir, brown, ferrous succinate 106 mg (37 mg iron)/5 mL. Net price 100 mL = £3.19
Dose: 5 mL 3 times daily; CHILD up to 2 years max. 1 mL twice daily, 2–5 years 2.5 mL 3 times daily, 5–10 years 5 mL twice daily

POLYSACCHARIDE-IRON COMPLEX

Indications; Cautions; Side-effects: see under Ferrous Sulphate
Dose: see under preparations below

Niferex® (Tillomed)
Elixir, brown, polysaccharide-iron complex equivalent to 100 mg of iron/5 mL. Net price 100 mL = £2.10; 30-mL dropper bottle for paediatric use = £1.80. Counselling, use of dropper
Dose: prophylactic, 2.5 mL daily; therapeutic, 5 mL daily; INFANT, 1 drop (from dropper bottle) per pound body-weight 3 times daily; CHILD 2–6 years, 2.5 mL daily, 6–12 years 5 mL daily

Niferex-150® (Tillomed)
Capsules, brown/orange, polysaccharide-iron complex equivalent to 150 mg of iron. Net price 20 = £1.90
Dose: 1–2 capsules daily

SODIUM IRONEDETATE

Indications; Cautions; Side-effects: see under Ferrous Sulphate
Dose: see under preparations below

Sytron® (P-D)
Elixir, sugar-free, sodium ironedetate 190 mg equivalent to 27.5 mg of iron/5 mL. Net price 100 mL = 34p
Dose: 5 mL increasing gradually to 10 mL 3 times daily; INFANT and PREMATURE INFANT 2.5 mL twice daily (smaller doses should be used initially); CHILD 1–5 years 2.5 mL 3 times daily, 6–12 years 5 mL 3 times daily

IRON AND FOLIC ACID

These preparations are used for the prevention of iron and folic acid deficiencies in pregnancy. The prophylactic dose in pregnancy is the equivalent of approximately 100 mg of iron with folic acid 200–500 micrograms daily.

It is important to note that the small doses of folic acid contained in these preparations are inadequate for the treatment of megaloblastic anaemias.

Fefol® (SK&F)
Spansule® (= capsules m/r), clear/green, enclosing red, yellow, and white pellets, dried ferrous sulphate 150 mg (47 mg iron), folic acid 500 micrograms. Net price 30-cap pack = £1.00. Label: 25
Dose: 1 capsule daily

Ferrocap-F 350® (Consolidated)
Capsules, m/r, pink, enclosing brown, white, and yellow granules, ferrous fumarate 330 mg (110 mg iron), folic acid 350 micrograms. Net price 30-cap pack = £1.25. Label: 25
Dose: 1 capsule daily

Ferrocontin Folic Continus® (ASTA Medica)
Tablets, orange, f/c, ferrous glycine sulphate equivalent to 100 mg iron for sustained release, folic acid 500 micrograms. Net price 30-tab pack = 79p. Label: 25
Dose: 1 tablet daily

Ferrograd Folic® (Abbott)
Filmtabs® (= tablets f/c), red/yellow, dried ferrous sulphate 325 mg (105 mg iron) for sustained release, folic acid 350 micrograms. Net price 150-tab pack = £4.21. Label: 25
Dose: 1 tablet daily before food

Folex-350® (Rybar)
Tablets, pink, s/c, ferrous fumarate 308 mg (100 mg iron), folic acid 350 micrograms. Net price 20 = 44p
Dose: 1 tablet daily

Galfer FA® (Galen)
Capsules, red/yellow, ferrous fumarate 290 mg (100 mg iron), folic acid 350 micrograms. Net price 20 = 53p
Dose: 1 capsule daily before food

PoM **Lexpec with Iron-M®** (RP Drugs)
Syrup, brown, sugar-free, ferric ammonium citrate equivalent to 80 mg iron, folic acid 500 micrograms/5 mL. Net price 125 mL = £5.30
Dose: 5–10 mL daily before food
Note. Lexpec with Iron-M® contains five times less folic acid than Lexpec with Iron®

PoM **Meterfolic®** (Sinclair)
Tablets, grey, f/c, ferrous fumarate equivalent to 100 mg iron, folic acid 350 micrograms. Net price 30-tab pack = £1.03
Dose: 1 tablet 1–2 times daily

PoM **Pregaday®** (Evans)
Tablets, brown, f/c, ferrous fumarate 304 mg (100 mg iron), folic acid 350 micrograms. Net price 28-tab pack = 51p
Dose: 1 tablet daily

Pregnavite Forte F, see compound iron preparations

PoM **Slow-Fe Folic®** (Ciba)
Tablets, m/r, ivory, f/c, dried ferrous sulphate 160 mg (50 mg iron), folic acid 400 micrograms. Net price 28-tab pack = 43p. Label: 25
Dose: 1–2 tablets daily

Higher folic acid content
The daily dose of folic acid in these preparations is unnecessarily high for the prevention of folate deficiency; it also has the theoretical disadvantage of masking anaemia due to vitamin-B_{12} deficiency (which could allow vitamin-B_{12} neuropathy to develop).

PoM **Ferfolic SV®** (Sinclair)
Tablets, pink, ferrous gluconate 250 mg (30 mg iron), folic acid 5 mg, ascorbic acid 10 mg. Net price 20 = 82p
Dose: anaemia, 1–3 tablets daily after food; prophylaxis of neural tube defects in women known to be at risk, 1 tablet daily started before conception and continued for at least first trimester

PoM **Lexpec with Iron®** (RP Drugs)
Syrup, brown, sugar-free, ferric ammonium citrate equivalent to 80 mg iron, folic acid 2.5 mg/5 mL. Net price 125 mL = £5.50
Dose: 5–10 mL daily before food
Note. Lexpec with Iron® contains five times as much folic acid as Lexpec with Iron-M®

COMPOUND IRON PREPARATIONS

There is no justification for prescribing compound iron preparations, except for preparations of iron and folic acid for prophylactic use in pregnancy (see above). Some of the preparations listed below only contain very small amounts of iron.

Ferrous Sulphate Tablets, Compound, green, s/c, dried ferrous sulphate equivalent to 170 mg of $FeSO_4$, copper sulphate 2.5 mg, manganese sulphate 2.5 mg. Net price 20 tabs = 9p
Dose: 1–2 tablets daily

NHS **Fefol-Vit**® (SK&F)
Spansule® (= capsules m/r), clear/white, enclosing red, orange, yellow, and white pellets, dried ferrous sulphate 150 mg (47 mg iron) with vitamins B group (including folic acid 500 micrograms) and C. Net price 30-cap pack = £1.82. Label: 25
Dose: 1 capsule daily during pregnancy

Fefol Z® (SK&F)
Spansule® (= capsules m/r), blue/clear, enclosing red, yellow, and white pellets, dried ferrous sulphate 150 mg (47 mg iron), folic acid 500 micrograms, zinc sulphate monohydrate 61.8 mg (22.5 mg zinc). Net price 30-cap pack = £1.79. Label: 25
Dose: 1 capsule daily during pregnancy

NHS **Ferrograd C**® (Abbott)
Filmtabs® (= tablets f/c), red, dried ferrous sulphate 325 mg (105 mg iron) for sustained release, ascorbic acid 500 mg (as sodium salt). Net price 30-tab pack = £1.48. Label: 25
Dose: 1 tablet daily before food

NHS **Fesovit**® (Smith Kline Beecham Brands)
Spansule® (= capsules m/r), colourless/yellow, enclosing red, orange, and white pellets, dried ferrous sulphate 150 mg (47 mg iron) with vitamins B group and C. Net price 30-cap pack = £1.82. Label: 25
Dose: 1–2 capsules daily; CHILD over 1 year 1 capsule daily

NHS **Fesovit Z**® (SK&F)
Spansule® (= capsules m/r), orange/clear, enclosing red, orange, and white pellets, dried ferrous sulphate 150 mg (47 mg iron), zinc sulphate monohydrate 61.8 mg (22.5 mg zinc) with vitamins B group and C. Net price 30-cap pack = £2.80. Label: 25
Dose: 1–2 capsules daily; CHILD over 1 year 1 capsule daily

PoM **Folicin**® (Paines & Byrne)
Tablets, s/c, dried ferrous sulphate 200 mg (60 mg iron), folic acid 2.5 mg with minerals. Net price 20 = 20p
Dose: 1–2 tablets daily during pregnancy

NHS **Givitol**® (Galen)
Capsules, red/maroon, ferrous fumarate 305 mg (100 mg iron) with vitamins B group and C. Net price 20 = 82p
Dose: 1 capsule daily before food

NHS **Octovit**® (SK&F)
Tablets, maroon, f/c, dried ferrous sulphate (10 mg iron) with vitamins A, B group, C, D, E, and minerals. Net price 14-tab pack = £2.03
Dose: 1 tablet daily

Unicap M® (Upjohn)
Tablets, yellow, f/c, ferrous fumarate equivalent to 10 mg iron with vitamins A, B group, C, D, and minerals. Net price 30-tab pack = £3.42, 90-tab pack = £8.90
Dose: dietary supplement, 1 tablet daily

Unicap T® (Upjohn)
Tablets, yellow, f/c, ferrous fumarate equivalent to 10 mg iron with vitamins A, B group, C, D, and minerals. Net price 30-tab pack = £4.79, 90-tab pack = £12.37
Dose: increased requirements for vitamins such as overt avitaminosis, catabolic states, severe chronic disease or malabsorption syndrome, 1 tablet daily

NHS *****Pregnavite Forte F**® (Bencard)
Tablets, lilac, s/c, dried ferrous sulphate 84 mg (25.2 mg iron), folic acid 120 micrograms, vitamin A 1333 units, thiamine hydrochloride 500 micrograms, riboflavine 500 micrograms, nicotinamide 5 mg, pyridoxine hydrochloride 330 micrograms, ascorbic acid 13.3 mg, vitamin D 133 units, calcium phosphate 160 mg. Net price 84-tab pack = £1.96
* except to reduce the risk of spina bifida or anencephaly in babies born to women who have previously given birth to one or more babies (or aborted a fetus) with a neural tube defect and endorsed 'SLS' ('S2B' in Scotland)
Dose: 1 tablet 3 times daily during or after food
Note. For prophylaxis of neural tube defects in pregnancy, dosage should be started not less than 28 days prior to conception and continue uninterrupted at least until the date of the second missed period

9.1.1.2 PARENTERAL IRON

The only valid reason for administering iron **parenterally** is failure of oral therapy due to lack of patient co-operation with oral treatment, severe gastro-intestinal side-effects, continuing severe blood loss or malabsorption. Provided that the oral iron preparation is taken reliably and is absorbed, then the haemoglobin response is not significantly faster with the parenteral route. The need for a rapid cure of the anaemia is therefore not met by parenteral administration of iron.

Preparations suitable for parenteral use contain iron either in the form of a complex of ferric hydroxide with dextrans of high molecular weight as **iron dextran injection** (Imferon®), or a complex of iron, sorbitol and citric acid as **iron sorbitol injection** (Jectofer®). Iron sorbitol injection is **not** suitable for intravenous injection and, although the low mean molecular weight allows rapid absorption from the injection site, excretion in the saliva and substantial urinary losses from each dose also occur.

It is usual to give a course of *deep intramuscular* injections. The manufacturer's dosage schedules should be consulted; these usually include a supplement for reconstitution of iron stores.

To prevent leakage along the needle track with subsequent staining of the skin, intramuscular injections should be deep for both preparations.

Iron dextran (Imferon®) may also be administered as a single dose by *slow intravenous infusion* over 6 to 8 hours provided that there is no reaction to a test dose. Although the incidence of side-effects is low, disquieting adverse reactions may occur, especially in allergic subjects, and intravenous infusion is contra-indicated in asthmatic patients. Therefore iron dextran (Imferon®) should only be administered *intravenously* in selected cases where proper indications exist for its use, that is, when continuing blood loss is likely to be permanent and oral prophylaxis cannot keep pace, when a patient requiring parenteral iron has a small muscle mass or a haemostatic defect contra-indicating intramuscular injection, or when psychological or social pressures make iron treatment by other means impracticable.

IRON DEXTRAN INJECTION
Contains 5% (50 mg/mL) of iron
Indications: iron deficiency anaemia (see notes above)
Cautions: risk of anaphylaxis especially in patients with history of allergy; test dose essential when given by intravenous infusion; patient should be under observation for entire period of infusion and 1 hour after; facilities to control allergic reactions including adrenaline should be available (see section 3.4.3)
Contra-indications: cardiac abnormalities (e.g. angina or arrhythmia), severe liver disease, acute kidney infections; intravenous infusion in asthmatic patients
Side-effects: staining of the skin if leakage along needle track occurs, transient nausea, vomiting, flushing; occasionally severe dyspnoea; rarely severe anaphylaxis (see Cautions)
Dose: see notes above and manufacturer's literature

PoM **Imferon**® (Fisons) [Not currently available]
Injection, iron dextran injection. Net price 2-mL amp = 54p; 5-mL amp = £1.08
Intravenous infusion, iron dextran injection. Net price 20-mL amp = £4.48 (hosp. only)

IRON SORBITOL INJECTION
Contains 5% (50 mg/mL) of iron
Indications: iron-deficiency anaemia
Cautions: oral administration of iron should be stopped at least 24 hours before giving iron sorbitol injection; administration of other injectable iron preparations should be stopped a week beforehand; urine may darken on standing
Contra-indications: cardiac abnormalities (e.g. angina or arrhythmia), liver disease, kidney disease (particularly pyelonephritis), untreated urinary-tract infections
Side-effects: occasionally severe arrhythmias
Dose: by deep intramuscular injection, see notes above and manufacturer's literature

PoM **Jectofer**® (Astra)
Injection, iron sorbitol injection. Net price 2-mL amp = 47p

9.1.2 Drugs used in megaloblastic anaemias

Most megaloblastic anaemias are due to lack of either vitamin B_{12} or folate and it is essential to establish in every case which deficiency is present and the underlying cause. In emergencies, where delay might be dangerous, it is sometimes necessary to administer both substances after the bone marrow test while plasma assay results are awaited. Normally, however, appropriate treatment should be instituted only when the results of tests are available.

The most common cause of megaloblastic anaemia in the UK is *pernicious anaemia* in which lack of gastric intrinsic factor due to an auto-immune gastritis causes malabsorption of vitamin B_{12}.

Vitamin B_{12} is also needed in the treatment of megaloblastosis due to *prolonged nitrous oxide anaesthesia*, which inactivates the vitamin, and in the rare syndrome of *congenital transcobalamin II deficiency*.

Vitamin B_{12} should be given prophylactically after *total gastrectomy* or *total ileal resection* (or after *partial gastrectomy* if a vitamin B_{12} absorption test shows vitamin B_{12} malabsorption).

Apart from dietary deficiency, all other causes of vitamin-B_{12} deficiency are attributable to *malabsorption* so there is little place for the use of vitamin B_{12} orally and none for vitamin B_{12} intrinsic factor complexes given by mouth.

Hydroxocobalamin has completely replaced cyanocobalamin as the form of vitamin B_{12} of choice for therapy; it is retained in the body longer than cyanocobalamin and thus for maintenance therapy need only be given at intervals of 3 months. Although a haematological response in vitamin-B_{12} deficiency may be obtained by small doses, it is customary to start treatment with 1 mg by intramuscular injection repeated 5 times at intervals of 2 to 3 days to replenish the depleted body stores. Thereafter, maintenance treatment, which is usually for life, can be instituted. There is no evidence that larger doses provide any additional benefit in vitamin-B_{12} neuropathy.

Folic acid has few indications for long-term therapy since most causes of folate deficiency are self-limiting or will yield to a short course of treatment. It should not be used in undiagnosed megaloblastic anaemia unless vitamin B_{12} is administered concurrently otherwise neuropathy may be precipitated (see above).

In *folate-deficient megaloblastic anaemia* (e.g. due to poor nutrition, pregnancy, or antiepileptics), standard treatment to bring about a haematological remission and replenish body stores, is oral administration of folic acid 5 mg daily for 4 months; up to 15 mg daily may be necessary in malabsorption states.

For *prophylaxis in chronic haemolytic states or in renal dialysis*, it is sufficient to give folic acid 5 mg daily or even weekly, depending on the diet and the rate of haemolysis.

For *prophylaxis in pregnancy* the dose of folic acid is 200–500 micrograms daily (see Iron and Folic Acid, section 9.1.1.1).

There is **no** justification for prescribing multiple-ingredient vitamin preparations containing vitamin B_{12} or folic acid.

HYDROXOCOBALAMIN
Indications: Pernicious anaemia, other causes of vitamin-B_{12} deficiency, subacute combined degeneration of the spinal cord
Cautions: should not be given before diagnosis fully established but see also notes above
Dose: by intramuscular injection, initially 1 mg repeated 5 times at intervals of 2–3 days; maintenance dose 1 mg every 3 months; CHILD, dosage as for adult

9.1 Anaemias and some other blood disorders

PoM Hydroxocobalamin Injection, hydroxocobalamin 1 mg/mL. Net price 1-mL amp = 36p
Note. The BP directs that when vitamin B$_{12}$ injection is prescribed or demanded hydroxocobalamin injection shall be dispensed or supplied
The brand names NHS Cobalin-H® (Paines & Byrne) and NHS Neo-Cytamen® (Evans) are used for hydroxocobalamin injection

CYANOCOBALAMIN
Indications: see notes above
Dose: by intramuscular injection, initially 1 mg repeated 10 times at intervals of 2–3 days, maintenance 1 mg every month, but see notes above

PoM Cyanocobalamin Injection, cyanocobalamin 1 mg/mL. Net price 1-mL amp = 34p
Note. The BP directs that when vitamin B$_{12}$ injection is prescribed or demanded hydroxocobalamin injection shall be dispensed or supplied
The brand name NHS Cytamen® (Evans) is used for cyanocobalamin injection
NHS **Cytacon®** (Evans)
Tablets, f/c, cyanocobalamin 50 micrograms. Net price 50-tab pack = £1.59
Liquid, red, cyanocobalamin 35 micrograms/5 mL. Net price 200 mL = £1.59

FOLIC ACID
Indications: see notes above
Cautions: should never be given alone in the treatment of Addisonian pernicious anaemia and other vitamin B$_{12}$-deficiency states because it may precipitate the onset of subacute combined degeneration of the spinal cord. Do not use in malignant disease unless megaloblastic anaemia due to folate deficiency is an important complication (some malignant tumours are folate-dependent); **interactions:** Appendix 1 (vitamins)
Dose: initially, 5 mg daily for 4 months (see notes above); maintenance, 5 mg every 1–7 days depending on underlying disease; CHILD up to 1 year, 500 micrograms/kg daily; over 1 year, as adult dose

PoM ¹Folic Acid Tablets, folic acid 5 mg, net price 20 = 7p; 100-microgram tablets also available
1. Can be sold to the public provided daily doses do not exceed 500 micrograms
PoM Lexpec® (RP Drugs)
Syrup, sugar-free, folic acid 2.5 mg/5 mL. Net price 125 mL = £4.85

9.1.3 Drugs used in hypoplastic, haemolytic, and renal anaemias

Anabolic steroids, pyridoxine, antilymphocyte immunoglobulin, and various corticosteroids are used in hypoplastic and haemolytic anaemias.

The place of **anabolic steroids** in the therapy of *aplastic anaemia* remains somewhat controversial and their effectiveness is unclear. There is a wide variation in the reported successful responses. Occasional patients, however, do seem to derive benefit. Since nandrolone decanoate requires intramuscular injection it is unsuitable in aplastic anaemia or cytotoxic aplasia because of the low platelet count; it is customary to prescribe oxymetholone in doses of the order of 2–3 mg/kg daily, and to continue therapy for at least 3 to 6 months. At these dose levels, virilising side-effects may be expected in female patients and in children. Controlled trials have shown that antilymphocyte immunoglobulin produces a response in 50% of acquired cases; higher response rates have been reported when cyclosporin is given as well.

It is unlikely that dietary deprivation of **pyridoxine** (section 9.6.2) produces haematological effects in man. However, certain forms of *sideroblastic anaemia* respond to pharmacological doses, possibly reflecting its role as a co-enzyme during haemoglobin synthesis. Pyridoxine is indicated in both *idiopathic acquired* and *hereditary sideroblastic anaemias*. Although complete cures have not been reported, some increase in haemoglobin may occur; the dose required is usually high, up to 400 mg daily. *Reversible sideroblastic anaemias* respond to treatment of the underlying cause but in pregnancy, haemolytic anaemias, and alcohol dependence, or during isoniazid treatment, pyridoxine is also indicated.

Corticosteroids (see section 6.3) have an important place in the management of a wide variety of haematological disorders. They include conditions with an immune basis such as *autoimmune haemolytic anaemia, immune thrombocytopenias* and *neutropenias,* and *major transfusion reactions*. They are also used in chemotherapy schedules for many types of *lymphoma, lymphoid leukaemias,* and *paraproteinaemias,* including *myelomatosis*. Corticosteroids are used in *aplastic anaemias,* where their value is more debatable.

NANDROLONE
Indications: aplastic anaemia but see notes above; postmenopausal osteoporosis, see section 6.4.3
Cautions; Contra-indications; Side-effects: see section 6.4.3
Dose: by deep intramuscular injection, aplastic anaemia (but not recommended, see notes above), nandrolone decanoate 50–100 mg weekly

PoM Deca-Durabolin 100® (Organon)
Injection (oily), nandrolone decanoate 100 mg/mL. Net price 1-mL amp = £6.68

OXYMETHOLONE
Indications: aplastic anaemia; see notes above
Cautions: cardiac and renal impairment, circulatory failure, hypertension, diabetes mellitus, epilepsy, migraine; monitor skeletal maturation in children for 6 months after treatment; **interactions:** Appendix 1 (anabolic steroids)

Cautionary label wordings, see inside back cover

Prices are **net**, see p. 1

Contra-indications: hepatic impairment, prostatic carcinoma, pregnancy, breast-feeding, porphyria (see section 9.8.2)
Side-effects: acne, oedema, jaundice and liver dysfunction, virilism with high doses, hypercalcaemia, menstrual irregularities; hyperglucagonaemia has also been reported with oxymetholone
Dose: aplastic anaemia, 2–3 mg/kg daily in divided doses; CHILD 2–3 mg/kg daily (less in Fanconi's anaemia)
See also notes above

PoM **Anapolon 50**® (Syntex)
Tablets, scored, oxymetholone 50 mg. Net price 20 = £14.83

ERYTHROPOIETIN

Epoetin (recombinant human erythropoietin) is used for the anaemia associated with erythropoietin deficiency in chronic renal failure. The clinical efficacy of epoetin alfa and epoetin beta is similar and they can be used interchangeably.

Other factors which contribute to the anaemia of chronic renal failure such as iron or folate deficiency should be corrected; aluminium toxicity, concurrent infection or other inflammatory disease may also impair the response to epoetin.

EPOETIN ALFA and BETA
Recombinant human erythropoietins
Indications: see under preparations, below
Cautions: inadequately treated or poorly controlled blood pressure (monitor closely blood pressure, haemoglobin, and electrolytes), interrupt treatment if blood pressure uncontrolled; exclude other causes of anaemia (e.g. folic acid, vitamin B_{12}) and give iron supplements if necessary; ischaemic vascular disease; thrombocytosis (monitor platelet count for first 8 weeks); history of convulsions; malignant disease; chronic liver failure; sudden stabbing migraine-like pain is warning of hypertensive crisis; increase in heparin dose may be needed; pregnancy and breast-feeding
Contra-indications: uncontrolled hypertension
Side-effects: dose-dependent increase in blood pressure or aggravation of hypertension; in isolated patients with normal or low blood pressure, hypertensive crisis with encephalopathy-like symptoms and generalised tonic-clonic seizures requiring immediate medical attention; dose-dependent increase in platelet count (but thrombocytosis rare) regressing during treatment; influenza-like symptoms (may be reduced if intravenous injection given over 5 minutes); shunt thrombosis especially if tendency to hypotension or arteriovenous shunt complications; isolated reports of hyperkalaemia, increase in plasma creatinine, urea and phosphate, convulsions, skin reactions, palpebral oedema, myocardial infarction, anaphylaxis

Dose: aimed at increasing haemoglobin concentration at rate not exceeding 2 g/100 mL/month to stable level of 10–12 g/100 mL; see under preparations, below
Note. Although epoetin alfa and beta are clinically indistinguishable the prescriber must specify which is required

Epoetin alfa
▼ PoM **Eprex**® (Cilag)
Injection, epoetin alfa 2000 units/mL, net price 1-mL amp = £18.00; 4000 units/mL, 1-mL amp = £36.00
Dose: anaemia associated with chronic renal failure in dialysis patients, *by subcutaneous injection* (max. 1 mL per injection site) or *by intravenous injection* over 2 minutes, initially 50 units/kg 3 times weekly increased according to response in steps of 25 units/kg at intervals of 4 weeks; omit one of the weekly doses if haemoglobin rise exceeds 2 g/100 mL with the initial dose; max. 600 units/kg weekly in 3 divided doses; maintenance dose (when haemoglobin concentration of 10–12 g/100 mL achieved), usually 100–300 units/kg weekly in 2–3 divided doses
Severe symptomatic anaemia of renal origin in patients with renal insufficiency not yet on dialysis, preferably *by subcutaneous injection* (max. 1 mL per injection site), initially 50 units/kg 3 times weekly increased according to response in steps of 25 units/kg at intervals of 4 weeks; max. 600 units/kg weekly in 3 divided doses; maintenance dose 50–100 units/kg weekly in 3 divided doses

Epoetin beta
▼ PoM **Recormon**® (Boehringer Mannheim)
Injection, powder for reconstitution, epoetin beta. Net price 1000-unit vial = £9.00; 2000-unit vial = £18.00; 5000-unit vial = £45.00 (all with water for injections)
Note. Avoid contact of reconstituted injection with glass; use only plastic materials
Dose: anaemia associated with chronic renal failure in dialysis patients, ADULT and CHILD over 2 years,
By subcutaneous injection, initially 20 units/kg 3 times weekly for 4 weeks, increased according to response at monthly intervals in steps of 20 units/kg; maintenance dose (when haemoglobin concentration of 10–12 g/100 mL achieved), initially reduce dose by half then adjust according to response at intervals of 1–2 weeks
By intravenous injection over 2 minutes, initially 40 units/kg 3 times weekly for 4 weeks, increased if initial haemoglobin rise less than 1 g/100 mL per month to 80 units/kg 3 times weekly with further increases if needed at monthly intervals in steps of 20 units/kg; maintenance dose (when haemoglobin concentration of 10–12 g/100 mL achieved), initially reduce dose by half then adjust according to response at intervals of 1–2 weeks
Max. by either route 720 units/kg weekly

IRON OVERLOAD

Severe tissue iron overload may occur in aplastic and other refractory anaemias, mainly as the result of repeated blood transfusions. It is a particular problem in refractory anaemias with hyperplastic bone marrow, especially *thalassaemia major*, where excessive iron absorption from the gut and inappropriate iron therapy may add to the tissue siderosis.

Venesection therapy is contra-indicated, but the long-term administration of the iron chelating compound **desferrioxamine mesylate** is useful. Subcutaneous infusions of desferrioxamine (20–40 mg/kg over 12 hours) are given on 5 to 7 nights each week. Desferrioxamine (up to 2 g per unit of blood) may also be given through the infusion line at the time of blood transfusion.

Iron excretion induced by desferrioxamine is enhanced by administration of vitamin C (section 9.6.3) in a dose of 200 mg daily (100 mg in infants); it should be given separately from food since it also enhances iron absorption. In patients with cardiac abnormalities vitamin C should be avoided for 1–2 weeks after starting desferrioxamine treatment.

Infusion of desferrioxamine may be used to treat *aluminium overload* in dialysis patients; theoretically 100 mg of desferrioxamine binds with 4.1 mg of aluminium.

Orally active iron chelators are under clinical study but are not available for general use.

DESFERRIOXAMINE MESYLATE

Indications: see notes above; iron poisoning, see Emergency Treatment of Poisoning

Cautions: renal impairment, eye and ear examinations; aluminium-related encephalopathy (may exacerbate neurological dysfunction), pregnancy, breast-feeding; **interactions:** Appendix 1 (desferrioxamine)

Side-effects: gastro-intestinal disturbances; arrhythmias, hypotension (especially when given too rapidly by intravenous injection); anaphylaxis; dizziness, convulsions; Yersinia infection more frequent; disturbances of hearing and vision (including lens opacity and retinopathy); skin reactions; pain on intramuscular injection

Dose: see notes above; iron poisoning, see Emergency Treatment of Poisoning

Note. For full details and warnings relating to administration, consult data sheet

Preparations
See under Emergency Treatment of Poisoning

9.1.4 Drugs used in autoimmune thrombocytopenic purpura

It is usual to commence the treatment of auto-immune (idiopathic) thrombocytopenic purpura with corticosteroids, e.g. prednisolone of the order of 1 mg/kg daily, gradually reducing the dosage over the subsequent weeks. In patients who fail to achieve a satisfactory platelet count or relapse when corticosteroid dosage is reduced or withdrawn, splenectomy is considered.

Other therapy that has been tried in refractory cases includes azathioprine (see section 8.2.1), cyclophosphamide (see section 8.1.1), vincristine or vinblastine (see section 8.1.4) (or vinblastine-loaded platelets), cyclosporin (see section 8.2.2), and danazol (section 6.7.3). Intravenous immuno-globulins (see section 14.5), have also been used in refractory cases or where a temporary rapid rise in platelets is needed, as in pregnancy or pre-operatively. For patients with chronic severe thrombocytopenia refractory to other therapy, tranexamic acid (see section 2.11) may be given to reduce the severity of haemorrhage.

9.1.5 G6PD deficiency

Glucose 6-phosphate dehydrogenase (G6PD) deficiency is highly prevalent in populations originating from most parts of Africa, from most parts of Asia, from Oceania, and from Southern Europe; it can also be encountered, rarely, in any other population.

When prescribing drugs for patients who are G6PD deficient, the following three points should be kept in mind:

1. G6PD deficiency is genetically heterogeneous; different genetic variants entail different susceptibility to the haemolytic risk from drugs; thus, a drug found to be safe in some G6PD-deficient subjects may not be equally safe in others;

2. no test specifically designed to identify potential risk in G6PD-deficient subjects is currently carried out by manufacturers;

3. the risk and severity of haemolysis is almost always dose-related.

The table below should be read with these points in mind. Whenever possible, a test for G6PD deficiency should be done before prescribing a drug in the list, especially if the patient belongs to a population group in which G6PD deficiency is common.

A very small group of G6PD-deficient individuals, with chronic non-spherocytic haemolytic anaemia, have haemolysis even in the absence of an exogenous trigger. These patients must be regarded as being at high risk of severe exacerbation of haemolysis following administration of any of the drugs listed below.

Drugs with definite risk of haemolysis in most G6PD-deficient subjects

Dapsone and other sulphones (higher doses for dermatitis herpetiformis more likely to cause problems)
Methylene blue
Niridazole [not on UK market]
Nitrofurantoin
Pamaquin [not on UK market]
Primaquine (30 mg weekly for 8 weeks has been found to be without undue harmful effects in Afro and Asian people, see section 5.4.1)
4-Quinolones (including ciprofloxacin and nalidixic acid)
Sulphonamides (including co-trimoxazole; some sulphonamides, e.g. sulphadiazine, have been tested and found not to be haemolytic in many G6PD-deficient subjects)

Drugs with possible risk of haemolysis in some G6PD-deficient subjects

Aspirin (acceptable in a dose of at least 1 g daily in most G6PD-deficient subjects)
Chloroquine (acceptable in acute malaria)
Menadione, water-soluble derivatives (e.g. menadiol sodium phosphate)
Probenecid
Quinidine (acceptable in acute malaria)
Quinine (acceptable in acute malaria)

Note. Mothballs may contain naphthalene which also causes haemolysis in subjects with G6PD-deficiency.

9.1.6 Drugs used in neutropenia

Filgrastim (recombinant human granulocyte-colony stimulating factor) may reduce the duration of neutropenia associated with the use of cancer chemotherapy and thereby reduce the incidence of associated sepsis. Filgrastim has, however, no routine indication at present and is expensive; it should only be administered by those experienced in its use.

FILGRASTIM

(Human granulocyte-colony stimulating factor, G-CSF)
Indications: reduction in duration of neutropenia and incidence of febrile neutropenia in cytotoxic chemotherapy of non-myeloid malignancy (specialist use only)
Cautions: tumours with myeloid characteristics (risk of tumour growth); pre-malignant myeloid conditions; reduced myeloid precursors (e.g. following extensive radiotherapy or chemotherapy); monitor leucocyte count (discontinue treatment if leucocytosis, see data sheet); monitor platelet count and haemoglobin; osteoporotic bone disease (monitor bone density if given for more than 6 months); does not prevent other toxic effects of high-dose chemotherapy; pregnancy, breast-feeding
Side-effects: musculoskeletal pain, transient hypotension, disturbances in liver enzymes and serum uric acid; urinary abnormalities including dysuria
Dose: by *subcutaneous injection* or by *intravenous infusion*, 500 000 units/kg daily started not less than 24 hours after cytotoxic chemotherapy, continued until neutrophil count in normal range, usually for up to 14 days

▼ PoM **Neupogen**® (Roche)
Injection, filgrastim 30 million units (300 micrograms)/mL; net price 1-mL vial = £79.00, 1.6-mL (48 million-unit) vial = £126.00

9.2 Fluids and electrolytes

9.2.1 Oral administration
9.2.2 Intravenous administration
9.2.3 Plasma and plasma substitutes

The following tables give a selection of useful electrolyte values:

Electrolyte concentrations—intravenous fluids

Intravenous infusion	Na⁺	K⁺	HCO₃⁻	Cl⁻	Ca²⁺
Normal Plasma Values	142	4.5	26	103	2.5
Sodium Chloride 0.9%	150	—	—	150	—
Compound Sodium Lactate (Hartmann's)	131	5	29	111	2
Sodium Chloride 0.18% and Glucose 4%	30	—	—	30	—
Potassium Chloride 0.3% and Glucose 5%	—	40	—	40	—
Potassium Chloride 0.3% and Sodium Chloride 0.9%	150	40	—	190	—
To correct metabolic acidosis					
Sodium Bicarbonate 1.26%	150	—	150	—	—
Sodium Bicarbonate 8.4% for cardiac arrest	1000	—	1000	—	—
Sodium Lactate (M/6)	167	—	—	167	—

Millimoles per litre

Millimoles of each ion in 1 gram of salt

Electrolyte	mmol/g approx.
Ammonium chloride	18.7
Calcium chloride (CaCl₂.2H₂O)	Ca 6.8 Cl 13.6
Potassium bicarbonate	10
Potassium chloride	13.4
Sodium bicarbonate	11.9
Sodium chloride	17.1
Sodium lactate	8.9

Electrolyte content—gastro-intestinal secretions

Type of fluid	H⁺	Na⁺	K⁺	HCO₃⁻	Cl⁻
Gastric	40–60	20–80	5–20	—	100–150
Biliary	—	120–140	5–15	30–50	80–120
Pancreatic	—	120–140	5–15	70–110	40–80
Small bowel	—	120–140	5–15	20–40	90–130

Millimoles per litre

Faeces, vomit, or aspiration should be saved and analysed where possible if abnormal losses are suspected; where this is impracticable the approximations above may be helpful in planning replacement therapy.

9.2.1 Oral administration

9.2.1.1 Oral potassium
9.2.1.2 Oral sodium and water
9.2.1.3 Oral bicarbonate

Sodium and potassium salts, which may be given by mouth to prevent deficiencies or to treat established deficiencies of mild or moderate degree, are discussed in this section. Oral preparations for removing excess potassium and preparations for oral rehydration therapy are also included

9.2 Fluids and electrolytes

here. Oral bicarbonate, for metabolic acidosis, is also described in this section.

For reference to calcium, magnesium, and phosphate, see section 9.5.

9.2.1.1 ORAL POTASSIUM

Compensation for potassium loss is especially necessary:
1. in those taking digoxin or anti-arrhythmic drugs, where potassium depletion may induce arrhythmias;
2. in patients in whom secondary hyperaldosteronism occurs, e.g. renal artery stenosis, cirrhosis of the liver, the nephrotic syndrome, and severe heart failure;
3. in patients with excessive losses of potassium in the faeces, e.g. chronic diarrhoea associated with intestinal malabsorption or laxative abuse.

Measures to compensate for potassium loss may also be required in the elderly since they frequently take inadequate amounts of potassium in the diet (but see below for warning on renal insufficiency). Measures may also be required during long-term administration of drugs known to induce potassium loss (e.g. corticosteroids). Potassium supplements are seldom required with the small doses of diuretics given to treat hypertension; potassium-sparing diuretics (rather than potassium supplements) are recommended for prevention of hypokalaemia due to diuretics such as frusemide or the thiazides when these are given to eliminate oedema.

DOSAGE. If potassium salts are used for the *prevention of hypokalaemia*, then doses of potassium chloride 2 to 4 g (approx. 25 to 50 mmol) daily by mouth are suitable in patients taking a normal diet. Smaller doses must be used if there is renal insufficiency (common in the elderly) otherwise there is danger of hyperkalaemia. Potassium salts cause nausea and vomiting therefore poor compliance is a major limitation to their effectiveness; where appropriate, potassium-sparing diuretics are preferable.

When there is *established potassium depletion* or when the plasma-potassium concentration is less than 3.5 mmol/litre, larger doses of 10 to 15 g (approx. 135 to 200 mmol) daily of potassium chloride may be required over periods of days or weeks. Potassium depletion is frequently associated with chloride depletion and with metabolic alkalosis, and these disorders require correction.

ADMINISTRATION. Potassium salts are preferably given as a liquid (or effervescent) preparation, rather than modified-release tablets; they should be given as the chloride (the use of effervescent potassium tablets BPC 1968 should be restricted to *hyperchloraemic states*, section 9.2.1.3).

Salt substitutes. A number of salt substitutes which contain significant amounts of potassium chloride are readily available as health food products (e.g. Losalt and Ruthmol). These should not be used by patients with renal failure as potassium intoxication may result.

POTASSIUM BICARBONATE
Section 9.2.1.3

POTASSIUM CHLORIDE
Indications: potassium depletion (see notes above)
Cautions: intestinal stricture, history of peptic ulcer, hiatus hernia (for sustained-release preparations); **interactions:** Appendix 1 (potassium salts)
Contra-indications: renal failure, plasma potassium concentrations above 5 mmol/litre
Side-effects: nausea and vomiting (severe symptoms may indicate obstruction), oesophageal or small bowel ulceration
Dose: see notes above

Note. Do not confuse Effervescent Potassium Tablets BPC 1968 (section 9.2.1.3) with effervescent potassium chloride tablets. Effervescent Potassium Tablets BPC 1968 do not contain chloride ions and their use should be restricted to hyperchloraemic states (section 9.2.1.3). Effervescent Potassium Chloride Tablets BP are usually available in two strengths, one containing 6.7 mmol each of K^+ and Cl^- (corresponding to Kloref®), the other containing 12 mmol K^+ and 8 mmol Cl^- (corresponding to Sando-K®). Generic prescriptions must specify the strength required.

Kay-Cee-L® (Geistlich)
Syrup, red, sugar-free, potassium chloride 7.5% (1 mmol/mL each of K^+ and Cl^-). Net price 200 mL = £2.05; 500 mL = £2.88. Label: 21

Kloref® (Cox)
Tablets, effervescent, betaine hydrochloride, potassium benzoate, bicarbonate, and chloride, equivalent to potassium chloride 500 mg (6.7 mmol each of K^+ and Cl^-). Net price 50 = £1.59. Label: 13, 21

Kloref-S® (Cox)
Granules, effervescent, sugar-free, betaine hydrochloride, potassium bicarbonate and chloride equivalent to potassium chloride 1.5 g (20 mmol each of K^+ and Cl^-)/sachet. Net price 30 sachets = £2.84. Label: 13, 21

Sando-K® (Sandoz)
Tablets, effervescent, potassium bicarbonate and chloride equivalent to potassium 470 mg (12 mmol of K^+) and chloride 285 mg (8 mmol of Cl^-). Net price 20 = 35p. Label: 13, 21

Modified-release preparations
Avoid unless effervescent tablets or liquid preparations inappropriate

Leo K® (Leo)
Tablets, m/r, f/c, potassium chloride 600 mg (8 mmol each of K^+ and Cl^-). Net price 20 = 20p. Label: 25, 27, counselling, swallow whole with fluid during meals while sitting or standing

Nu-K® (Consolidated)
Capsules, m/r, blue, potassium chloride 600 mg (8 mmol each of K^+ and Cl^-). Net price 20 = 43p. Label: 25, 27, counselling, swallow whole with fluid during meals while sitting or standing *or* open capsule and swallow enclosed granules with fluid or soft food

Slow-K® (Ciba)
Tablets, m/r, orange, s/c, potassium chloride 600 mg (8 mmol each of K^+ and Cl^-). Net price 20 = 10p. Label: 25, 27, counselling, swallow whole with fluid during meals while sitting or standing

POTASSIUM CITRATE
See section 7.4.3

POTASSIUM REMOVAL

Ion-exchange resins may be used to remove excess potassium in *mild hyperkalaemia* or in *moderate hyperkalaemia* when there are not ECG changes; intravenous therapy is required in emergencies (section 9.2.2).

POLYSTYRENE SULPHONATE RESINS
Indications: hyperkalaemia associated with anuria or severe oliguria, and in dialysis patients
Cautions: children (impaction of resin with excessive dosage or inadequate dilution)
Contra-indications: avoid calcium-containing resin in hyperparathyroidism, multiple myeloma, sarcoidosis, or metastatic carcinoma; avoid sodium-containing resin in congestive heart failure and severe renal impairment
Side-effects: rectal ulceration following rectal administration
Dose: by mouth, 15 g 3–4 times daily in water (not fruit juice which has a high K^+ content)
By rectum, as an enema, 30 g in methylcellulose solution, retained for 9 hours
CHILD, either route, 0.5–1 g/kg daily

Calcium Resonium® (Sanofi Winthrop)
Powder, buff, calcium polystyrene sulphonate. Net price 300 g = £44.34. Label: 13
Resonium A® (Sanofi Winthrop)
Powder, buff, sodium polystyrene sulphonate. Net price 454 g = £54.57. Label: 13

9.2.1.2 ORAL SODIUM AND WATER

Sodium chloride is indicated in states of sodium depletion and usually needs to be given intravenously (section 9.2.2). In chronic conditions associated with mild or moderate degrees of sodium depletion, e.g. in salt-losing bowel or renal disease, oral supplements of sodium chloride or bicarbonate (section 9.2.1.3), according to the acid-base status of the patient, may be sufficient.

SODIUM BICARBONATE
Section 9.2.1.3

SODIUM CHLORIDE
Indications: sodium depletion; see also section 9.2.2.

Sodium Chloride Tablets, sodium chloride 300 mg (approx 5 mmol each of Na^+ and Cl^-). Net price 20 = 19p. Label: 13
Slow Sodium® (Ciba)
Tablets, m/r, sodium chloride 600 mg (approx. 10 mmol each of Na^+ and Cl^-). Net price 20 = 11p. Label: 25

ORAL REHYDRATION THERAPY (ORT)

As a worldwide problem *diarrhoea* is by far the most important indication for fluid and electrolyte replacement. Intestinal absorption of sodium and water is enhanced by glucose, therefore replacement of fluid and electrolytes lost through diarrhoea can be achieved by giving solutions containing sodium, potassium, and glucose.

Oral rehydration solutions should:
enhance optimally the absorption of water and electrolytes;
replace the electrolyte deficit adequately and safely;
contain an alkalising agent to counter acidosis;
be simple to use in hospital and at home;
be palatable and acceptable, especially to children;
be readily available.

It is the policy of the World Health Organization (WHO) to promote a single oral rehydration solution but use it flexibly (e.g. by giving extra water between drinks of oral rehydration solution to moderately dehydrated infants).

Oral rehydration solutions used in the UK are lower in sodium (35–60 mmol/litre) and higher in glucose (up to 200 mmol/litre) than the WHO formulation. They are of benefit for *mild to moderate diarrhoea*, when the body's homoeostatic mechanisms are still working and will not be harmful, but they may be suboptimal in correction of fluid loss and electrolyte imbalance. In the *more severe diarrhoeas* the WHO formulation is marginally more effective in correcting dehydration; it carries no danger of hypernatraemia if used correctly.

For intravenous rehydration see section 9.2.2

ORAL REHYDRATION SALTS (ORS)
Indications: fluid and electrolyte loss in diarrhoea, see notes above
Dose: according to fluid loss, usually 200–400 mL solution after every loose motion; INFANT 1–1½ times usual feed volume; CHILD 200 mL after every loose motion

UK formulations
Note. After reconstitution any unused solution should be discarded no later than 1 hour after preparation unless stored in a refrigerator when it may be kept for up to 24 hours.

Dextrolyte® (Cow & Gate)
Oral solution, glucose, potassium chloride, sodium chloride, sodium lactate, providing Na^+ 35 mmol, K^+ 13.4 mmol, Cl^- 30.5 mmol, lactate 17.7 mmol, and glucose 200 mmol/litre. 100 mL (hosp. only)
Diocalm Junior® (SmithKline Beecham Brands)
Oral powder, sodium chloride 350 mg, potassium chloride 300 mg, sodium citrate 590 mg, anhydrous glucose 4 g/sachet. Net price 5-sachet pack (orange-flavoured) = £1.10
Reconstitute one sachet with 200 mL of water (freshly boiled and cooled for infants)
Note. Five sachets reconstituted with 1 litre of water provide Na^+ 60 mmol, K^+ 20 mmol, Cl^- 50 mmol, citrate 10 mmol, and glucose 111 mmol

9.2 Fluids and electrolytes

Dioralyte® (Rhône-Poulenc Rorer)
Effervescent tablets, sodium chloride 117 mg, sodium bicarbonate 336 mg, potassium chloride 186 mg, citric acid anhydrous 384 mg, anhydrous glucose 1.62 g. Net price 10-tab pack (blackcurrant- or citrus-flavoured) = £1.20
Reconstitute 2 tablets with 200 mL of water (only for adults and for children over 1 year)
Note. Ten tablets when reconstituted with 1 litre of water provide Na^+ 60 mmol, K^+ 25 mmol, Cl^- 45 mmol, citrate 20 mmol, and glucose 90 mmol
Oral powder, sodium chloride 470 mg, potassium chloride 300 mg, disodium hydrogen citrate 530 mg, glucose 3.56 g/sachet. Net price 20 sachet-pack (blackcurrant- or citrus-flavoured or plain) = £4.17
Reconstitute one sachet with 200 mL of water (freshly boiled and cooled for infants).
Note. Five sachets reconstituted with 1 litre of water provide Na^+ 60 mmol, K^+ 20 mmol, Cl^- 60 mmol, citrate 10 mmol, and glucose 90 mmol

Electrolade® (Nicholas)
Oral powder, sodium chloride 236 mg, potassium chloride 300 mg, sodium bicarbonate 500 mg, anhydrous glucose 4 g/sachet (banana- and melon-flavoured). Net price 4-sachet pack = 80p; 20-sachet pack = £3.99
Reconstitute one sachet with 200 mL of water (freshly boiled and cooled for infants)
Note. Five sachets when reconstituted with 1 litre of water provide Na^+ 50 mmol, K^+ 20 mmol, Cl^- 40 mmol, HCO_3^- 30 mmol, and glucose 111 mmol

Gluco-lyte® (Cupal)
Oral powder, sodium chloride 200 mg, potassium chloride 300 mg, sodium bicarbonate 300 mg, glucose 8 g/sachet. Net price 6 sachets = £1.35
Reconstitute one sachet with 200 mL of water (freshly boiled and cooled for infants)
Note. Five sachets when reconstituted with 1 litre of water provide Na^+ 35 mmol, K^+ 20 mmol, Cl^- 37 mmol, HCO_3^- 18 mmol, and glucose 200 mmol (corresponds to Oral Rehydration Salts—Formula A, BP)

Rapolyte® (Janssen)
Oral powder, sodium chloride 350 mg, potassium chloride 300 mg, sodium citrate 600 mg, anhydrous glucose 4 g/sachet. Net price 5-sachet pack (raspberry-flavoured) = £1.07
Reconstitute one sachet with 200 mL of water (freshly boiled and cooled for infants)
Note. Five sachets reconstituted with 1 litre of water provide Na^+ 60 mmol, K^+ 20 mmol, Cl^- 50 mmol, citrate 10 mmol, and glucose 111 mmol)

Rehidrat® (Searle)
Oral powder, sodium chloride 440 mg, potassium chloride 380 mg, sodium bicarbonate 420 mg, citric acid 440 mg, glucose 4.09 g, sucrose 8.07 g, fructose 70 mg/sachet. Net price 24-sachet pack (orange, blackcurrant or lemon and lime flavour) = £5.85; 16-sachet pack (mixed flavours) = £3.90
Note. Lemon and lime version stains vomit green
Reconstitute one sachet with 250 mL of water (freshly boiled and cooled for infants)
Note. Four sachets when reconstituted with one litre of water provide Na^+ 50 mmol, K^+ 20 mmol, Cl^- 50 mmol, HCO_3^- 20 mmol, citrate 9 mmol, glucose 91 mmol, sucrose 94 mmol, and fructose 2 mmol

WHO formulations
WHO Oral Rehydration Salts
Oral powder, sodium chloride 3.5 g, potassium chloride 1.5 g, sodium citrate 2.9 g, anhydrous glucose 20 g. To be dissolved in sufficient water to produce 1 litre (providing Na^+ 90 mmol, K^+ 20 mmol, Cl^- 80 mmol, citrate 10 mmol, glucose 111 mmol/litre)
Note. Recommended by the WHO and the United Nations Childrens Fund but not commonly used in the UK. Corresponds to Oral Rehydration Salts—Citrate (Formula C) BP; the alternative WHO formulation corresponds to Oral Rehydration Salts—Bicarbonate (Formula B) BP and is less stable

9.2.1.3 ORAL BICARBONATE

Sodium bicarbonate is given by mouth for *chronic acidotic states* such as uraemic acidosis or renal tubular acidosis. The dose for correction of metabolic acidosis is not predictable and the response must be assessed; 4.8 g daily (57 mmol each of Na^+ and HCO_3^-) or more may be required. For severe metabolic acidosis, sodium bicarbonate can be given intravenously (section 9.2.2).

Sodium bicarbonate may also be used to make the pH of the urine alkaline (see section 7.4.3); for use in dyspepsia see section 1.1.2.

Sodium supplements may increase blood pressure or cause fluid retention and pulmonary oedema in those at risk; hypokalaemia may be exacerbated.

Where *hyperchloraemic acidosis* is associated with potassium deficiency, as in some renal tubular and gastro-intestinal disorders it may be appropriate to give oral **potassium bicarbonate**, although acute or severe deficiency should be managed by intravenous therapy.

SODIUM BICARBONATE
Indications: see notes above
Cautions: see notes above; avoid in respiratory acidosis; **interactions:** Appendix 1 (antacids and adsorbents)
Dose: see notes above

Sodium Bicarbonate (Non-proprietary)
Capsules, sodium bicarbonate usual strengths 300 mg (approx. 3.6 mmol each of Na^+ and HCO_3^-), 500 mg (approx. 6 mmol each of Na^+ and HCO_3^-), 600 mg (approx. 7.1 mmol each of Na^+ and HCO_3^-)
Available from Martindale, Penn, etc (special order)
Tablets, sodium bicarbonate 300 mg, net price 20 tabs = 8p; 600 mg, 20 = 42p

POTASSIUM BICARBONATE
Indications: see notes above
Cautions: cardiac disease, renal impairment; interactions: Appendix 1 (potassium salts)
Contra-indications: hypochloraemia; plasma potassium concentration above 5 mmol/litre
Side-effects: nausea and vomiting
Dose: see notes above

Potassium Tablets, Effervescent, potassium bicarbonate 500 mg, potassium acid tartrate 300 mg, each tablet providing 6.5 mmol of K^+. To be dissolved in water before administration. Net price 100 = £2.71. Label: 13, 21

Note. These tablets do not contain chloride; for effervescent tablets containing potassium and chloride, see under Potassium Chloride, section 9.2.1.1

WATER

The term water used without qualification means either potable water freshly drawn direct from the public supply and suitable for drinking or freshly boiled and cooled purified water. The latter should be used if the public supply is from a local storage tank or if the potable water is unsuitable for a particular preparation. (Water for injections, section 9.2.2.)

9.2.2 Intravenous administration

Solutions of electrolytes are given intravenously, to meet normal fluid and electrolyte requirements or to replenish substantial deficits or continuing losses, when the patient is nauseated or vomiting and is unable to take adequate amounts by mouth.

In an individual patient the nature and severity of the electrolyte imbalance must be assessed from the history and clinical and biochemical examination. Sodium, potassium, chloride, magnesium, phosphate, and water depletion can occur singly and in combination with or without disturbances of acid-base balance; for reference to the use of magnesium and phosphates, see section 9.5.

Isotonic solutions may be infused safely into a peripheral vein. Solutions more concentrated than plasma, for example 20% glucose are best given through an indwelling catheter positioned in a large vein.

INTRAVENOUS SODIUM

Sodium chloride in isotonic solution provides the most important extracellular ions in near physiological concentration and is indicated in *sodium depletion* which may arise from such conditions as gastro-enteritis, diabetic ketoacidosis, ileus, and ascites. In a severe deficit of from 4 to 8 litres, 2 to 3 litres of isotonic sodium chloride may be given over 2 to 3 hours; thereafter infusion can usually be at a slower rate.

Excessive administration should be avoided; the jugular venous pressure should be assessed, the bases of the lungs should be examined for crepitations, and in elderly or seriously ill patients it is often helpful to monitor the right atrial (central) venous pressure.

Compound sodium lactate (Hartmann's solution) can be used instead of isotonic sodium chloride solution during surgery or in the initial management of the injured or wounded.

Sodium chloride and glucose solutions are indicated when there is combined *water and sodium depletion.* A 1:1 mixture of isotonic sodium chloride and 5% glucose allows some of the water (free of sodium) to enter body cells which suffer most from dehydration while the sodium salt with a volume of water determined by the normal plasma Na^+ remains extracellular. An example of combined sodium chloride and water depletion occurs in persistent vomiting.

SODIUM CHLORIDE
Indications: electrolyte imbalance, also section 9.2.1.2
Cautions: restrict intake in impaired renal function, cardiac failure, hypertension, peripheral and pulmonary oedema, toxaemia of pregnancy
Side-effects: administration of large doses may give rise to sodium accumulation and oedema
Dose: see notes above

PoM **Sodium Chloride Intravenous Infusion,** usual strength sodium chloride 0.9% (9 g, 150 mmol each of Na^+ and Cl^-/litre), this strength being supplied when normal saline for injection is requested. Net price 2-mL amp = 23p; 5-mL amp = 30p; 10-mL amp = 34p; 20-mL amp = 62p; 50-mL amp = £1.52
In hospitals, 500- and 1000-mL packs, and sometimes other sizes, are available

Note. The term 'normal saline' should **not** be used to describe sodium chloride intravenous infusion 0.9%; the term 'physiological saline' is acceptable but it is preferable to give the composition (i.e. sodium chloride intravenous infusion 0.9%).

With other ingredients

PoM **Sodium Chloride and Glucose Intravenous Infusion,** usual strength sodium chloride 0.18% (1.8 g, 30 mmol each of Na^+ and Cl^-/litre) and 4% of anhydrous glucose
In hospitals, 500- and 1000-mL packs, and sometimes other sizes are available

PoM **Ringer's Solution for Injection,** calcium chloride (dihydrate) 322 micrograms, potassium chloride 300 micrograms, sodium chloride 8.6 mg/mL, providing the following ions (in mmol/litre), Ca^{2+} 2.2, K^+ 4, Na^+ 147, Cl^- 156
In hospitals, 500- and 1000-mL packs, and sometimes other sizes, are available

PoM **Sodium Lactate Intravenous Infusion, Compound** (Hartmann's Solution for Injection; Ringer-Lactate Solution for Injection), sodium chloride 0.6%, sodium lactate 0.25%, potassium chloride 0.04%, calcium chloride 0.027% (containing Na^+ 131 mmol, K^+ 5 mmol, Ca^{2+} 2 mmol, HCO_3^- (as lactate) 29 mmol, Cl^- 111 mmol/litre)
In hospitals, 500- and 1000-mL packs, and sometimes other sizes are available

9.2 Fluids and electrolytes

INTRAVENOUS GLUCOSE

Glucose solutions (5%) are mainly used to replace water deficits and should be given alone when there is no significant loss of electrolytes. Average water requirements in a healthy adult are 1.5 to 2.5 litres daily and this is needed to balance unavoidable losses of water through the skin and lungs and to provide sufficient for urinary excretion. Water depletion (dehydration) tends to occur when these losses are not matched by a comparable intake, as for example may occur in coma or dysphagia or in the aged or apathetic who may not drink water in sufficient amount on their own initiative.

Excessive loss of water without loss of electrolytes is uncommon, occurring in fevers, hyperthyroidism, and in uncommon water-losing renal states such as diabetes insipidus or hypercalcaemia. The volume of glucose solution needed to replenish deficits varies with the severity of the disorder, but usually lies within the range of 2 to 10 litres.

Glucose solutions are also given in regimens with calcium, bicarbonate, and insulin for the emergency management of *hyperkalaemia*. They are also given, after correction of hyperglycaemia, during treatment of diabetic ketoacidosis, when they must be accompanied by continuing insulin infusion.

GLUCOSE
(Dextrose Monohydrate)
Note. Glucose BP is the monohydrate but Glucose Intravenous Infusion BP is a sterile solution of anhydrous glucose or glucose monohydrate, potency being expressed in terms of anhydrous glucose

Indications: fluid replacement (see notes above), provision of energy (section 9.3)

Side-effects: glucose injections especially if hypertonic may have a low pH and may cause venous irritation and thrombophlebitis

Dose: water replacement, see notes above; energy source, 1–3 litres daily of 20–50% solution

PoM **Glucose Intravenous Infusion,** glucose or anhydrous glucose (potency expressed in terms of anhydrous glucose), usual strength 5% (50 mg/mL). 20% solution, net price 20-mL amp = £1.30; 25% solution, 25-mL amp = £2.21; 50% solution, price 20-mL amp = £1.50; 25-mL amp = £3.11; 50-mL amp = £2.66
In hospitals, 500- and 1000-mL packs, and sometimes other sizes, are available; also available from IMS (Min-I-Jet® Glucose, 50% in 50-ml disposable syringe).

INTRAVENOUS POTASSIUM

Potassium chloride and sodium chloride intravenous infusion and **potassium chloride and glucose** intravenous infusion are used to correct severe *hypokalaemia* and depletion and when sufficient potassium cannot be taken by mouth. Potassium chloride, as ampoules containing 1.5 g (20 mmol K$^+$) in 10 mL[1], may be added to 500 mL of sodium chloride or glucose intravenous infusion; the solution then contains 40 mmol/litre and may be given slowly over 2 to 3 hours with ECG monitoring in difficult cases[2]. Repeated measurements of plasma potassium are necessary to determine whether further infusions are required and to avoid the development of hyperkalaemia; this is especially liable to occur in renal failure.

1. **Important:** mix infusion solution **thoroughly** after adding potassium chloride; use ready-prepared solutions when possible
2. Higher concentrations may be given in severe cases but require infusion pump control

POTASSIUM CHLORIDE
Indications: electrolyte imbalance; see also oral potassium supplements, section 9.2.1.1

Cautions: for intravenous infusion the concentration of solution should not usually exceed 3.2 g (43 mmol)/litre

Side-effects: rapid infusion toxic to heart

Dose: by slow intravenous infusion, depending on the deficit or the daily maintenance requirements, see also notes above

PoM **Potassium Chloride and Glucose Intravenous Infusion,** usual strength potassium chloride 0.3% (3 g, 40 mmol each of K$^+$ and Cl$^-$/litre) with 5% of anhydrous glucose
In hospitals, 500- and 1000-mL packs, and sometimes other sizes, are available

PoM **Potassium Chloride and Sodium Chloride Intravenous Infusion,** usual strength potassium chloride 0.3% (3 g/litre) and sodium chloride 0.9% (9 g/litre), containing 40 mmol of K$^+$, 150 mmol of Na$^+$, and 190 mmol of Cl$^-$/litre
In hospitals, 500- and 1000-mL packs, and sometimes other sizes, are available

PoM **Potassium Chloride, Sodium Chloride, and Glucose Intravenous Infusion,** sodium chloride 0.18% (1.8 g, 30 mmol of Na$^+$/litre) with 4% of anhydrous glucose and usually sufficient potassium chloride to provide 10–40 mmol of K$^+$/litre (to be specified by the prescriber)
In hospitals, 500- and 1000-mL packs, and sometimes other sizes, are available

PoM **Potassium Chloride Solution, Strong** (sterile), potassium chloride 15% (150 mg, approximately 2 mmol each of K$^+$ and Cl$^-$/mL). Net price 10-mL amp = 81p
IMPORTANT. Must be diluted with **not less** than 50 times its volume of sodium chloride intravenous infusion 0.9% or other suitable diluent and **mixed well**
Solutions containing 10 and 20% of potassium chloride are also available in both 5- and 10-mL ampoules.

BICARBONATE AND LACTATE

Sodium bicarbonate is used to control severe *metabolic acidosis* (as in renal failure or diabetic ketoacidosis). Since this condition is usually attended by sodium depletion, it is reasonable to correct this first by the administration of isotonic sodium chloride intravenous infusion, provided the kidneys are not primarily affected and the degree of acidosis is not so severe as to impair renal function. In these circumstances, isotonic sodium chloride alone is usually effective as it restores the ability of the kidneys to generate bicarbonate. In renal acidosis or in severe metabolic acidosis of any origin (for example blood pH<7.1) sodium bicarbonate (1.26%) may be infused with isotonic sodium chloride when the acidosis remains unresponsive to correction of anoxia or fluid depletion; a total volume of up to 6 litres (4 litres of sodium chloride and 2 litres of sodium bicarbonate) may be necessary in the adult. In severe shock due for example to cardiac arrest (see section 2.7), metabolic acidosis may develop without sodium depletion; in these circumstances sodium bicarbonate is best given in a small volume of hypertonic solution, such as 50 mL of 8.4% solution intravenously; plasma pH should be monitored.

Sodium bicarbonate infusion is also used in the emergency management of *hyperkalaemia* (see also under Glucose).

Sodium lactate intravenous infusion is obsolete in metabolic acidosis, and carries the risk of producing lactic acidosis, particularly in seriously ill patients with poor tissue perfusion or impaired hepatic function.

SODIUM BICARBONATE

Indications: metabolic acidosis

Dose: by slow intravenous injection, a strong solution (up to 8.4%), or *by continuous intravenous infusion*, a weaker solution (usually 1.26%), an amount appropriate to the body base deficit (see notes above)

PoM **Sodium Bicarbonate Intravenous Infusion,** usual strength sodium bicarbonate 1.26% (12.6 g, 150 mmol each of Na^+ and HCO_3^-/litre); various other strengths available
In hospitals, 500- and 1000-mL packs, and sometimes other sizes, are available

PoM **Min-I-Jet® Sodium Bicarbonate** (IMS)
Intravenous injection, sodium bicarbonate in disposable syringe, net price 4.2%, 10 mL = £4.19; 8.4%, 10 mL = £4.37, 50 mL = £7.09

SODIUM LACTATE

Indications: diabetic coma, diminished alkali reserve (but see notes above)

PoM **Sodium Lactate Intravenous Infusion,** sodium lactate M/6, contains the following ions (in mmol/litre), Na^+ 167, HCO_3^- (as lactate) 167

WATER

PoM **Water for Injections.** Net price 1-mL amp = 12p; 2-mL amp = 12p; 5-mL amp = 17p; 20-mL amp = 50p; 50-mL amp = £1.03

9.2.3 Plasma and plasma substitutes

Plasma and albumin solutions, prepared from whole blood, contain soluble proteins and electrolytes but no clotting factors, blood group antibodies, or pseudocholinesterases; they may be given without regard to the recipient's blood group.

Plasma and albumin solutions are used for the treatment of hypoproteinaemia and the low plasma volume associated with conditions such as burns, the complications of surgery, and pancreatitis. Plasma substitutes are more appropriate for acute blood loss (e.g. haematemesis).

ALBUMIN SOLUTION
(Human Albumin Solution)

A solution containing protein derived from plasma, serum, or normal placentas; at least 95% of the protein is albumin. The solution may be isotonic (containing 4–5% protein) or concentrated (containing 15–25% protein).

Indications: see under preparations, below

Cautions: history of cardiac or circulatory disease (administer slowly to avoid rapid rise in blood pressure and cardiac failure, and monitor cardiovascular and respiratory function); correct dehydration when administering concentrated solution

Contra-indications: cardiac failure; severe anaemia

Side-effects: allergic reactions with nausea, fever, and chills reported

Isotonic solutions

Indications: acute or sub-acute loss of plasma volume e.g. in burns, pancreatitis, trauma, and complications of surgery; plasma exchange

Available as: *Human Albumin Solution* 4.5% (50-, 100-, 250-, and 400-mL bottles—Immuno); *Albuminar-5®* (250-mL, 500-mL, and 1-litre vials—Armour); *Albutein®* 5% (250- and 500-mL vials—Alpha); *Buminate®* 5.0% (250- and 500-mL bottles—Baxter); *Zenalb®* 4.5 (50-, 100-, 250-, and 500-mL bottles—BPL)

Concentrated solutions (20–25%)

Indications: severe hypoalbuminaemia associated with low plasma volume and generalised oedema where salt and water restriction with plasma volume expansion are required; adjunct in the treatment of hyperbilirubinaemia by exchange transfusion in the newborn

Available as: *Albumin Solution 20%* (100-mL vials—SNBTS); *Human Albumin Solution 20%* (10-, 50- and 100-mL vials—Immuno); *Albuminar-20®* (50- and 100-mL vials—Armour); *Albuminar-25®* (20-, 50-, and 100-mL vials—Armour); *Albutein®* 20% (50- and 100-mL vials—Alpha); *Albutein®* 25% (20-, 50-, and 100-mL vials—Alpha); *Buminate®* 20% (50- and 100-mL vials—Baxter); *Zenalb®* 20 (5-, 50-, and 100-mL bottles—BPL)

9.2 Fluids and electrolytes 341

PLASMA PROTEIN SOLUTION
(Plasma Protein Fraction, PPF)
An isotonic solution containing 4–5% protein derived from plasma or serum; at least 85% of the protein is albumin.
Indications: see notes above
Cautions; Contra-indications; Side-effects: see under Albumin Solution

Available as: *Plasma Protein Solution* 4.5% (100- and 500-mL bottles—SNBTS); *Plasmatein®* 5% (250- and 500-mL vials—Alpha)

PLASMA SUBSTITUTES

Dextrans, **gelatin**, and **hetastarch** are macromolecular substances which are slowly metabolised; they may be used at the outset to expand and maintain blood volume in shock arising from conditions such as burns or septicaemia. They are rarely needed when shock is due to sodium and water depletion as, in these circumstances, the shock responds to water and electrolyte repletion. They should not be used to maintain plasma volume in conditions such as burns or peritonitis where there is loss of plasma protein, water and electrolytes over periods of several days or weeks. In these situations, plasma or plasma protein fractions containing large amounts of albumin should be given. Plasma substitutes should be used in haemorrhage if blood is not available as an immediate short-term measure until it is.

Dextrans may interfere with blood group cross-matching or biochemical measurements and these should be carried out before infusion is begun. Dextran 70 by intravenous infusion is used predominantly for volume expansion. Dextran 40 intravenous infusion is used in an attempt to improve peripheral blood flow in ischaemic disease of the limbs and peripheral thromboembolism.

Gelatin and **hetastarch** are also used for short-term volume expansion.

> **Dosage**. Because of the complex requirements relating to blood volume expansion and the primary significance of blood, plasma protein, and electrolyte replacement, detailed dose statements have been omitted. *In all cases specialist literature should be consulted.*

DEXTRAN 40 INTRAVENOUS INFUSION
Dextrans of weight average molecular weight about '40000' 10% in glucose intravenous infusion 5% or in sodium chloride intravenous infusion 0.9%
Indications: conditions associated with peripheral local slowing of the blood flow; prophylaxis of post-surgical thrombo-embolic disease
Cautions; Contra-indications; Side-effects: see under Dextran 70 Intravenous Infusion; correct dehydration before infusion and give adequate fluids during therapy; very special care in those at risk of vascular overloading
Dose: by intravenous infusion, initially 500–1000 mL; further doses are given according to the patient's condition (see notes above)

PoM **Gentran 40®** (Baxter)
Intravenous infusion, dextran 40 intravenous infusion in glucose intravenous infusion 5% or in sodium chloride intravenous infusion 0.9%. Net price 500-mL bottle (both) = £4.90
PoM **Lomodex 40®** (CP)
Intravenous infusion, dextran 40 intravenous infusion in glucose intravenous infusion 5% or in sodium chloride intravenous infusion 0.9%. Net price 500-mL bottle (both) = £5.77
PoM **Rheomacrodex®** (Kabi Pharmacia)
Intravenous infusion, dextran 40 intravenous infusion in glucose intravenous infusion 5% or in sodium chloride intravenous infusion 0.9%. Net price 500-mL bottle (both) = £6.51

DEXTRAN 70 INTRAVENOUS INFUSION
Dextrans of weight average molecular weight about '70000' 6% in glucose intravenous infusion 5% or in sodium chloride intravenous infusion 0.9%
Indications: short-term blood volume expansion; prophylaxis of post-surgical thrombo-embolic disease
Cautions: congestive heart failure, renal impairment; blood samples for cross-matching should ideally be taken before infusion
Contra-indications: severe congestive heart failure; renal failure; bleeding disorders such as thrombocytopenia and hypofibrinogenaemia
Side-effects: rarely anaphylactoid reactions
Dose: by intravenous infusion, after moderate to severe haemorrhage, 500–1000 mL rapidly initially followed by 500 mL later if necessary; severe burns, up to 3000 mL in the first few days with electrolytes (see also notes above)

PoM **Gentran 70®** (Baxter)
Intravenous infusion, dextran 70 intravenous infusion in glucose intravenous infusion 5% or in sodium chloride intravenous infusion 0.9%. Net price 500-mL bottle (both) = £4.90
PoM **Lomodex 70®** (CP)
Intravenous infusion, dextran 70 intravenous infusion in glucose intravenous infusion 5% or in sodium chloride intravenous infusion 0.9%. Net price 500-mL bottle (both) = £3.66
PoM **Macrodex®** (Kabi Pharmacia)
Intravenous infusion, dextran 70 intravenous infusion in glucose intravenous infusion 5% or in sodium chloride intravenous infusion 0.9%. Net price 500-mL bottle (both) = £4.11

DEXTRAN 110 INTRAVENOUS INFUSION
Dextrans of weight average molecular weight about '110000' 6% in glucose intravenous infusion 5% or in sodium chloride intravenous infusion 0.9%
Indications: see under Dextran 70 Intravenous Infusion
Cautions; Contra-indications; Side-effects: see under Dextran 70 Intravenous Infusion; blood samples for cross-matching should be taken before infusion
Dose: by intravenous infusion, see under Dextran 70 Intravenous Infusion

PoM **Dextraven 110®** (CP)
Intravenous infusion, dextran 110 intravenous infusion in sodium chloride intravenous infusion 0.9%. Net price 500-mL bottle = £5.77

GELATIN
Note. The gelatin is partially degraded
Indications: low blood volume
Cautions; Contra-indications; Side-effects: see under Dextran 70 Intravenous Infusion
Dose: by intravenous infusion, initially 500–1000 mL of a 3.5–4% solution (see notes above)

PoM **Gelofusine®** (Braun)
Intravenous infusion, succinylated gelatin (modified fluid gelatin, average molecular weight 30000) 4%, sodium chloride 0.9%. Net price 500-mL bottle = £3.56

PoM **Haemaccel®** (Hoechst)
Intravenous infusion, polygeline (degraded and modified gelatin, average molecular weight 35000) 35 g, Na$^+$ 145 mmol, K$^+$ 5.1 mmol, Ca^{2+} 6.25 mmol, Cl$^-$ 145 mmol/litre. Net price 500-mL bottle = £3.81

HETASTARCH
Indications: low blood volume (expansion)
Cautions; Contra-indications; Side-effects: see under Dextran 70 Intravenous Infusion
Dose: by intravenous infusion, 500–1000 mL; usual max. 1500 mL daily (see notes above)

PoM **Elohes® 6%** (Oxford Nutrition)
Intravenous infusion, hetastarch (weight average molecular weight 200000) 6% in sodium chloride intravenous infusion 0.9%. Net price 500-mL bottle = £9.75

PoM **Hespan®** (Du Pont)
Intravenous infusion, hetastarch (weight average molecular weight 450000) 6% in sodium chloride intravenous infusion 0.9%. Net price 500-mL Steriflex® bag = £16.72

9.3 Intravenous nutrition

When adequate feeding via the alimentary tract is not possible, nutrients may be given by intravenous infusion. This may be in addition to ordinary oral or tube feeding—**supplemental parenteral nutrition**, or may be the sole source of nutrition—**total parenteral nutrition** (TPN). Indications for this method include preparation of undernourished patients for surgery, chemotherapy, or radiation therapy; severe or prolonged disorders of the gastro-intestinal tract; major surgery, trauma, or burns; prolonged coma or refusal to eat; and some patients with renal or hepatic failure. The composition of proprietary preparations available is in the table below.

Protein is given as mixtures of essential and non-essential synthetic L-amino acids. Ideally, all essential amino acids should be included with a wide variety of non-essential ones to provide sufficient nitrogen together with electrolytes (see also section 9.2.2). Available solutions vary in their composition of amino acids; they often contain an energy source (usually glucose) and electrolytes.

Energy is provided in a ratio of 0.6 to 1.1 megajoules (150–250 kcals) per gram of protein nitrogen. Energy requirements must be met if amino acids are to be utilised for tissue maintenance. Although it has long been held that carbohydrate has a greater nitrogen-sparing effect than fat, recent studies have shown that a mixture of both energy sources, usually 30 to 50% as fat, gives better utilisation of amino acid solutions than glucose alone.

Glucose is the preferred source of carbohydrate, but if more than 180 g is given per day frequent monitoring of blood glucose is required, and insulin may be necessary. Glucose in various strengths from 10 to 50% must be infused through a central venous catheter to avoid thrombosis. Preparations are available with useful added ions and trace elements, e.g. Glucoplex®.

Fructose and sorbitol have been used in an attempt to avoid the problem of hyperosmolar hyperglycaemic non-ketotic acidosis but other metabolic problems may occur, as with xylitol and ethanol which are now rarely used.

Fat emulsions have the advantages of a high energy to fluid volume ratio, neutral pH, and iso-osmolarity with plasma, and provide essential fatty acids. Available preparations are soya bean oil emulsions. Several days of adaptation may be required to attain maximal utilisation. Reactions include occasional febrile episodes (usually only with 20% emulsions) and rare anaphylactic responses. Interference with biochemical measurements such as those for blood gases and calcium may occur if samples are taken before fat has been cleared. Daily checks are necessary to ensure complete clearance from the plasma in conditions where fat metabolism may be disturbed. **Additives may only be mixed with fat emulsions where compatibility is known.**

Total parenteral nutrition (TPN) requires the use of a solution containing amino acids, glucose, fat, electrolytes, trace elements, and vitamins. This is now commonly provided by the pharmacy in the form of the 3-litre bag. The solution is infused through a central venous catheter inserted under full surgical precautions. Only nutritional fluids should be given by this line. Loading doses of vitamin B$_{12}$ and folic acid are advised and other vitamins are given parenterally twice weekly.

Before starting, the patient should be well oxygenated with a near normal circulating blood volume, renal function, and acid-base status. Appropriate biochemical tests should have been carried out beforehand and serious deficits corrected. Nutritional and electrolyte status must be monitored throughout treatment.

9.3 Intravenous nutrition

Proprietary Infusion Fluids for Parenteral Feeding

Preparation	Nitrogen g/litre	[1]Energy kJ/litre	K$^+$	Mg^{2+}	Na$^+$	Acet$^-$	Cl$^-$	Other components/litre
Aminoplasmal L5 (Braun)	8.03		25	2.5	48	59	31	acid phosphate 9 mmol, malate 7.5 mmol
Net price 500 mL = £7.50								
Aminoplasmal L10 (Braun)	16.06		25	2.5	48	59	62	acid phosphate 9 mmol, malate 7.5 mmol
Net price 500 mL = £14.20								
Aminoplasmal Ped (Braun)	7.4		25	2.5	50	27	15	
Net price 100 mL = £5.25; 250 mL = £6.50								
Aminoplex 5 (Geistlich)	5.0	3600	28	4	35	28	43	ethanol 5%, sorbitol 125 g, malic acid 1.85 g
Net price 1000 mL = £11.95								
Aminoplex 12 (Geistlich)	12.44		30	2.5	35	5	67	malic acid 4.6 g
Net price 500 mL = £11.31; 1000 mL = £19.08								
Aminoplex 14 (Geistlich)	13.4		30		35		79	vitamins, malic acid 5.36 g
Net price 500 mL = £10.36								
Aminoplex 24 (Geistlich)	24.9		30	2.5	35	5	67	malic acid 4.5 g
Net price 250 mL = £9.79; 500 mL = £17.28								
Branched Chain Amino Acids (Clintec) 500-mL Viaflex® pack	4.4							
FreAmine III 8.5% (Fresenius)	13.0				10	72	<3	phosphate 10 mmol
Net price 500 mL = £10.20; 1000 mL = £18.95								
FreAmine III 10% (Fresenius)	15.3				10	88	<2	phosphate 20 mmol
Net price 500 mL = £13.95; 1000 mL = £24.10								
Glucoplex 1000 (Geistlich)		4200	30	2.5	50		67	acid phosphate 18 mmol, Zn^{2+} 0.046 mmol, anhydrous glucose 240 g
Net price 500 mL = £2.76; 1000 mL = £3.10								
Glucoplex 1600 (Geistlich)		6700	30	2.5	50		67	acid phosphate 18 mmol, Zn^{2+} 0.046 mmol, anhydrous glucose 400 g
Net price 500 mL = £2.90; 1000 mL = £3.35								
Hepanutrin (Geistlich)	15.6							
Net price 500 mL = £15.74								
HeplexAmine 8% (Fresenius)	12				10	61	<3	phosphate 10 mmol
Net price 500 mL = £16.70								
Intralipid 10% (Kabi Pharmacia)		4600						fractionated soya oil 100 g, glycerol 22.5 g
Net price 100 mL = £4.35; 500 mL = £9.65								
Intralipid 20% (Kabi Pharmacia)		8400						fractionated soya oil 200 g, glycerol 22.5 g
Net price 100 mL = £6.55; 500 mL = £14.40								
[2]Lipofundin MCT/LCT 10% (Braun)		4430						soya oil 50 g, medium chain triglycerides 50 g
Net price 100 mL = £6.40; 500 mL = £10.50								
[2]Lipofundin MCT/LCT 20% (Braun)		8000						soya oil 100 g, medium chain triglycerides 100 g
Net price 100 mL = £7.30; 500 mL = £16.00								
Lipofundin S 10% (Braun)		4470						soya oil 100 g
Net price 100 mL = £6.00; 500 mL = £9.80								
Lipofundin S 20% (Braun)		8520						soya oil 200 g
Net price 100 mL = £7.00; 500 mL = £15.30								
Nephramine 5.4% (Fresenius)	6.4				5	44	<3	essential amino acids only
Net price 250 mL = £24.99								
Nutracel 400 (Clintec)		3400		18		0.16	66	Ca^{2+} 15 mmol, Mn^{2+} 0.08 mmol, Zn^{2+} 0.08 mmol, anhydrous glucose 200 g
Net price 500 mL = £2.60								
Nutracel 800 (Clintec)		3400		9		0.08	33	Ca^{2+} 7.5 mmol, Mn^{2+} 0.04 mmol, Zn^{2+} 0.04 mmol, anhydrous glucose 200 g
Net price 1000 mL = £4.50								
Perifusin (Kabi Pharmacia)	5.0		30	5	40	10	9	malate 22.5 mmol
Net price 1000 mL = £7.20								
Plasma-Lyte 148 (water) (Baxter)			5	1.5	140	27	98	gluconate 23 mmol
Net price 1000 mL = £1.63								
Plasma-Lyte 148 (dextrose 5%) (Baxter)		840	5	1.5	140	27	98	gluconate 23 mmol, anhydrous glucose 50 g
Net price 1000 mL = £1.63								
Plasma-Lyte M (dextrose 5%) (Baxter)		840	16	1.5	40	12	40	Ca^{2+} 2.5 mmol, lactate 12 mmol, anhydrous glucose 50 g
Net price 1000 mL = £1.36								
[3]Primene 10% (Clintec)	15				25		15.5	
Net price 100 mL = £6.20; 250 mL = £8.50								

1. Excludes protein- or amino acid-derived energy
2. Treatment with Lipofundin MCT/LCT should be limited to up to 10 days
3. For use in neonates and children only

Note. 1000 kcal = 4.1868 MJ; 1 MJ (1000 kJ) = 238.8 kcal. All entries are PoM

Cautionary label wordings, see inside back cover   Prices are **net**, see p. 1

Proprietary Infusion Fluids for Parenteral Feeding (*continued*)

Preparation	Nitrogen g/litre	[1]Energy kJ/litre	K^+	Mg^{2+}	Na^+	$Acet^-$	Cl^-	Other components/litre
Soyacal 10% (Alpha)		4600						purified soya oil 100 g, glycerol 22.1 g
Net price 50 mL = £2.75; 100 mL = £4.25; 250 mL = £7.25; 500 mL = £9.50								
Soyacal 20% (Alpha)		8400						purified soya oil 200 g, glycerol 22.1 g
Net price 50 mL = £4.25; 100 mL = £6.50; 250 mL = £10.75; 500 mL = £14.00								
Synthamin 9 (Clintec)	9.1		60	5	70	100	70	acid phosphate 30 mmol
Net price 500 mL = £7.15; 1000 mL = £13.25								
Synthamin 14 (Clintec)	14.0		60	5	70	140	70	acid phosphate 30 mmol
Net price 500 mL = £10.35; 1000 mL = £18.40								
Synthamin 14 without electrolytes (Clintec)	14.0					68	34	
Net price 500 mL = £10.60; 1000 mL = £18.80								
Synthamin 17 (Clintec)	16.5		60	5	70	150	70	acid phosphate 30 mmol
Net price 500 mL = £13.60; 1000 mL = £24.70								
Synthamin 17 without electrolytes (Clintec)	16.5					82	40	
Net price 500 mL = £13.60; 1000 mL = £24.70								
Synthamix 9/800X (Clintec)	4.55	1680	30	7	35	50	51.5	acid phosphate 15 mmol, Zn^{2+} 0.02 mmol, Ca^{2+} 3.75 mmol, Mn^{2+} 0.02 mmol, anhydrous glucose 100 g
Net price 2000 mL = £35.00								
Synthamix 9/1800X (Clintec)	3.64	3024	24	5.6	28	40	41.2	acid phosphate 12 mmol, Zn^{2+} 0.016 mmol, Ca^{2+} 3 mmol, Mn^{2+} 0.016 mmol, anhydrous glucose 180 g
Net price 2500 mL = £36.50								
Synthamix 14/1200X (Clintec)	7	2520	30	7	35	70	51.5	acid phosphate 15 mmol, Zn^{2+} 0.02 mmol, Ca^{2+} 3.75 mmol, Mn^{2+} 0.02 mmol, anhydrous glucose 150 g
Net price 2000 mL = £38.50								
Synthamix 14/2200X (Clintec)	5.6	3696	24	5.6	28	56	41.2	acid phosphate 12 mmol, Zn^{2+} 0.016 mmol, Ca^{2+} 3 mmol, Mn^{2+} 0.016 mmol, anhydrous glucose 220 g
Net price 2500 mL = £40.00								
Vamin 9 (Kabi Pharmacia)	9.4		20	1.5	50		55	Ca^{2+} 2.5 mmol
Net price 500 mL = £6.60; 1000 mL = £11.90								
Vamin 9 glucose (Kabi Pharmacia)	9.4	1700	20	1.5	50		55	Ca^{2+} 2.5 mmol, anhydrous glucose 100 g
Net price 100 mL = £3.40; 500 mL = £7.10; 1000 mL = £12.80								
Vamin 14 (Kabi Pharmacia)	13.5		50	8	100	135	100	Ca^{2+} 5 mmol, SO_4^{2-} 8 mmol
Net price 500 mL = £9.55; 1000 mL = £16.95								
Vamin 14 (electrolyte-free) (Kabi Pharmacia)	13.5							
Net price 500 mL = £9.55; 1000 mL = £16.95								
Vamin 18 (electrolyte-free) (Kabi Pharmacia)	18.0							
Net price 500 mL = £12.70; 1000 mL = £22.80								
Vaminolact (Kabi Pharmacia)	9.3							
Net price 100 mL = £3.80; 500 mL = £8.70								
Vitrimix KV (Kabi Pharmacia)	7.0	3340	15	1.1	38		38	Ca^{2+} 1.9 mmol, anhydrous glucose 75 g
Net price (combined pack of Intralipid 20% 250 mL and Vamin 9 glucose 750 mL) = £19.90								

1. Excludes protein- or amino acid-derived energy

Note. 1000 kcal = 4.1868 MJ; 1 MJ (1000 kJ) = 238.8 kcal. All entries are PoM

SUPPLEMENTARY PREPARATIONS

PoM **Addamel**® (Kabi Pharmacia)
Solution, electrolytes and trace elements for addition to Vamin® solutions except Vamin 18®, Ca^{2+} 5 mmol, Mg^{2+} 1.5 mmol, Cl^- 13.3 mmol/10 mL; traces of Fe^{3+}, Zn^{2+}, Mn^{2+}, Cu^{2+}, F^-, I^-. For adult use. Net price 10-mL amp = £1.59

PoM **Addiphos**® (Kabi Pharmacia)
Solution, sterile, phosphate 40 mmol, K^+ 30 mmol, Na^+ 30 mmol/20 mL. For addition to Vamin® solutions and glucose intravenous infusions. Net price 20-mL vial = £1.18

PoM **Additrace**® (Kabi Pharmacia)
Solution, trace elements for addition to Vamin® solutions traces of Fe^{3+}, Zn^{2+}, Mn^{2+}, Cu^{2+}, Cr^{3+}, Se^{4+}, Mo^{6+}, F^-, I^-. For adult use. Net price 10-mL amp = £1.79

PoM **Multibionta**® (Merck)
Solution, ascorbic acid 500 mg, dexpanthenol 25 mg, nicotinamide 100 mg, pyridoxine hydrochloride 15 mg, riboflavine sodium phosphate 10 mg, thiamine hydrochloride 50 mg, tocopheryl acetate 5 mg, vitamin A 10 000 units. For addition to infusion solutions. Net price 10-mL amp = £1.47

PoM **Ped-El**® (Kabi Pharmacia)
Solution, sterile, Ca^{2+}, Cu^{2+}, Fe^{3+}, Mg^{2+}, Mn^{2+}, Zn^{2+}, Cl^-, F^-, I^-, P. For addition to Vamin® solutions. For paediatric use. Net price 20-mL vial = £1.59

PoM **Solivito N**® (Kabi Pharmacia)
Solution, powder for reconstitution, biotin 60 micrograms, cyanocobalamin 5 micrograms, folic acid 400 micrograms, glycine 100 mg, nicotinamide 40 mg, pyridoxine hydrochloride 4.9 mg, riboflavine sodium phosphate 4.9 mg, sodium ascorbate 113 mg, sodium pantothenate 16.5 mg, thiamine mononitrate 3.1 mg. Dissolve in water for injections or glucose intravenous infusion for adding to glucose intravenous infusion or Intralipid®; dissolve in Vitlipid N® or Intralipid® for adding to Intralipid® only. Net price per vial = £1.80

PoM **Vitlipid N**® (Kabi Pharmacia)
Emulsion, adult, vitamin A 330 units, ergocalciferol 20 units, dl-alpha tocopherol 1 unit, phytomenadione 15 micrograms/mL. For addition to Intralipid®. Net price 10-mL amp = £1.75
Emulsion, infant, vitamin A 230 units, ergocalciferol 40 units, dl-alpha tocopherol 0.7 unit, phytomenadione 20 micrograms/mL. For addition to Intralipid®. Net price 10-mL amp = £1.75

9.4 Oral nutrition

9.4.1 Foods for special diets
9.4.2 Enteral nutrition

9.4.1 Foods for special diets

These are preparations that have been modified to eliminate a particular constituent from a food or are nutrient mixtures formulated as substitutes for the food. They are for patients who either cannot tolerate or cannot metabolise certain common constituents of food. An example is the coeliac patient who cannot tolerate gluten which is present in wheat (and to a lesser extent other cereals). In other cases, for example, in patients with phenylketonuria who cannot metabolise phenylalanine, a small amount, sufficient for tissue building and repair, must be incorporated in the formulation.

ACBS. In certain clinical conditions some foods may have the characteristics of drugs and the Advisory Committee on Borderline Substances advises as to the circumstances in which such foods may be regarded as drugs and so can be prescribed in the NHS. Prescriptions for these foods issued in accordance with the advice of this committee and endorsed 'ACBS' will normally not be investigated.

See Appendix 7 for details of these foods and a listing by clinical condition (consult Drug Tariff for late amendments).

Preparations
See Appendix 7

9.4.2 Enteral nutrition

The body's reserves of protein rapidly become exhausted in severely ill patients, especially during chronic illness or in those with severe burns, extensive trauma, pancreatitis, or intestinal fistula. Much can be achieved by frequent meals and by persuading the patient to take supplementary snacks of ordinary food between the meals.

However, extra calories, protein, other nutrients, and vitamins are often best given by supplementing ordinary meals with sip or tube feeds of one of the nutritionally complete foods.

When patients cannot feed normally at all, for example patients with severe facial injury, oesophageal obstruction, or coma, a diet composed solely of nutritionally complete foods must be given. This is planned by a dietitian who will take into account the protein and total energy requirement of the patient and decide on the form and relative contribution of carbohydrate and fat to the energy requirements.

There are a number of nutritionally complete foods available and their use reduces an otherwise heavy workload in hospital or in the home. Most contain protein derived from milk or soya. Some contain protein hydrolysates or free amino acids and are only appropriate for patients who have diminished ability to break down protein, as may be the case in inflammatory bowel disease or pancreatic insufficiency.

Even when nutritionally complete feeds are being given it may be important to monitor water and electrolyte balance. Extra minerals (e.g. magnesium and zinc) may be needed in patients where gastro-intestinal secretions are being lost. Additional vitamins may also be needed. Regular haematological and biochemical tests may be needed particularly in the unstable patient.

Some feeds are supplemented with vitamin K; for drug interactions of vitamin K see Appendix 1 (vitamins).

CHILDREN. Infants and young children have special requirements and in most situations liquid feeds prepared for adults are totally unsuitable and should not be given. Expert advice should be sought.

Preparations
See Appendix 7

9.5 Minerals

9.5.1 Calcium and magnesium
9.5.2 Phosphorus
9.5.3 Fluoride
9.5.4 Zinc

See section 9.1.1 for iron salts.

9.5.1 Calcium and magnesium

9.5.1.1 Calcium supplements
9.5.1.2 Hypercalcaemia
9.5.1.3 Magnesium

9.5.1.1 CALCIUM SUPPLEMENTS

Calcium supplements are usually only required where dietary calcium intake is deficient. This dietary requirement varies with age and is relatively greater in childhood, pregnancy, and lactation, due to an increased demand, and in old age, due to impaired absorption. In osteoporosis a daily supplement of 800 mg (20 mmol) calcium may reduce the rate of bone loss, but larger doses have not been shown to be more effective. Patients with hypoparathyroidism rarely require calcium supplements after the early stages of stabilisation on vitamin D (section 9.6.4).

In hypocalcaemic tetany an initial intravenous injection of 10 mL (2.25 mmol) of calcium gluconate injection 10% may be followed by the continuous infusion of about 40 mL (9 mmol) daily, but plasma calcium should be monitored. This regimen can also be used, immediately but temporarily, to reduce the toxic effects of hyperkalaemia.

Calcium may also be used in cardiac resuscitation (see section 2.7).

CALCIUM SALTS

Indications: see notes above; calcium deficiency
Cautions: **interactions:** Appendix 1 (calcium salts)
Side-effects: bradycardia, arrhythmias, and irritation after intravenous injection
Dose: by mouth, daily in divided doses, as calcium gluconate or lactate, see notes above
By intramuscular or slow intravenous injection, acute hypocalcaemia, calcium gluconate 1–2 g (2.25–4.5 mmol of Ca^{2+}); avoid intramuscular route in children

Oral preparations
Calcium Gluconate Tablets, calcium gluconate 600 mg (1.35 mmol Ca^{2+}). To be chewed before swallowing. Net price 20 = 44p. Label: 24
Calcium Gluconate Tablets, Effervescent, calcium gluconate 1 g (2.25 mmol Ca^{2+}). Net price 100 = £5.32. Label: 13
Note. Each tablet usually contains sodium 102.6 mg (4.46 mmol Na^+)
Calcium Lactate Tablets, calcium lactate 300 mg (1 mmol Ca^{2+}), net price 20 = 25p
Cacit® (Norwich Eaton)
Tablets, effervescent, pink, calcium carbonate 1.25 g, providing calcium citrate when dispersed in water (500 mg calcium or 12.6 mmol Ca^{2+}). Net price 76-tab pack = £19.64. Label: 13
Calcichew® (Shire)
Tablets (chewable), calcium carbonate 1.26 g (500 mg calcium or 12.6 mmol Ca^{2+}). Net price 100 = £11.25. Label: 24
Calcidrink® (Shire)
Granules, effervescent, calcium carbonate 2.52 g (1 g calcium or 25 mmol Ca^{2+}). Net price 30-sachet pack = £8.70. Label: 13

Calcium-500 (Renacare)
Tablets, pink, f/c, calcium carbonate 1.25 g (500 mg calcium or 12.5 mmol Ca^{2+}). Net price 100-tab pack = £4.72. Label: 25
Calcium-Sandoz® (Sandoz)
Syrup, calcium glubionate 1.09 g, calcium lactobionate 723 mg (108.3 mg calcium or 2.7 mmol Ca^{2+})/5 mL. Net price 100 mL = 49p
Citrical® (Shire)
Granules, calcium carbonate 1.26 g (500 mg or 12.5 mmol Ca^{2+})/sachet. Net price 90-sachet pack = £24.00. Label: 13
Ossopan® (Sanofi Winthrop)
Tablets, buff, f/c, hydroxyapatite 830 mg (4.4 mmol Ca^{2+}). Net price 50 = £10.35
Granules, brown, hydroxyapatite 3.32 g (17.8 mmol Ca^{2+}). Net price 28-sachet pack = £18.50
Sandocal® (Sandoz)
Sandocal-400 tablets, effervescent, calcium lactate gluconate 930 mg, calcium carbonate 700 mg, anhydrous citric acid 1.189 g, providing calcium 400 mg (10 mmol Ca^{2+}). Net price 5 × 20-tab pack = £7.35. Label: 13
Sandocal-1000 tablets, effervescent, calcium lactate gluconate 2.327 g, calcium carbonate 1.75 g, anhydrous citric acid 2.973 g providing 1 g calcium (25 mmol Ca^{2+}). Net price 3 × 10-tab pack = £6.63. Label: 13
Titralac®: section 9.5.2.2

Parenteral preparations
PoM **Calcium Gluconate Injection,** calcium gluconate 10%. Net price 5-mL amp = 43p; 10-mL amp = 50p
Calcium Sandoz® (Sandoz)
PoM *Injection*, calcium glubionate equivalent to 10% of calcium gluconate (93 mg calcium or 2.32 mmol Ca^{2+}/10 mL). Net price 10-mL amp = 27p
PoM **Min-I-Jet**® **Calcium Chloride 10%** (IMS)
Injection, calcium chloride 100 mg/mL. Net price 10-mL disposable syringe = £3.30

9.5.1.2 HYPERCALCAEMIA

Severe hypercalcaemia calls for urgent treatment before detailed investigation of the cause. After rehydration (if necessary with intravenous infusion of **sodium chloride 0.9%**) a **loop diuretic** may be given to increase urinary calcium excretion. Drugs (such as thiazides and vitamin D compounds) which promote hypercalcaemia should be discontinued and dietary calcium should be restricted.

If *severe hypercalcaemia persists* drugs which inhibit mobilisation of calcium from the skeleton may be required. The **bisphosphonates** are useful and disodium pamidronate (see section 6.6.2) is probably the most effective; it is probably as effective as plicamycin, yet is less toxic and has a much longer effect. **Plicamycin** (see section 8.1.2) is probably the most rapidly effective drug but cannot be given continuously for more than a few days because of marrow toxicity; the duration of its hypocalcaemic effect is unpredictable but can last several days.

Corticosteroids (see section 6.3) are widely given, but may only be useful where hypercalcaemia is due to sarcoidosis or vitamin D intoxication; they often take several days to achieve the desired effect.

Calcitonin (see section 6.6.1) is relatively non-toxic but is expensive and its effect can wear off after a few days despite continued use; it is rarely effective where bisphosphonates have failed to reduce serum calcium adequately.

Intravenous chelating drugs such as **trisodium edetate** are rarely used; they usually cause pain in the limb receiving the infusion and may cause renal damage.

After treatment of severe hypercalcaemia the underlying cause must be established. *Further treatment* is governed by the same principles as for initial therapy. Salt and water depletion and drugs promoting hypercalcaemia should be avoided; oral administration of a bisphosphonate may be useful. **Sodium cellulose phosphate**, which binds calcium in the gut, is rarely helpful, and any associated increase in serum phosphate may be harmful. Similarly, oral and intravenous phosphate may only achieve a reduction in serum calcium by precipitating calcium phosphate in the tissues, resulting in nephrocalcinosis and impairment of renal function. Parathyroidectomy may be indicated for hyperparathyroidism.

BISPHOSPHONATES
See section 6.6.2

CALCITONIN
See section 6.6.1

CORTICOSTEROIDS
See section 6.3.4

PLICAMYCIN
See section 8.1.2

SODIUM CELLULOSE PHOSPHATE
Indications: hypercalcaemia (but see notes above), reduction of calcium absorption from food (in conjunction with low-calcium diet)
Contra-indications: congestive heart failure, renal impairment
Side-effects: occasional diarrhoea
Dose: 5 g 3 times daily with meals; CHILD 10 g daily in 3 divided doses with meals

Calcisorb® (3M)
Sachets, sodium cellulose phosphate 5 g. Net price 90-sachet pack = £19.71. Label: 13, 21, counselling, may be sprinkled on food

TRISODIUM EDETATE
Indications: hypercalcaemia (but see notes above); removal of lime burns in the eye (see under Preparations)
Cautions: plasma-calcium determinations required; caution in tuberculosis

Contra-indications: impaired renal function
Side-effects: nausea, diarrhoea, cramp; in overdosage renal damage
Dose: hypercalcaemia, *by slow intravenous infusion*, up to 70 mg/kg daily over 2–3 hours

PoM **Limclair**® (Sinclair)
Injection, trisodium edetate 200 mg/mL. Net price 5-mL amp = £3.81
For topical use in the eye, dilute 1 mL to 50 mL with sterile purified water

9.5.1.3 MAGNESIUM

Magnesium is an essential constituent of a vast number of enzyme systems, in particular those involved in energy generation. Most of it is found in the skeleton in the calcium apatite crystal lattice.

Magnesium salts are not well absorbed from the gastro-intestinal tract which explains the use of magnesium sulphate (section 1.6.4) as an osmotic laxative.

Magnesium is mainly excreted by the kidneys and is therefore retained in renal failure.

The effects of hypermagnesaemia and of hypomagnesaemia are similar to those of hyperkalaemia and hypokalaemia; hypocalcaemia is usually associated with hypomagnesaemia.

Oral magnesium salts are occasionally required on a long-term basis in patients with malabsorption.

Parenteral magnesium chloride or sulphate is occasionally needed to correct magnesium deficiency in alcoholism or that has arisen from prolonged diarrhoea or vomiting which has been treated with parenteral fluid and nutrition without magnesium supplements; 35–50 mmol of magnesium chloride (or sulphate) may be added to 1 litre of 5% glucose or other isotonic solution and given over a period of 12 to 24 hours. Repeated measurements of plasma magnesium are advisable to determine the rate and duration of the infusion. The dose should be reduced in renal failure. For maintenance (e.g. for intravenous nutrition) parenteral doses of magnesium are of the order of 10–20 mmol daily (often about 12 mmol daily).

9.5.2 Phosphorus
9.5.2.1 Phosphate supplements
9.5.2.2 Phosphate-binding agents

9.5.2.1 PHOSPHATE SUPPLEMENTS

Oral phosphate supplements may be required in addition to vitamin D in a small minority of patients with hypophosphataemic vitamin D-resistant rickets. Diarrhoea is a common side-effect and should prompt a reduction in dosage.

Phosphate infusion is occasionally needed in alcohol dependence or phosphate deficiency arising from parenteral fluid and nutrition deficient in phosphate supplements; phosphate depletion also occurs in severe diabetic ketoacidosis. A solution containing up to 50 mmol/litre can be infused in sodium chloride or glucose over 12 to 24 hours. Since potassium depletion is also commonly present the phosphate may be given as a mixture of the sodium and potassium salts.

Phosphate-Sandoz® (Sandoz)
Tablets, effervescent, anhydrous sodium acid phosphate 1.936 g, sodium bicarbonate 350 mg, potassium bicarbonate 315 mg, equivalent to phosphorus 500 mg (16.1 mmol phosphate), sodium 468.8 mg (20.4 mmol Na$^+$), potassium 123 mg (3.1 mmol K$^+$). Net price 20 = 75p. Label: 13

9.5.2.2 PHOSPHATE-BINDING AGENTS

Aluminium-containing and calcium-containing antacids are used as phosphate-binding agents in the management of hyperphosphataemia complicating renal failure. Calcium-containing phosphate-binding agents are contra-indicated in hypercalcaemia or hypercalciuria. Phosphate-binding agents which contain aluminium may increase plasma aluminium in dialysis patients.

ALUMINIUM HYDROXIDE
Indications: hyperphosphataemia
Cautions: hyperaluminaemia; see also notes above; **interactions:** Appendix 1 (antacids and adsorbents)

Aluminium Hydroxide (Non-proprietary)
Mixture (gel), about 4% w/w Al$_2$O$_3$ in water. Net price 200 mL = 36p.
Dose: hyperphosphataemia, 20–100 mL according to requirements of patient; antacid, see section 1.1.1
Note: The brand name NHS Aludrox® (Charwell) is used for aluminium hydroxide mixture, net price 200 mL = 69p. For NHS Aludrox® tablets see preparations with magnesium, section 1.1.1

Alu-Cap® (3M)
Capsules, green/red, dried aluminium hydroxide 475 mg (low Na$^+$). Net price 120-cap pack = £3.84
Dose: phosphate-binding agent in renal failure, 4–20 capsules daily in divided doses with meals; antacid, see section 1.1.1

CALCIUM CARBONATE
Indications: hyperphosphataemia
Cautions: see notes above; **interactions:** Appendix 1 (calcium salts)
Side-effects: hypercalcaemia

Calcichew®, section 9.5.1.1
Calcium-500, section 9.5.1.1
Titralac® (3M)
Tablets, calcium carbonate 420 mg, glycine 180 mg. Net price 180-tab pack = £2.23
Dose: calcium supplement, or phosphate-binding agent (with meals) in renal failure, according to the requirements of the patient

9.5.3 Fluoride

Availability of adequate fluoride confers significant resistance to dental caries. It is now considered that the topical action of fluoride on enamel and plaque is more important than the systemic effect.

Where the natural fluoride content of the drinking water is significantly less than 1 mg per litre (one part per million) artificial fluoridation is the most economical method of supplementing fluoride intake.

Daily administration of tablets or drops is a suitable alternative, but systemic fluoride supplements should not be prescribed without prior reference to the fluoride content of the local water supply; they are not advisable when the water contains more than 700 micrograms per litre (0.7 parts per million). In addition, the British Association for the Study of Community Dentistry now recommends that infants need not receive fluoride supplements until the age of 6 months.

Use of dentifrices which incorporate sodium fluoride and/or monofluorophosphate is also a convenient source of fluoride.

Individuals who are either particularly caries prone or medically compromised may be given additional protection by use of fluoride rinses or by application of fluoride gels. Rinses may be used daily or weekly; daily use of a less concentrated rinse is more effective than weekly use of a more concentrated one. Gels must be applied on a regular basis under professional supervision; extreme caution is necessary to prevent the child from swallowing any excess. Less concentrated gels have recently become available for home use. Varnishes are also available and are particularly valuable for young or handicapped children since they adhere to the teeth and set in the presence of moisture.

SODIUM FLUORIDE
Note. Sodium fluoride 2.2 mg provides approx. 1 mg fluoride ion
Indications: prophylaxis of dental caries—see notes above
Contra-indications: not for areas where drinking water is fluoridated
Side-effects: occasional white flecks on teeth with recommended doses; rarely yellowish-brown discoloration if recommended doses are exceeded
Dose: expressed as fluoride ion (F$^-$):
Water content less than 300 micrograms F$^-$/litre, CHILD up to 6 months none; 6 months–2 years 250 micrograms F$^-$ daily, 2–4 years 500 micrograms F$^-$ daily, over 4 years 1 mg F$^-$ daily
Water content between 300 and 700 micrograms F$^-$/litre, CHILD up to 2 years none, 2–4 years 250 micrograms F$^-$ daily, over 4 years 500 micrograms F$^-$ daily
Water content above 700 micrograms F$^-$/litre, supplements not advised (see notes above)

Tablets
COUNSELLING. Tablets should be sucked or dissolved in the mouth and taken preferably in the evening
There are arrangements for health authorities to supply fluoride tablets in the course of pre-school dental schemes, and they may also be supplied in school dental schemes.

En-De-Kay® (Stafford-Miller)
Fluotabs 2–4 years, natural orange-flavoured, scored, sodium fluoride 1.1 mg (500 micrograms F$^-$). Net price 200-tab pack = £1.73
Fluotabs 4+ years, natural orange-flavoured, scored, sodium fluoride 2.2 mg (1 mg F$^-$). Net price 200-tab pack = £1.73

Fluor-a-day® (Dental Health)
Tablets, buff, scored, sodium fluoride 2.2 mg (1 mg F$^-$). Net price 200-tab pack = £1.40

Fluorigard® (RMT)
Tablets 0.5, purple, sodium fluoride 1.1 mg (500 micrograms F$^-$). Net price 120-tab pack = £1.18
Tablets 1.0, sodium fluoride 2.2 mg (1 mg F$^-$). Net price 120-tab pack = £1.24 (available in 4 colours and flavours)

Oral-B Fluoride® (Oral-B Labs)
Tablets, sodium fluoride 1.1 mg (500 micrograms F$^-$), net price 200-tab pack = £1.80; 2.2 mg (1 mg F$^-$) (pink), 12-tab pack = £1.80

Zymafluor® (Zyma)
Tablets, sodium fluoride 550 micrograms (250 micrograms F$^-$), net price 400-tab pack = 75p

Oral drops
Note. Fluoride supplements no longer considered necessary below 6 months of age (see notes above)

En-De-Kay® (Stafford-Miller)
Fluodrops® (= paediatric drops), sugar-free, sodium fluoride 500 micrograms (250 micrograms F$^-$)/0.15 mL. Net price 60 mL = £1.31

Fluorigard® (RMT)
Paediatric drops, sodium fluoride 275 micrograms (125 micrograms F$^-$)/drop. Net price 30 mL = £1.33

Oral-B Fluoride® (Oral-B Labs)
Drops, sodium fluoride 0.15% (250 micrograms F$^-$/8 drops). Net price 48.7 mL = £1.43

Mouthwashes
Rinse mouth for 1 minute and spit out
COUNSELLING. Avoid eating, drinking, or rinsing mouth for 15 minutes after use

PoM **En-De-Kay®** (Stafford-Miller)
Fluorinse (= mouthwash), red, sodium fluoride 2%. Net price 100 mL = £2.50. Counselling, see above
CHILD 8 years and over, for *daily* use, dilute 5 drops to 10 mL of water; for *weekly* use, dilute 20 drops to 10 mL

Fluorigard® (RMT)
Daily dental rinse (= mouthwash), blue, sodium fluoride 0.05%. Net price 500 mL = £2.65. Counselling, see above
CHILD 6 years and over, for *daily* use, rinse with 5–10 mL
Weekly dental rinse (= mouthwash), blue, sodium fluoride 0.2%. Net price 150 mL = £1.76. Counselling, see above
CHILD 6 years and over, for *weekly* use, rinse with 5–10 mL

9.5.4 Zinc

Oral zinc therapy should only be given when there is good evidence of deficiency (hypoproteinaemia spuriously lowers plasma-zinc concentrations). Zinc deficiency can occur in individuals on inadequate diets, in malabsorption, with increased body loss due to trauma, burns and protein-losing conditions, and during intravenous feeding. Therapy should continue until clinical improvement occurs and be replaced by dietary measures unless there is severe malabsorption, metabolic disease, or continuing zinc loss. Side-effects of zinc salts are abdominal pain and dyspepsia.

ZINC SALTS
Indications; Cautions; Side-effects: see notes above; **interactions:** Appendix 1 (zinc)

Solvazinc® (Thames)
Effervescent tablets, yellow-white, zinc sulphate 200 mg (45 mg zinc). Net price 30 = £3.60. Label: 13, 21
Dose: 1 tablet in water 1–3 times daily after food

Zincomed® (Medo)
Capsules, blue/white, zinc sulphate 220 mg. Net price 30-cap pack = 99p. Label: 21
Dose: 1 capsule 3 times daily after food

Z Span® (SK&F)
Spansule® (= capsules m/r), blue/clear, enclosing white and grey pellets, zinc sulphate monohydrate 61.8 mg (22.5 mg zinc). Net price 30-cap pack = £1.38. Label: 25
Dose: adults and children over 1 year, 1–3 capsules daily as required; can be opened and pellets sprinkled on cool food; not to be chewed

9.6 Vitamins

9.6.1 Vitamin A
9.6.2 Vitamin B group
9.6.3 Vitamin C
9.6.4 Vitamin D
9.6.5 Vitamin E
9.6.6 Vitamin K
9.6.7 Multivitamin preparations

Vitamins are used for the prevention and treatment of specific deficiency states or where the diet is known to be inadequate; they may be prescribed in the NHS to prevent or treat deficiency but not as dietary supplements.

Their use as general 'pick-me-ups' is of unproven value and, in the case of preparations containing vitamin A or D, may actually be harmful if patients take more than the prescribed dose. The 'fad' for mega-vitamin therapy with water-soluble vitamins, such as ascorbic acid and pyridoxine, is unscientific and can be harmful.

Cautionary label wordings, see inside back cover   Prices are **net**, see p. 1

9.6.1 Vitamin A

Deficiency of vitamin A (retinol) is rare in Britain even in disorders of fat absorption.

Massive overdose can cause rough skin, dry hair, an enlarged liver, and a raised erythrocyte sedimentation rate and raised serum calcium and serum alkaline phosphatase concentrations. Use of excessive doses should be **avoided** in pregnancy (see below).

The Department of Health has advised that:
1. The recommended daily amount of vitamin A in the UK is 2250 units daily for adults, including pregnant women, increased to 4000 units daily for nursing mothers;
2. Several national and international organisations have proposed a maximum intake of vitamin A during pregnancy of 8000 to 10000 units daily;
3. Reports in the USA suggest that birth defects may follow an intake of vitamin A of 24000 to 30000 units daily.

In view of evidence suggesting that high levels of vitamin A may cause birth defects, women who are (or may become) pregnant are advised not to take vitamin A supplements (including tablets and fish-liver oil drops), except on the advice of a doctor or an antenatal clinic; nor should they eat liver or products such as liver paté or liver sausage.

VITAMIN A
(Retinol)
Indications; Cautions; Side-effects: see notes above
Dose: see notes above and under preparations

Vitamins A and D

Halibut-liver Oil Capsules, vitamin A 4000 units [also contains vitamin D]. Net price 20 = 15p

NHS **Halycitrol®** (LAB)
Emulsion, vitamin A 4600 units, vitamin D 380 units/5 mL. Net price 114 mL = £1.20
Dose: 5 mL daily but see notes above

Vitamins A, D, and C for children

Children's Vitamin Drops (Hough)
Oral drops, ascorbic acid (as sodium ascorbate) 20 mg, vitamin A 700 units, vitamin D 300 units/5 drops.
Recommended by Department of Health for routine supplementation in young children. Available direct to public under the Welfare Food Scheme from maternity and child health clinics and welfare food distribution centres; not available on prescription
Dose: CHILD 1 month–5 years, 5 drops daily
Note. The Department of Health recommends these drops for children aged 6 months to 2 years (preferably 5 years particularly in winter and early spring); some infants from 1 month of age may also benefit (for details see *Present Day Practice in Infant Feeding* 3rd Report)

Adexolin® (Seven Seas)
Oral drops, ascorbic acid 15 mg, vitamin A 750 units, vitamin D 200 units/0.14 mL. Net price 25-mL pack with pipette = £1.02, 50-mL pack with pipette = £1.80
Dose: INFANT and CHILD under 5 years, 0.28 mL (upper level on graduated pipette) daily; INFANT fed on vitamin D-fortified milk, CHILD over 5 years and ADULT, 0.14 mL (lower level on graduated pipette) daily

Vitamin A injection
PoM **Ro-A-Vit®** (Cambridge)
Injection, vitamin A (retinol) 50000 units (as palmitate)/mL. Net price 2-mL amp = 88p
Dose: by deep intramuscular injection, deficiency, 100000 units monthly, increased to weekly in acute deficiency states; courses no longer than 6 weeks with 2-week interval; Liver disease, 100000 units every 2–4 months; INFANT under 1 year and CHILD 50000 units monthly
Note. Contains polyethoxylated castor oil which has been associated with anaphylaxis; do **not** mix or dilute
Cautions: children, liver disease (specialist use); considerably enhanced bioavailability compared with previous formulation (dosage adjustment may be needed)

9.6.2 Vitamin B group

Deficiency of the B vitamins, other than deficiency of vitamin B_{12} (section 9.1.2) is rare in Britain and is usually treated by preparations containing thiamine (B_1), riboflavine (B_2), and nicotinamide, which is used in preference to nicotinic acid, as it does not cause vasodilatation. Other members (or substances traditionally classified as members) of the vitamin B complex such as aminobenzoic acid, biotin, choline, inositol, and pantothenic acid or panthenol may be included in vitamin B preparations but there is no evidence of their value.

The severe deficiency states Wernicke's encephalopathy and Korsakoff's psychosis, especially as seen in chronic alcoholism, are best treated by the parenteral administration of B vitamins (Parentrovite®); anaphylaxis has been reported with these preparations (see CSM advice, below).

As with other vitamins of the B group, pyridoxine (B_6) deficiency is rare, but it may occur during isoniazid therapy and is characterised by peripheral neuritis. High doses of pyridoxine are given in some metabolic disorders, such as hyperoxaluria, and it is also used in sideroblastic anaemia (section 9.1.3). Pyridoxine has been tried in a wide variety of other disorders, including the premenstrual syndrome, but there is little sound evidence to support the claims, and overdosage induces toxic effects.

THIAMINE
(Vitamin B_1)
Indications: see notes above
Cautions: anaphylactic shock may occasionally follow injection (see CSM advice below)
Dose: mild chronic deficiency, 10–25 mg daily; severe deficiency, 200–300 mg daily

Thiamine Hydrochloride Tablets, thiamine hydrochloride 25 mg, net price 20 = 15p; 50 mg, 20 = 24p; 100 mg, 20 = 42p; 300 mg, 20 = 68p

NHS **Benerva®** (Roche)
Tablets, thiamine hydrochloride 25 mg, net price 20 = 15p; 50 mg, 20 = 24p; 100 mg, 20 = 42p; 300 mg, 20 = 68p

Vitamins B and C injection

> **CSM advice**
> Since potentially serious allergic adverse reactions may occur during, or shortly after, administration, the CSM has recommended that:
> 1. Use be restricted to patients in whom parenteral treatment is essential;
> 2. Intravenous injections should be administered slowly (over 10 minutes);
> 3. Facilities for treating anaphylaxis should be available when administered.

PoM **Parentrovite**® (Bencard)
Parenteral vitamins B and C for confirmed or imminent acute Wernicke's encephalopathy and Korsakoff's psychosis when oral intake is impossible or inadequate
Dose: by intravenous injection (see CSM advice above) or infusion, 2–4 pairs of *IVHP* ampoules every 4–8 hours for up to 2 days, followed by 1 pair of *IMHP* ampoules by intramuscular injection *or* 1 pair of *IVHP* ampoules by intravenous injection or infusion daily for 5–7 days
IMHP Injection, for intramuscular use only, ascorbic acid 500 mg, nicotinamide 160 mg, pyridoxine hydrochloride 50 mg, riboflavine 4 mg, thiamine hydrochloride 250 mg/7 mL. Net price 7 mL (in 2 amps) = 43p
IVHP Injection, for intravenous use only, ascorbic acid 500 mg, anhydrous glucose 900 mg, nicotinamide 160 mg, pyridoxine hydrochloride 50 mg, riboflavine 4 mg, thiamine hydrochloride 250 mg/10 mL. Net price 10 mL (in 2 amps) = 43p

Oral vitamin B complex preparations, see below

RIBOFLAVINE
(Vitamin B$_2$)
Indications: see notes above

Preparations
Injections of vitamins B and C, see under Thiamine

Oral vitamin B complex preparations, see below

PYRIDOXINE HYDROCHLORIDE
(Vitamin B$_6$)
Indications: see under Dose
Cautions: interactions: Appendix 1 (vitamins)
Dose: deficiency states, 20–50 mg up to 3 times daily
Isoniazid neuropathy, prophylaxis 10 mg daily; therapeutic, 50 mg three times daily
Idiopathic sideroblastic anaemia, 100–400 mg daily in divided doses
Premenstrual syndrome, 50–100 mg daily (but see notes above)

Pyridoxine Tablets, pyridoxine hydrochloride 10 mg, net price 20 = 32p; 20 mg, 20 = 33p; 50 mg, 20 = 56p

Cautionary label wordings, see inside back cover

NHS **Benadon**® (Roche)
Tablets, pyridoxine hydrochloride 20 mg. Net price 20 = 33p
Tablets, scored, pyridoxine hydrochloride 50 mg. Net price 20 = 66p

NHS **Complement Continus**® (Napp)
Tablets, m/r, yellow, pyridoxine hydrochloride 100 mg. Net price 28-tab pack = £1.68. Label: 25

Injections of vitamins B and C, see under Thiamine

NICOTINAMIDE
Indications: see notes above

Nicotinamide Tablets, nicotinamide 50 mg. Net price 20 = 13p
Injections of vitamins B and C, see under Thiamine
Oral vitamin B complex preparations, see below

NICOTINIC ACID
See section 2.12

FOLIC ACID
See section 9.1.2

FOLINIC ACID
See section 8.1.3

VITAMIN B$_{12}$
See section 9.1.2

ORAL VITAMIN B COMPLEX PREPARATIONS

Note. Other multivitamin preparations are in section 9.6.7.

Vitamin B Tablets, Compound, nicotinamide 15 mg, riboflavine 1 mg, thiamine hydrochloride 1 mg. Net price 20 = 7p
Dose: prophylactic, 1–2 tablets daily
Vitamin B Tablets, Compound, Strong, brown, f/c or s/c, nicotinamide 20 mg, pyridoxine hydrochloride 2 mg, riboflavine 2 mg, thiamine hydrochloride 5 mg. Net price 20 = 9p
Dose: treatment of vitamin-B deficiency, 1–2 tablets 3 times daily

NHS **Becosym**® (Roche)
Tablets, brown, f/c, vitamin B tablets, compound, strong. Net price 20 = 15p
Forte tablets, brown, f/c, thiamine hydrochloride 15 mg, riboflavine 15 mg, nicotinamide 50 mg, pyridoxine hydrochloride 10 mg. Net price 25-tab pack = £1.14
Syrup, orange, thiamine hydrochloride 5 mg, riboflavine 2 mg, nicotinamide 20 mg, pyridoxine hydrochloride 2 mg/5 mL. Net price 100 mL = £1.10

NHS **Benerva Compound**® (Roche)
Tablets, yellow, vitamin B tablets, compound. Net price 20 = 11p

NHS **Vigranon B**® (Wallace Mfg)
Syrup, thiamine hydrochloride 5 mg, riboflavine 2 mg, nicotinamide 20 mg, pyridoxine hydrochloride 2 mg, panthenol 3 mg/5 mL. Net price 150 mL = £1.18

Prices are **net**, see p. 1

OTHER COMPOUNDS

Potassium aminobenzoate has been used in the treatment of various disorders associated with excessive fibrosis such as scleroderma but its therapeutic value is **doubtful**.

Potaba® (Glenwood)
Capsules, red/white, potassium aminobenzoate 500 mg. Net price 20 = £1.06. Label: 21
Tablets, potassium aminobenzoate 500 mg. Net price 20 = 83p. Label: 21
Dose: Peyronie's disease, scleroderma, 12 g daily in divided doses after food
Envules® (= powder in sachets), potassium aminobenzoate 3 g. Net price 40 sachets = £12.70. Label: 13, 21

9.6.3 Vitamin C
(Ascorbic acid)

Vitamin C therapy is essential in scurvy, but less florid manifestations of vitamin C deficiency are commonly found, especially in the elderly. It is rarely necessary to prescribe more than 100 mg daily except early in the treatment of scurvy.

Claims that vitamin C ameliorates colds or promotes wound healing have not been proved.

ASCORBIC ACID

Indications: prevention and treatment of scurvy
Dose: prophylactic, 25–75 mg daily; therapeutic, not less than 250 mg daily in divided doses

Ascorbic Acid Tablets, ascorbic acid 25 mg, net price 20 = 9p; 50 mg, 20 = 7p; 100 mg, 20 = 24p; 200 mg, 20 = 28p; 500 mg (label: 24), 20 = 68p
PoM **Ascorbic Acid Injection**, ascorbic acid 100 mg/mL. Net price 5-mL amp = £1.14
NHS **Redoxon®** (Roche)
Tablets, ascorbic acid 25 mg, net price 20 = 9p; 50 mg, 20 = 7p; 200 mg, 20 = 28p; 500 mg (label: 24), 50 = £1.69
Tablets, effervescent, ascorbic acid 1 g. Net price 10-tab pack = 81p. Label: 13
For children's welfare vitamin drops containing vitamin C with A and D, see vitamin A

9.6.4 Vitamin D

Note. The term Vitamin D is used for a range of compounds which possess the property of preventing or curing rickets. They include ergocalciferol (calciferol, vitamin D_2), cholecalciferol (vitamin D_3), dihydrotachysterol, alfacalcidol (1α-hydroxycholecalciferol), and calcitriol (1,25-dihydroxycholecalciferol).

Simple vitamin D *deficiency*, which is not uncommon in Asians consuming unleavened bread and in the elderly living alone, can be prevented by taking an oral supplement of only 10 micrograms (400 units) of **ergocalciferol** (calciferol, vitamin D_2) daily. Since there is no plain tablet of this strength available **calcium and ergocalciferol tablets** can be given (although the calcium is unnecessary).

Vitamin D deficiency caused by *intestinal malabsorption* or *chronic liver disease* usually requires vitamin D in pharmacological doses, such as **calciferol tablets** up to 1 mg (40 000 units) daily; the hypocalcaemia of *hypoparathyroidism* often requires doses of up to 2.5 mg (100 000 units) daily in order to achieve normocalcaemia. The newer vitamin D derivatives, **alfacalcidol** and **calcitriol**, have a shorter duration of action, and therefore have the advantage that problems associated with hypercalcaemia due to excessive dosage are shorter lasting and easier to treat.

Vitamin D requires hydroxylation by the kidney to its active form therefore the hydroxylated derivatives **alfacalcidol** or **calcitriol** should be prescribed if patients with *severe renal impairment* require vitamin D therapy.

Important. All patients receiving pharmacological doses of vitamin D should have the plasma calcium concentration checked at intervals (initially weekly) and whenever nausea or vomiting are present. Breast milk from women taking pharmacological doses of vitamin D may cause hypercalcaemia if given to an infant.

ERGOCALCIFEROL
(Calciferol, Vitamin D_2)
Indications: see notes above
Cautions: take care to ensure correct dose in infants; monitor plasma calcium in patients receiving high doses
Contra-indications: hypercalcaemia
Side-effects: symptoms of overdosage include anorexia, lassitude, nausea and vomiting, diarrhoea, weight loss, polyuria, sweating, headache, thirst, vertigo, and raised concentrations of calcium and phosphate in plasma and urine
Dose: see notes above

Daily supplements
Note. There is no plain vitamin D tablet available for treating simple deficiency (see notes above). Alternatives include vitamins capsules (see 9.6.7), preparations of vitamins A and D (see 9.6.1), and calcium and ergocalciferol tablets (see below).
Calcium and Ergocalciferol Tablets[1]
(Calcium and Vitamin D Tablets)
Tablets, calcium lactate 300 mg, calcium phosphate 150 mg (97 mg calcium or 2.4 mmol Ca^{2+}), ergocalciferol 10 micrograms (400 units). Net price 20 = 20p. Counselling, crush before administration or may be chewed
1. Calcium with Vitamin D Tablets (BPC) which contained ergocalciferol 12.5 micrograms (500 units) have been replaced by Calcium and Ergocalciferol Tablets
Calcichew D3® (Shire)
Tablets (chewable), calcium carbonate 1.26 g (500 mg calcium or 12.6 mmol Ca^{2+}), cholecalciferol 5 micrograms (200 units). Net price 100-tab pack = £14.00. Label: 24

9.6 Vitamins

Pharmacological strengths (see notes above)
Calciferol Tablets, BP
Tablets, cholecalciferol or ergocalciferol 250 micrograms (10 000 units), net price 20 = 49p; 1.25 mg (50 000 units), 20 = 64p
Note. May temporarily be unavailable
Note. The BP directs that when high-strength calciferol tablets are prescribed or demanded, tablets containing 250 micrograms shall be dispensed or supplied, and when strong calciferol tablets are prescribed or demanded it should be **confirmed** that tablets containing 1.25 mg are intended. To avoid **errors** arising from the use of these titles prescribers should **abandon** them and **specify strength required**
PoM **Calciferol Injection,** cholecalciferol or ergocalciferol, 7.5 mg (300 000 units)/mL in oil. Net price 1-mL amp = £2.96; 2-mL amp = £3.54

ALFACALCIDOL
(1α-Hydroxycholecalciferol)
Indications: see notes above
Cautions; Contra-indications; Side-effects: see under Ergocalciferol
Dose: by mouth or by intravenous injection over 30 seconds, ADULT and CHILD over 20 kg, initially 1 microgram daily (elderly 500 nanograms), adjusted to avoid hypercalcaemia; maintenance, usually 0.25–1 microgram daily; NEONATE and PREMATURE INFANT initially 50–100 nanograms/kg daily, CHILD under 20 kg initially 50 nanograms/kg daily

PoM **One-alpha**® (Leo)
Capsules, alfacalcidol 250 nanograms, net price 20 = £2.42; 1 microgram (brown), 20 = £7.20
Solution, sugar-free, alfacalcidol 200 nanograms/mL. Net price 60 mL = £15.58 (with oral syringe)
Injection, alfacalcidol 2 micrograms/mL, net price 0.5-mL amp = £2.49, 1-mL amp = £4.75
Note. Contains propylene glycol and should be used with caution in small premature infants

---

CALCITRIOL
(1,25-Dihydroxycholecalciferol)
Indications: see notes above
Cautions; Contra-indications; Side-effects: see under Ergocalciferol
Dose: see under preparation

PoM **Rocaltrol**® (Roche)
Capsules, calcitriol 250 nanograms (red/white), net price 20 = £3.92; 500 nanograms (red), 20 = £7.01
Dose: initially 1–2 micrograms daily, gradually increased to 2–3 micrograms daily

---

CHOLECALCIFEROL
(Vitamin D₃)
Indications; Cautions; Contra-indications; Side-effects: see under Ergocalciferol—alternative to ergocalciferol in calciferol tablets and injection

---

DIHYDROTACHYSTEROL
Cautions; Contra-indications; Side-effects: see under Ergocalciferol

AT 10® (Sanofi Winthrop)
Oral solution, dihydrotachysterol 250 micrograms/mL. Net price 15-mL dropper bottle = £19.84
Dose: acute, chronic, and latent forms of hypocalcaemic tetany due to hypoparathyroidism, consult data sheet

9.6.5 Vitamin E
(Tocopherols)

The daily requirement of vitamin E has not been well defined but is probably about 3 to 15 mg daily. There is little evidence that oral supplements of vitamin E are essential in adults, even where there is fat malabsorption secondary to cholestasis. In young children with congenital cholestasis, abnormally low vitamin E concentrations may be found in association with neuromuscular abnormalities, which usually respond only to the parenteral administration of vitamin E.

Vitamin E has been tried for various other conditions but there is no scientific evidence of its value. High doses have been associated with adverse effects.

ALPHA TOCOPHERYL ACETATE
Ephynal® (Roche)
Suspension, alpha tocopheryl acetate 500 mg/5 mL. Net price 100 mL = £3.64
Dose: cystic fibrosis, 100–200 mg daily; CHILD under 1 year 50 mg daily; 1 year and over 100 mg daily
Abetalipoproteinaemia, ADULT and CHILD 50–100 mg/kg daily

Vita-E® (Bioglan)
Gels (= capsules), *d*-α-tocopheryl acetate 75 units (yellow), net price 20 = 58p; 200 units (yellow), 20 = £1.37; 400 units (red), 20 = £2.19
Gelucaps® (= tablets), chewable, yellow, *d*-α-tocopheryl acetate 75 units. Net price 20 = 68p. Label: 24
Succinate tablets, yellow, *d*-α-tocopheryl succinate 50 units, net price 20 = 48p; 200 units, 20 = £1.44

9.6.6 Vitamin K

Vitamin K is necessary for the production of blood clotting factors and proteins necessary for the normal calcification of bone.

Because vitamin K is fat soluble, patients with *fat malabsorption,* especially if due to biliary obstruction or hepatic disease, may become deficient. For oral administration to prevent vitamin-K deficiency in malabsorption syndromes, a water-soluble preparation, **menadiol sodium phosphate** must be used; the usual dose is about 10 mg daily.

In *neonates* deficiency of vitamin K may occur because the gut is sterile and there is no synthesis of the vitamin by *Escherichia coli*. It may be treated with **phytomenadione** (vitamin K₁), 1 mg by intramuscular injection.

Oral coumarin *anticoagulants* act by interfering with vitamin K metabolism in the hepatic cells and their effects can be antagonised by giving vitamin K; for British Society for Haematology Guidelines, see section 2.8.2.

MENADIOL SODIUM PHOSPHATE

Indications; Dose: see notes above
Cautions: pregnancy; **interactions:** Appendix 1 (vitamins)

Synkavit® (Cambridge)
Tablets, scored, menadiol sodium phosphate equivalent to 10 mg of menadiol phosphate. Net price 20 = 41p

PHYTOMENADIONE
(Vitamin K_1)

Indications; Dose: see notes above
Cautions: intravenous injections (see section 2.8.2) should be given very slowly; **interactions:** Appendix 1 (vitamins)

Konakion® (Roche)
Tablets, s/c, phytomenadione 10 mg. Net price 25 = £4.20. To be chewed or allowed to dissolve slowly in the mouth (Label: 24)
PoM *Injection*, phytomenadione 2 mg/mL, net price 0.5-mL amp = 22p; 10 mg/mL, 1-mL amp = 41p
Note. Contains polyethoxylated castor oil which has been associated with anaphylaxis

9.6.7 Multivitamin preparations

Vitamins Capsules, ascorbic acid 15 mg, nicotinamide 7.5 mg, riboflavine 500 micrograms, thiamine hydrochloride 1 mg, vitamin A 2500 units, vitamin D 300 units. Net price 20 = 18p
Abidec® (W-L)
Drops, vitamins A, B group, C, and D. Net price 2 × 25 mL (with dropper) = £2.45
NHS **Allbee with C**® (Robins)
Capsules, yellow/green, vitamins B group and C. Net price 20 = £1.30
NHS **BC 500**® (Whitehall)
Tablets, orange, f/c, vitamins B group and C. Net price 30 = £1.45
NHS **Calcimax**® (Wallace Mfg)
Syrup, brown, vitamins B group, C, and D. Net price 150 mL = £1.41
NHS **Concavit**® (Wallace Mfg)
Capsules, vitamins A, B group, C, D, and E. Net price 20 = 93p
Drops and *syrup*, vitamins A, B group, C, and D. Net price drops 15 mL = £1.36; syrup 150 mL = £1.58
Dalivit® (Eastern)
NHS *Capsules*, red, vitamins A, B group, C, and D. Net price 20 = 31p
Oral drops, vitamins A, B group, C, and D. Net price 2 × 15 mL = £1.26
NHS **Orovite**® (SmithKline Beecham Brands)
Tablets, maroon, s/c, vitamins B group and C. Net price 25-tab pack = £1.66
NHS **Orovite 7**® (SmithKline Beecham Brands)
Granules, orange, vitamins A, B group, C, and D. Net price 10-sachet pack = £1.36, 30-sachet pack = £3.89. Label: 13
NHS **Surbex T**® (Abbott)
Tablets, orange, vitamins B group and C. Net price 20 = 58p

VITAMIN AND MINERAL SUPPLEMENTS AND ADJUNCTS TO SYNTHETIC DIETS

Forceval® (Unigreg)
Capsules, brown/red, vitamins (ascorbic acid 60 mg, biotin 100 micrograms, cyanocobalamin 3 micrograms, folic acid 300 micrograms, nicotinamide 18 mg, pantothenic acid 4 mg, pyridoxine 2 mg, riboflavine 1.6 mg, thiamine 1.2 mg, vitamin A 2500 units, vitamin D_2 400 units, vitamin E 10 mg, vitamin K_1 70 micrograms), minerals and trace elements (calcium 100 mg, chromium 200 micrograms, copper 2 mg, iodine 140 micrograms, iron 12 mg, magnesium 30 mg, manganese 3 mg, molybdenum 250 micrograms, phosphorus 77 mg, potassium 4 mg, selenium 50 micrograms, zinc 15 mg). Net price 15-cap pack = £2.57; 45-cap pack = £7.00
Dose: vitamin and mineral deficiency and as adjunct in synthetic diets, 1 capsule daily
Junior capsules, brown, vitamins (ascorbic acid 25 mg, biotin 50 micrograms, cyanocobalamin 2 micrograms, folic acid 100 micrograms, nicotinamide 7.5 mg, pantothenic acid 2 mg, pyridoxine 1 mg, riboflavine 1 mg, thiamine 1.5 mg, vitamin A 1250 units, vitamin D_2 200 units, vitamin E 5 mg, vitamin K_1 25 micrograms), minerals and trace elements (chromium 50 micrograms, copper 1 mg, iodine 75 micrograms, iron 5 mg, magnesium 1 mg, manganese 1.25 mg, molybdenum 50 micrograms, selenium 25 micrograms, zinc 5 mg). Net price 60-cap pack = £7.00
Dose: vitamin and mineral deficiency and as adjunct in synthetic diets, CHILD over 5 years, 2 capsules daily
Ketovite® (Paines & Byrne)
PoM *Tablets*, yellow, ascorbic acid 16.6 mg, riboflavine 1 mg, thiamine hydrochloride 1 mg, pyridoxine hydrochloride 330 micrograms, nicotinamide 3.3 mg, calcium pantothenate 1.16 mg, alpha tocopheryl acetate 5 mg, inositol 50 mg, biotin 170 micrograms, folic acid 250 micrograms, acetomenaphthone 500 micrograms. Net price 100-tab pack = £4.17
Dose: prevention of deficiency in disorders of carbohydrate or amino acid metabolism, 1 tablet 3 times daily; with Ketovite® Liquid as vitamin supplement with synthetic diets
Liquid, pink, sugar-free, vitamin A 2500 units, ergocalciferol 400 units, choline chloride 150 mg, cyanocobalamin 12.5 micrograms/5 mL. Net price 150-mL pack = £2.70
Dose: prevention of deficiency in disorders of carbohydrate or amino acid metabolism, 5 mL daily; with Ketovite® Tablets as vitamin supplement with synthetic diets
Supplementary Vitamin Tablets for Infants (Cow & Gate)
Tablets, ferrous sulphate 4.21 mg (850 micrograms iron), folic acid 63 micrograms, thiamine hydrochloride 250 micrograms, nicotinamide 830 micrograms, riboflavine 250 micrograms, pyridoxine hydrochloride 83 micrograms, cyanocobalamin 1 microgram, ascorbic acid 10 mg, d-α-tocopheryl acetate 1.24 mg, acetomenaphthone 125 micrograms, biotin 8 micrograms, calcium pantothenate 500 micrograms, copper 34 micrograms (as sulphate), iodine 12 micrograms (as potassium iodate), manganese 5 micrograms (as sulphate), molybdenum 6 micrograms (as ammonium molybdate), zinc 620 micrograms (as sulphate). Contains sucrose. Net price 100 = £3.88
Note. For infants on nutritionally incomplete synthetic foods
Dose: consult manufacturer's literature

9.7 Bitters and tonics

Mixtures containing simple and aromatic bitters, such as alkaline gentian mixture, are traditional remedies for loss of appetite. All depend on suggestion.

Gentian Mixture, Acid, BP
Mixture, concentrated compound gentian infusion 10%, dilute hydrochloric acid 5% in a suitable vehicle. Extemporaneous preparations should be recently prepared according to the following formula: concentrated compound gentian infusion 1 mL, dilute hydrochloric acid 0.5 mL, double-strength chloroform water 5 mL, water to 10 mL
Dose: 10 mL 3 times daily in water before meals

Gentian Mixture, Alkaline, BP
(Alkaline Gentian Oral Solution)
Mixture, concentrated compound gentian infusion 10%, sodium bicarbonate 5% in a suitable vehicle. Extemporaneous preparations should be recently prepared according to the following formula: concentrated compound gentian infusion 1 mL, sodium bicarbonate 500 mg, double-strength chloroform water 5 mL, water to 10 mL
Dose: 10 mL 3 times daily in water before meals

NHS **Effico**® (Pharmax)
Tonic, green, thiamine hydrochloride 180 micrograms, nicotinamide 2.1 mg, caffeine 20.2 mg, compound gentian infusion 0.31 mL/5 mL. Net price 300-mL pack = £1.47, 500-ml pack = £2.12

NHS **Labiton**® (LAB)
Tonic, brown, thiamine hydrochloride 375 micrograms, caffeine 3.5 mg, kola nut dried extract 3.025 mg, alcohol 1.4 mL/5 mL. Net price 200 mL = £1.63

NHS **Metatone**® (W-L)
Tonic, thiamine hydrochloride 500 micrograms, calcium glycerophosphate 45.6 mg, manganese glycerophosphate 5.7 mg, potassium glycerophosphate 45.6 mg, sodium glycerophosphate 22.8 mg/5 mL. Net price 300 mL = £1.79

9.8 Metabolic disorders

9.8.1 Wilson's disease
9.8.2 Acute porphyrias

This section covers drugs used in metabolic disorders and not readily classified elsewhere.

9.8.1 Wilson's disease

Penicillamine (see also section 10.1.3) is used in Wilson's disease (hepatolenticular degeneration) to aid the elimination of copper ions. For use in copper and lead poisoning, see p. 21.

Trientine is used for the treatment of Wilson's disease only, in patients intolerant of penicillamine; it is **not** an alternative to penicillamine for rheumatoid arthritis or cystinuria.

PENICILLAMINE

Indications: see under Dose below
Cautions; Contra-indications; Side-effects: see section 10.1.3

Dose: Wilson's disease, 1.5–2 g daily in divided doses before food; maintenance 0.75–1 g daily; ELDERLY, 20 mg/kg daily in divided doses; CHILD, up to 20 mg/kg daily in divided doses, min. 500 mg daily
Chronic active hepatitis (after disease is controlled), 500 mg daily in divided doses slowly increased over 3 months; usual maintenance dose 1.25 g daily
Cystinuria, therapeutic, 1–3 g daily in divided doses before food, adjusted to maintain urinary cystine below 200 mg/litre. Prophylactic (maintain urinary cystine below 300 mg/litre) 0.5–1 g at bedtime; maintain adequate fluid intake (at least 3 litres daily); CHILD minimum dose to maintain urinary cystine below 200 mg/litre

Preparations
See section 10.1.3

TRIENTINE DIHYDROCHLORIDE

Indications: Wilson's disease in patients intolerant of penicillamine
Cautions: see notes above; pregnancy; **interactions:** Appendix 1 (trientine)
Side-effects: nausea; penicillamine-induced systemic lupus erythematosus may not resolve on transfer to trientine
Dose: 1.2–2.4 g daily in 2–4 divided doses before food

▼ PoM **Trientine Dihydrochloride Capsules,** trientine dihydrochloride 300 mg. Label: 6, 22
Available from K & K Greeff

Note. The CSM has requested that in addition to the usual CSM reporting request special records should also be kept by the pharmacist

9.8.2 Acute porphyrias

The acute porphyrias (acute intermittent porphyria, variegate porphyria, hereditary coproporphyria and plumboporphyria) are hereditary disorders of haem biosynthesis; they have a prevalence of about 1 in 10 000 of the population.

Great care must be taken when prescribing for patients with acute porphyria since many drugs can induce acute porphyric crises. Since acute porphyrias are hereditary, relatives of affected individuals should be screened and advised about the potential danger of certain drugs.

The following list contains drugs on the UK market that have been classified as 'unsafe' in porphyria because they have been shown to be porphyrinogenic in animals or *in vitro*, or have been associated with acute attacks in patients.

Further information may be obtained from:

Porphyria Research Unit
Western Infirmary
Glasgow G11 6NT
Telephone 041-339 8822 Extn 4150

For a list of drugs unsafe for use in acute porphyrias, see p. 356.

Drugs unsafe for use in acute porphyrias

Note. Quite modest changes in chemical structure can lead to changes in porphyrinogenicity but where possible general statements have been made about groups of drugs; these should be checked first

Drug groups (please check **first**)

Amphetamines	Barbiturates[3]	Diuretics[6]	Menopausal Steroids[5]
Anabolic Steroids	Benzodiazepines[4]	Ergot Derivatives[7]	Progestogens
Antidepressants[1]	Cephalosporins	Hormone Replacement	Sulphonamides[8]
Antihistamines[2]	Contraceptives, steroid[5]	Therapy[5]	Sulphonylureas

Individual Drugs (please check groups above **first**)

Alcohol	Dexfenfluramine	Ketoconazole	Oxymetazoline
Alcuronium	Dextropropoxyphene[11]	Lignocaine	Oxyphenbutazone
Aluminium-containing	Diclofenac	Lisinopril	Oxytetracycline
Antacids[9]	Diethylpropion	Loxapine	Pentazocine[11]
Aminoglutethimide	Diltiazem	Mebeverine	Phenoxybenzamine
Amiodarone	Doxycycline	Mefenamic Acid	Phenylbutazone
Azapropazone	Econazole	Meprobamate	Phenytoin
Baclofen	Enalapril	Mercaptopurine	Piroxicam
Bromocriptine	Enflurane	Mercury Compounds	Pivampicillin[12]
Busulphan	Erythromycin	Methotrexate	Prilocaine
Captopril	Ethamsylate	Methyldopa	Probenecid
Carbamazepine	Ethionamide	Metoclopramide	Pyrazinamide
Carisoprodol	Ethosuximide	Metyrapone	Rifampicin
Chlorambucil	Etomidate	Miconazole	Simvastatin
Chloramphenicol	Fenfluramine	Mifepristone	Sulphinpyrazone
Chlormezanone	Flucloxacillin	Minoxidil	Sulpiride
Chloroform[10]	Flupenthixol	Nalidixic Acid	Tamoxifen
Clonidine	Gold salts	Natamycin	Theophylline
Cocaine	Griseofulvin	Nifedipine	Thioridazine
Colistin	Guaiphenesin	Nikethamide	Tinidazole
Cyclophosphamide	Halothane	Nitrofurantoin	Trimethoprim
Cycloserine	Hydralazine	Orphenadrine	Valproate[4]
Cyclosporin	Hyoscine Butylbromide	Oxpentifylline	Verapamil
Danazol	Isometheptene Mucate	Oxycodone	Zuclopenthixol
Dapsone	Isoniazid		

1. Includes tricyclic (and related) and MAOIs.
2. Most antihistamines should be avoided but chlorpheniramine and cyclizine thought to be safe.
3. Includes methohexitone, primidone, and thiopentone.
4. Status epilepticus has been treated successfully with intravenous diazepam; where essential, seizure prophylaxis has been undertaken with clonazepam or valproate.
5. Includes both progestogen-only and combined (progestogen content probably more hazardous than oestrogen).
6. Acetazolamide, amiloride, bumetanide, and triamterene have been used.
7. Includes ergometrine (oxytocin probably safe), lysuride and pergolide.
8. Includes co-trimoxazole and sulphasalazine.
9. Absorption limited but magnesium-containing antacids preferable.
10. Small amounts in medicines probably safe.
11. Morphine, diamorphine, codeine, dihydrocodeine, and pethidine are thought to be safe.
12. Ampicillin and amoxycillin probably safe.

10: Drugs used in the treatment of
MUSCULOSKELETAL and JOINT DISEASES

In this chapter, drug treatment is discussed under the following headings:
- 10.1 Drugs used in rheumatic diseases and gout
- 10.2 Drugs used in neuromuscular disorders
- 10.3 Drugs for the relief of soft-tissue inflammation

For treatment of septic arthritis see section 5.1, Table 1.

10.1 Drugs used in rheumatic diseases and gout

- 10.1.1 Non-steroidal anti-inflammatory drugs (NSAIDs)
- 10.1.2 Corticosteroids
- 10.1.3 Drugs which suppress the rheumatic disease process
- 10.1.4 Drugs used in the treatment of gout

Most rheumatic diseases require symptomatic treatment to relieve pain and stiffness. This applies to inflammatory diseases both in the adult and in the juvenile age group (juvenile arthritis—Still's disease). Suitable non-steroidal anti-inflammatory drugs (NSAIDs) are described in section 10.1.1; reference should also be made to section 10.1.4 for the treatment of acute gout.

In certain circumstances corticosteroids (section 10.1.2) may be used to suppress inflammation.

Drugs are also available which may affect the disease process itself and favourably influence the outcome. For *rheumatoid arthritis* these include penicillamine, gold salts, antimalarials (chloroquine and hydroxychloroquine), immunosuppressants (azathioprine, chlorambucil, cyclophosphamide, and methotrexate), and sulphasalazine; they are sometimes known as second-line or disease-modifying antirheumatic drugs. For *psoriatic arthritis* they include gold salts, azathioprine, and methotrexate, and for *gout* they include uricosuric drugs and allopurinol.

10.1.1 Non-steroidal anti-inflammatory drugs (NSAIDs)

In *single doses* NSAIDs have analgesic activity comparable to that of paracetamol (see section 4.7.1) and can therefore be taken on demand for mild or intermittent pain or as a supplement to regular treatment. In regular *full dosage* they have both a lasting analgesic and an anti-inflammatory effect. This combination makes them particularly useful for the treatment of continuous or regular pain associated with inflammation. NSAIDs are, therefore, more appropriate than paracetamol or the opioid analgesics in the *inflammatory arthritides* (e.g. rheumatoid arthritis) and in advanced osteoarthrosis (also termed osteoarthritis). They may also be of benefit in the less well defined conditions of *back pain* and *soft-tissue disorders*.

Differences in anti-inflammatory activity between different NSAIDs are small, but there is considerable variation in individual patient response. About 60% of patients will respond to any NSAID. Among the rest, those who do not respond to one may well respond to another. Therefore it is often necessary to try several drugs before finding one to suit a particular patient. Most NSAIDs should produce an effect within a few days. If used for analgesia alone they should be changed if no response is obtained after a week; if an anti-inflammatory action is also required they should be changed if no response is obtained after three weeks.

The main differences between NSAIDs are in the incidence and type of side-effects. Before treatment is started the prescriber should weigh efficacy against possible side-effects.

ASPIRIN AND THE SALICYLATES

Aspirin[1] was the traditional first choice anti-inflammatory analgesic but most physicians now prefer to start treatment with another NSAID which may be better tolerated and more convenient for the patient.

In regular high dosage aspirin has about the same anti-inflammatory effect as other NSAIDs. The required dose for active inflammatory joint disease is 3.6 g or more daily. There is little anti-inflammatory effect with less than 3 g daily. Gastro-intestinal side-effects such as nausea, dyspepsia, and gastro-intestinal bleeding may occur with any dosage of aspirin but anti-inflammatory doses are associated with a much higher incidence of side-effects. Gastro-intestinal side-effects may be minimised by taking the dose after food. Numerous formulations are available which improve gastric tolerance and minimise occult bleeding, including buffered, dispersible, and enteric-coated preparations.

Anti-inflammatory doses of aspirin may also cause mild chronic salicylate intoxication (salicylism) characterised by dizziness, tinnitus, and deafness; these symptoms may be controlled by reducing the dosage.

---

1. Owing to an association with Reye's syndrome the CSM has recommended that aspirin-containing preparations should no longer be given to children under the age of 12 years, unless specifically indicated, e.g. for juvenile arthritis (Still's disease).

Cautionary label wordings, see inside back cover   Prices are **net**, see p. 1

Benorylate[1], an aspirin-paracetamol ester, is broken down after absorption from the gastro-intestinal tract. It need only be given twice daily and gastric tolerance is slightly better than with aspirin.

ASPIRIN

Indications: pain and inflammation in rheumatic disease and other musculoskeletal disorders (including juvenile arthritis); see also section 4.7.1; antiplatelet, see section 2.9

Cautions: asthma, allergic disease, uncontrolled hypertension, hepatic or renal impairment (avoid if severe), dehydration, pregnancy (particularly at term) (see also Appendix 4), elderly; G6PD-deficiency (see section 9.1.5); *interactions:* Appendix 1 (aspirin)

Contra-indications: gastro-intestinal ulceration; children under 12 years (except for juvenile arthritis) and breast-feeding (association with Reye's syndrome, see section 4.7.1); haemophilia and other bleeding disorders; not for treatment of gout

Side-effects: common with anti-inflammatory doses; gastro-intestinal discomfort or nausea, ulceration with occult bleeding (but occasionally major haemorrhage); also other haemorrhage (e.g. subconjunctival); hearing disturbances such as tinnitus (leading rarely to deafness), vertigo, mental confusion, hypersensitivity reactions (angioedema, bronchospasm and rashes); increased bleeding time; rarely oedema, myocarditis, blood disorders, particularly thrombocytopenia; overdosage: see Emergency Treatment of Poisoning, p. 17

Dose: 0.3–1 g every 4 hours; max. in acute conditions 8 g daily; CHILD, juvenile arthritis, up to 80 mg/kg daily in 5–6 divided doses, increased in acute exacerbations to 130 mg/kg. Doses should be taken after food

Preparations
See section 4.7.1.

BENORYLATE

(Aspirin-paracetamol ester; 2 g benorylate is equivalent to approximately 1.15 g aspirin and 970 mg paracetamol)

Indications: pain and inflammation in rheumatic disease and other musculoskeletal disorders; see also section 4.7.1

Cautions; Contra-indications; Side-effects: see under Aspirin (above) and Paracetamol (section 4.7.1)

Dose: 4–8 g daily divided into 2–3 doses

Benorylate (Non-proprietary)
Tablets, benorylate 750 mg. Net price 100 = £8.58. Label: 21, 31
Available from APS, Norton, Sterwin
Suspension, benorylate 2 g/5 mL. Net price 100 mL = £4.05. Label: 21, 31
Available from APS, Berk, Hillcross, Sterwin

---

1. Owing to an association with Reye's syndrome the CSM has recommended that aspirin-containing preparations should no longer be given to children under the age of 12 years, unless specifically indicated, e.g. for juvenile arthritis (Still's disease).

Benoral® (Sanofi Winthrop)
Tablets, benorylate 750 mg. Net price 20 = £1.72. Label: 21, 31
Granules, benorylate 2 g/sachet. Net price 60 sachet-pack = £14.12. Label: 13, 21, 31
Suspension, sugar-free, benorylate 2 g/5 mL. Net price 300 mL = £12.16. Label: 21, 31

SALICYLATE COMPOUNDS

Indications: pain and inflammation in rheumatic disease and other musculoskeletal disorders

Cautions; Contra-indications; Side-effects: see under Aspirin (above)

PoM **Disalcid®** (3M)
Capsules, orange/grey, salsalate 500 mg, net price 120-cap pack = £6.88. Label: 21, 33
Dose: 2–4 g daily in 3–4 divided doses

Trilisate® (Napp)
Tablets, orange, scored, choline magnesium trisalicylate ≡ salicylate 500 mg, net price 60-tab pack = £4.95. Label: 21, 33
Dose: 0.5–1.5 g of salicylate twice daily; for maintenance, total daily dose may be taken once daily

---

OTHER NSAIDs

Ibuprofen is a propionic acid derivative with anti-inflammatory, analgesic, and antipyretic properties. It has fewer side-effects than other NSAIDs but its anti-inflammatory properties are weaker. Doses of 1.6 to 2.4 g daily are needed for rheumatoid arthritis and it is unsuitable for conditions where inflammation is prominent such as acute gout.

Other propionic acid derivatives:
Naproxen has emerged as one of the first choices as it combines good efficacy with a low incidence of side-effects and administration is only twice daily.
Fenbufen is claimed to be associated with less gastro-intestinal bleeding, but there is a high risk of rashes (see p. 361).
Fenoprofen is as effective as naproxen, and **flurbiprofen** may be slightly more effective. Both are associated with slightly more gastro-intestinal side-effects than ibuprofen.
Ketoprofen has anti-inflammatory properties similar to ibuprofen and has more side-effects.
Tiaprofenic acid is as effective as naproxen; it has more side-effects than ibuprofen.

Drugs with properties similar to those of propionic acid derivatives:
Azapropazone is similar in effect to naproxen; it has a tendency to cause rashes.
Diclofenac has an action similar to that of naproxen; its side-effects are also similar.
Diflunisal is an aspirin derivative but its clinical effect more closely resembles that of the propionic acid derivatives than that of its parent compound. Its long duration of action allows twice-daily administration.

10.1 Drugs used in rheumatic diseases and gout

Etodolac is comparable in effect to naproxen; side-effects appear to be comparable to those of ibuprofen but long-term data are awaited.

Indomethacin has an action equal to or superior to that of naproxen, but with a high incidence of side-effects including headaches, dizziness, and gastro-intestinal disturbances. It can also be used for acute gout.

Mefenamic acid is a related analgesic but its anti-inflammatory properties are minor and side-effects differ in that diarrhoea and occasionally haemolytic anaemia may occur which necessitate discontinuation of treatment.

Nabumetone is comparable in effect to naproxen; side-effects appear to be comparable to those of ibuprofen but long-term data are awaited.

Phenylbutazone is a potent anti-inflammatory drug but because of occasional serious side-effects its use is limited to the hospital treatment of ankylosing spondylitis. In addition to its gastric side-effects it has two rare but dangerous side-effects. It causes fluid retention and, in predisposed patients, may precipitate cardiac failure. It also causes agranulocytosis (which may occur within the first few days of treatment) and aplastic anaemia. In ankylosing spondylitis prolonged administration may be necessary but it should not be used unless other drugs have failed.

Piroxicam is as effective as naproxen and has a prolonged duration of action which permits once-daily administration. It has more gastro-intestinal side-effects than ibuprofen, especially in the elderly.

Sulindac is similar in tolerance to naproxen.

Tenoxicam is similar in effectiveness and tolerance to naproxen. Its long half-life allows once-daily administration.

Tolmetin is comparable in effect to ibuprofen.

CAUTIONS. NSAIDs should be used with caution in the *elderly*, in *allergic disorders* (particularly salicylate hypersensitivity and asthma, see **CSM warning** below), and during *pregnancy*.

In patients with *renal, cardiac, or hepatic impairment* caution is required since the use of NSAIDs may result in deterioration of renal function (see also under Side-effects, below); the dose should be kept as **low as possible** and renal function should be **monitored**.

NSAIDs should not be given to patients with *active peptic ulceration*, see also **CSM advice** below. While it is preferable to avoid them in patients with current or previous peptic ulceration, and to withdraw them if gastro-intestinal lesions develop, nevertheless patients with serious rheumatic diseases (e.g. rheumatoid arthritis) are usually dependent on NSAIDs for effective relief of pain and stiffness. Administration of histamine H$_2$-receptor blocking drugs or misoprostol (see section 1.3.4) may permit recommencement of a NSAID without further gastro-intestinal problems.

SIDE-EFFECTS. Side-effects are variable in severity and frequency. Gastro-intestinal discomfort, nausea, diarrhoea, and occasionally bleeding and ulceration occur; dyspepsia may be minimised by taking these drugs with food or milk. Other side-effects include hypersensitivity reactions (particularly angioedema, asthma, and rashes), headache, dizziness, vertigo, hearing disturbances such as tinnitus, and haematuria. Blood disorders have also occurred. Fluid retention may occur (rarely precipitating congestive heart failure in elderly patients). Reversible acute renal failure may be provoked by NSAIDs especially in patients with pre-existing renal impairment (**important**, see also under Cautions above). Rarely, papillary necrosis or interstitial fibrosis associated with NSAIDs may lead to renal failure. Aseptic meningitis has been reported rarely with NSAIDs; patients with connective tissue disorders such as systemic lupus erythematosus may be especially susceptible.

Overdosage: see Emergency Treatment of Poisoning, p. 18.

CSM advice (peptic ulceration).
1. NSAIDs should not be given to patients with active peptic ulceration.
2. In patients with a history of peptic ulcer disease and in the elderly they should be given only after other forms of treatment have been carefully considered.
3. In all patients it is prudent to start at the bottom end of the dose range.

CSM warning (asthma).
Any degree of worsening of asthma may be related to the ingestion of NSAIDs, either prescribed or (in the case of ibuprofen and others) purchased over the counter.

IBUPROFEN

Indications: pain and inflammation in rheumatic disease (including juvenile arthritis) and other musculoskeletal disorders; see also section 4.7.1

Cautions; Side-effects: see notes above; *interactions:* Appendix 1 (NSAIDs)

Dose: initially 1.2–1.8 g daily in 3–4 divided doses preferably after food; increased if necessary to max. of 2.4 g daily; maintenance dose of 0.6–1.2 g daily may be adequate; CHILD 20 mg/kg daily in divided doses (juvenile arthritis, up to 40 mg/kg daily), not recommended for children under 7 kg

PoM Ibuprofen (Non-proprietary)
Tablets, coated, ibuprofen 200 mg, net price 20 = 26p; 400 mg, 20 = 51p; 600 mg, 20 = £1.36. Label: 21
Various strengths available from APS (Apsifen®), Ashbourne (Arthrofen®), Berk (Lidifen®), Cox, DDSA (Ebufac®), Evans, Kerfoot, Lagap (Ibular®), Norton, Rima (Rimafen®), Upjohn (Motrin®, including an 800-mg strength)

Note. Proprietary brands of ibuprofen tablets are on sale to the public; brand names include Anadin Ibuprofen®, Contrapain Femafen®, Cuprofen®, Ibrufhalal®, Inoven®, Librofem®, Migrafen®, Novaprin®, Nurofen®, Pacifene®, PhorPain®, Proflex®, Relcofen®

PoM **Brufen®** (Boots)
Tablets, all magenta, ibuprofen 200 mg (s/c), net price 20 = 61p; 400 mg (s/c), 20 = £1.21; 600 mg (f/c), 20 = £1.93. Label: 21
Syrup, orange, ibuprofen 100 mg/5 mL. Net price 500 mL = £4.17. Label: 21
Dose: 20 mg/kg daily in divided doses *or* 1–2 years 2.5 mL 3–4 times daily, 3–7 years 5 mL 3–4 times daily, 8–12 years 10 mL 3–4 times daily; not recommended for children weighing less than 7 kg; juvenile rheumatoid arthritis up to 40 mg/kg daily in divided doses
Granules, effervescent, ibuprofen 600 mg/sachet. Net price 20-sachet pack = £4.68. Label: 13, 21
Note. Contains sodium approx. 9 mmol/sachet

PoM **Brufen Retard®** (Boots)
Tablets, m/r, f/c, ibuprofen 800 mg, net price 56-tab pack = £11.76. Label: 25, 27
Dose: 2 tablets daily, preferably in the early evening, increased in severe cases to 3 tablets daily in 2 divided doses

PoM **Fenbid®** (SK&F)
Spansule® (= capsule m/r), maroon/pink, enclosing off-white pellets, ibuprofen 300 mg. Net price 120-cap pack = £7.14. Label: 25
Dose: 1–3 capsules every 12 hours

PoM **Junifen®** : see section 4.7.1

With codeine
PoM **Codafen Continus®** (Napp)
Tablets, white/pink, ibuprofen 300 mg (m/r), codeine phosphate 20 mg. Net price 112-tab pack = £11.21. Label: 2, 21, 25
Dose: 1–2 tablets every 12 hours; max. 3 tablets every 12 hours

Topical preparations: section 10.3.2

ACEMETACIN
(Glycolic acid ester of indomethacin)
Indications: pain and inflammation in rheumatoid arthritis, osteoarthritis, and post-operatively
Cautions; Side-effects: see under Indomethacin
Dose: 120 mg daily in divided doses with food, increased if necessary to 180 mg daily

▼ PoM **Emflex®** (Merck)
Capsules, yellow/orange, acemetacin 60 mg, net price 90-cap pack = £22.50. Label: 21, counselling, driving

AZAPROPAZONE
Indications: pain and inflammation in rheumatic disease and other musculoskeletal disorders; gout
Cautions; Side-effects: see notes above; photosensitivity may occur. Avoid in porphyria (see section 9.8.2); **important:** recent reports of serious enhancement of effect of warfarin; other **interactions:** Appendix 1 (NSAIDs)

Dose: 1.2 g daily in 2 or 4 divided doses (elderly 300 mg twice daily, max. 900 mg daily)
Acute gout, initially 2.4 g in divided doses over 24 hours, then 1.8 g reducing to 1.2 g daily in divided doses
Chronic gout, 600 mg twice daily (elderly 300 mg twice daily, max. 900 mg daily)

PoM **Rheumox®** (Wyeth)
Capsules, orange, azapropazone 300 mg. Net price 20 = £3.37. Label: 21, counselling: in some patients direct sunlight may lead to a rash
Tablets, orange, f/c, scored, azapropazone 600 mg. Net price 20 = £5.85. Label: 21, counselling: in some patients direct sunlight may lead to a rash

DICLOFENAC SODIUM
Indications: pain and inflammation in rheumatic disease (including juvenile arthritis) and other musculoskeletal disorders; acute gout
Cautions; Side-effects: see notes above. Avoid in porphyria (see section 9.8.2); pain may occur at the injection site; suppositories may cause irritation; **interactions:** Appendix 1 (NSAIDs)
Dose: by mouth, 75–150 mg daily in 2–3 divided doses, preferably after food
By deep intramuscular injection into the gluteal region, acute exacerbations and post-operative, 75 mg once daily (twice daily in severe cases) for max. of 2 days
Ureteric colic, 75 mg then a further 75 mg after 30 minutes if necessary
By rectum in suppositories, 100 mg, usually at night
Max. total daily dose by any route 150 mg
CHILD 1 year or over, juvenile arthritis, *by mouth or by rectum*, 1–3 mg/kg daily in divided doses

PoM **Diclofenac Sodium** (Non-proprietary)
Tablets, both e/c, diclofenac sodium 25 mg, net price 20 = £1.88; 50 mg, 20 = £3.65. Label: 5, 25
Available from APS, Ashbourne (Diclozip®), Cox, Eastern (Volraman®), Evans, Kerfoot, Lagap (Rhumalgan®), Norton, Shire (Valenac®), Sterwin

PoM **Voltarol®** (Geigy)
Tablets, both e/c, diclofenac sodium 25 mg (yellow), net price 84-tab pack = £7.88; 50 mg (brown), 84-tab pack = £15.32. Label: 5, 25
Dispersible tablets, pink, diclofenac, equivalent to diclofenac sodium 50 mg, net price 21-tab pack = £4.68. Label: 13, 21
Injection, diclofenac sodium 25 mg/mL. Net price 3-mL amp = 79p
Suppositories, diclofenac sodium 100 mg. Net price 10 = £3.11
Paediatric suppositories, diclofenac sodium 12.5 mg. Net price 10 = 59p
Emulgel® gel, section 10.3.2

PoM **Voltarol® 75 mg SR** (Geigy)
Tablets, m/r, pink, diclofenac sodium 75 mg. Net price 56-tab pack = £18.74. Label: 21, 25
Dose: 1–2 tablets daily preferably with food

PoM Voltarol® Retard (Geigy)
Tablets, m/r, red, diclofenac sodium 100 mg. Net price 28-tab pack = £12.49. Label: 21, 25
Dose: 100 mg once daily preferably with food

DIFLUNISAL
Indications: pain and inflammation in rheumatic disease and other musculoskeletal disorders; see also section 4.7.1
Cautions; Side-effects: see notes above; breast-feeding; **interactions:** Appendix 1 (NSAIDs)
Dose: initially 1 g daily in 2 divided doses, then 0.5–1 g daily; max. 1.5 g daily
Osteoarthrosis, rheumatoid arthritis, 0.5–1 g daily as a single daily dose *or* in 2 divided doses

PoM Diflunisal (Non-proprietary)
Tablets, coated, diflunisal 250 mg, net price 20 = £1.80; 500 mg, 20 = £3.61. Label: 21, 25, counselling, avoid aluminium hydroxide
Available from APS

PoM Dolobid® (Morson)
Tablets, both f/c, diflunisal 250 mg (peach), net price 20 = £1.80; 500 mg (orange), 20 = £3.61. Label: 21, 25, counselling, avoid aluminium hydroxide

ETODOLAC
Indications: pain and inflammation in rheumatoid arthritis and osteoarthrosis
Cautions; Side-effects: see notes above; **interactions:** Appendix 1 (NSAIDs)
Dose: 200 mg or 300 mg twice daily *or* 400 mg or 600 mg once daily; max. 600 mg daily

PoM Lodine® (Wyeth)
Capsules, etodolac 200 mg (light- and dark-grey), net price 20 = £4.06; 300 mg (light-grey), 60-cap pack = £16.89. Label: 21
Tablets, brown, f/c, etodolac 200 mg. Net price 20 = £4.08. Label: 21

FENBUFEN
Indications: pain and inflammation in rheumatic disease and other musculoskeletal disorders
Cautions; Side-effects: see notes above, but high risk of rashes (discontinue immediately); erythema multiforme and Stevens-Johnson syndrome reported; also allergic interstitial lung disorders (may follow rashes); **interactions:** Appendix 1 (NSAIDs)
Dose: 300 mg in the morning and 600 mg at bedtime *or* 450 mg twice daily

PoM Lederfen® (Lederle)
Capsules, dark blue, fenbufen 300 mg. Net price 84-cap pack = £19.61. Label: 21
Tablets, both light blue, f/c, fenbufen 300 mg, net price 84-tab pack = £19.61; 450 mg, 56-tab pack = £19.61. Label: 21
PoM Lederfen F® (Lederle)
Effervescent tablets, fenbufen 450 mg. Net price 56-tab pack = £24.85. Label: 13, 21

FENOPROFEN
Indications: pain and inflammation in rheumatic disease and other musculoskeletal disorders; see also section 4.7.1
Cautions; Side-effects: see notes above; upper respiratory infection and nasopharyngitis reported; **interactions:** Appendix 1 (NSAIDs)
Dose: 300–600 mg 3–4 times daily with food; max. 3 g daily

PoM Fenopron® (Dista)
Fenopron 300 tablets, orange, fenoprofen 300 mg (as calcium salt). Net price 20 = £1.57. Label: 21
Fenopron 600 tablets, orange, scored, fenoprofen 600 mg (as calcium salt). Net price 20 = £3.03. Label: 21
PoM Progesic®: see section 4.7.1

FLURBIPROFEN
Indications: pain and inflammation in rheumatoid arthritis, osteoarthrosis, and ankylosing spondylitis; mild to moderate pain
Cautions; Side-effects: see notes above; local irritation on rectal administration; **interactions:** Appendix 1 (NSAIDs)
Dose: by mouth or by rectum in suppositories, 150–200 mg, daily in divided doses, increased in acute conditions to 300 mg daily

PoM Froben® (Boots)
Tablets, both yellow, s/c, flurbiprofen 50 mg, net price 20 = £1.77; 100 mg, 20 = £3.68. Label: 21
Suppositories, flurbiprofen 100 mg. Net price 12 = £2.90
PoM Froben SR® (Boots)
Capsules, m/r, yellow, enclosing white, off-white beads, flurbiprofen 200 mg. Net price 30-cap pack = £12.80. Label: 21, 25
Dose: 1 capsule daily, preferably in the evening

INDOMETHACIN
Indications: pain and moderate to severe inflammation in rheumatic disease and other acute musculoskeletal disorders; acute gout; dysmenorrhoea
Cautions: see notes above; breast-feeding, epilepsy, parkinsonism, psychiatric disturbances; during prolonged therapy ophthalmic and blood examinations are particularly advisable; avoid rectal administration in proctitis and haemorrhoids; **interactions:** Appendix 1 (NSAIDs)
DRIVING. Dizziness may affect performance of skilled tasks (e.g. driving)
Side-effects: see notes above; frequently gastro-intestinal disturbances (including diarrhoea), headache, dizziness, and light-headedness; gastro-intestinal ulceration and bleeding; rarely, drowsiness, confusion, insomnia, convulsions, psychiatric disturbances, depression, syncope, blood disorders (particularly throm-

bocytopenia), hypertension, hyperglycaemia, blurred vision, corneal deposits, peripheral neuropathy. On rectal administration pruritus, discomfort, bleeding

Dose: by mouth, 50–200 mg daily in divided doses, with food

Dysmenorrhoea, up to 75 mg daily

By rectum in suppositories, 100 mg at night and in the morning if required

Combined oral and rectal treatment, max. total daily dose 150–200 mg

PoM **Indomethacin** (Non-proprietary)
Capsules, indomethacin 25 mg, net price 20 = 18p; 50 mg, 20 = 55p. Label: 21, counselling, driving, see above
Available from APS, Ashbourne (Indomax®), Berk (Imbrilon®), Cox, DDSA (Artracin®), Evans, Galen (Mobilan®), Kerfoot, Rima (Rimacid®)
Suppositories, indomethacin 100 mg. Net price 10 = £1.83. Counselling, driving, see above
Available from Berk (Imbrilon®), Cox, Evans, Norton

PoM **Flexin®** (Napp)
Flexin-25 Continus®, tablets, m/r, green, indomethacin 25 mg, net price 56-tab pack = £7.33. Label: 21, 25, counselling, driving, see above
Flexin-LS Continus®, tablets, m/r, red, indomethacin 50 mg, net price 28-tab pack = £7.33. Label: 21, 25, counselling, driving, see above
Flexin Continus®, tablets, m/r, yellow, indomethacin 75 mg, net price 28-tab pack = £10.47. Label: 21, 25, counselling, driving, see above
Dose: initially 75 mg daily, adjusted in steps of 25–50 mg; range 25–200 mg daily in 1–2 divided doses
Dysmenorrhoea, up to 75 mg daily

PoM **Indocid®** (Morson)
Capsules, indomethacin 25 mg, net price 20 = 99p; 50 mg, 20 = £1.78. Label: 21, counselling, driving, see above
Suspension, sugar-free, indomethacin 25 mg/5 mL. Net price 200 mL = £3.12. Label: 21, counselling, driving, see above
Suppositories, indomethacin 100 mg. Net price 10 = £2.43. Counselling, driving, see above

PoM **Indocid-R®** (Morson)
Capsules, m/r, ivory/clear-blue, enclosing white and blue pellets, indomethacin 75 mg. Net price 20 = £5.71. Label: 21, 25, counselling, driving, see above
Dose: 1–2 capsules daily

PoM **Indomax 75 SR®** (Ashbourne)
Capsules, m/r, blue/clear, enclosing white pellets, indomethacin 75 mg. Net price 28-cap pack = £7.20. Label: 21, 25, counselling, driving, see above
Dose: 1 capsule 1–2 times daily

PoM **Indolar SR®** (Lagap)
Capsules, m/r, blue/clear, enclosing white pellets, indomethacin 75 mg. Net price 20 = £4.02. Label: 21, 25, counselling, driving, see above
Dose: 1 capsule 1–2 times daily

PoM **Indomod®** (Kabi Pharmacia)
Capsules, both m/r, enclosing e/c pellets, indomethacin 25 mg (orange), net price 20 = £2.24; 75 mg (brown), 30-cap pack = £7.71. Label: 25, counselling, driving, see above
Dose: initially 50–75 mg daily, adjusted in steps of 25–50 mg to max. 200 mg daily in divided doses

PoM **Rheumacin SR®** (CP)
Capsules, m/r, yellow/blue, enclosing off-white pellets, indomethacin 75 mg. Net price 20 = £3.34. Label: 21, 25, counselling, driving, see above
Dose: 1–2 capsules daily

PoM **Slo-Indo®** (Generics)
Capsules, m/r, red/yellow enclosing off-white pellets, indomethacin 75 mg. Net price 20 = £4.47. Label: 21, 25, counselling, driving, see above
Dose: 1–2 capsules daily

PoM **Indocid PDA®** : see section 7.1.1.1

KETOPROFEN

Indications: pain and mild inflammation in rheumatic disease and other musculoskeletal disorders, and after orthopaedic surgery; acute gout; dysmenorrhoea

Cautions; Side-effects: see notes above; suppositories may cause rectal irritation; **interactions:** Appendix 1 (NSAIDs)

Dose: by mouth, 100–200 mg daily in 2–4 divided doses with food

By rectum in suppositories, 100 mg at bedtime

Combined oral and rectal treatment, max. total daily dose 200 mg

By deep intramuscular injection into the gluteal muscle, 50–100 mg every 4 hours (max. 200 mg in 24 hours) for up to 3 days

PoM **Alrheumat®** (Bayer)
Capsules, off-white, ketoprofen 50 mg. Net price 20 = £1.22. Label: 21

PoM **Orudis®** (Rhône-Poulenc Rorer)
Capsules, ketoprofen 50 mg (green/purple), net price 112-cap pack = £8.07; 100 mg (pink), 56-cap pack = £8.09. Label: 21
Suppositories, ketoprofen 100 mg. Net price 10 = £3.54

PoM **Oruvail®** (Rhône-Poulenc Rorer)
Capsules, both m/r, enclosing white pellets, ketoprofen 100 mg (pink/purple), net price 56-cap pack = £16.14; 200 mg (pink/white), 28-cap pack = £16.41. Label: 21, 25
Dose: 100–200 mg once daily with food
Injection, ketoprofen 50 mg/mL. Net price 2-mL amp = 75p
Gel, section 10.3.2

KETOROLAC TROMETAMOL
Section 15.1.4.2

MEFENAMIC ACID
Indications: mild to moderate pain in rheumatoid arthritis (including juvenile arthritis), osteoarthrosis, and related conditions; see also section 4.7.1

Cautions: see notes above; blood tests required during long-term treatment; avoid in porphyria (see section 9.8.2); **interactions:** Appendix 1 (NSAIDs)
Side-effects: see notes above; drowsiness; diarrhoea or rashes (withdraw treatment); thrombocytopenia, haemolytic anaemia; convulsions in overdosage
Dose: 500 mg 3 times daily preferably after food; CHILD over 6 months, 25 mg/kg daily in divided doses for not longer than 7 days, except in juvenile arthritis

PoM **Mefenamic Acid** (Non-proprietary)
Capsules, mefenamic acid 250 mg. Net price 20 = £1.32. Label: 21
Available from APS, Ashbourne (Dysman 250®), Cox, Evans, Kerfoot, Norton, Sterwin
Tablets, mefenamic acid 500 mg, net price 20 = £2.46. Label: 21
Available from Ashbourne (Dysman 500®), Cox, Evans, Kerfoot, Norton

PoM **Ponstan**® (P-D)
Capsules, ivory/blue, mefenamic acid 250 mg. Net price 20 = £1.56. Label: 21
Dispersible tablets, blue, mefenamic acid 250 mg. Net price 20 = £1.71. Label: 13, 21
Tablets forte, yellow, f/c, mefenamic acid 500 mg. Net price 20 = £2.90. Label: 21
Paediatric suspension, mefenamic acid 50 mg/5 mL. Net price 125 mL = £3.37. Label: 21

NABUMETONE

Indications: pain and inflammation in osteoarthrosis and rheumatoid arthritis
Cautions; Side-effects: see notes above; **interactions:** Appendix 1 (NSAIDs)
Dose: 1 g at night, in severe conditions 0.5–1 g in morning as well; elderly 0.5–1 g daily

PoM **Relifex**® (Bencard)
Tablets, red, f/c, nabumetone 500 mg. Net price 56-tab pack = £15.68. Label: 21, 25
Suspension, nabumetone 500 mg/5 mL. Net price 300-mL pack = £21.84. Label: 21

NAPROXEN

Indications: pain and inflammation in rheumatic disease (including juvenile arthritis) and other musculoskeletal disorders; acute gout; see also Naproxen Sodium, section 4.7.1
Cautions; Side-effects: see notes above; suppositories may cause rectal irritation and occasional bleeding; **interactions:** Appendix 1 (NSAIDs)
Dose: by mouth, 0.5–1 g daily in 2 divided doses *or* 1 g once daily; CHILD (over 5 years), juvenile arthritis, 10 mg/kg daily in 2 divided doses
Acute musculoskeletal disorders, 500 mg initially, then 250 mg every 6–8 hours as required; max. dose after first day 1.25 g daily
Acute gout, 750 mg initially, then 250 mg every 8 hours until attack has passed
By rectum in suppositories, 500 mg at bedtime; if necessary 500 mg in morning as well

PoM **Naproxen** (Non-proprietary)
Tablets, naproxen 250 mg, net price 20 = £1.71; 500 mg, 20 = £3.30. Label: 21
Available from Ashbourne (Arthrosin®), BHR (Prosaid®), Cox, CP, Evans, Goldshield (Rheuflex®), Kerfoot, Lagap (Laraflex®), Norton, Shire (Valrox®), Sterwin

PoM **Naprosyn**® (Syntex)
Tablets, all scored, naproxen 250 mg (buff), net price 20 = £2.50; 375 mg (pink), 60-tab pack = £11.25; 500 mg (buff), 60-tab pack = £14.98. Label: 21
Suspension, orange, naproxen 125 mg/5 mL. Contains about 1.7 mmol Na$^+$/5 mL. Net price 100 mL = £2.18. Label: 21
Granules, naproxen 500 mg/sachet. Net price 60 sachets = £19.47. Label: 13, 21
Suppositories, naproxen 500 mg. Net price 10 = £3.26

PoM **Naprosyn**® **EC** (Syntex)
Tablets, all e/c, naproxen 250 mg, net price 56-tab pack = £7.00; 375 mg, 56-tab pack = £10.50; 500 mg, 56-tab pack = £14.00. Label: 5, 25

PoM **Nycopren**® (Nycomed)
Tablets, both e/c, naproxen 250 mg (scored), net price 20 = £2.07; 500 mg, 60-tab pack = £12.41. Label: 5, 25

PoM **Synflex**® : see section 4.7.1

With misoprostol
For cautions, contra-indications, and side-effects of misoprostol, see section 1.3.4

PoM **Napratec**® (Searle)
Combination pack, 56 yellow scored tablets, naproxen 500 mg; 56 white scored tablets, misoprostol 200 micrograms. Net price = £18.00. Label: 21
Dose: patients requiring naproxen for rheumatoid arthritis, osteoarthritis, or ankylosing spondylitis, with prophylaxis against NSAID-induced gastroduodenal ulceration, 1 naproxen 500-mg tablet and 1 misoprostol 200-microgram tablet taken together twice daily with food

PHENYLBUTAZONE

Indications: ankylosing spondylitis when other therapy is unsuitable
Cautions: blood counts before and during treatment if for more than 7 days; elderly (reduce dose); breast-feeding; withdraw treatment if acute pulmonary syndrome including fever and dyspnoea occurs; see also notes above; **interactions:** Appendix 1 (NSAIDs)
Contra-indications: cardiovascular disease, renal and hepatic impairment; pregnancy; history of peptic ulceration, gastro-intestinal haemorrhage, or blood disorders; porphyria (see section 9.8.2); thyroid disease; children under 14
Side-effects: see notes above; parotitis, stomatitis, goitre, pancreatitis, hepatitis, nephritis, visual disturbances; rarely leucopenia, thrombocytopenia, agranulocytosis, aplastic anaemia, erythema multiforme, toxic epidermal necrolysis
Dose: initially 200 mg 2–3 times daily for 2 days, with or after food, then reduced to minimum effective, usually 100 mg 2–3 times daily

PoM **Butacote**® (Geigy)
Tablets, violet, e/c, s/c, phenylbutazone 100 mg, net price 20 = 40p (hosp. only). Label: 5, 21, 25

PIROXICAM

Indications: pain and inflammation in rheumatic disease (including juvenile arthritis) and other musculoskeletal disorders; acute gout

Cautions: see notes above; avoid in porphyria (see section 9.8.2); **interactions:** Appendix 1 (NSAIDs)

Side-effects: see notes above

Dose: by mouth or by rectum, initially 20 mg daily, maintenance 10–30 mg daily, in single or divided doses

Acute musculoskeletal disorders, 40 mg daily in single or divided doses for 2 days, then 20 mg daily for 7–14 days

Acute gout, 40 mg initially, then 40 mg daily in single or divided doses for 4–6 days

CHILD (over 6 years) *by mouth,* juvenile arthritis, less than 15 kg, 5 mg daily; 16–25 kg, 10 mg; 26–45 kg, 15 mg; over 46 kg, 20 mg

PoM **Piroxicam** (Non-proprietary)
Capsules, piroxicam 10 mg, net price 20 = £2.96; 20 mg, 20 = £5.93. Label: 21
Available from APS, Ashbourne (Pirozip®), Cox, Evans, Kerfoot, Lagap, Norton

PoM **Feldene®** (Pfizer)
Capsules, piroxicam 10 mg (maroon/blue), net price 56-cap pack = £8.87; 20 mg (maroon), 28-cap pack = £8.87. Label: 21
Dispersible tablets, piroxicam 10 mg (scored), net price 56-tab pack = £9.75; 20 mg, 28-tab pack = £9.75. Label: 13, 21
Suppositories, piroxicam 20 mg. Net price 10 = £5.20
Gel, section 10.3.2

SULINDAC

Indications: pain and inflammation in rheumatic disease and other musculoskeletal disorders; acute gout

Cautions; Side-effects: see notes above; caution if history of renal stones; ensure adequate hydration; **interactions:** Appendix 1 (NSAIDs)

Dose: 200 mg twice daily with food (may be reduced according to response); max. 400 mg daily; acute gout should respond within 7 days; limit treatment of peri-articular disorders to 7–10 days

PoM **Clinoril®** (MSD)
Tablets, both yellow, scored, sulindac 100 mg, net price 20 = £2.24; 200 mg, 20 = £4.11. Label: 21
Note. Sulindac tablets also available from Generics

TENOXICAM

Indications: pain and inflammation in rheumatoid arthritis and osteoarthrosis

Cautions; Side-effects: see notes above; **interactions:** Appendix 1 (NSAIDs)

Dose: 20 mg daily

Note. Also indicated for short-term treatment (usually 7 days, max. 14 days) of acute musculoskeletal disorders.

PoM **Mobiflex®** (Roche)
Tablets, red-brown, f/c, tenoxicam 20 mg. Net price 28-tab pack = £16.52. Label: 21

TIAPROFENIC ACID

Indications: pain and inflammation in rheumatic disease and other musculoskeletal disorders

Cautions; Side-effects: see notes above; bladder irritation reported; **interactions:** Appendix 1 (NSAIDs)

Dose: 600 mg daily in 2–3 divided doses

PoM **Tiaprofenic Acid** (Non-proprietary)
Tablets, tiaprofenic acid 200 mg, net price 84-tab pack = £13.08; 300 mg, 56-tab pack = £14.37. Label: 21
Available from Cox

PoM **Surgam®** (Roussel)
Tablets, tiaprofenic acid 200 mg, net price 84-tab pack = £15.89; 300 mg, 56-tab pack = £15.89. Label: 21

PoM **Surgam SA®** (Roussel)
Capsules, m/r, maroon/pink enclosing white pellets, tiaprofenic acid 300 mg. Net price 56-cap pack = £15.89. Label: 21, 25
Dose: 2 capsules once daily

TOLMETIN

Indications: pain and inflammation in rheumatic disease (including juvenile arthritis) and other musculoskeletal disorders

Cautions; Side-effects: see notes above; **interactions:** Appendix 1 (NSAIDs)

Dose: 0.6–1.8 g daily in 2–4 divided doses; max. 30 mg/kg daily up to 1.8 g
CHILD, juvenile arthritis, 20–25 mg/kg daily in 3–4 divided doses; max. 30 mg/kg daily up to 1.8 g

PoM **Tolectin®** (Cilag)
Capsules, tolmetin (as sodium salt) 200 mg (ivory/orange), net price 90-cap pack = £15.97; 400 mg (orange), 90-cap pack = £23.97. Label: 21

10.1.2 Corticosteroids

10.1.2.1 Systemic corticosteroids
10.1.2.2 Local corticosteroid injections

10.1.2.1 SYSTEMIC CORTICOSTEROIDS

The general actions and uses of the corticosteroids are described in section 6.3. Treatment with corticosteroids in rheumatic diseases should be reserved for specific indications, e.g. when other anti-inflammatory drugs are unsuccessful.

In severe, possibly life-threatening, situations a high initial dose of corticosteroid is given to induce remission and the dose then gradually reduced to the lowest maintenance dose that will control the disease or, if possible, discontinued altogether. A major problem is that relapse may occur as dosage reduction is made, particularly if this is carried out too rapidly. The tendency is therefore to increase and maintain dosage and consequently the patient becomes dependent on corticosteroids. For this reason pulse doses of corticosteroids (e.g. methylprednisolone up to 1 g intravenously on three consecutive days) is in current use to suppress highly active inflammatory disease while longer term and slower acting medication is being commenced.

Prednisolone is used for most purposes; it has the advantage over the more potent corticosteroids (see section 6.3.2) of permitting finer dosage adjustments. To minimise side-effects the maintenance dose of prednisolone should be kept as low as possible, usually 7.5 mg daily and seldom exceeding 10 mg daily.

Polymyalgia rheumatica and *temporal (giant cell) arteritis* are always treated with corticosteroids. The usual initial dose of prednisolone in polymyalgia rheumatica is 10 to 15 mg daily and in temporal arteritis 40 to 60 mg daily (the higher dose being used if visual symptoms occur). Treatment should be continued until remission occurs and doses then gradually reduced. Relapse is common if therapy is stopped within 3 years but most patients can discontinue treatment after approximately 3 to 6 years after which recurrences become rare.

Polyarteritis nodosa and *polymyositis* are usually treated with corticosteroids. An initial dose of 60 mg of prednisolone daily is often used and reduced to a maintenance dose of 10 to 15 mg daily.

Systemic lupus erythematosus is treated with corticosteroids when necessary using a similar dosage regimen to that for polyarteritis nodosa and polymyositis (above). Patients with pleurisy, pericarditis, or other systemic manifestations will respond to corticosteroids. It may then be possible to reduce the dosage; alternate-day treatment is sometimes adequate, and the drug may be gradually withdrawn. In some mild cases corticosteroid treatment may be stopped after a few months. Many mild cases of systemic lupus erythematosus do not require corticosteroid treatment. Alternative treatment with anti-inflammatory analgesics, and possibly chloroquine, should be considered.

Since effective doses of systemic corticosteroids may cause Cushing's syndrome these drugs should **not** be used to suppress symptoms of *rheumatoid arthritis* unless alternative anti-inflammatory drugs and drugs which may affect the disease process (section 10.1.3) have proved unsuccessful, with increasing disability due to the inflammatory process. The smallest effective dose should be used and increased if necessary, but should not exceed the equivalent of prednisolone 7.5 to 10 mg daily. Attempts should always be made gradually to reduce the dose. Corticosteroids in low dosage may be useful in the elderly patient, and similar nocturnal doses may relieve morning stiffness.

Ankylosing spondylitis should not be treated with long-term corticosteroids; rarely, pulse doses may be needed and may be useful in extremely active disease that does not respond to conventional treatment.

10.1.2.2 LOCAL CORTICOSTEROID INJECTIONS

Corticosteroids are injected locally for an anti-inflammatory effect. In inflammatory conditions of the joints, particularly in rheumatoid arthritis, they are given by *intra-articular injection* to relieve pain, increase mobility, and reduce deformity in one or a few joints. Full aseptic precautions are essential. Infected areas should be avoided. An almost insoluble, long-acting compound such as triamcinolone hexacetonide is preferred for intra-articular injection.

Smaller amounts of corticosteroids may also be injected directly into soft tissues for the relief of inflammation in conditions such as *tennis* or *golfer's elbow* or *compression neuropathies*. In *tendinitis*, injections should be made into the tendon sheath and not directly into the tendon. A soluble, short-acting compound such as betamethasone is preferred for injection into the carpal tunnel.

Cortisone acetate is **not** effective for local injection and hydrocortisone acetate or one of the synthetic analogues such as triamcinolone hexacetonide is generally used. The risk of necrosis and muscle wasting may be slightly increased with triamcinolone; flushing has been reported with intra-articular corticosteroid injections.

Corticosteroid injections are also injected into soft tissues for the treatment of skin lesions (see section 13.4).

DEXAMETHASONE SODIUM PHOSPHATE

Indications: local inflammation of joints and soft tissues

Cautions; Contra-indications; Side-effects: see notes above and section 6.3.3

Dose: by intra-articular, intralesional, or soft-tissue injection, dexamethasone 0.4–4 mg, according to size of joint or amount of soft-tissue, at intervals of 3–21 days according to response

Note. 1.3 mg dexamethasone sodium phosphate ≡ 1.2 mg dexamethasone phosphate ≡ 1 mg dexamethasone

PoM **Dexamethasone** (Organon)
Injection, dexamethasone sodium phosphate 5 mg/mL (= 4 mg dexamethasone/mL). Net price 1-mL amp = 83p; 2-mL vial = £1.27

PoM **Decadron**® (MSD)
Injection, dexamethasone phosphate 4 mg/mL (as sodium salt) (≡ 3.33 mg/mL dexamethasone). Net price 2-mL vial = £1.76

HYDROCORTISONE ACETATE

Indications: local inflammation of joints and soft tissues

Cautions; Contra-indications; Side-effects: see notes above and section 6.3.3

Dose: by intra-articular or soft-tissue injection, 5–50 mg, according to joint size or amount of soft tissue; not more than 3 joints should be treated on any one day; CHILD, 5–30 mg (divided)

PoM Hydrocortisone Acetate Injection (aqueous suspension), hydrocortisone acetate 25 mg/mL. Net price 1-mL amp = 88p

PoM Hydrocortistab® (Boots)
Injection (aqueous suspension), hydrocortisone acetate 25 mg/mL. Net price 1-mL amp = 88p

METHYLPREDNISOLONE ACETATE

Indications: local inflammation of joints and soft-tissues
Cautions; Contra-indications; Side-effects: see notes above and section 6.3.3
Dose: by intra-articular or soft-tissue injection, 4–80 mg, according to joint size or amount of soft tissue, repeated every 1–5 weeks according to response

PoM Depo-Medrone® (Upjohn)
Injection (aqueous suspension), methylprednisolone acetate 40 mg/mL. Net price 1-mL vial = £2.59; 2-mL vial = £4.65; 3-mL vial = £6.75

PoM Depo-Medrone® with Lidocaine (Upjohn)
Injection (aqueous suspension), methylprednisolone acetate 40 mg, lignocaine hydrochloride 10 mg/mL. For injection into joints, bursae, or tendon sheaths. Net price 1-mL vial = £2.56; 2-mL vial = £4.65

PREDNISOLONE ACETATE

Indications: local inflammation of joints and soft tissues
Cautions; Contra-indications; Side-effects: see notes above and section 6.3.3
Dose: by intra-articular or soft-tissue injection, 5–25 mg according to joint size or amount of soft tissue; not more than 3 joints should be treated on any one day

PoM Deltastab® (Boots)
Injection (aqueous suspension), prednisolone acetate 25 mg/mL. Net price 1-mL amp = 88p

TRIAMCINOLONE ACETONIDE

Indications: local inflammation of joints and soft tissues
Cautions; Contra-indications; Side-effects: see notes above and section 6.3.3; not recommended for children under 6 years
Dose: by intra-articular injection, 2.5–40 mg according to joint size, to a max. of 80 mg in multiple injections
By intralesional injection, 2–3 mg; max. 30 mg (5 mg at any one site). Doses are repeated every 1–2 weeks according to response

PoM Adcortyl®   Intra-articular / Intradermal (Squibb)
Injection (aqueous suspension), triamcinolone acetonide 10 mg/mL. Net price 1-mL amp = £1.02; 5-mL vial = £4.14

PoM Kenalog®   Intra-articular / Intramuscular (Squibb)
Injection (aqueous suspension), triamcinolone acetonide 40 mg/mL. Net price 1-mL vial = £1.70

TRIAMCINOLONE HEXACETONIDE

Indications: local inflammation of joints and soft tissues
Cautions; Contra-indications; Side-effects: see notes above and section 6.3.3
Dose: by intra-articular, intrasynovial, or soft-tissue injection, 2–30 mg, according to joint size or amount of soft tissue, repeated at intervals of not less than 3–4 weeks according to the response
By intracutaneous injection of a suspension containing not more than 5 mg/mL, up to 500 micrograms/square inch of affected skin

PoM Lederspan® (Lederle)
Injection (aqueous suspension), triamcinolone hexacetonide 5 mg/mL. For intralesional or sublesional injection. Net price 5-mL vial = £2.92
Injection (aqueous suspension), triamcinolone hexacetonide 20 mg/mL. For intra-articular or intrasynovial injection. Net price 1-mL vial = £2.54; 5-mL vial = £9.90

10.1.3 Drugs which suppress the rheumatic disease process

Certain drugs such as gold, penicillamine, hydroxychloroquine, chloroquine, immunosuppressants, and sulphasalazine may affect the disease process in *rheumatoid arthritis*, as may gold and immunosuppressants in *psoriatic arthritis*. Unlike NSAIDs they do not produce an immediate therapeutic effect but require 4 to 6 months of treatment for a full response. If one of these drugs does not lead to objective benefit within 6 months, it should be discontinued.

These drugs may improve not only the symptoms and signs of inflammatory joint disease but also extra-articular manifestations such as vasculitis. They reduce the erythrocyte sedimentation rate and sometimes the titre of rheumatoid factor. Some (e.g. the immunosuppressants) may retard erosive damage as judged radiologically.

These drugs are used in rheumatoid arthritis where treatment with NSAIDs has been unsuccessful, so that there is evidence of disease progression including continuing active joint inflammation and worsening radiological changes. Since, in the first few months, the course of rheumatoid arthritis is unpredictable, it is usual to delay treatment for about 6 months depending on the progress of the disease, but treatment should be initiated before joint damage becomes irreversible.

Penicillamine and immunosuppressants are also sometimes used in rheumatoid arthritis where there are troublesome extra-articular features such as vasculitis, and in patients who are taking

10.1 Drugs used in rheumatic diseases and gout

excessive doses of corticosteroids. Where the response is satisfactory there is often a striking reduction in requirements of both corticosteroids and other drugs. Gold, penicillamine, and related drugs may also be used to treat *juvenile arthritis* (Still's disease) when indications are similar.

Gold and penicillamine are effective in *palindromic rheumatism* and chloroquine is sometimes used to treat *systemic* and *discoid lupus erythematosus*.

GOLD

Gold may be given by intramuscular injection as sodium aurothiomalate or by mouth as auranofin.

Sodium aurothiomalate must be given by deep intramuscular injection and the area gently massaged. A test dose of 10 mg must be given followed by doses of 50 mg at weekly intervals until there is definite evidence of remission. Benefit is not to be expected until about 300 to 500 mg has been given; if there is no remission after 1 g has been given it should be discontinued. In patients who do respond, the interval between injections is then gradually increased to 4 weeks and treatment is continued for up to 5 years after complete remission. If relapse occurs dosage may be immediately increased to 50 mg weekly and only once control has been obtained again should the dosage be reduced. It is important to avoid complete relapse since second courses of gold are not usually effective. Children may be given 1 mg/kg weekly to a maximum of 50 mg weekly, the intervals being gradually increased to 4 weeks according to response; an initial test dose is given corresponding to one-tenth to one-fifth of the calculated dose.

Auranofin is given by mouth. If there is no response after 9 months treatment should be discontinued.

Gold therapy should be discontinued in the presence of blood disorders or proteinuria (associated with immune complex nephritis) which is repeatedly above 300 mg/litre without other cause (such as urinary-tract infection). Urine tests and full blood counts (including total and differential white cell and platelet counts) must therefore be performed before each intramuscular injection; in the case of oral treatment the urine and blood tests should be carried out monthly. Rashes with pruritus often occur after 2 to 6 months of intramuscular treatment and may necessitate discontinuation of treatment; the most common side-effect of oral therapy, diarrhoea with or without nausea or abdominal pain, may respond to bulking agents (such as bran) or temporary reduction in dosage.

SODIUM AUROTHIOMALATE

Indications: active progressive rheumatoid arthritis, juvenile arthritis
Cautions: see notes above; patients should report pruritus, metallic taste, fever, sore throat or tongue, buccal ulceration, purpura, epistaxis, bleeding gums, bruising, menorrhagia, diarrhoea; renal and hepatic impairment, elderly, breast-feeding, history of urticaria, eczema, colitis, drugs which cause blood disorders; annual chest x-ray
Contra-indications: severe renal and hepatic disease (see notes above); history of blood disorders or bone marrow aplasia, exfoliative dermatitis, systemic lupus erythematosus, necrotising enterocolitis, pulmonary fibrosis; pregnancy (see Appendix 4); porphyria (see section 9.8.2)
Side-effects: severe reactions (occasionally fatal) in up to 5% of patients; mouth ulcers, skin reactions, proteinuria, blood disorders (sometimes sudden and fatal); rarely colitis, peripheral neuritis, pulmonary fibrosis, hepatotoxicity with cholestatic jaundice, alopecia
Dose: by deep intramuscular injection, administered on expert advice, see notes above

PoM **Myocrisin**® (Rhône-Poulenc Rorer)
Injection 10 mg, sodium aurothiomalate 20 mg/mL. Net price 0.5-mL amp = £1.34
Injection 20 mg, sodium aurothiomalate 40 mg/mL. Net price 0.5-mL amp = £1.95
Injection 50 mg, sodium aurothiomalate 100 mg/mL. Net price 0.5-mL amp = £3.97

AURANOFIN

Indications: active progressive rheumatoid arthritis when NSAIDs inadequate alone
Cautions; Contra-indications: see under Sodium Aurothiomalate
Side-effects: diarrhoea most common (reduced by bulking agents such as bran); see also under Sodium Aurothiomalate
Dose: administered on expert advice, 6 mg daily (initially in 2 divided doses then if tolerated as single dose), if response inadequate after 6 months, increase to 9 mg daily (in 3 divided doses), discontinue if no response after a further 3 months

PoM **Ridaura**® (Bencard)
Tablets, pale yellow, f/c, auranofin 3 mg. Net price 60-tab pack = £28.00. Label: 21

PENICILLAMINE

Penicillamine has a similar action to gold, and more patients are able to continue treatment than with gold but side-effects occur frequently. An initial dose of 125 to 250 mg daily before food is given for 1 month, increased by this amount every 4 to 12 weeks until remission occurs. Penicillamine should be discontinued if there is no improvement within 1 year. The usual maintenance dose is 500 to 750 mg daily, but up to 1.5 g may rarely be required.

Patients should be warned not to expect improvement for at least 6 to 12 weeks after treatment is initiated. If remission has been sustained for 6 months, reduction of dosage by 125 to 250 mg every 12 weeks may be attempted.

Cautionary label wordings, see inside back cover

Blood counts, including platelets, and urine examinations should be carried out every 1 or 2 weeks for the first 2 months then every 4 weeks to detect blood disorders and proteinuria. A reduction in platelet count indicates that treatment with penicillamine should be stopped, subsequently re-introduced at a lower dosage level and then, if possible, gradually increased. Proteinuria, associated with immune complex nephritis, occurs in up to 30% of patients, but may resolve despite continuation of treatment; treatment may be continued provided that renal function tests remain normal, oedema is absent, and the 24-hour urinary excretion of protein does not exceed 2 g.

Nausea may occur but is not usually a problem provided that penicillamine is taken before food or on retiring and that low initial doses are used and only gradually increased. Loss of taste may occur about 6 weeks after treatment is started but usually returns 6 weeks later irrespective of whether or not treatment is discontinued; mineral supplements are not recommended. Rashes are a common side-effect. Those which occur in the first few months of treatment disappear when the drug is stopped and treatment may then be re-introduced at a lower dose level and gradually increased. Late rashes are more resistant and often necessitate discontinuation of treatment.

PENICILLAMINE

Indications: severe active or progressive rheumatoid arthritis, juvenile arthritis. For use in Wilson's disease, see section 9.8
For use in copper and lead poisoning, see Emergency Treatment of Poisoning

Cautions: see notes above; renal impairment, pregnancy, and portal hypertension; avoid concurrent gold, chloroquine, hydroxychloroquine, or immunosuppressive treatment; **interactions:** Appendix 1 (penicillamine)

Contra-indications: lupus erythematosus

Side-effects: hypersensitivity reactions (may necessitate discontinuation of treatment); nausea, anorexia, taste loss, mouth ulcers, skin reactions (see notes above), oedema, proteinuria, agranulocytosis or severe thrombocytopenia (sometimes fatal); rarely myasthenia, febrile reactions, lupus erythematosus

Dose: rheumatoid arthritis, administered on expert advice, ADULT, see notes above; CHILD initial dose, 50 mg daily before food for 1 month, increased at 4-week intervals to a maintenance dose of 15–20 mg/kg daily

PoM **Penicillamine** (Non-proprietary)
Tablets, coated, penicillamine 125 mg, net price 20 = £2.88; 250 mg, 20 = £4.97. Label: 6, 22
Available from APS, Cox, Evans

PoM **Distamine®** (Dista)
Tablets, all f/c, penicillamine 50 mg (scored), net price 20 = £1.09; 125 mg, 20 = £2.17; 250 mg, 20 = £3.74. Label: 6, 22

PoM **Pendramine®** (ASTA Medica)
Tablets, both scored, f/c, penicillamine 125 mg, net price 20 = £2.98; 250 mg, 20 = £5.13. Label: 6, 22

ANTIMALARIALS

Chloroquine and **hydroxychloroquine** have a similar action to, and are better tolerated than, gold or penicillamine but their use is limited by their ocular toxicity. However, retinopathy is rare provided the doses given below are not exceeded.

These drugs should not be used for psoriatic arthritis and are best **avoided** in elderly patients as it is difficult to distinguish ageing changes from drug-induced retinopathy.

They are also used in systemic lupus erythematosus (section 10.1.2.1).

Mepacrine (see section 5.4.4) is sometimes used in discoid lupus erythematosus.

CHLOROQUINE

Indications: active rheumatoid arthritis (including juvenile arthritis), systemic and discoid lupus erythematosus; malaria, see section 5.4.1

Cautions: hepatic and renal impairment, pregnancy (but for malaria benefit outweighs risk, see Appendix 4, Antimalarials), porphyria, may exacerbate psoriasis, neurological disorders (especially history of epilepsy), severe gastro-intestinal disorders, G6PD deficiency (see section 9.1.5); elderly (see notes above); avoid concurrent therapy with hepatotoxic drugs—other **interactions:** Appendix 1 (chloroquine)

Advice of College of Ophthalmologists on long-term therapy.
1. Eye examination before long-term chloroquine or hydroxychloroquine to establish baseline;
2. Patient to stop taking and seek immediate advice if any disturbance of vision noted;
3. Prescribing medical practitioner to be responsible for monitoring if considered necessary.

Ocular toxicity very unlikely with chloroquine (base) less than 4 mg/kg daily or hydroxychloroquine sulphate less than 6.5 mg/kg daily.

Side-effects: gastro-intestinal disturbances, headache, visual disturbances, irreversible retinal damage, corneal opacities, depigmentation or loss of hair, skin reactions; rarely blood disorders (thrombocytopenia, agranulocytosis and aplastic anaemia)

Dose: administered on expert advice, chloroquine (base) 150 mg daily preferably after food; CHILD, 3 mg/kg daily

Note. Chloroquine base 150 mg ≡ chloroquine sulphate 200 mg ≡ chloroquine phosphate 250 mg (approx.).

Preparations
See section 5.4.1

HYDROXYCHLOROQUINE SULPHATE

Indications: active rheumatoid arthritis (including juvenile arthritis), systemic and discoid lupus erythematosus

Cautions; Side-effects: see under Chloroquine and notes (above)

Dose: administered on expert advice, initially 400 mg daily in divided doses; maintenance 200–400 mg daily; max. 6.5 mg/kg daily; CHILD, up to 6.5 mg/kg daily (dosage form not suitable for children who weigh less than 33 kg)

PoM **Plaquenil**® (Sanofi Winthrop)
Tablets, orange, s/c, hydroxychloroquine sulphate 200 mg. Net price 56-tab pack = £19.36. Label: 5

IMMUNOSUPPRESSANTS

When used in *rheumatoid arthritis* **immunosuppressants** have a similar action to gold and are useful alternatives in cases that have failed to respond to gold, penicillamine, chloroquine, or hydroxychloroquine.

Azathioprine (see section 8.2.1) is usually chosen and is given in a dose of 1.5 to 2.5 mg/kg daily in divided doses. Blood counts should be carried out every 4 weeks to detect possible neutropenia and/or thrombocytopenia which is usually resolved by reducing the dose. Nausea, vomiting, and diarrhoea may occur, usually starting early during the course of treatment, and may necessitate withdrawal of the drug; herpes zoster infection may also occur.

Methotrexate (see section 8.1.3) has also been shown to be effective. It is usually given in an initial dose of 2.5 mg by mouth once a week, increased slowly to a maximum of 15 mg once a week, subject to regular full blood counts (including differential white cell count and platelet count) and liver-function tests initially weekly and monthly thereafter.

Chlorambucil (see section 8.1.1) is another immunosuppressant which is used in rheumatoid arthritis; a dose of 100 to 200 micrograms/kg daily is usually given initially; most patients require between 2.5 and 7.5 mg daily. Regular blood counts including platelets should be carried out.

Cyclophosphamide (see section 8.1.1) is more toxic but may be used at a dose of 1 to 1.5 mg/kg daily for rheumatoid arthritis with severe systemic manifestations.

Immunosuppressants are also used in the management of severe cases of *systemic lupus erythematosus* and other connective tissue disorders. They are often given in conjunction with corticosteroids for patients with severe or progressive renal disease though the evidence for their benefit is doubtful. They may be used in cases of *polymyositis* which are resistant to corticosteroids. They are used for their corticosteroid-sparing effect in patients whose corticosteroid requirements are excessive. **Azathioprine** is usually used but **chlorambucil** is an alternative.

Azathioprine and methotrexate are used in the treatment of *psoriatic arthropathy* for severe or progressive cases which are not controlled with anti-inflammatory drugs. There is an impression that **azathioprine** is the more effective for psoriatic arthritis and that **methotrexate** is the more effective for skin manifestations. Methotrexate is usually given in a dose of 10–25 mg once a week by mouth. Regular full blood counts and liver-function tests should be carried out initially weekly and monthly thereafter.

SULPHASALAZINE

Sulphasalazine was initially introduced for the treatment of rheumatoid arthritis. Recent re-evaluation has confirmed that it has a beneficial effect in suppressing the inflammatory activity of rheumatoid arthritis. Side-effects include rashes, gastro-intestinal intolerance and, especially in patients with rheumatoid arthritis, occasional leucopenia, neutropenia, and thrombocytopenia. These haematological abnormalities occur usually in the first 3 to 6 months of treatment and are reversible on cessation of treatment. Close monitoring of full blood counts (including differential white cell count and platelet count) is necessary throughout treatment of rheumatoid arthritis, monthly during the first 6 months and 3-monthly thereafter, liver function tests being performed at the same time.

SULPHASALAZINE

Indications: active rheumatoid arthritis; ulcerative colitis, see section 1.5
Cautions; Contra-indications; Side-effects: see section 1.5
Dose: by mouth, administered on expert advice, as enteric-coated tablets, initially 500 mg daily, increased by 500 mg at intervals of 1 week to a max. of 2–3 g daily in divided doses

PoM **Salazopyrin EN-tabs**® (Kabi Pharmacia)
Tablets, e/c, yellow, f/c, sulphasalazine 500 mg. Net price 125-tab pack = £12.75. Label: 5, 14, 25, counselling, see lenses section 1.5

10.1.4 Drugs used in the treatment of gout

It is important to distinguish drugs used for the treatment of acute attacks of gout from those used in the long-term control of the disease. The latter exacerbate and prolong the acute manifestations if started during an attack.

ACUTE ATTACKS

Acute attacks of gout are usually treated with high doses of **NSAIDs** such as azapropazone, diclofenac, indomethacin, ketoprofen, naproxen, piroxicam, and sulindac (section 10.1.1). Colchicine is an alternative. Aspirin is **contra-indicated** in gout. Allopurinol and uricosurics are not effective in treating an acute attack and may prolong it indefinitely if started during the acute episode.

Indomethacin is often chosen in acute attacks. High doses are usually well tolerated for short periods (50 to 100 mg repeated after a few hours if necessary and followed by reducing doses every 6 hours as the patient improves). If courses of treatment last for less than one week side-effects are unusual despite the high doses used.

Colchicine is probably as effective as indomethacin. Its use is limited by the development of toxicity at higher doses, but it is of value in patients with heart failure since, unlike NSAIDs, it does not induce fluid retention; moreover it can be given to patients receiving anticoagulants.

COLCHICINE

Indications: acute gout, short-term prophylaxis during initial therapy with allopurinol and uricosuric drugs

Cautions: gastro-intestinal disease, renal impairment, pregnancy and breast-feeding

Side-effects: most common are nausea, vomiting, and abdominal pain; excessive doses may also cause profuse diarrhoea, gastro-intestinal haemorrhage, rashes, and renal damage. Rarely peripheral neuritis, alopecia, and with prolonged treatment blood disorders

Dose: 1 mg initially, followed by 500 micrograms every 2–3 hours until relief of pain is obtained or vomiting or diarrhoea occurs, or until a total dose of 10 mg has been reached. The course should not be repeated within 3 days
Prevention of attacks during initial treatment with allopurinol or uricosuric drugs, 500 micrograms 2–3 times daily

PoM **Colchicine** (Non-proprietary)
Tablets, colchicine 500 micrograms, net price 20 = 97p
Available from CP, Evans

INTERVAL TREATMENT

For long-term ('interval') control of gout the formation of uric acid from purines may be reduced with the **xanthine-oxidase inhibitor** allopurinol, or the **uricosuric drugs** probenecid or sulphinpyrazone may be used to increase the excretion of uric acid in the urine. Treatment should be continued indefinitely once the decision has been made to prevent further attacks of gout by correcting the hyperuricaemia. These drugs should never be started during an acute attack. The initiation of treatment may precipitate an acute attack therefore colchicine or an anti-inflammatory analgesic should be used as a prophylactic and continued for at least one month after the hyperuricaemia has been corrected (usually about 3 months of prophylaxis).

Allopurinol is a convenient well tolerated drug which is now widely used. It is especially useful in patients with renal impairment or urate stones where uricosuric drugs cannot be used. It is usually given once daily, as the active metabolite of allopurinol has a long half-life, but doses over 300 mg daily should be divided. Allopurinol treatment should not be started until an acute attack of gout has completely subsided, as further attacks may be precipitated. It is well tolerated in most patients but may occasionally cause rashes.

The uricosuric drugs include **probenecid** and **sulphinpyrazone**. They can be used instead of allopurinol, or in conjunction with it in cases that are resistant to treatment.

If an acute attack develops in a patient taking allopurinol or a uricosuric the treatment should continue at the same dosage while the acute attack is treated in its own right.

Azapropazone (section 10.1.1) also has a uricosuric effect and may be useful in the long-term treatment of chronic gout.

Aspirin and salicylates antagonise the uricosuric drugs; they do not antagonise allopurinol but are nevertheless **contra-indicated** in gout.

Crystallisation of urate in the urine may occur with the uricosuric drugs and it is important to ensure that there is an adequate urine output especially in the first few weeks of treatment. As an additional precaution the urine may be rendered alkaline.

The **NSAIDs** are described in section 10.1.1.

ALLOPURINOL

Indications: gout prophylaxis, hyperuricaemia

Cautions: administer prophylactic colchicine or NSAID (*not* aspirin or salicylates) until at least 1 month after hyperuricaemia corrected; ensure adequate fluid intake (2 litres/day); hepatic and renal impairment. In neoplastic conditions treatment with allopurinol (if required) should be commenced before cytotoxic drugs are given; interactions: Appendix 1 (allopurinol)

Contra-indications: not a treatment for acute gout but continue if attack develops when already receiving allopurinol, and treat attack separately (see notes above)

Side-effects: rashes, sometimes with fever (**withdraw** therapy; if rash mild re-introduce cautiously but **discontinue** immediately if recurrence); gastro-intestinal disorders. Rarely malaise, headache, vertigo, drowsiness, taste disturbances, hypertension, symptomless xanthine deposits in muscle, alopecia, hepatotoxicity

Dose: initially 100 mg daily as a single dose, after food, gradually increased over 1–3 weeks according to the plasma or urinary uric acid concentration, to about 300 mg daily; usual maintenance dose 200–600 mg, rarely 900 mg daily, divided into doses of not more than 300 mg; CHILD (in neoplastic conditions, enzyme disorders) 10–20 mg/kg daily

PoM **Allopurinol** (Non-proprietary)
Tablets, allopurinol 100 mg, net price 20 = 50p; 300 mg, 20 = £1.79. Label: 8, 21, 27
Available from APS, Ashbourne (Xanthomax®), Berk (Caplenal®), Cox, CP, DDSA (Cosuric®), Evans, Kerfoot, Nicholas (Hamarin®), Rima (Rimapurinol®)

PoM **Zyloric®** (Wellcome)
Tablets, allopurinol 100 mg, net price 20 = £4.06; 300 mg, 28-tab pack = £14.56. Label: 8, 21, 27

PROBENECID

Indications: gout prophylaxis (to correct hyperuricaemia); reduction of tubular excretion of penicillins and certain cephalosporins, see section 5.1

Cautions: during initial gout therapy administer prophylactic colchicine or NSAID (*not* aspirin or salicylates), ensure adequate fluid intake (about 2 litres daily), render urine alkaline if uric acid overload is high; peptic ulceration, renal impairment (avoid if severe); transient false-positive Benedict's test; G6PD-deficiency (see section 9.1.5); **interactions:** Appendix 1 (probenecid)

Contra-indications: history of blood disorders, nephrolithiasis, porphyria (see section 9.8.2), acute gout attack; avoid aspirin and salicylates

Side-effects: infrequent; occasionally nausea and vomiting, urinary frequency, headache, flushing, dizziness, rashes; rarely hypersensitivity, nephrotic syndrome, hepatic necrosis, aplastic anaemia

Dose: uricosuric therapy, initially 250 mg twice daily after food, increased after a week to 500 mg twice daily then up to 2 g daily in 2–4 divided doses according to plasma-uric acid concentration and reduced for maintenance

PoM **Benemid**® (MSD)
Tablets, scored, probenecid 500 mg. Net price 20 = 66p. Label: 12, 21, 27

SULPHINPYRAZONE

Indications: gout prophylaxis, hyperuricaemia
Cautions; Contra-indications: see under Probenecid; regular blood counts advisable; avoid in hypersensitivity to NSAIDs; **interactions:** Appendix 1 (sulphinpyrazone)

Side-effects: gastro-intestinal disturbances, occasionally allergic skin reactions; rarely blood disorders, gastro-intestinal ulceration and bleeding, acute renal failure, raised liver enzymes, jaundice and hepatitis

Dose: initially 100–200 mg daily with food (or milk) increasing over 2–3 weeks to 600 mg daily (rarely 800 mg daily), continued until serum uric acid concentration normal then reduced for maintenance (maintenance dose may be as low as 200 mg daily)

PoM **Anturan**® (Geigy)
Tablets, both yellow, s/c, sulphinpyrazone 100 mg, net price 20 = 94p; 200 mg, 84-tab pack = £7.82. Label: 12, 21

10.2 Drugs used in neuromuscular disorders

10.2.1 Drugs which enhance neuromuscular transmission
10.2.2 Skeletal muscle relaxants

Anticholinesterases are used as first-line treatment in *myasthenia gravis*.

Corticosteroids are only given concomitantly if anticholinesterase treatment is failing.

Plasmapheresis may produce temporary remission in otherwise unresponsive patients.

ANTICHOLINESTERASES

Anticholinesterase drugs are used to enhance neuromuscular transmission in voluntary and involuntary muscle in myasthenia gravis. They prolong the action of acetylcholine by inhibiting the action of the enzyme acetylcholinesterase. Excessive dosage of these drugs may impair neuromuscular transmission and precipitate 'cholinergic crises' by causing a depolarising block. This may be difficult to distinguish from a worsening myasthenic state.

Side-effects of anticholinesterases are due to their parasympathomimetic action. Muscarinic effects include increased sweating, salivary, and gastric secretion, also increased gastro-intestinal and uterine motility, and bradycardia. These effects are antagonised by atropine.

Edrophonium has a very brief action and is therefore used mainly for the diagnosis of myasthenia gravis. A single test-dose usually causes substantial improvement in muscle power (lasting about 5 minutes) in patients with the disease (if respiration already impaired, *only* in conjunction with someone skilled at intubation).

It can also be used to determine whether a patient with myasthenia is receiving inadequate or excessive treatment with cholinergic drugs. If treatment is excessive an injection of edrophonium will either have no effect or will intensify symptoms (if respiration already impaired, *only* in conjunction with someone skilled at intubation). Conversely, transient improvement may be seen if the patient is being inadequately treated. The test is best performed just before the next dose of anticholinesterase.

Neostigmine produces a therapeutic effect for up to 4 hours. Its pronounced muscarinic action is a disadvantage, and simultaneous administration of an antimuscarinic drug such as atropine or propantheline may be required to prevent colic, excessive salivation, or diarrhoea. In severe disease neostigmine may be given every 2 hours. The maximum that most patients can tolerate is 180 mg daily.

Pyridostigmine is less powerful and slower in action than neostigmine but it has a longer duration of action. It is preferable to neostigmine because of its smoother action and the need for less frequent dosage. It is particularly preferred in patients whose muscles are weak on wakening. It has a comparatively mild gastro-intestinal effect but an antimuscarinic drug may still be required. It is inadvisable to exceed a daily dose of 720 mg.

Distigmine has the most protracted action but the danger of a 'cholinergic crisis' caused by accumulation of the drug is greater than with shorter-acting drugs.

Neostigmine and edrophonium are also used to reverse the actions of the non-depolarising muscle relaxants (see section 15.1.6).

NEOSTIGMINE

Indications: myasthenia gravis; other indications, see section 15.1.6
Cautions: asthma, bradycardia, recent myocardial infarction, epilepsy, hypotension, parkinsonism, vagotonia, peptic ulceration, pregnancy. Atropine or other antidote to muscarinic effects may be necessary (particularly when neostigmine is given by injection), but it should not be given routinely as it may mask signs of overdosage; **interactions:** Appendix 1 (cholinergics)
Contra-indications: intestinal or urinary obstruction
Side-effects: nausea, vomiting, increased salivation, diarrhoea, abdominal cramps (more marked with higher doses). Signs of overdosage are increased gastro-intestinal discomfort, bronchial secretions, and sweating, involuntary defaecation and micturition, miosis, nystagmus, bradycardia, hypotension, agitation, excessive dreaming, and weakness eventually leading to fasciculation and paralysis
Dose: by mouth, neostigmine bromide 15–30 mg at suitable intervals throughout day, total daily dose 75–300 mg (but see also notes above); NEONATE 1–5 mg every 4 hours, half an hour before feeds; CHILD up to 6 years initially 7.5 mg, 6–12 years initially 15 mg, usual total daily dose 15–90 mg
By subcutaneous or intramuscular injection, neostigmine methylsulphate 1–2.5 mg at suitable intervals throughout day (usual total daily dose 5–20 mg); NEONATE 50–250 micrograms every 4 hours half an hour before feeds; CHILD 200–500 micrograms as required

PoM **Prostigmin**® (Roche)
Tablets, scored, neostigmine bromide 15 mg. Net price 20 = 53p
Injection, neostigmine methylsulphate 500 micrograms/mL, net price 1-mL amp = 16p; 2.5 mg/mL, 1-mL amp = 16p

DISTIGMINE BROMIDE

Indications: myasthenia gravis; urinary retention and other indications, see section 7.4.1
Cautions; Contra-indications; Side-effects: see under Neostigmine
Dose: initially 5 mg daily half an hour before breakfast, increased at intervals of 3–4 days if necessary to a max. of 20 mg daily; CHILD up to 10 mg daily according to age

Preparations
See section 7.4.1

EDROPHONIUM CHLORIDE

Indications: see under Dose and notes above; surgery, see section 15.1.6

Cautions; Contra-indications; Side-effects: see under Neostigmine; *great* caution in respiratory distress (see notes above)
Note. Severe cholinergic reactions can be counteracted by injection of atropine sulphate (which should always be available)
Dose: diagnosis of myasthenia gravis, *by intravenous injection,* 2 mg followed after 30 seconds (if no adverse reaction has occurred) by 8 mg; in adults without suitable veins, *by intramuscular injection,* 10 mg
Detection of overdosage or underdosage of cholinergic drugs, *by intravenous injection,* 2 mg (best before next dose of anticholinesterase, see notes above)
CHILD *by intravenous injection* 20 micrograms/kg followed after 30 seconds (if no adverse reaction has occurred) by 80 micrograms/kg

PoM **Tensilon**® (Cambridge)
Injection, edrophonium chloride 10 mg/mL. Net price 1-mL amp = 27p

PYRIDOSTIGMINE BROMIDE

Indications: myasthenia gravis
Cautions; Contra-indications; Side-effects: see under Neostigmine; weaker muscarinic action
Dose: by mouth, 30–120 mg at suitable intervals throughout day, total daily dose 0.3–1.2 g (but see also notes above); NEONATE 5–10 mg every 4 hours, ½–1 hour before feeds; CHILD up to 6 years initially 30 mg, 6–12 years initially 60 mg, usual total daily dose 30–360 mg

PoM **Mestinon**® (Roche)
Tablets, scored, pyridostigmine bromide 60 mg. Net price 20 = £1.01

IMMUNOSUPPRESSANT THERAPY

Corticosteroids (see section 6.3) are established as treatment for myasthenia gravis where *thymectomy* is inadvisable or to reduce the risk of surgery beforehand. The initial dose may be high (up to 100 mg **prednisolone** daily) but most advise starting with a smaller dose (20 mg prednisolone daily) and gradually increasing it. There is grave risk of exacerbation of the myasthenia during the initial stages of therapy, particularly in the first 2–3 weeks, therefore inpatient supervision is essential. Improvement usually begins after about 2 weeks on the high-dose regimen. In some patients a prolonged remission may be induced, but often patients need a maintenance dose of 10–40 mg of prednisolone daily; alternate-day therapy is popular. Patients who need a corticosteroid may benefit from the addition of **azathioprine** (see section 8.2.1) in a dose of 2 mg/kg daily which may allow a reduction in corticosteroid dosage.

10.2.2 Skeletal muscle relaxants

Drugs described below are used for the relief of chronic muscle spasm or spasticity; they are not indicated for spasm associated with minor injuries. They act principally on the central nervous system with the exception of dantrolene which has a peripheral site of action. They differ in action from the muscle relaxants used in anaesthesia (see section 15.1.5) which block transmission of impulses at the neuromuscular junction.

The underlying cause of spasticity should be treated and any aggravating factors (e.g. pressure sores, infection) remedied. Skeletal muscle relaxants are effective in most forms of spasticity except the rare alpha variety. The major disadvantage of treatment with these drugs is that reduction in muscle tone can cause a loss of splinting action of the spastic leg and trunk muscles and sometimes lead to an increase in disability.

Dantrolene acts directly on skeletal muscle and produces fewer central adverse effects making it a drug of choice. The dose should be increased slowly.

Baclofen inhibits transmission at spinal level and also depresses the central nervous system. The dose should be increased slowly to avoid the major side-effects of sedation and hypotonia (other adverse events are uncommon).

Diazepam may also be used. Sedation and, occasionally, extensor hypotonus are disadvantages. Other benzodiazepines also have muscle-relaxant properties. Muscle-relaxant doses of benzodiazepines are similar to anxiolytic doses (see section 4.1.2).

Clonazepam (see section 4.8) may sometimes help in myoclonus.

Quinine salts (see section 5.4.1) 200 to 300 mg at bedtime are effective in relieving nocturnal leg cramps. They are toxic in overdosage and accidental fatalities have occurred in children.

BACLOFEN

Indications: chronic severe spasticity of voluntary muscle
Cautions: psychiatric illness, cerebrovascular disease, elderly; respiratory, hepatic, or renal impairment; epilepsy; hypertonic bladder sphincter; pregnancy; avoid abrupt withdrawal; avoid in peptic ulceration and in porphyria (see section 9.8.2); **interactions:** Appendix 1 (muscle relaxants)
DRIVING. Drowsiness may affect performance of skilled tasks (e.g. driving); effects of alcohol enhanced
Side-effects: frequently sedation, drowsiness, nausea; occasionally lightheadedness, lassitude, confusion, dizziness, ataxia, hallucinations, headache, euphoria, insomnia, depression, tremor, nystagmus, paraesthesias, convulsions, muscular pain and weakness, respiratory or cardiovascular depression, hypotension, gastro-intestinal and urinary disturbances; rarely visual disorders, taste alterations, increased sweating, rash, altered liver function, and paradoxical increase in spasticity

Dose: 5 mg 3 times daily, preferably after food, gradually increased; max. 100 mg daily; CHILD 0.75–2 mg/kg daily (over 10 years, max. 2.5 mg/kg daily) *or* 2.5 mg 4 times daily increased gradually according to age to maintenance: 1–2 years 10–20 mg daily, 2–6 years 20–30 mg daily, 6–10 years 30–60 mg daily

PoM **Baclofen** (Non-proprietary)
Tablets, baclofen 10 mg. Net price 20 = £2.43. Label: 2, 8
Available from APS, Ashbourne (Baclospas®), Cox, Evans, Kerfoot, Norton
PoM **Lioresal**® (Geigy)
Tablets, scored, baclofen 10 mg. Net price 20 = £2.34. Label: 2, 8
Additives: include gluten
Liquid, sugar-free, baclofen 5 mg/5 mL. Net price 300 mL = £6.16. Label: 2, 8

DANTROLENE SODIUM

Indications: chronic severe spasticity of voluntary muscle
Cautions: impaired cardiac and pulmonary function; test liver function before and at intervals during therapy; therapeutic effect may take a few weeks to develop but if treatment is ineffective it should be discontinued after 4–6 weeks. Avoid in children or when spasticity is useful, for example, locomotion; **interactions:** Appendix 1 (muscle relaxants).
DRIVING. Drowsiness may affect performance of skilled tasks (e.g. driving); effects of alcohol enhanced
Contra-indications: hepatic impairment (may cause severe liver damage)
Side-effects: transient drowsiness, dizziness, weakness, malaise, fatigue, diarrhoea (withdraw if severe, discontinue treatment if recurs on re-introduction), anorexia, nausea, headache, rash; less frequently constipation, dysphagia, speech and visual disturbances, confusion, nervousness, insomnia, depression, seizures, chills, fever, increased urinary frequency; rarely, tachycardia, erratic blood pressure, dyspnoea, haematuria, possible crystalluria, urinary incontinence or retention, pleural effusion, pericarditis, dose-related hepatotoxicity (occasionally fatal) may be more common in women over 30 especially those taking oestrogens
Dose: initially 25 mg daily, may be increased at weekly intervals to max. of 100 mg 4 times daily; usual dose 75 mg 3 times daily

PoM **Dantrium**® (Norwich Eaton)
Capsules, both orange/brown, dantrolene sodium 25 mg, net price 20 = £3.11; 100 mg, 20 = £10.88. Label: 2
Injection—see section 15.1.8

DIAZEPAM

Indications: muscle spasm of varied aetiology, including tetanus; other indications, see sections 4.1.2, 4.8, 15.1.4.2

Cautions; Contra-indications; Side-effects: see section 4.1.2; also hypotonia; special precautions for intravenous injection (see section 4.8.2)
Dose: by mouth, 2–15 mg daily in divided doses, increased if necessary in spastic conditions to 60 mg daily according to response
Cerebral spasticity in selected cases, CHILD 2–40 mg daily in divided doses
By intramuscular or by slow intravenous injection (at a rate of 0.5 mL (2.5 mg) per 30 seconds), in acute muscle spasm, 10 mg repeated if necessary after 4 hours
Tetanus, ADULT and CHILD, *by intravenous injection,* 100–300 micrograms/kg repeated every 1–4 hours; *by intravenous infusion (or by nasoduodenal tube),* 3–10 mg/kg over 24 hours, adjusted according to response

Preparations
See section 4.1.2

OTHER MUSCLE RELAXANTS

The clinical efficacy of carisoprodol, chlormezanone and meprobamate (see section 4.1.2), methocarbamol, and orphenadrine as muscle relaxants is **not** well established although they have been included in compound analgesic preparations.

CARISOPRODOL
Indications: short-term symptomatic relief of muscle spasm (but see notes above)
Cautions; Contra-indications; Side-effects: see under Meprobamate, section 4.1.2. Drowsiness is common; avoid in porphyria (see section 9.8.2)
Dose: 350 mg 3 times daily; ELDERLY half adult dose or less

PoM **Carisoma**® (Pharmax)
Tablets, carisoprodol 125 mg, net price 20 = 76p; 350 mg, 20 = 84p. Label: 2

METHOCARBAMOL
Indications: short-term symptomatic relief of muscle spasm (but see notes above)
Cautions: hepatic and renal impairment (avoid injection in renal impairment)
DRIVING. Drowsiness may affect performance of skilled tasks (e.g. driving); effects of alcohol enhanced
Contra-indications: coma or pre-coma, brain damage, epilepsy, myasthenia gravis
Side-effects: lassitude, light-headedness, dizziness, restlessness, anxiety, confusion, drowsiness, nausea, allergic rash or angioedema, convulsions
Dose: by mouth, 1.5 g 4 times daily (elderly 750 mg or less); may be reduced to 750 mg 3 times daily
By slow intravenous injection or by infusion, 1–3 g (max. rate 300 mg/min.); max. dose 3 g (elderly, 1.5 g) daily for 3 days

PoM **Robaxin**® (Wyeth)
750 Tablets, scored, methocarbamol 750 mg. Net price 20 = £2.36. Label: 2
Injection, methocarbamol 100 mg/mL in aqueous macrogol '300'. Net price 10-mL amp = £1.39
PoM **Robaxisal Forte**®: see section 4.7.1

ORPHENADRINE CITRATE
Indications: short-term symptomatic relief of muscle spasm (but see notes above)
Cautions: see under Benzhexol Hydrochloride, section 4.9.2. Avoid in children and in porphyria (see section 9.8.2); reduce dose in elderly
Side-effects: dry mouth and other antimuscarinic side-effects; see also Orphenadrine Hydrochloride, section 4.9.2
Dose: by intramuscular or by slow intravenous injection (over 5 minutes), 60 mg repeated after 12 hours if necessary

PoM **Norflex**® (3M)
Injection, orphenadrine citrate 30 mg/mL. Net price 2-mL amp = 60p

10.3 Drugs for the relief of soft-tissue inflammation

10.3.1 Enzymes
10.3.2 Rubefacients and other topical antirheumatics

10.3.1 Enzymes

Hyaluronidase is used to render the tissues more easily permeable to injected fluids, e.g. for introduction of fluids by subcutaneous infusion (termed hypodermoclysis).

HYALURONIDASE
Indications: enhance permeation of subcutaneous or intramuscular injections; promote resorption of excess fluids and blood
Contra-indications: intravenous route, bites or stings, infection or malignancy at site
Dose: to enhance tissue permeability, *by subcutaneous or intramuscular injection,* usually 1500 units, either mixed with the injection fluid or injected into the site before injection is administered
By subcutaneous infusion, 1500 units administered before 500–1000 mL infusion fluid

PoM **Hyalase**® (CP)
Injection, powder for reconstitution, hyaluronidase (ovine). Net price 1500-unit amp = £1.98

10.3.2 Rubefacients and other topical antirheumatics

Rubefacients act by counter-irritation. Pain, whether superficial or deep-seated, is relieved by any method which itself produces irritation of the skin. Counter-irritation is comforting in painful lesions of the muscles, tendons, and joints, and in non-articular rheumatism. Rubefacients probably all act through the same essential mechanism and differ mainly in intensity and duration of action.

Topical **NSAIDs** (e.g. benzydamine, felbinac, ibuprofen, salicylamide) may provide some slight relief of pain in musculoskeletal conditions.

10.3 Drugs for the relief of soft-tissue inflammation

Cautions. Apply with gentle massage. Avoid contact with eyes, mucous membranes, and inflamed or broken skin. **Not** generally suitable for children. Liniments are very toxic if taken by mouth.

COUNTER-IRRITANTS

Algesal® (Duphar)
Cream, diethylamine salicylate 10%. Net price 50 g = 75p. Apply 3 times daily

Algipan® (Whitehall)
Cream, methyl nicotinate 1%, capsicum oleoresin (capsicin) 0.1%, glycol salicylate 10%. Net price 40 g = 77p; 80 g = £1.23
Spray application, methyl nicotinate 1.5%, glycol salicylate 10%. Net price 120-mL aerosol spray = £1.15. Label: 15

Aspellin® (Fisons)
Liniment, ammonium salicylate 1%, camphor 0.6%, menthol 1.4%, ethyl and methyl salicylate 0.54%. Net price 125 mL = 90p; 500 mL = £3.06; 150-mL spray can = 96p. Label: 15

Balmosa® (Pharmax)
Cream, camphor 4%, capsicum oleoresin 0.035%, menthol 2%, methyl salicylate 4%. Net price 40 g = 47p

Bayolin® (Bayer)
Cream, benzyl nicotinate 2.5%, glycol salicylate 10%, heparinoid 50 units/g. Net price 35 g = 70p. Apply 2–3 times daily

NHS **Bengué's Balsam**® (Bengué)
Ointment, menthol 20%, methyl salicylate 20% in a lanolin basis. Net price 25 g = 86p

NHS **Bengué's Balsam SG**® (Bengué)
Cream, menthol 10%, methyl salicylate 15% in a vanishing cream basis. Net price 25 g = 86p

Cremalgin® (Rhône-Poulenc Rorer)
Balm (= cream), capsicin 0.1%, glycol salicylate 10%, methyl nicotinate 1%. Net price 30 g = 71p. Apply 2–3 times daily

Dubam® (Norma)
Cream, methyl salicylate 20%, menthol 2%, cineole 1%. Net price 30 g = 70p
Spray application, glycol salicylate 5%, methyl nicotinate 1.6%, methyl salicylate 1%, ethyl salicylate 4%. Net price 50 g = £1.75; 113-g aerosol spray = £3.01

Salonair® (Eastern)
Spray application, glycol salicylate 1.75%, methyl salicylate 1.75%, menthol 3.2%, camphor 3.0%, squalane 0.5%, benzyl nicotinate 0.04%. Net price 80-mL aerosol spray = £4.90

Transvasin® (Seton)
Cream, ethyl nicotinate 2%, hexyl nicotinate 2%, tetrahydrofurfuryl salicylate 14%. Net price 40 g = 74p. Apply at least twice daily

POULTICES

Kaolin Poultice, heavy kaolin 52.7%, thymol 0.05%, boric acid 4.5%, peppermint oil 0.05%, methyl salicylate 0.2%, glycerol 42.5%. Net price 200 g = £1.43
Warm and apply directly or between layers of muslin; avoid application of overheated poultice
Kaolin Poultice K/L Pack® (K/L)
Kaolin poultice. Net price 4 × 100-g pouches = £4.16

TOPICAL NSAIDs

Note. For NSAID asthma warning, see p. 349.
Difflam® (3M)
Cream, benzydamine hydrochloride 3%. Net price 15 g = £1.29; 50 g = £4.83; 100 g = £8.86. Apply 3–6 times daily for up to 10 days

PoM **Feldene**® (Pfizer)
Gel, piroxicam 0.5%. Net price 60 g = £7.77; 112 g = £12.20
Apply 3–4 times daily; therapy should be reviewed after 4 weeks; 30-g (**Feldene**® **Sports Gel**) tube for short-term use, net price = £3.89

Ibugel® (Dermal)
Gel, ibuprofen 5%. Net price 100 g = £6.70
Apply up to 3 times daily

Ibuleve® (DDD)
Gel, ibuprofen 5%. Net price 30 g =£2.08
Apply up to 3 times daily

Intralgin® (3M)
Gel, benzocaine 2%, salicylamide 5% in an alcoholic vehicle. Net price 50 g = 51p

Movelat® (Panpharma)
Cream, heparinoid 0.2%, salicylic acid 2%. Net price 100 g = £3.90. Apply up to 4 times daily
Gel, ingredients as for cream but in a colourless gel basis. Net price 100 g = £3.90. Apply up to 4 times daily

PoM **Oruvail**® (Rhône-Poulenc Rorer)
Gel, ketoprofen 2.5%. Net price 100 g = £6.95
Apply 2–4 times daily for up to 7 days (usual recommended dose 15 g daily)

Proflex® (Zyma)
Cream, ibuprofen 5%. Net price 50 g = £4.23; 100 g = £8.70. Apply 3–4 times daily

PoM **Traxam**® (Lederle)
Aerosol application, felbinac 3·17%. Net price 100 g = £9.78. Label: 15
Gel, felbinac 3%. Net price 50 g = £8.72.
Apply 2–4 times daily; max. 25 g daily; therapy should be reviewed after 14 days
Note. Felbinac is an active metabolite of the NSAID fenbufen

PoM **Voltarol Emulgel**® (Geigy)
Gel, diclofenac diethylammonium salt 1.16% (equivalent to diclofenac sodium 1%). Net price 20 g (hosp. only) = £1.55; 100 g = £7.75. Apply 3–4 times daily; therapy should be reviewed after 14 days

11: Drugs acting on the
EYE

In this chapter, drug treatment is discussed under the following headings:
- 11.1 Administration of drugs to the eye
- 11.2 Control of microbial contamination
- 11.3 Anti-infective eye preparations
- 11.4 Corticosteroids and other anti-inflammatory preparations
- 11.5 Mydriatics and cycloplegics
- 11.6 Treatment of glaucoma
- 11.7 Local anaesthetics
- 11.8 Miscellaneous ophthalmic preparations
- 11.9 Contact lenses

The entries in this chapter generally relate only to local eye treatment. Systemic indications and side-effects of many of the drugs are given elsewhere (see index).

11.1 Administration of drugs to the eye

EYE-DROPS AND EYE OINTMENTS. When administered in the form of eye-drops, drugs penetrate the globe, probably through the cornea. However, systemic effects, which are usually undesirable, may well arise from absorption of drugs into the general circulation via conjunctival vessels or from the nasal mucosa after the excess of the preparation has drained down through the tear duct. For example, timolol (a beta-blocker), administered as eye-drops may induce bronchospasm or bradycardia in susceptible individuals.

Eye ointments are often applied to lid margins for blepharitis. They may also be used in the conjunctival sac for other conditions especially where a prolonged action is required.

When two different preparations in the form of eye-drops are required at the same time of day, for example pilocarpine and timolol in glaucoma, dilution and overflow may occur when one immediately follows the other. The patient should therefore leave an interval of a few minutes. At night, an eye ointment for the second drug will reduce the problem.

Generally it is inadvisable for patients to continue to wear contact lenses, particularly hydrophilic (soft) contact lenses when receiving eye-drops. For warnings relating to eye-drops and contact lenses, see section 11.9.

EYE LOTIONS. These are solutions for the irrigation of the conjuctival sac. They act mechanically to flush out irritants or foreign bodies as a first-aid treatment. Sterile sodium chloride 0.9% solution (section 11.8.2) is usually used. It should be used once only from a previously unopened container for first aid, while for treatment it should be used for no longer than 24 hours after the container is first opened. Single-application containers are available. In emergency, tap water drawn freshly from the main (not stored water) will suffice.

OTHER PREPARATIONS. Subconjunctival injection may be used to administer anti-infective drugs, mydriatics, or corticosteroids for conditions not responding to topical therapy. The drug diffuses through the sclera to the anterior and posterior chambers and vitreous humour in higher concentration than can be achieved by absorption from eye-drops. However, because the dose-volume is limited (usually not more than 1 mL), this route is suitable only for drugs which are readily soluble.

Drugs such as antibiotics and corticosteroids may be administered systemically to treat an eye condition.

Suitable plastic devices which gradually release a specified amount of drug over a period of, say, 1 week are also used (e.g. Ocuserts®).

11.2 Control of microbial contamination

Preparations for the eye should be sterile when issued. For routine domiciliary use they are supplied in multiple-application containers for individual use. Eye-drops contain a suitable preservative and provided that contamination is avoided they may be used for not more than 4 weeks (unless otherwise stated) after which a new container should be opened (if treatment is to be continued) and the old one discarded.

In eye surgery it is wise to use single-application containers. Preparations used during intra-ocular procedures and others that may penetrate into the anterior chamber must be isotonic and without preservatives and buffered if necessary to a neutral pH. Large volume intravenous infusion preparations are not suitable for this purpose. For all surgical procedures, a previously unopened container is used for each patient.

11.3 Anti-infective eye preparations

- 11.3.1 Antibacterials
- 11.3.2 Antifungals
- 11.3.3 Antivirals

Most acute eye infections can be treated topically. Ideally, eye-drops should be instilled very frequently (at least every 2 hours).

A useful addition for night-time use is an eye ointment because of its longer action. It will also soften crusts which cause the lids and eye lashes to adhere together when the patient is asleep. A

11.3 Anti-infective eye preparations

small quantity of eye ointment is applied to the eye or inside the lower lid.

In severe infections, *subconjunctival injection* of a suitable drug may help to achieve a high intra-ocular concentration. *Systemic* treatment is indicated in infective endophthalmitis and may also help in gonococcal conjunctivitis in the newborn. The blood-aqueous barrier usually breaks down in the latter case allowing intra-ocular penetration of systemically administered drugs.

11.3.1 Antibacterials

When prescribing antibiotics, in general, it is preferable to use topically in the eye antibiotics that are seldom or never used for systemic infections. However, the possibility of systemic absorption (section 11.1) must be taken into consideration. Examples of antibiotics with a wide spectrum of activity are **chloramphenicol, framycetin, gentamicin,** and **neomycin**. **Gentamicin** and **tobramycin** are effective for treating infections due to *Pseudomonas aeruginosa*; **norfloxacin** has a spectrum of activity similar to that of gentamicin. **Fusidic acid** is useful for staphylococcal infections.

Sulphacetamide should no longer be used topically to treat eye infections, since it is rarely of any value.

Propamidine isethionate eye-drops are of little value in bacterial infections but are specific for the rare but devastating condition of acanthamoeba keratitis.

The use of **mercuric oxide** eye ointment, even for short periods, is **not** recommended.

WITH CORTICOSTEROIDS. Many antibiotic preparations also incorporate a corticosteroid but such mixtures should **not** be used unless a patient is under close specialist supervision. In particular they should not be prescribed for undiagnosed 'red eye' which is sometimes caused by the herpes simplex virus and may be difficult to diagnose (section 11.4).

ADMINISTRATION
Eye-drops. Apply at least every 2 hours then reduce frequency as infection is controlled and continue for 48 hours after healing.
Eye ointment. Apply *either* at night (if eye-drops used during the day) *or* 3–4 times daily (if eye ointment used alone).

CHLORAMPHENICOL

Indications; Administration: see notes above
Side-effects: transient stinging; rare reports of aplastic anaemia

PoM **Chloramphenicol** (Non-proprietary)
Eye-drops, chloramphenicol 0.5%. Net price 10 mL = 67p
Eye ointment, chloramphenicol 1%. Net price 4 g = 68p

PoM **Chloromycetin**® (P-D)
Ophthalmic ointment (= eye ointment), chloramphenicol 1%. Net price 4 g = 67p

Redidrops (= eye-drops), chloramphenicol 0.5%. Net price 5 mL = £1.10; 10 mL = £1.18
Additives: include phenylmercuric acetate

PoM **Sno Phenicol**® (S&N Pharm.)
Eye-drops, chloramphenicol 0.5%, in a viscous vehicle. Net price 10 mL = £1.11
Additives: include chlorhexidine acetate

Single use
PoM **Minims**® **Chloramphenicol** (S&N Pharm.)
Eye-drops, chloramphenicol 0.5%. Net price 20 × 0.5 mL = £5.05

CHLORTETRACYCLINE

Indications: local treatment of infections, including trachoma (see notes above and under Tetracycline)
Administration: see notes above

PoM **Aureomycin**® (Lederle)
Ophthalmic ointment (= eye ointment), chlortetracycline hydrochloride 1%. Net price 3.5 g = 94p

FRAMYCETIN SULPHATE

Indications; Administration: see notes above

PoM **Soframycin**® (Roussel)
Eye-drops, framycetin sulphate 0.5%. Net price 8 mL = £2.97
Additives: include phenylmercuric nitrate
Eye ointment, framycetin sulphate 0.5%. Net price 5 g = £1.20
Ophthalmic powder, framycetin sulphate (sterile) for preparing subconjunctival injections. Net price 500-mg vial = £3.85

FUSIDIC ACID

Indications: see notes above

PoM **Fucithalmic**® (Leo)
Eye-drops, m/r, fusidic acid 1% in gel basis (liquifies on contact with eye). Net price 5 g = £2.25
Additives: include benzalkonium chloride
Apply twice daily

GENTAMICIN

Indications; Administration: see notes above

PoM **Cidomycin**® (Roussel)
Drops (for ear or eye), gentamicin 0.3% (as sulphate). Net price 8 mL = £1.34
Additives: include benzalkonium chloride, disodium edetate
Eye ointment, gentamicin 0.3% (as sulphate). Net price 3 g = £1.21

PoM **Garamycin**® (Schering-Plough)
Drops (for ear or eye), gentamicin 0.3% (as sulphate). Net price 10 mL = £1.79
Additives: include benzalkonium chloride

PoM **Genticin**® (Nicholas)
Eye-drops, gentamicin 0.3% (as sulphate). Net price 10 mL = £2.06
Additives: include benzalkonium chloride
Eye ointment, gentamicin 0.3% (as sulphate). Net price 3 g = £1.43
Additives: include hydroxybenzoates

Cautionary label wordings, see inside back cover

Single use
PoM **Minims**® **Gentamicin** (S&N Pharm.)
Eye-drops, gentamicin 0.3% (as sulphate). Net price 20 × 0.5 mL = £5.90

NEOMYCIN SULPHATE
Indications; Administration: see notes above

PoM **Neomycin** (Non-proprietary)
Eye-drops, neomycin sulphate 0.5% (3500 units/mL). Net price 10 mL = £1.52
Eye ointment, neomycin sulphate 0.5% (3500 units/g). Net price 3 g = 64p

PoM **Neosporin**® (Cusi)
Eye-drops, gramicidin 25 units, neomycin sulphate 1700 units, polymyxin B sulphate 5000 units/mL. Net price 5 mL = £5.50
Additives: include thiomersal
Apply 2–4 times daily or more frequently if required

Single use
PoM **Minims**® **Neomycin Sulphate** (S&N Pharm.)
Eye-drops, neomycin sulphate 0.5%. Net price 20 × 0.5 mL = £5.90

NORFLOXACIN
Indications; Administration: see notes above
Side-effects: local burning and smarting; rarely conjunctival hyperaemia, chemosis (conjunctival oedema) and photophobia, bitter taste

▼ PoM **Noroxin**® (MSD)
Ophthalmic solution (= eye-drops), norfloxacin 0.3%. Net price 5 mL = £1.97
Additives: include benzalkonium chloride

POLYMYXIN B SULPHATE
Indications; Administration: see notes above

PoM **Polyfax**® (Cusi)
Eye ointment, polymyxin B sulphate 10 000 units, bacitracin zinc 500 units/g. Net price 4 g = £3.50

PoM **Polytrim**® (Cusi)
Eye-drops, trimethoprim 0.1%, polymyxin B sulphate 10000 units/mL. Net price 5 mL = £3.27
Additives: include thiomersal
Eye ointment, trimethoprim 0.5%, polymyxin B sulphate 10000 units/g. Net price 4 g = £3.27

PROPAMIDINE ISETHIONATE
Indications: local treatment of infections (but see notes above)

Brolene® (Rhône-Poulenc Rorer)
Eye-drops, propamidine isethionate 0.1%. Net price 10 mL = £1.56
Apply 4 times daily
Eye ointment, dibromopropamidine isethionate 0.15%. Net price 5 g = £1.62
Apply 1–2 times daily

SULPHACETAMIDE SODIUM
Indications: not recommended, see notes above
Administration: apply eye-drops every 2–6 hours

PoM **Albucid**® (Nicholas)
Eye-drops, sulphacetamide sodium 10%, net price 10 mL = 85p
Additives: include cetrimide

Single use
PoM **Minims**® **Sulphacetamide Sodium** (S&N Pharm.)
Eye-drops, sulphacetamide sodium 10%. Net price 20 × 0.5 mL = £5.90

TETRACYCLINE HYDROCHLORIDE
Indications; Administration: see notes above

TRACHOMA. For mass antitrachoma treatment, the World Health Organization recommends **tetracycline hydrochloride** eye ointment applied to both eyes twice daily for 5 days in each month for 6 months. Chlortetracycline eye ointment may also be used but chloramphenicol is not as effective.

For active trachoma in the individual, one or both of the following are effective. (i) For adults, orally administered sulphonamides for 2 weeks or the long-acting sulphadimethoxine (no longer on UK market) 1 g initially followed by 500 mg daily for 10 days (see section 5.1.8). For children, erythromycin should be used (see section 5.1.5). (ii) Tetracycline eye ointment three times daily for 6 weeks.

PoM **Achromycin**® (Lederle)
Ointment (for ear or eye), tetracycline hydrochloride 1%. Net price 3.5 g = 70p

TOBRAMYCIN
Indications; Administration: see notes above

PoM **Tobralex**® (Alcon)
Eye-drops, tobramycin 0.3%. Net price 5 mL = £1.43
Additives: include benzalkonium chloride

11.3.2 Antifungals

Fungal infections of the cornea are rare but tend to occur after agricultural injuries, especially in hot and humid climates. Orbital mycosis is rare, and when it occurs is usually due to direct spread of infection from the paranasal sinuses. Increasing age, debility, or immunosuppression by drugs, for example, following renal transplantation, may encourage fungal proliferation in many parts of the body. The spread of infection via the bloodstream occasionally produces a metastatic endophthalmitis.

A wide range of fungi are capable of producing ocular mycosis and may be identified by appropriate laboratory procedures.

Antifungal preparations for the eye are not generally available. Treatment will normally be carried out at specialist centres, but requests for information about supplies of preparations not available commercially should be addressed to the District Pharmaceutical Officer (or equivalent in Scotland or Northern Ireland) or to Moorfields Eye Hospital, City Road, London EC1V 2PD (071-253 3411).

11.3.3 Antivirals

Herpes simplex infections producing, for example, dendritic corneal ulcer can be treated with **acyclovir**; alternatively **idoxuridine** may be used.

ACYCLOVIR
Indications: local treatment of herpes simplex infections
Administration: apply 5 times daily (continue for at least 3 days after complete healing)

PoM **Zovirax**® (Wellcome)
Eye ointment, acyclovir 3%. Net price 4.5 g = £10.67
Tablets and injection, see section 5.3

IDOXURIDINE
Indications: local treatment of herpes simplex infections
Contra-indications: pregnancy (toxicity in *animal* studies)
Administration: apply eye ointment every 4 hours Max. period of treatment 21 days

PoM **Idoxene**® (Spodefell)
Eye ointment, idoxuridine 0.5%. Net price 3 g = £1.35

11.4 Corticosteroids and other anti-inflammatory preparations

11.4.1 Corticosteroids
11.4.2 Other anti-inflammatory preparations

11.4.1 Corticosteroids

Corticosteroids administered topically, by subconjunctival injection, and systemically have an important place in treating uveitis and scleritis; they are also used to reduce post-operative inflammation following eye operations.

Topical corticosteroids should normally only be used under expert supervision; they should not be prescribed for undiagnosed 'red eye'. There are two main dangers from topical corticosteroids. First the 'red eye' may be caused by herpes simplex virus which produces a dendritic ulcer; corticosteroids aggravate the condition which may lead to loss of vision or even loss of the eye. Second, again arising from the use of eye-drop formulations, a 'steroid glaucoma' may be produced, after a few weeks treatment, in patients predisposed to chronic simple glaucoma. Use of a combination product containing a corticosteroid with an anti-infective is rarely justified.

Systemic corticosteroids can usefully be given on an alternate-day basis to minimise side-effects.

The risk of producing glaucoma is not great, but 'steroid cataract' is a very high risk (75%) if more than 15 mg of prednisolone or equivalent is given daily for several years. The longer the duration, the greater is the risk. A dose of less then 10 mg per day is usually safe.

BETAMETHASONE
Indications: local treatment of inflammation (short-term)
Cautions; Side-effects: see notes above
Administration: apply eye-drops every 1–2 hours until controlled then reduce frequency, eye ointment 2–4 times daily or at night when used with eye-drops

PoM **Betnesol**® (Evans)
Drops (for ear, eye, or nose), betamethasone sodium phosphate 0.1%. Net price 10 mL = £1.31
Additives: include benzalkonium chloride
Eye ointment, betamethasone sodium phosphate 0.1%. Net price 3 g = 56p
PoM **Betnesol-N**® (Evans)
Drops (for ear, eye, or nose), see section 12.1.1
Eye ointment, betamethasone sodium phosphate 0.1%, neomycin sulphate 0.5%. Net price 3 g = 64p
PoM **Vista-Methasone**® (Daniel)
Drops (for ear, eye, or nose), betamethasone sodium phosphate 0.1%. Net price 5 mL = 89p; 10 mL = £1.14
Additives: include benzalkonium chloride
PoM **Vista-Methasone N**® (Daniel)
Drops (for ear, eye, or nose), see section 12.1.1

CLOBETASONE BUTYRATE
Indications: local treatment of inflammation (short-term)
Cautions; Side-effects: see notes above; reduced tendency to raise intra-ocular pressure
Administration: apply eye-drops 4 times daily; severe conditions every 1–2 hours until controlled then reduce frequency

PoM **Eumovate**® (Glaxo)
Eye-drops, clobetasone butyrate 0.1%. Net price 10 mL = £3.04
Additives: include benzalkonium chloride
PoM **Eumovate-N**® (Glaxo)
Eye-drops, clobetasone butyrate 0.1%, neomycin sulphate 0.5%. Net price 10 mL = £2.70
Additives: include benzalkonium chloride

DEXAMETHASONE
Indications: local treatment of inflammation (short-term)
Cautions; Side-effects: see notes above
Administration: apply eye-drops 4–6 times daily; severe conditions every hour until controlled then reduce frequency

PoM **Maxidex**® (Alcon)
Eye-drops, dexamethasone 0.1%, hypromellose 0.5%. Net price 5 mL = £1.53; 10 mL = £3.03
Additives: include benzalkonium chloride

PoM **Maxitrol®** (Alcon)
Eye-drops, dexamethasone 0.1%, hypromellose 0.5%, neomycin 0.35% (as sulphate), polymyxin B sulphate 6000 units/mL. Net price 5 mL = £1.81
Additives: include benzalkonium chloride
Eye ointment, dexamethasone 0.1%, neomycin 0.35% (as sulphate), polymyxin B sulphate 6000 units/g. Net price 3.5 g = £1.56
Additives: include hydroxybenzoates

PoM **Sofradex®** (Roussel)
Drops and ointment (for ear or eye), see section 12.1.1

FLUOROMETHOLONE

Indications: local treatment of inflammation (short-term)

Cautions; Side-effects: see notes above; reduced tendency to raise intra-ocular pressure

Administration: apply eye-drops 2–4 times daily (initially every hour for 24–48 hours then reduce frequency)

PoM **FML®** (Allergan)
Ophthalmic suspension (= eye-drops), fluorometholone 0.1%, polyvinyl alcohol (Liquifilm®) 1.4%. Net price 5 mL = £1.78; 10 mL = £2.83
Additives: include benzalkonium chloride, disodium edetate, polysorbate 80

PoM **FML-Neo®** (Allergan)
Eye-drops, fluorometholone 0.1%, neomycin sulphate 0.5%, polyvinyl alcohol (Liquifilm®) 1.4%. Net price 5 mL = £1.90
Additives: include benzalkonium chloride, disodium edetate, polysorbate 80

HYDROCORTISONE ACETATE

Indications: local treatment of inflammation (short-term)

Cautions; Side-effects: see notes above

PoM **Hydrocortisone** (Non-proprietary)
Eye-drops, hydrocortisone acetate 1%. Net price 10 mL = £2.15
Eye ointment, hydrocortisone acetate 0.5%, net price 3 g = 85p; 1%, 3 g = £1.00; 2.5%, 3 g = £1.35

PoM **Chloromycetin Hydrocortisone®** (P-D)
Eye ointment, chloramphenicol 1%, hydrocortisone acetate 0.5%. Net price 4 g = 70p

PoM **Neo-Cortef®** (Cusi)
Drops and ointment (for ear or eye), see section 12.1.1
Note. Eye-drops containing hydrocortisone acetate 1.5% and neomycin sulphate 0.5% also available from CP

PREDNISOLONE

Indications: local treatment of inflammation (short-term)

Cautions; Side-effects: see notes above

Administration: apply eye-drops every 1–2 hours until controlled then reduce frequency

PoM **Pred Forte®** (Allergan)
Eye-drops, prednisolone acetate 1%. Net price 5 mL = £1.55; 10 mL = £3.09
Additives: include benzalkonium chloride, disodium edetate, polysorbate 80
Apply 2–4 times daily

PoM **Predsol®** (Glaxo)
Drops (for ear or eye), prednisolone sodium phosphate 0.5%. Net price 10 mL = £1.31
Additives: include benzalkonium chloride

PoM **Predsol-N®** (Glaxo)
Drops (for ear or eye), see section 12.1.1

Single use
PoM **Minims® Prednisolone** (S&N Pharm.)
Eye-drops, prednisolone sodium phosphate 0.5%. Net price 20 × 0.5 mL = £5.90

11.4.2 Other anti-inflammatory preparations

Other preparations used for the topical treatment of inflammation and allergic conjunctivitis include antihistamines, oxyphenbutazone, and sodium cromoglycate

Oxyphenbutazone eye ointment does not have the disadvantages of corticosteroids and has been used in the treatment of episcleritis.

Topical preparations of **antihistamines** such as eye-drops containing antazoline sulphate (with xylometazoline hydrochloride as Otrivine-Antistin®) may be used for short-term treatment of allergic conjunctivitis.

Sodium cromoglycate eye-drops may be useful for vernal catarrh and other allergic forms of conjunctivitis.

Lodoxamide eye-drops have been introduced for allergic conjunctival conditions including seasonal allergic conjunctivitis and vernal catarrh.

ANTAZOLINE

Indications: allergic conjunctivitis

Otrivine-Antistin® (Zyma)
Eye-drops, antazoline sulphate 0.5%, xylometazoline hydrochloride 0.05%. Net price 10 mL = £1.52
Additives: include benzalkonium chloride, disodium edetate
Apply 2–3 times daily

PoM **Vasocon A®** (Iolab)
Eye-drops, antazoline phosphate 0.5%, naphazoline hydrochloride 0.05%. Net price 10 mL = £2.41
Additives: include benzalkonium chloride, disodium edetate
Apply every 3–4 hours

LODOXAMIDE

Indications: allergic conjunctivitis
Side-effects: mild transient burning, stinging, itching, and lachrymation
Administration: ADULT and CHILD over 4 years, apply eye drops 4 times daily

▼ PoM **Alomide®** (Galen)
Ophthalmic solution (= eye-drops), lodoxamide 0.1% (as trometamol). Net price 10 mL = £4.98
Additives: include benzalkonium chloride, disodium edetate

OXYPHENBUTAZONE

Indications: local treatment of inflammation
Administration: apply eye ointment 2–5 times daily (discontinue if no improvement after 8 days)

PoM **Tanderil**® (Zyma)
Eye ointment, oxyphenbutazone 10%. Net price 5 g = 63p
Additives: include wool fat

SODIUM CROMOGLYCATE
Indications: allergic conjunctivitis
Administration: apply eye-drops 4 times daily, eye ointment 2–3 times daily

PoM **Opticrom**® (Fisons)
[1]*Aqueous eye-drops*, sodium cromoglycate 2%. Net price 13.5 mL = £6.06
Additives: include benzalkonium chloride, disodium edetate
1. Formerly called *Opticrom*® *Eye-drops*
Eye ointment, sodium cromoglycate 4%. Net price 5 g = £6.59
Additives: include wool fat

11.5 Mydriatics and cycloplegics

Antimuscarinics dilate the pupil and paralyse the ciliary muscle; they vary in potency and duration of action. The relative potencies and durations of action of the principal drugs, in ascending order, are:
tropicamide (3 hours)
cyclopentolate, hyoscine, homatropine (all up to 24 hours)
atropine (7 days or longer)

Short-acting, relatively weak mydriatics, such as **tropicamide 0.5%**, facilitate the examination of the fundus of the eye.

Cyclopentolate 1% or **atropine** are preferable for producing cycloplegia for refraction in young children. Atropine 1% (in ointment form) is sometimes preferred for children under 5 years of age. Atropine is also used for the treatment of iridocyclitis mainly to prevent posterior synechiae, often with phenylephrine 10% eye-drops (2.5% in children and those with cardiac disease).

CAUTIONS AND SIDE-EFFECTS. Contact dermatitis is not uncommon with the antimuscarinic mydriatic drugs, especially atropine. In addition, toxic systemic reactions to atropine (and hyoscine) and cyclopentolate may occur in the very young and the very old.

Darkly pigmented iris is more resistant to pupillary dilatation and caution should be exercised to avoid overdosage.

Mydriasis may precipitate acute closed-angle ('congestive') glaucoma in a few patients, usually aged over 60 years, who are predisposed to the condition because of a shallow anterior chamber.

Interactions. Phenylephrine may interact with systemically administered monoamine-oxidase inhibitors; see also Appendix 1 (sympathomimetics).

DRIVING. Patients should be warned not to drive for 1 to 2 hours after mydriasis.

Cautionary label wordings, see inside back cover

ANTIMUSCARINICS

ATROPINE SULPHATE
Indications: refraction procedures in young children; see also notes above
Cautions: action persistent, may precipitate glaucoma; see also notes above

PoM **Atropine Eye-drops**, atropine sulphate 1%. Net price 10 mL = 74p
PoM **Atropine Eye Ointment**, atropine sulphate 1%. Net price 3 g = £1.01
PoM **Isopto Atropine**® (Alcon)
Eye-drops, atropine sulphate 1%, hypromellose 0.5%. Net price 5 mL = £1.02
Additives: include benzalkonium chloride

Single use
PoM **Minims**® **Atropine Sulphate** (S&N Pharm.)
Eye-drops, atropine sulphate 1%. Net price 20 × 0.5 mL = £5.05

CYCLOPENTOLATE HYDROCHLORIDE
Indications: see notes above
Cautions: patients with raised intra-ocular pressure; see notes above

PoM **Alnide**® (Cusi)
Eye-drops, cyclopentolate hydrochloride 0.5%, net price 5 mL = £1.38; 1%, 5 mL = £1.76
Additives: include benzalkonium chloride
PoM **Mydrilate**® (Boehringer Ingelheim)
Eye-drops, cyclopentolate hydrochloride 0.5%, net price 5 mL = 73p; 1%, 5 mL = 98p
Additives: include benzalkonium chloride

Single use
PoM **Minims**® **Cyclopentolate** (S&N Pharm.)
Eye-drops, cyclopentolate hydrochloride 0.5 and 1%. Net price 20 × 0.5 mL (both) = £5.05

HOMATROPINE HYDROBROMIDE
Indications; Cautions: see notes above

PoM **Homatropine Eye-drops**, homatropine hydrobromide 1%, net price 10 mL = £1.68; 2%, 10 mL = £1.79

Single use
PoM **Minims**® **Homatropine Hydrobromide** (S&N Pharm.)
Eye-drops, homatropine hydrobromide 2%. Net price 20 × 0.5 mL = £5.90

HYOSCINE HYDROBROMIDE
Indications; Cautions: see notes above

PoM **Hyoscine Eye-drops**, usual strength hyoscine hydrobromide 0.25%. Net price 10 mL = 85p

Prices are **net**, see p. 1

TROPICAMIDE
Indications; Cautions: see notes above

PoM **Mydriacyl**® (Alcon)
Eye-drops, tropicamide 0.5%, net price 5 mL = £1.39; 1%, 5 mL = £1.72
Additives: include benzalkonium chloride

Single use
PoM **Minims**® **Tropicamide** (S&N Pharm.)
Eye-drops, tropicamide 0.5 and 1%. Net price 20 × 0.5 mL (both) = £5.90

SYMPATHOMIMETICS

ADRENALINE
Section 11.6

PHENYLEPHRINE HYDROCHLORIDE
Indications; Cautions: see notes above

Phenylephrine Eye-drops, phenylephrine hydrochloride 10%. Net price 10 mL = £1.75
See also under Hypromellose (section 11.8.1)

Single use
Minims® **Phenylephrine Hydrochloride** (S&N Pharm.)
Eye-drops, phenylephrine hydrochloride 2.5%, net price 20 × 0.5 mL = £5.90; 10%, 20 × 0.5 mL = £5.90

11.6 Treatment of glaucoma

An abnormally high intra-ocular pressure, glaucoma, may result in blindness. In virtually all cases, rise in pressure is due to reduced outflow of aqueous humour, the inflow remaining constant.

Glaucoma is treated by the application of eye-drops containing beta-blockers, miotics, or adrenaline (and guanethidine). Acetazolamide and dichlorphenamide are given by mouth and, in emergency or before surgery, mannitol may be given by intravenous infusion.

Probably the commonest condition is *chronic simple glaucoma* where the obstruction is in the trabecular meshwork. It is commonly first treated with a topical beta-blocker and other drugs added as necessary to control the intra-ocular pressure e.g. adrenaline or pilocarpine.

If supplementary topical treatment is required after *iridectomy* or a drainage operation in either open-angle or closed-angle glaucoma, a beta-blocker is preferred to pilocarpine. This is because of the risk that posterior synechiae will be formed as a result of the miotic effect of pilocarpine, especially in closed-angle glaucoma. It is then also advantageous to utilise the mydriatic side-effect of adrenaline.

MIOTICS

The small pupil is an unfortunate side-effect of these drugs (except when pilocarpine is used temporarily prior to operation for *closed-angle glaucoma*). The key factor is the opening up of the inefficient drainage channels in the trabecular meshwork resulting from contraction or spasm of the ciliary muscle. This also produces accommodation spasm that may result in blurring of vision and browache (a particular disadvantage in patients under 40 years of age).

Pilocarpine has a duration of action of 3 to 4 hours. **Physostigmine** is more potent; it is still used with pilocarpine but is not usually used alone. **Carbachol** is sometimes used to lower intra-ocular pressure, usually in conjunction with other miotics such as physostigmine.

Demecarium bromide (as *Tosmilen*®, Sinclair) and **ecothiopate iodide** (as *Phospholine Iodide*®, Cusi) are no longer on the UK market but are still available on a named-patient basis for use under expert supervision.

Generalised parasympathomimetic side effects such as sweating, bradycardia and intestinal colic may follow systemic absorption of these eye-drops; other effects may include hypersalivation and bronchospasm.

CARBACHOL
Indications: see notes above
Administration: apply eye-drops up to 4 times daily

PoM **Isopto Carbachol**® (Alcon)
Eye-drops, carbachol 3%, hypromellose 1%. Net price 10 mL = £1.80
Additives: include benzalkonium chloride

PHYSOSTIGMINE SULPHATE
(Eserine)
Indications; Side-effects: see notes above
Administration: apply eye-drops 2–6 times daily

PoM **Physostigmine** (Non-proprietary)
Eye-drops, physostigmine sulphate 0.25 and 0.5%. Net price 10 mL (both) = £1.90

PoM **Physostigmine and Pilocarpine** (Non-proprietary)
Eye-drops, physostigmine sulphate 0.25%, pilocarpine hydrochloride 2%. Net price 10 mL = £2.10
Eye-drops, physostigmine sulphate 0.25%, pilocarpine hydrochloride 4%. Net price 10 mL = £2.25
Eye-drops, physostigmine sulphate 0.5%, pilocarpine hydrochloride 4%. Net price 10 mL = £2.46

PILOCARPINE
Indications; Side-effects: see notes above
Administration: apply eye-drops 3–6 times daily

PoM **Pilocarpine** (Non-proprietary)
Eye-drops, pilocarpine hydrochloride 0.5 and 1%, net price 10 mL = £1.11; 2%, 10 mL = £1.20; 3%, 10 mL = £1.36; 4%, 10 mL = £1.51

11.6 Treatment of glaucoma

PoM **Isopto Carpine**® (Alcon)
Eye-drops, all with hypromellose 0.5%; pilocarpine hydrochloride 0.5%, net price 10 mL = 75p; 1%, 10 mL = 83p; 2%, 10 mL = 92p; 3%, 10 mL = 99p; 4%, 10 mL = £1.07
Additives: include benzalkonium chloride

PoM **Sno Pilo**® (S&N Pharm.)
Eye-drops, in a viscous vehicle, pilocarpine hydrochloride 1%, net price 10 mL = £1·07; 2%, 10 mL = £1.17; 4%, 10 mL = £1.39
Additives: include benzalkonium chloride

Single use
PoM **Minims**® **Pilocarpine Nitrate** (S&N Pharm.)
Eye-drops, pilocarpine nitrate 1, 2, and 4%. Net price 20 × 0.5 mL (all) = £5.05

Modified release
PoM **Ocusert**® (Cusi)
Pilo-20 ocular insert, m/r, pilocarpine 20 micrograms released per hour for 1 week. Net price pack of 8 inserts = £35.98. Counselling, method of use
Pilo-40 ocular insert, m/r, pilocarpine 40 micrograms released per hour for 1 week. Net price pack of 8 inserts = £41.95. Counselling, method of use

---

ADRENALINE/GUANETHIDINE

Adrenaline probably acts both by reducing the rate of production of aqueous humour and by increasing the outflow through the trabecular meshwork. It is contra-indicated in closed-angle glaucoma because it is a mydriatic, unless an iridectomy has been carried out. Side-effects include severe smarting and redness of the eye; adrenaline should be used with caution in patients with hypertension and heart disease.

Dipivefrine is a prodrug of adrenaline. It is stated to pass more rapidly through the cornea and is then converted to the active form.

Guanethidine enhances and prolongs the effects of adrenaline. It is also used alone and produces initial mydriasis with increased aqueous outflow followed by miosis with reduced aqueous secretion. Prolonged use, particularly of the higher strengths may result in conjunctival fibrosis with secondary corneal changes; the conjunctiva and cornea should be examined at least every six months.

ADRENALINE
Indications; Contra-indications: see notes above
Administration: apply eye-drops 1–2 times daily

Epifrin® (Allergan)
Eye-drops, adrenaline 1% (as hydrochloride). Net price 10 mL = £2.24
Additives: include benzalkonium chloride, disodium edetate

Eppy® (S&N Pharm.)
Eye-drops, adrenaline 1%. Net price 7.5 mL = £4.16
Additives: include phenylmercuric acetate

PoM **Simplene**® (S&N Pharm.)
Eye-drops, adrenaline, in a viscous vehicle, 0.5%, net price 7.5 mL = £3.54; 1%, 7.5 mL = £3.89
Additives: include benzalkonium chloride

DIPIVEFRINE HYDROCHLORIDE
Indications; Contra-indications: as for Adrenaline, see notes above
Administration: apply 1 drop twice daily

PoM **Propine**® (Allergan)
Eye-drops, dipivefrine hydrochloride 0.1%. Net price 5 mL = £4.29, 10 mL = £4.89
Additives: include benzalkonium chloride, disodium edetate

GUANETHIDINE MONOSULPHATE
Indications; Cautions: see notes above
Administration: apply eye-drops 1–2 times daily

PoM **Ganda**® (S&N Pharm.)
Eye-drops '1 + 0.2', guanethidine monosulphate 1%, adrenaline 0.2% in a viscous vehicle. Net price 7.5 mL = £4.60
Additives: include benzalkonium chloride
Eye-drops '3 + 0.5', guanethidine monosulphate 3%, adrenaline 0.5% in a viscous vehicle. Net price 7.5 mL = £6.01
Additives: include benzalkonium chloride

PoM **Ismelin**® (Zyma)
Eye-drops, guanethidine monosulphate 5%. Net price 5 mL = £1.87
Additives: include benzalkonium chloride

BETA-BLOCKERS

Topical application of a beta-blocker to the eye reduces intra-ocular pressure effectively in *chronic simple glaucoma*, probably by reducing the rate of production of aqueous humour. Administration by mouth also reduces intra-ocular pressure but this route is not used (see comment under Systemic Drugs).

Beta-blockers used as eye-drops include **timolol** and, more recently, **betaxolol**, **carteolol**, **levobunolol**, and **metipranolol**.

SIDE-EFFECTS. Systemic absorption may follow topical application, therefore beta-blocker eye-drops are contra-indicated in patients with asthma or a history of obstructive airways disease; the CSM has advised that both cardioselective *and* non-cardioselective beta-blocker eye-drops should be avoided. They may cause shortness of breath even in patients with no history of cardiac or respiratory problems.

Consider also other cautions, contra-indications and side-effects of beta-blockers (p. 77).

> **CSM advice.** The CSM has advised that beta-blockers, even those with apparent cardioselectivity, should not be used in patients with asthma or a history of obstructive airways disease, unless no alternative treatment is available. In such cases the risk of inducing bronchospasm should be appreciated and appropriate precautions taken.

Eye-drops containing a beta-blocker are also contra-indicated in patients with bradycardia, heart block, or heart failure.

Local side-effects of eye-drops containing a beta-blocker include transitory dry eyes and allergic blepharoconjunctivitis.

INTERACTIONS. Since systemic absorption may follow topical application the possibility of interactions, in particular, with drugs such as verapamil should be borne in mind. See also section 2.3.2 and Appendix 1 (beta-blockers).

BETAXOLOL HYDROCHLORIDE

Indications; Cautions; Contra-indications; Side-effects: see notes above
Administration: apply eye-drops twice daily

PoM **Betoptic**® (Alcon)
Eye-drops, betaxolol 0.5% (as hydrochloride). Net price 5 mL = £5.30
Additives: include benzalkonium chloride

CARTEOLOL HYDROCHLORIDE

Indications; Cautions; Contra-indications; Side-effects: see notes above
Administration: apply eye-drops twice daily

PoM **Teoptic**® (Dispersa)
Eye-drops, carteolol hydrochloride 1%, net price 5 mL = £5.05; 2%, 5 mL = £5.67
Additives: include benzalkonium chloride

LEVOBUNOLOL HYDROCHLORIDE

Indications; Cautions; Contra-indications; Side-effects: see notes above
Administration: apply eye-drops once or twice daily

PoM **Betagan**® (Allergan)
Eye-drops, levobunolol hydrochloride 0.5%, polyvinyl alcohol (Liquifilm®) 1.4%. Net price 5 mL = £5.05
Additives: include benzalkonium chloride, disodium edetate

METIPRANOLOL

Indications; Cautions; Contra-indications; Side-effects: see notes above but in chronic open angle glaucoma **restricted** to patients allergic to preservatives or to those wearing soft contact lenses (in whom benzalkonium chloride should be avoided); granulomatous anterior uveitis reported (discontinue treatment)
Administration: apply eye-drops twice daily

PoM **Minims**® **Metipranolol** (S&N Pharm.)
Eye-drops, metipranolol 0.1%, net price 20 × 0.5 mL = £10.45; 0.3%, 20 × 0.5 mL = £11.37

TIMOLOL MALEATE

Indications; Cautions; Contra-indications; Side-effects: see notes above
Administration: apply eye-drops twice daily

PoM **Timoptol**® (MSD)
Eye-drops, in Ocumeter® metered-dose unit, timolol (as maleate) 0.25%, net price 5 mL = £5.18; 0.5%, 5 mL = £5.82
Additives: include benzalkonium chloride

SYSTEMIC DRUGS

The side-effects of beta-blockers are probably sufficient to prevent their being prescribed by the ophthalmologist for administration by mouth. Hence **acetazolamide** will retain a significant place in treatment. It inhibits carbonic anhydrase, thus reducing the bicarbonate in aqueous humour and the water secreted with it, resulting in a fall in the intra-ocular pressure. **Dichlorphenamide** has a similar but more prolonged action. Both these drugs have a diuretic action and a moderate incidence of side-effects, giving rise, especially in the elderly, to paraesthesia, hypokalaemia, lack of appetite, drowsiness and depression; rashes and blood disorders occur rarely. Intravenous hypertonic **mannitol**, or **glycerol** by mouth, are useful short-term ocular hypotensive drugs. Acetazolamide by intramuscular or preferably intravenous injection is also useful in the pre-operative treatment of closed-angle glaucoma.

ACETAZOLAMIDE

Indications; Side-effects: see notes above
Cautions: avoid in severe renal impairment; pregnancy; not generally recommended for prolonged administration but if given blood counts needed; **interactions:** Appendix 1 (acetazolamide)
Dose: by mouth or by intravenous injection, 0.25–1 g daily in divided doses
By intramuscular injection, as for intravenous injection but preferably avoided because of alkaline pH

PoM **Diamox**® (Lederle)
Tablets, acetazolamide 250 mg. Net price 20 = £1.96. Label: 3
Sodium Parenteral (= injection), powder for reconstitution, acetazolamide (as sodium salt). Net price 500-mg vial = £15.14

PoM **Diamox**® **SR** (Storz)
Capsules, m/r, two-tone orange, enclosing orange f/c pellets, acetazolamide 250 mg. Net price 28-cap pack = £10.77. Label: 3, 25
Dose: 1–2 capsules daily

DICHLORPHENAMIDE

Indications; Cautions; Side-effects: see under Acetazolamide and notes above
Dose: initially 100–200 mg, then 100 mg every 12 hours, adjusted according to the patient's response

PoM **Daranide**® (MSD)
Tablets, yellow, scored, dichlorphenamide 50 mg. Net price 20 = 95p

11.7 Local anaesthetics

Oxybuprocaine and amethocaine are probably the most widely used topical local anaesthetics. Proxymetacaine causes less initial stinging and is useful for children. Cocaine produces useful vasoconstriction, but is now much less used in surgery. Oxybuprocaine or a combined preparation of lignocaine and fluorescein is used for tonometry. Lignocaine, with or without adrenaline, is injected into the eyelids for minor surgery, while a retrobulbar injection may be used for major eye surgery.

AMETHOCAINE HYDROCHLORIDE
Indications: local anaesthetic

PoM **Amethocaine Eye-drops,** amethocaine hydrochloride 0.5%, net price, 10 mL = £1.95; 1%, 10 mL = £1.46

Single use
PoM **Minims® Amethocaine Hydrochloride** (S&N Pharm.)
Eye-drops, amethocaine hydrochloride 0.5 and 1%. Net price 20 × 0.5 mL (both) = £5.90

COCAINE HYDROCHLORIDE
Indications: local anaesthetic

CD **Cocaine Eye-drops,** cocaine hydrochloride 4%. Net price 10 mL = £3.20
CD **Cocaine and Homatropine Eye-drops,** cocaine hydrochloride 2%, homatropine hydrobromide 2%.

LIGNOCAINE HYDROCHLORIDE
Indications: local anaesthetic

PoM **Minims® Lignocaine and Fluorescein** (S&N Pharm.)
Eye-drops, lignocaine hydrochloride 4%, fluorescein sodium 0.25%. Net price 20 × 0.5 mL = £7.11

OXYBUPROCAINE HYDROCHLORIDE
Indications: local anaesthetic

PoM **Minims® Benoxinate (Oxybuprocaine) Hydrochloride** (S&N Pharm.)
Eye-drops, oxybuprocaine hydrochloride 0.4%. Net price 20 × 0.5 mL = £5.05

PROXYMETACAINE HYDROCHLORIDE
Indications: local anaesthetic

PoM **Ophthaine®** (Squibb)
Eye-drops, proxymetacaine hydrochloride 0.5%. Net price 15 mL = £4.49
Additives: include benzalkonium chloride, chlorbutol

11.8 Miscellaneous ophthalmic preparations

11.8.1 Preparations for tear deficiency

Chronically sore eyes associated with reduced tear secretion, usually in cases of rheumatoid arthritis (Sjögren's syndrome), often respond to hypromellose eye-drops and mucolytic agents.

ACETYLCYSTEINE
Indications: tear deficiency, impaired mucus production
Administration: apply eye-drops 3–4 times daily

PoM **Ilube®** (Cusi)
Eye-drops, acetylcysteine 5%, hypromellose 0.35%. Net price 10 mL = £4.75
Additives: include benzalkonium chloride, disodium edetate

HYDROXYETHYLCELLULOSE
Indications: tear deficiency

Minims® Artifical Tears (S&N Pharm.)
Eye-drops, hydroxyethylcellulose 0.44%. Net price 20 × 0.5 mL = £5.90

HYPROMELLOSE
Indications: tear deficiency

Hypromellose Eye-drops, hypromellose '4000' (or '4500' or '5000') 0.3%. Net price 10 mL = 75p
BJ6® (Martindale; Thornton & Ross)
Eye-drops, hypromellose 0.25%. Net price 10 mL = 95p
Additives: include chlorhexidine (as acetate or gluconate), polysorbate 80
Isopto Alkaline® (Alcon)
Eye-drops, hypromellose 1%. Net price 10 mL = £1.02
Additives: include benzalkonium chloride
Isopto Plain® (Alcon)
Eye-drops, hypromellose 0.5%. Net price 10 mL = 87p
Additives: include benzalkonium chloride
Tears Naturale® (Alcon)
Eye-drops, dextran '70' 0.1%, hypromellose 0.3%. Net price 15 mL = £1.72
Additives: include benzalkonium chloride, disodium edetate

With phenylephrine
Isopto Frin® (Alcon)
Eye-drops, phenylephrine hydrochloride 0.12%, hypromellose 0.5%. Net price 10 mL = £1.17
Additives: include benzethonium chloride

LIQUID PARAFFIN
Indications: tear deficiency

Lacri-Lube® (Allergan)
Eye ointment, white soft paraffin, liquid paraffin. Net price 3.5 g = £1.97, 5 g = £2.49
Additives: include wool fat derivatives

POLYVINYL ALCOHOL
Indications: tear deficiency

Hypotears® (Iolab)
Eye-drops, macrogol '8000' 2%, polyvinyl alcohol 1%. Net price 10 mL = £1.85
Additives: include benzalkonium chloride, disodium edetate

Liquifilm Tears® (Allergan)
Ophthalmic solution (= eye-drops), polyvinyl alcohol 1.4%. Net price 15 mL = £1.72
Additives: include benzalkonium chloride, disodium edetate
Preservative-free ophthalmic solution (= eye-drops), polyvinyl alcohol 1.4%, povidone 0.6%. Net price 30 × 0.4 mL = £5.60

Sno Tears® (S&N Pharm.)
Eye-drops, polyvinyl alcohol 1.4%. Net price 10 mL = £1.13
Additives: include benzalkonium chloride, disodium edetate

11.8.2 Other preparations

Zinc sulphate is a traditional astringent which has been used in eye-drops for treatment of excessive lachrymation.

Simple eye ointment is a bland sterile preparation which may be used to soften crusts in blepharitis or as a bland lubricant at night.

Fluorescein sodium and **rose bengal** are used in diagnostic procedures and for locating damaged areas of the cornea due to injury or disease. Rose bengal is much more efficient for the diagnosis of conjunctival epithelial damage.

Certain eye-drops, e.g. benzylpenicillin, colistin, desferrioxamine, and trisodium edetate (see also section 9.5.1.2), may be prepared aseptically from material supplied for injection.

ACETYLCHOLINE CHLORIDE
Indications: cataract surgery, penetrating keratoplasty, iridectomy, and other anterior segment surgery requiring rapid miosis

PoM Miochol® (Iolab)
Solution for intra-ocular irrigation, acetylcholine chloride 1%, mannitol 3% when reconstituted. Net price 2 mL-vial = £7.78

CHYMOTRYPSIN
Indications: zonulolysis in intracapsular cataract extraction

PoM Zonulysin® (Henleys)
Injection, powder for reconstitution, alphachymotrypsin 300 USP units (≡ 1.5 microkatals). Net price per vial (with diluent) = £6.08

FLURBIPROFEN SODIUM
Indications: inhibition of intraoperative miosis (but does not possess intrinsic mydriatic properties)

▼ **PoM Ocufen**® (Allergan)
Ophthalmic solution (= eye-drops), flurbiprofen sodium 0.03%, polyvinyl alcohol (Liquifilm®) 1.4%. Net price 10 × 0.4 mL = £45.60

PARAFFIN, YELLOW, SOFT
Indications: see notes above

Simple Eye Ointment, liquid paraffin 10%, wool fat 10%, in yellow soft paraffin. Net price 3 g = £1.55

SODIUM CHLORIDE
Indications: irrigation, including first-aid removal of harmful substances

Balanced Salt Solution
Solution (sterile), sodium chloride 0.64%, sodium acetate 0.39%, sodium citrate 0.17%, calcium chloride 0.048%, magnesium chloride 0.03%, potassium chloride 0.075%.
Available from Alcon (15 mL and 30 mL) and from Iolab (15 mL)

Normasol® (Seton Prebbles)
Solution (sterile), sodium chloride 0.9%. Net price 25 mL sachet = 16p

Single use
Minims® **Sodium Chloride** (S&N Pharm.)
Eye-drops, sodium chloride 0.9%. Net price 20 × 0.5 mL = £5.05

SODIUM HYALURONATE
(a visco-elastic polymer normally present in the aqueous and vitreous humour)
Indications: used during surgical procedures on the eye
Side-effects: occasional hypersensitivity (avian origin); occasional transient rise in intra-ocular pressure

PoM Healonid® (Kabi Pharmacia)
Injection, sodium hyaluronate 10 mg/mL in disposable syringes, net price 0.5 mL = £41.10, 0.75 mL = £61.62

ZINC SULPHATE
Indications; Cautions: see notes above

Zinc Sulphate Eye-drops, zinc sulphate 0.25%. Net price 10 mL = £1.64

DIAGNOSTIC PREPARATIONS

FLUORESCEIN SODIUM
Indications: detection of lesions and foreign bodies

Minims® **Fluorescein Sodium** (S&N Pharm.)
Eye-drops, fluorescein sodium 1 or 2%. Net price 20 × 0.5 mL (both) = £5.05

ROSE BENGAL
Indications: detection of lesions and foreign bodies

Minims® **Rose Bengal** (S&N Pharm.)
Eye-drops, rose bengal 1%. Net price 20 × 0.5 mL = £5.90

11.9 Contact lenses

Many patients wear these lenses and special care is required in prescribing eye preparations for them. Unless medically indicated the lenses should not be worn during treatment. If the patient is wearing hard lenses the use of eye-drops containing anti-inflammatory drugs over long periods of time is to be deprecated. Some drugs can spoil hydrophilic soft lenses. Therefore unless eye-drops are specifically indicated as safe to use with hydrophilic contact lenses, the lenses should be removed before instillation and not worn during the period of treatment.

12: Drugs used in the treatment of diseases of the
EAR, NOSE, and OROPHARYNX

In this chapter, drug treatment is discussed under the following headings:
  12.1 Drugs acting on the ear
  12.2 Drugs acting on the nose
  12.3 Drugs acting on the oropharynx

12.1 Drugs acting on the ear
  12.1.1 Otitis externa
  12.1.2 Otitis media
  12.1.3 Removal of ear wax

For treatment of labyrinthine disorders see section 4.6.

12.1.1 Otitis externa

Otitis externa is an inflammatory reaction of the meatal skin. It is important to exclude an underlying chronic otitis media before treatment is commenced. Many cases recover after thorough cleansing of the external ear canal by suction, dry mopping, or gentle syringing. A frequent problem in resistant cases is the difficulty in applying lotions and ointments satisfactorily to the relatively inaccessible affected skin. The most effective method is to introduce a ribbon gauze dressing soaked with **corticosteroid** ear drops or with an astringent such as **aluminium acetate** solution. When this is not practical, the ear should be gently cleaned with a probe covered in cotton wool and the patient encouraged to lie with the affected ear uppermost for ten minutes after the canal has been filled with a liberal quantity of the appropriate solution.

If infection is present, a topical anti-infective which is not used systemically (such as **neomycin** or **clioquinol**) may be used, but for only about a week as excessive use may result in fungal infections; these may be difficult to treat and require expert advice. Sensitivity to the anti-infective or solvent may occur and resistance to antibacterials is a possibility with prolonged use. **Chloramphenicol** may also be used but the ear drops contain propylene glycol and cause sensitivity in about 10% of patients (the eye ointment can be used instead). Solutions containing an anti-infective and a corticosteroid (such as Locorten-Vioform®) are used for treating cases where infection is present with inflammation and eczema. The CSM has warned that when otitis externa is treated topically with preparations containing chlorhexidine, aminoglycosides (e.g. neomycin, framycetin), or polymyxins in patients who have a perforation of the tympanic membrane, there is an increased risk of drug-induced deafness. It is therefore important to ensure that there is no perforation in such patients before prescription of these preparations. In the presence of a perforation many specialists, however, do use these drops cautiously in patients with *otitis media*, see section 12.1.2.

An acute infection may cause severe pain and a systemic antibiotic is required with a simple analgesic such as paracetamol. When a resistant staphylococcal infection (a boil) is present in the external auditory meatus, **flucloxacillin** is the drug of choice (see section 5.1, Table 1).

The skin of the pinna adjacent to the ear canal is often affected by eczema, and topical corticosteroid creams and ointments (see section 13.4) are then required and should be applied five or six times daily. Prolonged use should be avoided.

Ear drops or **ointment** should be applied using 3–4 drops of a liquid preparation or a similar quantity of ointment, warmed if necessary, inserted into the affected ear. If discharge is profuse, ear drops applied directly may be washed away; in these circumstances the ear canal should be carefully cleaned and a 1 cm gauze wick impregnated with the ear drops should be introduced into it.

ASTRINGENT PREPARATIONS

ALUMINIUM ACETATE
Indications: inflammation in otitis externa

Aluminium Acetate Ear drops (13%) consists of aluminium acetate solution, BP.
Insert into the meatus or apply on a gauze wick which should be kept saturated with the ear-drops
Available from Martindale and Penn (special order)

Aluminium Acetate Ear drops (8%), prepared by diluting 8 parts of aluminium acetate solution, BP, with 5 parts of purified water, freshly boiled and cooled. It must be freshly prepared.
Directions as above

ANTI-INFLAMMATORY PREPARATIONS

BETAMETHASONE SODIUM PHOSPHATE
Indications: eczematous inflammation in otitis externa
Cautions: avoid prolonged use
Contra-indications: untreated infection

PoM **Betnesol**® (Evans)
Drops (for ear, eye, or nose), betamethasone sodium phosphate 0.1%. Net price 10 mL = £1.31
Additives: include benzalkonium chloride

Apply every 2–3 hours; reduce frequency of application when relief is obtained

12.1 Drugs acting on the ear

PoM Vista-Methasone® (Daniels)
Drops (for ear, eye, or nose), betamethasone sodium phosphate 0.1%. Net price 5 mL = 89p; 10 mL = £1.14
Additives: include benzalkonium chloride
Apply every 3–4 hours; reduce frequency of application when relief is obtained

PREDNISOLONE SODIUM PHOSPHATE
Indications: eczematous inflammation in otitis externa
Cautions: avoid prolonged use
Contra-indications: untreated infection

PoM Predsol® (Evans)
Drops (for ear or eye), prednisolone sodium phosphate 0.5%. Net price 10 mL = £1.31
Additives: include benzalkonium chloride
Apply every 2–3 hours; reduce frequency of application when relief is obtained

---

ANTI-INFECTIVE PREPARATIONS

CHLORAMPHENICOL
Indications: bacterial infection in otitis externa
Cautions: avoid prolonged use (see notes above)
Side-effects: high incidence of sensitivity reactions to vehicle
Administration: apply 2–3 times daily

PoM Chloramphenicol Ear drops 5% and **10%**, chloramphenicol in propylene glycol. Net price 10 mL (5%) = 95p; 10 mL (10%) = £1.00

CLIOQUINOL
Indications: mild bacterial or fungal infections in otitis externa
Cautions: avoid prolonged use (see notes above)
Side-effects: local sensitivity; stains skin and clothing

PoM Locorten-Vioform® (Zyma)
Ear drops, clioquinol 1%, flumethasone pivalate 0.02%. Net price 7.5 mL = £1.05
Apply 2–3 drops twice daily

CLOTRIMAZOLE
Indications: fungal infection in otitis externa
Side-effects: occasional skin irritation or sensitivity

Canesten® (Baypharm)
Solution, clotrimazole 1% in polyethylene glycol. Net price 20 mL = £2.38
Apply 2–3 times daily continuing for at least 14 days after disappearance of infection

FRAMYCETIN SULPHATE
Indications; Cautions; Side-effects: see under Gentamicin

Preparations
Ingredient of compound anti-infective ear preparations (see next page)

GENTAMICIN
Indications: bacterial infection in otitis externa
Cautions: avoid prolonged use; slight risk of ototoxicity increased if perforated eardrum (see notes above)
Side-effects: local sensitivity
Administration: apply 3–4 times daily and at night

PoM Cidomycin® (Roussel)
Drops (for ear or eye), gentamicin 0.3% (as sulphate). Net price 8 mL = £1.34
Additives: include benzalkonium chloride, disodium edetate

PoM Garamycin® (Schering-Plough)
Drops (for ear or eye), gentamicin 0.3% (as sulphate). Net price 10 mL = £1.79
Additives: include benzalkonium chloride

PoM Genticin® (Nicholas)
Drops (for ear or eye), gentamicin 0.3% (as sulphate). Net price 10 mL = £2.06
Additives: include benzalkonium chloride

PoM Gentisone HC® (Nicholas)
Ear drops, gentamicin 0.3% (as sulphate), hydrocortisone acetate 1%. Net price 10 mL = £4.27

NEOMYCIN SULPHATE
Indications: bacterial infection in otitis externa
Cautions: avoid prolonged use; slight risk of ototoxicity increased if perforated eardrum (see notes above)
Side-effects: local sensitivity
Administration: apply ear drops every 2–3 hours; ear ointment 2–4 times daily. Reduce frequency of application when relief is obtained

PoM Audicort® (Lederle)
Ear drops, neomycin (as neomycin undecenoate) 0.35%, triamcinolone acetonide 0.1%. Net price 10 mL = £7.50
Apply 3–4 times daily

PoM Betnesol-N® (Evans)
Drops (for ear, eye, or nose), betamethasone sodium phosphate 0.1%, neomycin sulphate 0.5%. Net price 10 mL = £1.35
Additives: include thiomersal

PoM Neo-Cortef® (Cusi)
Drops (for ear or eye), hydrocortisone acetate 1.5%, neomycin sulphate 0.5%. Net price 5 mL = £3.98
Ointment (for ear or eye), hydrocortisone acetate 1.5%, neomycin sulphate 0.5%. Net price 3.9 g = £2.98

PoM Otomize® (Stafford-Miller)
Ear spray, dexamethasone 0.1%, neomycin sulphate 3250 units/mL. Net price 5-mL pump-action aerosol unit = £3.95
Apply 1 metered spray 3 times daily

PoM Predsol-N® (Evans)
Drops (for ear or eye), neomycin sulphate 0.5%, prednisolone sodium phosphate 0.5%. Net price 10 mL = £1.20
Additives: include thiomersal

PoM Vista-Methasone N® (Daniels)
Drops (for ear, eye, or nose), betamethasone sodium phosphate 0.1%, neomycin sulphate 0.5%. Net price 5 mL = 96p; 10 mL = £1.20

Cautionary label wordings, see inside back cover   Prices are **net**, see p. 1

TETRACYCLINE HYDROCHLORIDE
Indications: susceptible bacterial infection in otitis externa
Cautions: avoid prolonged use
Side-effects: local sensitivity; stains skin and clothing
Administration: apply every 2 hours

PoM **Achromycin**® (Lederle)
Ointment (for ear or eye), tetracycline hydrochloride 1%. Net price 3.5 g = 70p

COMPOUND ANTI-INFECTIVE PREPARATIONS

PoM **Otosporin**® (Wellcome)
Ear drops, hydrocortisone 1%, neomycin sulphate 0.439%, polymyxin B sulphate 0.119%. Net price 5 mL = £4.58; 10 mL = £7.83
Apply 3–4 times daily

PoM **Sofradex**® (Roussel)
Drops (for ear or eye), dexamethasone (as sodium metasulphobenzoate) 0.05%, framycetin sulphate 0.5%, gramicidin 0.005%. Net price 10 mL = £5.50
Apply 3–4 times daily
Ointment (for ear or eye), dexamethasone 0.05%, framycetin sulphate 0.5%, gramicidin 0.005%. Net price 5 g = £3.64
Apply 2–3 times daily and at bedtime

PoM **Soframycin**® (Roussel)
Cream, framycetin sulphate 1.5%, gramicidin 0.005% in a water-miscible basis. Net price 15 g = £1.72
Ointment, ingredients as for cream, but in a greasy basis. Net price 15 g = £1.72
Apply 1–3 times daily

PoM **Terra-Cortril**® (Pfizer)
Ear suspension (= ear drops), hydrocortisone acetate 1.5%, oxytetracycline 0.5% (as hydrochloride), polymyxin B sulphate 0.119%. Net price 5 mL = £2.06
Apply 3 times daily

PoM **Tri-Adcortyl Otic**® (Squibb)
Ear ointment, gramicidin 0.025%, neomycin 0.25% (as sulphate), nystatin 3.33%, triamcinolone acetonide 0.1% in Plastibase®. Net price 10 g = £1.58
Apply 2–4 times daily

OTHER AURAL PREPARATIONS

Choline salicylate is a mild analgesic but it is of doubtful value when applied topically. There is no place for the use of local anaesthetics in ear drops.

Audax® (Napp)
Ear drops, choline salicylate 20%, glycerol 10%. Net price 8 mL = £1.45

12.1.2 Otitis media

Acute otitis media is the commonest cause of severe pain in small children and recurrent attacks, especially in infants, are particularly distressing. *Sero-mucinous otitis media* ('glue ear') is present in about 10% of the child population and in 90% of children with cleft palates; this condition should be referred to hospital because of the risk of permanent damage to middle ear function and impaired language development. Chronic otitis media is thought to be a legacy from untreated or resistant cases of sero-mucinous otitis media.

Local treatment of *acute otitis media* is ineffective and there is no place for drops containing a local anaesthetic. Many attacks are viral in origin and need only treatment with a **simple analgesic** such as paracetamol for pain. Severe attacks of bacterial origin should be treated with **systemic antibiotics**; bacterial examination of any discharge is helpful in selecting the appropriate treatment (see section 5.1, Table 1). Again, simple analgesics such as paracetamol are used to relieve pain. In *recurrent acute otitis media* a daily dose of a prophylactic antibiotic (trimethoprim or erythromycin) during the winter months can be tried.

The organisms recovered from patients with *chronic otitis media* are often opportunists living in the debris, keratin, and necrotic bone present in the middle ear and mastoid. Thorough cleansing with an aural suction tube may completely control infection of many years duration. Acute exacerbations of chronic infection may require systemic antibiotics (see section 5.1, Table 1). A swab should be taken to determine the organism present and its antibiotic sensitivity. Unfortunately the culture often produces *Pseudomonas aeruginosa* and *Proteus* spp. sensitive only to parenteral antibiotics. Local debridement of the meatal and middle ear contents may then be followed by topical treatment with ribbon gauze dressings as for otitis externa (section 12.1.1). This is particularly true with infections in mastoid cavities when dusting powders can also be tried.

In the presence of a perforation, however, many specialists use ear drops containing **aminoglycosides** (e.g. neomycin) or **polymyxins**, if the otitis media has failed to settle with systemic antibiotics; it is considered that the pus in the middle ear associated with otitis media carries a higher risk of ototoxicity than the drops themselves.

12.1.3 Removal of ear wax

Wax is a normal bodily secretion which provides a protective film on the meatal skin and need only be removed if it causes deafness or interferes with a proper view of the eardrum. As a general rule syringing is best avoided in patients with a history of recurring otitis externa, a perforated ear drum, or previous ear surgery. A person who has hearing only in one ear should not have that ear syringed because even a very slight risk of damage is unacceptable in this situation.

Wax may be removed by syringing with warm water. If necessary, wax can be softened before syringing with simple remedies such as **olive oil** or **almond oil**. The patient should lie with the affected ear uppermost for 5 to 10 minutes after a generous amount of the solution has been introduced into the ear. Some proprietary preparations containing organic solvents can cause irritation of the meatal skin, and in most cases the simple remedies which are indicated above are just as effective and less likely to cause irritation. **Docu-**

sate sodium is an ingredient in a number of proprietary preparations.

Almond Oil (warm before use)
Olive Oil (warm before use)
Sodium Bicarbonate Ear Drops, BP
Ear drops, sodium bicarbonate 5%. Extemporaneous preparations should be recently prepared according to the following formula: sodium bicarbonate 500 mg, glycerol 3 mL, freshly boiled and cooled purified water to 10 mL

Audinorm® (Carlton)
Ear drops, docusate sodium 5%, glycerol 10%. Net price 12 mL = 30p

Cerumol® (LAB)
Ear drops, chlorbutol 5%, paradichlorobenzene 2%, arachis oil 57%. Net price 11 mL = £1.07

Dioctyl® (Medo)
Ear drops, docusate sodium 5% in macrogol. Net price 10 mL = £1.12

Exterol® (Dermal)
Ear drops, urea-hydrogen peroxide complex 5% in glycerol. Net price 12 mL = £2.75

Molcer® (Wallace Mfg)
Ear drops, docusate sodium 5%. Net price 15 mL = £1.02

Waxsol® (Norgine)
Ear drops, docusate sodium 0.5%. Net price 10 mL = 98p

12.2 Drugs acting on the nose

12.2.1 Drugs used in nasal allergy
12.2.2 Topical nasal decongestants
12.2.3 Anti-infective nasal preparations

Rhinitis is often self-limiting and sinusitis best treated with antibiotics (see section 5.1, Table 1). There are few indications for the use of sprays and drops except in allergic rhinitis where topical preparations of corticosteroids or sodium cromoglycate have much to offer. Most other preparations contain sympathomimetic drugs which may damage the nasal cilia and their prolonged use causes mucosal oedema and severe nasal obstruction (rhinitis medicamentosa). Symptomatic relief in chronic nasal obstruction may be obtained with **systemic nasal decongestants** (see section 3.10). Douching the nose with salt and water is **not** recommended.

12.2.1 Drugs used in nasal allergy

Mild cases are controlled by **oral antihistamines** and **systemic nasal decongestants** (see sections 3.4.1 and 3.10). Many patients with severe symptoms can now expect relief from topical preparations of **corticosteroids** or **sodium cromoglycate**. Although sodium cromoglycate is less effective than a topical corticosteroid, it is often the first choice in children. Treatment should begin 2 to 3 weeks before the hay fever season commences and may have to be continued for months or even years in some patients. No significant side-effects have been reported. Very disabling symptoms occasionally justify the use of **systemic corticosteroids** for short periods (see section 6.3), for example in students taking important examinations. They may also be used at the beginning of a course of treatment with a corticosteroid spray to relieve severe mucosal oedema and allow the spray to penetrate the nasal cavity.

Azelastine is an antihistamine available as a nasal spray for allergic rhinitis.

For reference to injections of **allergen extracts** see section 3.4.2.

AZELASTINE HYDROCHLORIDE

Indications: allergic rhinitis
Side-effects: irritation of nasal mucosa; taste disturbance
Administration: apply 140 micrograms (1 spray) into each nostril twice daily; CHILD not yet recommended

▼ PoM **Rhinolast**® (ASTA Medica)
Nasal spray, azelastine hydrochloride 140 micrograms (0.14 mL)/metered spray. Net price 10 mL (with metered pump) = £6.40

BECLOMETHASONE DIPROPIONATE

Indications: allergic and vasomotor rhinitis
Cautions: untreated nasal infection, prolonged use in children, previous treatment with corticosteroids by mouth
Side-effects: sneezing after administration; rarely dryness and irritation of nose and throat, epistaxis
Administration: adults and children over 6 years, apply 100 micrograms (2 sprays) into each nostril twice daily *or* 50 micrograms (1 spray) 3–4 times daily; max. 8 sprays daily

PoM **Beconase**® (A&H)
Beconase® *nasal spray (aerosol)*, beclomethasone dipropionate 50 micrograms/metered inhalation. Net price 200-spray unit with applicator = £5.01
Beconase® *aqueous nasal spray (aqueous suspension)*, beclomethasone dipropionate 50 micrograms/metered spray. Net price 200-spray unit with applicator = £5.01

BETAMETHASONE SODIUM PHOSPHATE

Indications; Cautions; Side-effects: see under Beclomethasone Dipropionate
Administration: apply 2–3 drops into each nostril 2–3 times daily

PoM **Betnesol**® (Evans)
Drops (for ear, eye, or nose), section 12.1.1
PoM **Vista-Methasone**® (Daniels)
Drops (for ear, eye, or nose), section 12.1.1

BUDESONIDE
Indications: allergic and vasomotor rhinitis
Cautions: see under Beclomethasone Dipropionate; also patients with pulmonary tuberculosis
Side-effects: see under Beclomethasone Dipropionate

PoM **Rhinocort**® (Astra)
Rhinocort® *nasal aerosol*, budesonide 50 micrograms/metered inhalation, 200-spray unit with nasal adaptor. Net price complete unit = £5.66
Administration: apply 100 micrograms (2 sprays) into each nostril twice daily, reducing to 50 micrograms (1 spray) twice daily
Rhinocort Aqua® *nasal spray*, budesonide 100 micrograms/metered spray. Net price 100-spray unit = £6.00
Administration: adults and children over 12 years, apply 200 micrograms (2 sprays) into each nostril once daily in the morning *or* 100 micrograms (1 spray) into each nostril twice daily, reduced for maintenance

FLUNISOLIDE
Indications; Cautions; Side-effects: see under Beclomethasone Dipropionate
Administration: apply 50 micrograms (2 sprays) into each nostril 2–3 times daily; CHILD over 5 years 25 micrograms (1 spray) into each nostril 3 times daily, reduced for maintenance

PoM **Syntaris**® (Syntex)
Nasal spray, flunisolide 25 micrograms/0.1 mL metered spray. Net price 240-spray unit with pump and applicator = £5.64

FLUTICASONE PROPIONATE
Indications: allergic rhinitis
Cautions; Side-effects: see under Beclomethasone Dipropionate
Administration: adults and children over 12 years, 100 micrograms (2 sprays) into each nostril daily, preferably in the morning, increased to twice daily if required; max. 8 sprays daily

▼ PoM **Flixonase**® (A&H)
Aqueous nasal spray, fluticasone propionate 50 micrograms/metered spray. Net price 120-spray unit with applicator = £11.43

SODIUM CROMOGLYCATE
Indications: prophylaxis of allergic rhinitis (see notes above)
Side-effects: local irritation, particularly during initial treatment with insufflations; rarely transient bronchospasm

Rynacrom® (Fisons)
Nasal insufflation, cartridges, pink, sodium cromoglycate 10 mg for use with insufflator. Net price 20 cartridges = 86p; insufflator = £1.66
Adults and children, insufflate 10 mg into each nostril up to 4 times daily

Nasal drops, sodium cromoglycate 2%. Net price 15 mL = £4.53
Adults and children, instil 2 drops into each nostril 6 times daily
4% nasal spray, sodium cromoglycate 4% (5.2 mg/squeeze). Net price 22 mL with pump = £7.55
Adults and children, apply 1 squeeze into each nostril 2–4 times daily

Rynacrom Compound® (Fisons)
Nasal spray, sodium cromoglycate 2% (2.6 mg/metered spray) and xylometazoline hydrochloride 0.025% (32.5 micrograms/metered spray). Net price 26 mL with pump = £5.94
Apply 1 spray into each nostril 4 times daily
Note. A proprietary brand of sodium cromoglycate 2% and xylometazoline hydrochloride 0.025% (Resiston One®) is on sale to the public

12.2.2 Topical nasal decongestants

The nasal mucosa is sensitive to changes in the atmospheric temperature and humidity and these alone may cause slight nasal congestion. The nose and nasal sinuses produce a litre of mucus in 24 hours and much of this finds its way silently into the stomach via the nasopharynx. Slight changes in the nasal airway, accompanied by an awareness of mucus passing along the nasopharynx causes some patients to be inaccurately diagnosed as suffering from chronic sinusitis. These symptoms are particularly noticeable in the later stages of the common cold for which there is no effective treatment at the moment; the temptation to use nasal drops should be resisted. **Sodium chloride** 0.9% given as nasal drops may relieve nasal congestion by helping to liquefy mucous secretions.

Symptomatic relief from the nasal congestion associated with vasomotor rhinitis, nasal polypi, and the common cold can be obtained by the short-term use of decongestant nasal drops and sprays. These all contain sympathomimetic drugs which exert their effect by vasoconstriction of the mucosal blood vessels which in turn reduces the thickness of the nasal mucosa. They are of limited value as they can give rise to a rebound phenomenon as their effects wear off, due to a secondary vasodilatation with a subsequent temporary increase in nasal congestion. This in turn tempts the further use of the decongestant, leading to a vicious circle of events. **Ephedrine nasal drops** is the safest sympathomimetic preparation and can give relief for several hours. The more potent sympathomimetic drugs oxymetazoline, phenylephrine, and xylometazoline are more likely to cause a rebound effect. **All** of these preparations may cause a hypertensive crisis if used during treatment with a monoamine-oxidase inhibitor.

Non-allergic watery rhinorrhoea often responds well to treatment with **ipratropium bromide**.

Inhalations of **warm moist air** are useful in the treatment of symptoms of acute infective

12.2 Drugs acting on the nose

conditions, and the use of compounds containing volatile substances such as menthol and eucalyptus may encourage their use (see section 3.8). There is no evidence that nasal preparations containing antihistamines and anti-infective agents have any therapeutic effect.

Systemic nasal decongestants—see section 3.10.

SYMPATHOMIMETICS

EPHEDRINE HYDROCHLORIDE
Indications: nasal congestion
Cautions: avoid excessive use; caution in infants under 3 months (no good evidence of value—if irritation occurs might narrow nasal passage); **interactions:** Appendix 1 (sympathomimetics)
Side-effects: local irritation; after excessive use tolerance with diminished effect, rebound congestion
Administration: see below

Ephedrine Nasal Drops, BP
Nasal drops, ephedrine hydrochloride in a suitable aqueous vehicle
Note. The BP directs that if no strength is specified 0.5% drops should be supplied; net price 10 mL = 80p
Instil 1–2 drops into each nostril up to 3 or 4 times daily when required

OXYMETAZOLINE HYDROCHLORIDE
Indications: nasal congestion
Cautions; Side-effects: see under Ephedrine Hydrochloride; avoid in porphyria (see section 9.8.2)

NHS **Afrazine**® (Schering-Plough)
Nasal spray, oxymetazoline hydrochloride 0.05%. Net price 15 mL = 98p
Adults and children over 5 years, apply 2–3 times to each nostril every 12 hours when required

PHENYLEPHRINE HYDROCHLORIDE
Indications: nasal congestion
Cautions; Side-effects: see under Ephedrine Hydrochloride

Compound preparations
Section 12.2.3

XYLOMETAZOLINE HYDROCHLORIDE
Indications: nasal congestion
Cautions; Side-effects: see under Ephedrine Hydrochloride

Xylometazoline Nasal Drops, xylometazoline hydrochloride 0.1%, net price 10 mL = 97p
Instil 2–3 drops into each nostril 2–3 times daily when required; not recommended for children under 12 years

Xylometazoline Nasal Drops, Paediatric
xylometazoline hydrochloride 0.05%, net price 10 mL = 97p
CHILD over 3 months instil 1–2 drops into each nostril 1–2 times daily when required (not recommended for infants under 3 months of age)
Note. The brand name NHS Otrivine® (Zyma) is used for xylometazoline adult nasal drops 0.1%, children's nasal drops 0.05%, and adult nasal spray 0.1%.

ANTIMUSCARINIC

IPRATROPIUM BROMIDE
Indications: watery rhinorrhoea associated with perennial rhinitis
Cautions; Side-effects: see section 3.1.2; avoid spraying near eyes
Administration: apply 20–40 micrograms (1–2 puffs) into affected nostril up to 4 times daily; not recommended for children under 12 years

PoM **Rinatec**® (Boehringer Ingelheim)
Nasal spray, ipratropium bromide 20 micrograms/metered spray. Net price 200-dose unit = £4.21

12.2.3 Anti-infective nasal preparations

There is **no** evidence that topical anti-infective nasal preparations have any therapeutic value; for elimination of nasal staphylococci, see below.

Systemic treatment of sinusitis—see section 5.1, Table 1.

PoM **Betnesol-N**® (Evans)
Drops (for ear, eye, or nose), section 12.1.1
PoM **Dexa-Rhinaspray**® (Boehringer Ingelheim)
Nasal inhalation, dexamethasone 21-isonicotinate 20 micrograms, neomycin sulphate 100 micrograms, tramazoline hydrochloride 120 micrograms/metered inhalation. Net price 125-dose unit = £1.79
PoM **Locabiotal**® (Servier)
Nasal inhalation, fusafungine 125 micrograms/metered inhalation. Net price 200-dose unit = £1.59
PoM **Vibrocil**® (Zyma)
Nasal drops, dimethindene maleate 0.025%, neomycin sulphate 0.35%, phenylephrine 0.25%. Net price 15 mL = 52p
Nasal gel, dimethindene maleate 0.025%, neomycin sulphate 0.35%, phenylephrine 0.25%. Net price 12 g = 52p
Nasal spray, dimethindene maleate 0.025%, neomycin sulphate 0.35%, phenylephrine 0.25%. Net price 10 mL = 52p
PoM **Vista-Methasone N**® (Daniels)
Drops (for ear, eye, or nose), section 12.1.1

NASAL STAPHYLOCOCCI

Elimination of organisms such as staphylococci from the nasal vestibule can be achieved by the use of a cream containing **chlorhexidine and neomycin** (Naseptin®), but re-colonisation frequently occurs. Coagulase-positive staphylococci can be obtained from the noses of 40% of the population.

Cautionary label wordings, see inside back cover   Prices are **net**, see p. 1

A nasal ointment containing **mupirocin** is also available; it should probably be kept in reserve for resistant cases.

PoM **Bactroban**® **Nasal** (Beecham)
Nasal ointment, mupirocin 2% in white soft paraffin basis. Net price 3 g = £5.15
For eradication of nasal carriage of staphylococci, including methicillin-resistant *Staphylococcus aureus* (MRSA), apply 2–3 times daily to the inner surface of each nostril

PoM **Naseptin**® (ICI)
Cream, chlorhexidine hydrochloride 0.1%, neomycin sulphate 0.5%. Do not dilute. Net price 15 g = £1.02
For eradication of nasal carriage of staphylococci, apply to nostrils 4 times daily for 10 days; for preventing nasal carriage of staphylococci apply to nostrils twice daily

12.3 Drugs acting on the oropharynx

12.3.1 Drugs for oral ulceration and inflammation
12.3.2 Oropharyngeal anti-infective drugs
12.3.3 Lozenges, sprays, and gels
12.3.4 Mouthwashes, gargles, and dentifrices

12.3.1 Drugs for oral ulceration and inflammation

Ulceration of the oral mucosa may be caused by trauma (physical or chemical), recurrent aphthae, infections, carcinoma, dermatological disorders, nutritional deficiencies, gastro-intestinal disease, haematopoietic disorders, and drug therapy. It is important to establish the diagnosis in each case as the majority of these lesions require specific management in addition to local treatment. Local treatment aims at protecting the ulcerated area, or at relieving pain or reducing inflammation.

SIMPLE MOUTHWASHES. A **saline** or **compound thymol glycerin** mouthwash may relieve the pain of traumatic ulceration. The mouthwash is made up with warm water and used at frequent intervals until the discomfort and swelling subsides.

ANTISEPTIC MOUTHWASHES. Secondary bacterial infection may be a feature of any mucosal ulceration; it can increase discomfort and delay healing. Use of a **chlorhexidine** or **povidone-iodine** mouthwash is often beneficial and may accelerate healing of recurrent aphthae.

MECHANICAL PROTECTION. **Carmellose gelatin paste** may relieve some discomfort arising from ulceration by protecting the ulcer site. The paste adheres to the mucosa, but is difficult to apply effectively to some parts of the mouth.

CORTICOSTEROIDS. Topical corticosteroid therapy may be used for different forms of oral ulceration. In the case of aphthous ulcers it is most effective if applied in the 'prodromal' phase.

Thrush or other types of candidiasis are recognised complications of corticosteroid treatment.

Hydrocortisone lozenges are allowed to dissolve next to an ulcer and are useful in recurrent aphthae, erosive lichen planus, discoid lupus erythematosus, and benign mucous membrane pemphigoid.

Triamcinolone dental paste is designed to keep the corticosteroid in contact with the mucosa for long enough to permit penetration of the lesion, but is difficult for patients to apply properly.

Systemic corticosteroid therapy is reserved for severe conditions such as pemphigus vulgaris (see section 6.3.4).

LOCAL ANALGESICS. Local analgesics have a limited role in the management of oral ulceration. When applied topically their action is of a relatively short duration so that analgesia cannot be maintained continuously throughout the day. The main indication for a topical local analgesic is to relieve the pain of otherwise intractable oral ulceration particularly when it is due to major aphthae. For this purpose lignocaine 5% ointment or lozenges containing a local anaesthetic are applied to the ulcer. When local anaesthetics are used in the mouth care must be taken not to produce anaesthesia of the pharynx before meals as this might lead to choking.

Benzydamine mouthwash or spray may be useful in palliating the discomfort associated with a variety of ulcerative conditions. It has also been found to be effective in reducing the discomfort of post-irradiation mucositis. Some patients find the full-strength mouthwash causes some stinging and, for them, it should be diluted with an equal volume of water.

Choline salicylate dental gel has some analgesic action and may provide relief for recurrent aphthae, but excessive application or confinement under a denture irritates the mucosa and can itself cause ulceration. Benefit in teething may merely be due to pressure of application (comparable with biting a teething ring); excessive use can lead to salicylate poisoning.

OTHER PREPARATIONS. **Carbenoxolone** gel or mouthwash may be of some value. **Tetracycline** rinsed in the mouth may also be of value.

BENZYDAMINE HYDROCHLORIDE

Indications: painful inflammatory conditions of oropharynx
Side-effects: occasional numbness or stinging

Difflam® (3M)
Oral rinse, green, benzydamine hydrochloride 0.15%. Net price 300 mL = £4.25

Rinse or gargle, using 15 mL (diluted if stinging occurs) every 1½–3 hours as required, usually for not more than 7 days; not suitable for children under 12 years

Spray, benzydamine hydrochloride 0.15%. Net price 30-mL unit = £3.39

4–8 puffs onto affected area every 1½–3 hours; CHILD under 6 years 1 puff per 4 kg to max. 4 puffs every 1½–3 hours; 6–12 years 4 puffs every 1½–3 hours

12.3 Drugs acting on the oropharynx

CARBENOXOLONE SODIUM
Indications: mild oral and perioral lesions

Bioral Gel® (Sterling Health)
Gel, carbenoxolone sodium 2% in adhesive basis. Net price 5 g = £1.83
Apply after meals and at bedtime

PoM ¹**Bioplex®** (Thames)
Mouthwash granules, carbenoxolone sodium 1% (20 mg/sachet). Net price 24 × 2-g sachets = £9.60
For mouth ulcers, rinse with 1 sachet in 30–50 mL of warm water 3 times daily and at bedtime
1. Can be sold to the public for use as a mouthwash by adults and children over 12 years, provided it is labelled with a maximum single dose of 20 mg and a maximum daily dose of 80 mg

CARMELLOSE SODIUM
Indications: mechanical protection of oral and perioral lesions

Orabase® (Squibb)
Oral paste, carmellose sodium 16.58%, pectin 16.58%, gelatin 16.58%, in Plastibase®. Net price 30 g = £1.50; 100 g = £3.32
Apply a thin layer when necessary after meals

Orahesive® (Squibb)
Powder, carmellose sodium, pectin, gelatin, equal parts. Net price 25 g = £1.72
Sprinkle on the affected area

CORTICOSTEROIDS
Indications: oral and perioral lesions
Contra-indications: untreated oral infection
Side-effects: occasional exacerbation of local infection

PoM **Adcortyl in Orabase®** (Squibb)
Oral paste, triamcinolone acetonide 0.1% in adhesive basis. Net price 10 g = £1.27
ADULT and CHILD, apply a thin layer 2–4 times daily; do not rub in; use limited to 5 days for children and short-term use also advised for elderly

PoM **Corlan®** (Evans)
Pellets (= lozenges), hydrocortisone 2.5 mg (as sodium succinate). Net price 20 = £1.40
ADULT and CHILD, 1 lozenge 4 times daily, allowed to dissolve slowly in the mouth in contact with the ulcer; if ulcers recur rapidly treatment may be continued for a period at reduced dosage

LOCAL ANAESTHETICS
Indications: relief of pain in oral lesions
Cautions: avoid prolonged use; hypersensitivity

Standard strength lozenges
Available with antiseptics, section 12.3.2

High strength lozenges
Benzocaine Lozenges, Compound, BPC 1973,
benzocaine 100 mg, menthol 3 mg
Note. It is **essential** not to confuse these with benzocaine lozenges which contained one-tenth the amount of benzocaine and are no longer available
Available from Penn (**special order**, bulk quantities only)

SALICYLATES
Indications: mild oral and perioral lesions
Cautions: frequent application, especially in children, may give rise to salicylate poisoning
Note. CSM warning on aspirin and Reye's syndrome does not apply to non-aspirin salicylates or to topical preparations such as teething gels

Choline salicylate
Choline Salicylate Dental Gel (BP)
Oral gel, choline salicylate 8.7% in a flavoured gel basis
Available as Bonjela® (R&C), net price 15 g (sugar-free) = £1.11; Teejel® (Napp), 10 g = 72p
Apply ½-inch of gel with gentle massage not more often than every 3 hours; CHILD over 4 months ¼-inch of gel not more often than every 3 hours; max. 6 applications daily

Salicylic acid
Pyralvex® (Norgine)
Oral paint, brown, anthraquinone glycosides 5%, salicylic acid 1%. Net price 10 mL with brush = £1.27. Apply 3–4 times daily

TETRACYCLINE
Indications: severe recurrent aphthous ulceration; oral herpes (section 12.3.2)
Side-effects: fungal superinfection
For side-effects, cautions and contra-indications relating to systemic administration of tetracyclines see section 5.1.3

Local application
For preparation of a mouthwash, the contents of a 250-mg tetracycline capsule (see section 5.1.3) can be stirred into a small amount of water, then held in the mouth for 2–3 minutes 3 times daily for not longer than 3 days followed by a break of at least 3 days before treatment is recommenced (to avoid oral thrush); it should preferably not be swallowed
Note. Tetracycline stains teeth; avoid in children under 12 years of age

12.3.2 Oropharyngeal anti-infective drugs

The most common cause of a sore throat is a viral infection which does not benefit from anti-infective treatment. Streptococcal sore throats require systemic **penicillin** therapy (see section 5.1.1). Acute ulcerative gingivitis (Vincent's infection) responds to systemic **metronidazole** 200 mg 3 times daily for 3 days (see section 5.1.11) or **nimorazole** 500 mg twice daily for 2 days (see section 5.4.3).

FUNGAL INFECTIONS

Candida albicans may cause thrush and other forms of stomatitis which are sometimes a sequel to the use of broad-spectrum antibiotics or cytotoxics; withdrawing the causative drug may lead to rapid resolution. Otherwise, **nystatin**, **amphotericin**, or **miconazole** may be effective.

AMPHOTERICIN
Indications: oral and perioral fungal infections

PoM **Fungilin**® (Squibb)
Lozenges, yellow, amphotericin 10 mg. Net price 6 × 10 lozenge-pack = £3.95. Label: 9, 24, counselling, after food
Dissolve 1 lozenge slowly in the mouth 4 times daily, may require 10–15 days' treatment (continued for 48 hours after lesions have resolved); increase to 8 daily if infection severe
Suspension, yellow, sugar-free, amphotericin 100 mg/mL. Net price 12 mL with pipette = £2.31. Label: 9, counselling, use of pipette, hold in mouth, after food
Place 1 mL in the mouth after food and retain near lesions 4 times daily for 14 days (continued for 48 hours after lesions have resolved)

MICONAZOLE
Indications: oral fungal infections
Cautions: pregnancy; avoid in porphyria (see section 9.8.2); **interactions:** Appendix 1 (miconazole)

PoM[1] **Daktarin**® (Janssen)
Oral gel, sugar-free, miconazole 25 mg/mL. Net price 80 g = £5.00. Label: 9, counselling, hold in mouth, after food
Place 5–10 mL in the mouth after food 4 times daily; retain near lesions; CHILD under 2 years 2.5 mL twice daily, 2–6 years 5 mL twice daily, over 6 years 5 mL 4 times daily
Localised lesions, smear affected area with clean finger; a 15-g tube (net price £1.70) also available
1. 15-g tube can be sold to the public
Tablets—see section 5.2

NYSTATIN
Indications: oral and perioral fungal infections
Dose: (as pastilles or as suspension) 100 000 units 4 times daily after food, usually for 7 days (continued for 48 hours after lesions have resolved)
Note. Immunosuppressed patients may require higher doses (e.g. 500 000 units 4 times daily)

PoM **Nystan**® (Squibb)
Pastilles, yellow/brown, nystatin 100 000 units. Net price 28 pastille-pack = £3.95. Label: 9, 24, counselling, after food
Suspension, yellow, nystatin 100 000 units/mL. Net price 30 mL with pipette = £2.50. Label: 9, counselling, use of pipette, hold in mouth, after food
Suspension, gluten-, lactose-, and sugar-free, nystatin 100 000 units/mL when reconstituted with water. Measure with pipette. Net price 24 mL with pipette = £1.67. Label: 9, counselling, use of pipette, hold in mouth, after food

PoM **Nystatin-Dome**® (Lagap)
Suspension, yellow, nystatin 100 000 units/mL. Net price 30 mL with 1-mL spoon = £2.50. Label: 9, counselling, use of 1-mL spoon, hold in mouth, after food

VIRAL INFECTIONS

The management of herpes infections of the mouth is a soft diet, adequate fluid intake, analgesics as required, and the use of **chlorhexidine** mouthwash (Corsodyl®, section 12.3.4) to control plaque accumulation if toothbrushing is painful. In the case of severe herpetic stomatitis, systemic **acyclovir** is required (see section 5.3).

Herpes infections of the mouth may also respond to **tetracycline** (section 12.3.1) rinsed in the mouth.

Idoxuridine 0.1% paint has been superseded by more effective preparations.

ACYCLOVIR
See section 5.3

TETRACYCLINE
Section 12.3.1

12.3.3 Lozenges, sprays, and gels

There is no convincing evidence that antiseptic lozenges and sprays have a beneficial action and they sometimes irritate and cause sore tongue and sore lips. Some of these preparations also contain local anaesthetics which relieve pain but may cause sensitisation.

In particular preparations containing clioquinol are not recommended.

Benzalkonium Lozenges, benzalkonium chloride 500 micrograms. Net price 20 lozenges = 48p
Bradosol® (Zyma)
Lozenges, domiphen bromide 500 micrograms. Net price 24 lozenges = 66p
Dequadin® (Crookes)
Lozenges, orange, dequalinium chloride 250 micrograms. Net price 20 lozenges = 69p
Dissolve 1 lozenge slowly in the mouth when required
Labosept® (LAB)
Pastilles, red, dequalinium chloride 250 micrograms. Net price 20 pastilles = 68p
Suck 1 pastille slowly when required
PoM **Locabiotal**® (Servier)
Aerosol spray, fusafungine 125 micrograms/metered inhalation. Net price 200-dose unit with nasal and oral adaptor = £1.59
Merocets® (Merrell)
Lozenges, yellow, cetylpyridinium chloride 0.066%. Net price 24 lozenges = 83p

Clioquinol
Oralcer® (Vitabiotics)
Lozenges, ivory, ascorbic acid 6 mg, clioquinol 35 mg. Net price 20 lozenges = 73p

With local anaesthetic
AAA® (Rhône-Poulenc Rorer)
Mouth and throat spray, benzocaine 1.5 mg/metered dose. Net price 60-dose unit = £2.46
2 sprays every 2–3 hours (max. 16 sprays daily); CHILD 6–12 years, 1 spray every 2–3 hours (max. 8 sprays daily)
Bradosol Plus® (Zyma)
Lozenges, pink, lignocaine hydrochloride 5 mg, domiphen bromide 500 micrograms. Net price 24 = 89p
Adults and children over 12 years, 1 lozenge sucked every 2–3 hours; max. 8 lozenges daily

12.3 Drugs acting on the oropharynx 397

Dequacaine® (Crookes)
Lozenges, amber, benzocaine 10 mg, dequalinium chloride 250 micrograms. Net price 24 lozenges = 98p
Adults and children over 12 years, 1 lozenge sucked every 2 hours or as required; max. 8 lozenges daily

Eludril® (Fabre)
Aerosol spray, amethocaine hydrochloride 0.015%, chlorhexidine gluconate 0.05%. Net price 55 mL = £1.67
Adults and children over 12 years, 1 spray 3–4 times daily; not immediately before food

Medilave® (Martindale)
Gel, benzocaine 1%, cetylpyridinium chloride 0.01%. Net price 10 g = 61p
Adults, apply thin layer 3–4 times daily; no longer recommended for children under 12 years

Merocaine® (Merrell)
Lozenges, green, benzocaine 10 mg, cetylpyridinium chloride 1.4 mg. Net price 24 lozenges = 90p
Adults and children over 12 years, 1 lozenge sucked every 2 hours or as required; max. 8 lozenges daily

Tyrozets® (MSD)
Lozenges, pink, benzocaine 5 mg, tyrothricin 1 mg. Net price 24 lozenges = 66p
1 lozenge sucked every 3 hours (max. 8 lozenges daily); reduce dose in children (not for children under 3 years)

Vicks Ultra Chloraseptic® (Procter & Gamble)
Throat spray, benzocaine 1 mg/metered spray. Net price 15 mL = £2.47
Adults and children over 13 years, 3 sprays every 2–3 hours (max. 24 sprays daily); child 6–12 years, 1 spray every 2–3 hours (max. 8 sprays daily)

For teething

Calgel® (Wellcome)
Teething gel, lignocaine hydrochloride 0.33%, cetylpyridinium chloride 0.1%. Net price 10 g = 75p
Apply small quantity to gum up to 6 times daily

12.3.4 Mouthwashes, gargles, and dentifrices

Mouthwashes have a mechanical cleansing action and freshen the mouth. Warm **compound sodium chloride mouthwash** or **compound thymol glycerin** is as useful as any.

Hydrogen peroxide mouthwash has a mechanical cleansing effect due to frothing when in contact with oral debris. **Sodium perborate** is similar in effect to hydrogen peroxide.

There is evidence that **chlorhexidine** has a specific effect in inhibiting the formation of plaque on teeth. A chlorhexidine mouthwash may be useful as an adjunct to other oral hygiene measures in cases of oral infection or when toothbrushing is not possible.

There is no convincing evidence that gargles are effective.

CETYLPYRIDINIUM CHLORIDE
Indications: oral hygiene

Merocet® (Merrell)
Solution (= mouthwash or gargle), yellow, cetylpyridinium chloride 0.05%. Net price 200 mL = £1.12
To be used undiluted or diluted with an equal volume of warm water

CHLORHEXIDINE GLUCONATE
Indications: oral hygiene; plaque inhibition
Side-effects: idiosyncratic mucosal irritation; reversible brown staining of teeth

Corsodyl® (ICI)
Dental gel, chlorhexidine gluconate 1%. Net price 50 g = 83p
Brush on the teeth once or twice daily
Mouthwash, chlorhexidine gluconate 0.2% (aniseed or mint-flavoured). Net price 300 mL = £1.25; 60-mL spray pack (mint-flavoured) also available, net price = £2.80
Rinse the mouth with 10 mL for about 1 minute twice daily *or* spray with up to 12 actuations twice daily

Eludril® (Fabre)
Mouthwash, chlorhexidine gluconate 0.1%, chlorbutol 0.5%. Net price 90 mL = 89p; 250 mL = £1.76; 500 mL = £3.19
Use 10–15 mL in a third of a tumblerful of warm water 2–3 times daily

HEXETIDINE
Indications: oral hygiene

Oraldene® (W-L)
Mouthwash or *gargle*, red, hexetidine 0.1%. Net price 100 mL = 87p; 200 mL = £1.43
Use 15 mL undiluted 2–3 times daily

OXIDISING AGENTS
Indications: oral hygiene, see notes above

Hydrogen Peroxide Mouthwash, DPF, consists of Hydrogen Peroxide Solution (6% ≡ approx. 20 volume) BP
Rinse the mouth for 2–3 minutes with 15 mL in half a tumblerful of warm water 2–3 times daily

Bocasan® (Oral-B Labs)
Mouthwash, sodium perborate 68.6% (buffered). Net price 20 × 1.7-g sachet-pack = £1.40
Use 1 sachet in 30 mL of water 3 times daily after meals
Cautions: Do not use for longer than 7 days because of possible absorption of borate; not recommended in renal impairment or for children under 5 years

PHENOL
Indications: oral hygiene

Chloraseptic® (Procter & Gamble)
Mouthwash/gargle, green, phenol 1.4%. Net price 150 mL = £1.85
Use every 2 hours if necessary, undiluted or diluted with an equal volume of water as a mouthwash or gargle (CHILD 6–12 years on doctor's advice only; under 6 years not recommended)

Vicks Ultra Chloraseptic, see section 12.3.3

POVIDONE-IODINE

Indications: oral hygiene
Cautions: pregnancy; breast-feeding
Side-effects: idiosyncratic mucosal irritation and hypersensitivity reactions

Betadine® (Napp)
Mouthwash or *gargle*, amber, povidone-iodine 1%. Net price 250 mL = 82p
Adults and children over 6 years, up to 10 mL undiluted or diluted with an equal quantity of warm water up to 4 times daily for up to 14 days

SODIUM CHLORIDE

Indications: oral hygiene, see notes above

Sodium Chloride Mouthwash, Compound, BP
Mouthwash, sodium bicarbonate 1%, sodium chloride 1.5% in a suitable vehicle with a peppermint flavour.
Extemporaneous preparations should be prepared according to the following formula: sodium chloride 1.5 g, sodium bicarbonate 1 g, concentrated peppermint emulsion 2.5 mL, double-strength chloroform water 50 mL, water to 100 mL
To be diluted with an equal volume of warm water

THYMOL

Indications: oral hygiene, see notes above

Compound Thymol Glycerin, glycerol 10%, thymol 0.05% with colouring and flavouring
To be used undiluted or diluted with 3 volumes of warm water

Mouthwash Solution-tablets, consist of tablets which may contain antimicrobial, colouring, and flavouring agents in a suitable soluble effervescent basis to make a mouthwash suitable for dental purposes. Net price 20 solution-tablets = 32p
Dissolve 1 tablet in a tumblerful of warm water

OTHER PREPARATIONS FOR OROPHARYNGEAL USE

Artificial saliva may be indicated for dry mouth. Of the proprietary preparations available, Luborant® is licensed for any condition giving rise to a dry mouth; Saliva Orthana® and Glandosane® have ACBS approval for dry mouth associated only with radiotherapy or sicca syndrome.

Glandosane® (Fresenius)
Aerosol spray, carmellose sodium 500 mg, sorbitol 1.5 g, potassium chloride 60 mg, sodium chloride 42.2 mg, magnesium chloride 2.6 mg, calcium chloride 7.3 mg, and dipotassium hydrogen phosphate 17.1 mg/50 g. Net price 50-mL unit (neutral or lemon flavoured) = £3.95
ACBS: patients suffering from dry mouth as a result of having (or having undergone) radiotherapy, or sicca syndrome, spray onto oral and pharyngeal mucosa as required

Luborant® (Antigen)
Oral spray, pink, sorbitol 1.8 g, carmellose sodium (sodium carboxymethylcellulose) 390 mg, dibasic potassium phosphate 48.23 mg, potassium chloride 37.5 mg, monobasic potassium phosphate 21.97 mg, calcium chloride 9.972 mg, magnesium chloride 3.528 mg, sodium fluoride 258 micrograms/60 mL, with preservatives and colouring agents. Net price 60-mL unit = £3.96
Saliva deficiency, 2–3 sprays onto oral mucosa up to 4 times daily, or as directed

Saliva Orthana® (Nycomed)
Aerosol spray, gastric mucin (porcine) 3.5%, with preservatives and flavouring agents. Net price 450 mL bottle (with empty 50-mL spray bottle) = £25.10; 450 mL refill = £24.68; also 50-mL spray bottle (hosp. only)
Lozenges, mucin 63 mg, xylitol 39 mg, in a sorbitol basis. Net price 10 × 45-lozenge pack = £21.80
ACBS: patients suffering from dry mouth as a result of having (or having undergone) radiotherapy, or sicca syndrome, spray 2–3 times onto oral and pharyngeal mucosa, when required
Note. Saliva Orthana aerosol spray is available with (sodium fluoride 4.2 mg/litre) and without fluoride; the lozenges do not contain fluoride

13: Drugs acting on the
SKIN

In this chapter, drug treatment is discussed under the following headings:
- 13.1 Vehicles
- 13.2 Emollient and barrier preparations
- 13.3 Local anaesthetics and antipruritics
- 13.4 Topical corticosteroids
- 13.5 Preparations for psoriasis and eczema
- 13.6 Preparations for acne
- 13.7 Preparations for warts and calluses
- 13.8 Sunscreens and camouflagers
- 13.9 Shampoos and some other scalp preparations
- 13.10 Anti-infective skin preparations
- 13.11 Disinfectants and cleansers
- 13.12 Antiperspirants
- 13.13 Wound management products
- 13.14 Topical circulatory preparations

Suitable quantities of dermatological preparations to be prescribed for specific areas of the body are:

	Creams and Ointments	Lotions
Face	5 to 15 g	100 mL
Both hands	25 to 50 g	200 mL
Scalp	50 to 100 g	200 mL
Both arms or both legs	100 to 200 g	200 mL
Body	200 g	500 mL
Groins and genitalia	15 to 25 g	100 mL
Dusting powders	50 to 100 g	
Paints	10 to 25 mL	

These amounts are usually suitable for 2 to 4 weeks. The recommendations do not apply to corticosteroid preparations which should be applied thinly. Corticosteroid creams and ointments are available in various pack sizes, commonly 15 g or 30 g, while corticosteroid lotions are usually packed in 20- or 100-mL sizes.

13.1 Vehicles

Both vehicle and active ingredients are important in the treatment of skin conditions; it is being increasingly recognised that the vehicle alone may have more than a mere placebo effect. The vehicle affects the degree of hydration of the skin, has a mild anti-inflammatory effect, and aids the penetration of active drug in the preparation.

The vehicle may take the form of a cream, ointment, lotion, paste, dusting powder, application, collodion, or paint basis.

DILUTION. The BP directs that creams and ointments should **not** normally be diluted but that should dilution be necessary care should be taken, in particular, to prevent microbial contamination. The appropriate diluent should be used and heating should be avoided during mixing; excessive dilution may affect the stability of some creams. Diluted creams should normally be used within 2 weeks of their preparation.

ADDITIVES. The following additives in topical preparations may be associated with sensitisation, particularly of eczematous skin. Details of whether they are contained in preparations listed in the BNF are given after the preparation entry.

Most commonly	Less commonly	Rarely[1]
Wool fat and related substances	Benzyl alcohol	Beeswax
Chlorocresol	Butylated hydroxyanisole	Edetic acid (EDTA)
Ethylenediamine	Butylated hydroxytoluene	Isopropyl palmitate
Fragrances	Hydroxybenzoates (parabens)	
	Polysorbates	
	Propylene glycol	
	Sorbic acid	

1. Non-dermatologists can reasonably disregard the substances in this category

APPLICATIONS are usually viscous solutions, emulsions, or suspensions for application to the skin.

COLLODIONS are painted on the skin and allowed to dry to leave a flexible film over the site of application. Flexible collodion may be used to seal minor cuts and wounds. Collodions may also be used to provide a means of holding a dissolved drug in contact with the skin for a long period, e.g. salicylic acid collodion (section 13.7).

CREAMS are essentially miscible with the skin secretion. They may contain an antimicrobial preservative unless the active ingredient or basis has sufficient intrinsic bactericidal or fungicidal activity. Generally, creams are cosmetically more acceptable than ointments as they are less greasy and easier to apply.

DUSTING POWDERS are finely divided powders that contain one or more active ingredients with or without auxiliary substances. They are intended to be applied to skin for therapeutic, prophylactic or lubricant purposes. If dusting powder is intended for large open wounds or severely injured skin it should be sterile.

LINIMENTS are liquid preparations for external application and may contain analgesics and rubefacients, see section 10.3.2.

LOTIONS are usually aqueous solutions or suspensions which cool diffusely inflamed unbroken skin. They cool by evaporation and should be reapplied frequently. Volatile solvents increase the cooling effect but are liable to cause stinging. Lotions are also used to apply drugs to the skin and may be preferred to ointments or creams when it is intended to apply a thin layer of the

---

Cautionary label wordings, see inside back cover   Prices are **net**, see p. 1

preparation over a large or hairy area. *Shake lotions* (such as calamine lotion) containing insoluble powders are applied to less acute, scabbed, dry lesions. In addition to cooling they leave a deposit of inert powder on the skin surface.

OINTMENTS are greasy preparations which are normally anhydrous and insoluble in water, and are more occlusive than creams. The most commonly used ointment bases consist of soft paraffin or a combination of soft paraffin with liquid paraffin and hard paraffin. Some modern ointment bases have both hydrophilic and lipophilic properties; they may have occlusive properties on the skin surface, encourage hydration, and be miscible with water; they often have a mild anti-inflammatory effect. Water-soluble ointments contain macrogols which are freely soluble in water and are therefore readily washed off; they have a limited but useful application in circumstances where ready removal is desirable. Ointments are particularly suitable for chronic, dry lesions.

PAINTS are liquid preparations intended for application with a brush to the skin or mucous surfaces.

PASTES are stiff preparations containing a high proportion of finely powdered solids such as zinc oxide and starch. They are used for circumscribed lesions such as those which occur in lichen simplex, chronic eczema, or psoriasis. They are less occlusive than ointments and can be used to protect sub-acute, lichenified, or excoriated skin.

13.2 Emollient and barrier preparations

13.2.1 Emollients
13.2.2 Barrier preparations
13.2.3 Dusting powders

> BORDERLINE SUBSTANCES. The preparations marked 'ACBS' are regarded as drugs when prescribed in accordance with the advice of the Advisory Committee on Borderline Substances for the clinical conditions listed. Prescriptions issued in accordance with this advice and endorsed 'ACBS' will normally not be investigated. See Appendix 7 for listing by clinical condition.

13.2.1 Emollients

Emollients soothe, smooth and hydrate the skin and are indicated for all dry scaling disorders (such as ichthyosis). Their effects are short-lived and they should be applied frequently even after improvement occurs. They are useful in dry eczematous disorders, and to a lesser extent in psoriasis (section 13.5). Simple preparations such as **aqueous cream** are often as effective as the more complex proprietary formulations; sprays offer little advantage but, in general, the choice depends on patient preference. Some ingredients may cause sensitisation, notably hydrous wool fat (lanolin) or antibacterials and this should be suspected if an eczematous reaction occurs.

Camphor, menthol, and phenol have a mild antipruritic effect when used in emollient preparations. Calamine and zinc oxide may also be included as they slightly enhance therapeutic efficacy; they are particularly useful in dry eczema. Zinc and titanium preparations have mild astringent properties. Thickening agents such as talc and kaolin may also be included. Preparations containing an antibacterial should be avoided unless infection is present (section 13.10).

Urea is employed as a hydrating agent. It is used in scaling conditions and may be useful in elderly patients and infantile eczemas. It is often used with other topical agents such as corticosteroids to enhance penetration.

Aqueous Cream, BP, emulsifying ointment 30%, phenoxyethanol 1%, in freshly boiled and cooled purified water. Net price 100 g = 28p
Available from APS, Cox, Evans

Emulsifying Ointment, BP, emulsifying wax 30%, white soft paraffin 50%, liquid paraffin 20%. Net price 100 g = 30p
Available from APS, Cox, CP, Evans

Hydrous Ointment, BP (oily cream), dried magnesium sulphate 0.5%, phenoxyethanol 1%, wool alcohols ointment 50%, in freshly boiled and cooled purified water. Net price 100 g = 34p
Available from CP, Evans

Paraffin, White Soft, BP (white petroleum jelly). Net price 100 g = 36p
Available from APS, CP, Evans

Paraffin, Yellow Soft, BP (yellow petroleum jelly). Net price 100 g = 38p
Available from CP, Evans

Zinc Cream, BP, zinc oxide 32%, arachis oil 32%, calcium hydroxide 0.045%, oleic acid 0.5%, wool fat 8%, in freshly boiled and cooled purified water. Net price 50 g = 34p. For napkin and urinary rash and eczematous conditions
Available from Evans

Zinc Ointment, BP, zinc oxide 15%, in simple ointment. Net price 25 g = 20p. For napkin and urinary rash and eczematous conditions
Available from Evans

Zinc and Castor Oil Ointment, BP, zinc oxide 7.5%, castor oil 50%, arachis oil 30.5%, white beeswax 10%, cetostearyl alcohol 2%. Net price 25 g = 14p. For napkin and urinary rash
Available from CP, Evans

Alcoderm® (Galderma)
Cream, containing liquid paraffin, cetyl alcohol, stearyl alcohol, sodium lauryl sulphate, carbomer, triethanolamine, sorbitan monosterate, sorbitol, spermaceti, silicone fluid. Net price 60 g = £2.40
Additives: hydroxybenzoates (parabens), isopropyl palmitate

Lotion, water-miscible, ingredients as above. Net price 120 mL = £2.86

Aveeno® (Bioglan)
Cream, colloidal oat fraction in emollient basis containing allantoin. Net price 75 mL = £2.17. ACBS: For endogenous and exogenous eczema, xeroderma, ichthyosis, and senile pruritus associated with dry skin
Additives: benzyl alcohol

13.2 Emollient and barrier preparations

Diprobase® (Schering-Plough)
Cream, cetomacrogol 2.25%, cetostearyl alcohol 7.2%, liquid paraffin 6%, white soft paraffin 15%, water-miscible basis used for Diprosone® cream. Net price 50 g = £1.65; 500-g dispenser = £7.10
Additives: chlorocresol
Ointment, liquid paraffin 5%, white soft paraffin 95%, basis used for Diprosone® ointment. Net price 50 g = £1.65
Additives: none as listed in section 13.1

Dermalex®—section 13.10.5

Drapolene®—section 13.10.5

E45® (Crookes)
Cream, light liquid paraffin 12.6%, white soft paraffin 13.5%, wool fat 1% self-emulsifying monostearin. Net price 50 g = 98p; 125 g = £2.03; 500 g = £4.82
Additives: hydroxybenzoates (parabens)
Wash E45, soap substitute, zinc oxide 5% in an emollient basis. Net price 150 mL = £2.17. ACBS: endogenous and exogenous eczema, xeroderma, ichthyosis and senile pruritus associated with dry skin
Additives: butylated hydroxytoluene

Eczederm®—section 13.3

Hewletts Cream® (Bioglan)
Cream, hydrous wool fat 4%, zinc oxide 8%. Net price 35 g = 67p; 400 g = £3.30. For nursing hygiene and care of skin
Additives: fragrance

Humiderm® (BritCair)
Cream, pyrrolidone carboxylic acid 5% (as sodium salt). Net price 60 g = £3.71. For dry skin conditions
Additives: hydroxybenzoates (parabens), propylene glycol

Hydromol® (Quinoderm Ltd)
Cream, arachis oil 10%, isopropyl myristate 5%, liquid paraffin 10%, sodium pyrrolidone carboxylate 2.5%, sodium lactate 1%. Net price 50 g = £2.04; 100 g = £3.40; 500 g = £10.94. For dry skin conditions
Additives: hydroxybenzoates (parabens)

Kamillosan® (Norgine)
Ointment, chamomile extracts 10.5%. Net price 5 g = 57p (hosp. only); 24 g = £1.49. For napkin rash, cracked nipples and chapped hands
Additives: beeswax, hydroxybenzoates (parabens), wool fat

Keri® (Bristol-Myers)
Lotion, mineral oil 16%, with lanolin oil. Net price 190-mL pump pack = £3.65; 380-mL pump pack = £5.96. For dry skin conditions and napkin rash
Additives: hydroxybenzoates (parabens), propylene glycol, fragrance

Lacticare® (Stiefel)
Lotion, lactic acid 5%, sodium pyrrolidone carboxylate 2.5%. Net price 150 mL = £3.19. For dry skin conditions
Additives: isopropyl palmitate, fragrance

Lipobase® (Brocades)
Cream, fatty cream basis used for Locoid Lipocream®. Net price 50 g = £2.05
Additives: hydroxybenzoates (parabens)

Massé Breast Cream® (Cilag)
Cream (water-miscible), containing arachis oil, cetyl alcohol, glycerol, glyceryl monostearate, wool fat, polysorbate 60, potassium hydroxide, sorbitan monostearate, stearic acid. Net price 28 g = £1.40. For pre- and post-natal nipple care
Additives: hydroxybenzoates (parabens)

Morhulin® (Napp)
Ointment, cod-liver oil 11.4%, zinc oxide 38%, in a basis containing wool fat and paraffin. Net price 50 g = 93p; 350 g = £4.53. For minor wounds, varicose ulcers, and pressure sores

Morsep® (Napp)
Cream, cetrimide 0.5%, ergocalciferol 10 units/g, vitamin A 70 units/g. Net price 40 g = £1.00; 300 g = £3.87. For urinary rash
Additives: wool fat derivative, fragrance

Natuderm® (Burgess)
Cream (hydrophilic and lipophilic), free fatty acids 5%, glycerides 15.5%, glycerol 3.7%, phospholipids 0.2%, polysorbate '60' 1.1%, sorbitan monostearate 1%, squalane 0.5%, squalene 3.3%, free sterols 0.8%, sterol esters 1.3%, α-tocopherol 0.003%, waxes 7%, butylated hydroxyanisole 0.003%. Net price 100 g = £2.08; 450 g = £8.19

Oilatum® (Stiefel)
Cream, arachis oil 21%, povidone (polyvinylpyrrolidone) 1%. Net price 40 g = £1.79; 80 g = £2.78
Additives: fragrance
Shower emollient (gel), light liquid paraffin 70%. Net price 125 g = £4.84
Additives: fragrance
Apply daily

Sudocrem® (Tosara)
Cream, benzyl alcohol 0.39%, benzyl benzoate 1.01%, benzyl cinnamate 0.15%, wool fat 4%, zinc oxide 15.25%. Net price 30 g = 60p; 60 g = 66p; 125 g = £1.15; 250 g = £2.07; 400 g = £2.98. For napkin rash and pressure sores
Additives: beeswax (synthetic), polysorbates, propylene glycol, fragrance

Ultrabase® (Schering Health Care)
Cream, water-miscible, containing liquid paraffin and white soft paraffin. Net price 50 g = £1.05; 500 g = £5.70
Additives: hydroxybenzoates (parabens), disodium edetate, fragrance

Unguentum Merck® (Merck)
Cream (hydrophilic and lipophilic), cetostearyl alcohol 9%, glyceryl monostearate 3%, saturated neutral oil 2%, liquid paraffin 3%, white soft paraffin 32%, propylene glycol 5%, polysorbate '40' 8%, silicic acid 0.1%, sorbic acid 0.2%. Net price 50 g = £1.63; 100 g = £3.21; 200 mL = £6.35; 500 g = £9.80

Vaseline Dermacare® (Elida Gibbs)
Cream, dimethicone 1%, white soft paraffin 15%. Net price 100 mL = £1.45. ACBS: for endogenous and exogenous eczema, xeroderma, ichthyosis and senile pruritus associated with dry skin
Additives: hydroxybenzoates (parabens)
Lotion, dimethicone 1%, liquid paraffin 4%, white soft paraffin 5% in an emollient basis. Net price 75 mL = £1.10; 200 mL = £2.09. ACBS: for endogenous and exogenous eczema, xero-

derma, ichthyosis and senile pruritus associated with dry skin
Additives: disodium edetate, hydroxybenzoates (parabens), wool fat

Vita-E® (Bioglan)
Ointment, d-α-tocopheryl acetate 30 units/g in yellow soft paraffin. Net price 50 g = £2.50. For pressure sores and related conditions
Additives: none as listed in section 13.1

Preparations containing urea
Aquadrate® (Norwich Eaton)
Cream, urea 10%. Net price 30 g = £1.63; 100 g = £4.91
Additives: none as listed in section 13.1
Apply thinly and rub into area when required

Calmurid® (Kabi Pharmacia)
Cream, urea 10%, lactic acid 5%. Diluent aqueous cream, life of diluted cream 14 days. Net price 100 g = £3.49; 400-g dispenser = £12.50
Additives: none as listed in section 13.1
Apply a thick layer for 3–5 minutes, massage into area, and remove excess, usually twice daily. Use half-strength cream for 1 week if stinging occurs with undiluted preparation

Nutraplus® (Galderma)
Cream, urea 10%. Net price 60 g = £2.62
Additives: hydroxybenzoates (parabens), propylene glycol
Apply 2–3 times daily

Sential E® (Kabi Pharmacia)
Cream, urea 4%, sodium chloride 4%. Net price 100 g = £2.97
Additives: hydroxybenzoates (parabens)
For dry, scaling and itching skin, apply twice daily after washing

---

13.2.1.1 EMOLLIENT BATH ADDITIVES

For bath additives containing tar, see section 13.5 and for antiseptic bath additives, see section 13.11.

Alpha Keri Bath® (Bristol-Myers)
Bath oil, liquid paraffin 91.7%, oil-soluble fraction of wool fat 3%. Net price 240 mL = £3.54; 480 mL = £6.59
Additives: fragrance
Add 10–20 mL/bath (infants 5 mL)

Aveeno Oilated® (Bioglan)
Bath additive, oat (protein fraction) 41%, liquid paraffin 35%. Net price 10 × 50-g sachets = £5.29. ACBS: for endogenous and exogenous eczema, xeroderma, ichthyosis, and senile pruritus associated with dry skin
Additives: none as listed in section 13.1
Add 1 sachet/bath

Aveeno Regular® (Bioglan)
Bath additive, oat (protein fraction). Net price 10 × 50-g sachets = £5.29. ACBS: as for Aveeno Oilated
Additives: none as listed in section 13.1
Add 1 sachet/bath

Balmandol® (S&N Pharm.)
Bath oil, almond oil 30%, light liquid paraffin 69.6%. Net price 225 mL = £3.68; 500 mL = £7.36
Additives: butylated hydroxyanisole, fragrance
Add 15–30 mL/bath

Balneum® (Merck)
Balneum® bath oil, soya oil 84.75%. Net price 200 mL = £2.86; 500 mL = £6.22; 1 litre = £12.00
Additives: butylated hydroxytoluene, propylene glycol, fragrance
Add 20 mL/bath
Balneum Plus® bath oil, soya oil 82.95%, mixed lauromacrogols 15%. Net price 500 mL = £8.55
Additives: butylated hydroxytoluene, propylene glycol, fragrance
Add 20 mL/bath

Balneum with Tar®—section 13.5

Bath E45® (Crookes)
Bath oil, cetyl dimethicone 5%. Net price 150 mL = £2.17. ACBS: for endogenous and exogenous eczema, xeroderma, ichthyosis, and senile pruritus associated with dry skin
Additives: butylated hydroxyanisole
Add 15 mL/bath

Diprobath® (Schering-Plough)
Bath additive, isopropyl myristate 39%, light liquid paraffin 46%. Net price 500 mL = £8.55.
Additives: none as listed in section 13.1
Add 25 mL/bath (infants 10 mL)

Emmolate® (Bio-Medical)
Bath oil, acetylated wool alcohols 5%, liquid paraffin 65%. Net price 200 mL = £1.95 (hosp. only)
Additives: none as listed in section 13.1
Add 15–20 mL/bath

Emulsiderm® (Dermal)
Liquid emulsion, liquid paraffin 25%, isopropyl myristate 25%, benzalkonium chloride 0.5%. Net price 250 mL (with 10-mL measure) = £4.44; 1 litre (with 30-mL measure) = £11.87
Additives: polysorbate 60
Add 30 mL/bath (infants 15 mL)

Hydromol Emollient® (Quinoderm Ltd)
Bath additive, isopropyl myristate 13%, light liquid paraffin 37.8%. Net price 150 mL = £1.64; 350 mL = £3.06; 1 litre = £7.09
Additives: none as listed in section 13.1
Add 1–3 capfuls/bath (infants ½–2 capfuls)

Oilatum Emollient® (Stiefel)
Bath additive (emulsion), acetylated wool alcohols 5%, liquid paraffin 63.7%. Net price 150 mL = £1.65; 350 mL = £3.20
Additives: isopropyl palmitate, fragrance
Add 5–15 mL/bath

13.2.2 Barrier preparations

Barrier preparations often contain water-repellent substances such as **dimethicone** or other silicones. They are used to give protection against irritation or repeated hydration (areas around stomata, sore areas in the elderly, bedsores, etc.). They are no substitute for adequate nursing care, and it is doubtful if they are any more effective than the traditional compound **zinc ointments**.

For stoma care preparations, see section 1.8.

NAPKIN RASH. Barrier creams and ointments are also used to give protection against napkin rash which is usually a local dermatitis. The first line of treatment is to ensure that napkins are changed frequently, and that tightly fitting rubber pants are avoided. The rash may clear when left exposed to the air and an emollient, or an antimicrobial preparation (e.g. clotrimazole cream), may be helpful. A mild corticosteroid such as hydrocortisone may be useful but treatment should be limited to a week or less and it should be remembered that napkins and plastic pants may act as an occlusive dressing and increase absorption (for cautions see hydrocortisone p. 405).

Conotrane® (Boehringer Ingelheim)
Cream, benzalkonium chloride 0.1%, dimethicone '350' 22%. Net price 50 g = 59p; 100 g = 96p; 500 g = £3.66. For napkin and urinary rash and pressure sores
Additives: fragrance

Metanium® (Bengué)
Ointment, titanium dioxide 20%, titanium peroxide 5%, titanium salicylate 3%, titanium tannate 0.1%, in a silicone basis. Net price 25 g = 72p. For napkin rash and related disorders
Additives: none as listed in section 13.1

Siopel® (ICI)
Barrier cream, dimethicone '1000' 10%, cetrimide 0.3%. Net price 50 g = 63p. For dermatoses, colostomy and ileostomy care, urinary rash, and related conditions
Additives: butylated hydroxytoluene, hydroxybenzoates (parabens)

Sprilon® (Kabi Pharmacia)
Spray application, dimethicone 1.04%, zinc oxide 12.5%, in a basis containing wool fat, wool alcohols, cetostearyl alcohol, dextran, white soft paraffin, liquid paraffin, propellants. Net price 115-g pressurised aerosol unit = £3.81. For urinary rash, pressure sores, and ileostomy
Caution: flammable

Vasogen® (Pharmax)
Barrier cream, dimethicone 20%, calamine 1.5%, zinc oxide 7.5%. Net price 50 g = 63p; 100 g = £1.07. For napkin and urinary rash, pressure sores, and pruritus ani
Additives: hydroxybenzoates (parabens), wool fat

13.2.3 Dusting powders

Dusting powders are used in folds where friction may occur between opposing skin surfaces. They should not be applied in areas that are very moist as they tend to cake and abrade the skin. **Talc** acts as a lubricant powder but does not absorb moisture whereas **starch** is less lubricant but absorbs water. Other inert powders such as kaolin or zinc oxide may also be used in the formulation of dusting powders.

See also section 13.11 for antiseptic dusting powders.

Talc Dusting Powder, BP, starch 10% in sterilised purified talc. Net price 100 g = 33p
Zinc, Starch and Talc Dusting-powder, BPC, zinc oxide 25%, starch 25%, sterilised purified talc 50%. Net price 50 g = 16p
ZeaSORB® (Stiefel)
Dusting powder, aldioxa 0.2%, chloroxylenol 0.5%, pulverised maize core 45%. Net price 50 g = £2.15
Additives: fragrance

13.3 Local anaesthetics and antipruritics

Pruritus may be caused by systemic disease (such as drug hypersensitivity, obstructive jaundice, endocrine disease, and certain malignant diseases) as well as by skin disease (e.g. psoriasis, eczema, urticaria, and scabies). Where possible the underlying causes should be treated.

There is no really effective antipruritic. **Calamine** preparations are widely prescribed. **Emollient** preparations (section 13.2.1) may also be of value. **Oral antihistamines** (section 3.4.1) should be used in allergic rashes.

Some topical antihistamines and local anaesthetics may cause sensitisation. Topical antihistamines are only marginally effective. Insect bites and stings, though often treated with such preparations, are best treated with calamine preparations or emollients.

Crotamiton shows little evidence of greater effectiveness than calamine in the relief of pruritus.

For preparations used in pruritus ani, see section 1.7.1.

CALAMINE
Indications: pruritus

Calamine Cream, Aqueous, BP, calamine 4%, zinc oxide 3%, liquid paraffin 20%, self-emulsifying glyceryl monostearate 5%, cetomacrogol emulsifying wax 5%, phenoxyethanol 0.5%, freshly boiled and cooled purified water 62.5%. Net price 50 g = 33p
Calamine Lotion, BP, calamine 15%, zinc oxide 5%, glycerol 5%, bentonite 3%, sodium citrate 0.5%, liquefied phenol 0.5%, in freshly boiled and cooled purified water. Net price 200 mL = 50p
Calamine Lotion, Oily, BP1980, calamine 5%, arachis oil 50%, oleic acid 0.5%, wool fat 1%, in calcium hydroxide solution. Net price 200 mL = 78p
Calamine Ointment, BP, calamine 15%, in white soft paraffin
Eczederm® (Quinoderm Ltd)
Cream, calamine 20.88%, arachis oil 12.5%. Net price 30 g = £1.12; 60 g = £1.92; 500 g = £10.20. For mild dermatoses including eczema
Additives: hydroxybenzoates (parabens), fragrance

CROTAMITON
Indications: pruritus (including pruritus after scabies)
Cautions: avoid use near eyes and broken skin
Contra-indications: acute exudative dermatoses

Eurax® (Zyma)
Cream, crotamiton 10%. Net price 30 g = £1.49; 100 g = £2.58
Additives: beeswax, hydroxybenzoates (parabens), fragrance
Lotion, crotamiton 10%. Net price 100 mL = £1.82
Additives: propylene glycol, sorbic acid, fragrance

LOCAL ANAESTHETICS

Indications: relief of local pain, see notes above. See section 15.2 for use in surface anaesthesia
Cautions: may cause hypersensitivity

Note. Topical local anaesthetic preparations may be absorbed, especially through mucosal surfaces, therefore excessive application should be avoided, particularly in infants and children.

Anethaine® (Crookes)
Cream, amethocaine hydrochloride 1%. Net price 25 g = £1.14
Additives: fragrance

Solarcaine® (Schering-Plough)
Cream, benzocaine 1%, triclosan 0.2%. Net price 25 mL = £1.31
Additives: benzyl alcohol, disodium edetate
Lotion, benzocaine 0.5%, triclosan 0.2%. Net price 75 mL = £1.76
Additives: disodium edetate, hydroxybenzoates (parabens)
Spray (= application), benzocaine 2.86%, triclosan 0.057%, pressurised aerosol unit. Net price 95 g = £2.26
Additives: propylene glycol

Xylocaine® (Astra)
Ointment, see section 15.2

TOPICAL ANTIHISTAMINES

Indications: pruritus, urticaria, see notes above
Cautions: may cause hypersensitivity; avoid in eczema; photosensitivity (diphenhydramine)

Anthisan® (Rhône-Poulenc Rorer)
Cream, mepyramine maleate 2%. Net price 25 g = £1.29
Additives: hydroxybenzoates (parabens), fragrance
Apply 2–3 times daily for up to 3 days

Caladryl® (W-L)
Cream, diphenhydramine hydrochloride 1%, calamine 8%, camphor 0.1%. Net price 42 g = £1.43
Additives: hydroxybenzoates (parabens), polysorbate 60, propylene glycol
Lotion, ingredients as for cream. Net price 125 mL = £1.43
Additives: fragrance
Apply 3–4 times daily for up to 3 days

R.B.C.® (Rybar)
Cream, antazoline hydrochloride 1.8%, calamine 8%, camphor 0.1%, cetrimide 0.5%. Net price 25 g = £1.15
Additives: propylene glycol
Apply when required for up to 3 days

13.4 Topical corticosteroids

Topical corticosteroids are used for the treatment of inflammatory conditions of the skin other than those due to an infection, in particular the eczematous disorders. Corticosteroids suppress various components of the inflammatory reaction while in use; they are in no sense curative, and when treatment is discontinued a rebound exacerbation of the condition may occur. They are indicated for the relief of symptoms and for the suppression of signs of the disorder when potentially less harmful measures are ineffective.

Corticosteroids are of no value in the treatment of urticaria and are **contra-indicated** in rosacea and in ulcerative conditions as they worsen the condition. They should not be used indiscriminately in pruritus.

CHOICE OF PREPARATION. The preparation containing the **least potent** drug at the **lowest strength** which is effective is the one of choice, but extemporaneous dilution should be avoided whenever possible.

There is no good evidence that it is of any benefit to prescribe a potent corticosteroid for initial treatment; it is probably just as useful to 'ascend' in potency as it is to 'descend'. It should be noted that if a patient ceases to respond to a particular corticosteroid another of similar potency ought to be prescribed, not a more potent one. In general, the most potent corticosteroids should be reserved for recalcitrant dermatoses such as *chronic discoid lupus erythematosus, lichen simplex chronicus, hypertrophic lichen planus,* and *palmar plantar pustulosis*. With rare exceptions, potent corticosteroids should not be used on the face as they may precipitate a rosacea-like disorder and aggravate pre-existing rosacea.

Considerable caution must be exercised in the use of potent corticosteroids in children (see below).

Topical corticosteroid preparations are divided into four groups in respect of potency. In ascending order these are:

	Potency	Examples
IV	Mild	Hydrocortisone 1%
III	Moderately potent	Clobetasone butyrate 0.05% (Eumovate®)
II	Potent	Betamethasone 0.1% (as valerate) (Betnovate®); hydrocortisone butyrate (Locoid®)
I	Very potent	Clobetasol propionate 0.05% (Dermovate®)

Intradermal corticosteroid injections (see section 10.1.2.2) are more effective than the very potent topical corticosteroid preparations and they should be reserved for severe cases where there are localised lesions and topical treatment has failed. Their effects may last for several weeks or even months.

SIDE-EFFECTS. Unlike groups I and II, groups III and IV are rarely associated with side-effects. The more potent the preparation the more care is required, as absorption through the skin can cause severe pituitary-adrenal-axis suppression and hypercorticism (see section 6.3.3), both of which depend on the area of the body treated and the duration of the treatment. It must also be remembered that absorption is greatest from areas of thin skin, raw surfaces, and intertriginous areas, and is increased by occlusion.

Local side-effects from the use of corticosteroids topically include:
(a) spread and worsening of untreated infection;
(b) thinning of the skin which may be restored over a period of time although the original structure may never return;
(c) irreversible striae atrophicae;
(d) increased hair growth;

(e) perioral dermatitis, an inflammatory papular disorder on the face of young women;
(f) acne at the site of application in some patients;
(g) mild depigmentation and vellus hair.

CHOICE OF FORMULATION. Water-miscible creams are suitable for moist or weeping lesions whereas ointments are generally chosen for dry, lichenified or scaly lesions or where a more occlusive effect is required. Lotions may be useful when minimal application to a large area is required. Occlusive polythene dressings have been used to increase the effect, but also increase the risk of side-effects. The inclusion of urea increases the penetration of the corticosteroid.

USE IN CHILDREN. Children, especially babies, are particularly susceptible to side-effects. The more potent corticosteroids should be **avoided** in paediatric treatment or if necessary used with great care for short periods; a mild corticosteroid such as hydrocortisone is useful for treating napkin rash (see section 13.2.2) and infantile eczemas (but see caution below).

COMPOUND PREPARATIONS. The advantages of including other substances with corticosteroids in topical preparations are debatable. The commonest ones are the **antibacterials**.

HYDROCORTISONE

Indications: mild inflammatory skin disorders
Cautions: see notes above and in section 13.5 (psoriasis); also avoid prolonged use in infants and children (extreme caution in dermatoses of infancy including napkin rash—where possible treatment should be limited to 5–7 days), and on the face; more potent corticosteroids contra-indicated in infants and young children
Contra-indications: untreated bacterial, fungal, or viral skin lesions
Side-effects: see notes above
Administration: apply thinly 2–3 times daily, reducing strength and frequency as condition responds

---

Over-the-counter sales. Proprietary brands of hydrocortisone cream (0.1 and 1%) and ointment (1%) are on sale to the public for treatment of allergic contact dermatitis, irritant dermatitis, and insect bite reactions only
Cautions: not for children under 10 years or in pregnancy, without medical advice
Contra-indications: eyes/face, anogenital region, broken or infected skin (including cold sores, acne, and athlete's foot)
Administration: apply sparingly over small area 1–2 times daily for max. of 1 week
Labelling must state. If the condition is not improved, consult your doctor.

PoM **Hydrocortisone** (Non-proprietary)
Cream, hydrocortisone 0.5%, net price, 15 g = 38p; 30 g = 60p; 1%, 15 g = 47p. Label: 28. Potency IV
When hydrocortisone cream is prescribed and no strength is stated, the 1% strength should be supplied
Ointment, hydrocortisone 0.5%, net price 15 g = 36p; 30 g = 60p; 1%, 15 g = 47p. Label: 28. Potency IV
When hydrocortisone ointment is prescribed and no strength is stated, the 1% strength should be supplied

PoM **Cobadex**® (Cox Pharmaceuticals)
Cream, hydrocortisone 0.5 or 1%, dimethicone '350' 20%. Net price 20 g (0.5%) = £1.29; 20 g (1%) = £1.85. Label: 28. Potency IV
Additives: hydroxybenzoates (parabens), polysorbate 80, propylene glycol

PoM **Dioderm**® (Dermal)
Cream, hydrocortisone 0.1%. Net price 30 g = £2.66. Label: 28. Potency IV
Additives: propylene glycol

PoM **Efcortelan**® (Glaxo)
Cream, hydrocortisone 0.5%, net price, 30 g = 60p; 1%, 30 g = 74p; 2.5%, 30 g = £1.66. Label: 28. Potency IV
Additives: chlorocresol
Ointment, hydrocortisone 0.5%, net price, 30 g = 60p; 1%, 30 g = 74p; 2.5%, 30 g = £1.66. Label: 28. Potency IV
Additives: none as listed in section 13.1

PoM **Hydrocortistab**® (Boots)
Cream, hydrocortisone acetate 1%. Net price 15 g = 33p. Label: 28. Potency IV
Additives: chlorocresol
Ointment, hydrocortisone 1%. Net price 15 g = 33p. Label: 28. Potency IV
Additives: none as listed in section 13.1

PoM **Hydrocortisyl**® (Roussel)
Cream, hydrocortisone 1%. Net price 15 g = 28p. Label: 28. Potency IV
Additives: chlorocresol
Ointment, hydrocortisone 1%. Net price 15 g = 28p. Label: 28. Potency IV
Additives: wool fat

PoM **Mildison**® (Brocades)
Lipocream, hydrocortisone 1%. Net price 30 g = £2.19. Label: 28. Potency IV
Additives: hydroxybenzoates (parabens)

Compound preparations
Note. Compound preparations with coal tar, section 13.5
PoM **Alphaderm**® (Norwich Eaton)
Cream, hydrocortisone 1%, urea 10%. Net price 30 g = £2.42; 100 g = £7.51. Label: 28. Potency III
Additives: none as listed in section 13.1
Apply thinly twice daily

PoM **Calmurid HC**® (Kabi Pharmacia)
Cream, hydrocortisone 1%, urea 10%, lactic acid 5%. Diluent aqueous cream, life of diluted cream 14 days. Net price 30 g = £2.33; 100 g = £6.75. Label: 28. Potency III
Additives: none as listed in section 13.1
Apply thinly twice daily.
Note. Dilute to half-strength with aqueous cream for 1 week if stinging occurs then transfer to undiluted preparation

PoM Epifoam® (Stafford-Miller)
Foam (= application), hydrocortisone acetate 1%, pramoxine hydrochloride 1%, in a muco-adherent basis (pressurised aerosol pack). Net price 12-g unit (approx. 20 applications of 5 mL) = £2.81. Label: 28. Potency IV
Additives: hydroxybenzoates (parabens), propylene glycol
For perineal trauma including post-episiotomy pain and dermatoses
Apply on a pad 3–4 times daily

Eurax-Hydrocortisone® (Zyma)
Cream, hydrocortisone 0.25%, crotamiton 10%. Net price 30 g = 93p. Label: 28. Potency IV
Additives: hydroxybenzoates (parabens), propylene glycol, fragrance
Apply thinly 2–3 times daily

PoM Hydrocal® (Bioglan)
Cream, hydrocortisone acetate 1%, in a basis containing calamine. Net price 25 g = £3.69. Label: 28. Potency IV
Additives: hydroxybenzoates (parabens), polysorbates
Apply thinly 2–3 times daily

PoM Sential® (Kabi Pharmacia)
Cream, hydrocortisone 0.5%, urea 4%, sodium chloride 4%. Net price 30 g = £2.40. Label: 28. Potency IV
Additives: sorbic acid
Apply thinly twice daily

With antimicrobials

PoM Canesten HC® (Baypharm)
Cream, hydrocortisone 1%, clotrimazole 1%. Net price 30 g = £3.18. Label: 28. Potency IV
Additives: benzyl alcohol
Apply thinly twice daily

PoM Daktacort® (Janssen)
Cream, hydrocortisone 1%, miconazole nitrate 2%. Net price 30 g = £2.24. Label: 28. Potency IV
Additives: butylated hydroxyanisole, disodium edetate
Ointment, hydrocortisone 1%, miconazole nitrate 2%. Net price 30 g = £3.10. Label: 28. Potency IV
Additives: none as listed in section 13.1
Apply thinly 2–3 times daily

PoM Econacort® (Squibb)
Cream, hydrocortisone 1%, econazole nitrate 1%. Net price 30 g = £2.85. Label: 28. Potency IV
Additives: butylated hydroxyanisole
Apply thinly twice daily

PoM Fucidin H® (Leo)
Cream, hydrocortisone acetate 1%, fusidic acid 2%. Net price 15 g = £3.30; 30 g = £5.69. Label: 28. Potency IV
Additives: butylated hydroxyanisole, potassium sorbate
Gel, hydrocortisone acetate 1%, fusidic acid 2%. Net price 15 g = £2.91; 30 g = £5.06. Label: 28. Potency IV
Additives: hydroxybenzoates (parabens), polysorbate 80
Ointment, hydrocortisone acetate 1%, sodium fusidate 2%. Net price 15 g = £2.70; 30 g = £4.68. Label: 28. Potency IV
Additives: wool fat
Apply thinly 3–4 times daily

PoM ¹Gentisone® HC (Nicholas)
Cream, hydrocortisone acetate 1%, gentamicin 0.3% (as sulphate). Net price 15 g = £2.05. Label: 28. Potency IV
Additives: hydroxybenzoates (parabens), polysorbates, propylene glycol
Ointment, ingredients as for cream but greasy basis. Net price 15 g = £2.05. Label: 28. Potency IV
Additives: none as listed in section 13.1
Apply thinly 3–4 times daily
1. Formerly Genticin® HC

PoM Gregoderm® (Unigreg)
Ointment, hydrocortisone 1%, neomycin sulphate 0.4%, nystatin 100 000 units/g, polymyxin B sulphate 7250 units/g. Net price 15 g = £2.24. Label: 28. Potency IV
Additives: none as listed in section 13.1
Apply thinly 2–3 times daily

PoM Nystaform-HC® (Bayer)
Cream, hydrocortisone 0.5%, nystatin 100 000 units/g, chlorhexidine hydrochloride 1%. Net price 30 g = £2.73. Label: 28. Potency IV
Additives: benzyl alcohol, polysorbate 60
Ointment, hydrocortisone 1%, nystatin 100 000 units/g, chlorhexidine acetate 1%. Net price 30 g = £2.73. Label: 28. Potency IV
Additives: none as listed in section 13.1
Apply thinly 2–3 times daily

PoM Quinocort® (Quinoderm Ltd)
Cream, hydrocortisone 1%, potassium hydroxyquinoline sulphate 0.5%. Net price 30 g = £2.59. Label: 28. Potency IV
Additives: edetic acid (EDTA), chlorocresol
Apply thinly 2–3 times daily

PoM Terra-Cortril® (Pfizer)
Topical ointment, hydrocortisone 1%, oxytetracycline 3% (as hydrochloride). Net price 15 g = £1.01; 30 g = £1.82. Label: 28. Potency IV
Additives: none as listed in section 13.1
Apply thinly 2–4 times daily
Spray application, hydrocortisone 50 mg, oxytetracycline 150 mg (as hydrochloride) in a pressurised aerosol unit, net price 30-mL = £1.44; double these amounts in 60-mL unit, net price = £2.50. Label: 28. Potency IV
Additives: none as listed in section 13.1
Spray area thinly 2–4 times daily

PoM Terra-Cortril Nystatin® (Pfizer)
Cream, hydrocortisone 1%, nystatin 100 000 units/g, oxytetracycline 3% (as calcium salt). Net price 30 g = £2.01. Label: 28. Potency IV
Additives: hydroxybenzoates (parabens), polysorbate, propylene glycol, fragrance
Apply thinly 2–4 times daily

PoM Timodine® (R&C)
Cream, hydrocortisone 0.5%, nystatin 100 000 units/g, benzalkonium chloride solution 0.2%, dimethicone '350' 10%. Net price 30 g = £2.38. Label: 28. Potency IV
Additives: butylated hydroxyanisole, hydroxybenzoates (parabens), sorbic acid
Apply thinly 3 times daily (napkin rash, after each change)

13.4 Topical corticosteroids

PoM **Tri-Cicatrin**® (Wellcome)
Ointment, hydrocortisone 1%, bacitracin zinc 250 units/g, neomycin sulphate 3400 units/g, nystatin 100 000 units/g. Net price 15 g = £5.23; 30 g = £9.50. Label: 28. Potency IV
Additives: none as listed in section 13.1
Apply thinly 1–3 times daily

PoM **Vioform-Hydrocortisone**® (Zyma)
Cream, hydrocortisone 1%, clioquinol 3%. Net price 30 g = £1.57. Label: 28. Potency IV
Additives: none as listed in section 13.1
Ointment, hydrocortisone 1%, clioquinol 3%. Net price 30 g = £1.57. Label: 28. Potency IV
Additives: none as listed in section 13.1
Apply thinly 1–3 times daily
Caution: stains clothing

HYDROCORTISONE BUTYRATE

Indications: severe inflammatory skin disorders such as eczema unresponsive to less potent corticosteroids
Cautions; Contra-indications; Side-effects: see under Hydrocortisone and notes above
Administration: apply thinly 2–4 times daily, reducing frequency as condition responds

PoM **Locoid**® (Brocades)
Cream, hydrocortisone butyrate 0.1%. Net price 30 g = £2.27; 100 g = £6.95. Label: 28. Potency II
Additives: hydroxybenzoates (parabens)
Lipocream, hydrocortisone butyrate 0.1%. Net price 30 g = £2.38; 100 g = £7.29. Label: 28. Potency II
Additives: hydroxybenzoates (parabens)
Note. For bland cream basis see Lipobase®, section 13.2.1
Ointment, hydrocortisone butyrate 0.1%. Net price 30 g = £2.27; 100 g = £6.95. Label: 28. Potency II
Additives: none as listed in section 13.1
Scalp lotion, hydrocortisone butyrate 0.1%, in an aqueous isopropyl alcohol basis. Net price 30 mL = £3.20; 100 mL = £9.81. Label: 15, 28. Potency II
Additives: none as listed in section 13.1
Apply 1–2 times daily, reducing frequency as condition responds

With antimicrobials
PoM **Locoid C**® (Brocades)
Cream, hydrocortisone butyrate 0.1%, chlorquinaldol 3%. Net price 30 g = £2.97. Label: 28. Potency II
Additives: none as listed in section 13.1
Ointment, ingredients as for cream, in a greasy basis. Net price 30 g = £2.97. Label: 28. Potency II
Additives: none as listed in section 13.1
Apply thinly 2–4 times daily.
Max. 60 g for up to 14 days

ALCLOMETASONE DIPROPIONATE

Indications: inflammatory skin disorders such as eczema
Cautions; Contra-indications; Side-effects: see under Hydrocortisone and notes above
Administration: apply thinly 2–3 times daily, reducing frequency as condition responds

PoM **Modrasone**® (Schering-Plough)
Cream, alclometasone dipropionate 0.05%. Net price 15 g = £1.70; 50 g = £4.80. Label: 28. Potency III
Additives: chlorocresol, propylene glycol
Ointment, alclometasone dipropionate 0.05%. Net price 15 g = £1.70; 50 g = £4.80. Label: 28. Potency III
Additives: beeswax, propylene glycol

BECLOMETHASONE DIPROPIONATE

Indications: severe inflammatory skin disorders such as eczema unresponsive to less potent corticosteroids
Cautions; Contra-indications; Side-effects: see under Hydrocortisone and notes above
Administration: apply thinly twice daily, reducing strength and frequency as condition responds

PoM **Propaderm**® (Glaxo)
Cream, beclomethasone dipropionate 0.025%. Net price 30 g = £1.58. Label: 28. Potency II
Additives: chlorocresol
Ointment, beclomethasone dipropionate 0.025%. Net price 30 g = £1.58. Label: 28. Potency II
Additives: propylene glycol

BETAMETHASONE ESTERS

Indications: severe inflammatory skin disorders such as eczema unresponsive to less potent corticosteroids
Cautions; Contra-indications; Side-effects: see under Hydrocortisone and notes above. Application of more than 100 g per week of 0.1% preparation is likely to cause adrenal suppression
Administration: apply thinly 2–3 times daily, reducing strength and frequency as condition responds

PoM **Betamethasone Valerate** (Non-proprietary)
Cream, betamethasone 0.1% (as valerate). Net price 30 g = £1.40. Label: 28. Potency II
Ointment, betamethasone 0.1% (as valerate). Net price 30 g = £1.40. Label: 28. Potency II

PoM **Betnovate**® (Glaxo)
Cream, betamethasone 0.1% (as valerate), in a water-miscible basis. Net price 30 g = £1.40; 100 g = £3.95; 100 g pump-dispenser = £4.45. Label: 28. Potency II
Additives: chlorocresol

Ointment, betamethasone 0.1% (as valerate), in an anhydrous paraffin basis. Net price 30 g = £1.40; 100 g = £3.95; 100 g pump-dispenser = £4.45. Label: 28. Potency II
Additives: none as listed in section 13.1

Lotion, betamethasone 0.1% (as valerate). Net price 100 mL = £4.75. Label: 28. Potency II
Additives: hydroxybenzoates (parabens)

Scalp application, betamethasone 0.1% (as valerate). Net price 100 mL = £5.18. Label: 15, 28. Potency II
Additives: none as listed in section 13.1

Apply thinly 1–2 times daily, then reduce

PoM **Betnovate-RD**® (Glaxo)
Cream, betamethasone 0.025% (as valerate) in a water-miscible basis (1 in 4 dilution of Betnovate cream). Net price 100 g = £3.26. Label: 28. Potency III
Additives: chlorocresol

Ointment, betamethasone 0.025% (as valerate) in an anhydrous paraffin basis (1 in 4 dilution of Betnovate ointment). Net price 100 g = £3.26. Label: 28. Potency III
Additives: none as listed in section 13.1

PoM **Diprosone**® (Schering-Plough)
Cream, betamethasone 0.05% (as dipropionate). Net price 30 g = £2.57; 100 g = £7.30. Label: 28. Potency II
Additives: chlorocresol
Note. For bland cream basis see Diprobase®, section 13.2.1

Ointment, betamethasone 0.05% (as dipropionate). Net price 30 g = £2.57; 100 g = £7.30. Label: 28. Potency II
Additives: none as listed in section 13.1
Note. For bland ointment basis see Diprobase®, section 13.2.1

Apply thinly once or twice daily

Lotion, betamethasone 0.05% (as dipropionate). Net price 30 mL = £3.25; 100 mL = £9.30. Label: 28. Potency II
Additives: none as listed in section 13.1

Apply twice daily, then reduce

With salicylic acid
PoM **Diprosalic**® (Schering-Plough)
Ointment, betamethasone 0.05% (as dipropionate), salicylic acid 3%. Net price 30 g = £3.30; 100 g = £9.50. Label: 28. Potency II
Additives: none as listed in section 13.1

Scalp application, betamethasone 0.05% (as dipropionate), salicylic acid 2%, in an alcoholic basis. Net price 100 mL = £10.50. Label: 28. Potency II
Additives: disodium edetate

Apply thinly 1–2 times daily; max. 60 g per week

With antimicrobials
PoM **Betnovate-C**® (Glaxo)
Cream, betamethasone 0.1% (as valerate), clioquinol 3%. Net price 30 g = £1.72. Label: 28. Potency II
Additives: chlorocresol

Ointment, betamethasone 0.1% (as valerate), clioquinol 3%. Net price 30 g = £1.72. Label: 28. Potency II
Additives: none as listed in section 13.1

Apply thinly 2–3 times daily
Caution: stains clothing

PoM **Betnovate-N**® (Glaxo)
Cream, betamethasone 0.1% (as valerate), neomycin sulphate 0.5%. Net price 30 g = £1.72; 100 g = £4.77. Label: 28. Potency II
Additives: chlorocresol

Ointment, betamethasone 0.1% (as valerate), neomycin sulphate 0.5%. Net price 30 g = £1.72; 100 g = £4.77. Label: 28. Potency II
Additives: none as listed in section 13.1

Apply thinly 2–3 times daily

PoM **Fucibet**® (Leo)
Cream, betamethasone 0.1% (as valerate), fusidic acid 2%. Net price 15 g = £3.84; 30 g = £6.48. Label: 28. Potency II
Additives: chlorocresol

Apply thinly 2–3 times daily

PoM **Lotriderm**® (Schering-Plough)
Cream, betamethasone 0.05% (as dipropionate), clotrimazole 1%. Net price 15 g = £3.49. Label: 28. Potency II
Additives: benzyl alcohol, propylene glycol

Apply thinly twice daily

BUDESONIDE

Indications: severe inflammatory skin disorders such as eczema

Cautions; Contra-indications; Side-effects: see under Hydrocortisone and notes above

Administration: apply thinly 2–3 times daily

PoM **Preferid**® (Brocades)
Cream, budesonide 0.025%. Net price 30 g = £2.96; 100 g = £9.06. Label: 28. Potency II
Additives: sorbic acid

Ointment, budesonide 0.025%. Net price 30 g = £2.96; 100 g = £9.06. Label: 28. Potency II
Additives: white beeswax, propylene glycol

CLOBETASOL PROPIONATE

Indications: short-term treatment only of severe resistant inflammatory skin disorders such as psoriasis (excluding widespread plaque psoriasis), recalcitrant eczemas, lichen planus, discoid lupus erythematosus unresponsive to less potent corticosteroids

Cautions; Contra-indications; Side-effects: see under Hydrocortisone and notes above. Not more than 50 g of 0.05% preparation should be applied per week

Administration: apply thinly 1–2 times daily for up to 4 weeks, reducing frequency as condition responds

PoM **Dermovate**® (Glaxo)
Cream, clobetasol propionate 0.05%. Net price 30 g = £2.56; 100 g = £7.52. Label: 28. Potency I
Additives: beeswax (or beeswax substitute), chlorocresol, propylene glycol

Ointment, clobetasol propionate 0.05%. Net price 30 g = £2.56; 100 g = £7.52. Label: 28. Potency I
Additives: propylene glycol

Scalp application, clobetasol propionate 0.05%, in a thickened alcoholic basis. Net price 30 mL = £2.93; 100 mL = £9.91. Label: 15, 28. Potency I
Additives: none as listed in section 13.1

13.4 Topical corticosteroids

With antimicrobials
PoM Dermovate-NN® (Glaxo)
Cream, clobetasol propionate 0.05%, neomycin sulphate 0.5%, nystatin 100 000 units/g. Net price 30 g = £3.50. Label: 28. Potency I
Additives: beeswax substitute
Ointment, ingredients as for cream, in a paraffin basis. Net price 30 g = £3.50. Label: 28. Potency I
Additives: none as listed in section 13.1
Apply thinly once or twice daily, for up to 4 weeks reducing as condition responds

CLOBETASONE BUTYRATE
Indications: eczema and dermatitis of all types; maintenance between courses of more potent corticosteroids
Cautions; Contra-indications; Side-effects: see under Hydrocortisone and notes above
Administration: apply thinly up to 4 times daily, reducing frequency as condition responds

PoM Eumovate® (Glaxo)
Cream, clobetasone butyrate 0.05%. Net price 30 g = £1.76; 100 g = £5.16. Label: 28. Potency III
Additives: beeswax substitute, chlorocresol
Ointment, clobetasone butyrate 0.05%. Net price 30 g = £1.76; 100 g = £5.16. Label: 28. Potency III
Additives: none as listed in section 13.1

With antimicrobials
PoM Trimovate® (Glaxo)
Cream, clobetasone butyrate 0.05%, oxytetracycline 3% (as calcium salt), nystatin 100 000 units/g. Net price 30 g = £3.13. Label: 28. Potency III
Additives: chlorocresol

DESOXYMETHASONE
Indications: severe acute inflammatory, allergic, and chronic skin disorders
Cautions; Contra-indications; Side-effects: see under Hydrocortisone and notes above
Administration: apply thinly 2–3 times daily reducing frequency as condition responds

PoM Stiedex® (Stiefel)
Oily cream, desoxymethasone 0.25%. Net price 30 g = £3.43. Label: 28. Potency II
Additives: wool fat
LP Oily cream, desoxymethasone 0.05%. Net price 30 g = £2.86. Label: 28. Potency III
Additives: edetic acid (EDTA), wool fat
Lotion, desoxymethasone 0.25%, salicylic acid 1%. Net price 50 mL = £8.05. Label: 28. Potency II
Additives: disodium edetate, propylene glycol

DIFLUCORTOLONE VALERATE
Indications: severe inflammatory skin disorders such as eczema unresponsive to less potent corticosteroids; high strength (0.3%), short-term treatment of severe exacerbations
Cautions; Contra-indications; Side-effects: see under Hydrocortisone and notes above; not more than 50 g of 0.3% applied per week
Administration: apply thinly 2–3 times daily for up to 4 weeks (0.1% preparations) or 2 weeks (0.3% preparations), reducing strength and frequency as condition responds

PoM Nerisone® (Schering Health Care)
Cream, diflucortolone valerate 0.1%. Net price 30 g = £2.56. Label: 28. Potency II
Additives: disodium edetate, hydroxybenzoates (parabens)
Note. For bland cream basis see Ultrabase®, section 13.2.1
Oily cream, diflucortolone valerate 0.1%. Net price 30 g = £2.56. Label: 28. Potency II
Additives: none as listed in section 13.1
Ointment, diflucortolone valerate 0.1%. Net price 30 g = £2.56. Label: 28. Potency II
Additives: none as listed in section 13.1

PoM Nerisone Forte® (Schering Health Care)
Oily cream, diflucortolone valerate 0.3%. Net price 15 g = £2.09. Label: 28. Potency I
Additives: none as listed in section 13.1
Ointment, diflucortolone valerate 0.3%. Net price 15 g = £2.09. Label: 28. Potency I
Additives: none as listed in section 13.1

FLUCLOROLONE ACETONIDE
Indications: severe inflammatory skin disorders such as eczema unresponsive to less potent corticosteroids
Cautions; Contra-indications; Side-effects: see under Hydrocortisone and notes above
Administration: apply thinly twice daily, reducing frequency as condition responds

PoM Topilar® (Bioglan)
Cream, fluclorolone acetonide 0.025%. Net price 30 g = £2.80; 100 g = £8.39. Label: 28. Potency II
Additives: propylene glycol
Ointment, fluclorolone acetonide 0.025%. Net price 30 g = £2.80; 100 g = £8.39. Label: 28. Potency II
Additives: propylene glycol, wool fat

FLUOCINOLONE ACETONIDE
Indications: inflammatory skin disorders such as eczema, 0.0025–0.01% in milder conditions, 0.025% in severe conditions
Cautions; Contra-indications; Side-effects: see under Hydrocortisone and notes above
Administration: apply thinly 2–3 times daily, reducing strength and frequency as condition responds

Chapter 13: Skin

PoM Synalar® (ICI)
Cream, fluocinolone acetonide 0.025%. Net price 15 g = 78p; 30 g = £1.40; 50 g = £2.10. Label: 28. Potency II
Additives: benzyl alcohol, polysorbates, propylene glycol

Gel, fluocinolone acetonide 0.025%. Net price 30 g = £1.49. For use on scalp and other hairy areas. Label: 28. Potency II
Additives: hydroxybenzoates (parabens), propylene glycol

Ointment, fluocinolone acetonide 0.025%. Net price 15 g = 78p; 30 g = £1.40; 50 g = £2.10. Label: 28. Potency II
Additives: propylene glycol, wool fat

PoM Synalar 1 in 4 Dilution® (ICI)
Cream, fluocinolone acetonide 0.00625%. Net price 50 g = £1.60. Label: 28. Potency III
Additives: benzyl alcohol, polysorbates, propylene glycol

Ointment, fluocinolone acetonide 0.00625%. Net price 50 g = £1.88. Label: 28. Potency III
Additives: propylene glycol, wool fat

PoM Synalar 1 in 10 Dilution® (ICI)
Cream, fluocinolone acetonide 0.0025%. Net price 50 g = £1.52. Label: 28. Potency IV
Additives: benzyl alcohol, polysorbates, propylene glycol

With antibacterials

PoM Synalar C® (ICI)
Cream, fluocinolone acetonide 0.025%, clioquinol 3%. Net price 15 g = 96p. Label: 28. Potency II
Additives: disodium edetate, hydroxybenzoates (parabens), polysorbates, propylene glycol

Ointment, ingredients as for cream. Net price 15 g = 96p. Label: 28. Potency II. *Caution:* stains clothing
Additives: propylene glycol, wool fat

Apply thinly 2–3 times daily

PoM Synalar N® (ICI)
Cream, fluocinolone acetonide 0.025%, neomycin sulphate 0.5%. Net price 15 g = 83p; 30 g = £1.45. Label: 28. Potency II
Additives: hydroxybenzoates (parabens), polysorbates, propylene glycol

Ointment, ingredients as for cream, in a greasy basis. Net price 15 g = 83p; 30 g = £1.45. Label: 28. Potency II
Additives: propylene glycol, wool fat

Apply thinly 2–3 times daily

FLUOCINONIDE

Indications: severe inflammatory skin disorders such as eczema unresponsive to less potent corticosteroids

Cautions; Contra-indications; Side-effects: see under Hydrocortisone and notes above

Administration: apply thinly 3–4 times daily, reducing frequency as condition responds

PoM Metosyn® (Stuart)
FAPG cream, fluocinonide 0.05%. Net price 25 g = £1.25; 100 g = £4.71. Label: 28. Potency II
Additives: propylene glycol

Ointment, fluocinonide 0.05%. Net price 25 g = £1.25; 100 g = £4.71. Label: 28. Potency II
Additives: propylene glycol, wool fat

Scalp lotion, fluocinonide 0.05% in a propylene glycol-alcohol basis. Net price 30 mL (with applicator) = £2.59. Label: 15, 28. Potency II
Additives: propylene glycol

Apply 1–2 times daily, reducing frequency as condition responds

FLUOCORTOLONE

Indications: 0.25%—severe inflammatory skin disorders such as eczema unresponsive to less potent corticosteroids; 0.1%—milder inflammatory skin disorders

Cautions; Contra-indications; Side-effects: see under Hydrocortisone and notes above

Administration: apply thinly 2–3 times daily, reducing strength and frequency as condition responds

PoM Ultradil Plain® (Schering Health Care)
Cream, fluocortolone hexanoate 0.1%, fluocortolone pivalate 0.1%. Net price 50 g = £2.86. Label: 28. Potency III
Additives: disodium edetate, hydroxybenzoates (parabens), fragrance
Note. For bland cream basis see Ultrabase®, section 13.2.1

Ointment, fluocortolone hexanoate 0.1%, fluocortolone pivalate 0.1%. Net price 50 g = £2.86. Label: 28. Potency III
Additives: wool fat, fragrance

PoM Ultralanum Plain® (Schering Health Care)
Cream, fluocortolone hexanoate 0.25%, fluocortolone pivalate 0.25%. Net price 50 g = £4.65. Label: 28. Potency III
Additives: disodium edetate, hydroxybenzoates (parabens), fragrance
Note. For bland cream basis see Ultrabase®, section 13.2.1

Ointment, fluocortolone 0.25%, fluocortolone pivalate 0.25%. Net price 50 g = £4.65. Label: 28. Potency III
Additives: wool fat, fragrance

FLURANDRENOLONE

Indications: eczema and dermatitis of all types

Cautions; Contra-indications; Side-effects: see under Hydrocortisone and notes above

Administration: apply thinly 2–3 times daily, reducing strength and frequency as condition responds

PoM Haelan® (Dista)
Cream, flurandrenolone 0.0125%. Net price 60 g = £2.97. Label: 28. Potency III
Additives: propylene glycol

Ointment, flurandrenolone 0.0125%. Net price 60 g = £2.97. Label: 28. Potency III
Additives: beeswax, polysorbate

With antibacterials

PoM Haelan-C® (Dista)
Cream, flurandrenolone 0.0125%, clioquinol 3%. Net price 30 g = £2.02. Label: 28. Potency III
Additives: hydroxybenzoates (parabens), disodium edetate

Ointment, flurandrenolone 0.0125%, clioquinol 3%. Net price 30 g = £2.02. Label: 28. Potency III
Additives: none as listed in section 13.1
Apply thinly 2–3 times daily
Caution: stains clothing

HALCINONIDE
Indications: severe inflammatory skin disorders such as eczema unresponsive to less potent corticosteroids
Cautions; Contra-indications; Side-effects: see under Hydrocortisone and notes above
Administration: apply thinly 2–3 times daily, reducing frequency as condition responds

PoM **Halciderm Topical**® (Squibb)
Cream, halcinonide 0.1%. Net price 30 g = £3.40. Label: 28. Potency I
Additives: propylene glycol

METHYLPREDNISOLONE ACETATE
Indications: see notes above
Cautions; Contra-indications; Side-effects: see under Hydrocortisone

PoM **Neo-Medrone**® (Upjohn)
Cream, methylprednisolone acetate 0.25%, neomycin sulphate 0.5%. Net price 15 g = £1.44. Label: 28. Potency IV
Additives: butylated hydroxyanisole, butylated hydroxytoluene, hydroxybenzoates (parabens), fragrance
Apply thinly 1–3 times daily

TRIAMCINOLONE ACETONIDE
Indications: severe inflammatory skin disorders such as eczema unresponsive to less potent corticosteroids
Cautions; Contra-indications; Side-effects: see under Hydrocortisone and notes above
Administration: apply thinly 2–4 times daily, reducing frequency as condition responds

PoM **Adcortyl**® (Squibb)
Cream, triamcinolone acetonide 0.1%. Net price 30 g = £1.98. Label: 28. Potency II
Additives: benzyl alcohol, propylene glycol
Ointment, triamcinolone acetonide 0.1%. Net price 30 g = £1.98. Label: 28. Potency II
Additives: none as listed in section 13.1

PoM **Ledercort**® (Lederle)
Cream, triamcinolone acetonide 0.1%. Net price 15 g = £1.72. Label: 28. Potency II
Additives: benzyl alcohol

With antimicrobials
PoM **Adcortyl with Graneodin**® (Squibb)
Cream, triamcinolone acetonide 0.1%, gramicidin 0.025%, neomycin 0.25% (as sulphate). Net price 25 g = £3.00. Label: 28. Potency II
Additives: benzyl alcohol, propylene glycol
Apply thinly 2–4 times daily

PoM **Aureocort**® (Lederle)
Cream, triamcinolone acetonide 0.1%, chlortetracycline hydrochloride 3% (as chlortetracycline), in a water-miscible basis. Net price 15 g = £2.77. Label: 28. Potency II
Additives: chlorocresol
Ointment, triamcinolone acetonide 0.1%, chlortetracycline hydrochloride 3%, in an anhydrous greasy basis containing wool fat and white soft paraffin. Net price 15 g = £2.77. Label: 28. Potency II
Additives: hydroxybenzoates (parabens), wool fat
Caution: stains clothing
Apply thinly 2–3 times daily

PoM **Nystadermal**® (Squibb)
Cream, triamcinolone acetonide 0.1%, nystatin 100 000 units/g. Net price 15 g = £2.27. Label: 28. Potency II
Additives: benzyl alcohol, propylene glycol, fragrance
Apply thinly 2–4 times daily on moist weeping lesions

PoM **Pevaryl TC**® (Cilag)
Cream, triamcinolone 0.1%, econazole nitrate 1%. Net price 15 g = £4.00. Label: 28. Potency II
Additives: butylated hydroxyanisole, disodium edetate, benzoic acid
Apply thinly twice daily for 14 days

PoM **Tri-Adcortyl**® (Squibb)
Cream, triamcinolone acetonide 0.1%, gramicidin 0.025%, neomycin 0.25% (as sulphate), nystatin 100 000 units/g. Net price 30 g = £3.23. Label: 28. Potency II
Additives: benzyl alcohol, ethylenediamine, propylene glycol, fragrance
Ointment, ingredients as for cream, in an ointment basis. Net price 30 g = £3.23. Label: 28. Potency II
Additives: none as listed in section 13.1
Apply thinly 2–4 times daily

13.5 Preparations for psoriasis and eczema

ECZEMA

Eczema ('dermatitis') is due to a particular type of epidermal inflammation and is caused by a wide variety of factors; where possible the causative factors should be established and removed. In many cases no underlying factor can be identified (atopic eczema).

Dry, fissured, scaly lesions are treated with bland **emollients** (section 13.2.1) which are often all that is necessary to allay irritation and permit healing. Preparations containing zinc oxide and calamine are sometimes useful; zinc may have a weak anti-eczematous action. Preparations such as **emulsifying ointment** are used as soap substitutes and in the bath. **Keratolytics** such as salicylic acid, followed by coal tar (see p. 413) are used in chronic eczematous conditions where there is marked thickening of the skin and pronounced scaling.

Weeping eczemas may be treated with corticosteroids (section 13.4) ; they are, however, commonly secondarily infected. Wet dressings of **potassium permanganate** (0.01%) (section 13.11.6) are applied; if a large area is involved, potassium permanganate baths are taken. When necessary **topical antibacterials** are used (section 13.10.1) but those which are not given systemically should be chosen.

Coal tar is more active than salicylic acid and has anti-inflammatory, antipruritic and keratolytic properties. It is used in psoriasis and eczema. Coal tar has superseded wood tar as it is more active. The formulation and strength chosen depends on patient acceptability and severity of the condition; the 'thicker' the patch of eczema or psoriasis the stronger the concentration of coal tar required. **Coal tar paste** or **zinc and coal tar paste** are generally suitable for most cases but are limited by their unpleasant appearance and smell and they may not be used on the face. Some of the newer preparations are less unsightly and may be preferred. Preparations such as Carbo-Dome® are suitable for treating the face. **Zinc paste and coal tar bandage** (section 13.13.1) is useful for treating the limbs. **Tar shampoos** are described in section 13.9. When lesions are extensive coal tar baths are useful. Combinations of coal tar with zinc or salicylic acid have no advantage over the simpler preparations. Preparations containing hydrocortisone and coal tar are useful in eczemas.

Ichthammol has a milder action than coal tar and has been used in the less acute forms of eczema. It can be applied conveniently to flexures of the limbs as **zinc paste and ichthammol bandage** (section 13.13.1).

Gamolenic acid has been claimed to improve patients with eczema and in particular atopic dermatitis. However, the evidence in favour of a useful therapeutic effect is slim.

PSORIASIS

Psoriasis is characterised by epidermal thickening and scaling. It has less tendency to heal spontaneously than eczema. For mild conditions, treatment, other than reassurance and an emollient, may be unnecessary. In more troublesome cases, local application of **salicylic acid**, **coal tar**, or **dithranol** may have a beneficial effect. Topical and systemic corticosteroids should be avoided or given under specialist supervision because, although they may be effective, subsequent treatment becomes more difficult, as tachyphylaxis may occur and they may induce or precipitate severe pustular psoriasis. In resistant cases an antimetabolite, usually methotrexate (see section 8.1.3), may be used for its antimitotic activity but this must always be done under hospital supervision and the dose adjusted according to severity of the condition and in accordance with haematological and biochemical measurements; the usual dose is 10 to 25 mg of methotrexate weekly, usually by mouth.

Salicylic acid may be used in all hyperkeratotic and scaling conditions to enhance the rate of loss of surface scale. Preparations containing salicylic acid 2% are used initially and then gradually increased to concentrations of 3 to 6%. Side-effects are few but include allergic contact sensitivity, or, when large areas are treated, salicylism (see section 10.1.1).

Dithranol is used in psoriasis and is the most potent topical preparation available for this condition. The preparation is applied carefully to the lesion, covered with a dressing, and left for one hour. Traditionally applications have been left on the skin overnight but this has now been shown to be unnecessary as short contact applications of one hour or less are equally effective. Usual concentrations are 0.1–2% although in individual patients 5% or more may be used. Dithranol must be used with caution as it can cause quite severe skin irritation. For this reason it must be applied only to the lesions and it is customary to start with low concentrations and gradually build up to the maximum concentration which produces a therapeutic effect without irritation. Hands should be washed thoroughly after use. Some patients are intolerant to dithranol even in low concentrations; it is important to recognise them early in treatment. Fair skin is more sensitive than dark skin. Proprietary preparations such as Dithrocream® are most commonly used as they may cause less staining and irritation than dithranol paste. Dithranol and urea combinations (Psoradrate®) may improve skin texture by rehydration. **Dithranol triacetate** has no advantage over traditional preparations.

Ingram's method of applying dithranol is sometimes used in hospital. The patient soaks in a warm bath containing coal tar solution 1 in 800 and after drying is exposed to ultraviolet radiation B (UVB) to produce a slight erythema. **Dithranol paste** is applied to the lesions and the normal skin protected by applying talc and stockinette dressings. The procedure is repeated daily.

PUVA, photochemotherapy using psoralens with long-wave ultraviolet irradiation (UVA), is an effective method of treating some patients with psoriasis. Special lamps are required, and a psoralen, generally methoxsalen (available on named-patient basis only) is given by mouth about 2 hours beforehand, to sensitise the skin to the effects of irradiation. A course of PUVA may last 4 to 6 weeks and requires a variable number of treatments. Treatment is only available in specialist centres; it has to be carefully regulated, owing to the short-term hazard of severe burning and the long-term hazards of cataract formation, accelerated ageing, and the development of skin cancer.

Calcipotriol is a vitamin D derivative that has been newly introduced for topical application for mild to moderate psoriasis affecting up to 40% of skin area.

Etretinate is given by mouth for the treatment of severe resistant or complicated psoriasis and some of the congenital disorders of keratinisation including Darier's disease (keratosis follicularis). It should be prescribed **only** by, or under the supervision of, a consultant dermatologist and is available to hospitals **only**. It is a retinoid compound with marked effects on keratinising epithelia. A therapeutic effect occurs after 2 to 4 weeks with maximum benefit after 4 to 6 weeks. Etretinate treats only manifestations not the ultimate causes of these diseases, but treatment should be limited to a period of 6 to 9 months with a 3- to 4-month rest period before repeating treatment, as experience with this drug is limited. Most patients suffer from dryness and cracking of the lips. Other side-effects include a mild transient increase in the rate of hair fall (reversible on withdrawal), occasional generalised pruritus, paronychia, and nose bleeds. There is a tendency for the plasma lipids to rise in some patients. Etretinate is **teratogenic** and must be **avoided** in pregnancy. Contraceptive measures must be taken at least **1 month before** and during treatment by women who may become pregnant and for at least **two years after** a course of the drug.

TOPICAL PREPARATIONS FOR PSORIASIS OR ECZEMA

COAL TAR

Indications: chronic eczema and psoriasis
Cautions: avoid broken or inflamed skin
Side-effects: skin irritation and acne-like eruptions, photosensitivity; stains skin, hair, and fabric
Administration: apply 1–3 times daily starting with low-strength preparations

Note. For shampoo preparations see section 13.9; impregnated dressings see section 13.13.1

Ointments and similar preparations
Calamine and Coal Tar Ointment, BP, calamine 12.5 g, strong coal tar solution 2.5 g, zinc oxide 12.5 g, hydrous wool fat 25 g, white soft paraffin 47.5 g
Coal Tar and Salicylic Acid Ointment, BP, coal tar 2 g, salicylic acid 2 g, emulsifying wax 11.4 g, white soft paraffin 19 g, coconut oil 54 g, polysorbate '80' 4 g, liquid paraffin 7.6 g
Coal Tar Paste, BP, strong coal tar solution 7.5%, in compound zinc paste
Zinc and Coal Tar Paste, BP, zinc oxide 6%, coal tar 6%, emulsifying wax 5%, starch 38%, yellow soft paraffin 45%
Alphosyl® (Stafford-Miller)
Cream, coal tar extract 5%, allantoin 2%, in a vanishing-cream basis. Net price 100 g = £2.50
Additives: beeswax, hydroxybenzoates (parabens), isopropyl palmitate, propylene glycol
For application to skin particularly intertriginous areas, 2–4 times daily
Lotion, coal tar extract 5%, allantoin 2%. Net price 250 mL = £2.27
Additives: isopropyl palmitate, propylene glycol
For application to skin or scalp, 2–4 times daily

Carbo-Dome® (Lagap)
Cream, coal tar solution 10%, in a water-miscible basis. Net price 30 g = £1.97; 100 g = £5.95
Additives: beeswax, hydroxybenzoates (parabens)
Apply 2–3 times daily
Clinitar® (Shire)
Cream, coal tar extract 1%. Net price 100 g = £5.51
Additives: isopropyl palmitate, propylene glycol
Apply 1–2 times daily
Cocois® (Bioglan)
Ointment, coal tar solution 12%, salicylic acid 2%, precipitated sulphur 4%, and coconut oil. Net price 40 g (with applicator nozzle) = £3.41
Additives: none as listed in section 13.1
For dry and scaly scalp conditions, apply at night and remove by washing in the morning
Gelcosal® (Quinoderm Ltd)
Gel, strong coal tar solution 5%, pine tar 5%, salicylic acid 2%. Net price 50 g = £3.12
Additives: none as listed in section 13.1
Apply twice daily
Gelcotar® (Quinoderm Ltd)
Gel, strong coal tar solution 5%, pine tar 5%. Net price 50 g = £2.83; 500 g = £14.74
Additives: none as listed in section 13.1
Apply twice daily
Liquid, see section 13.9
Pragmatar® (Bioglan)
Cream, cetyl alcohol-coal tar distillate 4%, salicylic acid 3%, sulphur (precipitated) 3%. Net price 25 g = £1.90; 100 g = £6.37
Additives: fragrance
Apply thinly daily; for scalp apply weekly to clean hair or in severe cases daily. Dilute with a few drops of water before application to infants
Psoriderm® (Dermal)
Cream, coal tar 6%, lecithin 0.4%. Net price 225 mL = £3.32
Additives: hydroxybenzoates (parabens), isopropyl palmitate, propylene glycol
Apply 1–2 times daily
PsoriGel® (Galderma)
Gel, coal tar solution USP 7.5% in an alcoholic emollient basis. Net price 90 g = £3.81
Additives: propylene glycol
Apply 1–2 times daily

Bath preparations
Coal Tar Solution, BP, coal tar 20%, polysorbate '80' 5%, in alcohol (96%). Net price 100 mL = 56p
Use 100 mL in a bath
Note. Strong Coal Tar Solution BP contains coal tar 40%
Balneum with Tar® (Merck)
Bath oil, coal tar distillate 30%, soya oil 55%. Net price 225 mL = £3.72. For psoriasis and eczema
Additives, none as listed in section 13.1
Use 1 measure (20 mL) in bath (infants 10 mL)
Polytar Emollient® (Stiefel)
Bath additive, coal tar solution 2.5%, arachis oil extract of coal tar 7.5%, tar 7.5%, cade oil 7.5%, liquid paraffin 35%. Net price 350 mL = £4.87. ACBS: for psoriasis, eczema, atopic and pruritic dermatoses
Additives: isopropyl palmitate
Use 2–4 capfuls in bath and soak for 20 minutes

Psoriderm® (Dermal)
Bath emulsion, coal tar 40%. Net price 200 mL = £2.95. For psoriasis
Additives: polysorbate 20
Use 30 mL in a bath and soak for 5 minutes

Coal tar and corticosteroid preparations
PoM **Alphosyl HC®** (Stafford-Miller)
Cream, coal tar extract 5%, hydrocortisone 0.5%, allantoin 2%. Net price 30 g = £1.70; 100 g = £4.85. Label: 28. Potency IV
Additives: beeswax, hydroxybenzoates (parabens), isopropyl palmitate, wool fat
Apply thinly twice daily

PoM **Carbo-Cort®** (Lagap)
Cream, coal tar solution 3%, hydrocortisone 0.25%. Net price 30 g = £3.61. Label: 28. Potency IV
Additives: beeswax, hydroxybenzoates (parabens)
Apply thinly 2–3 times daily

PoM **Tarcortin®** (Stafford-Miller)
Cream, coal tar extract 5%, hydrocortisone 0.5%. Net price 100 g = £3.88. Label: 28. Potency IV
Additives: hydroxybenzoates (parabens), isopropyl palmitate, propylene glycol, polysorbates, fragrance
Apply thinly 2–4 times daily

BUFEXAMAC
Indications: mild inflammatory skin disorders
Cautions: avoid broken skin
Side-effects: skin irritation

PoM **Parfenac®** (Lederle)
Cream, bufexamac 5%. Net price 30 g = £2.16
Additives: hydroxybenzoates (parabens)
Apply thinly 2–3 times daily (not indicated for infants)

CALCIPOTRIOL
Indications: mild to moderate psoriasis
Cautions: pregnancy; avoid use on face and inadvertent transfer to other body areas; wash hands thoroughly after application
Contra-indications: disorders of calcium metabolism
Side-effects: transient local irritation; rarely facial or perioral dermatitis
Administration: apply twice daily; max. 100 g weekly, period of treatment should not exceed 6 weeks

▼ PoM **Dovonex®** (Leo)
Ointment, calcipotriol 50 micrograms/g. Net price 30 g = £7.95; 100 g = £22.85
Additives: disodium edetate, propylene glycol

DITHRANOL
Indications: subacute and chronic psoriasis, see notes above
Cautions: avoid use near eyes; see also notes above
Contra-indications: hypersensitivity; acute psoriasis
Side-effects: local burning sensation and irritation; stains skin, hair, and fabrics
Administration: see notes above

*PoM **Dithranol Ointment, BP,** dithranol, in yellow soft paraffin; usual strengths 0.1–2%. Part of basis may be replaced by hard paraffin if a stiffer preparation is required. Label: 28
*PoM if dithranol content more than 1%, otherwise P

Dithranol Paste, BP, dithranol in zinc and salicylic acid (Lassar's) paste. Usual strengths 0.1–1% of dithranol. Label: 28

Alphodith® (Stafford-Miller)
Ointment, dithranol 0.4%, net price 50 g = £3.50; 1%, 50 g = £4.25; PoM 2%, 50 g = £6.00; PoM 3%, 50 g = £8.50. Label: 10 patient information leaflet, 28. For application to skin or scalp
Additives: none as listed in section 13.1

Anthranol® (Stiefel)
Ointment, dithranol 0.4%, net price 50 g = £3.50; 1%, 50 g = £4.25; PoM 2%, 50 g = £6.00. Label: 28. For application to skin or scalp
Additives: contains salicylic acid 0.5% as an antioxidant

Dithrocream® (Dermal)
Cream, dithranol 0.1%, net price 50 g = £3.96; 0.25%, 50 g = £4.25; 0.5% (Forte), 50 g = £4.89; 1% (HP); 50 g = £5.69; PoM 2%, 50 g = £7.13. Label: 28. For application to skin or scalp
Additives: chlorocresol

Dithrolan® (Dermal)
Ointment, dithranol 0.5%, salicylic acid 0.5%. Net price 90 g = £5.49. Label: 28
Additives: none as listed in section 13.1

Psoradrate® (Norwich Eaton)
Cream, dithranol in a powder-in-cream basis containing urea. 0.1%, net price 30 g = £2.54, 100 g = £7.59; 0.2%, 30 g = £2.81, 100 g = £8.72. Label: 28
Additives: polysorbate 40

Psorin® (Thames)
Ointment, dithranol 0.11%, crude coal tar 1%, salicylic acid 1.6%. Net price 25 g = £2.79; 50 g = £5.30; 100 g = £10.50. Label: 28
Additives: beeswax, wool fat

Dithranol triacetate
Exolan® (Dermal)
Cream, dithranol triacetate 1%. Net price 50 g = £3.00. Label: 28
Additives: chlorocresol
Apply daily to skin and scalp

ICHTHAMMOL
Indications: chronic eczema
Side-effects: skin irritation and sensitisation
Administration: apply 1–3 times daily

Ichthammol Ointment, BP 1980, ichthammol 10%, yellow soft paraffin 45%, wool fat 45%. Net price 25 g = 17p

Zinc and Ichthammol Cream, BP, ichthammol 5%, cetostearyl alcohol 3%, wool fat 10%, in zinc cream. Net price 100 g = 60p

Zinc Paste and Ichthammol Bandage, BP (Ichthopaste®, Icthaband®), see section 13.13.1

SALICYLIC ACID

Indications: hyperkeratoses
Cautions: see notes above; avoid broken or inflamed skin
Side-effects: sensitivity, excessive drying, irritation, systemic effects after prolonged use (see section 10.1.1)

Salicylic Acid Collodion, BP—section 13.7
Salicylic Acid Ointment, BP, salicylic acid 2%, in wool alcohols ointment. Net price 25 g = 16p
Apply twice daily
Zinc and Salicylic Acid Paste, BP (Lassar's Paste), zinc oxide 24%, salicylic acid 2%, starch 24%, white soft paraffin 50%. Net price 25 g = 15p
Apply twice daily

ORAL PREPARATIONS FOR
PSORIASIS OR ECZEMA

ETRETINATE

Indications: severe extensive psoriasis resistant to other forms of therapy; palmo-plantar pustular psoriasis; severe congenital ichthyosis; severe Darier's disease (keratosis follicularis)
Cautions: exclude pregnancy before starting—patients should avoid pregnancy at least 1 month before, during, and for at least 2 years after treatment, should avoid concomitant high doses of vitamin A and use of keratolytics, and should not donate blood during or for 2 years after stopping therapy (teratogenic risk); monitor hepatic function and plasma lipids (especially in hypertriglyceridaemia) at start, 1 month after initiating treatment, and then at intervals of 3 months; diabetes (can alter glucose tolerance); radiographic assessment on long-term treatment; investigate atypical musculoskeletal symptoms; avoid long-term use in children (skeletal hyperostosis and extra-osseous calcification); **interactions:** Appendix 1 (etretinate)
Contra-indications: hepatic and renal impairment; pregnancy (**important teratogenic risk:** see Cautions and Appendix 4); breast-feeding
Side-effects: (mainly dose-related) dryness of mucous membranes (sometimes erosion), of skin (sometimes scaling, thinning, erythema, and pruritus), and of conjunctiva (sometimes conjunctivitis); palmar and plantar exfoliation, epistaxis, and epidermal fragility reported, also paronychia; granulomatous lesions reported; reversible alopecia; myalgia and arthralgia; occasional nausea, headache, malaise, drowsiness and sweating; benign intracranial hypertension reported (avoid concomitant tetracyclines); raised liver enzymes, rarely jaundice and hepatitis (avoid concomitant methotrexate); raised triglycerides; decreased night vision reported
Dose: administered in accordance with expert advice, adults and children, initially up to 750 micrograms/kg daily in divided doses for 2–4 weeks, increased to 1 mg/kg daily if necessary (max. daily dose 75 mg), then reduced to 500 micrograms/kg daily for a further 6–8 weeks, then intermittently as necessary; usual maintenance dose 250–500 micrograms/kg daily (**important:** see Cautions and notes above)

PoM **Tigason®** (Roche)
Capsules, etretinate 10 mg (yellow), net price 56-cap pack = £20.40; 25 mg (orange/yellow), 56-cap pack = £44.05 (**hosp. only,** specialist dermatological supervision). Label: 10, patient information card, 21

GAMOLENIC ACID

Indications: see under preparations
Cautions: history of epilepsy, concomitant treatment with epileptogenic drugs e.g. phenothiazines
Side-effects: occasional nausea, indigestion, headache
Dose: see below

PoM **Epogam®** (Searle)
Capsules, gamolenic acid 40 mg in evening primrose oil. Net price 240-cap pack = £25.04. Counselling, see below
Additives: include vitamin E 10 mg as *in vivo* antioxidant
Dose: symptomatic relief of atopic eczema 4–6 capsules twice daily; CHILD 1–12 years 2–4 capsules twice daily
Paediatric capsules, gamolenic acid 80 mg in evening primrose oil. Net price 60-cap pack = £15.80. Counselling, see below
Additives: include vitamin E 20 mg as *in vivo* antioxidant
Dose: symptomatic relief of atopic eczema CHILD over 1 year, 1–2 capsules twice daily
COUNSELLING. Capsules may be cut open and contents swallowed or taken on bread; paediatric capsules have 'snip-off' neck for convenience of administration

Mastalgia (for advice see p. 283)
PoM **Efamast®** (Searle)
Capsules, gamolenic acid 40 mg in evening primrose. Net price 224-cap pack = £24.33
Additives: include vitamin E 10 mg as *in vivo* antioxidant
Dose: symptomatic relief of cyclical and non-cyclical mastalgia, 3–4 capsules twice daily

13.6 Preparations for acne

TOPICAL TREATMENT. Most topical preparations are intended for removing follicular plugs and reducing skin flora. The skin is cleansed regularly with detergent solutions, for example cetrimide solution (section 13.11.3). Abrasive agents may also be used but their effectiveness is uncertain.

Cleansing is followed by application of **antiseptics** and **keratolytics**; thick greasy preparations should not be used. Preparations usually contain benzoyl peroxide, hydroxyquinoline, sulphur, salicylic acid, or tretinoin. Many of these irritate the skin but it is doubtful if a therapeutic effect can be obtained without some degree of irritation (which subsides with continued treatment). Topical application of **tretinoin** (Retin-A®) a vitamin

A derivative has been shown to be useful in treating acne but patients should be warned that some redness and skin peeling may occur after application for several days.

Topical antibiotics are also used for mild to moderately severe acne. Topical preparations of erythromycin, tetracycline, and clindamycin seem to be quite useful for many patients with the milder forms of acne; they can produce mild irritation of the skin but rarely sensitise. It has been suggested that percutaneous absorption of clindamycin can cause pseudomembranous colitis. Chloramphenicol is included in some preparations but can sensitise the skin; topical neomycin is not suitable owing to sensitisation. Antibiotics cause resistant strains of micro-organisms to appear but as yet no adverse clinical effects have resulted.

Topical **corticosteroids** should **not** be used in acne.

SYSTEMIC TREATMENT. Systemic antibacterial treatment is useful. **Tetracycline** (see section 5.1.3), **erythromycin** (see section 5.1.5), and occasionally other antibacterials are used. The usual dosage regimen for tetracycline and erythromycin, taken before meals, is 250 mg 3 times daily for 1–4 weeks and then reduced to twice daily until improvement occurs. Higher doses are sometimes indicated when there is a poor response to the usual regimen; in general the dose of the antibiotic used should be matched to the patient's condition. Maximum improvement usually occurs after three or four months but in resistant cases treatment may need to be continued for two or more years. As there have been some reports of pseudomembranous colitis with tetracycline, caution is necessary in long-term administration.

Cyproterone acetate with **ethinyloestradiol** (Dianette®) contains an anti-androgen and is used to treat women with severe acne refractory to prolonged oral antibacterial therapy. Improvement of acne probably occurs because of decreased sebum secretion which is under androgen control. Some women with mild to moderate idiopathic hirsutism may also benefit as hair growth is also androgen-dependent (see also section 6.4.2). Dianette® may also be used as an oral contraceptive but should be reserved for women who are being treated for androgen-dependent skin conditions. It is contra-indicated in pregnancy and in a predisposition to thrombosis.

Isotretinoin (Roaccutane®) is used for the systemic treatment of cystic and conglobate acne and severe acne which has failed to respond to an adequate course of a systemic antimicrobial agent. It should be prescribed **only** by, or under the supervision of, a consultant dermatologist, and is available to hospitals **only**. It is given in doses of 500 micrograms/kg/day for 12–16 weeks but doses may be adjusted if necessary after 4 weeks. Repeat courses should not normally be given. An exacerbation is common some 2–4 weeks after starting treatment but usually subsides after a few weeks.

Side-effects include dry lips, sore eyes, nose bleeds, mild transient hair loss, and joint pains. Plasma lipids and liver function should be checked by investigation monthly as there is a tendency for the plasma lipids to rise in some patients. The drug is **teratogenic** and must **not** be given to women who are pregnant or those who may become pregnant unless there is concomitant effective contraception and then only after detailed explanation by the physician. The contraceptive measures must continue for at least **one month** after ceasing treatment with the drug.

TOPICAL ACNE PREPARATIONS

ABRASIVE AGENTS

Indications: cleansing in acne vulgaris
Cautions: avoid contact with eyes; discontinue use temporarily if skin becomes irritated
Contra-indications: superficial venules, telangiectasia

Brasivol® (Stiefel)
Paste No. 1, aluminium oxide 38.09% in fine particles, in a soap-detergent basis. Net price 75 g = £2.49
Additives: fragrance
Paste No. 2, aluminium oxide 52.2% in medium particles, in a soap-detergent basis. Net price 75 g = £2.49
Additives: fragrance
Use instead of soap 1–3 times daily, starting with fine grade

Ionax Scrub® (Galderma)
Gel, polyethylene granules 21.9%, benzalkonium chloride 0.25% in a foaming aqueous alcoholic basis. Net price 60 g = £3.13. ACBS: for control and hygiene of acne and cleansing of the skin prior to acne treatment
Additives: propylene glycol
Use instead of soap 1–2 times daily

ANTIBIOTICS

Indications: acne vulgaris
Cautions: alcoholic preparations are not suitable for use with benzoyl peroxide; max. duration of treatment 10–12 weeks

PoM **Dalacin T®** (Upjohn)
Topical solution, clindamycin (as phosphate) 1%, in an aqueous alcoholic basis. Net price 30 mL (with applicator) = £6.05
Additives: propylene glycol
Apply to clean skin twice daily
Lotion, clindamycin (as phosphate) 1% in an aqueous basis. Net price 30 mL = £6.65
Additives: hydroxybenzoates (parabens)
Apply to clean skin twice daily

PoM **Stiemycin®** (Stiefel)
Solution, erythromycin 2% in an alcoholic basis. Net price 2 × 25 mL applicator bottles = £9.00
Additives: propylene glycol
Apply to clean skin twice daily

13.6 Preparations for acne 417

PoM **Topicycline**® (Norwich Eaton)
Solution, powder for reconstitution, tetracycline hydrochloride, 4-epitetracycline hydrochloride, providing tetracycline hydrochloride 2.2 mg/mL when reconstituted with solvent containing n-decyl methyl sulphoxide and citric acid in 40% alcohol. Net price per pack of powder and solvent to provide 70 mL = £7.90
Additives: none as listed in section 13.1
Apply to clean skin twice daily

PoM **Zineryt**® (Brocades)
Topical solution, powder for reconstitution, erythromycin 40 mg, zinc acetate 12 mg/mL when reconstituted with solvent containing ethanol. Net price per pack of powder and solvent to provide 30 mL = £8.04
Additives: none as listed in section 13.1
Apply to clean skin twice daily

BENZOYL PEROXIDE

Indications: acne vulgaris
Cautions: avoid contact with eyes, mouth, and mucous membranes; may bleach fabrics
Side-effects: skin irritation
Administration: apply 1–2 times daily to clean skin, starting treatment with lower-strength preparations

Acetoxyl® (Stiefel)
'2.5' Gel, benzoyl peroxide 2.5%, in an aqueous-acetone-gel basis. Net price 40 g = £1.59
Additives: propylene glycol
'5' Gel, benzoyl peroxide 5%, in an aqueous-acetone-gel basis. Net price 40 g = £1.76
Additives: propylene glycol

Acnegel® (Stiefel)
Gel, benzoyl peroxide 5%, in an aqueous alcoholic basis. Net price 50 g = £2.17
Additives: none as listed in section 13.1
Forte gel, benzoyl peroxide 10%, in an aqueous alcoholic basis. Net price 50 g = £2.38
Additives: none as listed in section 13.1

Acnidazil® (Cilag)
Cream, benzoyl peroxide 5%, miconazole nitrate 2%. Net price 15 g = £2.10; 30 g = £3.40
Additives: polysorbate 20, propylene glycol

Benoxyl® (Stiefel)
'5' Cream, benzoyl peroxide 5%, in a non-greasy basis. Net price 40 g = £1.29
Additives: isopropyl palmitate, propylene glycol
'5' Lotion, benzoyl peroxide 5%, in a non-greasy basis. Net price 30 mL = £1.03
Additives: isopropyl palmitate, propylene glycol
'10' Lotion, benzoyl peroxide 10%, in a water-miscible basis. Net price 30 mL = £1.09
Additives: isopropyl palmitate, propylene glycol

Benzagel® (Bioglan)
'5' Gel, benzoyl peroxide 5%. Net price 40 g = £2.40
Additives: fragrance
'10' Gel, benzoyl peroxide 10%. Net price 40 g = £2.74
Additives: fragrance

Nericur® (Schering Health Care)
Gel 5, benzoyl peroxide 5%, in an aqueous gel basis. Net price 30 g = £1.45
Additives: propylene glycol
Gel 10, benzoyl peroxide 10%, in an aqueous gel basis. Net price 30 g = £1.60
Additives: propylene glycol

Panoxyl® (Stiefel)
'2.5' Aquagel (= aqueous gel), benzoyl peroxide 2.5%. Net price 40 g = £1.72
Additives: propylene glycol
'5' Gel, benzoyl peroxide 5%, in an aqueous alcoholic basis. Net price 40 g = £1.44
Additives: fragrance
'5' Aquagel (= aqueous gel), benzoyl peroxide 5%. Net price 40 g = £1.92
Additives: propylene glycol
'10' Gel, benzoyl peroxide 10%, in an aqueous alcoholic basis. Net price 40 g = £1.63
Additives: fragrance
'10' Aquagel (= aqueous gel), benzoyl peroxide 10%. Net price 40 g = £2.12
Additives: propylene glycol
'10' Wash, benzoyl peroxide 10%, in a detergent basis. Net price 150 mL = £3.50
Additives: none as listed in section 13.1

With antimicrobials
Quinoderm® (Quinoderm Ltd)
Cream, benzoyl peroxide 10%, potassium hydroxyquinoline sulphate 0.5%, in an astringent vanishing-cream basis. Net price 25 g = £1.24; 50 g = £1.86
Additives: edetic acid (EDTA)
Cream 5, benzoyl peroxide 5%, potassium hydroxyquinoline sulphate 0.5%, in an astringent vanishing-cream basis. Net price 50 g = £1.69
Additives: edetic acid (EDTA)
Lotio-gel 5%, benzoyl peroxide 5%, potassium hydroxyquinoline sulphate 0.5%, in an astringent creamy basis. Net price 30 mL = £1.47
Additives: edetic acid (EDTA)

CORTICOSTEROIDS

Indications: not recommended (see notes above)
Cautions; Contra-indications; Side-effects: section 13.4 and notes above

PoM **Actinac**® (Roussel)
Lotion (powder for reconstitution), chloramphenicol 1.25%, hydrocortisone acetate 1.25%, allantoin 0.75%, butoxyethyl nicotinate 0.75%, precipitated sulphur 10%, when reconstituted with solvent. Discard after 21 days. Net price 2 × 6.25 g bottles powder with 2 × 20-mL bottles solvent = £9.54. Label: 28. Potency IV
Additives: fragrance

PoM **Quinoderm with Hydrocortisone**® (Quinoderm Ltd)
Cream, hydrocortisone 1%, benzoyl peroxide 10%, potassium hydroxyquinoline sulphate 0.5%, in an astringent vanishing-cream basis. Net price 30 g = £1.77. Label: 28. Potency IV
Additives: edetic acid (EDTA)

SULPHUR

Cautions: avoid contact with eyes, mouth, and mucous membranes; causes skin irritation

With resorcinol
Prolonged application of resorcinol may interfere with thyroid function therefore not recommended

Eskamel® (SK&F)
Cream, resorcinol 2%, sulphur 8%, in a non-greasy flesh-coloured basis. Net price 25 g = £1.26
Additives: propylene glycol, fragrance

Cautionary label wordings, see inside back cover
Prices are **net**, see p. 1

With salicylic acid
Salicylic Acid and Sulphur Cream, BP 1980, salicylic acid 2%, precipitated sulphur 2%, in aqueous cream
Salicylic Acid and Sulphur Ointment, BPC, salicylic acid 3%, precipitated sulphur 3%, in hydrous ointment (oily cream). Net price 25 g = 21p

TRETINOIN

Indications: acne vulgaris

Cautions: avoid contact with eyes, mouth, and mucous membranes; do not use simultaneously with other peeling agents (can be alternated every 12 hours with benzoyl peroxide); do not use with ultra-violet lamps

Contra-indications: eczema, broken skin

Side-effects: irritation, erythema, peeling, with excessive use; changes in pigmentation, photosensitivity

Administration: apply to clean skin 1–2 times daily

PoM **Retin-A**® (Cilag)
Cream, tretinoin 0.025%, net price 60 g = £6.03; 0.05% (cream forte), 60 g = £6.03. For dry or fair skin
Additives: butylated hydroxytoluene, sorbic acid
Gel, tretinoin 0.01%, net price 60 g = £6.03; 0.025% (gel forte), 60 g = £6.03. For severe acne, initial treatment, or dark and oily skins
Additives: butylated hydroxytoluene
Lotion, tretinoin 0.025%. Net price 100 mL = £6.94. For application to large areas such as the back
Additives: butylated hydroxytoluene

ORAL PREPARATIONS

CYPROTERONE ACETATE

Indications: see notes above

Cautions; Contra-indications; Side-effects: see under Combined Oral Contraceptives (section 7.3.1)

PoM **Dianette**® (Schering Health Care)
Tablets, beige, s/c, cyproterone acetate 2 mg, ethinyloestradiol 35 micrograms. Net price 21-tab pack = £4.80
Dose: 1 tablet daily for 21 days starting on 1st day of menstrual cycle and repeated after a 7-day interval, usually for several months; withdraw when acne or hirsutism completely resolved (repeat courses may be given if recurrence)

ISOTRETINOIN

Indications: see notes above

Cautions: exclude pregnancy before starting—pregnancy must be avoided at least 1 month before, during, and for at least 1 month after treatment; avoid donating blood during and for at least 1 month after treatment; monitor hepatic function and plasma lipids at start, 1 month after initiating treatment, then at intervals; avoid high doses of vitamin A and use of keratolytics during treatment; monitor blood glucose in diabetic patients

Contra-indications: pregnancy (**important teratogenic risk:** see Cautions and Appendix 4); breast-feeding; renal or hepatic impairment

Side-effects: (mainly dose-related) dryness of skin (with scaling, thinning, erythema, pruritus), epidermal fragility (trauma may cause blistering); dryness of nasal mucosa (with mild epistaxis), dryness of conjunctiva (sometimes conjunctivitis), decreased tolerance to contact lenses; visual disturbances (papilloedema, optic neuritis, corneal opacities, decreased night vision, blurred vision); hair thinning (reversible on withdrawal); nausea, headache, malaise, drowsiness, sweating; benign intracranial hypertension (avoid concomitant tetracyclines); myalgia and arthralgia; raised liver enzymes; raised plasma triglycerides and cholesterol; allergic vasculitis and granulomatous lesions reported

Dose: initially 500 micrograms/kg daily in 1–2 divided doses with food for 4 weeks; if good response continue for further 8–12 weeks; if little response, up to 1 mg/kg daily for 8–12 weeks; if intolerant, reduce dose to 100–200 micrograms/kg daily

PoM **Roaccutane**® (Roche)
Capsules, isotretinoin 5 mg (red-violet/white), net price 56-cap pack = £19.08; 20 mg (red-violet/white), 56-cap pack = £54.98 (**hosp. only,** specialist dermatological supervision). Label: 10, patient information card, 21

13.7 Preparations for warts and calluses

The least destructive method possible should be chosen to treat these lesions as they are self-limiting and all viral warts including those on the soles of the feet (verrucas) eventually disappear spontaneously. The preparations used are keratolytics which slowly remove the hyperkeratotic layers and destroy the underlying epidermis.

Salicylic acid preparations are useful but can cause considerable irritation of the treated area. They are suitable for the removal of *warts and calluses.* An ointment containing podophyllum resin with salicylic acid (*Posalfilin*®) is available for treating *plantar warts.*

Podophyllum preparations may also be useful but again can cause considerable irritation of the treated area and podophyllum treatment may be painful. Podophyllum resin made into a paint, in concentrations of between 5 and 20% is employed for the treatment of *anogenital warts.* The paint should be allowed to stay on the treated area for not longer than 6 hours and then washed off. Care should be taken to avoid splashing the surrounding skin during application; it must be covered with soft paraffin as a protection. Where there are a large number of warts only a few should be treated at any one time as **severe toxicity** caused by absorption of podophyllin has been reported. It should also be avoided in pregnancy.

13.7 Preparations for warts and calluses

Preparations containing the standardised active ingredient **podophyllotoxin** (*Condyline®*, *Warticon®*) are also available for *anogenital warts*.

Preparations containing **formaldehyde, glutaraldehyde**, and **bromine** are also available but their effects are unpredictable. Formaldehyde and glutaraldehyde preparations may both irritate and sensitise the skin.

SALICYLIC ACID

Indications: see under preparations
Cautions: protect surrounding skin and avoid broken skin; not suitable for application to face, anogenital region, or large areas
Contra-indications: diabetes or if peripheral blood circulation impaired
Side-effects: skin irritation, see notes above
ADMINISTRATION. Instructions in proprietary packs generally incorporate advice to remove dead skin by gentle rubbing with a pumice stone and to cover with plaster after application (unless in collodion basis)

Salicylic Acid Collodion, BP, salicylic acid 12%, in flexible collodion. Label: 15. For warts and calluses, apply daily or on alternate days
Cuplex® (S&N Pharm.)
Gel, salicylic acid 11%, lactic acid 4%, copper acetate (= Cu²⁺ 0.0011%), in a collodion basis. Net price 5 g = £2.39. Label: 15. For plantar and mosaic warts, corns, and calluses, apply twice daily
Duofilm® (Stiefel)
Paint, salicylic acid 16.7%, lactic acid 16.7%, in flexible collodion. Net price 15 mL (with applicator) = £1.95. Label: 15. For plantar and mosaic warts, apply daily
Salactol® (Dermal)
Paint, salicylic acid 16.7%, lactic acid 16.7%, in flexible collodion. Net price 10 mL (with applicator) = £1.98. Label: 15. For warts, particularly plantar warts, verrucas, corns, and calluses, apply daily
Salatac® (Dermal)
Gel, salicylic acid 12%, lactic acid 4% in a collodion basis. Net price 8 g (with applicator) = £3.45. Label: 15. For warts, verrucas, corns, and calluses, apply daily
Verrugon® (Pickles)
Ointment, salicylic acid 50% in a paraffin basis. Net price 6 g = £1.35. For plantar warts daily

With podophyllum
Posalfilin® (Norgine)
Ointment, podophyllum resin 20%, salicylic acid 25%. Net price 10 g = £3.20. For plantar warts only, apply 2–3 times weekly
Note. Not suitable for anogenital warts

BROMINE COMPLEXES

Indications: see under preparations
Cautions; Contra-indications; Side-effects: see under Salicylic Acid

Callusolve® (Dermal)
Paint, benzalkonium chloride-bromine adduct 25%. Net price 10 mL (with applicator) = £2.44. For warts, particularly plantar and mosaic warts, apply daily

FORMALDEHYDE

Indications: see under preparations
Cautions; Contra-indications; Side-effects: see under Salicylic Acid

Formaldehyde Lotion, formaldehyde solution, BP, 3 mL, water to 100 mL. For plantar warts, applied at night as a soak
Veracur® (Typharm)
Gel, formaldehyde solution 1.5% in a water-miscible gel basis. Net price 15 g = £1.15. For warts, particularly plantar warts, apply twice daily

GLUTARALDEHYDE

Indications: see under preparations
Cautions; Contra-indications; Side-effects: see under Salicylic Acid, stains skin brown

Glutarol® (Dermal)
Solution (= application), glutaraldehyde 10%. Net price 10 mL (with applicator) = £2.25. For warts, particularly plantar warts, apply twice daily
Novaruca® (Bioglan)
Gel, glutaraldehyde 10%. Net price 15 g = £1.95. For warts, particularly plantar warts, apply twice daily
Verucasep® (Galen)
Gel, glutaraldehyde 10%. Net price 15 g = £1.95. For warts, particularly plantar warts, apply twice daily

PODOPHYLLUM RESIN

Indications: see under preparations
Cautions: avoid normal skin and open wounds; keep away from face; very irritant to eyes; **important:** see also notes above
Contra-indications: pregnancy
Side-effects: may cause pain on application; see also notes above

PoM **Podophyllin Paint, Compound, BP,** (podophyllum resin 15% in compound benzoin tincture), podophyllum resin 1.5 g, compound benzoin tincture to 10 mL; 5 mL to be dispensed unless otherwise directed. Label: 15.
External anogenital warts, applied weekly in genito-urinary clinic (**important cautions**, see notes above)

Podophyllotoxin
PoM **Condyline®** (Brocades)
Solution, podophyllotoxin 0.5% in alcoholic basis. Net price 3.5 mL (with applicators) = £16.00. Label: 15
External anogenital warts (condylomata acuminata), apply twice daily for 3 consecutive days; treatment may be repeated after 7 days if necessary; max. 5 treatment courses; direct medical supervision for lesions in the female and for lesions greater than 4 cm² in the male

PoM **Warticon**® (Perstorp)
Solution, podophyllotoxin 0.5% in alcoholic basis. Net price 3 mL (with applicators) = £16.00. Label: 15
Penile warts in preputial space (condylomata acuminata), apply twice daily for 3 consecutive days; treatment may be repeated after 7 days if necessary; max. 5 treatment courses; direct medical supervision for lesions greater than 4 cm^2

CRYOTHERAPY

Histofreezer® (Thames, direct mail), an aerosol kit consisting of ether (diethyl ether) and propane, is available as an alternative to liquid nitrogen for cryotherapy of warts. The kit includes 40 cotton bud applicators and a detailed instruction booklet. It is not available on the NHS but a claim can be made for removal of warts as a minor surgical procedure.

13.8 Sunscreens and camouflagers

13.8.1 Sunscreening preparations
13.8.2 Camouflaging preparations

> BORDERLINE SUBSTANCES. The preparations marked 'ACBS' are regarded as drugs when prescribed for skin protection against ultraviolet radiation in photodermatoses, including those resulting from radiotherapy. Prescriptions issued in accordance with this advice and endorsed 'ACBS' will normally not be investigated. Preparations with SPF less than 15 are no longer prescribable. See Appendix 7 for listing by clinical condition.

13.8.1 Sunscreening preparations

Solar ultraviolet irradiation is harmful to the skin. It is responsible for disorders such as polymorphic light eruption, Hutchinson's summer prurigo, and the various cutaneous porphyrias. It also provokes (or at least aggravates) disorders such as rosacea and lupus erythematosus. It may also contribute to serious skin disorders in patients sensitised by drugs such as demeclocycline, phenothiazines, or amiodarone. All these conditions (as well as sunburn) may occur after relatively short periods of exposure to the sun. Exposure over longer periods may cause more serious problems. Both melanoma and non-melanoma skin cancer are now thought to be caused in many instances by solar ultraviolet irradiation. It is now also believed that exposure to the sun causes the skin to wrinkle and develop other signs associated with aging.

Solar ultraviolet radiation is approximately 200–400 nm in wavelength. The medium wavelengths (280–310 nm, known as UVB) cause sunburn and contribute to the long-term changes responsible for skin cancer and aging. The long wavelengths (310–400 nm, known as UVA) do not cause sunburn but are responsible for many photosensitivity reactions and photodermatoses; they also seem to contribute to long-term damage and to be involved in the pathogenesis of skin cancer and aging.

Sunscreen preparations that contain substances such as aminobenzoic acid protect the skin against UVB and hence against sunburn. The sun protection factor (SPF, usually indicated in the preparation title) provides guidance on the degree of protection offered against UVB; it indicates the multiples of protection provided against burning, compared with unprotected skin; for example, an SPF of 8 should enable a person to remain 8 times longer in the sun without burning. Such preparations, however, do not prevent long-term damage associated with UVA, which might not become apparent for 10 to 20 years. Preparations that also contain reflective substances, such as titanium dioxide, provide the most effective protection against UVA. Some products now indicate the degree of protection offered against UVA with a star rating system. This system does not refer to an absolute measure but indicates the protection against UVA relative to protection against UVB for the same product. Four stars indicate that the product offers a balanced amount of UVA and UVB protection; products with three, two, or one star rating indicate that the protection offered is greater against UVB than UVA. However the usefulness of the star rating system remains controversial.

Some sunscreens, particularly aminobenzoates, may rarely cause photosensitivity reactions. Bergamot oil (which contains 5-methoxypsoralen) occasionally causes photosensitisation with subsequent pigmentation; it is suspected of increasing the incidence of skin cancers, but this has not been established.

Almay Total Sunbloc® (Sara Lee)
Cream, (SPF 15), padimate-O 7%, oxybenzone 3%, titanium dioxide. Net price 50 mL = £2.87. ACBS
Additives: disodium edetate, hydroxybenzoates (parabens), propylene glycol
Lip protector, (SPF 15), padimate-O 7%, oxybenzone 3%. Net price 10 mL = £1.71. ACBS
Additives: butylated hydroxyanisole, hydroxybenzoates (parabens), propylene glycol

Coppertone® (Scholl)
Sunstick 15, titanium dioxide 17.6% in wax-based stick. Net price 6 g = £2.46. ACBS
Additives: butylated hydroxytoluene, hydroxybenzoates (parabens), wool fat, fragrance
Supershade 15 lotion, padimate-O 7%, oxybenzone 3%. Net price 125 mL = £4.21. ACBS
Additives: wool fat, fragrance
Ultrashade 23 lotion, ethylhexyl p-methoxycinnamate 7.5%, oxybenzone 3%, padimate-O 2.5%. Net price 150 mL = £4.46. ACBS
Additives: hydroxybenzoates (parabens), wool fat, fragrance

Piz Buin® (Zyma)
Sunblock lotion, (SPF 24), ethylhexyl p-methoxycinnamate 7.5%, butyl methoxydibenzoylmethane 2%, titanium dioxide 3%. Net price 125 mL = £6.13. ACBS
Additives: hydroxybenzoates (parabens), propylene glycol, fragrance

RoC® (RoC)
Total sunblock cream, (SPF over 15), colourless or tinted, ethylhexyl *p*-methoxycinnamate 5%, oxybenzone 4%, dibenzoylmethane 2%, titanium dioxide 4%. Net price 50 mL = £3.57. ACBS
Additives: beeswax, hydroxybenzoates (parabens)
Sunscreen stick, (SPF 10–15), cinnamic ester 7.5%, dibenzoylmethane 4%. Net price 3-g stick = £2.07. ACBS
Additives: none as listed in section 13.1

Spectraban® (Stiefel)
Lotion, (SPF 15) aminobenzoic acid 5%, padimate-O 3.2%, in an alcoholic basis. Net price 150 mL = £2.49. ACBS
Additives: fragrance
Caution: flammable; stains clothing
Ultra lotion, (SPF 17), water resistant, butyl methoxydibenzoylmethane 2%, oxybenzone 3%, padimate-O 8%, titanium dioxide 2%. Net price 150 mL = £4.32. ACBS
Additives: benzyl alcohol, disodium edetate, sorbic acid, fragrance

Sun E45® (Crookes)
Sunblock cream, (SPF 25), water resistant, titanium dioxide 18%. Net price 75 mL = £3.91. ACBS.
Additives: butylated hydroxytoluene, isopropyl palmitate
Ultra protection lotion, (SPF 15), water resistant, titanium dioxide 13.4%. Net price 150 mL = £4.89. ACBS
Additives: butylated hydroxytoluene, isopropyl palmitate

Uvistat® (Windsor)
Cream (SPF 15), water-resistant, mexenone 4%, ethylhexyl *p*-methoxycinnamate 7.5%, butyl methoxydibenzoylmethane 2%. Net price 100 g = £4.14. ACBS
Additives: Hydroxybenzoates (parabens), fragrance
Lipscreen, (SPF 15), mexenone 2%, ethylhexyl *p*-methoxycinnamate 6%, butyl methoxydibenzoylmethane 2%. Net price 5-g stick = £1.24. ACBS (also sunlight-provoked chronic or recurrent herpes labialis)
Additives: fragrance
Cream (SPF 20), water-resistant, ethylhexyl *p*-methoxycinnamate 7%, mexenone 2%, butyl methoxydibenzoylmethane 2%, titanium dioxide 4.5%. Net price 50 g = £3.11, 100 g = £4.70. ACBS
Additives: hydroxybenzoates (parabens), fragrance
Ultrablock cream, (SPF 30), mexenone 2%, ethylhexyl *p*-methoxycinnamate 7.5%, butyl methoxydibenzoylmethane 4%, titanium dioxide 6%. Net price 50 g = £3.74. ACBS
Additives: hydroxybenzoates (parabens), fragrance

13.8.2 Camouflagers

Disfigurement of the skin can be very distressing to patients and have a marked psychological effect. In skilled hands, or with experience, these preparations can be very effective in concealing scars, areas of discoloration, and birthmarks.

Boots Covering Cream® (Boots)
Cream (4 shades). 20 g. ACBS
Additives: hydroxybenzoates (parabens)

Covermark® (Stiefel)
Additives: beeswax, hydroxybenzoates (parabens), fragrance
Cream rouge, (3 shades). Net price 4.5 g = £2.96. ACBS
Grey toner (= cream). Net price 4.5 g = £2.96. ACBS
Masking cream (covering cream, 10 shades). Net price 25 g = £4.35. ACBS
Shading cream. Net price 4.5 g = £2.96. ACBS
Finishing powder. Net price 50 g = £2.62; 250 g = £9.37. ACBS

Dermablend® (DDC)
Cover creme, (10 shades). Net price 10.7 g = £5.95; 28.4 g = £10.22. ACBS
Additives: beeswax, hydroxybenzoates (parabens)
Leg cover, (6 shades). Net price 64 g = £8.85. ACBS
Additives: beeswax, hydroxybenzoates (parabens)
Setting powder. Net price 28 g = £8.24. ACBS
Additives: hydroxybenzoates (parabens)

Dermacolor® (Fox)
Camouflage creme, (30 shades). Net price 30 g = £5.80. ACBS
Additives: beeswax, wool fat, fragrance
Fixing powder, (5 shades). Net price 60 g = £4.64. ACBS
Additives: fragrance

Keromask® (Network Management)
Masking cream, (2 shades). Net price 15 mL = £3.56. ACBS
Additives: butylated hydroxyanisole, hydroxybenzoates (parabens), wool fat
Finishing powder. Net price 25 g = £3.56. ACBS
Additives: none as listed in section 13.1

Veil® (Blake)
Cover cream, (19 shades). Net price 19 g = £3.41; 44 g = £4.82; 70 g = £6.53. ACBS
Additives: hydroxybenzoates (parabens), wool fat derivative
Finishing powder, translucent. Net price 35 g = £3.41. ACBS
Additives: butylated hydroxyanisole, hydroxybenzoates (parabens)

13.9 Shampoos and some other scalp preparations

> BORDERLINE SUBSTANCES. The preparations marked 'ACBS' are regarded as drugs when prescribed in accordance with the advice of the Advisory Committee on Borderline Substances for the clinical conditions listed. Prescriptions issued in accordance with this advice and endorsed 'ACBS' will normally not be investigated. See Appendix 7 for listing by clinical condition.

Dandruff (*pityriasis capitis*) is believed to be caused by follicular overgrowth with pityrosporum yeasts; it often increases at puberty. The treatment of choice is the frequent use of a mild detergent shampoo generally once or twice weekly; this rids the scalp of scale but does not have a therapeutic effect in itself. Shampoos containing antimicrobial agents such as **pyrithione zinc** have beneficial effects and are on sale to the general public. Shampoos containing **tar** extracts may be useful and they are also used in *psoriasis*, both as adjunctive treatment and for the removal of pastes etc. Shampoos containing **selenium sulphide** are of no more value than the other shampoos and should not be used within 48 hours of applying hair colouring or permanent waving preparations. **Ketoconazole** is also useful as a shampoo (see section 13.10.2) and **lithium succinate** has been shown to be effective in shampoo form.

For more severe conditions, weak **corticosteroid** gels and lotions (section 13.4), applied to the scalp may be helpful.

Cradle cap in infants may be treated with **olive oil** or **arachis oil** applications before shampooing. See also sections 13.5 (psoriasis and eczema), 13.10.4 (lice), and 13.10.2 (ringworm).

ADMINISTRATION. Shampoos should be used once or twice weekly

Alphosyl® (Stafford-Miller)
Shampoo, allantoin 0.2%, refined coal tar extract 5%. Net price 125 mL = £1.30; 250 mL = £2.41. ACBS: for psoriasis and other scaly disorders of the scalp
Additives: hydroxybenzoates (parabens), fragrance

Baltar® (Merck)
Shampoo, coal tar distillate 1.5% in soap-free basis. Net price 225 mL = £2.63; 500 mL = £4.60
Additives: fragrance

Betadine® (Napp)
Scalp and skin cleanser—section 13.11.4
Shampoo solution, povidone-iodine 4%, in a surfactant solution. Net price 250 mL = £1.74. ACBS: for seborrhoeic scalp conditions associated with excessive dandruff, pruritic scaling, seborrhoeic dermatitis, pityriasis capitis, infected lesions of the scalp, pyodermas (recurrent furunculosis, infective folliculitis, impetigo)
Additives: wool fat, fragrance

Calmurid® (Kabi Pharmacia)
Solution, urea 20%, lactic acid 5%, in an aqueous vehicle. Net price 125 mL = £4.10
Additives: polysorbate 20
Apply twice daily to scalp

Capasal® (Dermal)
Shampoo, coal tar 1%, coconut oil 1%, salicylic acid 0.5%. Net price 250 mL = £4.95
Additives: none as listed in section 13.1

Capitol® (Dermal)
Gel, benzalkonium chloride 0.5%. Net price 120 g = £3.13. ACBS: for pityriasis capitis and seborrhoeic dermatitis of the scalp
Additives: none as listed in section 13.1

Ceanel Concentrate® (Quinoderm Ltd)
Shampoo, cetrimide 10%, undecenoic acid 1%, phenethyl alcohol 7.5%. Net price 50 mL = £1.07; 150 mL = £2.83; 500 mL = £8.33. ACBS: for psoriasis or seborrhoeic conditions
Additives: none as listed in section 13.1

Clinitar® (Shire)
Shampoo solution, coal tar extract 2%. Net price 100 g = £4.12
Additives: polysorbate, fragrance

PoM **Efalith**® (Scotia)
Ointment, lithium succinate 8%, zinc sulphate 0.05%. Net price 20 g = £12.50
Additives: wool fat derivative
Cautions: psoriasis
Seborrhoeic dermatitis, apply thinly twice daily initially, then reduce

Gelcotar® (Quinoderm Ltd)
Liquid, strong coal tar solution 1.25%, cade oil 0.5%, in a shampoo basis. Net price 150 mL = £1.41; 350 mL = £2.83. ACBS: for psoriasis of the scalp, seborrhoeic dermatitis, and dandruff
Additives: chlorocresol, fragrance
Gel, see section 13.5

Genisol® (Fisons)
Liquid, prepared coal tar 2% (as purified coal tar fractions), sodium sulphosuccinated undecylenic monoalkylolamide 1%. Net price 58 mL = £1.22; 250 mL = £3.98; 600 mL = £8.29. ACBS: for psoriasis, eczema, and scaling of the scalp (psoriasis, dandruff, or eczema)
Additives: fragrance

Ionil T® (Galderma)
Shampoo application, benzalkonium chloride 0.2%, coal tar solution 5%, salicylic acid 2% in an alcoholic basis. Net price 200 mL = £2.56. ACBS: for seborrhoeic dermatitis of the scalp
Additives: tetrasodium edetate

Lenium® (Cilag)
Cream, selenium sulphide 2.5%. Net price 42 g = 88p; 100 g = £1.50
Additives: fragrance

PoM **Nizoral**® shampoo—section 13.10.2

Polytar® (Stiefel)
Liquid, arachis oil extract of crude coal tar 0.3%, cade oil 0.3%, coal tar solution 0.1%, oleyl alcohol 1%, tar 0.3%. Net price 150 mL = £1.34; 350 mL = £2.37. ACBS: for psoriasis, eczema, and scaling of the scalp (psoriasis, dandruff, and eczema)
Additives: polysorbate 80, fragrance

Polytar Plus® (Stiefel)
Liquid, ingredients as above with hydrolysed animal protein 3%. Net price 350 mL = £3.29. ACBS: for scalp disorders such as scaling (psoriasis, dandruff, eczema), pruritus, and in the removal of pastes and pomades used in psoriasis
Additives: fragrance

Pragmatar®—section 13.5

Psoriderm® (Dermal)
Scalp lotion (= shampoo), coal tar 2.5%, lecithin 0.3%. Net price 250 mL = £4.97
Additives: disodium edetate

Selsun® (Abbott)
Shampoo application, selenium sulphide 2.5%. Net price 50 mL = 92p; 100 mL = £1.49; 150 mL = £2.02
Additives: fragrance

T/Gel® (Neutrogena)
Shampoo, coal tar extract 2%. Net price 125 mL = £2.36. ACBS: for psoriasis, eczema, and scaling of the scalp (psoriasis, dandruff, and eczema)
Additives: hydroxybenzoates (parabens), tetrasodium edetate, fragrance

MALE-PATTERN BALDNESS

Topical application of minoxidil may stimulate limited hair growth in a small proportion of patients but only for as long as it is used

MINOXIDIL

Indications: male-pattern baldness (men and women)
Cautions; Contra-indications; Side-effects: see section 2.5.1 (about 1.4% absorbed); local side-effects: itching, dermatitis

NHS PoM **Regaine**® (Upjohn)
Topical solution, minoxidil 2% in an aqueous alcoholic basis. Net price 60-mL bottle = £20.00
Additives: propylene glycol
Cautions: flammable; wash hands after application
Note. The Royal Pharmaceutical Society's Law Department has reminded pharmacists that neither the safety nor the stability of mixtures of Minoxidil lotion with other products has been established, and that this fact should be drawn to the prescriber's attention before any such mixture is dispensed.

13.10 Anti-infective skin preparations

13.10.1 Antibacterial preparations

13.10.1.1 Antibacterial preparations only used topically
13.10.1.2 Antibacterial preparations also used systemically

For many skin infections such as *erysipelas* and *cellulitis* systemic antibacterial treatment is the method of choice because the infection is too deeply sited for adequate penetration of topical preparations. For details of suitable treatment see section 5.1, table 1.

Impetigo may be treated by topical application of **fusidic acid** or **mupirocin** or, if widespread, with oral administration of **flucloxacillin** or **erythromycin** (see section 5.1, table 1). Mild antiseptics such as **povidone-iodine** (section 13.11.4) are used to remove crusts and exudate.

Although there are a great many antibacterial drugs presented in topical preparations they are potentially hazardous and frequently their use is not necessary if adequate hygienic measures can be taken. Moreover not all skin conditions that are oozing, crusted, or characterised by pustules are actually infected.

To minimise the development of resistant organisms it is advisable to limit the choice of drugs applied topically to those not used systemically. Unfortunately some of these drugs, for example neomycin, may cause sensitisation and, if large areas of skin are being treated, ototoxicity may be a hazard, particularly in children and the elderly. Resistant organisms are more common in hospitals, and whenever possible swabs for examination should be taken before beginning treatment.

Mupirocin is not related to any other antibiotic in use. Its use should be restricted as it is particularly useful when there is resistant infection.
Silver sulphadiazine is used in the treatment of infected burns.

13.10.1.1 ANTIBACTERIAL PREPARATIONS ONLY USED TOPICALLY

FRAMYCETIN SULPHATE
Indications; Cautions; Side-effects: see under Neomycin Sulphate

PoM **Soframycin**® (Roussel)
Cream, framycetin sulphate 1.5%, gramicidin 0.005%. Net price 15 g = £1.72
Additives: hydroxybenzoates (parabens)
Ointment, ingredients as for cream, in a wool fat and paraffin basis. Net price 15 g = £1.72
Additives: wool fat
Sterile powder for preparing topical solutions, framycetin sulphate. Net price 500-mg vial = £3.85
Sofra-Tulle® *see* Framycetin Gauze Dressing, section 13.13.6

MUPIROCIN
Indications: bacterial skin infections
Cautions: see below
Administration: apply up to 3 times daily for up to 10 days

PoM **Bactroban**® (Beecham)
Ointment, mupirocin 2%. Net price 15 g = £4.08
Additives: none as listed in section 13.1
Note. Contains macrogol therefore caution in renal impairment; may sting
Nasal ointment, see section 12.2.3

NEOMYCIN SULPHATE
Indications: skin infections
Cautions: see notes above; large open wounds, sensitivity to other aminoglycosides
Side-effects: local hypersensitivity reactions

PoM **Neomycin Cream, BPC,** neomycin sulphate 0.5%, cetomacrogol emulsifying ointment 30%, chlorocresol 0.1%, disodium edetate 0.01%, in freshly boiled and cooled purified water. Net price 15 g = 52p
Apply up to 3 times daily; max. 60 g daily for 3 weeks; do not repeat for at least 3 months

PoM **Cicatrin**® (Wellcome)
Cream, neomycin sulphate 3300 units, bacitracin zinc 250 units, cysteine 2 mg, glycine 10 mg, threonine 1 mg/g. Net price 15 g = £4.52; 30 g = £8.22
Additives: wool fat derivative
Apply up to 3 times daily; max. 60 g daily for 3 weeks; do not repeat for at least 3 months
Dusting powder, neomycin sulphate 3300 units, bacitracin zinc 250 units, cysteine 2 mg, glycine 10 mg, threonine 1 mg/g. Net price 15 g = £4.87; 50 g = £12.31. Max. 50 g daily for 4 weeks; do not repeat for at least 3 months
Additives: none as listed in section 13.1

Cautionary label wordings, see inside back cover Prices are **net**, see p. 1

Powder spray, neomycin sulphate 16 500 units, bacitracin zinc 1250 units, cysteine 12 mg, glycine 60 mg/g; pressurised aerosol unit. Net price 103 g = £11.74. Max. 3 g daily for 12 weeks; do not repeat for at least 3 months
Additives: none as listed in section 13.1

PoM **Graneodin**® (Squibb)
Ointment, neomycin sulphate 0.25%, gramicidin 0.025%. Net price 25 g = £1.47
Additives: none as listed in section 13.1
Apply 2–4 times daily

PoM **Polybactrin**® (Wellcome)
Powder spray, neomycin sulphate 495 000 units, bacitracin zinc 37 500 units, polymyxin B sulphate 150 000 units/pressurised aerosol unit. Net price per unit (115 mL) = £21.51. Max. 1 unit daily for 7 days; do not repeat for at least 3 months
Additives: none as listed in section 13.1

PoM **Tribiotic**® (3M)
Spray application, neomycin sulphate 500 000 units, bacitracin zinc 10 000 units, polymyxin B sulphate 150 000 units/pressurised aerosol unit. Net price per unit (110 g) = £5.72. Max. 1 unit daily for 7 days; do not repeat for at least 3 months
Additives: none as listed in section 13.1

POLYMYXINS

(Includes colistin sulphate and polymyxin B sulphate)
Indications: skin infections
Cautions: see notes above; large open wounds
Side-effects: transient irritation; local hypersensitivity reactions

PoM **Polyfax**® (Cusi)
Ointment, polymyxin B sulphate 10 000 units, bacitracin zinc 500 units/g. Net price 20 g = £8.95
Apply 3 times daily

PoM **Colomycin**® (Pharmax)
Powder, sterile, for making topical preparations (usually 1%), colistin sulphate. Net price 1 g vial = £19.73

Other preparations
Ingredient of Polybactrin® and Tribiotic®

SILVER SULPHADIAZINE

Indications: skin infection, particularly Gram-negative infections such as pseudomonal infections in second- and third-degree burns, infected leg ulcers, and pressure sores
Cautions: hepatic and renal impairment
Contra-indications: sensitivity to sulphonamides
Side-effects: rarely allergic reactions including rashes

PoM **Flamazine**® (S&N Pharm.)
Cream, silver sulphadiazine 1%. Net price 50 g = £4.41; 250 g = £11.82; 500 g = £20.92
Additives: polysorbates, propylene glycol
Note. Silver sulphadiazine 1% cream is also available from Norton, net price 50 g = £4.19; 250 g = £11.23; 500 g = £19.87
In burns apply daily with sterile applicator; in leg ulcers apply at least 3 times a week

13.10.1.2 ANTIBACTERIAL PREPARATIONS ALSO USED SYSTEMICALLY

CHLORTETRACYCLINE HYDROCHLORIDE

Indications: susceptible skin infections; impetigo, see section 5.1, Table 1
Cautions: see notes above; overgrowth with non-susceptible organisms; stains clothing
Side-effects: rarely local hypersensitivity reactions
Administration: apply 1 to 3 times daily

PoM **Aureomycin**® (Lederle)
Cream, chlortetracycline hydrochloride 3% (as chlortetracycline). Net price 30 g = £1.82
Additives: chlorocresol
Ointment, chlortetracycline hydrochloride 3%. Net price 30 g = £1.82
Additives: hydroxybenzoates (parabens), wool fat

FUSIDIC ACID

Indications: staphylococcal skin infections and abscesses
Cautions: see notes above; avoid contact with eyes
Side-effects: rarely local hypersensitivity reactions
Administration: skin infections apply 3–4 times daily; abscesses see under *Caviject gel*

PoM **Fucidin**® (Leo)
Cream, fusidic acid 2%. Net price 15 g = £2.94; 30 g = £4.96
Additives: butylated hydroxyanisole
Gel, fusidic acid 2%. Net price 15 g = £2.54; 30 g = £4.40
Additives: hydroxybenzoates (parabens), polysorbate 80
Caviject gel, sterile fusidic acid 2%, in a single-dose unit (7 g) fitted with elongated nozzle. For treatment of abscesses. Net price 1 unit = £1.49
Inject once only into curetted abscess and apply dressing
Ointment, sodium fusidate 2%. Net price 15 g = £2.40; 30 g = £4.07
Additives: wool fat

PoM **Fucidin Intertulle**® see section 13.13.6

GENTAMICIN

Indications: skin infections
Cautions: see notes above; large open wounds, sensitivity to other aminoglycosides
Administration: apply 3 times daily

PoM **Cidomycin Topical**® (Roussel)
Cream, gentamicin 0.3% (as sulphate). Do not dilute. Net price 15 g = £1.75; 30 g = £3.40
Additives: hydroxybenzoates (parabens), propylene glycol
Ointment, gentamicin 0.3% (as sulphate). Do not dilute. Net price 15 g = £1.75; 30 g = £3.40
Additives: none as listed in section 13.1

PoM **Genticin**® (Nicholas)
Cream, gentamicin 0.3% (as sulphate). Net price 15 g = £1.37; 100 g = £9.15
Additives: hydroxybenzoates (parabens)
Ointment, gentamicin 0.3% (as sulphate). Net price 15 g = £1.37
Additives: hydroxybenzoates (parabens)

METRONIDAZOLE
Indications: see under preparations

PoM **Metrogel**® (Sandoz)
Gel, metronidazole 0.75%. Net price 40 g = £17.80. Label: 10 patient information leaflet
Additives: propylene glycol
Administration: acute inflammatory exacerbations of acne rosacea, apply thinly twice daily for 8–9 weeks; avoid contact with eyes

PoM **Metrotop**® (Farmitalia Carlo Erba)
Gel, metronidazole 0.8%. Net price 30 g = £6.95
Additives: none as listed in section 13.1
Administration: de-odourisation of fungating malodorous tumours, apply to clean wound 1 to 2 times daily and cover (flat wounds, apply liberally; cavities, smear on paraffin gauze and pack loosely); use tube once only

TETRACYCLINE HYDROCHLORIDE
Indications; Cautions; Side-effects: see under Chlortetracycline Hydrochloride

PoM **Achromycin Topical**® (Lederle)
Ointment, tetracycline hydrochloride 3%. Net price 30 g = £1.48
Additives: hydroxybenzoates (parabens), wool fat
Apply 1–3 times daily

13.10.2 Antifungal preparations
Ideally skin scrapings should be examined to confirm diagnosis before treatment is begun. Widespread or intractable fungal infections are treated systemically (see section 5.2). Most localised infections are treated with the topical preparations described below.

Nail ringworm (tinea unguium) and scalp ringworm (*T. capitis*) are best treated systemically (see section 5.2). Most other ringworm infections, including tinea pedis, may be adequately treated with topical preparations. The imidazoles **clotrimazole**, **econazole**, and **miconazole** are all effective and commonly used. **Sulconazole** is a recently introduced imidazole with similar properties. Combinations of imidazoles and weak corticosteroids may be of use in the treatment of some eczematous disorders and, in the first few days only, of a severely inflamed patch of ringworm. **Compound benzoic acid ointment** (Whitfield's ointment) is also quite effective but cosmetically less acceptable than the proprietary preparations. It is generally used to treat patches of ringworm (tinea) on the trunk, limbs, palms, or soles. The **undecenoates** are less effective in treating ringworm infections.

Candidal skin infections may also be treated by topical application with the broad-spectrum antifungals, clotrimazole, econazole, and miconazole. **Nystatin** preparations are also equally as effective in candidiasis although they are ineffective against infections due to dermatophyte fungi (tinea).

Lotions are generally chosen for application to large and hairy areas. Ointments are best avoided on moist surfaces because of their occlusive properties. Dusting-powders have no place in the treatment of fungal infections, except for toiletry or cosmetic purposes, as they are therapeutically ineffective and may cause skin irritation.

Amorolfine is a newly introduced antifungal that differs chemically from other antifungals. It is available as a cream for fungal skin infections and a lacquer for fungal nail infections.

AMOROLFINE
Indications: see under preparations
Cautions: pregnancy, breast-feeding; avoid eyes, ears, and mucous membranes
Side-effects: occasional transient burning sensation, erythema, pruritus

▼ PoM **Loceryl**® (Roche)
Cream, amorolfine (as hydrochloride) 0.25%. Net price 20 g = £4.95. Label: 10 patient information leaflet
Administration: fungal skin infections, apply once daily after cleansing in the evening for at least 2–3 weeks (up to 6 weeks for foot mycosis)
Nail lacquer, amorolfine (as hydrochloride) 5%. Net price 5-mL pack (with nail files, spatulas and cleansing swabs) = £34.38. Label: 10 patient information leaflet
Administration: fungal nail infections, apply to infected nails 1–2 times weekly after filing and cleansing; allow to dry (approx. 3 minutes); treat finger nails for 6 months, toe nails for 9–12 months (review at intervals of 3 months)

BENZOIC ACID
Indications: ringworm (tinea)

Benzoic Acid Ointment, Compound, BP (Whitfield's ointment), benzoic acid 6%, salicylic acid 3%, in emulsifying ointment. Net price 25 g = 16p
Apply twice daily

BENZOYL PEROXIDE
Indications: fungal skin infections, particularly tinea pedis

Quinoped® (Quinoderm Ltd)
Cream, benzoyl peroxide 5%, potassium hydroxyquinoline sulphate 0.5%, in an astringent basis. Net price 25 g = 96p
Additives: edetic acid (EDTA)
Apply twice daily

CLOTRIMAZOLE

Indications: fungal skin infections
Side-effects: occasional skin irritation or sensitivity
Administration: apply 2–3 times daily continuing for 14 days after lesions have healed

Canesten® (Baypharm)
Cream, clotrimazole 1%. Net price 20 g = £1.82; 50 g = £4.26
Additives: benzyl alcohol, polysorbate 60
Solution, clotrimazole 1% in macrogol 400. Net price 20 mL = £2.38. For hairy areas
Additives: none as listed in section 13.1
Spray, clotrimazole 1%, in 30% isopropyl alcohol. Net price 40-mL atomiser = £5.12. Label: 15. For large or hairy areas
Additives: propylene glycol
Dusting powder, clotrimazole 1%. Net price 30 g = £1.56
Additives: none as listed in section 13.1

ECONAZOLE NITRATE

Indications; Side-effects: see under Clotrimazole
Administration: apply 2–3 times daily continuing for 14 days after lesions have healed; nail infections, apply daily under occlusive dressing

Ecostatin® (Squibb)
Cream, econazole nitrate 1%. Net price 15 g = £1.49; 30 g = £2.75
Additives: butylated hydroxyanisole, fragrance
Lotion, econazole nitrate 1%. Net price 30 mL = £2.75
Additives: butylated hydroxyanisole, fragrance
Spray solution, econazole nitrate 1% in an alcoholic solution. Net price 150 g = £3.48. Label: 15
Additives: propylene glycol, fragrance
Dusting powder, econazole nitrate 1%. Net price 30 g = £2.90
Additives: fragrance
Spray powder, econazole nitrate 1%. Net price 200-g unit = £2.64
Additives: fragrance

Pevaryl® (Cilag)
Cream, econazole nitrate 1%. Net price 30 g = £2.65
Additives: butylated hydroxyanisole, fragrance
Lotion, econazole nitrate 1%. Net price 30 mL = £3.33
Additives: butylated hydroxyanisole, fragrance
Spray powder, econazole nitrate 1%. Net price 200-g pressurised aerosol unit (20 g powder) = £3.33
Additives: fragrance

KETOCONAZOLE

Indications; Side-effects: see under Clotrimazole

PoM **Nizoral®** (Janssen)
Cream, ketoconazole 2%. Net price 30 g = £3.81
Additives: polysorbates, propylene glycol
Apply 1–2 times daily, continuing for a few days after lesions have healed

Shampoo, ketoconazole 2%. Net price 100 mL = £8.75
Additives: none as listed in section 13.1
For seborrhoeic dermatitis and dandruff apply twice weekly for 2–4 weeks, for pityriasis versicolor once daily for max. 5 days; avoid for 2 weeks following topical corticosteroid treatment

MICONAZOLE NITRATE

Indications; Side-effects: see under Clotrimazole
Administration: apply twice daily continuing for 10 days after lesions have healed; nail infections, apply daily under occlusive dressing

Daktarin® (Janssen)
Cream, miconazole nitrate 2%. Net price 30 g = £2.07
Additives: butylated hydroxyanisole
Note. A generic version of miconazole nitrate 2% cream is also available from Hillcross, net price 30 g = £2.04
Dusting powder, miconazole nitrate 2%. Net price 20 g = £1.50
Additives: none as listed in section 13.1
Spray powder, miconazole nitrate 0.16%, in an aerosol basis. Net price 100 g = £1.50
Additives: none as listed in section 13.1
Twin pack, 1 × 30 g pack of cream miconazole nitrate 2%, with 1 × 30 g dusting-powder miconazole nitrate 2%. Net price (complete pack) = £3.80

NYSTATIN

Indications: skin infections due to *Candida* spp.
Administration: apply 2–4 times daily, continuing for 7 days after lesions have healed

PoM **Nystaform®** (Bayer)
Cream, nystatin 100 000 units/g, chlorhexidine hydrochloride 1%. Net price 30 g = £2.69
Additives: benzyl alcohol, polysorbate 60
Ointment, nystatin 100 000 units/g, chlorhexidine acetate 1%. Net price 30 g = £2.69
Additives: none as listed in section 13.1

PoM **Nystan®** (Squibb)
Cream, nystatin 100 000 units/g. Net price 30 g = £2.66
Additives: benzyl alcohol, propylene glycol, fragrance
Gel, nystatin 100 000 units/g. Net price 30 g = £2.66
Additives: chlorocresol, fragrance
Ointment, nystatin 100 000 units/g, in Plastibase®. Net price 30 g = £2.14
Additives: none as listed in section 13.1

PoM **Tinaderm-M®** (Schering-Plough)
Cream, nystatin 100 000 units/g, tolnaftate 1%. Net price 20 g = £1.83. For *Candida* infections and tinea
Additives: butylated hydroxytoluene, hydroxybenzoates (parabens), fragrance
Apply 2–3 times daily

SALICYLIC ACID

Indications: fungal skin infections, particularly tinea
Side-effects: hypersensitivity reactions

Phytex® (Pharmax)
Paint, salicylic acid 1.46% (total combined), tannic acid 4.89% and boric acid 3.12% (as borotannic complex), in a vehicle containing alcohol and ethyl acetate. Net price 25 mL (with brush) = £1.33. For fungal nail infections (onychomycosis)
Additives: none as listed in section 13.1
Apply twice daily
Caution: flammable; avoid in pregnancy and children under 5 years

Phytocil® (Fisons)
Cream, salicylic acid 1.5%, 2-*p*-chlorophenoxyethanol 1%, menthol 1%, 1-phenoxypropan-2-ol 2%. Net price 25 g = 66p. For tinea pedis, tinea cruris, and tinea circinata
Additives: none as listed in section 13.1
Apply 2–3 times daily

SULCONAZOLE NITRATE
Indications; Side-effects: see under Clotrimazole
Cautions: avoid contact with eyes (lens changes in *animals* after high oral doses)
Administration: apply 1–2 times daily continuing for 2–3 weeks after lesions have healed

PoM **Exelderm®** (ICI)
Cream, sulconazole nitrate 1%. Net price 30 g = £3.90
Additives: polysorbates, propylene glycol

TIOCONAZOLE
Indications: see under preparations
Side-effects: local irritation, usually during first week of treatment; discontinue if sensitivity reaction develops

Trosyl® (Pfizer)
PoM *Nail solution*, tioconazole 28%. Net price 12 mL (with applicator brush) = £25.00
Additives: none as listed in section 13.1
Administration: fungal nail infections, apply to nails and surrounding skin twice daily for up to 6 months (may be extended to 12 months)
Cream, tioconazole 1%. Net price 15 g = £1.51; 30 g = £2.78
Additives: benzyl alcohol, polysorbate 60
Administration: fungal skin infections, apply once or twice daily for 2–4 weeks (up to 6 weeks for foot mycosis)

UNDECENOATES
Indications: skin infections, particularly tinea pedis

Monphytol® (LAB)
Paint, methyl undecenoate 5%, propyl undecenoate 0.7%, salicylic acid 3%, methyl salicylate 25%, propyl salicylate 5%, chlorbutol 3%. Net price 18 mL (with brush) = £1.17. For fungal (particularly nail) infections
Additives: none as listed in section 13.1
Apply 4 times daily

Mycota® (Crookes)
Cream, zinc undecenoate 20%, undecenoic acid 5%. Net price 25 g = 83p
Additives: fragrance
Dusting powder, zinc undecenoate 20%, undecenoic acid 2%. Net price 70 g = £1.33
Additives: fragrance

Spray application, undecenoic acid 2.5%, dichlorophen 0.25% (pressurised aerosol pack). Net price 113 g = £1.33
Additives: fragrance
Apply 1–2 times daily

Phytocil® (Fisons)
Dusting powder, zinc undecenoate 5.8%, 2-*p*-chlorophenoxyethanol 1%, 1-phenoxypropan-2-ol 2%. Net price 50 g = 91p. For use with cream
Additives: none as listed in section 13.1

13.10.3 Antiviral preparations

Acyclovir cream is indicated for the treatment of initial and recurrent labial and genital herpes simplex infections; treatment should begin as early as possible. Systemic treatment is necessary for buccal or vaginal infections; herpes zoster (shingles) also requires systemic treatment (for details of systemic use see section 5.3).

Idoxuridine solution (5% in dimethyl sulphoxide) is used less frequently for herpetic infections of the skin since acyclovir is more effective. Herpes simplex seems to respond to frequent applications if started early and continued for 3 to 4 days, but may be less successful if delayed. Evidence of its value in herpes zoster infections is conflicting.

ACYCLOVIR
Indications: see notes above
Side-effects: transient stinging or burning on application; occasionally erythema or drying of the skin
Cautions: avoid contact with eyes and mucous membranes
Administration: apply to lesions every 4 hours (5 times daily) for 5 days, started at first sign of attack

PoM **Zovirax®** (Wellcome)
Cream, acyclovir 5%. Net price 2 g = £8.37; 10 g = £25.22
Additives: propylene glycol
Eye ointment, see section 11.3.3
Tablets, see section 5.3

IDOXURIDINE IN DIMETHYL SULPHOXIDE
Indications: see notes above
Cautions: avoid contact with the eyes, mucous membranes, and textiles; breast-feeding
Contra-indications: pregnancy (toxicity in *animal* studies)
Side-effects: stinging on application, changes in taste; overuse may cause maceration
Administration: apply 5% solution to lesions 4 times daily for 3–4 days; in severe zoster (shingles) apply 40% solution over affected area daily for 4 days
Note. Not to be used in mouth

PoM **Herpid®** (Boehringer Ingelheim)
Application, idoxuridine 5% in dimethyl sulphoxide. Net price 5 mL (with applicator) = £7.04
Additives: none as listed in section 13.1

PoM **Iduridin**® (Ferring)
Application, idoxuridine 5% in dimethyl sulphoxide. Net price 5 mL (with applicator) = £4.90
Additives: none as listed in section 13.1

Application, idoxuridine 40% in dimethyl sulphoxide. Net price 5 mL (with applicator) = £19.00; 20 mL with dropper = £39.00. For severe herpes zoster
Additives: none as listed in section 13.1

PoM **Virudox**® (Bioglan)
Application, idoxuridine 5% in dimethyl sulphoxide. Net price 5 mL (with applicator) = £5.95
Additives: none as listed in section 13.1

13.10.4 Parasiticidal preparations

SCABIES (*Sarcoptes scabiei*). **Lindane** and **malathion** are the treatments of choice for scabies, but lindane should be avoided during pregnancy or breast-feeding, in young children, and in patients with low body-weight or a history of epilepsy. **Permethrin**, a recently introduced pyrethroid, is also indicated for scabies.

Older preparations include benzyl benzoate, which is an irritant and should be avoided in children, and monosulfiram, which may induce disulfiram-like reactions with alcohol. Evidence that monosulfiram is particularly suitable for children is inconclusive.

Aqueous lotions are preferable to creams as they give better coverage; alcoholic lotions are not recommended owing to irritation of excoriated skin and the genitalia. Although the preparations have traditionally been applied after a hot bath there is evidence that this may increase absorption of the acaricide into the bloodstream.

All members of the affected household should be treated. Treatment should be applied to the whole body paying particular attention to the webs of the fingers and toes and brushing lotion under the ends of the nails. In the case of infants and young children (up to the age of about 2 years) the lotion (preferably malathion, see notes above) should also be applied on the scalp, neck, face, and ears. Providing the application is done properly lindane, malathion and permethrin need only be applied once; in the case of benzyl benzoate up to three applications on consecutive days may be needed.

The itch of scabies persists for some days after the infestation has been eliminated and antipruritic treatment may be required. Application of **crotamiton** can be used to control itching after treatment with more effective acaricides, but caution is necessary if the skin is excoriated. **Calamine** is probably more suitable. Oral administration of a sedative antihistamine at night may also be useful.

HEAD LICE (*Pediculus humanus capitis*). **Malathion** and **carbaryl** are the treatments of choice for *head lice*. **Lindane** is no longer recommended because of resistant strains. Lotions should be used in preference to shampoos, which are not in contact with the hair long enough and are normally diluted too much in use to be effective; aqueous lotions are preferred for asthmatic patients and small children, to avoid alcoholic fumes. A contact time of 12 hours or overnight treatment is recommended. A 2-hour treatment is no longer regarded as sufficient to ensure death of eggs. **Permethrin** and **phenothrin** are two recently introduced pyrethroids, both of which are very effective if formulated in a good carrier basis.

In general, treatment for head lice should preferably be repeated after 7 days to kill lice emerging from any eggs that might have survived the first application.

> **Rotational policies.** Most health districts operate a rotating policy for head lice treatment. Details of the drugs which are currently recommended for use in the different health districts can be obtained from District Pharmaceutical Officers.

CRAB (PUBIC) LICE (*Pthirus pubis*). **Malathion**, **lindane** and **carbaryl** are effective for *crab lice*. Aqueous lotions should be applied to all hairy parts of the body for 12 hours or overnight; a second treatment is preferable after 7 days to kill lice emerging from surviving eggs. Alcoholic lotions are not recommended (owing to irritation of excoriated skin and the genitalia). Aqueous malathion lotion should be used for *crab lice of the eye lashes*.

BENZYL BENZOATE

Indications: scabies, pediculosis (but see notes above)

Cautions: children (see notes above), avoid contact with eyes and mucous membranes

Side-effects: skin irritation, burning sensation especially on genitalia and excoriations, occasionally rashes

Benzyl Benzoate Application, BP, benzyl benzoate 25% in an emulsion basis.

Administration: scabies—apply 25% application over the whole body, omitting the head and neck; repeat without bathing on the following day and wash off 24 hours later; a third application may be required in some cases
Note. Not recommended for children—dilution to reduce irritant effect also reduces efficacy (see notes above)
Available from CP, Evans, Rhône-Poulenc Rorer (Ascabiol®, net price 100 mL = £1.17)

CARBARYL

Indications: pediculosis

Cautions: avoid contact with eyes; alcoholic lotions **not** recommended for pediculosis in asthmatics or small children, or for crab lice (see notes above); do not use more than once a week for 3 weeks at a time

13.10 Anti-infective skin preparations

Side-effects: skin irritation
Administration: lotion—apply to dry hair and rub into the hair and scalp or affected areas, allow to dry, comb, and remove by washing 12 hours later (see also notes above); shampoo—shampoo in, leave on hair for 5 minutes, rinse, repeat, rinse, allow to dry, comb, repeat twice at intervals of 3 days

Carylderm® (Napp)
Lotion, carbaryl 0.5%, in an alcoholic basis. Net price 55 mL = £1.23; 160 mL = £2.51. Label: 15
Additives: none as listed in section 13.1
Shampoo, carbaryl 1%. Net price 100 mL = £1.88
Additives: wool fat derivative, fragrance

Clinicide® (De Witt)
Lotion, carbaryl 0.5% in an aqueous basis containing 10% alcohol. Net price 50 mL = £1.04
Additives: none as listed in section 13.1

Derbac® C (Napp)
Liquid (= lotion), carbaryl 1% in an aqueous basis. Net price 50 mL = £1.30; 200 mL = £3.04. Label: 10 patient information leaflet
Additives: hydroxybenzoates (parabens)
Shampoo solution, carbaryl 0.5% in an aqueous basis. Net price 75 mL = £1.26. Label: 10 patient information leaflet
Additives: hydroxybenzoates (parabens), fragrance

Suleo-C® (Napp)
Lotion, carbaryl 0.5%, in an alcoholic basis. Net price 55 mL = £1.14; 210 mL = £2.64. Label: 15
Additives: fragrance
Shampoo, carbaryl 0.5%. Net price 75 mL = £1.16
Additives: fragrance

LINDANE

Indications: scabies, pediculosis (but see notes above)
Cautions: avoid contact with eyes and mucous membranes; do not use more than twice for one course of treatment; see also above (under Scabies)
Side-effects: skin irritation
Administration: see preparations

Quellada® (Stafford-Miller)
Lotion, lindane 1%, in a lotion basis. Net price 100 mL = 63p; 500 mL = £2.08. For scabies
Additives: hydroxybenzoates (parabens), fragrance
Administration: scabies, apply thinly over whole body, omitting head and neck, wash off using cool water after 24 hours; repeat if necessary after 7 days
Application PC, lindane 1%, in a shampoo basis. Net price 100 mL = 71p; 500 mL = £2.54. For pediculosis (but see notes above)
Additives: polysorbates
Administration: pediculosis (but see notes above), apply to dry hair, leave for 4 minutes, add water to produce lather, rinse, towel dry, comb

MALATHION

Indications: pediculosis, scabies
Cautions: avoid contact with eyes; alcoholic lotions **not** recommended for pediculosis in asthmatics or small children, or for scabies or crab lice (see notes above); do not use more than once a week for 3 weeks at a time
Side-effects: skin irritation
Administration: pediculosis—rub 0.5% lotion into dry hair, scalp, and affected area, comb, allow to dry naturally, remove by washing after 12 hours (see also notes above); apply 1% shampoo to hair for 5 minutes, rinse, repeat, rinse again, comb, repeat twice at intervals of 3 days
Scabies—apply 0.5% preparation over whole body, omitting the head and neck, and wash off after 24 hours, see also notes above

Derbac-M® (Napp)
Liquid, malathion 0.5% in an aqueous basis. Net price 55 mL = £1.19; 200 mL = £3.04
Additives: hydroxybenzoates (parabens), fragrance

Prioderm® (Napp)
Lotion, malathion 0.5%, in an alcoholic basis. Net price 55 mL = £1.23; 160 mL = £2·51. Label: 15
Additives: fragrance
Cream shampoo, malathion 1%. Net price 40 g = £1.23
Additives: disodium edetate, hydroxybenzoates (parabens), propylene glycol, wool fat derivative, fragrance

Suleo-M® (Napp)
Lotion, malathion 0.5%, in an alcoholic basis. Net price 55 mL = £1.14; 210 mL = £2.64. Label: 15
Additives: fragrance

MONOSULFIRAM

Indications: scabies, but see notes above
Cautions: avoid contact with eyes; avoid alcohol; **interactions:** Appendix 1 (monosulfiram)
Side-effects: hypersensitivity, rashes
Administration: apply diluted solution over whole body omitting head and neck; repeat if necessary for 2–3 consecutive days; discard diluted solution after single use

Tetmosol® (ICI)
Solution, monosulfiram 25%, in industrial methylated spirit. Dilute with 2–3 parts of water before use. Net price 100 mL = £1.32. Label: 4, 15. ACBS: for control of scabies (clinic use preferred)
Additives: none as listed in section 13.1

PERMETHRIN

Indications: see under preparations
Cautions: avoid contact with eyes; use in children under 2 years only under medical supervision
Side-effects: pruritus, erythema, and stinging; rarely rashes and oedema

Lyclear® (Wellcome)
Cream rinse, permethrin 1% in basis containing isopropyl alcohol 20%. Net price 59 mL = £1.83
Additives: hydroxybenzoates (parabens), propylene glycol, fragrance
Administration: pediculosis, apply to clean damp hair, leave on for 10 minutes, rinse and dry

Dermal cream, permethrin 5%. Net price 30 g = £5.50. Label: 10 patient information leaflet
Additives: butylated hydroxytoluene, wool fat
Administration: scabies, apply over whole body, omitting head and neck, and wash off after 8–24 hours. If hands are washed with soap and water within 8 hours of application, cream should be reapplied

PHENOTHRIN

Indications: pediculosis
Cautions: avoid contact with eyes; children under 6 months (medical supervision required)
Side-effects: skin irritation

Full Marks® (Napp)
Shampoo, phenothrin 0.2%. Net price 125 mL = £2.63
Additives: fragrance
Administration: shampoo hair, leave on for at least 5 minutes, rinse, repeat once, comb

Lotion, phenothrin 0.2% in basis containing isopropyl alcohol 69.3%. Net price 55 mL = £1.30; 160 mL = £2.60. Label: 15
Additives: fragrance
Administration: apply to dry hair, allow to dry naturally; shampoo after 2 hours, comb while still wet

13.10.5 Preparations for minor cuts and abrasions

Some of the preparations listed are used in minor burns, and abrasions. They are applied as necessary. Preparations containing camphor, hydrargaphen, and sulphonamides should be **avoided**. Preparations such as magnesium sulphate paste are also listed but are now rarely used to treat carbuncles and boils as these are best treated with antibiotics (see section 5.1.1.2).

Cetrimide Cream, BP, cetrimide 0.5% in a suitable water-miscible basis such as cetostearyl alcohol 5%, liquid paraffin 50% in freshly boiled and cooled purified water. Net price 50 g = 20p

Chlorhexidine Cream, BP, chlorhexidine gluconate solution usually 5% (≡ chlorhexidine gluconate 1%), cetomacrogol emulsifying wax 25%, liquid paraffin 10%, in purified water, freshly boiled and cooled

Proflavine Cream, BPC, proflavine hemisulphate 0.1%, yellow beeswax 2.5%, chlorocresol 0.1%, liquid paraffin 67.3%, freshly boiled and cooled purified water 25%, wool fat 5%. Net price 100 mL = 33p
Caution: stains clothing

Anaflex® (Geistlich)
Cream, polynoxylin 10%, in a water-miscible basis. Net price 50 g = £2.71

Betadine® (Napp)
Ointment, povidone-iodine 10%, in a water-miscible basis. Net price 80 g = £2.03
Additives: none as listed in section 13.1

Brulidine® (Rhône-Poulenc Rorer)
Cream, dibromopropamidine isethionate 0.15%, in a water-miscible basis. Net price 25 g = 76p
Additives: hydroxybenzoates (parabens), fragrance

Cetavlex® (ICI)
Cream, cetrimide 0.5%, in a water-miscible basis. Net price 50 g = 55p
Additives: hydroxybenzoates (parabens)

Dermalex® (Sanofi Winthrop)
Skin lotion, allantoin 0.25%, hexachlorophane 0.5%, squalane 3% in an emulsion basis. Net price 100 mL = £2.05; 250 mL = £5.35. For prevention of pressure sores and prevention and treatment of urinary rash. Avoid in children under 2 years
Additives: butylated hydroxyanisole, edetic acid, hydroxybenzoates (parabens), wool fat, fragrance

Drapolene® (Wellcome)
Cream, benzalkonium chloride 0.01%, cetrimide 0.2% in a water-miscible basis. Net price 55 g = 70p; 100 g = £1.08. For urinary rash and minor wounds
Additives: chlorocresol, wool fat

Vesagex® (Rybar)
Cream, cetrimide 1%. Net price 500 g = £4.60
Additives: chlorocresol, fragrance

Preparations for boils
Magnesium Sulphate Paste, BP, dried magnesium sulphate 45 g, glycerol 55 g, phenol 500 mg
Should be stirred before use
Apply under dressing

Secaderm®—section 13.14

COLLODION

Flexible collodion may be used to seal minor cuts and wounds that have partially healed.

Collodion, Flexible, BP, castor oil 2.5%, colophony 2.5% in a collodion basis, prepared by dissolving pyroxylin (10%) in a mixture of 3 volumes of ether and 1 volume of alcohol (90%). Net price 10 mL = 12p. Label: 15

SURGICAL TISSUE ADHESIVE

Enbucrilate is used as a tissue adhesive for closure of minor skin wounds and sealing sutured skin wounds. Within 20 seconds of contact with tissue moisture it polymerises with an exothermic reaction into a firm adhesive bond. It must therefore by applied very thinly (to avoid heat damage) and with proper technique (poor alignment cannot be corrected). Contact with eyes, internal organs, blood vessels, and nervous tissue should be **avoided**.

Histoacryl® (Davis & Geck)
Tissue adhesive, sterile, enbucrilate with blue dye. Net price (both single use) 200-mg vial = £8.00; 500-mg vial (hosp. use only)

13.11 Disinfectants and cleansers

13.11.1 Alcohols and saline
13.11.2 Chlorhexidine salts
13.11.3 Cationic surfactants and soaps
13.11.4 Chlorine and iodine
13.11.5 Phenolics
13.11.6 Astringents, oxidisers, and dyes
13.11.7 Desloughing agents

The choice of *cleanser* is an important factor in treating skin conditions. For example, scaling disorders are best treated with **emulsifying ointment** (section 13.2.1) or other cleansers that do not irritate the skin.

Sodium chloride solution 0.9% is suitable for general cleansing of skin and wounds.

Useful *disinfectants* for skin cleansing include **cetrimide** (which has useful detergent properties), **chlorhexidine** and **potassium permanganate solution** 1 in 8000. **Povidone-iodine** is preferred to chlorinated solutions (such as dilute sodium hypochlorite solution) which are too irritant and are no longer recommended. Topical preparations of **hexachlorophane** should be used with caution in neonates and should **not** be used on large raw surfaces.

Astringent preparations, such as **potassium permanganate** solution are useful for treating eczematous reactions (section 13.5). Silver nitrate lotion is now rarely used as it stains the skin black and may cause toxic effects if used for prolonged periods.

> BORDERLINE SUBSTANCES. The preparations marked 'ACBS' are regarded as drugs when prescribed in accordance with the advice of the Advisory Committee on Borderline Substances for the clinical conditions listed. Prescriptions issued in accordance with this advice and endorsed 'ACBS' will normally not be investigated. See Appendix 7 for listing by clinical condition.

13.11.1 Alcohols and saline

ALCOHOL
Indications: skin preparation before injection
Cautions: flammable; avoid broken skin; patients have suffered severe burns when diathermy has been preceded by application of alcoholic skin disinfectants.

Industrial Methylated Spirit, BP
Mixture of 19 volumes of ethanol (absolute alcohol) of an appropriate strength with 1 volume of approved wood naphtha and is Industrial Methylated Spirit of the quality known either as '66 OP' or as '74 OP'
Net price 100 mL = 15p. Label: 15

Surgical Spirit, BP, methyl salicylate 0.5 mL, diethyl phthalate 2%, castor oil 2.5%, in industrial methylated spirit. Net price 100 mL = 17p. Label: 15

SODIUM CHLORIDE
Indications: see notes above

Normasol® (Seton)
Solution (sterile), sodium chloride 0.9%. Net price 25 × 25-mL sachet = £3.98; 6 × 100-mL sachet = £2.97. To be used undiluted for topical irrigation of burns, wounds, and eyes
See also section 11.8.2

Sterac® **Sodium Chloride** (Galen)
Solution (sterile), sodium chloride 0.9%. Net price 150 mL = 83p; 1000 mL = £1.10. For irrigation of eyes and wounds

13.11.2 Chlorhexidine salts

CHLORHEXIDINE
Indications: see under preparations; bladder irrigation and catheter patency solutions (see section 7.4.4)
Cautions: avoid contact with eyes, brain, meninges and middle ear; not for use in body cavities; alcoholic solutions not suitable before diathermy
Side-effects: occasional sensitivity

Chlorasept® (Baxter)
2000 Solution (sterile), pink, chlorhexidine acetate 0.05%. Net price 500 mL = 74p; 1000 mL = 79p. For cleansing and disinfecting wounds and burns

CX Antiseptic Dusting Powder® (Bio-Medical)
Dusting powder, sterile, chlorhexidine acetate 1%. Net price 15 g = £2.00. For skin disinfection and antisepsis
Note. Chlorhexidine Dusting Powder BP contains chlorhexidine hydrochloride 0.5% but no preparation is available commercially

Hibiscrub® (ICI)
Cleansing solution, red, chlorhexidine gluconate solution 20% (≡4% chlorhexidine gluconate), perfumed, in a surfactant solution. Net price 12 × 100-mL sachets = £11.16; 250 mL = £1.13; 500 mL = £1.65. Use instead of soap for pre-operative hand and skin preparation and for general hand and skin antisepsis

Hibisol® (ICI)
Solution, chlorhexidine gluconate solution 2.5% (≡0.5% chlorhexidine gluconate), in isopropyl alcohol 70% with emollients. Net price 250 mL = £1.04; 500 mL = £1.72. To be used undiluted for hand and skin disinfection

Hibitane Obstetric® (ICI)
Cream, chlorhexidine gluconate solution 5% (≡1% chlorhexidine gluconate), in a pourable water-miscible basis. Net price 250 mL = 91p. For use in obstetrics and gynaecology as an antiseptic and lubricant (for application to skin around vulva and perineum and to hands of midwife or doctor)

Phiso-med® (Sanofi Winthrop)
Solution, chlorhexidine gluconate 4% in an emulsion basis. Net price 150 mL = £4.76. For use as a soap substitute in acne and seborrhoeic conditions; for bathing mothers and babies in maternity units (as 1 in 10 dilution) to prevent cross-infection and for pre-operative hand and skin preparation

Rotersept® (Roterpharma)
Spray application, chlorhexidine gluconate 0.2% in a pressurised aerosol unit. Net price 284-g unit = £1.99. For prevention and treatment of sore cracked nipples

Sterexidine® (Galen)
Solution (sterile), chlorhexidine gluconate 0.02%. Net price 150 mL = 83p; 1000 mL = £1.10. For disinfection and wound cleansing

Unisept® (Seton)
Solution (sterile), pink, chlorhexidine gluconate 0.05%. Net price 25 × 25-mL sachet = £2.20; 6 × 100-mL sachet = £1.26. For cleansing and disinfecting wounds and burns and swabbing in obstetrics

With cetrimide
Tisept® (Seton)
Solution (sterile), yellow, chlorhexidine gluconate 0.015%, cetrimide 0.15%. Net price 25 × 25-mL sachet = £1.45; 6 × 100-mL sachet = 99p. To be used undiluted for general skin disinfection and wound cleansing

Travasept 100® (Baxter)
Solution (sterile), yellow, chlorhexidine acetate 0.015%, cetrimide 0.15%. Net price 500 mL = 74p; 1000 mL = 79p. To be used undiluted in skin disinfection such as wound cleansing and obstetrics

---

CONCENTRATES

Hibitane 5% Concentrate® (ICI)
Solution, red, chlorhexidine gluconate solution 25% (≡ 5% chlorhexidine gluconate), in a perfumed aqueous solution. Net price 5 litres = £11.75. To be used diluted 1 in 10 (0.5%) with alcohol 70% for pre-operative skin preparation, or 1 in 100 (0.05%) with water for general skin disinfection
Note. Alcoholic solutions not suitable before diathermy (see Alcohol, above)

Hibitane Gluconate 20%® (ICI)
Solution, chlorhexidine gluconate 20% in an aqueous solution. Net price 500 mL = £5.01. To be used diluted as above in body cavity and bladder irrigation, urethral disinfection and catheter lubrication

With cetrimide
Savlon Hospital Concentrate® (ICI)
Solution, orange, chlorhexidine gluconate solution 7.5% (≡ chlorhexidine gluconate 1.5%), cetrimide 15%. Net price 1 litre = £2.24. To be used diluted 1 in 100 (1%) to 1 in 30 with water for skin disinfection and wound cleansing, and diluted 1 in 30 in alcohol 70% for pre-operative skin preparation
Note. Alcoholic solutions not suitable before diathermy (see Alcohol, above)

13.11.3 Cationic surfactants and soaps

BENZALKONIUM CHLORIDE
Indications: skin disinfection such as pre-operative skin preparation
Cautions: avoid contact with eyes

Roccal® (Sterling-Winthrop)
Solution, blue, benzalkonium chloride 1%. Net price 2.25 litres = £10.99. To be used diluted 1 in 10 to 1 in 200
Additives: fragrance

Roccal Concentrate 10X® (Sterling-Winthrop)
Concentrate, blue, benzalkonium chloride 10%. Net price 2.25 litres = £44.99. For preparation of Roccal Solution with freshly boiled and cooled purified water
Additives: fragrance

CETRIMIDE
Indications: skin disinfection
Cautions: avoid contact with eyes; avoid use in body cavities
Side-effects: skin irritation and occasionally sensitisation

Preparations
Ingredient of Savlon Hospital Concentrate®, Tisept®, and Travasept® 100, see above

SOFT SOAP
Indications: removal of adherent crusts

Soap Spirit, BP, soft soap 65% in alcohol (90%). Net price 100 mL = 54p

SUBSTITUTE SOAPS
See section 13.2.1 (emulsifying ointment); section 13.2.1.1 (emollient bath additives)

13.11.4 Chlorine and iodine

CHLORINATED SOLUTIONS
Cautions: bleaches fabric; irritant (protect surrounding tissues with soft paraffin)

Chlorinated Lime and Boric Acid Solution, BP, (Eusol), chlorinated lime 1.25%, boric acid 1.25%, in purified water, freshly boiled and cooled. Contains not less than 0.25% available chlorine. It must be freshly prepared. Has been used undiluted for skin disinfection, particularly in wound and ulcer cleansing but no longer recommended (too irritant)

13.11 Disinfectants and cleansers

Chlorinated Soda Solution, Surgical, BPC, (Dakin's Solution), boric acid, chlorinated lime, sodium carbonate, sufficient of each to provide a solution containing 0.5% of available chlorine in purified water, freshly boiled and cooled. Net price 500 mL = 68p. Has been used undiluted for cleansing wounds and ulcers but no longer recommended (too irritant)

Chlorasol® (Seton)
Solution (sterile), sodium hypochlorite, containing 0.3–0.4% available chlorine. Net price 25 × 25-mL sachets = £6.61
Additives: none as listed in section 13.1
Irritant therefore no longer recommended

IODINE COMPOUNDS

Indications: skin disinfection
Cautions: pregnancy, breast-feeding; broken skin; thyroid disorders, renal impairment (see appendix 3)
Side-effects: rarely sensitivity; may interfere with thyroid function tests

Betadine® (Napp)
Antiseptic paint, povidone-iodine 10% in an alcoholic solution. Net price 8 mL (with applicator brush) = 69p. Apply undiluted to minor wounds and infections, twice daily
Additives: none as listed in section 13.1

Alcoholic solution, povidone-iodine 10%. Net price 500 mL = £1.24. To be applied undiluted in pre- and post-operative skin disinfection
Additives: none as listed in section 13.1
Note. Flammable—caution in procedures involving hot wire cautery and diathermy

Antiseptic solution, povidone-iodine 10% in aqueous solution. Net price 500 mL = £1.09. To be applied undiluted in pre- and post-operative skin disinfection
Additives: none as listed in section 13.1

Dry powder spray, povidone-iodine 2.5% in a pressurised aerosol unit. Net price 150-g unit = £2.36. For skin disinfection, particularly minor wounds and infections

Scalp and skin cleanser solution, povidone-iodine 7.5%, in a surfactant basis. Net price 250 mL = £2.06. ACBS: for infective conditions of the skin. Retain on scalp for 5 minutes before rinsing

Skin cleanser solution, povidone-iodine 4%, in a surfactant basis. Net price 250 mL = £1.74. ACBS: for infective conditions of the skin. Retain on skin for 3–5 minutes before rinsing; repeat twice daily

Surgical scrub, povidone-iodine 7.5%, in a non-ionic surfactant basis. Net price 500 mL = 96p. To be used as a pre-operative scrub for hands and skin
Additives: wool fat derivative

Savlon Dry® (Ciba)
Dry powder spray, povidone-iodine 0.5% in a pressurised aerosol unit. Net price 55-g unit = £1.59. For minor wounds

Videne® (Beta)
Dusting powder, povidone-iodine 5%. Net price 15 g = £2.60. For minor wounds

13.11.5 Phenolics

HEXACHLOROPHANE

Indications: see under preparations (below)
Contra-indications: avoid use on badly burned or excoriated skin; pregnancy; children under 2 years except on medical advice
Side-effects: sensitivity; rarely photosensitivity

PoM **Ster-Zac DC Skin Cleanser®** (Hough)
Cream, hexachlorophane 3%. Net price 150 mL = £3.55. Use 3–5 mL instead of soap as pre-operative scrub for hands
Additives: information not disclosed for BNF

Ster-Zac Powder® (Hough)
Dusting-powder, hexachlorophane 0.33%, zinc oxide 3%, talc 88.67%, starch 8% (sterile). Net price 30 g = 66p
Additives: information not disclosed for BNF
Prevention of neonatal staphylococcal sepsis, after ligature of cord sprinkle on perineum, groin, front of abdomen, and axillas; after cutting cord and spraying with plastic dressing, powder stump and adjacent skin; after every napkin change powder stump, adjacent skin, perineum, groin, axillas, buttocks, and front of abdomen; continue until stump drops away and wound healed
Adjunct for treatment of recurrent furunculosis, powder daily area of skin normally subject to furunculosis

TRICLOSAN

Indications: skin disinfection
Cautions: avoid contact with eyes

Manusept® (Hough)
Antibacterial hand rub, blue, triclosan 0.5%, isopropyl alcohol 70%. Net price 250 mL = 96p; 500 mL = £1.47. For disinfection and pre-operative hand preparation
Additives: information not disclosed for BNF

Ster-Zac Bath Concentrate® (Hough)
Solution, triclosan 2%. Net price 28.5 mL = 38p; 500 mL = £3.64. ACBS: for staphylococcal skin infections. For prevention of cross-infection use 1 sachet/bath
Additives: information not disclosed for BNF

13.11.6 Astringents, oxidisers, and dyes

ALUMINIUM ACETATE

Indications: exudative eczematous reactions and wounds

Aluminium Acetate Lotion, aluminium acetate solution 5 mL, purified water, freshly boiled and cooled, to 100 mL. It should be freshly prepared. To be used undiluted as a wet dressing
Note. Aluminium acetate solution (13%) for the preparation of aluminium acetate lotion (0.65%) is available from Martindale, Penn, etc. (special order)

Cautionary label wordings, see inside back cover   Prices are **net**, see p. 1

CRYSTAL VIOLET
(Gentian violet)
Indications: see below
Cautions: stains clothes and skin
Side-effects: mucosal ulcerations

Crystal Violet Paint, BP 1980, crystal violet 0.5%, in purified water, freshly boiled and cooled. To be used undiluted
Note. Licensed for topical application on unbroken skin only; no longer recommended for application to mucous membranes or open wounds; restrictions do not apply to use for skin marking prior to surgery

HYDROGEN PEROXIDE
Indications: skin disinfection, particularly cleansing and deodorising wounds and ulcers
Cautions: large or deep wounds; avoid normal skin; bleaches fabric

Hydrogen Peroxide Solution, BP
Solution 6% (20 vols). Net price 100 mL = 20p
Solution 3% (10 vols). Net price 100 mL = 16p
Note. The BP directs that when hydrogen peroxide is prescribed, hydrogen peroxide solution 6% (20 vols) should be dispensed.
IMPORTANT. Strong solutions of hydrogen peroxide which contain 27% (90 vols) and 30% (100 vols) are only for the preparation of weaker solutions

Hioxyl® see Desloughing Agents (below)

POTASSIUM PERMANGANATE
Indications: cleansing and deodorising suppurating eczematous reactions and wounds
Cautions: irritant to mucous membranes; stains skin and clothing
Administration: wet dressings or baths, approx. 0.01% solution

Potassium Permanganate Solution, potassium permanganate 0.1% (1 in 1000) in water
To be diluted 1 in 10 to provide a 0.01% (1 in 10 000) solution

Permitabs® (Bioglan)
Solution tablets, for preparation of topical solution, potassium permanganate 400 mg. Net price 30-tab pack = £2.49
1 tablet dissolved in 4 litres of water provides a 0.01% (1 in 10 000) solution

13.11.7 Desloughing agents
Desloughing agents for ulcers are second-line treatment and the underlying causes should be treated. The main beneficial effect is removal of slough and clot and the ablation of local infection. Preparations which absorb or help promote the removal of exudate may also help (section 13.13.8). It should be noted that substances applied to an open area are easily absorbed and perilesional skin is easily sensitised. Gravitational dermatitis may be due to neomycin or lanolin sensitivity. Enzyme preparations such as streptokinase-streptodornase or alternatively dextranomer (section 13.13.8) are designed for sloughing ulcers and may help.

Aserbine® (Bencard)
Cream, benzoic acid 0.024%, malic acid 0.36%, propylene glycol 1.7%, salicylic acid 0.006%. Net price 100 g = £1.20
Additives: hydroxybenzoates (parabens)

Solution, benzoic acid 0.15%, malic acid 2.25%, propylene glycol 40%, salicylic acid 0.0375%. Net price 500 mL = £1.81
Additives: fragrance

Hioxyl® (Quinoderm Ltd)
Cream, hydrogen peroxide (stabilised) 1.5%. Net price 25 g = £1.81; 100 g = £5.66. For leg ulcers and pressure sores
Additives: none as listed in section 13.1
Apply when necessary and if necessary cover with a dressing

Variclene® (Dermal)
Gel, brilliant green 0.5%, lactic acid 0.5%, in an aqueous basis. Net price 50 g = £4.58. For venous and other skin ulcers
Additives: none as listed in section 13.1
Apply to cleaned and dried lesion with a sterile applicator avoiding surrounding skin; in severe ulceration apply on dressing and repeat as required at intervals of not more than 7 days

PoM Varidase Topical® (Lederle)
Powder, streptokinase 100 000 units, streptodornase 25 000 units. For preparing solutions for topical use. Net price per vial = £7.80
Additives: none as listed in section 13.1
Apply as wet dressing usually 1–2 times daily Also used to dissolve clots in the bladder or urinary catheters

13.12 Antiperspirants
Aluminium chloride is a potent antiperspirant used in the treatment of severe hyperhidrosis.
Dusting powders are described in section 13.2.3.

ALUMINIUM CHLORIDE
Indications: hyperhidrosis
Cautions: avoid contact with eyes; do not shave axilla or use depilatories within 12 hours of use
Side-effects: skin irritation—may be less with hydroxychloride
Administration: apply at night to dry skin, wash off on following morning, initially daily then reduce frequency as condition improves—do not bathe immediately before use

PoM Anhydrol Forte® (Dermal)
Solution (= application), aluminium chloride hexahydrate 20%. Net price 10-mL bottle with roll-on applicator = £2.75. Label: 15
Additives: none as listed in section 13.1

PoM Driclor® (Stiefel)
Application, aluminium chloride hexahydrate 20% in an alcoholic basis. Net price 60-mL bottle with roll-on applicator = £2.82. Label: 15
Additives: none as listed in section 13.1

13.13 Wound management products

13.13.1 Bandages
13.13.2 Surgical adhesive tapes
13.13.3 Adhesive dressings
13.13.4 Surgical absorbents
13.13.5 Wound dressing pads
13.13.6 Tulle dressings
13.13.7 Semipermeable adhesive film
13.13.8 Gel and colloid dressings
13.13.9 Foam dressings
13.13.10 Elastic hosiery

13.13.1 Bandages

RETENTION BANDAGES

Non-stretch fabric retention bandages
Open-wove Bandage, BP (types 1, 2 and 3). Cotton cloth, plain weave, warp of cotton, weft of cotton, viscose, or combination, one continuous length. Type 1, 5 m (all): 2.5 cm, net price = 25p; 5 cm = 42p; 7.5 cm = 60p; 10 cm = 78p (most suppliers) 5 m × 5 cm supplied when size not stated
Uses: protection and retention of absorbent dressings; support for minor strains, sprains; securing splints
Note. Type 1 bandage formerly described as Open-Wove Bandage BPC 1973; Type 2 formerly described as 'medium quality'; Type 3 formerly described as 'hospital quality'
Triangular Calico Bandage, BP. Unbleached calico rt. angle triangle. 90 cm × 90 cm × 1.27 m, net price = 92p (most suppliers)
Uses: sling
NHS Domette Bandage, BP. Fabric, plain weave, cotton warp and wool weft (hospital quality also available, all cotton). 5 m (all): 5 cm, net price = 54p; 7.5 cm = 81p; 10 cm = £1.08; 15 cm = £1.61 (Robert Bailey, Vernon-Carus)
Uses: protection and support where warmth required
Multiple Pack Dressing No. 1 (Drug Tariff). Contains absorbent cotton, absorbent cotton gauze type 13 light (sterile), open-wove bandages (banded). Net price per pack = £2.66
Multiple Pack Dressing No. 2 (Drug Tariff). As for No. 1 (above) but with larger quantities of cotton and cotton gauze and two sizes of bandages. Net price per pack = £4.74

Stretch fabric retention bandages
Cotton Conforming Bandage, BP. Cotton fabric, plain weave, treated to impart some elasticity to warp and weft. 3.5 m (all):
type A, 5 cm, net price = 50p; 7.5 cm = 63p; 10 cm = 78p, 15 cm = £1.06 (S&N—*Crinx*®)
type B, 5 cm = 51p; 7.5 cm = 65p; 10 cm = 80p; 15 cm = £1.07 (J&J—*Kling*®)
Uses: retention of dressings in difficult positions (e.g. over joints)

Polyamide and Cellulose Contour Bandage, BP (formerly Nylon and Viscose Stretch Bandage). Fabric, plain weave, warp of polyamide filament, weft of cotton or viscose, fast edges, one continuous length. 4 m stretched (all): Robinsons—*Stayform*® (5 cm = 29p, 7.5 cm = 37p, 10 cm = 42p, 15 cm = 71p); Seton—*Slinky*® (net price 5 cm = 33p, 7.5 cm = 46p, 10 cm = 56p, 15 cm = 79p); S&N—*Easifix*® (5 cm = 27p, 7.5 cm = 34p, 10 cm = 38p, 15 cm = 65p)
Uses: retention of dressings
NHS Tubular Gauze Bandage, Seamless. Unbleached cotton yarn, positioned with applicators. 20 m roll (all): 00, net price = £1.70; 01 = £1.74; 12 = £2.33; 34 = £3.42; 56 = £4.73; 78 = £5.54; T1 = £7.98; T2 = £10.29 (Seton—*Tubegauz*®)
Uses: retention of dressings on limbs, abdomen, trunk
Elasticated Tubular Bandage, BP (formerly Elasticated Surgical Tubular Stockinette). Knitted fabric, elasticated threads of rubber-cored polyamide or polyester with cotton or cotton and viscose yarn, tubular. Lengths 50 cm and 1 m, various widths 6.25 cm–12 cm, net price 45p–£1.43 (JLB Textiles—*Textube*® (formerly called *Lastogrip*®); Salt—*Rediform*®; S&N—*Tensogrip*®; Seton—*Tubigrip*®; Texlastic—*Texagrip*®). Where no brand stated by prescriber, net price of stockinette supplied not to exceed: length 50 cm, 6.25 cm = 51p, 6.75 cm = 55p, 7.5 cm = 56p, 8.75 cm = 62p, 10 cm = 63p, 12 cm = 64p; length 1 m, 6.25 cm = 92p, 6.75 cm = 98p, 7.5 cm = £1.00, 8.75 cm = £1.05, 10 cm = £1.05, 12 cm = £1.21
Uses: retention of dressings on limbs, abdomen, trunk
Foam Padded Elasticated Surgical Tubular Stockinette (Drug Tariff). Fabric as for Elasticated Tubular Bandage with polyurethane lining. Heel, elbow, knee, small, net price = £1.95, medium = £2.10, large = £2.26; sacral, small, medium, and large (all) = £10.03 (Seton—*Tubipad*®)
Uses: relief of pressure and elimination of friction in relevant area; porosity of foam lining allows normal water loss from skin surface
Elasticated Viscose Stockinette (Drug Tariff). Lightweight plain-knitted elasticated tubular bandage. Length 1 m (all): net price 5 cm (medium limb) = 63p; 7.5 cm (large limb) = 83p; 10.75 cm (OS limb, head, child trunk) = £1.34; 17.5 cm (adult trunk) = £1.68 (Seton—*Tubifast*®)
Uses: retention of dressings
Elastic Net Surgical Tubular Stockinette (Drug Tariff). Lightweight elastic open-work net tubular fabric.
type A: arm/leg, 40 cm × 1.8 cm (size C), net price = 32p; thigh/head, 60 cm × 2.5 cm (size E) = 58p; trunk (adult), 60 cm × 4.5 cm (size F) = 85p; trunk (OS adult) 60 cm × 5.4 cm (size G) = £1.14 (Brevit—*Netelast*®)
type B: withdrawn
type C: arm/leg, 40 cm × 1.8 cm (size C) = 25p; thigh/head, 60 cm × 2.7 cm (size E) = 48p; trunk (adult), 60 cm × 5.5 cm (size F) = 67p; trunk (OS adult) 60 cm × 6 cm (size G) = 85p (Martindale—*Macrofix*®)
Drug Tariff requires size and type to be specified by prescriber
Uses: retention of dressings, particularly on awkward sites
Cotton Stockinette, BP (formerly Cotton Surgical Tubular Stockinette). Knitted fabric, cotton yarn, tubular. 1 m × 2.5 cm, net price = 22p; 5 cm = 34p; 7.5 cm = 40p; 6 m × 10 cm = £2.78 (J&J, Seton)
Uses: 1 m lengths, basis (with wadding) for Plaster of Paris bandages etc.; 6 m length, compression bandage
Ribbed Cotton and Viscose Surgical Tubular Stockinette, BP. Knitted fabric of 1:1 ribbed structure, singles yarn spun from blend of two-thirds cotton and one third viscose fibres, tubular. Length 5 m (all):
type A (lightweight): arm/leg (child), arm (adult) 5 cm, net price = £1.70; arm (OS adult), leg (adult) 7.5 cm = £2.21; leg (OS adult) 10 cm = £2.94; trunk (child)

15 cm = £4.23; trunk (adult) 20 cm = £4.88; trunk (OS adult) 25 cm = £5.85 (Seton)
type B (heavyweight): sizes as for type A, net price £1.70–£5.85 (Sallis—*Eesiban*®)
Drug Tariff specifies various combinations of sizes to provide sufficient material for part or full body coverage
Uses: protective dressings with tar-based and other non-steroid ointments

SUPPORT AND COMPRESSION BANDAGES

Non-adhesive woven extensible bandages
Crepe Bandage, BP. Fabric, plain weave, warp of wool threads and crepe-twisted cotton threads, weft of cotton threads; stretch bandage. 4.5 m stretched (all): 5 cm, net price = 71p; 7.5 cm = 99p; 10 cm = £1.32; 15 cm = £1.88 (most suppliers)
Uses: light support system for strains, sprains, compression over paste bandages for varicose veins

Cotton Crepe Bandage, BP. Fabric, plain weave, warp of crepe-twisted cotton threads, weft of cotton and/or viscose threads; stretch bandage. 4.5 m stretched (both): 7.5 cm, net price = £2.24; 10 cm = £2.89; other sizes NHS (most suppliers)
Uses: light support system for strains, sprains, compression over paste bandages for varicose ulcers

NHS **Cotton Stretch Bandage**, BP. Fabric, plain weave, warp of crepe-twisted cotton threads, weft of cotton threads; stretch bandage, lighter than cotton crepe. 4.5 m stretched (all): 5 cm, net price = 30p; 7.5 cm = 41p; 10 cm = 54p; 15 cm = 76p (most suppliers)
Uses: light support system for strains, sprains, compression over paste bandages for varicose veins

Cotton Suspensory Bandage (Drug Tariff). Type 1: cotton net bag with draw tapes and webbing waistband; net price small, medium, and large (all) = £1.21, extra large = £1.27. Type 2: cotton net bag with elastic edge and webbing waistband; small = £1.37, medium = £1.37, large = £1.42, extra large = £1.48. Type 3: cotton net bag with elastic edge and webbing waistband with elastic insertion; small, medium, and large (all) = £1.43; extra large = £1.49
Type supplied to be endorsed
Uses: support of scrotum

NHS **Cotton and Rubber Elastic Bandage**, BP. Fabric, plain weave, warp of combined cotton and rubber threads, weft of cotton threads (S&N)
Uses: provision of high compression and medium support

Heavy Cotton and Rubber Elastic Bandage, BP. Heavy version of above with one end folded as foot loop; fastener also supplied. 1.8 m unstretched × 7.5 cm, net price = £9.60 (Marlow, Seton, S&N—*Elastoweb*®).
Uses: provision of high even compression over large surface

Elastic Web Bandage, BP. (also termed Blue Line Webbing). Characteristic fabric woven ribbon fashion, warp threads of cotton and rubber with mid-line threads coloured blue, weft threads of cotton or combined cotton and viscose; may be dyed skin colour; with or without foot loop. Per m (both): 7.5 cm, net price = 65p; 10 cm = 90p; with foot loop 7.5 cm each = £3.46 (Marlow, Seton)
Uses: provision of support and high compression over large surface

Elastic Web Bandage without Foot Loop (also termed Red Line Webbing) (Scott-Curwen). Characteristic fabric woven ribbon fashion, warp threads of cotton and rubber with mid-line threads coloured red, weft threads of cotton or combined cotton and viscose. 7.5 cm × 2.75 m (2.5 m approx. unstretched), net price = £3.03; 7.5 cm × 3.75 m (3.5 m approx. unstretched) = £3.66
Uses: provision of support and high compression over large surfaces

High compression extensible bandages
PEC High Compression Bandage (Drug Tariff). Polymide, elastane, and cotton compression (high) extensible bandage, 3 m unstreatched (both): 7.5 cm, net price = £1.98; 10 cm = £2.56 (Seton—*Setopress*®)
Uses: high compression for varicose ulcers

VEC High Compression Bandage (Drug Tariff). Viscose, elastane, and cotton compression (high) extensible bandage, 3 m unstretched (both); 7.5 cm, net price = £2.09; 10 cm = £2.70 (S&N—*Tensopress*®)
Uses: high compression for varicose ulcers

Adhesive woven extensible bandages
Titanium Dioxide Elastic Adhesive Bandage, BP. (Drug Tariff title: Porous Flexible Adhesive Bandage). Woven fabric, elastic in warp (crepe-twisted cotton threads), weft of cotton and/or viscose threads, spread with adhesive mass containing titanium dioxide but free from rubber and zinc oxide. 4.5 m stretched × 7.5 cm, net price = £3.20 (Scholl—*Poroplast*®)
Uses: compression for chronic leg ulcers; continuous pressure and support in patients hypersensitive to rubber and zinc oxide.

Elastic Adhesive Bandage, BP. Woven fabric, elastic in warp (crepe-twisted cotton threads), weft of cotton and/or viscose threads spread with adhesive mass containing zinc oxide. 4.5 m stretched (all): 5 cm, net price = £2.65; 7.5 cm = £3.83; 10 cm = £5.10 (Robinsons—*Flexoplast*®; S&N—*Elastoplast*® Bandage). 7.5 cm width supplied when size not stated
Uses: compression for chronic leg ulcers; compression and support for fractured ribs, clavicles, swollen or sprained joints

NHS **Half-spread Elastic Adhesive Bandage**, BP. Fabric as for elastic adhesive bandage but only partially spread with adhesive. (S&N)
Uses: compression for leg ulcers; compression and support for fractured ribs, clavicles, swollen/sprained joints

NHS **Ventilated Elastic Adhesive Bandage**, BP. Fabric as for elastic adhesive bandage but adhesive spread such that there are regular strips of unspread fabric along length. (S&N)
Uses: compression for leg ulcers; compression and support for fractured ribs, clavicles, swollen/sprained joints

NHS **Extension Plaster**, BP. Woven fabric, elastic in weft, spread with adhesive mass containing zinc oxide, warp threads cotton and/or viscose, weft threads crepe-twisted cotton. (S&N)
Uses: support of light strains, joints and limbs removed from plaster casts, fractured ribs; traction bandaging

NHS Cohesive extensible bandages.
These elastic bandages adhere to themselves and not to the patient's skin, which prevents slipping during use. 2.25 m (both): 5 cm, 10 cm; 4.5 m (all): 5 cm, 7.5 cm, 10 cm, 15 cm (Boots, 3M—*Coban*®, J&J—*Secure*®, Seton, Steriseal—*Cohepress*®)
Uses: support of sprained joints

MEDICATED BANDAGES

Zinc Paste Bandage, BP. Cotton fabric, plain weave, impregnated with suitable paste containing zinc oxide; requires additional bandaging. Net price 6 m × 7.5 cm = £2.48 (Seton—*Zincaband*® (15%)); £2.53 (S&N—*Viscopaste PB7*® (10%), *additives*:hydroxybenzoates)

Zinc Paste and Calamine Bandage (Drug Tariff). Cotton fabric, plain weave, impregnated with suitable paste containing calamine and zinc oxide; requires additional bandaging. Net price 6 m × 7.5 cm = £2.55 (Seton—*Calaband*®)

13.13 Wound management products

Zinc Paste, Calamine, and Clioquinol Bandage, BP. Cotton fabric, plain weave, impregnated with suitable paste containing calamine, clioquinol, and zinc oxide; requires additional bandaging. Net price 6 m × 7.5 cm = £2.55 (Seton—*Quinaband*®, *additives*: hydroxybenzoates)

Zinc Paste and Coal Tar Bandage, BP. Cotton fabric, plain weave, impregnated with a suitable paste containing coal tar and zinc oxide; requires additional bandaging. Net price 6 m × 7.5 cm = £2.48 (Seton—*Tarband*®, *additives*: hydroxybenzoates; S&N—*Coltapaste*®, *additives*: wool fat)
Uses: see section 13.5

Zinc Paste and Ichthammol Bandage, BP. Cotton fabric, plain weave, impregnated with suitable paste containing zinc oxide and ichthammol; requires additional bandaging. Net price 6 m × 7.5 cm = £2.48 (Seton—*Icthaband*® (15/2%), *additives*: hydroxybenzoates; S&N—*Ichthopaste*® (6/2%), *additives*: none as listed in section 13.1)
Uses: see section 13.5

13.13.2 Surgical adhesive tapes

PERMEABLE SURGICAL ADHESIVE TAPES

Zinc Oxide Surgical Adhesive Tape, BP. (Zinc Oxide Plaster). Fabric, plain weave, warp and weft of cotton and/or viscose, spread with an adhesive containing zinc oxide. 1.25 cm, net price 1 m = 22p, 3 m = 48p, 5 m = 68p; 2.5 cm, 1 m = 31p, 3 m = 73p, 5 m = 99p; 5 cm × 5 m = £1.67; 7.5 cm × 5 m = £2.37 (most suppliers)
Drug Tariff specifies 1 m × 2.5 cm supplied when size not stated
Uses: securing dressings and immobilising small areas

Permeable Woven Surgical Synthetic Adhesive Tape, BP. Non-extensible closely woven fabric, spread with a polymeric adhesive. 5 m (all): 1.25 cm, net price = 55p; 2.5 cm = 80p; 5 cm = £1.40 (Beiersdorf—*Leukosilk*®)
Uses: securing dressings
For patients with skin reaction to other plasters and strapping, requiring use for long periods

Elastic Surgical Adhesive Tape, BP (Elastic Adhesive Plaster). Woven fabric, elastic in warp (crepe-twisted cotton threads), weft of cotton and/or viscose threads, spread with adhesive mass containing zinc oxide. 1.5 m stretched × 2.5 cm, net price = 62p; 4.5 m stretched × 2.5 cm = £1.18 (Robinsons—*Flexoplast*®; S&N—*Elastoplast* ®)
Uses: securing dressings
For 5 cm width, see Elastic Adhesive Bandage, section 13.13.1

Permeable Non-woven Surgical Synthetic Adhesive Tape, BP. Backing of paper-based or non-woven textile material spread with a polymeric adhesive mass. 5 m (all): BioDiagnostics—*Scanpor*® (net price 1.25 cm = 38p, 2.5 cm = 60p, 5 cm = £1.06); Beiersdorf—*Leukopor*® (1.25 cm = 39p, 2.5 cm = 61p, 5 cm = £1.07); 3M—*Micropore*® (1.25 cm = 48p, 2.5 cm = 74p, 5 cm = £1.34); S&N—*Hypal 2*® (1.25 cm = 52p, 2.5 cm = 80p, 5 cm = £1.47)
Where no brand stated by prescriber, net price of tape supplied not to exceed 34p (1.25 cm), 54p (2.5 cm), 96p (5 cm)
Uses: securing dressings; skin closures for small incisions
For patients with skin reaction to other plasters and strapping, requiring use for long periods

OCCLUSIVE SURGICAL ADHESIVE TAPES

Impermeable Plastic Surgical Adhesive Tape, BP. Extensible water-impermeable plastic film spread with an adhesive mass. 2.5 cm × 3 m, net price = 92p; 5 m = £1.38; 5 cm × 5 m = £1.77; 7.5 cm × 5 m = £2.55 (Robinsons; Seton; S&N)
Uses: securing dressings; covering site of infection where exclusion of air, water, and water vapour is required

Impermeable Plastic Surgical Synthetic Adhesive Tape, BP. Extensible water-impermeable plastic film spread with a polymeric adhesive mass. 5 m (both): net price, 2.5 cm = £1.27; 5 cm = £2.42 (3M—*Blenderm*®)
Uses: isolating wounds from external environment; covering sites where total exclusion of water and water vapour required; securing dressings and appliances

13.13.3 Adhesive dressings
(also termed Island dressings)

PERMEABLE ADHESIVE DRESSINGS

NHS **Elastic Adhesive Dressing**, BP. Wound dressing or dressing strip, pad attached to piece of extension plaster, leaving suitable adhesive margin; both pad and margin covered with suitable protector; pad may be dyed yellow and may be impregnated with suitable antiseptic (see below); extension plaster may be perforated or ventilated (most suppliers)
Uses: general purpose wound dressing
Note. Permitted antiseptics are aminacrine hydrochloride, chlorhexidine hydrochloride (both 0.07–0.13%), chlorhexidine gluconate (0.11–0.20%); domiphen bromide (0.05–0.25%)

NHS **Permeable Plastic Wound Dressing**, BP. Consisting of an absorbent pad, which may be dyed and impregnated with a suitable antiseptic (see under Elastic Adhesive Dressing), attached to a piece of permeable plastic surgical adhesive tape, to leave a suitable adhesive margin; both pad and margin covered with suitable protector (most suppliers)
Uses: general purpose wound dressing, permeable to air and water

VAPOUR-PERMEABLE (SEMIPERMEABLE) ADHESIVE DRESSINGS

Vapour-permeable Waterproof Plastic Wound Dressing, BP (former Drug Tariff title: Semipermeable Waterproof Plastic Wound Dressing). Consists of absorbent pad, may be dyed and impregnated with suitable antiseptic (see under Elastic Adhesive Dressing), attached to piece of semipermeable waterproof surgical adhesive tape, to leave a suitable adhesive margin; both pad and margin covered with suitable protector. 8.5 cm × 6 cm, net price = 27p (S&N—*Airstrip*®)
Uses: general purpose waterproof wound dressing, permeable to air and water vapour

OCCLUSIVE ADHESIVE DRESSINGS

NHS **Impermeable Plastic Wound Dressing**, BP. Consists of absorbent pad, may be dyed and impregnated with suitable antiseptic (see under Elastic Adhesive Dressing), attached to piece of impermeable plastic surgical adhesive tape, to leave suitable adhesive margin; both pad and margin covered with suitable protector (most suppliers)
Uses: protective covering for wounds requiring an occlusive dressing

---

Cautionary label wordings, see inside back cover   Prices are **net**, see p. 1

13.13.4 Surgical absorbents

Absorbent Cotton, BP. Carded cotton fibres of not less than 10 mm average staple length, available in rolls and balls. 25 g, net price = 48p; 100 g = £1.12; 500 g = £3.87 (most suppliers). 25-g pack to be supplied when weight not stated
Uses: general purpose cleansing and swabbing, pre-operative skin preparation, application of medicaments; supplementary absorbent pad to absorb excess wound exudate

Absorbent Cotton, Hospital Quality. As for absorbent cotton but lower quality materials, shorter staple length etc. 100 g, net price = 80p; 500 g = £2.64 (most suppliers)
Drug Tariff specifies to be supplied only where specifically ordered
Uses: suitable only as general purpose absorbent, for swabbing, and routine cleansing of incontinent patients; not for wound cleansing

Gauze and Cotton Tissue, BP. Consists of absorbent cotton enclosed in absorbent cotton gauze type 12 or absorbent cotton and viscose gauze type 2. 500 g, net price = £5.08 (most suppliers)
Uses: absorbent and protective pad, as burns dressing on non-adherent layer

Gauze and Cotton Tissue (Drug Tariff). Similar to above. 500 g, net price = £3.75 (most suppliers)
Drug Tariff specifies to be supplied only where specifically ordered
Uses: absorbent and protective pad, as burns dressing on non-adherent layer

Absorbent Lint, BPC. Cotton cloth of plain weave with nap raised on one side from warp yarns. 25 g, net price = 63p; 100 g = £1.94; 500 g = £8.16 (most suppliers). 25-g pack supplied where no quantity stated
Uses: external absorbent protective dressing

Absorbent Cotton Gauze, BP. Cotton fabric of plain weave, in rolls and as swabs (see below), usually Type 13 light, sterile. 90 cm (all) × 1 m, net price = 77p; 3 m = £1.62; 5 m = £2.52; 10 m = £4.88 (most suppliers). 1-m packet supplied when no size stated
Uses: pre-operative preparation, for cleansing and swabbing
Note. Drug Tariff also includes unsterilised absorbent cotton gauze, 25 m roll, net price = £10.53

Cellulose Wadding, BP. Delignified wood pulp bleached white, in multiple laminate form. 500 g, net price = £2.08 (most suppliers, including Robinsons—*Cellosene*®)
Uses: absorbing large volumes of fluid

Gauze and Cellulose Wadding Tissue, BP. Consists of thick layer of cellulose wadding enclosed in absorbent cotton gauze type 12 or absorbent cotton and viscose gauze type 2. 500 g, net price = £2.87 (most suppliers)
Uses: absorbing large volumes of fluid

NHS **Absorbent Muslin**, BP. Fabric of plain weave, warp threads of cotton, weft threads of cotton and/or viscose (most suppliers)
Uses: wet dressing, soaked in 0.9% sterile sodium chloride solution

NHS **Absorbent Cotton Ribbon Gauze**, BP. Cotton fabric of plain weave in ribbon form with fast selvedge edges (most suppliers)
Uses: post-surgery cavity packing for sinus, dental, throat cavities etc.

Absorbent Cotton and Viscose Ribbon Gauze, BP. Woven fabric in ribbon form with fast selvedge edges, warp threads of cotton, weft threads of viscose or combined cotton and viscose yarn, sterile. 5 m (both) × 1.25 cm, net price = 55p; 2.5 cm = 62p (most suppliers)
Uses: post-surgery cavity packing for sinus, dental, throat cavities etc.

Gauze Swab, BP. Consists of absorbent cotton gauze type 13 light or absorbent cotton and viscose gauze type 1 folded into squares or rectangles of 8-ply with no cut edges exposed. Sterile, 7.5 cm square, net price 5-pad packet = 27p; non-sterile, 10 cm square 100-pad packet = £4.57 (most suppliers)

Filmated Gauze Swab, BP. As for Gauze Swab, but with thin layer of Absorbent Cotton enclosed within. Non-sterile, 10 cm × 10 cm, net price 100-pad packet = £5.51 (Vernon-Carus—*Cotfil*®)
Uses: general swabbing and cleansing

Non-woven Swab (Drug Tariff). Consists of non-woven viscose fabric folded 4-ply; alternative to gauze swabs, type 13 light. Sterile, 7.5 cm square, net price 5-pad packet = 25p; non-sterile, 10 cm square, 100-pad packet = £3.20 (J&J—*Topper 8*®)
Uses: general purpose swabbing and cleansing; absorbs more quickly than gauze

Non-woven Filmated Swab (Drug Tariff). Film of viscose fibres enclosed within non-woven viscose fabric folded 8-ply. Non-sterile, 10 cm square, net price 100-pad packet = £4.38 (J&J—*Regal*®)
Uses: general purpose swabbing and cleansing

13.13.5 Wound dressing pads

Perforated Film Absorbent Dressing, BP. Low-adherence dressing consisting of 3 layers; wound-facing layer, film of poly-(ethylene terephthalate) perforated in regular pattern; middle layer of type 1 consists of non-woven bleached cotton and viscose fibres or mixture of these with polyacrylonitrile fibres; in type 2 (NHS) middle layer consists of bleached cotton fibres; backing layer of type 1 is apertured non-woven cellulose material; in type 2, the backing layer is identical with wound-facing layer. Type 1, 5 cm × 5 cm, net price, each = 11p; 10 cm × 10 cm = 19p; 20 × 10 cm = 37p (S&N—*Melolin*® (type 1); Kendall—*Telfa*® (type 2)). 5 cm size supplied where size not stated
Uses: dressing for post-operative and low exudate wounds; low adherence property and low absorption capacity

Knitted Viscose Primary Dressing, BP. (Drug Tariff title: Sterile Knitted Viscose Dressing). Warp knitted fabric manufactured from a bright viscose monofilament. 9.5 cm × 9.5 cm (both): net price = 25p (J&J—*N-A Dressing*®); net price = 21p (S&N—*Tricotex*®)
Uses: low adherence wound contact layer for use on ulcerative and other granulating wounds with superimposed absorbent pad

Sterile Dressing Pack (Drug Tariff specification 10). Contains gauze and cotton tissue pad, gauze swabs, absorbent cotton balls, absorbent paper towel, water repellent inner wrapper. Net price per pack = 64p

Sterile Dressing Pack with Non-woven Pads (Drug Tariff specification 35). Contains non-woven fabric covered dressing pad (*Surgipad*®), non-woven fabric swabs (*Topper 8*®), absorbent cotton wool balls, absorbent paper towel, water repellent inner wrapper. Net price per pack = 65p

NHS* **Surgipad**®. Absorbent pad of absorbent cotton and viscose in sleeve of non-woven viscose fabric (J&J)
Uses: for heavily exuding wounds requiring frequent dressing changes

* Except in Sterile Dressing Pack with Non-woven Pads (see above)

NHS Perfron®. Absorbent pad consisting of alternate layers of absorbent cotton and crepe cellulose tissue, in sleeve of non-woven viscose fabric with coating of polypropylene (J&J)
Uses: low adherence pad for heavily exuding wounds; laminate structure delays strike through
NHS Melolite®. Absorbent fabric pad covered on both sides by polyethylene net (S&N)
Uses: primary dressing over clean sutured wounds, lacerations, and abrasions
NHS Mesorb®. Cellulose wadding pad with gauze wound contact layer and non-woven water repellent backing (Molnlycke)
Uses: post-operative dressing for heavily exuding wounds
NHS Ete®. Wound pad of rayon wadding with rayon silk wound contact layer stitched in chequered pattern (Molnlycke)
Uses: leg wounds, decubitus ulcers, minor burns, donor sites
NHS Release II®. Two layered knitted construction of bright viscose in non-woven, non-adherent sleeve. Pack of 100 (all): 5 cm × 5 cm, net price = £5.23; 10 cm × 10 cm = £11.50; 10 cm × 20 cm = £18.93 (J&J)
Uses: high absorbency, low adherence wound contact dressing

Charcoal cloth dressings
Uses: to deodorise discharging, infected, malodorous wounds and ulcers
NHS Actisorb Plus®. Knitted fabric of activated charcoal, with one-way stretch, with silver residues, within spun-bonded nylon sleeve. Net price (each) 10.5 cm × 10.5 cm = £1.37; 19 cm × 10.5 cm = £2.66 (J&J)
NHS Carbonet®. Activated charcoal dressing. 10 cm × 10 cm, net price, each = £1.56; 10 cm × 20 cm = £3.05 (S&N)
NHS Carbosorb®. Outer cover of non-woven polyester-nylon fabric, activated charcoal cloth layer bonded to outer cover and semipermeable polyurethane film contact layer (Seton)
NHS CliniFlex® Odour Control Dressings. Layer of activated charcoal cloth between viscose rayon with outer polyamide coating. Net price 10 cm × 10 cm, 10 = £12.00; 10 cm × 20 cm, 10 = £16.00; 15 cm × 25 cm, 10 = £26.00 (CliniFlex)
NHS Lyofoam C®. Lyofoam sheet with layer of activated charcoal cloth and additional outer envelope of polyurethane foam. 10 cm × 10 cm, net price, each = £1.26; 15 cm × 20 cm = £2.80 (Ultra)

13.13.6 Tulle dressings

Non-medicated tulle dressings
Paraffin Gauze Dressing, BP. Fabric of leno weave, weft and warp threads of cotton and/or viscose yarn, impregnated with white or yellow soft paraffin; sterile. 10 cm × 10 cm, net price, each = 27p; pack of 10 pieces = £1.90 (most suppliers including Seton—*Paratulle®*; Roussel—*Unitulle®*; S&N—*Jelonet®*)
Uses: treatment of abrasions, burns, and other injuries of skin, and ulcerative conditions; post-operatively as penial and vaginal dressing and for sinus packing; heavier loading for skin graft transfer

Medicated tulle dressings
Chlorhexidine Gauze Dressing, BP. Fabric of leno weave, weft and warp threads of cotton and/or viscose yarn, impregnated with ointment containing chlorhexidine acetate; sterile. 5 cm × 5 cm, net price = 19p; 10 cm × 10 cm = 41p (Seton—*Serotulle®*; Roussel—*Clorhexitulle®*; S&N—*Bactigras®*)

PoM Framycetin Gauze Dressing, BP. Fabric of leno weave, weft and warp threads of cotton, impregnated with ointment containing framycetin sulphate 1% in white soft paraffin containing 10% wool fat; sterile. 10 cm × 10 cm, net price = 24p; NHS 10 cm × 30 cm, 10 = £8.45 (Roussel—*Sofra-Tulle®*)
PoM Sodium Fusidate Gauze Dressing, BP. Leno weave cotton gauze impregnated with ointment containing sodium fusidate 2% in white soft paraffin and wool fat. 10 cm × 10 cm, net price = 22p (Leo—*Fucidin Intertulle®*)
Povidone-Iodine Fabric Dressing. Knitted viscose primary dressing impregnated with povidone-iodine ointment 10%. 5 cm × 5 cm, net price, each = 20p; 9.5 cm × 9.5 cm = 34p (J&J—*Inadine®*)
Uses: wound contact layer for abrasions and superficial burns; max. 4 dressings at same time

13.13.7 Semipermeable films and membranes

Vapour-permeable Adhesive Film Dressing, BP. (Semi-permeable Adhesive Dressing.) Sterile, extensible, waterproof, water vapour-permeable polyurethane film coated with synthetic adhesive mass; transparent. Supplied in single-use pieces. Type 1: 10 cm × 10 cm, net price = £1.10 (S&N—*Opsite® Flexigrid*), Type 2: 10 cm × 12 cm, net price = £1.04 (3M—*Tegaderm®*). Type 3: 10.2 cm × 12.7 cm, net price = £1.10 (J&J—*Bioclusive®*)
Uses: post-operative dressing, donor sites, IV sites, superficial decubitus ulcers, amputation stumps, stoma care; protective cover to prevent skin breakdown
NHS Omiderm®. Sterile, adherent, water-vapour permeable polyurethane film. Net price 5 cm × 7 cm, net price 20 = £23.00; 8 cm × 10 cm, 20 = £49.00; 18 cm × 10 cm, 25 = £121.25; 60 cm × 10 cm, 10 = £138.00; 21 cm × 31 cm, 5 = £72.50 (Perstorp)
Uses: donor sites; superficial and partial thickness burns
NHS Spyroflex® (formerly Flexipore 6000). Sterile, semi-permeable, polyurethane membrane with hydrophilic adhesive. Net price 10 cm × 10 cm, 25 = £46.25 (BritCair).
Uses: minor trauma, skin closure (alternative to skin sutures)
NHS Spyrosorb®. Sterile, semipermeable, absorbent polyurethane membrane with polyurethane film and hydrophilic adhesive. Net price 10 cm × 10 cm, 25 = £49.50 (BritCair).
Uses: leg ulcers, pressure sores
NHS Transite Film Dressing®. Primary exudate transfer film composed of two layers which allow excess exudate to pass to secondary absorbent dressing through fine slits which narrow again when exudation decreases. Pack of 10 (all): 10 cm × 10 cm, net price = 79p; 15 cm × 20 cm = £1.24; 30 cm × 40 cm = £2.36 (S&N)
Uses: donor sites; partial and full thickness burns

13.13.8 Gel and colloid dressings

Occlusive or semi-occlusive dressings which adhere to dry skin and interact with moisture in the wound to form a gel; may remain on a wound for up to 7 days.

Hydrogels
NHS Bard Absorption Dressing®. A dry polysaccharide derivative in flake form which is mixed with water and applied directly into the wound. 60-g pack
Uses: treatment of wounds and ulcers.

Debrisan®. Spherical beads of dextranomer packed in plastic castors, single-use sachets, paste or pads. Beads sprinkled onto cleansed wound and covered with a suitable non-woven, adhesive, semi-occlusive covering, or sterile dressing. Alternatively paste or pad is applied and covered in similar manner. Beads, net price 4-g sachet = £1.99, 60 g = £29.75; paste in sachets, 4 × 10 g = £20.40; pads, 3 g sachet = £2.36 (Kabi Pharmacia)
Uses: debriding agent to remove necrotic tissue

NHS Fibracol®. Calcium alginate with collagen matrix. Net price 9.5 cm × 9.5 cm, 10 = £13.00 (J & J)
Uses: moderate to heavily exuding wounds, leg ulcers, pressure sores

NHS Geliperm®. Gel sheets, dry and wet forms; tubed granulated gel. Dry, 11 cm × 25 cm, net price, 6 sheets = £51.23; granulate, 20 g, 6 tubes = £20.82, 50 g, 6 tubes = £52.04. Wet, 10 cm × 10 cm, net price, 20 sheets = £44.85, 12 cm × 13 cm, 6 sheets = £25.62; 12 cm × 26 cm, 6 sheets = £51.23 (Geistlich)
Uses: wound and ulcer dressing, burns, donor sites

Intrasite® Gel (formerly Scherisorb). A ready-mixed hydrogel containing Graft T® starch copolymer applied directly into the wound. 15-g sachet, net price = £1.62 (S&N)

PoM Iodosorb®. Powder, microbeads of cadexomer iodine (modified starch gel containing iodine 0.9%). Net price 3-g sachet = £2.07; also Iodosorb® Ointment, 4 × 10 g = £19.05; 2 × 20 g = £19.05; also Iodoflex® Paste, 5 × 5-g units = £20.55 (Perstorp)
Uses: for venous leg ulcers and pressure sores apply 3 mm layer to wound surface and renew daily (3 times weekly for ointment or paste) or when saturated with exudate; *caution:* thyroid disorders

NHS Kaltocarb®. Dressing in 3 layers: wound-facing layer of calcium alginate fibre; absorbent middle layer of activated charcoal cloth; backing layer of bonded polyester and viscose non-woven material. Net price 7.5 cm × 12 cm, 25 = £47.50; 15 cm × 15 cm, 15 = £65.25 (BritCair)
Uses: discharging infected malodorous wounds and ulcers

NHS Kaltoclude®. Calcium alginate fibre bonded to semipermeable copolymer adhesive film. Pack of 25 (both); 10 cm × 10 cm, net price per pack = £42.50; 15 cm × 20 cm = £127.00 (BritCair)
Uses: light to moderately exuding wounds such as leg ulcers and pressure sores

Kaltostat®. (Drug Tariff title: Calcium Alginate Dressing, type 2). Calcium alginate fibre, flat non-woven pads, 5 cm × 5 cm, net price, each = 66p; 7.5 cm × 12 cm = £1.46; other sizes (NHS) 10 cm × 20 cm, 25 = £82.50; 15 cm × 25 cm, 25 = £143.75; 30 cm × 60 cm, 5 = £113.00; wound packing, 2 g, 25 = £70.00; also (NHS) Kaltostat® Fortex, 10 cm × 10 cm, 10 = £38.50 (BritCair)
Uses: haemostatic

Sorbsan® (Drug Tariff title: Calcium Alginate Dressing, type 1). Calcium alginate fibre, highly absorbent, flat non-woven pads, 5 cm × 5 cm, net price, each = 78p; 10 cm × 10 cm = £1.38; other sizes (NHS) 10 cm × 20 cm, 5 = £19.75; surgical packing 30 cm, 5 = £19.50; ribbon, 40 cm (+12.5-cm probe), 5 = £14.75; also (bonded to a secondary absorbent viscose pad) Sorbsan® Plus (NHS), 7.5 cm × 10 cm, 5 = £9.95; 10 cm × 15 cm, 5 = £20.75 (Steriseal)
Uses: heavily to moderately exuding wounds

NHS Sorbsan® SA Calcium alginate fibre, highly absorbent flat non-woven pads for wound contact bonded to adhesive semipermeable polyurethane foam. Net price 9 cm × 11 cm, 5 = £9.95 (Steriseal)
Uses: moderately to lightly exuding shallow wounds

NHS Tielle®. Semi-permeable, foamed gel with non-woven wicking layer and polyurethane backing layer. Net price 11 cm × 11 cm, 10 = £22.50 (J&J)
Uses: light to moderately exuding wounds, leg ulcers

NHS Vigilon®. Semi-permeable hydrogel sheets on a polyethylene mesh support. Sterile, 3 in × 6 in, net price 10 = £35.50, 4 in × 4 in, 10 = £35.50; non-sterile, 4 in × 4 in, 10 = £24.75, 13 in × 24 in, 2 = £43.00 (Seton)

Hydrocolloids

NHS Biofilm®. Hydrocolloid dressing with non-woven fibre backing; also in powder form for direct application into wound: 10 cm × 10 cm, net price 10 = £16.50; 20 cm × 20 cm, 5 = £28.50; powder, 10 sachets = £18.20 (CliniMed)

Comfeel®. Soft elastic pad consisting of carmellose (carboxymethylcellulose) sodium particles embedded in adhesive mass; smooth outer layer and polyurethane film backing; available as sheets, powder in plastic blister units and paste for direct application into the wound: ulcer dressing, 10 cm × 10 cm, net price each = £1.88; 15 cm × 15 cm = £3.76; 20 cm × 20 cm = £5.64; other sizes (NHS) 4 cm × 6 cm, 30 = £22.20; transparent dressing, 5 cm × 7 cm, 10 = £9.70; 9 cm × 14 cm, 10 = £28.80; 15 cm × 20 cm, 5 = £32.15; powder 6 g, 10 = £24.80; paste 12-g sachet, 10 = £10.40, 50-g tube, 10 = £36.60 (Coloplast)

NHS Dermiflex®. Hydrocolloid dressing bonded to PVC foam 10.2 cm × 10.2 cm, net price, each = £1.95 (J&J)

Granuflex®. Hydrocolloid wound contact layer bonded to plastic foam layer, with outer impermeable plastic film. 10 cm × 10 cm, net price each = £2.00; 15 cm × 20 cm = £4.26; other sizes (NHS), 10 cm × 10 cm, 10 = £21.50, 20 cm × 20 cm, 3 = £22.50; also Granuflex® Extra Thin (NHS), 7.5 cm × 7.5 cm, 5 = £5.05; 10 cm × 10 cm, 5 = £6.26; 15 cm × 15 cm, 5 = £13.27; 5 cm × 10 cm, 10 = £6.92; 5 cm × 20 cm, 10 = £13.82; also Granuflex® Compression Bandage (NHS), 10 cm × 6.5 m (stretched), 6 = £32.64; also Granuflex Paste (NHS), net price 30 g = £2.68; also Granuflex® Granules (NHS), 5 g, 5 = £9.40; also Granuflex® E (NHS), 10 cm × 10 cm, 5 = £10.55; 15 cm × 15 cm, 5 = £22.88; 15 cm × 20 cm, 3 = £17.19; 20 cm × 20 cm, 3 = £22.11; 20 cm × 30 cm, 3 = £33.46; bordered dressing, 6 cm × 6 cm, 5 = £7.38; 10 cm × 10 cm, 5 = £15.61; 15 cm × 15 cm, 5 = £30.98; triangular dressing, 10 cm × 13 cm, 5 = £15.61; 15 cm × 18 cm, 5 = £26.55 (Convatec)
Uses: chronic ulcers, pressure sores, open wounds, debridement of wounds; powders and pastes used with sheet dressings to fill deep or heavily exudating wounds

Tegasorb®. Hydrocolloid dressing bordered with adhesive film edge, 10 cm × 12 cm (oval), net price each = £1.76; other sizes (NHS) 13 cm × 15 cm (oval), 5 = £23.14; 17 cm × 20 cm (oval), 3 = £20.15 (3M)
Uses: chronic wounds such as leg ulcers and pressure sores

13.13.9 Foam dressings

Polyurethane Foam Dressing, BP. Absorbent foam dressing of low adherence; sterile. 7.5 cm × 7.5 cm, net price, each = 69p; 10 cm × 10 cm, each = 82p; other sizes (NHS) 10 cm × 17.5 cm, 25 = £31.68; 15 cm × 20 cm, 20 = £34.46; 10 cm × 25 cm, 35 = £58.05; 25 cm × 30 cm, each = £3.91 (Ultra—Lyofoam®)
Uses: treatment of burns, decubitus ulcers, donor sites, granulating wounds

NHS Allevyn®. Hydrophilic polyurethane dressing; foam sheets with trilaminate structure, non-adherent wound contact layer, foam based central layer, bacteria and waterproof outer layer. 10 cm × 10 cm, each = £2.95 (S&N)
Uses: treatment of heavily exuding wounds, specifically venous leg ulcers

NHS Silicone Foam Cavity Wound Dressing, BP. Soft slightly absorbent wound dressing of low adherence prepared from fluid silicone elastomer base and tin (II) 2-ethylhexanoate by mixing thoroughly for 15 seconds immediately before use and allowing to expand to about 4 times its volume within the wound. Foam dressing, 20 g, net price = £5.10; 500 g = £83.43; gel sheeting, 12 cm × 15 cm, 10 = £77.50 (Dow Corning—*Silastic*®)
Uses: in the managament of open granulating wounds such as pressure sores, abdominal wall breakdown, pilonidal sinus excision

13.13.10 Elastic hosiery

Before elastic hosiery can be dispensed, the quantity (single or pair), article (including accessories), and compression class (I, II or III) must be specified by the prescriber; for further details see Drug Tariff

Graduated compression hosiery
Class 1 Light Support
Hosiery, compression at ankle 14–17 mm Hg, thigh length or below knee with knitted in heel. Net price per pair, circular knit (standard), thigh length = £5.50, below knee = £5.00; light weight elastic net (made-to-measure), thigh length = £13.98, below knee = £10.90
Uses: superficial or early varices, varicosis during pregnancy

Class 2 Medium Support
Hosiery, compression at ankle 18–24 mm Hg, thigh length or below knee with knitted in heel. Net price per pair, circular knit (standard), thigh length = £8.20, below knee = £7.30, (made-to-measure), thigh length = £26.40, below knee = £16.50; net (made-to-measure), thigh length = £13.98, below knee = £10.90; flat bed (made-to-measure, only with closed heel and open toe), thigh length = £26.40, below knee = £16.50
Uses: varices of medium severity, ulcer treatment and prophylaxis, mild oedema, varicosis during pregnancy

Class 3 Strong Support
Hosiery, compression at ankle 25–35 mm Hg, thigh length or below knee with open or knitted in heel. Net price per pair, circular knit (standard), thigh length = £9.70, below knee = £8.30, (made-to-measure) thigh length = £26.40, below knee = £16.50; one way stretch (made-to-measure, only with open heel and open toe), thigh length = £26.40, below knee = £16.50
Uses: gross varices, post thrombotic venous insufficiency, gross oedema, ulcer treatment and prophylaxis

Accessories
Suspender, for thigh stockings, net price = 46p, belt (specification 13), = £3.50, fitted (additional price) = 46p

Anklets
Class 2 Medium Support
Anklets, compression 18–24 mm Hg, circular knit (standard and made-to-measure), net price per pair = £4.62; flat bed (standard and made-to-measure) = £9.68; net (made-to-measure) = £8.98
Uses: soft tissue support

Class 3 Strong Support
Anklets, compression 25–35 mm Hg, circular knit (standard and made-to-measure), net price per pair = £6.42; one way stretch (standard and made-to-measure) = £6.42
Uses: soft tissue support

Kneecaps
Class 2 Medium Support
Kneecaps, circular knit (standard and made-to-measure), net price per pair = £4.62; flat bed (standard and made-to-measure) = £9.68; net (made-to-measure) = £7.46
Uses: soft tissue support

Class 3 Strong Support
Kneecaps, circular knit (standard and made-to-measure), net price per pair = £6.18; one way stretch (standard and made-to-measure) = £6.18
Uses: soft tissue support

13.14 Topical circulatory preparations

These preparations are used to improve circulation in conditions such as bruising, superficial thrombophlebitis, chilblains and varicose veins but are of little value. Chilblains are best managed by avoidance of exposure to cold; neither systemic nor topical vasodilator therapy is established as being effective. Sclerotherapy of varicose veins is described in section 2.13.

Rubefacients are described in section 10.3.2.

Hirudoid® (Panpharma)
Cream, heparinoid 0.3% in a vanishing-cream basis. Net price 40 g = £1.90
 Additives: hydroxybenzoates (parabens)
Gel, heparinoid 0.3%. Net price 40 g = £1.90
 Additives: propylene glycol, fragrance
Apply up to 4 times daily in superficial soft-tissue injuries and superficial thrombophlebitis

Lasonil® (Bayer)
Ointment, heparinoid 50 units, hyaluronidase 150 units/g. Net price 14 g = 38p; 40 g = £1.08
 Additives: wool fat derivative
Apply 2–3 times daily in superficial soft-tissue injuries

Secaderm® (Fisons)
Salve (= ointment), colophony 26%, melaleuca oil 5.6%, phenol 2.4%, terebene 5.25%, turpentine oil 6%. For boils and chilblains. Net price 15 g = 85p
 Additives: beeswax
Apply 1–2 times daily and cover with dressing

14: Immunological products and
VACCINES

In this chapter, immunisation is discussed under the following headings:

14.1 Active immunity
14.2 Passive immunity
14.3 Storage and use
14.4 Vaccines and antisera
14.5 Immunoglobulins
14.6 International travel

14.1 Active immunity

Vaccines may consist of:

1. an attenuated form of an infective agent, as in the vaccines which are used against virus diseases such as rubella and measles, or BCG used against tuberculosis,
2. inactivated preparations of the virus (e.g. influenza vaccine) or bacteria (e.g. typhoid vaccine), or
3. extracts of or detoxified exotoxins produced by a micro-organism (e.g. tetanus vaccine).

Vaccines stimulate the production of protective antibodies and other components of the immune mechanism.

For **live** vaccines, immunisation is generally achieved with a single dose, but 3 doses are required with oral poliomyelitis vaccine. Live virus multiplies in the body and usually produces a durable immunity but not always as long as that of the natural infection. When two live virus vaccines are required (and are not available as a combined preparation) they should be given either simultaneously at different sites or with an interval of at least 3 weeks.

Inactivated vaccines usually require a primary series of doses of vaccine to produce an adequate antibody response and in most cases reinforcing or 'booster' injections are required. The duration of immunity following the use of inactivated vaccines varies from months to many years.

The health departments of the UK have issued a memorandum, *Immunisation against Infectious Disease 1992* which describes the vaccines, immunoglobulins, and antisera in routine use in the UK; recommended schemes for immunisation in childhood are included and advice is given on storage, technique, and record keeping.

Immunisation against Infectious Disease can be obtained from:

HMSO Publications Centre
PO Box 276, London SW8 5DT
Telephone orders, 071-873 9090
or from HMSO bookshops and through all good booksellers.

SIDE-EFFECTS. Some vaccines (e.g. poliomyelitis vaccines) produce very few reactions, while others (e.g. measles and rubella vaccines) may produce a very mild form of the disease. Some vaccines may produce discomfort at the site of injection and mild fever and malaise. Occasionally there are more serious untoward reactions and these should always be reported in the usual way to the CSM. Anaphylactic reactions are very rare but can be fatal (see section 3.4.3 for the management of allergic emergencies).

CONTRA-INDICATIONS. Most vaccines have some basic contra-indication to their use, and the manufacturer's leaflet should always be consulted. In general, vaccination should be postponed if the subject is suffering from an *acute illness*. Minor infections without fever or systemic upset are not contra-indications.

Some viral vaccines contain small quantities of antibiotics such as neomycin or polymyxin (or both); such vaccines may need to be withheld from individuals who are *sensitive to the antibiotic*. *Hypersensitivity to egg* contra-indicates influenza vaccine (residual egg protein present) and, if evidence of previous anaphylactic reaction, also MMR and yellow fever vaccines.

Live vaccines should not be routinely administered to *pregnant women* because of possible harm to the fetus but where there is a significant risk of exposure (e.g. to poliomyelitis or yellow fever), the need for vaccination outweighs any possible risk to the fetus. Live vaccines should not be given to individuals with *impaired immune responsiveness*, whether caused by disease (for special reference to *AIDS*, see below) or as a result of radiotherapy or treatment with high doses of corticosteroids or other immunosuppressive drugs[1,2]. They should not be given to those suffering from *malignant conditions* or other tumours of the reticulo-endothelial system[2].

VACCINES AND AIDS. The Department of Health has advised that HIV-positive subjects with or without symptoms can receive the following live vaccines as appropriate:
measles[2] (or MMR), mumps, poliomyelitis[3], rubella;
and the following inactivated vaccines:
cholera, diphtheria, hepatitis B, haemophilus influenzae, pertussis, poliomyelitis[3], tetanus, typhoid (injection).
HIV-positive subjects should **not** receive:
BCG, yellow fever[4], typhoid (oral)

Note. The above advice differs from that for other immunocompromised patients.

---

1. Live vaccines should be postponed until at least 3 months after stopping corticosteroids and 6 months after stopping chemotherapy.
2. Consideration should be given to use of normal immunoglobulin after exposure to measles and to varicella-zoster immunoglobulin after exposure to varicella.
3. Virus may be excreted for longer periods than in normal subjects; contacts should be warned of this and of need for washing hands after changing a vaccinated infant's nappies; HIV-positive contacts are at greater risk than normal contacts. For HIV-positive symptomatic subjects inactivated poliomyelitis vaccine can be used at discretion of clinician.
4. Because insufficient evidence of safety.

14.1 Active immunity

Vaccination programmes

There is no contra-indication to administration of pertussis vaccine to unimmunised older children in order to protect infants and siblings. Since a course of 3 injections is required to protect against whooping cough, vaccine cannot be used to control an outbreak.

If the pertussis component has been omitted from earlier vaccinations 3 doses of pertussis vaccine can be given at monthly intervals to provide protection.

Where the basic course against diphtheria and tetanus is incomplete triple vaccine may be used to begin or complete the course against whooping-cough so that the infant is not given more injections than necessary.

Measles/mumps/rubella vaccine can be given at the time of the reinforcing dose of diphtheria/tetanus vaccine and poliomyelitis vaccine; because the diphtheria/tetanus vaccine can be more painful, measles/mumps/rubella vaccine should be injected first; the diphtheria/tetanus should then be given with a separate syringe and needle in the opposite limb (or a second appointment can be made).

Vaccines for the childhood immunisation programme should be obtained via local Health Authorities rather than by FP10 prescription.

Age	Vaccine	Interval	Notes
During the first year of life	DTPer/Vac/Ads *and* Haemophilus influenzae *and* Pol/Vac (Oral)	3 doses at intervals of 4 weeks	The first doses should be given at 2 months of age
During the second year of life	Meas/Mump/Rub (MMR) Vac (Live) Haemophilis influenzae		At 12–15 months of age One dose at 13 months–4 years of age if not previously immunised
At school entry or entry to nursery school	DT/Vac/Ads *and* Pol/Vac (Oral)	Preferable to allow an interval of at least 3 years after completing basic course	
	Meas/Mump/Rub (MMR) Vac (Live)		Unless documented history of measles/mumps/rubella vaccination *or* valid contra-indication *or* laboratory evidence of immunity to measles, mumps, and rubella
Between 10th and 14th birthdays	BCG	Leave an interval of not less than 3 weeks between BCG and rubella vaccination	For tuberculin-negative children. For tuberculin-negative contacts at any age
Between 10th and 14th birthdays (girls only)	Rub/Vac (Live)		All girls of this age should be offered rubella vaccine regardless of a past history of an attack of rubella (unless documented history of Meas/Mump/Rub Vac)
On leaving school or before employment or further education	Pol/Vac (Oral) *and* Tet/Vac/Ads		
Adult life	Pol/Vac (Oral) if previously unvaccinated	3 doses at intervals of 4 weeks	No adult should remain unimmunised; reinforcing doses for travellers to countries where polio endemic and for health care workers in possible contact with polio
	Rub/Vac (Live) for susceptible women of child-bearing age		Women of child-bearing age should be tested for rubella antibodies and if sero-negative offered rubella vaccination. Pregnancy must be excluded and patient warned not to become pregnant for 1 month after
	Tet/Vac/Ads if previously unvaccinated	For previously unvaccinated adults: 2 doses at an interval of 4 weeks followed by a third dose 4 weeks later	A reinforcing dose 10 years after primary course and again 10 years later maintains a satisfactory level of protection
	Hepatitis A and B, Influenza, Pneumococcal		All for individuals in high-risk groups, see under individual vaccines

> **Post-immunisation pyrexia—Joint Committee on Vaccination and Immunisation recommendation.** The doctor should advise the parent that if pyrexia develops after immunisation the child can be given a dose of paracetamol followed, if necessary, by a second dose 4 to 6 hours later. The dose of paracetamol for post-immunisation pyrexia in an infant aged 2–3 months is 60 mg; an oral syringe can be obtained from any pharmacy to give the small dose-volume required. The doctor should warn the parent that if the pyrexia persists after the second dose medical advice should be sought.
>
> For full range of doses of paracetamol, see p. 174.

14.2 Passive immunity

Immunity with immediate protection against certain infective organisms can be obtained by injecting preparations made from the plasma of immune individuals with adequate levels of antibody to the disease for which protection is sought (see under Immunoglobulins, section 14.5). This passive immunity lasts only a few weeks; where necessary passive immunisation can be repeated.

Antibodies of human origin are usually termed *immunoglobulins*. The term *antiserum* is applied to material prepared in animals. Because of serum sickness and other allergic-type reactions that may follow injections of antisera, this therapy has been replaced wherever possible by the use of immunoglobulins. Reactions are theoretically possible after injection of human immunoglobulins but reports of such reactions are very rare.

14.3 Storage and use

Care must be taken to store all vaccines and other immunological products under the conditions recommended in the manufacturer's leaflet, otherwise the preparation may become denatured and totally ineffective. **Refrigerated storage** is usually necessary; many vaccines need to be stored at 2–8°C and not allowed to freeze. Opened multidose vials which have not been fully used should be discarded within one hour if no preservative is present (most live virus vaccines) or within 3 hours or at the end of a session (when vaccines containing a preservative are used but also including oral poliomyelitis vaccine).

Particular attention must be paid to the instructions on the use of diluents and ampoules of vaccine should always be adequately shaken before use to ensure uniformity of the material to be injected.

Note. The Department of Health has advised against the use of jet guns for vaccination owing to the risk of transmitting blood-borne infections, such as HIV.

14.4 Vaccines and antisera

AVAILABILITY. Anthrax, rabies, smallpox, and yellow fever vaccines, botulism antitoxin, and snake venom antitoxin are available from local designated holding centres. Details of current arrangements with names, addresses, and telephone numbers of holding centres are given in:
The Health Service Supply Purchasing Guide, section D pp. 1101–1199
and
The Pharmaceutical Supplies Bulletin, volume 8, no. 5, Oct. 1985, 63/85.

For telephone numbers for information on supply of antivenom, see also p. 22.

Enquiries for vaccines not available commercially can also be made to
Department of Health
Room 222
14 Russell Square
London WC1B 5EP
telephone 071-636 6811 extn 3117/3236.

In Scotland information about availability of vaccines can be obtained from the Chief Administrative Pharmaceutical Officer of the local Health Board. In Wales enquiries should be directed to the Welsh Office, Cathays Park, Cardiff CF1 3NQ, telephone 0222 825111, extn 4658 and in Northern Ireland to the Department of Health and Social Services, Dundonald House, Belfast BT4 3FS, telephone 0232 63939 extn 2841.

For further details of availability, see under individual vaccines.

ANTHRAX VACCINE

Anthrax vaccine is available for anyone subject to heavy exposure to anthrax, such as those exposed to infected hides and carcasses and to imported bonemeal, fishmeal, and feeding stuffs. The vaccine is the alum precipitate of an antigen from *Bacillus anthracis* and, following the primary course of injections, reinforcing doses should be given at about yearly intervals.

PoM **Anthrax Vaccine**
Dose: initial course 3 doses of 0.5 mL by intramuscular injection at intervals of 3 weeks followed by a 4th dose after an interval of 6 months
Reinforcing doses: 0.5 mL annually
Available from local designated centres

BCG VACCINES

BCG (Bacillus Calmette-Guérin) is a live attenuated strain derived from *Mycobacterium bovis* which stimulates the development of hypersensitivity to *M. tuberculosis*. BCG vaccine should be given intradermally by operators skilled in the technique (see below); the percutaneous multiple puncture technique is an acceptable alternative **only** for young children in whom the technique of intradermal injection may be difficult (18–20 puncture points are required).

Within 2–6 weeks a small swelling appears at the injection site which progresses to a papule or to a benign ulcer about 10 mm in diameter and heals in 6–12 weeks. A dry dressing may be used if the ulcer discharges, but the air should **not** be excluded. The CSM has reported that serious reactions with BCG are uncommon and most often consist of prolonged ulceration or subcutaneous abscess formation due to faulty injection technique.

14.4 Vaccines and antisera

BCG is recommended for the following groups if they are negative for tuberculoprotein hypersensitivity:

contacts of those with active respiratory tuberculosis (immigrants in whose communities there is a high incidence of tuberculosis may be regarded as contacts—newborn infants need not be tested for sensitivity but should be vaccinated without delay);

health service staff (including medical students, hospital medical staff, nurses, and anybody who comes into contact with patients, including physiotherapists and radiographers, technical staff in pathology departments and any others considered to be at special risk because of the likelihood of contact with infective patients or their sputum; particularly important to test staff in maternity and paediatric departments);

children between their tenth and fourteenth birthdays (see schedule, section 14.1);

students (including those in teacher training colleges);

veterinary and other staff who handle animal species known to be susceptible to tuberculosis;

those travelling to countries with a high incidence of tuberculosis (section 14.6)

Apart from newborn infants any person being considered for BCG vaccination must first be given a skin test for hypersensitivity to tuberculoprotein (see under Diagnostic agents, below).

It is recommended that an interval of at least 3 weeks should be allowed between the administration of a live virus vaccine and BCG. However, when BCG is given to infants, there is no need to delay the primary immunisations, including poliomyelitis.

See section 14.1 for general contra-indications. BCG is also contra-indicated in subjects with generalised septic skin conditions (in the case of eczema, a vaccination site free from lesions should be chosen).

PoM **Bacillus Calmette-Guérin Vaccine.** BCG Vaccine, Dried Tub/Vac/BCG. A freeze-dried preparation of live bacteria of a strain derived from the bacillus of Calmette and Guérin.
Dose: 0.1 mL (INFANT under 3 months 0.05 mL) by intradermal injection
Available from District Health Authorities (also from Evans)
INTRADERMAL INJECTION TECHNIQUE. After swabbing with spirit and allowing to dry, skin is stretched between thumb and forefinger and needle (size 25G or 26G) inserted (bevel upwards) for about 2 mm into superficial layers of dermis (almost parallel with surface). Needle should be short with short bevel (can usually be seen through epidermis during insertion). Raised blanched bleb showing tips of hair follicles is sign of correct injection; 7 mm bleb ≡ 0.1 mL injection; if considerable resistance not felt, needle is removed and reinserted before giving more vaccine.
Injection site is at insertion of deltoid muscle onto humerus (sites higher on arm more likely to lead to keloid formation); tip of shoulder should be **avoided**; in girls, for cosmetic reasons, upper and lateral surface of thigh may be preferred.

PoM **Bacillus Calmette-Guérin Vaccine, Isoniazid-Resistant.** A freeze-dried preparation of live bacteria of an isoniazid-resistant strain derived from the bacillus of Calmette and Guérin.
Dose: 0.1 mL (INFANT under 3 months 0.05 mL) by intradermal injection; for active immunisation of tuberculosis contacts receiving prophylactic treatment with isoniazid.
Available from Evans
PoM **Bacillus Calmette-Guérin Vaccine, Percutaneous** Tub/Vac/BCG(Perc). A preparation of live bacteria of a strain derived from the bacillus of Calmette and Guérin.
Dose: 0.02 mL by percutaneous administration but not recommended, see notes above.
Available from District Health Authorities (also from Evans)

DIAGNOSTIC AGENTS. In the *Mantoux test* the initial diagnostic dose in patients in whom tuberculosis is suspected (or who are known to be hypersensitive to tuberculin) is 1 unit of tuberculin PPD in 0.1 mL by intradermal injection and in subsequent tests 10 and finally 100 units in 0.1 mL may be given. For routine pre-BCG skin-testing the 10-unit dose of tuberculin PPD is used. In the *Heaf test* (multiple puncture) a solution containing 100 000 units in 1 mL is used.

PoM **Tuberculin PPD.** Prepared from the heat-treated products of growth and lysis of the appropriate species of mycobacterium, and containing 100 000 units/mL. Net price 1-mL amp = £5.89. Also available diluted 1 in 100 (1000 units/mL), 1 in 1000 (100 units/mL), and 1 in 10000 (10 units/mL). Net price 1 mL (all) = £2.22
Available from District Health Authorities (also from Evans)

BOTULISM ANTITOXIN

A trivalent botulism antitoxin is available for the post-exposure prophylaxis of botulism and for the treatment of persons thought to be suffering from botulism. It specifically neutralises the toxins produced by *Clostridium botulinum* types A, B, and E. It is not effective against infantile botulism as the toxin (type A) is seldom, if ever, found in the blood in this type of infection.

Hypersensitivity reactions are a problem. It is essential to read the contra-indications, warnings, and details of sensitivity tests on the package insert. Prior to treatment checks should be made regarding previous administration of any antitoxin and history of any allergic condition, e.g. asthma, hay fever, etc. All patients should be tested for sensitivity (diluting the antitoxin if history of allergy).

PoM **Botulism Antitoxin.** A preparation containing the specific antitoxic globulins that have the power of neutralising the toxins formed by types A, B, and E of *Clostridium botulinum*.
Note. The BP title Botulinum Antitoxin is not used because the preparation currently available has a higher phenol content (0.45% against 0.25%).
Dose: prophylaxis, 20 mL by intramuscular injection as soon as possible after exposure; treatment, 20 mL by slow intravenous infusion followed by 10 mL 2–4 hours later if necessary, and further doses at intervals of 12–24 hours.

Available from local designated centres

CHOLERA VACCINE
Cholera vaccine contains heat-killed Inaba and Ogawa sub-types of *Vibrio cholerae*, Serovar O1. Cholera vaccine provides little protection and cannot control the spread of the disease. The Department of Health has therefore advised that:

> immunisation against cholera is no longer a legal requirement for entry into any foreign country and should not be required of any traveller. However, border officials in some countries may still ask people travelling from endemic or epidemic areas for evidence of immunisation. Travellers who are likely to cross borders from such areas, especially overland, should therefore be advised to have the vaccine here before travel rather than risk injections abroad. For this purpose one injection is sufficient.

Patients who travel to a country where cholera exists should be warned that attention to food and water and personal hygiene is **essential**, even after vaccination.

PoM **Cholera Vaccine** Cho/Vac. Net price 1.5-mL vial = £4.51; 10-mL vial = £7.18
Dose: 0.5 mL by deep subcutaneous or by intramuscular injection; CHILD under 1 year, not recommended, 1–5 years 0.1 mL, 5–10 years 0.3 mL
Available from Evans

DIPHTHERIA VACCINES
Protection against diphtheria is essentially due to antitoxin, the production of which is stimulated by vaccines prepared from the toxin of *Corynebacterium diphtheriae*. These are more effective and cause fewer reactions if adsorbed onto a mineral carrier. Adsorbed diphtheria vaccines are recommended for the routine immunisation of babies and given in the form of a triple vaccine, **adsorbed diphtheria, tetanus, and pertussis vaccine**. A dose of poliomyelitis vaccine, live (oral) is generally given at the same time as each of the doses of the triple vaccine (see 14.1). Adsorbed diphtheria and tetanus vaccine is used in place of the triple vaccine when immunisation against whooping-cough is contra-indicated.

A reinforcing dose of adsorbed diphtheria and tetanus vaccine is recommended at school entry (4–5 years of age). This should preferably be given after an interval of at least 3 years from the last dose of the basic course.

Further reinforcing doses of diphtheria vaccine are not recommended as a routine except in the case of those who work in units where there is a potentially high risk of infection such as those employed in infectious disease units or microbiology laboratories. A dilute vaccine, adsorbed diphtheria vaccine for adults, is available for this purpose. The small quantity of diphtheria toxoid present in the preparation is sufficient to recall immunity in individuals previously immunised against diphtheria but whose immunity may have diminished with time; it is insufficient to cause the serious reactions that may occur when diphtheria vaccine of conventional formulation is used in an individual who is already immune. The dilute vaccine must be used when immunising adults and children over 10 years; it may be given without prior Schick testing.

Diphtheria antitoxin is used for passive immunisation; it is prepared in horses therefore reactions are common after administration.

It is now only used in suspected cases of diphtheria (without waiting for bacteriological confirmation); tests for hypersensitivity should be first carried out.

It is no longer used for prophylaxis because of the risk of hypersensitivity; unimmunised contacts should be promptly investigated and given erythromycin prophylaxis (see section 5.1, table 2) and vaccine (see below).

Combined vaccines
With tetanus and pertussis (triple vaccine)
PoM **Adsorbed Diphtheria, Tetanus, and Pertussis Vaccine** DTPer/Vac/Ads. Prepared from diphtheria formol toxoid, tetanus formol toxoid, and pertussis vaccine with a mineral carrier (aluminium hydroxide).
Dose: primary immunisation of children, 0.5 mL by intramuscular or deep subcutaneous injection at 2 months followed by second dose after 4 weeks and third dose after another 4 weeks (see schedule, section 14.1)
Available as **Trivax-AD**® (Evans). Net price 0.5-mL amp = £1.32; 5-mL vial = £7.02

PoM **Diphtheria, Tetanus, and Pertussis Vaccine** DTPer/Vac. A mixture of diphtheria formol toxoid, tetanus formol toxoid, and pertussis vaccine. The adsorbed vaccine is preferred
Available as **Trivax**® (Evans). Net price 0.5-mL amp = £1.32; 5-mL vial = £7.02

With tetanus only
PoM **Adsorbed Diphtheria and Tetanus Vaccine** DT/Vac/Ads. Prepared from diphtheria formol toxoid and tetanus formol toxoid with a mineral carrier (aluminium hydroxide).
Dose: primary immunisation of children omitting pertussis component, 0.5 mL by intramuscular or deep subcutaneous injection at 2 months followed by second dose after 4 weeks and third dose after another 4 weeks (see schedule, section 14.1); reinforcement at school entry, 0.5 mL (see schedule, section 14.1)
Available from Evans (net price 0.5-mL amp = £1.14), Merieux (net price 0.5-mL amp = £1.11; 0.5-mL pre-filled syringe = £1.95)

PoM **Diphtheria and Tetanus Vaccine** DT/Vac/FT. A mixture of diphtheria formol toxoid and tetanus formol toxoid. The adsorbed vaccine is preferred
Available from Evans. Net price 5-mL vial = £4.95

Single antigen vaccines
For children
PoM **Diphtheria Vaccine, Adsorbed** Dip/Vac/Ads. Prepared from diphtheria formol toxoid with a mineral carrier (aluminium hydroxide). Net price 0.5-mL amp = £1.12
Note. Used only for contacts of a diphtheria case or carrier; immunised children under 10 years are given one dose of 0.5 mL by intramuscular or by deep subcutaneous injection, unimmunised children under 10 years are given three doses of 0.5 mL with an interval of 4 weeks between first and second doses and another 4 weeks between second and third; adults and children over 10 years must be given diphtheria vaccine for adults, adsorbed (see below).
Available from Evans

14.4 Vaccines and antisera

Low dose vaccine for adults
PoM Diphtheria Vaccine for Adults, Adsorbed.
Dip/Vac/Ads for Adults. Net price 0.5-mL amp = £3.00
Dose: primary immunisation in patients over 10 years without prior Schick testing, three doses each of 0.5 mL by intramuscular or deep subcutaneous injection separated by intervals of 1 month; reinforcement, 0.5 mL
Note. Unimmunised adults and children over 10 years who are contacts of a diphtheria case or carrier are given the primary immunisation course; immunised adults and children over 10 years are given the reinforcement dose.
Available from distributor (Regent)

Antisera
PoM Diphtheria Antitoxin Dip/Ser.
Dose: prophylactic 500 to 2000 units by intramuscular injection (but **not** used, see notes above); therapeutic 10 000 to 30 000 units increased to 40 000 to 100 000 units in severe cases; doses of up to 30 000 units should be given intramuscularly but for those over 40 000 units a portion is given intramuscularly followed by the bulk of the dose intravenously after an interval of ½–2 hours
Note. Children require the same dose as adults, depending on the severity of the case.
Available from distributor (Regent) or stocks may be held by hospital pharmacies

DIAGNOSTIC AGENTS. The *Schick test* is recommended for individuals who may be exposed to diphtheria in the course of their work. In such cases immunity to diphtheria is confirmed by means of a Schick test carried out at least 3 months after completion of immunisation. A dose of 0.2 mL of Schick Test Toxin is injected intradermally into the flexor surface of the left forearm and 0.2 mL of Schick Control into the corresponding position on the right arm. Readings are made at 24–48 hours and 5–7 days.

PoM Schick Test Toxin and **Control**. Sterile diluted filtrate from a culture of *Corynebacterium diphtheriae*. The control is the same material heated to inactivate the toxin. Net price 2-mL toxin and control set = £15.71
Available from Evans

HAEMOPHILUS INFLUENZAE TYPE B VACCINE

Haemophilus influenzae type B vaccine (Hib) is given in a course of 3 doses at monthly intervals usually at the same time as routine childhood immunisation against diphtheria, tetanus, pertussis and poliomyelitis (see schedule, section 14.1) in infants from 2 months of age. Children under 13 months of age who have already commenced or completed their primary routine immunisation should still receive 3 doses of Hib vaccine at monthly intervals. Children between 13 months and 4 years of age are at lower risk of infection, therefore a single dose is sufficient. The risk of infection falls sharply after the age of 4 years therefore the vaccine is not recommended for adults and children over 4 years.
See section 14.1 for general contra-indications

▼ **PoM Haemophilus influenzae type B** Hib.
Capsular conjugated polysaccharide vaccine
Dose: 0.5 mL by intramuscular or deep subcutaneous injection in a different limb from other concurrently administered vaccines; for primary immunisation 3 doses are required at intervals of 1 month (see schedule, section 14.1)
Available from District Health Authorities (Cyanamid, Merieux or MSD brand). Each company's vaccine is prepared by conjugation to a different type of protein therefore the different brands are not interchangeable. If it is necessary to change brands during a primary immunisation course the entire course should be repeated

HEPATITIS A VACCINE

Hepatitis A vaccine is a formaldehyde inactivated hepatitis A virus (HAV) vaccine prepared from HM 175 strain grown in human diploid cells. The vaccine is an alternative to human normal immunoglobulin for frequent travellers to moderate to high risk areas or those who stay for more than 3 months.

Vaccination should be considered for those travelling to destinations outside Northern and Western Europe, North America, Australia and New Zealand. Travellers who require vaccination less than two weeks before departure may be given a single dose of vaccine plus normal immunoglobulin, and should receive the second dose of vaccine on their return. Administration of human normal immunoglobulin at the same time as the vaccine, at different injection sites, does not affect rate of seroconversion but the level of antibody may be reduced. In the UK some occupational groups such as sewerage workers may be at risk from infection.

Side-effects, usually mild, include transient soreness, erythema, and induration at the injection site. Less common effects include fever, malaise, fatigue, headache, nausea, and loss of appetite.
See section 14.1 for general contra-indications

▼ **PoM Havrix**® (SmithKline Beecham)
A suspension of formaldehyde-inactivated hepatitis virus (HM 175 grown in human diploid cells) 720 ELISA units/mL adsorbed onto aluminium hydroxide. Net price 1-mL pre-filled syringe = £13.60
Dose: by intramuscular injection (see note below), 2 doses of 1-mL, the second 2–4 weeks after the first dose; booster dose, 1-mL 6–12 months following the initial dose. CHILD not yet recommended
Note. The deltoid region is the preferred site of injection in adults. The subcutaneous route may be used for patients with haemophilia

HEPATITIS B VACCINE

Hepatitis B vaccine contains inactivated hepatitis B virus surface antigen (HBsAg) adsorbed on aluminium hydroxide adjuvant. It is made biosynthetically using recombinant DNA technology. The vaccine is used in individuals at high risk of contracting hepatitis B.

In the UK, high-risk groups include health care personnel and patients in units where there is a high incidence of hepatitis B or a direct risk of contact with contaminated human blood, and also certain family contacts of carriers. Similar persons in indirect contact with a source of infection and at a lower risk would be considered a lower priority group. Another group for whom vaccination is recommended is infants born to mothers who are hepatitis B carriers or HBsAg-positive (particularly if they are e antigen-positive or are without anti-e antibody). Active immunisation combined with hepatitis B immunoglobulin is started immediately after delivery.

It should be borne in mind that immunisation takes up to 6 months to confer adequate protection; the duration of immunity is thought to last for 3 to 5 years.

More detailed guidance is given in the memorandum *Immunisation against Infectious Disease 1992*. Vaccination does not eliminate the need for commonsense precautions for avoiding the risk of infection from known carriers by the routes of infection which have been clearly established, see *Guidance for Clinical Health Care Workers: Protection against Infection with HIV and Hepatitis Viruses*. Accidental inoculation of hepatitis B virus-infected blood into a wound, incision, needle-prick, or abrasion may lead to infection, whereas it is unlikely that indirect exposure to a carrier will do so.

Specific hepatitis B immunoglobulin ('HBIG') is available for use with the vaccine in those accidentally infected and in infants (section 14.5).

See section 14.1 for general contra-indications.

PoM **Engerix B**® (SK&F)
A suspension of hepatitis B surface antigen (rby, prepared from yeast cells by recombinant DNA technique) 20 micrograms/mL adsorbed onto aluminium hydroxide. Net price 0.5 mL (paediatric) vial = £8.66; 1-mL vial =£11.55
Dose: by intramuscular injection (see note below), 3 doses of 1 mL, the second 1 month and the third 6 months after the first dose; more rapid (e.g. for travellers), third dose 2 months after first dose with booster at 12 months; CHILD birth to 12 years 3 doses of 0.5 mL; INFANTS born to HBsAg-positive mothers, 3 doses of 0.5 mL, first dose at birth with hepatitis B immunoglobulin injection (separate site)

Note. The deltoid muscle is the preferred site of injection in adults; the anterolateral thigh is the preferred site in infants and children; the buttock must not be used because vaccine efficacy may be reduced. The subcutaneous route is used for patients with haemophilia.

INFLUENZA VACCINES

While most viruses are antigenically stable, the influenza viruses A and B (especially A) are constantly altering their antigenic structure as indicated by changes in the haemagglutinins (H) and neuraminidases (N) on the surface of the viruses.

It is essential that influenza vaccines in use contain the H and N components of the prevalent strain or strains. Every year the World Health Organization recommends which strains should be included.

The recommended strains are grown in the allantoic cavity of chick embryos (therefore **contra-indicated** in those hypersensitive to eggs).

Since influenza vaccines will not control epidemics they are recommended *only for persons at high risk*. Immunisation is strongly recommended for those of all ages with the following conditions:
chronic respiratory disease, including asthma;
chronic heart disease;
chronic renal failure;
diabetes mellitus, and other endocrine disorders;
immunosuppression due to disease or treatment.
Influenza vaccination is also recommended for residents of nursing homes, old peoples homes, and other long-stay facilities.

In non-pandemic years immunisation is not recommended for Health Service staff, except for those at high risk (owing to medical disorders).
Interactions: Appendix 1 (influenza vaccine).
See section 14.1 for general contra-indications.

PoM **Fluvirin**® (Evans)
Inactivated influenza vaccine, surface antigen. Net price 0.5-mL disposable syringe = £5.09
Dose: 0.5 mL by deep subcutaneous or intramuscular injection; CHILD 4–13 years, 0.5 mL repeated once after 4–6 weeks

PoM **Fluzone**® (Servier)
Inactivated influenza vaccine (split virion vaccine). Net price 0.5-mL disposable syringe = £5.31
Dose: 0.5 mL by intramuscular injection; CHILD 6 months to 3 years, 0.25 mL repeated once after 4–6 weeks; 4–13 years, 0.5 mL repeated once after 4–6 weeks

PoM **Influvac Sub-unit**® (Duphar)
Inactivated influenza vaccine, surface antigen. Net price 0.5-mL disposable syringe = £5.08
Dose: 0.5 mL by deep subcutaneous or intramuscular injection; CHILD 4–13 years, 0.5 mL repeated once after 4–6 weeks

PoM **MFV-Ject**® (Merieux)
Inactivated influenza vaccine (split virion vaccine). Net price 0.5-mL disposable syringe = £5.10
Dose: 0.5 mL by deep subcutaneous or intramuscular injection; CHILD 6–35 months, 0.25 mL repeated once after 4–6 weeks; 3–12 years, 0.5 mL repeated once after 4–6 weeks

Note. A generic version is also available from Merieux at the same price

MEASLES VACCINE

Measles vaccine has been replaced by a combined measles/mumps/rubella vaccine (MMR vaccine) for all eligible children.

Administration of a measles-containing vaccine to children may be associated with a mild measles-like syndrome with a measles-like rash and pyrexia about a week after injection. Much less commonly, convulsions and, very rarely, encephalitis have been reported. Convulsions in infants are much less frequently associated with measles vaccines than with other conditions leading to febrile episodes.

MMR vaccine may be used in the control of outbreaks of measles (see under MMR vaccine, below).

Single antigen vaccine
Available from Merieux on named patient basis

Combined vaccines
With mumps and rubella
See below

MMR VACCINE

A combined measles/mumps/rubella vaccine (MMR vaccine) has been introduced with the aim of eliminating rubella (and congenital rubella syndrome), measles, and mumps. Health authorities have an obligation to ensure that every child has received MMR vaccine by entry to primary school, unless there is a valid contra-indication, parental refusal, or laboratory evidence of previous infection. Vaccination records should be checked; where there is no record of MMR vaccination or where the child has received single-antigen measles vaccine, parents should be advised that their children should receive MMR.

MMR vaccine has replaced measles vaccine for children of both sexes aged 12 to 15 months (or after this age if appointments have been missed).

MMR vaccine should be given to children of both sexes aged 4 to 5 years before starting primary school (irrespective of previous measles vaccine or of a history of measles, mumps, or rubella) unless there is:
 a documented history of MMR vaccination;
 a valid contra-indication (see below);
 laboratory evidence of immunity to measles, mumps, and rubella.

MMR vaccine may also be used in the control of outbreaks of measles and should be offered to susceptible children within 3 days of exposure to infection (**important**: MMR vaccine is not suitable for prophylaxis following exposure to mumps or rubella since the antibody response to the mumps and rubella components is too slow for effective prophylaxis).

Children with partially or totally impaired immune responsiveness should not receive live vaccines (for advice on AIDS see section 14.1). If they have been exposed to measles infection they should be given immunoglobulin (section 14.5).

As with measles vaccine, malaise, fever and/or a rash may occur with MMR vaccine, most commonly about a week after vaccination and lasting about 2 to 3 days. Parents should be given written information and advice for reducing fever (including the use of paracetamol). Parotid swelling occasionally occurs, usually in the third week. Post-vaccination meningoencephalitis has been reported very rarely (with complete recovery). Children with post-vaccination symptoms are not infectious.

Contra-indications to MMR include:
 children with untreated malignant disease or altered immunity, and those receiving immunosuppressive drugs or radiotherapy, or high-dose corticosteroids;
 children who have received another live vaccine by injection within 3 weeks;
 children with allergies to neomycin or kanamycin, or a history of anaphylaxis due to any cause;
 children with acute febrile illness (vaccination should be deferred);
 if given to adult women, pregnancy should be avoided for 1 month (as for rubella vaccine);
 should not be given within 3 months of an immunoglobulin injection.

It should be noted that:
 children with a personal or close family history of convulsions should be given MMR vaccine, provided the parents understand that there may be a febrile response;
 immunoglobulin must not be given with MMR vaccine since the immune response to rubella and mumps may be inhibited; doctors should seek specialist paediatric advice rather than refuse vaccination;
 allergy to egg is only a contra-indication if the child has had an anaphylactic reaction to food containing egg (dislike of egg or refusal to eat is not a contra-indication).

PoM MMR Vaccine
Live, measles, mumps, and rubella vaccine
Dose: 0.5 mL by deep subcutaneous or by intramuscular injection
Available from District Health Authorities as *Immravax*® (Merieux), *MMR II*® (MSD), *Pluserix MMR*® (SmithKline Beecham)

MENINGOCOCCAL POLYSACCHARIDE VACCINE

Meningococcal polysaccharide vaccine is indicated for areas of the world where the risk of acquiring meningococcal infection is much higher than in the UK, particularly for travellers proposing to travel 'rough'.

These areas include New Delhi, Nepal, Mecca (see below), and the meningitis belt of Africa, which encompasses southern sub-Saharan parts of Senegal, Mali, Niger, Chad, and Sudan; all of Gambia, Guinea, Togo, and Benin; South-west Ethiopia; northern parts of Sierra Leone, Liberia, Ivory Coast, Nigeria, Cameroon, Central African Republic, Uganda, and Kenya.

Saudi Arabia requires vaccination of pilgrims to Mecca during the Haj annual pilgrimage; this may apply to others visiting Saudi Arabia in the months leading up to August.

For advice on the immunisation of *close contacts* of disease cases of Group A and Group C meningococcal meningitis in the UK and on the role of the vaccine in the control of *local outbreaks*, see the memorandum *Immunisation against Infectious Disease, 1992*.

PoM AC Vax® (SmithKline Beecham)
Meningococcal polysaccharide vaccine prepared from *Neisseria meningitidis* (meningococcus) groups A and C. Net price single-dose vial (with diluent) = £6.86; 10-dose vial = £61.74
Dose: ADULT and CHILD aged 2 months and over, 0.5 mL by deep subcutaneous or intramuscular injection

---

Cautionary label wordings, see inside back cover   Prices are **net**, see p. 1

Chapter 14: Vaccines

PoM Mengivac (A+C)® (Merieux)
Meningococcal polysaccharide vaccine prepared from *Neisseria meningitidis* (meningococcus) groups A and C. Net price single-dose vial (with syringe containing diluent) = £6.86
Dose: ADULT and CHILD aged over 18 months, 0.5 mL by deep subcutaneous or intramuscular injection
Note. The lower age range for AC Vax® and Mengivac (A+C)® differ; in the case of Mengivac (A+C)® the data sheet states that young children and infants respond less well to the vaccine than older children and adults, with little response to the Group C polysaccharide under 18 months of age and a poor response to Group A polysaccharide under 3 months of age. Additionally, protection in infants under 18 months of age is of shorter duration

MUMPS VACCINE

Mumps vaccine consists of a live attenuated strain of virus grown in chick-embryo tissue culture.
See under MMR vaccine and section 14.1 for contra-indications.

PoM Mumpsvax® (Morson)
Mumps vaccine (Jeryl Lynn strain). Net price single-dose vial (with diluent) = £4.00
Dose: ADULT and CHILD over 1 year, 0.5 mL by subcutaneous injection

Combined vaccines
With measles and rubella
See MMR Vaccine

PERTUSSIS VACCINE

(Whooping-cough vaccine)
Pertussis vaccine is usually given combined with diphtheria and tetanus vaccine (in triple vaccine) starting at 2 months of age (see schedule, section 14.1) but may also be given as a single antigen vaccine.

With some vaccines available in the early 1960s persistent screaming and collapse were reported but these reactions are rarely observed with the vaccines now available.

Convulsions and encephalopathy have been reported as rare complications, but such conditions may arise from other causes and be falsely attributed to the vaccine. Neurological complications after whooping cough itself are considerably more common than after the vaccine.

As with any other elective immunisation procedure it is advisable to postpone vaccination if the child is suffering from any acute illness, until fully recovered. Minor infections without fever or systemic upset are not reasons to delay immunisation. Vaccination should not be carried out in children who have a history of severe local or general reaction to a preceding dose; the following reactions should be regarded as severe:

Local—an extensive area of redness and swelling which becomes indurated and involves most of the anterolateral surface of the thigh or a major part of the circumference of the upper arm.

General—fever equal to or more than 39.5°C within 48 hours of vaccine, anaphylaxis, bronchospasm, laryngeal oedema, generalised collapse, prolonged unresponsiveness, prolonged inconsolable screaming, and convulsions occurring within 72 hours.

A personal or family history of allergy is **not** a contra-indication to immunisation against whooping cough; nor are stable neurological conditions such as cerebral palsy or spina bifida.

Children with problem histories. When there is a personal or family history of *febrile* convulsions, there is an increased risk of these occurring after pertussis immunisation. In such children, immunisation is *recommended* but advice on the *prevention of fever* (see p. 444) should be given at the time of immunisation.

In a recent British study, children with a family history of epilepsy were immunised with pertussis vaccine without any significant adverse events. These childrens' developmental progress has been normal. In children with a close family history (first degree relatives) of *idiopathic epilepsy*, there may be a risk of developing a similar condition, irrespective of vaccine. Immunisation is *recommended* for these children.

Where there is a *still evolving neurological problem*, immunisation should be *deferred* until the condition is stable. When there has been a documented history of *cerebral damage in the neonatal period*, immunisation should be *carried out unless there is evidence of an evolving neurological abnormality*. If immunisation is to be deferred, this should be stated on the neonatal discharge summary. Where there is doubt, appropriate advice should be sought from a consultant paediatrician, district immunisation co-ordinator or consultant in public health medicine *rather than withholding vaccine*.

PoM Pertussis Vaccine Per/Vac. A sterile suspension of killed *Bordetella pertussis*. Net price 0.5-mL amp = £1.31
Dose: primary immunisation if pertussis component has been omitted from earlier vaccinations, three doses each of 0.5 mL by intramuscular or deep subcutaneous injection, separated by intervals of 1 month (see section 14.1)
Available from Evans

Combined vaccines, see under Diphtheria Vaccines

PNEUMOCOCCAL VACCINE

A polyvalent pneumococcal vaccine is available for the immunisation of persons for whom the risk of contracting pneumococcal pneumonia is unusually high. For example in patients who require a splenectomy it should preferably be given at least 2 weeks before surgery or as soon as possible after an emergency splenectomy. It is effective in a single dose if the types of pneumonia in the community are reflected in the polysaccharides contained in the vaccine. Studies with other pneumococcal vaccines suggest that protection may last for 5 years. Revaccination should not be carried out because of the risk of adverse reactions. The vaccine should not be given to children under 2 years, in pregnancy, or when there is infection. It should be used with caution in cardiovascular or respiratory disease. Hypersensitivity reactions may occur.

See section 14.1 for general contra-indications.

PoM **Pneumovax® II** (Morson)
Polysaccharide from each of 23 capsular types of pneumococcus
Dose: 0.5 mL by subcutaneous or intramuscular injection

POLIOMYELITIS VACCINES

There are two types of poliomyelitis vaccine, poliomyelitis vaccine, live (oral) (Sabin) and poliomyelitis vaccine, inactivated (Salk). The oral vaccine, consisting of a mixture of attenuated strains of virus types 1, 2, and 3 is at present generally used in the UK.

INITIAL COURSE. **Poliomyelitis vaccine, live (oral)** is given on 3 occasions, usually at the same time as routine immunisation against diphtheria, tetanus, and pertussis (see schedule, section 14.1).

The initial course of 3 doses should also be given to all unimmunised adults.

REINFORCEMENT. A reinforcing dose of oral poliomyelitis vaccine is recommended at school entry at which time children should also receive a reinforcing dose of diphtheria and tetanus vaccine, and a dose of MMR vaccine if this has not already been given. Oral poliomyelitis vaccine is also recommended at school leaving.

Vaccine-associated poliomyelitis and poliomyelitis in contacts of vaccinees are both rare. In England and Wales there is an annual average of 1 recipient and 1 contact case in relation to over 2 million doses of oral vaccine. The need for strict personal hygiene must be stressed; the contacts of a recently vaccinated baby should be advised of the necessity for personal hygiene, particularly of the need to wash their hands after changing the baby's napkins.

Contra-indications to the use of oral poliomyelitis vaccine include vomiting and diarrhoea, and immunodeficiency disorders (or household contacts of patients with immunodeficiency disorders). See section 14.1 for further contra-indications.

Poliomyelitis vaccine (inactivated) may be used for those in whom poliomyelitis vaccine (oral) is contra-indicated because of immunosuppressive disorders (for advice on AIDS see section 14.1).

TRAVELLERS. Travellers to areas other than Australia, New Zealand, Europe, and North America should be given a full course of oral poliomyelitis vaccine if they have not been immunised in the past. Those who have not received immunisation within the last 10 years should be given a booster dose of oral poliomyelitis vaccine.

Live (oral) (Sabin)
PoM **Poliomyelitis Vaccine, Live (Oral)** Pol/Vac (Oral)[1]. A suspension of suitable live attenuated strains of poliomyelitis virus, types 1, 2, and 3. Available in single-dose and 10-dose containers
Dose: 3 drops from a multidose container or the total contents of a single-dose container; for primary immunisation 3 doses are required (see schedule, section 14.1)

Available from District Health Authorities (private purchases from SmithKline Beecham and Evans)

1. BP permits code OPV for vaccine in single doses provided it also appears on pack.

Note. Poliomyelitis vaccine loses potency once the container has been opened, therefore any vaccine remaining at the end of an immunisation session should be discarded; whenever possible sessions should be arranged to avoid undue wastage.

Inactivated (Salk)
PoM **Poliomyelitis Vaccine, Inactivated** Pol/Vac (Inact). An inactivated suspension of suitable strains of poliomyelitis virus, types 1, 2, and 3.
Dose: 0.5 mL or as stated on the label by deep subcutaneous or intramuscular injection; for primary immunisation 3 doses are required (see schedule, section 14.1)

Available from Department of Health, Room 222, 14 Russell Square, London WC1B 5EP, telephone 071-636 6811, extn 3117/3236 *and*
Scottish Home and Health Department, telephone 031-552 6255, extn 2162 *and*
Welsh Health Common Services Authority, Heron House, 35–43 Newport Road, Cardiff CF2 1SB, telephone 0222 471234. Central Services Agency, 25 Adelaide St, Belfast BT2 8FH, telephone 0232 324431

Note. Should be ordered one dose at a time and only when required for use.

RABIES VACCINE

A human diploid cell **rabies vaccine** is now in use. It should be offered prophylactically to those at high risk—those working in quarantine stations, animal handlers, veterinary surgeons, and field workers who may be exposed to bites of wild animals.

The Department of Health has advised that for *prophylactic use* the vaccine produces a good antibody response when given in a 3-dose schedule on days 0, 7, and 28, with a reinforcing dose every 2–3 years depending on the risk of exposure.

For *post-exposure treatment of previously vaccinated patients* two reinforcing doses are needed (one on day 0 and one on day 3–7).

For *post-exposure treatment of previously unvaccinated patients* a course of injections should be started as soon as possible after exposure (days 0, 3, 7, 14, 30, and 90). The course may be discontinued if it is proved that the patient was not at risk. There are no specific contra-indications to this diploid cell vaccine and its use should be considered whenever a patient has been attacked by an animal in a country where rabies is endemic, even if there is no direct evidence of rabies in the attacking animal. Rabies immunoglobulin (section 14.5) should also be given.

Staff in attendance on a patient who is highly suspected of, or known to be suffering from, rabies should be offered vaccination. Four intradermal doses of 0.1 mL of human diploid cell vaccine (Merieux) given on the same day at different sites has been suggested for this purpose (ensuring correct intradermal technique).

Advice on post-exposure vaccination and treatment of rabies is available from the Virus Reference Laboratory, Central Public Health Laboratory, Colindale, London NW9 5HT, tel 081-200 4400.

PoM **Merieux Inactivated Rabies Vaccine** (Merieux)
Freeze-dried human diploid cell rabies vaccine prepared from Wistar strain PM/WI 38 1503-3M. Single-dose vial with syringe containing diluent

Note. Studies have shown that when this vaccine is injected into the gluteal region there is a poor response. Concomitant administration of chloroquine may also affect the antibody response.

Dose: prophylactic, 1 mL by deep subcutaneous or intramuscular injection in the deltoid region, followed by a second dose after 1 month and a third after 6–12 months; also further reinforcing doses every 1–3 years depending on the risk of infection

Note. Department of Health now recommends a prophylactic schedule of doses on days 0, 7 and 28, see notes above.

Post-exposure, see notes above
Staff in attendance, see notes above
Also available from local designated centres (special workers and post-exposure treatment)

RUBELLA VACCINE

The selective policy of protecting women of child-bearing age from the risks of rubella (German measles) in pregnancy has been extended to a policy of eliminating the circulation of rubella among young children. The existing rubella vaccination policy will therefore be reinforced by the mass vaccination of children of both sexes, using combined measles, mumps, and rubella vaccine.

Rubella vaccine is still recommended for pre-pubertal girls between their tenth and fourteenth birthdays (unless there is documented evidence that they have received MMR) and for seronegative women of child-bearing age (see schedule, section 14.1) as well as those who might put pregnant women at risk of infection (e.g. nurses and doctors in obstetric units).

Rubella vaccination should be avoided in early pregnancy, and women of child-bearing age should be advised not to become pregnant within 1 month of vaccination. However, despite active surveillance in the UK, the USA, and Germany, no case of congenital rubella syndrome has been reported following inadvertent vaccination shortly before or during pregnancy. There is thus no evidence that the vaccine is teratogenic, and termination of pregnancy following inadvertent vaccination should not be routinely recommended; potential parents should be given this information before making a decision about termination.

Vaccine may conveniently be offered to previously unvaccinated and seronegative post-partum women. Again they must avoid pregnancy for 1 month. Immunising susceptible post-partum women a few days after delivery is important as far as the overall reduction of congenital abnormalities in the UK is concerned, for about 60% of these abnormalities occur in the babies of multiparous women.

Susceptible pregnant women who are exposed to rubella and who do not want therapeutic abortion may be offered normal immunoglobulin injection (section 14.5).

See section 14.1 for general contra-indications.

PoM **Rubella Vaccine, Live** Rub/Vac (Live). A freeze-dried suspension of a suitable live attenuated strain of rubella virus grown in suitable cell cultures.
Dose: 0.5 mL by deep subcutaneous or by intramuscular injection (see schedule, section 14.1 and notes above)
Available as
PoM **Almevax®** (Evans)
Rubella vaccine, live, prepared from Wistar RA 27/3 strain propagated in human diploid cells. Net price single-dose amp with diluent = £2.61; 10-dose vial with diluent = £21.64
PoM **Ervevax®** (SmithKline Beecham)
Rubella vaccine, live, prepared from Wistar RA 27/3 strain propagated in human diploid cells. Net price single-dose vial = £2.30; 10-dose vial = £19.10 (both with diluent)
PoM **Rubavax®** (Merieux)
Rubella vaccine, live, prepared from Wistar RA27/3 strain propagated in human diploid cells. Net price single-dose vial with syringe containing diluent = £2.61

With measles and mumps, see MMR Vaccine

SMALLPOX VACCINE

Smallpox vaccination is no longer required routinely in the UK and other countries because global eradication of smallpox has now been achieved. Workers in laboratories where pox viruses (such as vaccinia) are handled, and others whose work involves an identifiable risk of exposure to pox virus, should be advised of the possible risk and vaccination should be considered. Detailed guidance for laboratory staff has been prepared by the Advisory Committee on Dangerous Pathogens and the Advisory Committee on Genetic Manipulation. There is no requirement for smallpox vaccination of travellers.

PoM **Smallpox Vaccine** Var/Vac. Consists of a suspension of live vaccinia virus grown in the skin of living animals, supplied in freeze-dried form with diluent

Advice on the need for vaccination and on contra-indications should be obtained from the Virus Reference Laboratory, Central Public Health Laboratory, Colindale (081-200 4400) who will also supply the vaccine (free of charge)

TETANUS VACCINES
(Tetanus toxoids)
Tetanus vaccines stimulate the production of the protective antitoxin. In general, adsorption on aluminium hydroxide, aluminium phosphate, or calcium phosphate improves antigenicity. Adsorbed tetanus vaccine is offered routinely to babies in combination with adsorbed diphtheria vaccine (DT/Vac/Ads) and more usually also combined with killed *Bordetella pertussis* organisms as a triple vaccine, adsorbed diphtheria, tetanus, and pertussis vaccine (DT Per/Vac/Ads), see schedule, section 14.1.

Of the single antigen tetanus vaccines adsorbed tetanus vaccine is again preferred to the plain vaccine. Adsorbed vaccine must not be given intradermally.

In children, the triple vaccine not only gives protection against tetanus in childhood but also gives the basic immunity for subsequent reinforcing doses of tetanus vaccine at school entry and at school leaving and also when a potentially tetanus-contaminated injury has been received. Normally, tetanus vaccine should not be given unless more than 10 years have elapsed since the last reinforcing dose because of the possibility that hypersensitivity reactions may develop.

Active immunisation is important for persons in older age groups who may never have had a routine or complete course of immunisation when younger. In these persons a course of adsorbed tetanus vaccine may be given. Very rarely, tetanus has developed after abdominal surgery; patients awaiting elective surgery should be asked about tetanus immunisation and immunised if necessary.

See section 14.1 for general contra-indications.

For serious, potentially contaminated wounds tetanus immunoglobulin injection (section 14.5) should be selectively used in addition to wound toilet, adsorbed tetanus vaccine, and benzylpenicillin or another appropriate antibiotic.

Single antigen vaccines
The BP directs that when Tetanus Vaccine is prescribed or demanded and the form is not stated, Adsorbed Tetanus Vaccine may be dispensed or supplied.

PoM **Adsorbed Tetanus Vaccine** Tet/Vac/Ads. Prepared from tetanus formol toxoid with a mineral carrier (aluminium hydroxide).
Dose: 0.5 mL or as stated on the label, by intramuscular or deep subcutaneous injection followed after 4 weeks by a second dose and after a further 4 weeks by a third
Note. This dose reflects the guidelines of the Joint Committee on Vaccination and Immunisation, see *Immunisation against Infectious Disease* 1990
Available from Evans (net price 0.5-mL amp = 71p, and as **Clostet**®, net price 0.5-mL single-dose syringe = £1.40), Merieux (as **Tetavax**®, net price 0.5-mL amp = 55p; 0.5-mL single-dose syringe = £1.20; 5-mL vial = £2.80), and from Servier (net price 0.5-mL amp = 64p; 5-mL vial = £2.89)

PoM **Tetanus Vaccine** Tet/Vac/FT. Tetanus formol toxoid. 0.5-mL amp and 5-mL vial
Dose: as for Adsorbed Tetanus Vaccine which is preferred (see notes above)
Available from Evans

Combined vaccines, see Diphtheria Vaccines

TYPHOID VACCINES
There are now three types of typhoid vaccine available, two given by injection and a third given by mouth. **None** of these typhoid vaccines is a substitute for personal hygiene (see section 14.6).

The original **typhoid vaccine**, **a whole cell** vaccine is normally given in 2 doses at intervals of 4–6 weeks for primary immunisation, with reinforcing doses about every 3 years on continued exposure. Local reactions to this vaccine, which consist of swelling, pain, and tenderness appear about every 2–3 hours after *intramuscular or deep subcutaneous injection*. Systemic reactions, which consist of fever, malaise, and headache, may also occur and usually last for about 36 hours after injection. If severe reactions are experienced after the first dose *intradermal injection* may be preferred for the second dose, as these reactions are virtually absent when the intradermal route is used.

A capsular **polysaccharide typhoid vaccine** is now available for single dose administration by *intramuscular or deep subcutaneous injection* with a reinforcing dose every 3 years on continued exposure. Local reactions, including pain, swelling or erythema, may appear 48–72 hours after administration.

An **oral typhoid vaccine** is now also available. It is **live attenuated** vaccine contained in an enteric-coated capsule. It is taken *by mouth* as three doses of one capsule on alternate days, providing protection 7–10 days after the last dose. Protection may persist for up to 3 years in those constantly (or repeatedly) exposed to *S. typhi*, but occasional travellers require a booster course at intervals of 1 year. Oral typhoid vaccine is **contra-indicated** in individuals who are immunosuppressed (whether due to disease or its treatment) and is inactivated by concomitant administration of antibiotics of sulphonamides, administration of a dose should be coordinated so that mefloquine is not taken for at least 12 hours before or after a dose.

For general contra-indications to vaccines, see section 14.1.

Whole cell vaccine for injection
PoM **Typhoid Vaccine** Typhoid/Vac. A suspension of killed *Salmonella typhi* organisms. Net price 1.5-mL vial = £4.11
Dose: 0.5 mL by deep subcutaneous or intramuscular injection; CHILD 1–10 years 0.25 mL
Second dose after 4–6 weeks, 0.5 mL (or 0.1 mL by intradermal injection); CHILD 1–10 years 0.25 mL (or 0.1 mL by intradermal injection)
Note. The Department of Health now recommends that the second dose of typhoid vaccine and subsequent boosters can be given intradermally to reduce reactions
Available from Evans

Polysaccharide vaccine
▼ PoM **Typhim Vi**® (Merieux)
Vi capsular polysaccharide typhoid vaccine, 50 micrograms/mL virulence polysaccharide antigen of *Salmonella typhi*. Net price 0.5-mL single-dose prefilled syringe = £10.95
Dose: 0.5 mL by deep subcutaneous or intramuscular injection; CHILD under 18 months, may show suboptimal response; under 12 months not recommended

Live oral vaccine
▼ PoM **Vivotif**® (Evans)
Capsules, e/c, live attenuated *Salmonella typhi* (Ty 21a). Net price 3-cap pack = £24.81. Label: 23, 25, C, administration
Dose: ADULT and CHILD over 6 years, 1 capsule on days 1, 3, and 5; under 6 years, not recommended
COUNSELLING. Swallow as soon as possible after placing in mouth with a cold or lukewarm drink; it is important to store in refrigerator

YELLOW FEVER VACCINE

Yellow fever vaccine consists of a live attenuated yellow fever virus (17D strain) grown in developing chick embryos. Infants under 9 months of age should only be vaccinated if the risk of yellow fever is unavoidable since there is a small risk of encephalitis. The vaccine should not be given to those with impaired immune responsiveness, or who have had an anaphylactic reaction to egg; it should not be given during pregnancy (but where there is a significant risk of exposure the need for vaccination outweighs any risk to the fetus). See section 14.1 for further contra-indications. Reactions are few. The immunity which probably lasts for life is officially accepted for 10 years starting from 10 days after primary vaccination and for a further 10 years immediately after revaccination.

PoM **Yellow Fever Vaccine, Live** Yel/Vac. A suspension of chick embryo proteins containing attenuated 17D strain virus
Dose: 0.5 mL by subcutaneous injection
Available (only to designated Yellow Fever Vaccination centres) as
PoM **Arilvax**® (Evans)
Freeze-dried yellow fever vaccine, live. 1-, 5-, and 10-dose vials (with diluent)

14.5 Immunoglobulins

Injection of immunoglobulins produces immediate protection lasting about 4–6 weeks. Immunoglobulins of animal origin (antisera) were frequently associated with hypersensitivity which led to their virtual abandonment; human immunoglobulins took their place.

The two types of human immunoglobulin preparation are **normal immunoglobulin** and **specific immunoglobulins**.

Further information about immunoglobulins is included in *Immunisation against Infectious Disease* (see section 14.1).

AVAILABILITY. **Normal immunoglobulin** is now only available from the Public Health Laboratory Service laboratories for contacts and the control of outbreaks. It is available commercially for other purposes.

Specific immunoglobulins are available from the *Public Health Laboratory Service laboratories* and *Regional Blood Transfusion Centres* in England and Wales with the exception of **tetanus immunoglobulin** which is distributed through *Regional Blood Transfusion Centres* to hospital pharmacies or blood transfusion departments and is also available to general medical practitioners. **Rabies immunoglobulin** is available from the *Central Public Health Laboratory, London*. The large amounts of **hepatitis B immunoglobulin** required by transplant centres should be obtained commercially.

In Scotland all immunoglobulins are available from the *Blood Transfusion Service*. **Tetanus immunoglobulin** is distributed by the *Blood Transfusion Service* to hospitals and general medical practitioners on demand.

NORMAL IMMUNOGLOBULIN
(Gamma Globulin)

Human **normal immunoglobulin** ('HNIG') is prepared from pools of at least 1000 donations of human plasma; it contains antibody to measles, mumps, varicella, hepatitis A, and other viruses that are currently prevalent in the general population. It is administered by intramuscular injection for the protection of susceptible contacts against hepatitis A virus (infectious hepatitis), measles and, to a lesser extent, rubella. Injection of human immunoglobulin produces immediate passive immunity lasting about 4–6 weeks. Intravenous administration is used for replacement therapy (see below).

Side-effects of immunoglobulins include malaise, chills, fever, and rarely anaphylaxis. Human normal immunoglobulin is **contra-indicated** in patients with known class specific antibody to immunoglobulin A (IgA).

Interference with live virus vaccines
Normal immunoglobulin may interfere with the immune response to live virus vaccines which should therefore only be given at least 3 weeks before or 3 months after an injection of normal immunoglobulin. This does not apply to yellow fever vaccine since normal immunoglobulin does not contain antibody to this virus. For travellers, if there is insufficient time, the recommended interval may have to be ignored.

HEPATITIS A. Control of hepatitis A depends on good hygiene and many studies have also shown the value of **normal immunoglobulin** in the prevention and control of outbreaks of this disease. It is recommended for controlling infection in contacts in closed institutions and also, under certain conditions, in school and home contacts and for travellers going to areas where the disease is highly endemic (all countries excluding Northern and Western Europe, North America, Australia, and New Zealand). Alternatively, **hepatitis A vaccine** may be used for those aged 16 years or over visiting such countries frequently or who stay for longer than 3 months.

MEASLES. Normal immunoglobulin may be given for prophylaxis in children with compromised immunity (and in adults with compromised immunity who have no measles antibodies); it should be given as soon as possible after contact with measles. It should also be given to children under 12 months with recent severe illness for whom measles should be avoided; MMR vaccine should then be given (after an interval of **at least 3 months**) at around the usual age.

RUBELLA. Immunoglobulin after exposure does **not** prevent infection in non-immune contacts and is **not** recommended for protection of pregnant women exposed to rubella. It may however reduce the likelihood of a clinical attack which may possibly reduce the risk to the fetus. It should only be used when termination of pregnancy would be unacceptable when it should be given as soon as possible after exposure. Serological follow-up of recipients is essential.

For routine prophylaxis, see Rubella Vaccine.

For intramuscular use

PoM **Human Normal Immunoglobulin** Human normal immunoglobulin injection. 250-mg vial; 750-mg vial

Available from BPL and SNBTS and from Public Health Laboratory Service (for contacts and control of outbreaks only, see p. 454)

Dose: by intramuscular injection, Hepatitis A travel prophylaxis (2 months or less abroad), 250 mg; CHILD under 10 years 125 mg; longer travel prophylaxis (3–5 months abroad) and to control outbreaks, 500 mg; CHILD under 10 years 250 mg

Measles prophylaxis, CHILD under 1 year 250 mg, 1–2 years 500 mg, 3 years and over 750 mg; to allow attenuated attack, CHILD under 1 year 100 mg, 1 year and over 250 mg

Rubella in pregnancy, prevention of clinical attack, 750 mg

¹PoM **Gammabulin**® (Immuno)

Human normal immunoglobulin injection. Net price 2-mL vial = £3.20; 5-mL vial = £6.50; 10-mL vial = £11.00; 320-mg vial with 2 mL water for injections = £3.50

¹PoM **Kabiglobulin**® (Kabi Pharmacia)

Human normal immunoglobulin injection 16%. Net price 2-mL amp = £2.85; 5-mL amp = £6.15

1. Doses for these preparations are expressed in terms of volume:
   Dose: by intramuscular injection,
   Hepatitis A prophylaxis, ADULT and CHILD 0.02–0.04 mL/kg; greater exposure risk, 0.06–0.12 mL/kg
   Measles prophylaxis, 0.2 mL/kg; to allow attenuated attack, 0.04 mL/kg
   Rubella in pregnancy, prevention of clinical attack, 20 mL

REPLACEMENT THERAPY

Special formulations for intravenous administration are available for replacement therapy for patients with congenital agammaglobulinaemia and hypogammaglobulinaemia, for the treatment of idiopathic thrombocytopenic purpura and Kawasaki syndrome, and for the prophylaxis of infection following bone marrow transplantation.

For intravenous use

Available as: *Endobulin*® (500 mg, 1 g, 2.5 g, 5 g, 7.5 g, 10 g—Immuno); *Gamimune-N*® (500 mg, 2.5 g, 5 g—Cutter); Human Immunoglobulin (3 g—SNBTS); *Sandoglobulin*® (1 g, 3 g, 6 g—Sandoz); *Venoglobulin*® (500 mg, 2.5 g, 5g—Alpha); *Vigam*® (2.5 g, 5 g—BPL)

SPECIFIC IMMUNOGLOBULINS

Specific immunoglobulins are prepared by pooling the plasma of selected donors with high levels of the specific antibody required.

Although a hepatitis B vaccine is now available for those at high risk of infection, specific **hepatitis B immunoglobulin** ('HBIG') is available for use in association with the vaccine for the prevention of infection in laboratory and other personnel who have accidentally become contaminated with hepatitis B virus, and in infants born to mothers who have become infected with this virus in pregnancy or who are high-risk carriers.

Following exposure to a rabid animal, specific **rabies immunoglobulin**, if possible of human origin, should be injected at the site of the bite and also given intramuscularly. Rabies vaccine should also be given.

Tetanus immunoglobulin of human origin ('HTIG') should be used selectively in addition to wound toilet, vaccine, and benzylpenicillin (or another appropriate antibiotic) for the more seriously contaminated wounds; it is rarely required for those with an established immunity in whom protection may be achieved by a reinforcing dose of vaccine if considered advisable. The administration of tetanus immunoglobulin should be considered for patients not known to have received active immunisation (a) whose wound was sustained more than 6 hours before treatment was received and (b) with puncture wounds or wounds potentially heavily contaminated with tetanus spores, septic, or with much devitalised tissue. A dose of adsorbed tetanus vaccine should be given at the same time as the tetanus immunoglobulin and the course of vaccine subsequently completed.

Other specific immunoglobulins include varicella-zoster immunoglobulin ('ZIG') and are in limited supply. Others are under study, but their availability and evaluation requires the cooperation of general practitioners to provide blood from patients who are convalescent from these and other specific viral infections in order to prepare specific immunoglobulin preparations.

PoM **Hepatitis B Immunoglobulin** (Antihepatitis B Immunoglobulin). See notes above
Available from Public Health Laboratory Service (except for Transplant Centres, see p. 454)
Also available from BPL and SNBTS

PoM **Rabies Immunoglobulin** (Antirabies Immunoglobulin Injection). Used for protection of persons who have been bitten by rabid animals or otherwise exposed to infection (see notes above)
Dose: 20 units/kg, half by intramuscular injection and half by infiltration around wound
Available from Public Health Laboratory Service (also from BPL and SNBTS)

PoM **Tetanus Immunoglobulin** (Antitetanus Immunoglobulin Injection). Used for the protection of unimmunised persons when there is a specific risk of tetanus
Dose: by intramuscular injection, prophylactic 250 units, increased to 500 units if more than 24 hours have elapsed or there is risk of heavy contamination
Therapeutic, 150 units/kg (multiple sites)
Available from BPL, SNBTS, and Evans (as *Humotet*®; net price 1-mL vial = £18.94)

PoM **Tetanus Immunoglobulin for Intravenous Use.** Used for proven or suspected clinical tetanus
Dose: by intravenous infusion, 5000–10000 units
Available from SNBTS (2500-unit vial)

PoM **Varicella-Zoster Immunoglobulin** (Antivaricella-zoster Immunoglobulin). Used for protection of immunosuppressed persons and neonates at risk.
Available from Public Health Laboratory Service (also from BPL and SNBTS)

ANTI-D (Rh₀) IMMUNOGLOBULIN

Anti-D immunoglobulin is available to prevent a rhesus-negative mother from forming antibodies to fetal rhesus-positive cells which may pass into the maternal circulation during childbirth or abortion. It should be injected within 72 hours of the birth or abortion but even if a longer period has elapsed it may still give protection and should be administered. The objective is to protect any subsequent child from the hazard of haemolytic disease of the newborn.

PoM **Anti-D (Rh₀) Immunoglobulin Injection.**
See notes above
Available from Regional Blood Transfusion Centres and from BPL and SNBTS
Dose: for rhesus-negative women, 500 units by intramuscular injection following birth of rhesus-positive infant; 250 units if before 20 weeks gestation; after transfusion, consult literature (5000 units capable of neutralising 40–50 mL packed red cells)

Note. Rubella vaccine may be administered in the postpartum period simultaneously with anti-D (Rh₀) immunoglobulin injection providing separate syringes are used and the products are administered into contralateral limbs. A blood test should be done not sooner than 8 weeks later to ensure that rubella antibodies have been produced. If blood transfusion was necessary vaccination should be delayed for 3 months.

PoM **Partobulin**® (Immuno)
Anti-D (Rh₀) immunoglobulin injection 1250 units/mL, net price 1-mL vial = £15.90; 1-mL prefilled syringe = £16.90
Dose: by intramuscular injection, Rhesus negative women, 1250 units immediately or within 72 hours following abortion, miscarriage, or birth of rhesus positive infant. Macrotransfusion (transplacental haemorrhage), 5000 units *or* 50 units/mL of fetal blood
Rh₀(D) incompatible blood transfusion, 50–100 units/mL of transfused blood

---

MONOCLONAL ANTIBODY

The cell line used to produce the human monoclonal IgM antibody HA-1A was prepared from cells derived from a patient immunised with a heat-inactivated J5 mutant *Escherichia coli* 0111:B4 vaccine.

HA-1A

Indications: sepsis syndrome and Gram-negative bacteraemia, especially with septic shock
Cautions: use in meningococcal septicaemia and in patients with burns not recommended; pregnancy and breast-feeding
Contra-indications: hypersensitivity to mouse proteins; previous exposure to HA-1A
Side-effects: rarely, transient flushing, localised urticaria, and hypotension
Dose: by intravenous infusion, 100 mg; not to be repeated

▼ PoM **Centoxin**® (Centocor)
Intravenous solution, HA-1A 5 mg/mL, net price 20-mL vial = £2200.00. For dilution and use as an infusion

14.6 International travel

Note. For advice on **malaria chemoprophylaxis**, see section 5.4.1.

No particular immunisation is required for travellers to the United States, Europe, Australia, or New Zealand although the traveller should have immunity to tetanus and poliomyelitis. In Non-European areas surrounding the Mediterranean, in Africa, the Middle East, Asia, and South America, certain special precautions are required.

Typhoid vaccine is indicated for travellers to those countries where typhoid is endemic but is no substitute for personal precautions. Green salads and uncooked vegetables should be avoided and only fruits which can be peeled should be eaten. Only suitable bottled water, or water that has been boiled, or treated with sterilising tablets should be used for drinking purposes. This advice also applies to cholera and other diarrhoeal diseases (including travellers' diarrhoea).

Cholera vaccine is no substitute for personal hygiene and has little value in preventing infections. For current advice, see p. 446.

Long-term travellers to areas that have a high incidence of **poliomyelitis** or **tuberculosis** should be immunised with the appropriate vaccine; in the case of poliomyelitis previously vaccinated adults may be given a reinforcing dose of oral poliomyelitis vaccine. BCG vaccination is recommended for travellers proposing to stay for longer than one month in Asia, Africa, or Central and South America; it should preferably be given three months or more before departure.

International Certificates of vaccination against **yellow fever** (section 14.4) are still required for travel to much of Africa and South America.

Vaccination against **meningococcal meningitis** is required for a number of areas of the world (for details, section 14.4).

Overland travellers to Asia and Africa and others at high risk may be given **normal immunoglobulin injection** (section 14.5) for protection against hepatitis A; **hepatitis A vaccine** (section 14.2) is now available and is preferable for those planning to go for more than 3–5 months. It is preferable to complete active immunisation and wait 4 weeks before administering the immunoglobulin. An interval of 2 weeks is acceptable provided the immunoglobulin is given just before departure. If time is short, it can be given with any vaccine (including polio).

The Department of Health has issued a booklet, *Health Advice For Travellers* (code: T4) which can be obtained from travel agents, post offices, or by telephoning 0800 555 777 (24-hour service); bulk copies may be ordered from:

Health Publications Unit
No. 2 Site, Heywood Stores
Manchester Road
Heywood
Lancs OL10 2PZ

It provides details of vaccination requirements or recommendations country-by-country, health insurance, and reciprocal agreements. Further advice (including details of a **rapid schedule** for travellers required to go abroad at short notice and details of requirements in relation to **Japanese** and **tick-borne encephalitis**) may be obtained from the Department of Health memorandum, *Immunisation against Infectious Disease* (for details, section 14.1).

Vaccination requirements change from time to time, and information on the current requirements for any particular country may be obtained from:

Department of Health
Friars House
London SE1 8EU
telephone 071-972 2000

Communicable Disease Surveillance Centre Travel Unit
61 Colindale Avenue
London NW9 5EQ
telephone 081-200 6868

Scottish Home and Health Department
St. Andrew's House
Edinburgh EH1 3DE
telephone 031-556 8400

Welsh Office
Cathays Park,
Cardiff CF1 3NQ
telephone 0222 825111

Department of Health and Social Services
Dundonald House
Upper Newtownards Road
Belfast BT4 3FS
telephone 0232 63939;

or from the embassy or legation of the appropriate country.

15: Drugs used in
ANAESTHESIA

This chapter describes briefly drugs used in anaesthesia; the reader is referred to other sources for more detailed information. The chapter is divided into two sections:
- **15.1** General anaesthesia
- **15.2** Local anaesthesia

15.1 General anaesthesia

- **15.1.1** Intravenous anaesthetics
- **15.1.2** Inhalational anaesthetics
- **15.1.3** Antimuscarinic premedication drugs
- **15.1.4** Sedative and analgesic peri-operative drugs
- **15.1.5** Muscle relaxants
- **15.1.6** Anticholinesterases used in surgery
- **15.1.7** Antagonists for central and respiratory depression
- **15.1.8** Antagonists for malignant hyperthermia

Note. The drugs in section 15.1 should be used only by experienced personnel and where adequate resuscitative equipment is available.

ANAESTHESIA AND DRIVING. Patients given sedatives and analgesics during minor outpatient procedures should be very carefully warned about the risk of driving afterwards. For intravenous benzodiazepines and for a short general anaesthetic the risk extends to **at least 24 hours** after administration. Responsible persons should be available to take patients home. The dangers of taking **alcohol** should also be emphasised.

MODERN ANAESTHETIC TECHNIQUE. It is now common practice to administer several drugs with different actions to produce a state of surgical anaesthesia with minimal risk of toxic effects. An intravenous anaesthetic is frequently used for induction, followed by maintenance with inhalational anaesthetics, perhaps supplemented by other drugs administered intravenously. Specific drugs are often used to produce muscular relaxation. Many of the drugs used interfere with the reflex maintenance of spontaneous respiration and intermittent positive pressure ventilation by manual or mechanical means is commonly employed.

For certain procedures controlled hypotension may be required. Labetalol (see section 2.4), sodium nitroprusside (see section 2.5.1), and trimetaphan camsylate (see section 2.5.6) are used.

Beta-blockers (see section 2.4) or verapamil (see section 2.6.2) may be used to control arrhythmias during anaesthesia.

Prazosin (see section 2.5.4) is also used to control hypertension, particularly postoperatively.

GAS CYLINDERS

Each gas cylinder bears a label with the name of the gas contained in the cylinder. The name or chemical symbol of the gas is stencilled in paint on the shoulder of the cylinder; the letters are not less than 9 mm high on cylinders up to and including 80 mm diameter, not less than 12 mm high on cylinders over 80 mm and up to and including 105 mm diameter, and 19 mm high on cylinders above 105 mm diameter. The name or chemical symbol of the gas is also clearly and indelibly stamped on the cylinder valve. The colours applied to the valve end of the cylinder extend down the cylinder to the shoulder; in the case of mixed gases the colours for the individual gases are applied in four segments, two for each colour. See table below.

Gas cylinders should be stored in a cool well-ventilated room, free from materials of a flammable nature.

No lubricant of any description should be used.

Name of gas	Symbol	Colour of cylinder body	Colour of valve end where different from body
Oxygen	O_2	Black	White
Nitrous oxide	N_2O	Blue	—
Cyclopropane	C_3H_6	Orange	—
Carbon dioxide	CO_2	Grey	—
Ethylene	C_2H_4	Violet	—
Helium	He	Brown	—
Nitrogen	N_2	Grey	Black
Oxygen and carbon dioxide mixture	$O_2 + CO_2$	Black	White and Grey
Oxygen and helium mixture	$O_2 + He$	Black	White and Brown
Oxygen and nitrous oxide mixture	$O_2 + N_2O$	Blue	Blue and White
Air (medical)	AIR	Grey	White and Black

British Standard 1319:1976; Medical gas cylinders, valves and yoke connections. The colours used for gas cylinders comply with specifications in British Standards 4800 and 5252.

Abbreviations and symbols, see inside front cover

Prices are **net**, see p. 1

15.1.1 Intravenous anaesthetics

SURGERY AND LONG-TERM MEDICATION. The risk of stopping long-term medication before surgery is often greater than the risk of continuing it during surgery. This applies particularly to corticosteroids, since patients with adrenal atrophy (see section 6.3.3) may experience a precipitous fall in blood pressure unless corticosteroid cover is provided during anaesthesia or in the immediate postoperative period. Anaesthetists must therefore know whether a patient is, or has been, taking corticosteroids. Other drugs that should not normally be stopped before surgery include analgesics, antiepileptics, antiparkinsonian drugs, bronchodilators, cardiovascular drugs, glaucoma drugs, and thyroid or antithyroid drugs. Although it is preferable to discontinue oral anticoagulants electively before operation, this is not possible in patients requiring long-term treatment (e.g. for valve prostheses). The haematologist or physician should be consulted for further advice.

Drugs that should be stopped before surgery include oestrogens and combined oral contraceptives, which should be discontinued (and adequate alternative contraceptive arrangements made) 4 weeks before major elective surgery (for details see Surgery, section 7.3.1). In view of their hazardous interactions MAOIs should normally be stopped 2 weeks before surgery. Tricyclic antidepressants need not be stopped, but there may be an increased risk of arrhythmias and hypotension, therefore the anaesthetist should be informed if they are not. Lithium should be stopped 2 days before major surgery but the normal dose can be continued for minor surgery (with careful monitoring of fluids and electrolytes). To avoid withdrawal symptoms antidepressants need to be withdrawn gradually (see section 4.3.1).

In all cases it is vital that the anaesthetist should know of all drugs that a patient is, or has been, taking.

15.1.1 Intravenous anaesthetics

Intravenous anaesthetics may be used alone to produce anaesthesia for short surgical procedures but are more commonly used for induction only. Intravenous anaesthetics are potent drugs which nearly all produce their effect in one arm-brain circulation time and can cause apnoea and hypotension, and so adequate resuscitative facilities **must** be available. Large doses should be avoided in obstetrics, as the drug may cross the placental barrier. The drugs are **contra-indicated** in any dose in patients in whom the anaesthetist is not confident to maintain the airway, for example if there are tumours in the pharynx or larynx. Extreme care is required in surgery of the mouth, pharynx, or larynx and in patients with acute cardiovascular failure (shock) or fixed cardiac output. Patients with a full stomach present a hazard during induction since there is a danger of regurgitation and pulmonary aspiration. This may cause Mendelson's syndrome, particularly in the pregnant patient. Cricoid pressure is applied until the lungs have been protected by a cuffed endotracheal tube.

Individual requirements vary considerably and the recommended dosage is only a guide. Smaller dosage is indicated in ill, shocked, or debilitated patients, while robust individuals may require more. The estimated dosage should be injected over 20 seconds and a further 20 to 30 seconds allowed to assess the effect before a supplementary dose is given. For tracheal intubation, induction should be followed by inhalational anaesthesia or by a neuromuscular blocking drug.

TOTAL INTRAVENOUS ANAESTHESIA. This is a technique in which major surgery is carried out with all anaesthetic drugs being given intravenously. Respiration is controlled, the lungs being inflated with oxygen-enriched air. Muscle relaxant drugs are used to provide relaxation and prevent reflex muscle movements. The main problem to be overcome is the assessment of depth of anaesthesia in the paralysed ventilated patient.

DRIVING. For advice on anaesthesia and driving, see previous page.

BARBITURATES

Thiopentone sodium is the most widely used intravenous anaesthetic, but has no analgesic properties. Induction is generally smooth and rapid, but owing to the potency of the drug, overdosage with cardiorespiratory depression may occur. Aqueous solutions are unstable, particularly when exposed to air. The solution is alkaline and therefore irritant on misplaced injection outside the vein, while arterial injection is particularly dangerous. The usual strength used is a 2.5% solution in water for injections.

Awakening from a moderate dose of thiopentone is rapid due to redistribution of the drug in the whole body tissues. Metabolism is, however, slow and some sedative effects may persist for up to 24 hours during which time the subject is particularly susceptible to the effects of alcohol. Repeated doses have a cumulative effect.

Methohexitone sodium is less irritant to tissues than thiopentone; it is usually used as a 1% solution. Recovery is marginally more rapid than in the case of thiopentone. Induction is less smooth with an incidence of hiccup, tremor, involuntary movements, and pain on injection.

Both thiopentone and methohexitone are **contra-indicated** in porphyria (see section 9.8.2).

OTHER INTRAVENOUS ANAESTHETICS

Etomidate is an induction agent associated with rapid recovery without hangover effect. It causes less hypotension than other drugs used for induction. There is a high incidence of extraneous muscle movement and pain on injection. These effects can be minimised by premedication with an opioid analgesic and the use of larger veins. There is evidence that repeated doses of etomidate have an undesirable suppressant effect on adrenocortical function.

Propofol is associated with rapid recovery without hangover effect. There is sometimes pain on intravenous injection, but significant extraneous muscle movements do not occur. The CSM have received reports of convulsions, anaphylaxis, and delayed recovery from anaesthesia after propofol administration. Propofol has been associated with bradycardia, occasionally profound; intravenous administration of an antimuscarinic may be necessary to prevent this.

Ketamine can be given by the intravenous or the intramuscular route, and has good analgesic properties when used in sub-anaesthetic dosage. The maximum effect occurs in more than one arm-brain circulation time. Muscle tone is increased and the airway is usually well maintained. There is cardiovascular stimulation and arterial pressure may rise with tachycardia. The main disadvantage is the high incidence of hallucinations and other transient psychotic sequelae, though it is believed that these are much less significant in children. The incidence can be reduced when drugs such as diazepam are also used. Ketamine is **contra-indicated** in patients with hypertension and is best avoided in those prone to hallucinations. It is used mainly for paediatric anaesthesia, particularly when repeated administrations are required. Recovery is relatively slow.

Midazolam (section 15.1.4.1) is in increasing use as an induction agent.

THIOPENTONE SODIUM

Indications: induction of general anaesthesia; anaesthesia of short duration

Cautions; Contra-indications; Side-effects: see notes above; reduce induction dose in severe liver disease; avoid in porphyria (see section 9.8.2); **interactions:** Appendix 1 (anaesthetics)

Dose: by intravenous injection, in fit premedicated adults, initially 100–150 mg (4–6 mL of 2.5% solution) over 10–15 seconds, repeated if necessary according to response after 20–30 seconds; *or* up to 4 mg/kg; CHILD induction 2–7 mg/kg

PoM **Thiopentone Sodium** (Non-proprietary)
Injection, powder for reconstitution, thiopentone sodium. Net price 500-mg vial = £1.10

PoM **Thiopentone Sodium** (IMS)
Dispensing kit, thiopentone sodium 2.5 g with 100 mL diluent to provide a 2.5% solution, net price 1 unit = £7.75; 5 g with 200 mL diluent to provide a 2.5% solution, 1 unit = £12.90

PoM **Intraval Sodium®** (Rhône-Poulenc Rorer)
Injection 2.5%, powder for reconstitution, thiopentone sodium. Net price 500-mg amp = £1.10 (with water for injections £1.49); 2.5-g vial = £4.10 (with water for injections £4.80)

ETOMIDATE

Indications: induction of anaesthesia

Cautions; Contra-indications; Side-effects: see notes above; avoid in porphyria (see section 9.8.2); **interactions:** Appendix 1 (anaesthetics)

Dose: by slow intravenous injection, 300 micrograms/kg; high-risk patients, 100 micrograms/kg/minute until anaesthetised (about 3 minutes)

PoM **Hypnomidate®** (Janssen)
Injection, etomidate 2 mg/mL in propylene glycol 35%. Net price 10-mL amp = £1.62
Concentrate injection, etomidate 125 mg (as hydrochloride)/mL. To be diluted before use. Net price 1-mL amp = £5.47
Note. With the concentrate use only glass syringes, avoid contact with plastics

KETAMINE

Indications: induction and maintenance of anaesthesia

Cautions; Contra-indications; Side-effects: see notes above; **interactions:** Appendix 1 (anaesthetics)

Dose: by intramuscular injection, short procedures, initially 6.5–13 mg/kg (10 mg/kg usually produces 12–25 minutes of surgical anaesthesia)

Diagnostic manoeuvres and procedures not involving intense pain, initially 4 mg/kg

By intravenous injection over at least 60 seconds, short procedures, initially 1–4.5 mg/kg (2 mg/kg usually produces 5–10 minutes of surgical anaesthesia)

By intravenous infusion of a solution containing 1 mg/mL, longer procedures, induction, total dose of 0.5–2 mg/kg; maintenance (using microdrip infusion), 10–45 micrograms/kg/minute, rate adjusted according to response

PoM **Ketalar®** (P-D)
Injection, ketamine (as hydrochloride) 10 mg/mL, net price 20-mL vial = £3.52; 50 mg/mL, 10-mL vial = £7.31; 100 mg/mL, 5-mL vial = £6.71

METHOHEXITONE SODIUM

Indications: induction and maintenance of anaesthesia for short procedures; with other anaesthetics for more prolonged anaesthesia

Cautions; Contra-indications; Side-effects: avoid or reduce dose in liver disease; see also under Thiopentone Sodium and notes above

Dose: by intravenous injection, usually as a 1% solution, 50–120 mg according to response at rate of 10 mg in 5 seconds; maintenance, 20–40 mg (2–4 mL of 1% solution) every 4–7 minutes; CHILD induction approx. 1 mg/kg

PoM **Brietal Sodium®** (Lilly)
Injection, powder for reconstitution, methohexitone sodium, net price 100 mg in 10-mL vial = 83p; 500 mg in 50-mL vial = £2.14

PROPOFOL

Indications: induction and maintenance of general anaesthesia; sedation of ventilated patients receiving intensive care, for up to 3 days

Cautions; Contra-indications; Side-effects: see notes above; monitor blood lipid concentrations in patients at risk of fat overload; contra-indicated if history of propofol allergy (see CSM warning above); **interactions:** Appendix 1 (anaesthetics)

Dose: induction, *by intravenous injection*, 2–2.5 mg/kg (less in elderly) at a rate of 20–40 mg every 10 seconds; CHILD over 3 years 2.5 mg/kg adjusted as necessary

Maintenance, *by intravenous infusion*, 4–12 mg/kg/hour; CHILD over 3 years 9–15 mg/kg/hour

Sedation during intensive care (with assisted ventilation), *by intravenous infusion*, 1–4 mg/kg/hour for up to 3 days; CHILD not recommended

PoM **Diprivan®** (ICI)
Injection (emulsion), propofol 10 mg/mL, net price 20-mL amp = £3.98; 50-mL vial = £9.95; 100-mL vial = £19.90

15.1.2 Inhalational anaesthetics

Inhalational anaesthetics may be gases or volatile liquids. They can be used both for induction and maintenance of anaesthesia and may be used following induction with an intravenous anaesthetic (section 15.1.1).

Gaseous anaesthetics require suitable equipment for storage and administration. They may be supplied via hospital pipelines or from metal cylinders. In clinical use it is necessary to monitor flow rate. Volatile anaesthetics are usually administered using calibrated vaporisers, using air, oxygen, or nitrous oxide–oxygen mixtures as the carrier gas.

To prevent hypoxia gaseous anaesthetics must be given with adequate concentrations of oxygen.

DRIVING. For advice on outpatient anaesthesia and driving, see section 15.1.

HALOGENATED ANAESTHETICS

Halothane is a volatile anaesthetic. Its advantages are that it is potent, induction is smooth, the vapour is non-irritant, pleasant to inhale, and seldom induces coughing or breath-holding. The incidence of postoperative vomiting is low.

It is indicated for induction and maintenance of anaesthesia in major surgery with oxygen or nitrous oxide–oxygen mixtures, but is much less widely used than previously owing to its association with severe hepatotoxicity (see CSM recommendations, below).

Halothane causes cardiorespiratory depression and because of its potency is administered from calibrated vaporisers. Respiratory depression results in elevation of arterial carbon dioxide tension and perhaps ventricular dysrhythmias. Intermittent positive-pressure ventilation must be carried out with care as myocardial depression may follow increase in blood concentrations. Halothane depresses the cardiac muscle fibres and may cause bradycardia. The result is diminished cardiac output and fall of arterial pressure. There is also peripheral vasodilatation. Adrenaline infiltrations should be used with care as ventricular dysrhythmias may result.

Halothane produces moderate muscle relaxation, but this may be inadequate for major abdominal surgery and specific muscle relaxants are then used.

In a publication on findings confirming that *severe hepatotoxicity* can follow halothane anaesthesia the CSM has reported that this occurs more frequently after repeated exposures to halothane and has a high mortality. The risk of severe hepatotoxicity appears to be increased by repeated exposures within a short time interval, but even after a long interval (sometimes of several years) susceptible patients have been reported to develop jaundice. Since there is no reliable way of identifying susceptible patients the CSM recommends the following precautions prior to use of halothane:

1. a careful anaesthetic history should be taken to determine previous exposure and previous reactions to halothane;
2. repeated exposure to halothane within a period of at least 3 months should be avoided unless there are overriding clinical circumstances;
3. a history of unexplained jaundice or pyrexia in a patient following exposure to halothane is an absolute **contra-indication** to its future use in that patient.

Enflurane is a volatile anaesthetic similar to halothane, but it is less potent, about twice the concentration being necessary for induction and maintenance. Administration from a calibrated vaporiser is recommended.

Enflurane is a powerful cardiorespiratory depressant. Shallow respiration is likely to result in a rise of arterial carbon dioxide tension, but ventricular dysrhythmias are uncommon and it is probably safe to use adrenaline infiltrations. Myocardial depression may result in a fall in cardiac output and in arterial hypotension.

Enflurane is usually given to supplement nitrous oxide–oxygen mixtures in concentrations of 1 to 3%. The drug is often used in preference to halothane when repeated anaesthesia is required.

Isoflurane is an isomer of enflurane. It has a potency intermediate between that of halothane and enflurane, and even less of an inhaled dose is metabolised than with enflurane. Heart rhythm is generally stable during isoflurane anaesthesia, but heart-rate may rise, particularly in younger patients. Systemic arterial pressure may fall, due to a decrease in systemic vascular resistance and with less decrease in cardiac output than occurs with halothane. Respiration is depressed. Muscle relaxation is produced and muscle relaxant drugs potentiated.

ENFLURANE

Indications; Cautions; Side-effects: see notes above; avoid in porphyria (see section 9.8.2); **interactions:** Appendix 1 (anaesthetics)
Dose: using a specifically calibrated vaporiser, *induction*, increased gradually from 0.4% to max. of 4.5% in air, oxygen, or nitrous oxide–oxygen, according to response
Maintenance, 0.5–3% in nitrous oxide–oxygen

Enflurane (Abbott)
Enflurane. 250 mL

HALOTHANE

Indications; Cautions; Contra-indications; Side-effects: see notes above; avoid in porphyria (see section 9.8.2); **interactions:** Appendix 1 (anaesthetics)
Dose: using a suitable vaporiser, *induction*, increased gradually to 2–4% in oxygen or nitrous oxide–oxygen; CHILD 1.5–2%
Maintenance, 0.5–2%

Halothane (Rhône-Poulenc Rorer)
Net price 250 mL = £10.49
Fluothane® (ICI)
Halothane. Net price 250 mL = £10.49

ISOFLURANE

Indications; Cautions; Side-effects: see notes above; **interactions:** Appendix 1 (anaesthetics)
Dose: using a specifically calibrated vaporiser, *induction*, increased gradually from 0.5% to 3%, in oxygen or nitrous oxide–oxygen
Maintenance, 1–2.5% in nitrous oxide–oxygen; an additional 0.5–1% may be required when given with oxygen alone; caesarean section, 0.5–0.75% in nitrous oxide–oxygen

Isoflurane (Abbott)
Isoflurane. Net price 100 mL = £35.95

NITROUS OXIDE

Nitrous oxide is used for induction and maintenance of anaesthesia and, in sub-anaesthetic concentrations, for analgesia in a variety of situations. For anaesthesia it is commonly used in a concentration of 50 to 70% in oxygen as part of a balanced technique in association with other inhalational or intravenous agents. Nitrous oxide is unsatisfactory as a sole anaesthetic owing to lack of potency, but is useful as part of a sequence of drugs since it allows a significant reduction in dosage.

A mixture of nitrous oxide and oxygen containing 50% of each gas (Entonox®) is used to produce analgesia without loss of consciousness. Self-administration using a demand valve is popular and may be appropriate in obstetric practice, for changing painful dressings, as an aid to postoperative physiotherapy, and in emergency ambulances.

Nitrous oxide may have a deleterious effect if used in patients with an air-containing closed space since nitrous oxide diffuses into such a space with a resulting build up of pressure. This effect may be dangerous in the presence of a pneumothorax which may enlarge to compromise respiration. Exposure of patients to nitrous oxide for prolonged periods, either by continuous or intermittent administration, may result in megaloblastic anaemia due to interference with the action of vitamin B_{12}. For the same reason, exposure of anaesthetists and theatre staff to nitrous oxide should be minimised. Depression of white cell formation may also occur.

NITROUS OXIDE

Indications; Cautions; Side-effects: see notes above; **interactions:** Appendix 1 (anaesthetics)
Dose: using a suitable anaesthetic apparatus, a mixture with 20–30% oxygen for *induction* and *maintenance* of light anaesthesia
Analgesic, as a mixture with 50% oxygen, according to the patient's needs

15.1.3 Antimuscarinic premedication drugs

Antimuscarinic premedication drugs are used (less commonly nowadays) to dry bronchial and salivary secretions which are increased by intubation and the inhalational anaesthetics. They are also used before or with neostigmine (section 15.1.6) to prevent bradycardia, excessive salivation, and other muscarinic actions of neostigmine. They are also used to prevent bradycardia and hypotension associated with agents such as halothane, propofol, and suxamethonium.

Atropine is the most commonly used. Intravenous administration immediately before anaesthesia or intramuscular injection (which should be given 30–60 minutes before the operation) is satisfactory.

Hyoscine effectively reduces secretions and also provides a degree of amnesia. It produces less tachycardia than atropine. In some patients, especially the elderly, hyoscine may cause the central anticholinergic syndrome (excitement, ataxia, hallucinations, behavioural abnormalities, and drowsiness).

Glycopyrronium bromide produces good drying of salivary secretions. When given intravenously it produces less tachycardia than atropine.

Phenothiazines have too little drying activity to be effective when used alone.

ATROPINE SULPHATE

Indications: drying secretions, reversal of excessive bradycardia; with neostigmine for reversal of competitive neuromuscular block; other indications, see sections 1.2, 2.3.1, 11.5
Cautions: cardiovascular disease; **interactions:** Appendix 1 (antimuscarinics)
Side-effects: tachycardia; see also section 1.2

Dose: premedication, *by intravenous injection*, 300–600 micrograms immediately before induction of anaesthesia, and in incremental doses of 100 micrograms for the treatment of bradycardia
By intramuscular injection, 300–600 micrograms 30–60 minutes before induction; CHILD 20 micrograms/kg
For control of muscarinic side-effects of neostigmine in reversal of competitive neuromuscular block, *by intravenous injection*, 0.6–1.2 mg
Acute arrhythmias after myocardial infarction, see section 2.3.1; see also Cardiopulmonary Resuscitation algorithm, section 2.7

PoM **Atropine** (Non-proprietary)
Tablets, atropine sulphate 600 micrograms. Net price 20 = £2.49
Injection, atropine sulphate 600 micrograms/mL. Net price 1-mL amp = 33p
Note. Other strengths also available

PoM **Min-I-Jet® Atropine Sulphate** (IMS)
Injection, atropine sulphate 100 micrograms/mL, net price 5-mL disposable syringe = £3.51; 10-mL disposable syringe = £3.51

CD **Morphine and Atropine Injection** see under Morphine Salts (section 15.1.4.3)

GLYCOPYRRONIUM BROMIDE
Indications; Cautions; Side-effects: see under Atropine Sulphate
Dose: premedication, *by intramuscular or intravenous injection*, 200–400 micrograms, *or* 4–5 micrograms/kg to a max. of 400 micrograms; CHILD, *by intramuscular or intravenous injection*, 4–8 micrograms/kg to a max. of 200 micrograms; intra-operative use, *by intravenous injection*, as for premedication
For control of muscarinic side-effects of neostigmine in reversal of competitive neuromuscular block, *by intravenous injection*, 10–15 micrograms/kg with 50 micrograms/kg neostigmine; CHILD, 10 micrograms/kg with 50 micrograms/kg neostigmine

PoM **Robinul®** (Wyeth)
Injection, glycopyrronium bromide 200 micrograms/mL. Net price 1-mL amp = 63p; 3-mL amp = £1.06
PoM **Robinul-Neostigmine®**: section 15.1.6

HYOSCINE HYDROBROMIDE
(Scopolamine Hydrobromide)
Indications: drying secretions, amnesia; other indications, see sections 4.6, 11.5
Cautions; Side-effects: see under Atropine Sulphate; may slow heart; avoid in the elderly (see notes above)
Dose: premedication, *by subcutaneous or intramuscular injection*, 200–600 micrograms 30–60 minutes before induction of anaesthesia, usually with papaveretum; CHILD 15 micrograms/kg

PoM **Hyoscine** (Non-proprietary)
Injection, hyoscine hydrobromide 400 micrograms/mL, net price 1-mL amp = £1.34; 600 micrograms/mL, 1-mL amp = £1.08
CD **Papaveretum and Hyoscine Injection,** see under Papaveretum (section 15.1.4.3)

15.1.4 Sedative and analgesic peri-operative drugs
15.1.4.1 Anxiolytics and neuroleptics
15.1.4.2 Non-opioid analgesics
15.1.4.3 Opioid analgesics

These drugs are given to allay the apprehension of the patient in the pre-operative period (including the night before operation), to relieve pain and discomfort when present, and to augment the action of subsequent anaesthetic agents. A number of the drugs used also provide some degree of pre-operative amnesia. The choice will vary with the individual patient, the nature of the operative procedure, the anaesthetic to be used and other prevailing circumstances such as out-patients, obstetrics, recovery facilities etc. The choice would also vary in elective and emergency operations.

PREMEDICATION IN CHILDREN. Oral or rectal administration is preferred to injections where possible but is not altogether satisfactory. Oral **trimeprazine** is still used but when given alone it may cause postoperative restlessness when pain is present. An alternative is **diazepam**. Some anaesthetists prefer the use of adult regimens, with dosage on a weight basis. (For guidelines on dose calculation in children, see Prescribing for Children, p. 11.)

Atropine or hyoscine is often given orally to children, but may be given intravenously immediately before induction.

DRIVING. For advice on outpatient anaesthesia and driving, see section 15.1.

15.1.4.1 ANXIOLYTICS AND NEUROLEPTICS

Oral premedication is increasing in popularity using benzodiazepines such as diazepam, lorazepam, and temazepam. A short-acting oral benzodiazepine is the most common premedicant.

Diazepam is used to produce light sedation with amnesia. The 'sleep' dose shows too great an individual variation to recommend it for induction of anaesthesia, and while this variation exists with regard to its sedative effect, it is probably less marked with lower doses and of little clinical significance. It is particularly valuable in sub-anaesthetic doses to produce light sedation for unpleasant procedures or for operations under local anaesthesia, including dentistry; sub-anaesthetic doses allow retention of the pharyngeal reflexes while a local block is performed, and the resultant amnesia is such that the patient is unlikely to have any unpleasant memories of the procedure (however, benzodiazepines, particularly when used for deep sedation, can sometimes induce sexual fantasies). Diazepam can also be used in a similar manner for endoscopy, with or without an opioid analgesic.

Preparations of diazepam in organic solvents are painful on intravenous injection and followed by a high incidence of venous thrombosis which may not be noticed until a week after the injection. They are also painful on intramuscular injection, and absorption from the injection site is erratic. An emulsion preparation of diazepam (Diazemuls®) is less irritant on intravenous injection and is followed by a negligible incidence of venous thrombosis, but it should not be given intramuscularly. Diazepam is also available as a rectal solution (Stesolid®).

Diazepam and related drugs are of particular value for sedation of patients in an intensive care unit, particularly those on ventilators. It can be given 4–6 hourly but dosage should be gradually reduced after some days to prevent delay in recovery, which can be caused by a build up of its metabolite. Since it has no analgesic action it is often given in conjunction with small doses of opioid analgesics.

Diazepam may on occasions cause marked respiratory depression and facilities for treatment of this are essential. Dental patients who are sitting in one position for a long time may develop hypotonia after diazepam and they should be warned about this possibility. Outpatients should be advised that this is a long-acting drug, and that a second period of drowsiness can occur 4–6 hours after its administration.

By virtue of its physical characteristics, diazepam can accumulate in the fetus and, particularly after the mother has been given large doses, babies can be born in a depressed state, with hypotonia and a tendency to develop hypothermia.

Temazepam has a shorter action and relatively more rapid onset than diazepam. Used orally as a premedicant, anxiolytic and sedative effects are produced which continue for one and a half hours. After this period patients are usually fully alert but there may be residual drowsiness. It has proved useful as a premedicant in inpatient and day-case surgery.

Lorazepam produces more prolonged sedation than temazepam. In addition amnesia is commonplace. It is particularly useful when used as a premedicant the night prior to major surgery; sound sleep is assured when an oral dose of 1 to 5 mg is given. A further, smaller, dose the following morning will be required if any delay in the commencement of surgery is anticipated. Alternatively the first dose may be given in the early morning of the day of operation.

Midazolam is a water-soluble benzodiazepine which is often used in preference to diazepam. Recovery is faster than with diazepam. The incidence of side-effects is low but the CSM has received reports of respiratory depression (sometimes associated with severe hypotension) following intravenous administration. A preparation containing 2 mg/mL is available to ensure easier titration of dosage.

Chlormethiazole has been used as an intravenous infusion to maintain sleep during surgery carried out under regional analgesia, including extradural block. It has no analgesic effect, little cardiac and respiratory depression, and may be used in elderly patients.

CHLORMETHIAZOLE EDISYLATE

Indications: sedative during regional anaesthesia; other indications, see sections 4.1.1, 4.8.2
Cautions: see section 4.1.1 for special cautions for intravenous infusion
Contra-indications; Side-effects: see section 4.1.1
Dose: by intravenous infusion, as a 0.8% solution, induction 25 mL (200 mg)/minute for 1–2 minutes; maintenance 1–4 mL (8–32 mg)/minute
Note. Special care on prolonged intravenous administration since accumulation may occur; also, contains no electrolytes

PoM **Heminevrin®** (Astra)
Intravenous infusion 0.8%, chlormethiazole edisylate 8 mg/mL. Net price 500-mL bottle = £5.25

CHLORPROMAZINE HYDROCHLORIDE

Indications: see under Dose; other indications, see section 4.2.1
Cautions; Contra-indications; Side-effects: see section 4.2.1
Dose: induction of hypothermia (to prevent shivering), *by deep intramuscular injection,* 25–50 mg every 6–8 hours; CHILD 1–12 years, initially 0.5–1 mg/kg, maintenance 500 micrograms/kg every 4–6 hours

PoM **Chlorpromazine** (Non-proprietary)
Injection, chlorpromazine hydrochloride 25 mg/mL, net price 1-mL amp = 21p; 2-mL amp = 27p

PoM **Largactil®** (Rhône-Poulenc Rorer)
Injection, chlorpromazine hydrochloride 25 mg/mL. Net price 2-mL amp = 28p

DIAZEPAM

Indications: premedication; sedation with amnesia, and in conjunction with local anaesthesia; other indications, see sections 4.1.2, 4.8, 10.2.2
Cautions; Contra-indications; Side-effects: see notes above and sections 4.1.2, 4.8.2

Dose: by mouth, 5 mg at night, 5 mg on waking, and 5 mg 2 hours before minor or dental surgery
By intravenous injection, 10–20 mg over 2–4 minutes as sedative cover for minor surgical and medical procedures; premedication 100–200 micrograms/kg
By rectum in solution, ADULT and CHILD over 3 years 10 mg; CHILD 1–3 years and elderly 5 mg

Oral and rectal preparations: see section 4.1.2

Parenteral preparations
PoM **Diazepam** (Non-proprietary)
Injection (solution), diazepam 5 mg/mL. See Appendix 6. Net price 2-mL amp = 25p
Available from CP
PoM **Diazemuls**® (Dumex)
Injection (emulsion), diazepam 5 mg/mL. For intravenous injection or infusion. See Appendix 6. Net price 2-mL amp = 69p
PoM **Valium**® (Roche)
Injection (solution), diazepam 5 mg/mL. See Appendix 6. Net price 2-mL amp = 30p

DROPERIDOL

Indications: anti-emetic, pre-operative sedation; neuroleptanalgesia; other indications, see section 4.2.1
Cautions; Contra-indications; Side-effects: see section 4.2.1
Dose: premedication, *by intramuscular injection*, up to 10 mg 60 minutes before operation; CHILD 200–500 micrograms/kg
Neuroleptanalgesia, *by intravenous injection*, 5–15 mg at induction with an opioid analgesic; CHILD 200–300 micrograms/kg

PoM **Droleptan**® (Janssen)
Injection, droperidol 5 mg/mL. Net price 2-mL amp = 92p
CD **Thalamonal**® — see under Fentanyl (section 15.1.4.1)

LORAZEPAM

Indications: sedation with amnesia; as pre-medication; other indications, see sections 4.1.2, 4.8.2
Cautions; Contra-indications; Side-effects: see under Diazepam
Dose: by mouth, 2–3 mg the night before operation; 2–4 mg 1–2 hours before surgery
By slow intravenous injection, preferably diluted with an equal volume of sodium chloride intravenous infusion 0.9% or water for injections, 50 micrograms/kg 30–45 minutes before operation
By intramuscular injection, diluted as above, 50 micrograms/kg 1–1½ hours before operation

PoM **Ativan**® (Wyeth)
Injection, lorazepam 4 mg/mL. Net price 1-mL amp = 40p
Tablets, see section 4.1.2

MIDAZOLAM

Indications: sedation with amnesia, and in conjunction with local anaesthesia; premedication, induction
Cautions; Contra-indications; Side-effects: see under Diazepam; see notes above for CSM warning; **important:** plasma concentration increased by erythromycin—profound sedation reported with oral midazolam (not on UK market); other **interactions:** Appendix 1 (benzodiazepines)
Dose: sedation, *by intravenous injection* over 30 seconds, 2 mg (elderly 1–1.5 mg) followed after 2 minutes by increments of 0.5–1 mg if sedation not adequate; usual range 2.5–7.5 mg (about 70 micrograms/kg), elderly 1–2 mg
Premedication, *by intramuscular injection*, 70–100 micrograms/kg 30–60 minutes before surgery; usual dose 5 mg (2.5 mg in elderly)
Induction, *by slow intravenous injection*, 200–300 micrograms/kg (elderly 100–200 micrograms/kg)
Sedation of patients receiving intensive care, *by intravenous infusion*, initially 30–300 micrograms/kg given over 5 minutes, then 30–200 micrograms/kg/hour; reduce dose (or omit initial dose) in hypovolaemia, vasoconstriction, or hypothermia; low doses may be adequate if opioid analgesic also used; avoid abrupt withdrawal after prolonged administration (safety after more than 14 days not established)

PoM **Hypnovel**® (Roche)
Injection, midazolam (as hydrochloride) 2 mg/mL, net price 5-mL amp = 92p; 5 mg/mL, 2-mL amp = 77p

PROMETHAZINE HYDROCHLORIDE

Indications: anti-emetic, pre-operative sedative and antimuscarinic; other indications, see sections 3.4.1, 3.4.3
Cautions; Side-effects: see section 4.6
Dose: premedication, *by mouth*, CHILD 1–5 years 15–20 mg, 6–10 years 20–25 mg
By deep intramuscular injection, 25–50 mg 1 hour before operation; CHILD 5–10 years, 6.25–12.5 mg

Preparations
See sections 3.4.1 and 15.1.4.3 (with pethidine)

TEMAZEPAM

Indications: premedication before minor surgery; anxiety before investigatory procedures; hypnotic, see section 4.1.1
Cautions; Contra-indications; Side-effects: see under Diazepam
Dose: by mouth, premedication, 20–40 mg (elderly, 10–20 mg) 1 hour before operation; CHILD 1 mg/kg (max. 30 mg)

Preparations
See section 4.1.1

TRIMEPRAZINE TARTRATE

Indications: pre-operative sedation, anti-emetic; other indications, see section 3.4.1

Cautions; Side-effects: see notes above and section 3.4.1

Dose: by mouth, premedication, 3 mg/kg 1–2 hours before operation; CHILD 2–7 years up to 2 mg/kg

Preparations
See section 3.4.1

15.1.4.2 NON-OPIOID ANALGESICS

DICLOFENAC SODIUM
See section 10.1.1

KETOPROFEN
See section 10.1.1

KETOROLAC TROMETAMOL

Indications: pain associated with surgical procedures

Cautions; Contra-indications; Side-effects: as for other NSAIDs, see section 10.1.1; postoperative wound haemorrhage and pain at injection site reported; **interactions:** Appendix 1 (NSAIDs)

Dose: by intramuscular injection, initially 30 mg, then 10–30 mg every 4–6 hours when required (every 2 hours in initial postoperative period); max. 120 mg daily; max. duration of treatment 5 days; ADOLESCENT and CHILD under 16 years not recommended

▼ PoM **Toradol**® (Syntex)
Injection, ketorolac trometamol 30 mg/mL, net price 1-mL amp = £1.31

15.1.4.3 OPIOID ANALGESICS

An opioid analgesic is commonly used as a premedicant, e.g. morphine or pethidine given intramuscularly about an hour before operation, usually combined with an antisialogogue. Sometimes they are combined with a phenothiazine or droperidol. The main side-effects are respiratory depression, cardiovascular depression, and nausea and vomiting. The principal advantages are that opioid analgesics provide analgesia persisting into the operative period giving a reduced chance of awareness during anaesthesia with full doses of muscle relaxants.

INTRA-OPERATIVE ANALGESIA. Many of the conventional opioid analgesics are used to supplement general anaesthesia, usually in combination with nitrous oxide–oxygen and a muscle relaxant. Pethidine was the first to be used for this purpose but other drugs now available include alfentanil, fentanyl, meptazinol, nalbuphine, and phenoperidine. The longer-acting drugs morphine and papaveretum, although equally effective for this purpose, are not commonly used because of the problems of respiratory depression in the postoperative period.

Small doses of opioids given immediately before or with thiopentone will reduce the induction dose of the barbiturate and this is a popular technique in poor-risk patients. **Alfentanil** and **fentanyl** are particularly useful in this respect because of their short duration of action although there may be some cumulation with large doses. Alfentanil may be preferable for short operations because of its very brief duration of action; for long procedures it can be given as a continuous infusion.

Repeated doses of intra-operative analgesics should be given with care, since not only may the respiratory depression persist into the postoperative period but it may become apparent for the first time postoperatively when the patient is away from immediate nursing attention. The specific opioid antagonist, naloxone (section 15.1.7), will immediately reverse this respiratory depression but the dose may have to be repeated. In clinical doses it will also reverse most of the analgesia. An alternative and equally acceptable approach is to use the specific respiratory stimulant, doxapram (see section 3.5.1), which can be given in an infusion and which will not affect the opioid analgesia. The use of intra-operative opioids should be borne in mind when prescribing postoperative analgesics. In many instances they will delay the need for the first dose but caution is necessary since there may be some residual respiratory depression potentiated by the postoperative analgesic.

Fentanyl may produce severe respiratory depression, especially in patients with decreased respiratory function or when other respiratory depressant drugs have been given. Respiratory depression may be treated by artificial ventilation or be reversed by naloxone or doxapram (see above). Alfentanil may also cause severe respiratory depression, especially when other respiratory depressant drugs have already been given; this may be reversed with naloxone (see above).

Meptazinol can be used for analgesia during or after operation. It is associated with nausea and vomiting, but is claimed to have a reduced incidence of respiratory depression.

For general notes on analgesics see section 4.7.

ALFENTANIL

Indications: analgesia especially during short operative procedure and outpatient surgery; enhancement of anaesthesia; analgesic and respiratory depressant in assisted respiration

Cautions; Contra-indications; Side-effects: see under Fentanyl and notes above

Dose: by intravenous injection, spontaneous respiration, ADULT, initially up to 500 micrograms over 30 seconds; supplemental, 250 micrograms
With assisted ventilation, ADULT and CHILD, initially 30–50 micrograms/kg; supplemental, 15 micrograms/kg
By intravenous infusion, with assisted ventilation, ADULT and CHILD, initially 50–100 micrograms/kg over 10 minutes *or* as a bolus, followed by maintenance of 0.5–1 micrograms/kg/minute

CD **Rapifen**® (Janssen)
Injection, alfentanil 500 micrograms (as hydrochloride)/mL. Net price 2-mL amp = 74p; 10-mL amp = £3.39
Intensive care injection, alfentanil 5 mg (as hydrochloride)/mL. To be diluted before use. Net price 1-mL amp = £2.72

BUPRENORPHINE

Indications: peri-operative analgesia; premedication; analgesia in other situations, see section 4.7.2; effects only partially reversed by naloxone
Cautions; Contra-indications; Side-effects: see section 4.7.2
Dose: pain, *by slow intravenous injection*, 300–450 micrograms
Premedication, *by sublingual administration*, 400 micrograms
By intramuscular injection, 300 micrograms

Preparations
See section 4.7.2

FENTANYL

Indications: analgesia during operation, neuroleptanalgesia, enhancement of anaesthesia; respiratory depressant in assisted respiration
Cautions: chronic respiratory disease, myasthenia gravis; reduce dose in elderly, hypothyroidism, chronic liver disease; obstetric use may cause respiratory depression in neonate; see also notes above; **interactions:** Appendix 1 (opioid analgesics)
Contra-indications: respiratory depression or obstructive airways disease unless patient ventilated
Side-effects: respiratory depression, transient hypotension, bradycardia, nausea and vomiting
Dose: by intravenous injection, with spontaneous respiration, 50–200 micrograms, then 50 micrograms as required; CHILD 3–5 micrograms/kg, then 1 microgram/kg as required
With assisted ventilation, 0.3–3.5 mg, then 100–200 micrograms as required; CHILD 15 micrograms/kg, then 1–3 micrograms/kg as required

CD **Fentanyl Citrate** (Non-proprietary)
Injection, fentanyl 50 micrograms (as citrate)/mL, net price 2-mL amp = 45p; 10-mL amp = £2.05
Available from David Bull, Evans

CD **Sublimaze**® (Janssen)
Injection, fentanyl 50 micrograms (as citrate)/mL. Net price 2-mL amp = 25p; 10-mL amp = £1.20

CD **Thalamonal**® (Janssen)
Injection, fentanyl 50 micrograms (as citrate), droperidol 2.5 mg/mL. Net price 2-mL amp = 95p
Dose: premedication, neuroleptanalgesia, by intramuscular injection 1–2 mL 5–15 minutes before operation; induction, by intravenous injection 6–8 mL followed by assisted ventilation; maintenance, by intravenous injection, 1–2 mL as required; CHILD premedication, neuroleptanalgesia, by intramuscular injection 0.4–1.5 mL

MEPTAZINOL

Indications: analgesia during and after operation; analgesia in other situations, see section 4.7.2
Cautions; Contra-indications; Side-effects: see section 4.7.2 and notes above
Dose: by mouth, 200 mg every 3–6 hours as required
By intramuscular injection, 75–100 mg, repeated every 2–4 hours as required
By slow intravenous injection, 50–100 mg, repeated every 2–4 hours as required
See also section 4.7.2 for analgesia

PoM **Meptid**® (Monmouth)
Tablets, orange, f/c, meptazinol 200 mg. Net price 20 = £1.80. Label: 2
Injection, meptazinol 100 mg (as hydrochloride)/mL. Net price 1-mL amp = 79p

MORPHINE SALTS

Indications: analgesia during and after operation; enhancement of anaesthesia; pre-operative sedation; analgesia in other situations, see section 4.7.2
Cautions; Contra-indications; Side-effects: see section 4.7.2 and notes above
Dose: by subcutaneous or intramuscular injection, up to 10 mg 1–1½ hours before operation; CHILD, *by intramuscular injection*, 150 micrograms/kg.
See also section 4.7.2 for analgesia

CD **Morphine Sulphate Injection,** morphine sulphate, 10, 15 and 30 mg/mL. Net price 1- and 2-mL amp (all) = 51–86p

CD **Morphine and Atropine Injection,** morphine sulphate 10 mg, atropine sulphate 600 micrograms/mL. Net price 1-mL amp = 53p
Dose: premedication, by subcutaneous injection, 0.5–1 mL

NALBUPHINE HYDROCHLORIDE

Indications: peri-operative analgesia; premedication; analgesia in other situations, see section 4.7.2
Cautions; Contra-indications; Side-effects: see section 4.7.2 and notes above; also caution in ambulant patients (impairment of mental and physical ability)

Dose: acute pain, by subcutaneous, intramuscular, or intravenous injection, 10–20 mg, adjusted according to response; CHILD up to 300 micrograms/kg repeated once or twice as necessary. See also section 4.7.2. for analgesia
Premedication, *by subcutaneous, intramuscular, or intravenous injection*, 100–200 micrograms/kg
Induction, *by intravenous injection*, 0.3–1 mg/kg over 10–15 minutes
Intra-operative analgesia, *by intravenous injection*, 250–500 micrograms/kg at 30-minute intervals

PoM **Nubain**® (Du Pont)
Injection, nalbuphine hydrochloride 10 mg/mL. Net price 1-mL amp = 75p; 2-mL amp = £1.16

PAPAVERETUM and OTHER MIXED OPIUM ALKALOIDS
Indications: analgesia during and after operation; pre-medication; see also under preparations
Cautions; Contra-indications; Side-effects: see section 4.7.2 and notes above; noscapine in papaveretum contra-indicated in women of child-bearing potential (see Appendix 4)
Dose: see under preparations, below

Papaveretum
The hydrochlorides of alkaloids of opium, containing the equivalent of anhydrous morphine 47.5–52.5%, anhydrous codeine 2.5–5%, noscapine 16–22%, and papaverine 2.5–7%
Note. Papaveretum 20 mg is approximately equivalent to morphine 12.5 mg
IMPORTANT. Do **not** confuse with papaverine (see section 7.4.5)

CD Papaveretum Injection, papaveretum 10 mg/mL, net price 1-mL amp = 31p; 20 mg/mL, 1-mL amp = 36p
Dose: acute pain, by subcutaneous or intramuscular injection, 20 mg repeated every 4 hours if necessary (10 mg for elderly or lighter patients); CHILD up to 1 month 150 micrograms/kg, 1–12 months 200 micrograms/kg, 1–12 years 200–300 micrograms/kg
By slow intravenous injection, quarter to half corresponding subcutaneous or intramuscular dose
Pre-operative sedation, *by subcutaneous or intramuscular injection*, 10–20 mg 45–60 minutes before anaesthesia; CHILD single doses as above

CD Papaveretum and Hyoscine Injection, papaveretum 20 mg, hyoscine hydrobromide 400 micrograms/mL. Net price 1-mL amp = 36p
Dose: premedication, by subcutaneous or intramuscular injection, 0.5–1 mL

Other mixed opium alkaloids
Note. Do not contain noscapine
CD Omnopon® (Roche) [New formulation]
Injection, morphine hydrochloride 13.44 mg (≡ anhydrous morphine 10 mg), codeine hydrochloride 1.04 mg, papaverine hydrochloride 1.2 mg/mL. Net price 1-mL amp = 17p
Dose: postoperative analgesia, premedication, severe chronic pain, and pain in myocardial infarction, by subcutaneous, intramuscular, or intravenous[1] injection, ADULT 0.5–1 mL repeated every 4 hours if necessary in chronic pain (0.5 mL for elderly); CHILD 1–12 years 0.01–0.015 mL/kg
Paediatric injection, morphine hydrochloride 6.72 mg (≡ anhydrous morphine 5 mg), codeine hydrochloride 520 micrograms, papaverine hydrochloride 600 micrograms/mL. Net price 1-mL amp = 16p
Dose: postoperative analgesia, premedication, severe chronic pain, and pain in myocardial infarction, by subcutaneous, intramuscular, or intravenous[1] injection, ADULT 1–2 mL repeated every 4 hours if necessary in chronic pain (1 mL for elderly); CHILD up to 1 month 0.015 mL/kg, 1–12 months 0.015–0.02 mL/kg, 1–12 years 0.02–0.03 mL/kg

1. In general the intravenous dose should be quarter to half corresponding subcutaneous or intramuscular dose

---

PETHIDINE HYDROCHLORIDE
Indications: peri-operative analgesia, enhancement of anaesthesia, for basal narcosis with phenothiazines; premedication; analgesia in other situations, see section 4.7.2
Cautions; Contra-indications; Side-effects: see section 4.7.2 and notes above
Dose: premedication, *by intramuscular injection*, 25–100 mg 1 hour before operation; CHILD 0.5–2 mg/kg
Adjunct to nitrous oxide–oxygen, *by slow intravenous injection*, 10–25 mg repeated when required
See also section 4.7.2 for analgesia

CD Pethidine (Roche)
Injection, pethidine hydrochloride 50 mg/mL, net price 1-mL amp = 11p; 2-mL amp = 14p; 10 mg/mL, 5-mL amp = 66p; 10-mL amp = 69p
Tablets, see section 4.7.2

CD Pamergan P100® (Martindale)
Injection, pethidine hydrochloride 50 mg, promethazine hydrochloride 25 mg/mL. Net price 2-mL amp = 45p
Dose: premedication, 2 mL by intramuscular injection 1–1½ hours before operation; CHILD, by intramuscular injection, 8–12 years 0.75 mL, 13–16 years 1 mL

PHENOPERIDINE HYDROCHLORIDE
Indications: analgesia during operation, neuroleptanalgesia, enhancement of anaesthetics; respiratory depressant in prolonged assisted respiration
Cautions; Contra-indications; Side-effects: see under Pethidine Hydrochloride and Fentanyl. Doses above 1 mg cause respiratory depression and require assisted ventilation (effects may be terminated with naloxone)

Dose: by intravenous injection, with spontaneous respiration, up to 1 mg, then 500 micrograms every 40–60 minutes as required; CHILD 30–50 micrograms/kg
With assisted ventilation, 2–5 mg, then 1 mg as required; CHILD 100–150 micrograms/kg

CD **Operidine**® (Janssen)
Injection, phenoperidine hydrochloride 1 mg/mL. Net price 2-mL amp = 77p; 10-mL amp = £4.05

15.1.5 Muscle relaxants

Muscle relaxants used in anaesthesia are also known as **neuromuscular blocking drugs** or **myoneural blocking drugs**. By specific blockade of the neuromuscular junction they enable light levels of anaesthesia to be employed with adequate relaxation of the muscles of the abdomen and diaphragm. They also relax the vocal cords and allow the passage of a tracheal tube. Their action differs from the muscle relaxants acting on the spinal cord or brain which are used in musculoskeletal disorders (see section 10.2.2).

Patients who have received a muscle relaxant should **always** have their respiration assisted or controlled until the drug has been inactivated or antagonised (section 15.1.6).

NON-DEPOLARISING MUSCLE RELAXANTS

Drugs of this group (also known as competitive muscle relaxants) cause blockade by competing with acetylcholine at the receptor site at the neuromuscular junction. These drugs are best suited to the production of paralysis of long duration. They have a slower, less complete action than the depolarising muscle relaxants and should be avoided in myasthenia gravis.

These drugs may be used during surgical operations and for patients receiving long-term ventilation in intensive care units, when larger total doses will be appropriate.

The action of the competitive muscle relaxants may be reversed with anticholinesterases such as neostigmine (section 15.1.6).

Atracurium and **vecuronium** are much more widely employed than the other muscle relaxants, atracurium because of its non-enzymatic elimination and vecuronium because it has the fewest side-effects.

Atracurium has a duration of action of 15 to 35 minutes. Histamine release may occur. The drug is without vagolytic or sympatholytic properties. It has an advantage over other non-depolarising muscle relaxants in patients with renal or hepatic impairment, as it is degraded by non-enzymatic Hofmann elimination, which is independent of liver and kidney function. It is non-cumulative on repeated dosage. Its action is reversed by neostigmine. Duration of action may be prolonged in hypothermia.

Vecuronium has a duration of action of 20 to 30 minutes. Large doses may have a cumulative effect. The drug does not cause histamine release, sympathetic blockade, or vagolytic effects.

Pancuronium does not cause ganglionic blockade or significant changes in blood pressure and may therefore be favoured when it is important to maintain cardiac output.

Tubocurarine starts to act between 3–5 minutes and lasts for about 30 minutes after injection. It may cause an erythematous rash on the chest and neck and this is probably due to histamine release. Onset of blockade may be associated with hypotension and this, though transient, may be important in poor-risk patients.

Gallamine has a more rapid onset of action and recovery than tubocurarine or pancuronium. It causes undesirable tachycardia by its vagolytic action. It should be avoided in patients with severe renal disease.

Alcuronium appears to have no significant advantages over other muscle relaxants. Its duration of action is similar to that of tubocurarine.

ALCURONIUM CHLORIDE

Indications: non-depolarising muscle relaxant of medium duration
Cautions; Contra-indications; Side-effects: see notes above. Reduce dose in renal impairment; avoid in porphyria (see section 9.8.2); **interactions:** Appendix 1 (muscle relaxants)
Dose: by intravenous injection, initially 200–250 micrograms/kg, then incremental doses of one-sixth to one-quarter of the initial dose, as required; CHILD over 1 month, 125–200 micrograms/kg

PoM **Alloferin**® (Roche)
Injection, alcuronium chloride 5 mg/mL. Net price 2-mL amp = 58p

ATRACURIUM BESYLATE

Indications: non-depolarising muscle relaxant of short to medium duration
Cautions; Contra-indications; Side-effects: see notes above; **interactions:** Appendix 1 (muscle relaxants)
Dose: by intravenous injection, ADULT and CHILD over 1 month initially 300–600 micrograms/kg, then 100–200 micrograms/kg as required
By intravenous infusion, 5–10 micrograms/kg/minute (300–600 micrograms/kg/hour)

PoM **Tracrium**® (Wellcome)
Injection, atracurium besylate 10 mg/mL. Net price 2.5-mL amp = £1.86; 5-mL amp = £3.38; 25-mL amp = £14.53

GALLAMINE TRIETHIODIDE

Indications: non-depolarising muscle relaxant of medium duration

Cautions; Contra-indications; Side-effects: see notes above; reduce dose in renal impairment (avoid if severe); **interactions:** Appendix 1 (muscle relaxants)

Dose: by intravenous injection, 80–120 mg, then 20–40 mg as required; CHILD, 1.5 mg/kg

PoM **Flaxedil**® (Rhône-Poulenc Rorer)
Injection, gallamine triethiodide 40 mg/mL. Net price 2-mL amp = 74p

---

PANCURONIUM BROMIDE

Indications: non-depolarising muscle relaxant of medium duration

Cautions; Contra-indications; Side-effects: see notes above; caution in hepatic impairment; reduce dose in renal impairment; **interactions:** Appendix 1 (muscle relaxants)

Dose: by intravenous injection, initially for intubation 50–100 micrograms/kg then 10–20 micrograms/kg as required; CHILD initially 60–100 micrograms/kg, then 10–20 micrograms/kg, NEONATE 30–40 micrograms/kg initially then 10–20 micrograms/kg

Intensive care, *by intravenous injection,* 60 micrograms/kg every 1–1½ hours

PoM **Pancuronium** (Non-proprietary)
Injection, pancuronium bromide 2 mg/mL. Net price 2-mL amp = 79p
Available from David Bull

PoM **Pavulon**® (Organon-Teknika)
Injection, pancuronium bromide 2 mg/mL. Net price 2-mL amp = 67p

---

TUBOCURARINE CHLORIDE

Indications: non-depolarising muscle relaxant of medium to long duration

Cautions; Contra-indications; Side-effects: see notes above. Reduce dose in renal impairment; **interactions:** Appendix 1 (muscle relaxants)

Dose: by intravenous injection, initially 15–30 mg according to circumstances then 5–10 mg as required; CHILD, initially 300–500 micrograms/kg then 60–100 micrograms/kg as required; NEONATE initially 200–250 micrograms/kg then 40–50 micrograms/kg as required

PoM **Jexin**® (Evans)
Injection, tubocurarine chloride 10 mg/mL. Net price 1.5-mL amp = 71p

PoM **Tubarine**® (Wellcome)
Injection, tubocurarine chloride 10 mg/mL. Net price 1.5-mL amp = £1.86

VECURONIUM BROMIDE

Indications: non-depolarising muscle relaxant of short to medium duration

Cautions; Contra-indications; Side-effects: see notes above; reduce dose in renal impairment; **interactions:** Appendix 1 (muscle relaxants)

Dose: by intravenous injection, initially 80–100 micrograms/kg (max. 250 micrograms/kg), then 30–50 micrograms/kg as required; CHILD, as adult dose (onset more rapid)

By intravenous infusion, 50–80 micrograms/kg/hour

PoM **Norcuron**® (Organon-Teknika)
Injection, powder for reconstitution, vecuronium bromide. Net price 10-mg vial = £3.77 (with water for injections)

DEPOLARISING MUSCLE RELAXANTS

Suxamethonium is the only commonly used drug of this group. With a 5-minute duration of action it is ideal for passage of a tracheal tube but may be used in repeated dosage for longer procedures.

It acts by mimicking acetylcholine at the neuromuscular junction but disengagement from the receptor site and subsequent breakdown is slower than for acetylcholine; depolarisation is therefore prolonged and neuromuscular blockade results.

It produces rapid, complete, and predictable paralysis, and recovery is spontaneous. Unlike the non-depolarising muscle relaxants its action cannot be reversed and clinical application is therefore limited.

Suxamethonium should be given after induction of anaesthesia because paralysis is usually preceded by painful muscle fasciculation. There is a transient rise in plasma potassium and creatine phosphokinase and there may be muscle pains postoperatively. Suxamethonium is **contra-indicated** in severe liver disease and in burned patients. Premedication with atropine is desirable.

Prolonged muscle paralysis may occur in patients with low or atypical plasma pseudocholinesterase enzymes. Prolonged paralysis may also occur in **dual block**, which occurs after repeated doses of suxamethonium have been used and is caused by the development of a non-depolarising block following the primary depolarising block. Artificial ventilation should be continued until muscle function is restored. Dual block is diagnosed by giving a short-acting anticholinesterase such as edrophonium; if an improvement occurs the block is treated with neostigmine (section 15.1.6).

SUXAMETHONIUM CHLORIDE

Indications: depolarising muscle relaxant of short duration

Cautions; Contra-indications; Side-effects: see notes above; **interactions:** Appendix 1 (muscle relaxants)

Dose: by *intravenous injection*, 600 micrograms/kg (range 0.3–1.1 mg/kg depending on degree of relaxation required); usual range 20–100 mg
By *intravenous infusion*, as a 0.1% solution, 2–5 mg/minute (2–5 mL/minute)

PoM **Anectine**® (Wellcome)
Injection, suxamethonium chloride 50 mg/mL. Net price 2-mL amp = 73p

PoM **Scoline**® (Evans)
Injection, suxamethonium chloride 50 mg/mL. Net price 2-mL amp = 31p

15.1.6 Anticholinesterases used in surgery

Anticholinesterases reverse the effects of the non-depolarising (competitive) muscle relaxant drugs such as tubocurarine but they prolong the action of the depolarising muscle relaxant drug suxamethonium.

Edrophonium has a transient action and is used to diagnose dual block caused by suxamethonium (section 15.1.5).

Neostigmine has a longer duration of action than edrophonium. It is the specific drug for reversal of non-depolarising (competitive) blockade. It acts within one minute of intravenous injection and lasts for 20 to 30 minutes; a second dose may then be necessary. It is also used in the treatment of dual block. Atropine or glycopyrronium (section 15.1.3) should be given before or with neostigmine in order to prevent bradycardia, excessive salivation, and other muscarinic actions of neostigmine.

For anticholinesterases used in myasthenia gravis see section 10.2.1.

EDROPHONIUM CHLORIDE
Indications: see under Dose
Cautions; Contra-indications; Side-effects: see section 10.2.1 and notes above. Atropine should also be given
Dose: brief reversal of non-depolarising neuromuscular blockade, by *intravenous injection* over several minutes, 500–700 micrograms/kg (after or with atropine sulphate 0.6–1.2 mg)
Diagnosis of dual block, by *intravenous injection*, 10 mg (with atropine)
Diagnosis of myasthenia gravis, see section 10.2.1

PoM **Tensilon**® (Cambridge)
Injection, edrophonium chloride 10 mg/mL. Net price 1-mL amp = 27p

NEOSTIGMINE METHYLSULPHATE
Indications: see under Dose
Cautions; Contra-indications; Side-effects: see section 10.2.1 and notes above. Atropine should also be given

Dose: reversal of non-depolarising neuromuscular blockade, by *intravenous injection* over 1 minute, 50–70 micrograms/kg (max. 5 mg) after or with atropine sulphate 0.6–1.2 mg
Myasthenia gravis, see section 10.2.1

PoM **Prostigmin**® (Roche)
Injection, neostigmine methylsulphate 500 micrograms/mL, net price 1-mL amp = 16p; 2.5 mg/mL, 1-mL amp = 16p

PoM **Robinul-Neostigmine**® (Wyeth)
Injection, neostigmine methylsulphate 2.5 mg, glycopyrronium bromide 500 micrograms/mL. Net price 1-mL amp = £1.06
Dose: by *intravenous injection* over 10–30 seconds, 1–2 mL *or* 0.02 mL/kg;
CHILD 0.02 mL/kg (*or* 0.2 mL/kg of a 1 in 10 dilution using water for injections or sodium chloride injection 0.9%)

15.1.7 Antagonists for central and respiratory depression

The opioid antagonist **naloxone** can be used at the end of an operation to reverse respiratory depression caused by opioid analgesics. Unless the dosage is carefully adjusted, analgesia may also be reversed. For respiratory stimulants see section 3.5.1. **Doxapram** is a respiratory stimulant which does not reverse the other effects of opioid analgesics.

Flumazenil is a benzodiazepine antagonist for the reversal of the central sedative effects of benzodiazepines in anaesthetic and similar procedures. It is important to recognize that the half-life of flumazenil is shorter than those of diazepam and midazolam, in order to avoid the risk of patients becoming resedated.

DOXAPRAM HYDROCHLORIDE
Indications: see under Dose
Cautions; Contra-indications; Side-effects: see section 3.5.1
Dose: postoperative respiratory depression, by *intravenous injection* over at least 30 seconds, 1–1.5 mg/kg repeated if necessary after intervals of 1 hour
By *intravenous infusion*, 2–3 mg/minute
Ventilatory failure, see section 3.5.1

PoM **Dopram**® (Wyeth)
Injection, doxapram hydrochloride 20 mg/mL. Net price 5-mL amp = £2.14
Intravenous infusion: see section 3.5.1

FLUMAZENIL
Indications: reversal of sedative effects of benzodiazepines in anaesthetic, intensive care, and diagnostic procedures

Cautions: short-acting (repeat doses may be necessary); benzodiazepine effects may persist for at least 24 hours; benzodiazepine dependence; ensure neuromuscular blockade cleared before giving; avoid rapid injection in high-risk or anxious patients and following major surgery; hepatic impairment; severe head injury (rapid reversal of benzodiazepine sedation may increase risk of raised intracranial pressure)

Contra-indications: epileptics who have received prolonged benzodiazepine therapy

Side-effects: nausea, vomiting, and flushing; if wakening too rapid, agitation, anxiety, and fear; transient increase in blood pressure and heart-rate in intensive care patients; very rarely convulsions (particularly in epileptics)

Dose: by intravenous injection, 200 micrograms over 15 seconds, then 100 micrograms at 60-second intervals if required; usual dose range, 300–600 micrograms; max. total dose 1 mg (2 mg in intensive care); question aetiology if no response to repeated doses

By intravenous infusion, if drowsiness recurs after injection, 100–400 micrograms/hour, adjusted according to level of arousal

PoM **Anexate**® (Roche)
Injection, flumazenil 100 micrograms/mL. Net price 5-mL amp = £16.32

NALOXONE HYDROCHLORIDE

Indications: reversal of opioid-induced respiratory depression

Cautions: see under Emergency Treatment of Poisoning

Dose: by intravenous injection, 100–200 micrograms (1.5–3 micrograms/kg); if response inadequate, increments of 100 micrograms every 2 minutes; further doses *by intramuscular injection* after 1–2 hours if required

CHILD, *by intravenous injection*, 10 micrograms/kg; subsequent dose of 100 micrograms/kg if no response; if intravenous route not possible, may be given in divided doses by *intramuscular or subcutaneous injection*

NEONATE, *by subcutaneous, intramuscular, or intravenous injection*, 10 micrograms/kg, repeated every 2 to 3 minutes *or* 200 micrograms (60 micrograms/kg) *by intramuscular injection* as a single dose at birth (onset of action slower)

PoM **Naloxone Hydrochloride** (Non-proprietary)
Injection, naloxone hydrochloride 20 micrograms/mL. Net price 2-mL amp = £3.57
Injection, naloxone hydrochloride 400 micrograms/mL—see under Emergency Treatment of Poisoning

PoM **Narcan**®—see under Emergency Treatment of Poisoning

PoM **Narcan Neonatal**® (Du Pont)
Injection, naloxone hydrochloride 20 micrograms/mL. Net price 2-mL amp = £3.57

15.1.8 Antagonists for malignant hyperthermia

Dantrolene is used in the treatment of malignant hyperthermia which is a rare but lethal complication of anaesthesia. It is characterised by a rapid rise in temperature, increasing muscle rigidity, tachycardia, and acidosis and can be triggered off by volatile anaesthetics, especially halothane, and suxamethonium. Dantrolene acts on skeletal muscle by interfering with calcium efflux in the muscle cell and stopping the contractile process. Known trigger agents should be avoided during anaesthesia.

DANTROLENE SODIUM

Indications: malignant hyperthermia
Cautions: avoid extravasation; **interactions:** Appendix 1 (muscle relaxants)
Dose: by rapid intravenous injection, 1 mg/kg, repeated as required to a cumulative max. of 10 mg/kg

PoM **Dantrium Intravenous**® (Norwich Eaton)
Injection, powder for reconstitution, dantrolene sodium. Net price 20-mg vial = £22.52 (hosp. only)

15.2 Local anaesthesia

The use of local anaesthetics by injection or by application to mucous membranes to produce local analgesia is discussed in this section.

See also section 1.7 (colon and rectum), section 11.7 (eye), section 12.3 (oropharynx), and section 13.3 (skin).

USE OF LOCAL ANAESTHETICS. Local anaesthetic drugs act by causing a reversible block to conduction along nerve fibres. The smaller the nerve fibre the more sensitive it is so that a differential block may occur where the smaller fibres carrying pain sensation and automatic impulses are blocked, sparing coarse touch and movement. The drugs used vary widely in their potency, toxicity, duration of action, stability, solubility in water, and ability to penetrate mucous membranes. These variations determine their suitability for use by various routes, e.g. topical (surface), infiltration, plexus, epidural (extradural) or spinal block.

ADMINISTRATION. In estimating the safe dosage of these drugs it is important to take account of the rate at which they are absorbed and excreted as well as their potency. The patient's age, weight, physique, and clinical condition, the degree of vascularity of the area to which the drug is to be applied, and the duration of administration are other factors which must be taken into account.

Local anaesthetics do not rely on the circulation to transport them to their sites of action, but

15.2 Local anaesthesia

uptake into the general circulation is important in terminating their action. Following most regional anaesthetic procedures, maximum arterial plasma concentrations of anaesthetic develop within about 10 to 25 minutes, so careful surveillance for toxic effects is necessary during the first 30 minutes after injection.

Epidural anaesthesia is commonly used during surgery, often combined with general anaesthesia, because of its protective effect against the stress response of surgery. It is often used when good postoperative pain relief is essential (e.g. aortic aneurysm surgery or major gut surgery).

TOXICITY. Toxic effects associated with the local anaesthetics are usually a result of excessively high plasma concentrations. The main effects are excitation of the central nervous system (nervousness, nausea, and convulsions) followed by depression. Less commonly the cardiovascular system is depressed. Hypersensitivity reactions occur mainly with the ester-type local anaesthetics such as amethocaine, benzocaine, cocaine, and procaine; reactions are less frequent with the amide types such as lignocaine, bupivacaine, and prilocaine.

USE OF VASOCONSTRICTORS. Toxicity may occur with repeated dosages due to accumulation of the drug, and reducing doses should therefore be given. Toxic effects may also occur if the injection is too rapid. Local anaesthetics should **not** be injected into inflamed or infected tissues nor should they be applied to the traumatised urethra. Under these conditions the drug may be so rapidly absorbed that a systemic rather than a local reaction is produced.

Most local anaesthetics, with the exception of cocaine, cause dilatation of blood vessels. The addition of a vasoconstrictor such as **adrenaline** diminishes local blood flow, slows the rate of absorption of the local anaesthetic, and prolongs its local effect. Care is necessary when using adrenaline for this purpose because, in excess, it may produce ischaemic necrosis.

Adrenaline should **not** be added to injections used in digits and appendages. When adrenaline is included in an injection of lignocaine or procaine the final concentration should be 1 in 200000. In dental surgery, up to 1 in 80000 of adrenaline is used with local anaesthetics. There is no justification for using higher concentrations.

The total dose of adrenaline should **not** exceed 500 micrograms and it is essential not to exceed a concentration of 1 in 200000 if more than 50 mL of the mixture is to be injected. For cautions associated with the use of adrenaline, see section 2.7. For drug interactions, see Appendix 1 (sympathomimetics).

LIGNOCAINE

Lignocaine is the most widely used local anaesthetic drug. It acts more rapidly and is more stable than most other local anaesthetics. It is effectively absorbed from mucous membranes and is a useful surface anaesthetic in concentrations of 2 to 4%. Except for surface anaesthesia, solutions should not usually exceed 1% in strength. The duration of the block (with adrenaline) is about 1½ hours. Concentrations of 1.5% are used for epidural (extradural) block, and for spinal anaesthesia a 5% solution in glucose intravenous infusion is used as a hyperbaric solution.

LIGNOCAINE HYDROCHLORIDE
(Lidocaine hydrochloride)

Indications: see under Dose; also dental anaesthesia; ventricular arrhythmias (section 2.3.2)

Cautions: epilepsy, hepatic or respiratory impairment, impaired cardiac conduction, bradycardia; reduce dose in elderly or debilitated; resuscitative equipment should be available; see section 2.3.2 for effects on heart

Contra-indications: hypovolaemia, complete heart block; avoid in porphyria (see section 9.8.2); do not use solutions containing adrenaline for anaesthesia in appendages

Side-effects: hypotension, bradycardia, cardiac arrest. CNS effects include agitation, euphoria, respiratory depression, convulsions. See also notes above

Dose: adjusted according to site of operation and response of patient

By injection, max. dose 200 mg, or 500 mg with solutions which also contain adrenaline. Max. dose of adrenaline 500 micrograms (see also notes above)

Infiltration anaesthesia, 0.25–0.5%, with adrenaline 1 in 200000, using 2–50 mL of a 0.5% solution in minor surgery and up to 60 mL in more extensive surgery

Nerve blocks, with adrenaline 1 in 200000, 1% to a max. of 50 mL, 2% to a max. of 25 mL

Epidural and caudal block, with adrenaline 1 in 200000, 1% to a max. of 50 mL, 2% to a max. of 25 mL

Surface anaesthesia, usual strengths 2–4%. Mouth, throat, and upper gastro-intestinal tract, max. 200 mg

Lignocaine hydrochloride injections
PoM **Lignocaine** (Non-proprietary)
Injection 0.5%, lignocaine hydrochloride 5 mg/mL, net price 10-mL amp = 22p
Injection 1%, lignocaine hydrochloride 10 mg/mL, net price 2-mL amp = 14p; 5-mL amp = 21p; 10-mL amp = 40p; 20-mL amp = 42p
Injection 2%, lignocaine hydrochloride 20 mg/mL, net price 2-mL amp = 22p; 5-mL amp = 25p

PoM **Min-I-Jet® Lignocaine Hydrochloride with Adrenaline** (IMS)
Injection, lignocaine hydrochloride 5 mg/mL, adrenaline 1 in 200000 (500 micrograms/100 mL). Net price 5-mL disposable syringe = £3.03

474 Chapter 15: Anaesthesia

PoM Xylocaine® (Astra)
Injection 0.5%, anhydrous lignocaine hydrochloride 5 mg/mL. Net price 20-mL vial = 67p
Injection 0.5% with adrenaline 1 in 200 000, anhydrous lignocaine hydrochloride 5 mg/mL, adrenaline 1 in 200 000. Net price 20-mL vial = 69p
Injection 1%, anhydrous lignocaine hydrochloride 10 mg/mL. Net price 20-mL vial = 69p
Injection 1% with adrenaline 1 in 200 000, anhydrous lignocaine hydrochloride 10 mg/mL, adrenaline 1 in 200 000. Net price 20-mL vial = 71p
Injection 1.5%, for epidural use, anhydrous lignocaine hydrochloride 15 mg/mL. Net price 25-mL amp = £1.21
Injection 2%, anhydrous lignocaine hydrochloride 20 mg/mL. Net price 20-mL vial = 73p
Injection 2% with adrenaline 1 in 200 000, anhydrous lignocaine hydrochloride 20 mg/mL, adrenaline 1 in 200 000. Net price 20-mL vial = 75p

Lignocaine injections for dental use
A large variety of lignocaine injections, plain or with adrenaline or noradrenaline, is also available in dental cartridges under the names **Lidocaton, Lignostab, Neo-Lidocaton, Xylocaine,** and **Xylotox.**

Lignocaine for surface anaesthesia
Note. Local anaesthetic ointments can be absorbed through the rectal mucosa therefore excessive application should be avoided, particularly in infants and children

PoM Emla® (Astra)
Drug Tariff cream, lignocaine 2.5%, prilocaine 2.5%. Net price 5-g tube = £1.73
Surgical pack cream, lignocaine 2.5%, prilocaine 2.5%. Net price 30-g tube (with spatula) = £10.25
NHS *Hospital pack cream*, lignocaine 2.5%, prilocaine 2.5%. Net price 10 × 5-g tube with 25 occlusive dressings = £19.50
Anaesthesia before e.g. venepuncture (not for infants), apply a thick layer under an occlusive dressing 1–5 hours before procedure; split skin grafting, apply a thick layer under an occlusive dressing 2–5 hours before procedure; genital warts (not for children), apply up to 10 g 5–10 minutes before removal
Cautions: not for wounds, mucous membranes (except genital warts in adults) or atopic dermatitis; avoid use near eyes or middle ear; side-effects include transient paleness, redness, and oedema

Instillagel® (CliniMed)
Gel, lignocaine hydrochloride 2%, chlorhexidine gluconate solution 0.25%, in a sterile lubricant basis in disposable syringe. Net price 6-mL syringe = £1.12; 11-mL syringe = £1.26
Dose: 6–11 mL into urethra

Xylocaine® (Astra)
Antiseptic gel, lignocaine hydrochloride 2%, chlorhexidine gluconate solution 0.25% in a sterile lubricant water-miscible basis. Net price 20 g = £1.09
Dose: into urethra, men 10 mL followed by 3–5 mL; women 3–5 mL

Gel, anhydrous lignocaine hydrochloride 2%, in a sterile lubricant water-miscible basis. Net price 20 g = 78p; 20-g single-use syringe (Accordion®) = £1.00
Dose: into urethra, men 10 mL followed by 3–5 mL; women 3–5 mL
Ointment, lignocaine 5% in a water-miscible basis. Net price 15 g = 83p
Dose: max. 35 g in 24 hours
Spray (= pump spray), lignocaine 10% (100 mg/g) supplying 10 mg lignocaine/dose; 500 spray doses per container. Net price 50-mL bottle = £3.21
Dose: dental practice, 1–5 doses; maxillary sinus puncture, 3 doses; during delivery in obstetrics, up to 20 doses; procedures in pharynx, larynx, and trachea, up to 20 doses
Topical 4%, anhydrous lignocaine hydrochloride 40 mg/mL. Net price 30-mL bottle = £1.24
Dose: bronchoscopy, 2–3 mL with suitable spray; biopsy in mouth, 3–4 mL with suitable spray *or* swab (with adrenaline if necessary); max. 7.5 mL

BUPIVACAINE

The great advantage of bupivacaine over other local anaesthetics is its duration of action of up to 8 hours when used for nerve blocks. It has a slow onset of action, taking up to 30 minutes for full effect. It is often used in lumbar epidural blockade and is particularly suitable for continuous epidural analgesia in labour; it then has a 2- to 3-hour duration of action. It is **contra-indicated** in intravenous regional anaesthesia (Bier's block). It is the principal drug for spinal anaesthesia in the UK.

BUPIVACAINE HYDROCHLORIDE

Indications: see under Dose
Cautions; Contra-indications; Side-effects: see under Lignocaine Hydrochloride and notes above; myocardial depression may be more severe and more resistant to treatment; contra-indicated in intravenous regional anaesthesia (Bier's block)
Dose: adjusted according to site of operation and response of patient
Local infiltration, 0.25% (up to 60 mL)
Peripheral nerve block, 0.25% (max. 60 mL), 0.5% (max. 30 mL)
Epidural block,
 Surgery, *lumbar*, 0.5–0.75% (max. 20 mL of either)
 caudal, 0.5% (max. 30 mL)
 Labour, *lumbar*, 0.25–0.5% (max. 12 mL of either)
 caudal, 0.25% (max. 30 mL), 0.5% (max. 20 mL)
Note. 0.75% **contra-indicated** for epidural use in obstetrics.

PoM Marcain Heavy® (Astra)
Injection, bupivacaine hydrochloride 5 mg, glucose 80 mg/mL. Net price 4-ml amp = £1.00
Dose: spinal anaesthesia, 2–4 mL

15.2 Local anaesthesia 475

PoM **Marcain**® (Astra)
Injection 0.25%, bupivacaine hydrochloride 2.5 mg/mL. Net price 10-mL amp = £1.13
Injection 0.5%, bupivacaine hydrochloride 5 mg/mL. Net price 10-mL amp = £1.30
Injection 0.75%, bupivacaine hydrochloride 7.5 mg/mL. Net price 10-mL amp = £1.95

PoM **Marcain with Adrenaline**® (Astra)
Injection 0.25%, bupivacaine hydrochloride 2.5 mg/mL, adrenaline 1 in 200 000. Net price 10-mL amp = £1.27
Injection 0.5%, bupivacaine hydrochloride 5 mg/mL, adrenaline 1 in 200 000. Net price 10-mL amp = £1.43

PRILOCAINE

Prilocaine is a local anaesthetic of low toxicity which is similar to lignocaine. It can be used for infiltration, regional nerve block, and spinal anaesthesia and regional intravenous analgesia. If used in high doses, methaemoglobinaemia may occur which can be treated with intravenous injection of methylene blue 1% using a dose of 75–100 mg.

PRILOCAINE HYDROCHLORIDE

Indications: see under Dose; also dental anaesthesia
Cautions; Contra-indications; Side-effects: see under Lignocaine Hydrochloride and notes above; avoid in anaemia or congenital or acquired methaemoglobinaemia
Dose: adjusted according to site of operation and response of patient, to max. 400 mg used alone, or 600 mg if used with adrenaline or felypressin

PoM **Citanest**® (Astra)
Injection 0.5%, prilocaine hydrochloride 5 mg/mL. Net price 20-mL multidose vial = 73p; 50-mL multidose vial = £1.02; 50-mL single dose vial = £1.30
Injection 1%, prilocaine hydrochloride 10 mg/mL. Net price 20-mL vial = 75p; 50-mL vial = £1.06
Injection 2%, prilocaine hydrochloride 20 mg/mL. Net price 10-mL single dose vial = 75p
Injection 4%, prilocaine hydrochloride 40 mg/mL. Net price 2-mL cartridge = 13p

PoM **Citanest with Octapressin**® (Astra)
Injection 3%, prilocaine hydrochloride 30 mg/mL, felypressin 0.03 unit/mL. Net price 2-mL cartridge and self-aspirating cartridge (both) = 13p

PROCAINE

Procaine is now seldom used. It is as potent an anaesthetic as lignocaine but has a shorter duration of action. It provides less intense analgesia because it has less tendency to spread through the tissues. It is poorly absorbed from mucous membranes and is of no value as a surface anaesthetic. When used for infiltration or regional anaesthesia, adrenaline 1 in 200 000 is generally added. Its metabolite para-aminobenzoic acid inhibits the action of the sulphonamides.

PROCAINE HYDROCHLORIDE

Indications: local anaesthesia by infiltration and regional routes
Cautions; Side-effects: see notes above
Dose: adjusted according to site of operation and patient's response
By injection, up to 1 g (200 mL of 0.5% solution or 100 mL of 1%) with adrenaline 1 in 200 000

PoM **Procaine Injection,** procaine hydrochloride 2% (20 mg/mL) in sodium chloride intravenous infusion. Net price 2-mL amp = 57p; 1% in 2-mL amp also available

OTHER LOCAL ANAESTHETICS

Amethocaine is an effective local anaesthetic for topical application. It is rapidly absorbed from mucous membranes and should **never** be applied to inflamed, traumatised, or highly vascular surfaces. It should **never** be used to provide anaesthesia for bronchoscopy or cystoscopy, as lignocaine is a safer alternative. It is used in ophthalmology (see section 11.7) and in skin preparations (see section 13.3). Hypersensitivity to amethocaine has been reported.

Benzocaine is a local anaesthetic of low potency and toxicity. Its only use is in surface anaesthesia for the relief of pain and irritation in the oropharynx (see section 12.3.1).

Cocaine readily penetrates mucous membranes and is an effective surface anaesthetic but, apart from its use in otolaryngology (see below), it has now been replaced by less toxic alternatives. It potentiates the action of adrenaline and possesses vasoconstrictor and mydriatic properties and should therefore **not** be used with adrenaline. It should **never** be given by injection because of its toxicity and doses not exceeding 3 mg/kg should be applied to mucous membranes. It stimulates the central nervous system and is a drug of addiction. It should be avoided in porphyria (see section 9.8.2). In otolaryngology concentrations of 4 to 10% (40–100 mg/mL) are applied to the nose. For the use of cocaine in ophthalmology see section 11.7.

Cautionary label wordings, see inside back cover

Prices are **net**, see p. 1

Appendix 1: Interactions

Two or more drugs given at the same time may exert their effects independently or may interact. The interaction may be potentiation or antagonism of one drug by another, or occasionally some other effect. Adverse drug interactions should be reported to the CSM as for other adverse drug reactions.

Drug interactions may be **pharmacodynamic** or **pharmacokinetic**.

PHARMACODYNAMIC INTERACTIONS

These are interactions between drugs which have similar or antagonistic pharmacological effects or side-effects. They may be due to competition at receptor sites, or occur between drugs acting on the same physiological system. They are usually predictable from a knowledge of the pharmacology of the interacting drugs; in general, those demonstrated with one drug are likely to occur with related drugs. They occur to a greater or lesser extent in most patients who receive the interacting drugs.

PHARMACOKINETIC INTERACTIONS

These occur when one drug alters the absorption, distribution, metabolism, or excretion of another, thus increasing or reducing the amount of drug available to produce its pharmacological effects. They are not easily predicted and many of them affect only a small proportion of patients taking the combination of drugs. Pharmacokinetic interactions occurring with one drug cannot be assumed to occur with related drugs unless their pharmacokinetic properties are known to be similar.

Pharmacokinetic interactions are of several types:

AFFECTING ABSORPTION. The rate of absorption or the total amount absorbed can both be altered by drug interactions. Delayed absorption is rarely of clinical importance unless high peak plasma concentrations are required (e.g. when giving an analgesic). Reduction in the total amount absorbed, however, may result in ineffective therapy.

DUE TO CHANGES IN PROTEIN BINDING. To a variable extent most drugs are loosely bound to plasma proteins. Protein-binding sites are non-specific and one drug can displace another thereby increasing its proportion free to diffuse from plasma to its site of action. This only produces a detectable increase in effect if it is an extensively bound drug (more than 90%) that is not widely distributed throughout the body. Even so displacement rarely produces more than transient potentiation because this increased concentration of free drug results in an increased rate of elimination.

Displacement from protein binding plays a part in the potentiation of warfarin by phenylbutazone, sulphonamides, and tolbutamide but the importance of these interactions is due mainly to the fact that warfarin metabolism is also inhibited.

AFFECTING METABOLISM. Many drugs are metabolised in the liver. Induction of the hepatic microsomal enzyme system by one drug can gradually increase the rate of metabolism of another, resulting in lower plasma concentrations and a reduced effect. On withdrawal of the inducer plasma concentrations increase and toxicity may occur. Barbiturates, griseofulvin, most antiepileptics, and rifampicin are the most important enzyme inducers in man. Drugs affected include warfarin and the oral contraceptives.

Conversely when one drug inhibits the metabolism of another higher plasma concentrations are produced, rapidly resulting in an increased effect with risk of toxicity. Some drugs which potentiate warfarin and phenytoin do so by this mechanism.

AFFECTING RENAL EXCRETION. Drugs are eliminated through the kidney both by glomerular filtration and by active tubular secretion. Competition occurs between those which share active transport mechanisms in the proximal tubule. Thus probenecid delays the excretion of many drugs including penicillins, some cephalosporins, indomethacin, and dapsone; aspirin may increase the toxicity of methotrexate by a similar mechanism.

RELATIVE IMPORTANCE OF INTERACTIONS

Many drug interactions are harmless and many of those which are potentially harmful only occur in a small proportion of patients; moreover, the severity of an interaction varies from one patient to another. Drugs with a small therapeutic ratio (e.g. phenytoin) and those which require careful control of dosage (e.g. anticoagulants, antihypertensives, and antidiabetics) are most often involved.

Patients at increased risk from drug interactions include the elderly and those with impaired renal or liver function.

HAZARDOUS INTERACTIONS. The symbol • has been placed against interactions that are **potentially hazardous** and where combined administration of the drugs involved should be **avoided** (or only undertaken with caution and appropriate monitoring).

Interactions that have no symbol do not usually have serious consequences.

List of drug interactions

The following is an alphabetical list of drugs and their interactions; to avoid excessive cross-referencing each drug or group is listed twice: in the alphabetical list and also against the drug or group with which it interacts; changes in the interactions lists since BNF No. 23 (March 1992) are underlined.
For explanation of symbol • see previous page

ACE Inhibitors
  Alcohol: enhanced hypotensive effect
• Anaesthetics: enhanced hypotensive effect
  Analgesics: antagonism of hypotensive effect and increased risk of renal failure with *NSAIDs*; hyperkalaemia with *indomethacin* and possibly other *NSAIDs*
  Antacids: absorption of *fosinopril* reduced
  Antibacterials: absorption of *tetracyclines* reduced by *quinapril* (tablets contain magnesium carbonate excipient)
  Antidepressants: enhanced hypotensive effect
  other Antihypertensives: enhanced hypotensive effect
  Antipsychotics: severe postural hypotension with *chlorpromazine* and possibly other *phenothiazines*
  Anxiolytics and Hypnotics: enhanced hypotensive effect
  Beta-blockers: enhanced hypotensive effect
  Calcium-channel Blockers: enhanced hypotensive effect
  Cardiac Glycosides: plasma concentration of *digoxin* possibly increased by *captopril*
  Corticosteroids: antagonism of hypotensive effect
  Cyclosporin: increased risk of hyperkalaemia
• Diuretics: enhanced hypotensive effect (can be extreme); hyperkalaemia with *potassium-sparing diuretics*
  Dopaminergics: *levodopa* enhances hypotensive effect
• Lithium: *ACE inhibitors* reduce excretion of *lithium* (increased plasma-lithium concentration)
  Muscle Relaxants: *baclofen* enhances hypotensive effect
  Nitrates: enhance hypotensive effect
• Potassium Salts: hyperkalaemia
  Sex Hormones: *oestrogens* and combined oral contraceptives antagonise hypotensive effect
  Sympathomimetics: *see* Sympathomimetics (main list)
  Ulcer-healing Drugs: *carbenoxolone* antagonises hypotensive effect
  Uricosurics: *probenecid* reduces excretion of *captopril*
Acebutolol *see* Beta-blockers
Acemetacin *see* NSAIDs
Acetazolamide (general hypokalaemic interactions as for Diuretics)
  Analgesics: *aspirin* reduces excretion of *acetazolamide* (risk of toxicity)
  Anti-arrhythmics: excretion of *quinidine* reduced in alkaline urine (occasionally increased plasma-concentrations); interaction with *flecainide* and with *mexiletine* no longer considered significant
  Antiepileptics: *phenytoin* possibly increases risk of osteomalacia
  Lithium: *lithium* excretion increased
Acrivastine *see* Antihistamines
Acrosoxacin *see* 4-Quinolones

Acyclovir
  other Antivirals: extreme lethargy reported on administration of *zidovudine* with *intravenous acyclovir*
  Uricosurics: *probenecid* reduces *acyclovir* excretion (increased plasma concentrations and risk of toxicity)
Adenosine
• Antiplatelet Drugs: effect enhanced by *dipyridamole* (risk of toxicity)
  Theophylline: antagonism of anti-arrhythmic effect
Adrenaline *see* Sympathomimetics
Adrenergic Neurone Blockers (*see also* Bretylium)
  Alcohol: enhanced hypotensive effect
• Anaesthetics: enhanced hypotensive effect
  Analgesics: *NSAIDs* antagonise hypotensive effect
  Antidepressants: *tricyclics* antagonise hypotensive effect
  other Antihypertensives: enhanced hypotensive effect
  Antipsychotics: *phenothiazines* enhance hypotensive effect (antagonism of hypotensive effect with higher doses of *chlorpromazine*)
  Anxiolytics and Hypnotics: enhanced hypotensive effect
  Beta-blockers: enhanced hypotensive effect
  Calcium-channel Blockers: enhanced hypotensive effect
  Corticosteroids: antagonism of hypotensive effect
  Diuretics: enhanced hypotensive effect
  Dopaminergics: *levodopa* enhances hypotensive effect
  Nitrates: enhance hypotensive effect
  Pizotifen: antagonism of hypotensive effect
  Sex Hormones: *oestrogens* and combined oral contraceptives antagonise hypotensive effect
• Sympathomimetics: *some anorectics* (e.g. *mazindol*) and some cough and cold remedies (e.g. *ephedrine*) antagonise hypotensive effect
  Ulcer-healing Drugs: *carbenoxolone* antagonises hypotensive effect
Alcohol
  Antibacterials: disulfiram-like reaction with *cephamandole, metronidazole, nimorazole* and *tinidazole*
• Anticoagulants: anticoagulant effects of *warfarin* and *nicoumalone* enhanced
• Antidepressants: sedative effect of *tricyclic* and related antidepressants enhanced; *tyramine* contained in some alcoholic and dealcoholised beverages interacts with *MAOIs* (hypertensive crisis)
  Antidiabetics: enhanced hypoglycaemic effect; flushing with *chlorpropamide* (in susceptible subjects); increased risk of lactic acidosis with *metformin*
  Antihistamines: enhanced sedative effect
  Antihypertensives: enhanced hypotensive effect; sedative effect of *indoramin* enhanced
  Antipsychotics: enhanced sedative effect
  Anxiolytics and Hypnotics: enhanced sedative effect
  Beta-blockers: enhanced hypotensive effect

Alcohol (*continued*)
  Cytotoxics: disulfiram-like reaction with *procarbazine*
  Dopaminergics: reduced tolerance to *bromocriptine*
  Monosulfiram: disulfiram-like reaction
  Muscle Relaxants: *baclofen* enhances sedative effect
  Nabilone: enhanced sedative effect
  Nitrates: enhanced hypotensive effect
Alcuronium *see* Muscle Relaxants (non-depolarising)
Alfentanil *see* Opioid Analgesics
Allopurinol
  Anticoagulants: effects of *nicoumalone and warfarin* may be enhanced
• Cytotoxics: effects of *azathioprine, cyclophosphamide, and mercaptopurine* enhanced with increased toxicity
Allyloestrenol *see* Progestogens
Alpha-blockers (general hypotensive interactions *as for* Hydralazine)
  Alcohol: sedative effect of *indoramin* enhanced
  Anxiolytics and Hypnotics: enhanced sedative effect
• Beta-blockers: increased risk of first-dose hypotensive effect of *post-synaptic alpha-blockers such as prazosin and terazosin*
• Diuretics: increased risk of first-dose hypotensive effect of *post-synaptic alpha-blockers such as prazosin and terazosin*
Alprazolam *see* Benzodiazepines and other Anxiolytics and Hypnotics
Aluminium Hydroxide *see* Antacids and Adsorbents
Amantadine
  Antihypertensives: *methyldopa* and *metirosine* have extrapyramidal side-effects
  Antimuscarinics: increased antimuscarinic side-effects
  Antipsychotics: all have extrapyramidal side-effects
  Domperidone and Metoclopramide: have extrapyramidal side-effects
  Tetrabenazine: has extrapyramidal side-effects
Ambutonium *see* Antimuscarinics
Amikacin *see* Aminoglycosides
Amiloride *see* Diuretics (potassium-sparing)
Aminoglutethimide
• Anticoagulants: metabolism of *nicoumalone and warfarin* accelerated (reduced anticoagulant effect)
  Cardiac glycosides: metabolism of *digitoxin* only accelerated (reduced effect)
  Corticosteroids: metabolism of *dexamethasone* accelerated (reduced effect)
  Theophylline: metabolism of *theophylline* accelerated (reduced effect)
Aminoglycosides
  other Antibacterials: increased risk of nephrotoxicity with *colistin and polymyxin*; increased risk of ototoxicity and nephrotoxicity with *capreomycin and vancomycin*
  Anticoagulants: *see* Phenindione and Warfarin
  Antifungals: increased risk of nephrotoxicity with *amphotericin*
  Bisphosphonates: severe hypocalcaemia
• Cholinergics: antagonism of effect of *neostigmine and pyridostigmine*
• Cyclosporin: increased risk of nephrotoxicity
• Cytotoxics: increased risk of nephrotoxicity and possibly of ototoxicity with *cisplatin*
  Diuretics: increased risk of ototoxicity with *loop diuretics*
• Muscle Relaxants: effect of *non-depolarising muscle relaxants such as tubocurarine* enhanced

Aminophylline *see* Theophylline
Amiodarone
• *other* Anti-arrhythmics: additive effect with *disopyramide, flecainide, procainamide, and quinidine* (increased risk of ventricular arrhythmias); increased plasma concentrations of *flecainide and procainamide*; increased myocardial depression with any anti-arrhythmic
• Anticoagulants: metabolism of *nicoumalone and warfarin* inhibited (enhanced anticoagulant effect)
• Antiepileptics: metabolism of *phenytoin* inhibited (increased plasma concentration)
• Beta-blockers: increased risk of bradycardia, AV block, and myocardial depression
• Calcium-channel Blockers: *diltiazem and verapamil* increase risk of bradycardia, AV block, and myocardial depression
• Cardiac Glycosides: increased plasma concentration of *digoxin* (halve digoxin maintenance dose)
  Cyclosporin: plasma concentration of cyclosporin possibly increased
  Diuretics: toxicity increased if hypokalaemia occurs with *acetazolamide, loop diuretics, and thiazides*
  Ulcer-healing Drugs: *cimetidine* increases plasma concentrations of *amiodarone*
Amitriptyline *see* Antidepressants, Tricyclic
Amlodipine *see* Calcium-channel Blockers
Amoxapine *see* Antidepressants, Tricyclic
Amoxycillin *see* Penicillins
Amphetamines *see* Sympathomimetics
Amphotericin
  Antibacterials: increased risk of nephrotoxicity with *aminoglycosides*
  other Antifungals: antagonises *miconazole*
• Cyclosporin: increased risk of nephrotoxicity
Ampicillin *see* Penicillins
Amylobarbitone *see* Barbiturates and Primidone
Anabolic Steroids
• Anticoagulants: anticoagulant effect of *nicoumalone, phenindione, and warfarin* enhanced
Anaesthetics (*see also* Surgery and Long-term Medication, section 15.1)
  Antibacterials: effect of *thiopentone* enhanced by *sulphonamides*
  Antidepressants: risk of arrhythmias and hypotension increased with *tricyclics*
• Antihypertensives: enhanced hypotensive effect
• Antipsychotics: enhanced hypotensive effect
  Anxiolytics and Hypnotics: enhanced sedative effect
• Beta-blockers: enhanced hypotensive effect
• Calcium-channel Blockers: enhanced hypotensive effect and AV delay with *verapamil*
• Dopaminergics: risk of arrhythmias if *volatile anaesthetics such as halothane* given with *levodopa*
• Sympathomimetics: risk of arrhythmias if *adrenaline or isoprenaline* given with *volatile anaesthetics such as halothane*
  Theophylline: increased risk of arrhythmias with *halothane*
Analgesics *see* Aspirin, Nefopam, NSAIDs, Opioid Analgesics, and Paracetamol
Anion-exchange Resins *see* Cholestyramine and Colestipol
Antacids and Adsorbents
  Analgesics: excretion of *aspirin* increased in alkaline urine; *antacids* reduce absorption of *diflunisal*
  Anti-arrhythmics: excretion of *quinidine* reduced in alkaline urine (may occasionally increase plasma concentrations)

Antacids and Adsorbents (*continued*)
 Antibacterials: *antacids* reduce absorption of *azithromycin, ciprofloxacin, isoniazid, norfloxacin, ofloxacin, pivampicillin, rifampicin, and most tetracyclines*
 Antiepileptics: *antacids* reduce *phenytoin* absorption
 Antifungals: *antacids* reduce absorption of *itraconazole* and *ketoconazole*
 Antihypertensives: *antacids* reduce absorption of *fosinopril*
 Antiplatelet Drugs: *dipyridamole* patient information leaflet advises avoidance of *antacids*
 Antimalarials: *antacids* reduce absorption of *chloroquine* and *hydroxychloroquine*
 Antipsychotics: *antacids* reduce absorption of *phenothiazines*
 Bisphosphonates: *antacids* reduce absorption (give at least 2 hours apart)
 Iron: *magnesium trisilicate* reduces absorption of *oral iron*
 Lithium: *sodium bicarbonate* increases excretion (reduced plasma-lithium concentration)
 Penicillamine: *antacids* reduce absorption
Antazoline see Antihistamines
Anti-arrhythmics see individual drugs
Anticholinergics see Antimuscarinics
Anticoagulants see Heparin, Phenindione, and Warfarin
Antidepressants see individual entries for Antidepressants, Serotonin-uptake Inhibitor; Antidepressants, Tricyclic; MAOIs; Mianserin; Trazodone; Tryptophan; and Viloxazine
Antidepressants, Serotonin-uptake Inhibitor
• Anticoagulants: effect of *nicoumalone and warfarin* possibly enhanced by *fluvoxamine* and *paroxetine*
• *other* Antidepressants: CNS effects of *MAOIs* increased (risk of toxicity); avoid *MAOIs* for at least 2 weeks before *serotonin-uptake inhibitor*; avoid *fluoxetine* for at least 5 weeks and *sertraline* for at least 7 days before *MAOIs*; *fluoxetine* increases plasma concentrations of some *tricyclics*; agitation and nausea with *tryptophan*
 Antiepileptics: antagonism (convulsive threshold lowered); plasma concentration of *carbamazepine* increased by *fluoxetine* and *fluvoxamine*; *phenytoin and possibly other antiepileptics* reduce plasma concentration of *paroxetine*
 Antipsychotics: plasma concentration of *haloperidol* increased by *fluoxetine*
 Beta-blockers: plasma concentration of *propranolol* increased by *fluvoxamine*
• Lithium: increased risk of CNS toxicity
• Sumatriptan: risk of CNS toxicity
Antidepressants, Tricyclic
• Alcohol: enhanced sedative effect
 Anaesthetics: risk of arrhythmias and hypotension increased
• *other* Antidepressants: CNS excitation and hypertension with *MAOIs* (avoid for at least 2 weeks after stopping MAOIs); *fluoxetine* increases plasma concentrations of some *tricyclics*
• Antiepileptics: antagonism (convulsive threshold lowered); plasma concentrations of *tricyclics* reduced (reduced antidepressant effect)
 Antihistamines: increased antimuscarinic and sedative effects
 Antihypertensives: in general, hypotensive effect enhanced, but antagonism of effect of *adrenergic neurone blockers* and of *clonidine* (and increased risk of hypertension on clonidine withdrawal)

Antidepressants, Tricyclic (*continued*)
 Antimuscarinics: increased antimuscarinic side-effects
 Antipsychotics: increased plasma concentrations of *tricyclic antidepressants* and increased antimuscarinic side-effects with *phenothiazines*
 Anxiolytics and Hypnotics: enhanced sedative effect
 Barbiturates: *see under* Antiepileptics, above
 Calcium-channel Blockers: *diltiazem* and *verapamil* increase plasma concentration of *imipramine* and possibly *other tricyclics*
 Disulfiram: inhibition of metabolism of *tricyclics* (increased plasma concentrations and increased disulfiram reaction reported with *alcohol with amitriptyline*)
 Diuretics: increased risk of postural hypotension
 Nitrates: reduced effect of *sublingual nitrates* (owing to dry mouth)
 Sex Hormones: *oral contraceptives* antagonise antidepressant effect (but side-effects may be increased due to increased plasma concentrations of *tricyclics*)
• Sympathomimetics: hypertension and arrhythmias with *adrenaline* (but local anaesthetics with adrenaline appear to be safe); hypertension with *noradrenaline*
 Ulcer-healing Drugs: plasma concentrations of *amitriptyline, desipramine, doxepin, imipramine, nortriptyline, and probably other tricyclics* increased by *cimetidine* (inhibition of metabolism)
Antidiabetics (includes Insulin, Metformin, and Sulphonylureas)
 Alcohol: enhanced hypoglycaemic effect; flushing with *chlorpropamide* (in susceptible subjects); risk of lactic acidosis with *metformin*
• Analgesics: *azapropazone* and *phenylbutazone* enhance effect of *sulphonylureas*
• Antibacterials: *chloramphenicol, co-trimoxazole, sulphonamides,* and *trimethoprim* enhance effect of *sulphonylureas*; *rifampicin* reduces effect of *sulphonylureas* (accelerates metabolism)
 Antidepressants: *MAOIs* enhance hypoglycaemic effect
 Antiepileptics: plasma-*phenytoin* concentration transiently increased by *tolbutamide* (possibility of toxicity)
• Antifungals: *miconazole* and possibly *fluconazole* enhance effect of *sulphonylureas*
 Antihypertensives: hypoglycaemic effect antagonised by *diazoxide*
 Beta-blockers: enhanced hypoglycaemic effect (and masking of warning signs such as tremor)
 Calcium-channel Blockers: *nifedipine* may occasionally impair glucose tolerance
 Clofibrate Group: may improve glucose tolerance and have an additive effect
 Corticosteroids: antagonism of hypoglycaemic effect
 Diuretics: hypoglycaemic effect antagonised by *loop and thiazide diuretics*; *chlorpropamide* increases risk of hyponatraemia with *thiazides in combination with potassium-sparing diuretics*
 Hormone Antagonists: *octreotide* may reduce *insulin and antidiabetic drug* requirements in diabetes mellitus
 Lithium: may occasionally impair glucose tolerance
 Sex Hormones: *oral contraceptives* antagonise hypoglycaemic effect

Antidiabetics (*continued*)
 Ulcer-healing Drugs: *cimetidine* inhibits renal excretion of *metformin* (increased plasma-metformin concentrations)
• Uricosurics: *sulphinpyrazone* enhances effect of *sulphonylureas*
Antiepileptics *see* individual drugs
Antifungals *see* individual drugs
Antihistamines
 Note. The following interactions apply to a lesser extent to the non-sedative antihistamines, and they do not appear to potentiate the effects of alcohol
 Alcohol: enhanced sedative effect
• Antibacterials: *erythromycin* inhibits *terfenadine* metabolism (see p. 127)
 Antidepressants: *tricyclics* increase antimuscarinic and sedative effects
• Antifungals: *ketoconazole* inhibits *terfenadine* metabolism (cardiac toxicity reported)
 Antimuscarinics: increased antimuscarinic side-effects
 Anxiolytics and Hypnotics: enhanced sedative effect
 Betahistine: antagonism (theoretical)
Antihypertensives *see* individual drugs or groups
Antimalarials *see* individual drugs
Antimuscarinics
 Note. Many drugs have antimuscarinic effects; concomitant use of two or three such drugs can increase side-effects such as dry mouth, urine retention, and constipation; concomitant use can also lead to confusion in the elderly
 Analgesics: increased antimuscarinic effects with *nefopam*
 Anti-arrhythmics: increased antimuscarinic effects with *disopyramide*; *atropine* delays absorption of *mexiletine*
 Antidepressants: increased antimuscarinic side-effects with *tricyclics and MAOIs*
 Antifungals: reduced absorption of *ketoconazole*
 Antihistamines: increased antimuscarinic side-effects
 Antipsychotics: increased antimuscarinic side-effects of *phenothiazines* (but reduced plasma concentrations)
 Cisapride: antagonism of gastro-intestinal effect
 Domperidone and Metoclopramide: *antimuscarinics* such as *propantheline* antagonise gastro-intestinal effects
 Dopaminergics: increased antimuscarinic side-effects with *amantadine*
 Nitrates: reduced effect of *sublingual nitrates* (failure to dissolve under tongue owing to dry mouth)
Antiplatelet Drugs *see* Aspirin and Dipyridamole
Antipsychotics *see* Phenothiazines and other Antipsychotics
Antivirals *see* individual drugs
Anxiolytics *see* Benzodiazepines and other Anxiolytics and Hypnotics
Appetite Suppressants *see* Sympathomimetics
Aspirin
 Antacids and Adsorbents: excretion of *aspirin* increased in alkaline urine
• Anticoagulants: increased risk of bleeding due to antiplatelet effect
 Antiepileptics: enhancement of effect of *phenytoin* and *sodium valproate*
• Cytotoxics: reduced excretion of *methotrexate* (increased toxicity)
 Diuretics: antagonism of diuretic effect of *spironolactone*; reduced excretion of *acetazolamide* (risk of toxicity)

Aspirin (*continued*)
 Domperidone and Metoclopramide: *metoclopramide* enhances effect of *aspirin* (increased rate of absorption)
 Mifepristone: manufacturer recommends avoid *aspirin* until 8–12 days after *mifepristone*
 Uricosurics: effect of *probenecid* and *sulphinpyrazone* reduced
Astemizole *see* Antihistamines
Atenolol *see* Beta-blockers
Atracurium *see* Muscle Relaxants (non-depolarising)
Atropine *see* Antimuscarinics
Azapropazone *see* NSAIDs
Azatadine *see* Antihistamines
Azathioprine
• Allopurinol: enhancement of effect with increased toxicity
Azithromycin
 Antacids and Adsorbents: *antacids* reduce absorption of *azithromycin*
 Anticoagulants: effect of *warfarin* possibly enhanced
 Cardiac Glycosides: effect of *digoxin* possibly enhanced
 Ergotamine: ergotism possible
Azlocillin *see* Penicillins
Aztreonam
• Anticoagulants: anticoagulant effect of *nicoumalone and warfarin* enhanced
Baclofen *see* Muscle Relaxants
Barbiturates and Primidone
 Anti-arrhythmics: metabolism of *disopyramide and quinidine* increased (reduced plasma concentrations)
 Antibacterials: metabolism of *chloramphenicol, doxycycline, and metronidazole* accelerated (reduced effect); *sulphonamides* enhance effect of *thiopentone*
• Anticoagulants: metabolism of *nicoumalone and warfarin* accelerated (reduced anticoagulant effect)
• Antidepressants: antagonism of anticonvulsant effect (convulsive threshold lowered); metabolism of *mianserin* and *tricyclics* accelerated (reduced plasma concentrations)
• Antiepileptics: concomitant administration of *phenobarbitone or primidone* with other antiepileptics may enhance toxicity without a corresponding increase in antiepileptic effect; moreover interactions can complicate monitoring of treatment; interactions include enhanced effects, increased sedation, and reductions in plasma concentrations; metabolism of *clonazepam* accelerated
 Antifungals: *phenobarbitone* accelerates metabolism of *griseofulvin* (reduced effect)
• Antipsychotics: antagonism of anticonvulsant effect (convulsive threshold lowered)
• Calcium-channel Blockers: effect of *felodipine, isradipine* and probably *nicardipine* and *nifedipine* reduced
 Cardiac Glycosides: metabolism of *digitoxin* only accelerated (reduced effect)
• Corticosteroids: metabolism of *corticosteroids* accelerated (reduced effect)
• Cyclosporin: metabolism of *cyclosporin* accelerated (reduced effect)
• Sex Hormones: metabolism of *gestrinone, tibolone,* and *oral contraceptives* accelerated (reduced contraceptive effect, important: see p. 291)
 Theophylline: metabolism of *theophylline* accelerated (reduced effect)

Appendix 1: Interactions 481

Barbiturates and Primidone (*continued*)
    Thyroxine: metabolism of thyroxine accelerated (may increase thyroxine requirements in hypothyroidism)
    Vitamins: vitamin D requirements possibly increased
Beclomethasone see Corticosteroids
Bendrofluazide see Diuretics (thiazide)
Benorylate see Aspirin *and* Paracetamol
Benperidol see Phenothiazines and other Antipsychotics
Benzhexol see Antimuscarinics
Benzodiazepines and other Anxiolytics and Hypnotics
    Alcohol: enhanced sedative effect
    Anaesthetics: enhanced sedative effect
    Analgesics: *opioid analgesics* enhance sedative effect
    Antibacterials: *erythromycin* inhibits metabolism of *midazolam* (increased plasma concentration, see also p. 465); *isoniazid* inhibits metabolism of *diazepam*; *rifampicin* increases metabolism of *diazepam*
    Anticoagulants: *chloral hydrate* may transiently enhance effect of *nicoumalone and warfarin*
    Antidepressants: enhanced sedative effect; manufacturer contra-indicates *buspirone* with *MAOIs*
    Antiepileptics: metabolism of *clonazepam* accelerated (reduced effect)
    Antihistamines: enhanced sedative effect
    Antihypertensives: enhanced hypotensive effect; enhanced sedative effect with *alpha-blockers*
    Antipsychotics: enhanced sedative effect
    Disulfiram: metabolism of *diazepam and chlordiazepoxide* inhibited (enhanced sedative effect)
    Dopaminergics: *benzodiazepines* occasionally antagonise effect of *levodopa*
    Muscle Relaxants: *baclofen* enhances sedative effect
    Nabilone: enhanced sedative effect
    Ulcer-healing Drugs: *cimetidine* inhibits metabolism of *benzodiazepines and chlormethiazole* (increased plasma concentrations); *omeprazole* inhibits metabolism of *diazepam* (increased plasma concentrations)
Benzthiazide see Diuretics (thiazide)
Benztropine see Antimuscarinics
Beta-blockers
    Alcohol: enhanced hypotensive effect
    • Anaesthetics: enhanced hypotensive effect
    Analgesics: *NSAIDs* antagonise hypotensive effect
    • Anti-arrhythmics: increased risk of myocardial depression and bradycardia; with *amiodarone* increased risk of bradycardia and AV block; increased risk of *lignocaine* toxicity with *propranolol*
    Antibacterials: *rifampicin* accelerates metabolism of *bisoprolol* and *propranolol* (reduced plasma concentration)
    Antidepressants: *fluvoxamine* increases plasma concentration of *propranolol*
    Antidiabetics: enhanced hypoglycaemic effect (and masking of warning signs such as tremor)
    • Antihypertensives: enhanced hypotensive effect; increased risk of withdrawal hypertension with *clonidine*; increased risk of first-dose hypotensive effect with *post-synaptic alpha-blockers* such as *prazosin* and *terazosin*
    Antimalarials: increased risk of bradycardia with *mefloquine*
    Antipsychotics: plasma concentration of *chlorpromazine* increased by *propranolol*

Beta-blockers (*continued*)
    Anxiolytics and Hypnotics: enhanced hypotensive effect
    • Calcium-channel Blockers: increased risk of bradycardia and AV block with *diltiazem*; severe hypotension and heart failure occasionally with *nifedipine*; asystole, severe hypotension, and heart failure with *verapamil* (see section 2.3.2)
    Cardiac Glycosides: increased AV block and bradycardia
    Cholinergics: *propranolol* antagonises effect of *neostigmine and pyridostigmine*
    Corticosteroids: antagonism of hypotensive effect
    Diuretics: enhanced hypotensive effect; risk of ventricular arrhythmias associated with *sotalol* increased by hypokalaemia
    Ergotamine: increased peripheral vasoconstriction
    Muscle Relaxants: *propranolol* enhances effect
    Sex Hormones: *oestrogens* and *combined oral contraceptives* antagonise hypotensive effect
    • Sympathomimetics: severe hypertension with *adrenaline* and *noradrenaline* (especially with *non-selective beta-blockers*); severe hypertension also possible with *sympathomimetics in anorectics and cough and cold remedies*
    Theophylline: *beta-blockers* should be avoided on pharmacological grounds (bronchospasm)
    Thyroxine: metabolism of *propranolol* accelerated (reduced effect)
    Ulcer-healing Drugs: plasma concentrations of *labetalol and propranolol* increased by *cimetidine*; hypotensive effect antagonised by *carbenoxolone*
    Xamoterol: antagonism of effect of xamoterol and reduction in beta-blockade
Betahistine
    Antihistamines: antagonism (theoretical)
Betamethasone see Corticosteroids
Betaxolol see Beta-blockers
Bethanechol see Cholinergics
Bethanidine see Adrenergic Neurone Blockers
Bezafibrate see Clofibrate Group
Biperiden see Antimuscarinics
Bisphosphonates
    Antacids: reduced absorption (give at least 2 hours apart)
    Antibacterials: severe hypocalcaemia reported with *aminoglycosides*
    Calcium Salts: reduced absorption (give at least 2 hours apart)
Bismuth Chelate
    Antibacterials: reduced absorption of *tetracyclines*
Bisoprolol see Beta-blockers
Bretylium (see also Adrenergic Neurone Blockers) other Antiarrhythmics: increased myocardial depression with any combination of two or more anti-arrhythmics
Bromazepam see Benzodiazepines and other Anxiolytics and Hypnotics
Bromocriptine
    Alcohol: reduced tolerance to *bromocriptine*
    Antibacterials: *erythromycin* increases plasma concentration
    Antipsychotics: antagonism of hypoprolactinaemic and antiparkinsonian effects
    Domperidone and Metoclopramide: antagonise hypoprolactinaemic effect
Budesonide see Corticosteroids
Bumetanide see Diuretics (loop)
Buprenorphine see Opioid Analgesics
Buspirone (general sedative interactions as for Benzodiazepines and other Anxiolytics and Hypnotics)
    Antidepressants: *MAOIs* contra-indicated by manufacturer

Butobarbitone see Barbiturates
Butriptyline see Antidepressants, Tricyclic
Calcium Salts
   Antibacterials: reduced absorption of *tetracyclines*
   Bisphosphonates: reduce absorption
   Cardiac Glycosides: large intravenous doses of *calcium* can precipitate arrhythmias
   Diuretics: increased risk of hypercalcaemia with *thiazides*

Calcium-channel Blockers
- Anaesthetics: *verapamil* increases hypotensive effect of *general anaesthetics* and risk of AV delay
- Anti-arrhythmics: *amiodarone-induced risk* of bradycardia, AV block, and myocardial depression increased by *diltiazem and verapamil*; with *verapamil* raised plasma concentration of *quinidine* (extreme hypotension may occur)
   Antibacterials: *rifampicin* increases metabolism of *verapamil and possibly isradipine* and *nifedipine* (reduced plasma concentrations)
   Antidepressants: *diltiazem and verapamil* increase plasma concentration of *imipramine and possibly other tricyclics*
   Antidiabetics: *nifedipine* may occasionally impair glucose tolerance
- Antiepileptics: effect of *carbamazepine* enhanced by *diltiazem and verapamil*; *diltiazem* increases plasma concentration of *phenytoin*; effect of *felodipine* and *isradipine* and probably *nicardipine and nifedipine* reduced by *carbamazepine, phenobarbitone, phenytoin,* and *primidone*; effect of *verapamil* reduced by *phenytoin*
   Antihypertensives: enhanced hypotensive effect
   Antimalarials: possible increased risk of bradycardia with some *calcium-channel blockers* and *mefloquine*
   Antipsychotics: enhanced hypotensive effect
   Barbiturates: see under Antiepileptics, above
- Beta-blockers: increased risk of bradycardia and AV block with *diltiazem;* occasionally severe hypotension and heart failure with *nifedipine;* asystole, severe hypotension, and heart failure with *verapamil* (see section 2.3.2)
- Cardiac Glycosides: plasma concentration of *digoxin* increased by *diltiazem, nicardipine,* and *verapamil;* increased AV block and bradycardia with *verapamil*
   Cyclosporin: plasma-cyclosporin concentrations increased by *diltiazem, nicardipine,* and *verapamil;* possibly increases plasma concentration of *nifedipine*
   Lithium: neurotoxicity may occur without increased plasma-lithium concentrations in patients given *diltiazem and verapamil*
   Muscle Relaxants: *nifedipine* and *verapamil* enhance effect of *non-depolarising muscle relaxants such as tubocurarine;* hypotension, myocardial depression, and hyperkalaemia with *verapamil* and intravenous *dantrolene*
   Sympathomimetics: see Sympathomimetics (main list)
- Theophylline: *diltiazem and verapamil* enhance effect
   Ulcer-healing Drugs: *cimetidine* inhibits metabolism of *some calcium-channel blockers* (increased plasma concentrations)

Canrenoate see Diuretics (as for spironolactone)
Capreomycin
   other Antibacterials: increased risk of nephrotoxicity with *colistin and polymyxin;* increased risk of nephrotoxicity and ototoxicity with *aminoglycosides and vancomycin*

Capreomycin (*continued*)
   Cytotoxics: increased risk of nephrotoxicity and ototoxicity with *cisplatin*
Captopril see ACE Inhibitors
Carbachol see Cholinergics
Carbamazepine
- Analgesics: *dextropropoxyphene* enhances effect of *carbamazepine*
- Antibacterials: metabolism of *doxycycline* accelerated (reduced effect); plasma-*carbamazepine* concentration increased by *erythromycin* and *isoniazid*
- Anticoagulants: metabolism of *nicoumalone* and *warfarin* accelerated (reduced anticoagulant effect)
- <u>Antidepressants:</u> antagonism of anticonvulsant effect (convulsive threshold lowered); plasma concentration of *carbamazepine* increased by *fluoxetine, fluvoxamine,* and *viloxazine;* metabolism of *mianserin* and *tricyclics* accelerated (reduced plasma concentrations); manufacturer advises avoid with *MAOIs* or within 2 weeks of *MAOIs*
- *other* Antiepileptics: concomitant administration of two or more antiepileptics may enhance toxicity without a corresponding increase in antiepileptic effect; moreover interactions between individual antiepileptics can complicate monitoring of treatment; interactions include enhanced effects, increased sedation, and reductions in plasma concentrations
- Antipsychotics: antagonism of anticonvulsant effect (convulsive threshold lowered); metabolism of *haloperidol* accelerated (reduced plasma-haloperidol concentration)
- Calcium-channel Blockers: *diltiazem and verapamil* enhance effect of *carbamazepine;* effect of *felodipine, isradipine* and probably *nicardipine* and *nifedipine* reduced
   Cardiac Glycosides: metabolism of *digitoxin only* accelerated (reduced effect)
- Corticosteroids: metabolism accelerated (reduced effect)
- Cyclosporin: metabolism accelerated (reduced plasma-cyclosporin concentration)
- Hormone Antagonists: *danazol* inhibits metabolism of *carbamazepine* (enhanced effect)
   Lithium: neurotoxicity may occur without increased plasma-lithium concentration
- Sex Hormones: *carbamazepine* accelerates metabolism of *oral contraceptives* (reduced contraceptive effect, important: see p. 291) and of *gestrinone* and *tibolone*
   Theophylline: metabolism of *theophylline* accelerated (reduced effect)
   Thyroxine: metabolism accelerated (may increase thyroxine requirements in hypothyroidism)
- Ulcer-healing Drugs: metabolism inhibited by *cimetidine* (increased plasma-carbamazepine concentration)
   <u>Vitamins:</u> *carbamazepine* (possibly increases *vitamin D* requirements)
Carbenicillin see Penicillins
Carbenoxolone
   Note. Do not apply to small amounts used topically on oral mucosa
   Antihypertensives: antagonism of hypotensive effect
   Cardiac Glycosides: toxicity increased if hypokalaemia occurs
   Corticosteroids: increased risk of hypokalaemia

Appendix 1: Interactions 483

Carbenoxolone (*continued*)
Diuretics: antagonism of diuretic effect; increased risk of hypokalaemia with *acetazolamide, thiazides,* and *loop diuretics;* inhibition of ulcer healing with *amiloride* and *spironolactone*

Cardiac Glycosides
Analgesics: *NSAIDs* may exacerbate heart failure, reduce GFR and increase plasma-cardiac glycoside concentrations
Anion-exchange Resins: absorption reduced by *cholestyramine* and *colestipol*
• Anti-arrhythmics: plasma concentration of *digoxin* increased by *amiodarone, propafenone,* and *quinidine* (halve maintenance dose of digoxin)
Antibacterials: *erythromycin* and possibly *azithromycin* enhance effect of *digoxin; rifampicin* accelerates metabolism of *digitoxin only* (reduced effect)
Antiepileptics: metabolism of *digitoxin only* accelerated (reduced effect)
<u>Antihypertensives:</u> *captopril* possibly increases plasma concentration of *digoxin*
• Antimalarials: *quinine* (includes use of quinine for cramp) and possibly *chloroquine* and *hydroxychloroquine* raises plasma concentration of *digoxin* (halve maintenance dose of digoxin); possible increased risk of bradycardia with *mefloquine*
Barbiturates: see under Antiepileptics, above
Beta-blockers: increased AV block and bradycardia
Calcium Salts: large intravenous doses of *calcium* can precipitate arrhythmias
• Calcium-channel Blockers: plasma concentration of *digoxin* increased by *diltiazem, nicardipine,* and *verapamil;* increased AV block and bradycardia with *verapamil*
• Diuretics: increased toxicity if hypokalaemia occurs with *acetazolamide, loop diuretics,* and *thiazides;* effects of *digoxin* enhanced by *spironolactone*
Hormone Antagonists: *aminoglutethimide* accelerates metabolism of *digitoxin only* (reduced effect)
Muscle Relaxants: arrhythmias with *suxamethonium*
Ulcer-healing Drugs: increased toxicity if hypokalaemia occurs with *carbenoxolone;* absorption possibly reduced by *sucralfate*
Carfecillin see Penicillins
Carteolol see Beta-blockers
Celiprolol see Beta-blockers
Cephalosporins
Alcohol: disulfiram-like reaction with *cephamandole*
• Anticoagulants: anticoagulant effect of *warfarin* and *nicoumalone* enhanced by *cephamandole* and possibly others
Probenecid: reduced excretion of *cephalosporins* (increased plasma concentrations)
Cetirizine see Antihistamines
Chloral (general sedative interactions *as for* Benzodiazepines and other Anxiolytics and Hypnotics)
Anticoagulants: may transiently enhance anticoagulant effect of *nicoumalone* and *warfarin*
Chloramphenicol
other Antibacterials: *rifampicin* accelerates metabolism (reduced chloramphenicol-plasma concentration)
• Anticoagulants: anticoagulant effect of *nicoumalone* and *warfarin* enhanced
• Antidiabetics: effect of *sulphonylureas* enhanced

Chloramphenicol (*continued*)
• Antiepileptics: metabolism accelerated by *phenobarbitone* (reduced chloramphenicol-plasma concentration); increased plasma concentration of *phenytoin* (risk of toxicity)
Barbiturates: see under Antiepileptics, above
Chlordiazepoxide see Benzodiazepines
Chlormethiazole (for general sedative interactions *see also* Benzodiazepines and other Anxiolytics and Hypnotics)
Ulcer-healing Drugs: *cimetidine* inhibits metabolism (increased plasma-chlormethiazole concentration)
Chlormezanone see Benzodiazepines and other Anxiolytics and Hypnotics
Chloroquine and Hydroxychloroquine
Antacids: reduced absorption
other Antimalarials: increased risk of convulsions with *mefloquine*
• Cardiac Glycosides: *chloroquine* and *hydroxychloroquine* possibly increases plasma concentration of *digoxin*
Ulcer-healing Drugs: *cimetidine* inhibits metabolism of *chloroquine* (increased plasma concentration)
<u>Vaccines:</u> see Rabies Vaccine p. 452
Chlorothiazide see Diuretics (thiazide)
Chlorpheniramine see Antihistamines
Chlorpromazine see Phenothiazines and other Antipsychotics
Chlorpropamide see Antidiabetics (sulphonylurea)
Chlorprothixene see Phenothiazines and other Antipsychotics
Chlortetracycline see Tetracyclines
Chlorthalidone see Diuretics (thiazide-related)
Cholestyramine and Colestipol
Analgesics: reduced absorption of *paracetamol* and *phenylbutazone*
Antibacterials: antagonism of effect of oral *vancomycin*
• Anticoagulants: anticoagulant effect of *nicoumalone, phenindione,* and *warfarin* may be enhanced or reduced
Cardiac Glycosides: reduced absorption
Diuretics: reduced absorption of *thiazides* (give at least 2 hours apart)
Thyroxine: reduced absorption
Cholinergics
Anti-arrhythmics: *procainamide, quinidine* and possibly *propafenone* antagonise effect of *neostigmine* and *pyridostigmine*
• Antibacterials: *aminoglycosides, clindamycin* and *polymyxins* antagonise effect of *neostigmine* and *pyridostigmine*
Beta-blockers: *propranolol* antagonises effect of *neostigmine* and *pyridostigmine*
Lithium: antagonism of effect of *neostigmine* and *pyridostigmine*
Muscle Relaxants: *demecarium* and *ecothiopate* eye-drops, and *neostigmine* and *pyridostigmine* enhance effect of *suxamethonium,* but antagonise effect of *non-depolarising muscle relaxants* such as *tubocurarine*
Cilazapril see ACE Inhibitors
Cimetidine see Histamine H2-antagonists
Cinnarizine see Antihistamines
Cinoxacin see 4-Quinolones
Ciprofloxacin see 4-Quinolones
Cisapride
Analgesics: *opioid analgesics* possibly antagonise effect on gastro-intestinal motility
Antimuscarinics: antagonism of effect on gastro-intestinal motility

Cisplatin
- Antibacterials: *aminoglycosides and capreomycin* increase risk of nephrotoxicity and possibly of ototoxicity

Clarithromycin *see* Erythromycin
Clemastine *see* Antihistamines

Clindamycin
Cholinergics: antagonism of effect of *neostigmine and pyridostigmine*
Muscle relaxants: enhancement of effect of *non-depolarising muscle relaxants such as tubocurarine*

Clobazam *see* Benzodiazepines and other Anxiolytics and Hypnotics
Clodronate Sodium *see* Bisphosphonates

Clofibrate Group
- Anticoagulants: enhancement of effect of *nicoumalone, phenindione, and warfarin*
Antidiabetics: may improve glucose tolerance and have additive effect
other Lipid-lowering Drugs: increased risk of myopathy with *pravastatin and simvastatin*

Clomipramine *see* Antidepressants, Tricyclic
Clomocycline *see* Tetracyclines

Clonazepam (general sedative interactions *as for* Benzodiazepines and other Anxiolytics and Hypnotics)
other Antiepileptics: metabolism of *clonazepam* accelerated by *carbamazepine, phenobarbitone and phenytoin*

Clonidine (for general hypotensive interactions *see also* Hydralazine)
- Antidepressants: *tricyclics* antagonise hypotensive effect and also increase risk of rebound hypertension on *clonidine* withdrawal
- Beta-blockers: increased risk of hypertension on *clonidine withdrawal*

Clopamide *see* Diuretics (thiazide)
Clorazepate *see* Benzodiazepines and other Anxiolytics and Hypnotics
Cloxacillin *see* Penicillins

Clozapine
Note. Clozapine should not be used concurrently with drugs associated with a substantial potential for causing agranulocytosis, such as co-trimoxazole, chloramphenicol, sulphonamides, penicillamine, or cytotoxics
see also Phenothiazines and other Antipsychotics

Codeine *see* Opioid Analgesics
Cold and Cough Remedies *see* Antihistamines and Sympathomimetics
Colestipol *see* Cholestyramine and Colestipol
Colistin *see* Polymyxins

Contraceptives, Oral
Note. Also covers oestrogens taken alone; in case of hormone replacement therapy low dose unlikely to induce interactions
- Antibacterials: *rifampicin* accelerates metabolism of both *combined and progestogen-only oral contraceptives* (reduced contraceptive effect, important: see p. 291); when broad-spectrum antibiotics such as ampicillin and tetracycline given with *combined oral contraceptives* possibility of reduced contraceptive effect (risk probably small, but see p. 291)
- Anticoagulants: antagonism of anticoagulant effect of *nicoumalone, phenindione, and warfarin*
Antidepressants: antagonism of antidepressant effect has been reported, but side-effects of *tricyclics* may be increased due to higher plasma concentrations
Antidiabetics: antagonism of hypoglycaemic effect
- Antiepileptics: *carbamazepine, phenobarbitone, phenytoin, and primidone* accelerate metabolism (reduced contraceptive effect, important: see p. 291)

Contraceptives, Oral (continued)
- Antifungals: *griseofulvin* accelerates metabolism (reduced contraceptive effect, important: see p. 291)
Antihypertensives: *combined oral contraceptives* antagonise hypotensive effect
Barbiturates: *see under* Antiepileptics, above
Beta-blockers: *oestrogens* and *combined oral contraceptives* antagonise hypotensive effect
- Cyclosporin: increased plasma-cyclosporin concentration
Diuretics: *combined oral contraceptives* antagonise diuretic effect
Theophylline: *combined oral contraceptives* delay excretion (increased plasma-theophylline concentration)

Corticosteroids
Note. Do not generally apply to corticosteroids used for topical action (including inhalation)
- Antibacterials: *rifampicin* accelerates metabolism of *corticosteroids* (reduced effect)
Antidiabetics: antagonism of hypoglycaemic effect
- Antiepileptics: *carbamazepine, phenobarbitone, phenytoin, and primidone* accelerate metabolism of *corticosteroids* (reduced effect)
Antihypertensives: antagonism of hypotensive effect
Barbiturates: *see under* Antiepileptics, above
Diuretics: antagonism of diuretic effect; *acetazolamide, loop diuretics, and thiazides* increase risk of hypokalaemia
Hormone Antagonists: *aminoglutethimide* accelerates metabolism of *dexamethasone* (reduced effect)
Sympathomimetics *see* Sympathomimetics, Beta$_2$ (main list)
Ulcer-healing Drugs: *carbenoxolone* increases risk of hypokalaemia

Co-trimoxazole and Sulphonamides
Anaesthetics: effect of *thiopentone* enhanced
- Anticoagulants: effect of *nicoumalone and warfarin* enhanced
- Antidiabetics: effect of *sulphonylureas* enhanced
- Antiepileptics: antifolate effect and plasma concentration of *phenytoin* increased by *co-trimoxazole*
Antimalarials: increased risk of antifolate effect with *pyrimethamine* (includes *Fansidar®* and *Maloprim®*)
Cyclosporin: increased risk of nephrotoxicity
Cytotoxics: antifolate effect of *methotrexate* increased by *co-trimoxazole*

Cyclizine *see* Antihistamines
Cyclobarbitone *see* Barbiturates
Cyclopenthiazide *see* Diuretics (thiazide)
Cyclopentolate *see* Antimuscarinics

Cyclophosphamide
- Allopurinol: toxicity of *cyclophosphamide* increased
Muscle Relaxants: *cyclophosphamide* enhances effect of *suxamethonium*

Cycloserine
other Antibacterials: increased CNS toxicity with *isoniazid*
- Antiepileptics: increased plasma concentration of *phenytoin* (risk of toxicity)

Cyclosporin
- Analgesics: increased risk of nephrotoxicity with *NSAIDs*
Anti-arrhythmics: *amiodarone* possibly increases plasma-cyclosporin concentration

Cyclosporin (continued)

- Antibacterials: *aminoglycosides, co-trimoxazole,* and *4-quinolones* increase risk of nephrotoxicity; *erythromycin* increases plasma-cyclosporin concentration; *rifampicin* reduces plasma-cyclosporin concentration
- Antiepileptics: *carbamazepine, phenobarbitone, phenytoin,* and *primidone* accelerate metabolism (reduced plasma-cyclosporin concentration)
- Antifungals: *amphotericin* increases risk of nephrotoxicity; *griseofulvin* possibly reduces plasma-cyclosporin concentration; *itraconazole, ketoconazole* and possibly *fluconazole* inhibit metabolism (increased plasma-cyclosporin concentration)

Antihypertensives: increased risk of hyperkalaemia with *ACE inhibitors*

Barbiturates: *see under* Antiepileptics, above

- Calcium-channel Blockers: *diltiazem, nicardipine,* and *verapamil* increase plasma-cyclosporin concentration; *cyclosporin* possibly increases plasma concentration of *nifedipine*
- Cytotoxics: increased toxicity with *methotrexate*
- Diuretics: *potassium-sparing diuretics* increase risk of hyperkalaemia
- Hormone Antagonists: *danazol* inhibits metabolism (increased plasma-cyclosporin concentration); *octreotide* reduces absorption (reduced plasma-cyclosporin concentration)

Lipid-lowering Drugs: increased risk of myopathy with *pravastatin and simvastatin*

- Potassium Salts: increased risk of hyperkalaemia
- Sex Hormones: *progestogens* inhibit metabolism (increased plasma-cyclosporin concentration)

Cyproheptadine *see* Antihistamines
Cytotoxics *see under* individual drugs
Dalteparin *see* Heparin
Danazol

- Anticoagulants: effect of *nicoumalone and warfarin* enhanced (inhibits metabolism)
- Antiepileptics: inhibits metabolism of *carbamazepine* (increased plasma-carbamazepine concentration)
- Cyclosporin: inhibits metabolism (increased plasma-cyclosporin concentration)

Dantrolene *see* Muscle Relaxants
Dapsone

Antibacterials: plasma concentration reduced by *rifampicin*

Probenecid: *dapsone* excretion reduced (increased risk of side-effects)

Debrisoquine *see* Adrenergic Neurone Blockers
Demecarium *see* Cholinergics
Demeclocycline *see* Tetracyclines
Desferrioxamine

Antipsychotics: manufacturer advises avoid *prochlorperazine*

Desipramine *see* Antidepressants, Tricyclic
Dexamethasone *see* Corticosteroids
Dexamphetamine *see* Sympathomimetics
Dexfenfluramine *see* Sympathomimetics
Dextromoramide *see* Opioid Analgesics
Dextropropoxyphene *see* Opioid Analgesics
Diamorphine *see* Opioid Analgesics
Diazepam *see* Benzodiazepines and other Anxiolytics and Hypnotics
Diazoxide (general hypotensive interactions *as for* Hydralazine)

Antidiabetics: antagonism of hypoglycaemic effect

Dichlorphenamide *see* Acetazolamide
Diclofenac *see* NSAIDs
Dicyclomine *see* Antimuscarinics
Diethylpropion *see* Sympathomimetics
Diflunisal *see* NSAIDs
Digitoxin *see* Cardiac Glycosides
Digoxin *see* Cardiac Glycosides
Dihydrocodeine *see* Opioid Analgesics
Dihydroergotamine *see* Ergotamine
Diltiazem *see* Calcium-channel Blockers
Dimenhydrinate *see* Antihistamines
Dimethindene *see* Antihistamines
Diphenhydramine *see* Antihistamines
Diphenylpyraline *see* Antihistamines
Diphenoxylate *see* Opioid Analgesics
Dipipanone *see* Opioid Analgesics
Dipivefrine *see* Sympathomimetics (*as for* adrenaline)
Dipyridamole

Antacids: patient information leaflet advises avoidance of *antacids*

- Anti-arrhythmics: effect of *adenosine* enhanced (risk of toxicity)
- Anticoagulants: enhanced effect due to antiplatelet action of *dipyridamole*

Disodium Etidronate *see* Bisphosphonates
Disodium Pamidronate *see* Bisphosphonates
Disopyramide

- *other* Anti-arrhythmics: *amiodarone* increases risk of ventricular arrhythmias; increased myocardial depression with any *anti-arrhythmic*
- Antibacterials: plasma concentration of *disopyramide* reduced by *rifampicin* but increased by *erythromycin* (risk of toxicity)

Antiepileptics: plasma concentration of *disopyramide* reduced by *phenobarbitone, phenytoin, and primidone*

Antimuscarinics: increased antimuscarinic side-effects

Barbiturates: *see under* Antiepileptics, above

- Diuretics: toxicity of *disopyramide* increased if hypokalaemia occurs with *acetazolamide, loop diuretics, and thiazides*

Nitrates: reduced effect of *sublingual nitrates* (failure to dissolve under tongue owing to dry mouth)

Distigmine *see* Cholinergics
Disulfiram

Alcohol: disulfiram reaction (*see* section 4.10)

Antibacterials: psychotic reaction with *metronidazole* reported

- Anticoagulants: effect of *nicoumalone and warfarin* enhanced

Antidepressants: inhibition of metabolism of *tricyclic antidepressants* (increased plasma concentrations); increased disulfiram reaction with alcohol reported if *amitriptyline* also taken

- Antiepileptics: inhibition of metabolism of *phenytoin* (increased risk of toxicity)

Anxiolytics and Hypnotics: inhibition of metabolism of *chlordiazepoxide and diazepam* (enhanced sedative effect)

Theophylline: inhibition of metabolism (increased risk of toxicity)

Diuretics

Analgesics: *diuretics* increase risk of nephrotoxicity of *NSAIDs*; *NSAIDs* notably *indomethacin* antagonise diuretic effect; *indomethacin and possibly other NSAIDs* increase risk of hyperkalaemia with *potassium-sparing diuretics*; diuretic effect of *spironolactone* antagonised by *aspirin*; *aspirin* reduces excretion of *acetazolamide* (risk of toxicity)

Anion-exchange Resins: *cholestyramine and colestipol* reduce absorption of *thiazides* (give at least 2 hours apart)

Diuretics (*continued*)
- Anti-arrhythmics: toxicity of *amiodarone, disopyramide, flecainide,* and *quinidine* increased if hypokalaemia occurs; action of *lignocaine, mexiletine,* and *tocainide* antagonised by hypokalaemia; *acetazolamide* reduces excretion of *quinidine* (increased plasma concentration)

  Antibacterials: *loop diuretics* increase ototoxicity of *aminoglycosides, polymyxins, and vancomycin*

  Antidepressants: increased risk of postural hypotension with *tricyclics*

  Antidiabetics: hypoglycaemic effect antagonised by *loop* and *thiazide diuretics; chlorpropamide* increases risk of hyponatraemia associated with *thiazides in combination with potassium-sparing diuretics*

- Antihypertensives: enhanced hypotensive effect; enhancement of effect of *ACE inhibitors* (risk of extreme hypotension, also risk of hyperkalaemia with *potassium-sparing diuretics);* increased risk of first-dose hypotensive effect of post-synaptic *alpha-blockers* such as *prazosin* and *terazosin;* increased risk of hypokalaemia with *indapamide*

  Antipsychotics: in hypokalaemia increased risk of ventricular arrhythmias with *pimozide*

  Beta-blockers: in hypokalaemia increased risk of ventricular arrhythmias with *sotalol*

  Calcium Salts: risk of hypercalcaemia with *thiazides*

- Cardiac Glycosides: increased toxicity if hypokalaemia occurs with *acetazolamide, loop diuretics, and thiazides;* effect enhanced by *spironolactone*

  Corticosteroids: increased risk of hypokalaemia with *acetazolamide, loop diuretics, and thiazides;* antagonism of diuretic effect

- Cyclosporin: increased risk of hyperkalaemia with *potassium-sparing* diuretics

  other Diuretics: increased risk of hypokalaemia if *acetazolamide, loop diuretics or thiazides* given together; profound diuresis possible if *metolazone* given with *frusemide* (section 2.2.1)

  Hormone Antagonists: *trilostane* increases risk of hyperkalaemia with *potassium-sparing diuretics*

- Lithium: lithium excretion reduced by *loop diuretics* and *thiazides* (increased plasma-lithium concentration and risk of toxicity—*loop diuretics* safer than *thiazides);* lithium excretion increased by *acetazolamide*

- Potassium Salts: hyperkalaemia with *potassium-sparing diuretics*

  Sex Hormones: *oestrogens* and *combined oral contraceptives* antagonise diuretic effect

  Ulcer-healing Drugs: increased risk of hypokalaemia if *acetazolamide, loop diuretics,* and *thiazides* given with *carbenoxolone; carbenoxolone* antagonises diuretic effect; *amiloride* and *spironolactone* antagonise ulcer-healing effect of *carbenoxolone*

Domperidone
Analgesics: *opioid analgesics* antagonise effect on gastro-intestinal activity

Antimuscarinics: antagonism of effect on gastro-intestinal activity

Dopaminergics: antagonism of hypoprolactinaemic effect of *bromocriptine*

Dopamine *see* Sympathomimetics
Dopaminergics *see* Amantadine, Bromocriptine, Levodopa, and Lysuride
Dopexamine *see* Sympathomimetics
Dothiepin *see* Antidepressants, Tricyclic
Doxapram
Sympathomimetics: risk of hypertension
Theophylline: increased CNS stimulation

Doxazosin *see* Alpha-blockers (post-synaptic)
Doxepin *see* Antidepressants, Tricyclic
Doxycycline *see* Tetracyclines
Droperidol *see* Phenothiazines and other Antipsychotics
Ecothiopate *see* Cholinergics
Edrophonium *see* Cholinergics
Enalapril *see* ACE Inhibitors
Enoxacin *see* 4-Quinolines
Enoxaparin *see* Heparin
Ephedrine *see* Sympathomimetics
Ergotamine
Antibacterials: ergotism with *erythromycin* and possibly *azithromycin*

Beta-blockers: increased peripheral vasoconstriction
- Sumatriptan: increased risk of vasospasm

Erythromycin
Analgesics: plasma concentration of *alfentanil* increased

- Anti-arrhythmics: plasma concentration of *disopyramide* increased (risk of toxicity)
- Anticoagulants: effect of *nicoumalone* and *warfarin* enhanced
- Antiepileptics: inhibition of metabolism of *carbamazepine* (increased plasma-carbamazepine concentration)
- Antihistamines: inhibition of metabolism of *terfenadine* (see p. 127)

  Anxiolytics and Hypnotics: inhibition of metabolism of *midazolam* (increased plasma concentration, see also p. 465)

  Cardiac Glycosides: effect of *digoxin* enhanced
- Cyclosporin: inhibition of metabolism (increased plasma-cyclosporin concentration)

  Dopaminergics: plasma concentration of *bromocriptine* increased

  Ergotamine: ergotism reported
- Theophylline: inhibition of metabolism (increased plasma-theophylline concentration)

Ethacrynic Acid *see* Diuretics (loop)
Ethosuximide
- Antibacterials: *isoniazid* increases plasma concentrations (increased risk of toxicity)
- Antidepressants: antagonism (convulsive threshold lowered)
- *other* Antiepileptics: concomitant administration of two or more antiepileptics may enhance toxicity without a corresponding increase in antiepileptic effect; moreover interactions between individual antiepileptics can complicate monitoring of treatment; interactions include enhanced effects, increased sedation, and reductions in plasma concentrations
- Antipsychotics: antagonism (convulsive threshold lowered)

Etidronate Disodium *see* Bisphosphonates
Etodolac *see* NSAIDs
Etretinate
Cytotoxics: increased plasma concentration of *methotrexate*

Famotidine *see* Histamine H2-antagonists
Fansidar® *contains* Sulfadoxine and Pyrimethamine
Felodipine *see* Calcium-channel Blockers
Fenbufen *see* NSAIDs
Fenfluramine *see* Sympathomimetics
Fenofibrate *see* Clofibrate Group
Fenoprofen *see* NSAIDs
Fenoterol *see* Sympathomimetics, Beta$_2$
Fentanyl *see* Opioid Analgesics
Ferrous Salts *see* Iron
Flavoxate *see* Antimuscarinics

Flecainide
- *other* Anti-arrhythmics: *amiodarone* increases plasma-flecainide concentration (and increases risk of ventricular arrhythmias); increased myocardial depression with any *anti-arrhythmic*
- Diuretics: toxicity increased if hypokalaemia occurs; interaction with *acetazolamide* no longer considered significant

Ulcer-healing Drugs: *cimetidine* inhibits metabolism of *flecainide* (increased plasma-flecainide concentration)

Flucloxacillin *see* Penicillins

Fluconazole
Antibacterials: *rifampicin* reduces plasma concentration
- Anticoagulants: effect of *nicoumalone and warfarin* enhanced
Antidiabetics: plasma concentrations of *sulphonylureas* possibly increased
- Antiepileptics: effect of *phenytoin* enhanced
Cyclosporin: possible inhibition of metabolism and increased plasma-cyclosporin concentration
Theophylline: plasma-theophylline concentration possibly increased

Fludrocortisone *see* Corticosteroids
Flunitrazepam *see* Benzodiazepines and other Anxiolytics and Hypnotics

Fluorouracil
Ulcer-healing Drugs: *cimetidine* inhibits metabolism (increased plasma-fluorouracil concentration)

Fluoxetine *see* Antidepressants, Serotonin-uptake Inhibitor
Flupenthixol *see* Phenothiazines and other Antipsychotics
Fluphenazine *see* Phenothiazines and other Antipsychotics
Flurazepam *see* Benzodiazepines and other Anxiolytics and Hypnotics
Flurbiprofen *see* NSAIDs
Fluspirilene *see* Phenothiazines and other Antipsychotics

Flutamide
- Anticoagulants: effect of *warfarin* enhanced

Fluvoxamine *see* Antidepressants, Serotonin-uptake Inhibitor
Folic Acid *see* Vitamins
Fosinopril *see* ACE Inhibitors
Framycetin *see* Aminoglycosides
Frusemide *see* Diuretics (loop)
Gallamine *see* Muscle Relaxants (non-depolarising)

Ganciclovir
Note: increased risk of myelosuppression with other *myelosuppressive drugs*
other Antivirals: profound myelosuppression with *zidovudine*

Gemfibrozil *see* Clofibrate Group
Gentamicin *see* Aminoglycosides

Gestrinone
Antibacterials: *rifampicin* accelerates metabolism (reduced plasma concentration)
Antiepileptics: *carbamazepine, phenobarbitone, phenytoin,* and *primidone* accelerate metabolism (reduced plasma concentration)

Glibenclamide *see* Antidiabetics (sulphonylurea)
Gliclazide *see* Antidiabetics (sulphonylurea)
Glipizide *see* Antidiabetics (sulphonylurea)
Gliquidone *see* Antidiabetics (sulphonylurea)

Glyceryl Trinitrate (general hypotensive interactions as for Hydralazine)
Anti-arrhythmics: *disopyramide* may reduce effect of *sublingual nitrates* (owing to dry mouth)

Glyceryl Trinitrate (continued)
Antidepressants: *tricyclics* may reduce effect of *sublingual nitrates* (owing to dry mouth)
Antimuscarinics: *antimuscarinics such as atropine and propantheline* may reduce effect of *sublingual nitrates* (owing to dry mouth)

Griseofulvin
- Anticoagulants: metabolism of *nicoumalone and warfarin* accelerated (reduced anticoagulant effect)
Antiepileptics: metabolism accelerated by *phenobarbitone* (reduced effect)
Cyclosporin: plasma-cyclosporin concentration possibly reduced
- Sex Hormones: metabolism of *oral contraceptives* accelerated (reduced contraceptive effect, important: see p. 291)

Guanethidine *see* Adrenergic Neurone Blockers

Guar Gum
Antibacterials: absorption of *phenoxymethylpenicillin* reduced

Haloperidol *see* Phenothiazines and other Antipsychotics
Halothane *see* Anaesthetics (volatile)

Heparin
Analgesics: *aspirin* enhances anticoagulant effect
Antiplatelet Drugs: *aspirin and dipyridamole* enhance anticoagulant effect

Hexamine
Potassium Citrate: urine should be acid

Histamine H1-antagonists *see* Antihistamines

Histamine H2-antagonists
Analgesics: *cimetidine* inhibits metabolism of *opioid analgesics* notably *pethidine* (increased plasma concentrations)
- Anti-arrhythmics: *cimetidine* increases plasma concentrations of *amiodarone, flecainide, lignocaine, procainamide, propafenone, and quinidine*
Antibacterials: *rifampicin* accelerates metabolism of *cimetidine* (reduced plasma-cimetidine concentration); *cimetidine* inhibits metabolism of *metronidazole* (increased plasma-metronidazole concentration)
- Anticoagulants: *cimetidine* enhances anticoagulant effect of *nicoumalone and warfarin* (inhibits metabolism)
Antidepressants: *cimetidine* inhibits metabolism of *amitriptyline, desipramine, doxepin, imipramine, and nortriptyline* (increased plasma concentrations)
Antidiabetics: *cimetidine* inhibits renal excretion of *metformin* (increased plasma concentration)
- Antiepileptics: *cimetidine* inhibits metabolism of *carbamazepine and phenytoin* (increased plasma concentrations)
Antifungals: absorption of *itraconazole and ketoconazole* reduced; plasma concentration of *terbinafine* increased by *cimetidine*
Antimalarials: *cimetidine* inhibits metabolism of *chloroquine and quinine* (increased plasma concentrations)
Antipsychotics: *cimetidine* may enhance effect of *chlorpromazine, clozapine, and possibly other antipsychotics*
Anxiolytics and Hypnotics: *cimetidine* inhibits metabolism of *benzodiazepines and chlormethiazole* (increased plasma concentrations)
Beta-blockers: *cimetidine* inhibits metabolism of *beta-blockers such as labetalol and propranolol* (increased plasma concentrations)
Calcium-channel Blockers: *cimetidine* inhibits metabolism of *some calcium-channel blockers* (increased plasma concentrations)

Histamine H2-antagonists (*continued*)
Cytotoxics: *cimetidine* increases plasma concentration of *fluorouracil*
• Theophylline: *cimetidine* inhibits metabolism (increased plasma-theophylline concentration)

Homatropine *see* Antimuscarinics

Hydralazine
Alcohol: enhanced hypotensive effect
• Anaesthetics: enhanced hypotensive effect
Analgesics: *NSAIDs* antagonise hypotensive effect
Antidepressants: enhanced hypotensive effect
other Antihypertensives: additive hypotensive effect
Antipsychotics: enhanced hypotensive effect
Anxiolytics and Hypnotics: enhanced hypotensive effect
Beta-blockers: enhanced hypotensive effect
Calcium-channel Blockers: enhanced hypotensive effect
Corticosteroids: antagonism of hypotensive effect
Diuretics: enhanced hypotensive effect
Dopaminergics: *levodopa* enhances hypotensive effect
Muscle Relaxants: *baclofen* enhances hypotensive effect
Nitrates: enhance hypotensive effect
Sex Hormones: *oestrogens and combined oral contraceptives* antagonise hypotensive effect
Ulcer-healing Drugs: *carbenoxolone* antagonises hypotensive effect

Hydrochlorothiazide *see* Diuretics (thiazide)
Hydrocortisone *see* Corticosteroids
Hydroflumethiazide *see* Diuretics (thiazide)
Hydroxychloroquine *see* Chloroquine and Hydroxychloroquine
Hydroxyzine *see* Antihistamines
Hyoscine *see* Antimuscarinics
Hypnotics *see* Benzodiazepines and other Anxiolytics and Hypnotics
Ibuprofen *see* NSAIDs

Ifosfamide
• Anticoagulants: effect of *warfarin* possibly enhanced

Imipramine *see* Antidepressants, Tricyclic
Indapamide *see* Diuretics (thiazide-related)
Indomethacin *see* NSAIDs
Indoramin *see* Alpha-blockers

Influenza Vaccine
Anticoagulants: effect of *warfarin* occasionally enhanced
Antiepileptics: effect of *phenytoin* enhanced
Theophylline: effect occasionally enhanced

Insulin *see* Antidiabetics

Interferons
Theophylline: metabolism of *theophylline* inhibited (enhanced effect)

Iprindole *see* Antidepressants, Tricyclic

Iron
Antacids: *magnesium trisilicate* reduces absorption of *oral iron*
Antibacterials: *tetracyclines* reduce absorption of *oral iron* (and *vice versa*); absorption of *ciprofloxacin, norfloxacin,* and *ofloxacin* reduced by *oral iron*
Dopaminergics: absorption of *levodopa* may be reduced
Penicillamine: reduced absorption of *penicillamine*
Trientine: reduced absorption of *oral iron*
Zinc: reduced absorption of *oral iron* (and *vice versa*)

Isocarboxazid *see* MAOIs
Isometheptene *see* Sympathomimetics

Isoniazid
Antacids and Adsorbents: *antacids* reduce absorption
other Antibacterials: increased CNS toxicity with *cycloserine*
• Antiepileptics: metabolism of *carbamazepine, ethosuximide, and phenytoin* inhibited (enhanced effect)
Anxiolytics and Hypnotics: metabolism of *diazepam* inhibited
Theophylline: *isoniazid* possibly increases plasma-theophylline concentration

Isoprenaline *see* Sympathomimetics
Isosorbide Dinitrate *see* Glyceryl Trinitrate
Isosorbide Mononitrate *see* Glyceryl Trinitrate
Isradipine *see* Calcium-channel Blockers

Itraconazole
Antacids and Adsorbents: *antacids* reduce absorption
Antibacterials: metabolism accelerated by *rifampicin* (reduced plasma-itraconazole concentration)
• Anticoagulants: effect of *warfarin* enhanced
• Cyclosporin: metabolism inhibited (increased plasma-cyclosporin concentration)
Ulcer-healing Drugs: *histamine H2-antagonists* reduce absorption

Kanamycin *see* Aminoglycosides
Kaolin *see* Antacids and Adsorbents

Ketoconazole
Antacids and Adsorbents: *antacids* reduce absorption
Antibacterials: metabolism accelerated by *rifampicin* (reduced plasma-ketoconazole concentration)
• Anticoagulants: effect of *nicoumalone and warfarin* enhanced
• Antiepileptics: plasma-ketoconazole concentration reduced by *phenytoin* and effect of *phenytoin* enhanced
• Antihistamines: *terfenadine* metabolism inhibited (risk of cardiac toxicity)
Antimuscarinics: reduced absorption
• Cyclosporin: metabolism inhibited (increased plasma-cyclosporin concentration)
Ulcer-healing Drugs: *histamine H2-antagonists* reduce absorption

Ketoprofen *see* NSAIDs
Ketorolac *see* NSAIDs
Ketotifen *see* Antihistamines
Labetalol *see* Beta-blockers

Lamotrigine
• *other* Antiepileptics: concomitant administration of *two or more antiepileptics* may enhance toxicity without a corresponding increase in antiepileptic effect; moreover interactions between individual antiepileptics can complicate monitoring of treatment; interactions include enhanced effects, increased sedation, and reductions in plasma concentrations

Lanatoside C *see* Cardiac Glycosides

Levodopa
• Anaesthetics: risk of arrhythmias with *volatile anaesthetics such as halothane*
• Antidepressants: hypertensive crisis with *MAOIs*
Antihypertensives: enhanced hypotensive effect
Antipsychotics: antagonism of effect
Anxiolytics and Hypnotics: occasional antagonism of effect by *chlordiazepoxide, diazepam, lorazepam and possibly other benzodiazepines*

Levodopa (*continued*)
　Domperidone and Metoclopramide: levodopa-plasma concentrations increased by *metoclopramide*
　Iron: absorption of *levodopa* may be reduced
　Vitamins: effect of *levodopa* antagonised by *pyridoxine* unless a *dopa decarboxylase inhibitor* also given
Lignocaine
　other Anti-arrhythmics: increased myocardial depression
　Beta-blockers: increased risk of myocardial depression; increased risk of *lignocaine* toxicity with *propranolol*
　Diuretics: effect of *lignocaine* antagonised by hypokalaemia with *acetazolamide, loop diuretics, and thiazides*
　Ulcer-healing Drugs: *cimetidine* inhibits metabolism of *lignocaine* (increased risk of toxicity)
Lisinopril *see* ACE Inhibitors
Lithium
● Analgesics: *NSAIDs* reduce excretion of *lithium* (possibility of toxicity)
　Antacids and Adsorbents: *sodium bicarbonate* increases excretion of *lithium* (reduced plasma-lithium concentrations)
　Antibacterials: *lithium* toxicity reported with *metronidazole* and *spectinomycin*
● Antidepressants: *fluoxetine, fluvoxamine, paroxetine, and sertraline* increase risk of CNS toxicity
　Antidiabetics: *lithium* may occasionally impair glucose tolerance
　Antiepileptics: neurotoxicity may occur with *carbamazepine and phenytoin* without increased plasma-lithium concentration
● Antihypertensives: *ACE inhibitors* reduce excretion of *lithium* (increased plasma-lithium concentration); neurotoxicity may occur with *methyldopa* without increased plasma-lithium concentration
　Antipsychotics: increased risk of extrapyramidal effects and possibility of neurotoxicity (notably with *haloperidol*)
　Calcium-channel Blockers: neurotoxicity may occur with *diltiazem and verapamil* without increased plasma-lithium concentration
　Cholinergics: *lithium* antagonises effect of *neostigmine and pyridostigmine*
● Diuretics: *lithium* excretion reduced by *loop diuretics and thiazides* (increased plasma-lithium concentration and risk of toxicity—*loop diuretics* safer than *thiazides)*; *lithium* excretion increased by *acetazolamide*
　Domperidone and Metoclopramide: increased risk of extrapyramidal effects and possibility of neurotoxicity with *metoclopramide*
　Muscle Relaxants: muscle relaxant effect enhanced
● Sumatriptan: risk of CNS toxicity
　Theophylline: *lithium* excretion increased (reduced plasma-lithium concentration)
Lofepramine *see* Antidepressants, Tricyclic
Loprazolam *see* Benzodiazepines and other Anxiolytics and Hypnotics
Loratadine *see* Antihistamines
Lorazepam *see* Benzodiazepines and other Anxiolytics and Hypnotics
Lormetazepam *see* Benzodiazepines and other Anxiolytics and Hypnotics
Loxapine *see* Phenothiazines and other Antipsychotics
Lymecycline *see* Tetracyclines

Lysuride
　Antipsychotics: antagonism of effect
Magnesium Salts (*see also* Antacids and Adsorbents)
　Muscle Relaxants: effect of *non-depolarising muscle relaxants such as tubocurarine* enhanced by *parenteral magnesium salts*
Magnesium Trisilicate *see* Antacids and Adsorbents
Maloprim® *contains* Dapsone and Pyrimethamine
MAOIs
● Alcohol: some *alcoholic and dealcoholised beverages contain tyramine* which interacts with *MAOIs* (hypertensive crisis); foods, *see* MAOI card, section 4.3.2
● Analgesics: CNS excitation or depression (hypertension or hypotension) with *pethidine and possibly other opioid analgesics;* manufacturer advises avoid *nefopam*
　Anorectics: *see* Sympathomimetics, below
● *other* Antidepressants: enhancement of CNS effects and toxicity with *other MAOIs* (avoid for at least a week after stopping *previous MAOIs* then start with reduced dose); CNS excitation and hypertension with most *tricyclics and related antidepressants* (avoid for at least 2 weeeks after stopping MAOIs); enhancement of CNS effects and toxicity possible with *serotonin-uptake inhibitors* (avoid *MAOIs* for at least 2 weeks before *serotonin-uptake inhibitors* and avoid *fluoxetine* for at least 5 weeks and *sertraline* for 7 days before *MAOIs*); CNS excitation and confusion with *tryptophan* (reduce tryptophan dose)
　Antidiabetics: effect of *insulin, metformin, and sulphonylureas* enhanced
● Antiepileptics: antagonism of anticonvulsant effect (convulsive threshold lowered); manufacturer advises avoid *carbamazepine* with or within 2 weeks of *MAOIs*
● Antihypertensives: hypotensive effect enhanced
　Antimuscarinics: increased side-effects
● Antipsychotics: CNS excitation and hypertension with *oxypertine*
　Anxiolytics and Hypnotics: manufacturer advises avoidance of *buspirone*
● Dopaminergics: hypertensive crisis with *levodopa*
● Sumatriptan: risk of CNS toxicity
● Sympathomimetics: hypertensive crisis with *sympathomimetics such as dexamphetamine and other amphetamines, dexfenfluramine, diethylpropion, dopamine, dopexamine, ephedrine, fenfluramine, isometheptene, mazindol, pemoline, phentermine, phenylephrine, phenylpropanolamine, and pseudoephedrine*
● Tetrabenazine: CNS excitation and hypertension
Maprotiline *see* Antidepressants, Tricyclic
Mazindol *see* Sympathomimetics
Mebhydrolin *see* Antihistamines
Medazepam *see* Benzodiazepines and other Anxiolytics and Hypnotics
Mefenamic Acid *see* NSAIDs
Mefloquine
　other Antimalarials: increased risk of convulsions with *chloroquine* and *quinine*, but should not prevent use of intravenous quinine in severe cases; for full precautions see footnote on p. 240 (also applies to *quinidine*)
　Cardioactive drugs: possible increased risk of bradycardia with *beta-blockers*, *digoxin*, and *some calcium-channel blockers*
　Vaccines: *see* Typhoid Vaccine, p. 453
Mefruside *see* Diuretics (thiazide)
Mepacrine
　other Antimalarials: increased plasma concentration of *primaquine* (risk of toxicity)

Mepenzolate see Antimuscarinics
Meprobamate see Benzodiazepines and other Anxiolytics and Hypnotics
Meptazinol see Opioid Analgesics
Mequitazine see Antihistamines
Mercaptopurine
- Allopurinol: enhancement of effect (increased toxicity)

Metaraminol see Sympathomimetics (*as* noradrenaline)
Metformin see Antidiabetics
Methadone see Opioid Analgesics
Methixene see Antimuscarinics
Methocarbamol see Muscle Relaxants
Methotrexate
- Analgesics: excretion reduced by *aspirin, azapropazone, diclofenac, indomethacin, ketoprofen, naproxen, phenylbutazone, and probably other NSAIDs* (increased risk of toxicity)

  Antibacterials: antifolate effect increased by *co-trimoxazole and trimethoprim*

  Antiepileptics: *phenytoin* increases antifolate effect

  Antimalarials: antifolate effect increased by *pyrimethamine* (ingredient of *Fansidar*® and *Maloprim*®)
- Cyclosporin: increased toxicity

  Etretinate: increased plasma concentration of *methotrexate*
- Uricosurics: excretion reduced by *probenecid* (increased risk of toxicity)

Methotrimeprazine see Phenothiazines and other Antipsychotics
Methoxamine see Sympathomimetics (*as* noradrenaline)
Methyclothiazide see Diuretics (thiazide)
Methyldopa
Alcohol: enhanced hypotensive effect
- Anaesthetics: enhanced hypotensive effect

  Analgesics: *NSAIDs* antagonise hypotensive effect

  Antidepressants: enhanced hypotensive effect

  other Antihypertensives: enhanced hypotensive effect

  Antipsychotics: increased risk of extrapyramidal effects; enhanced hypotensive effect

  Anxiolytics and Hypnotics: enhanced hypotensive effect

  Beta-blockers: enhanced hypotensive effect

  Calcium-channel Blockers: enhanced hypotensive effect

  Corticosteroids: antagonism of hypotensive effect

  Diuretics: enhanced hypotensive effect

  Dopaminergics: antagonism of antiparkinsonian effect; *levodopa* enhances hypotensive effect

  Lithium: neurotoxicity may occur without increased plasma-lithium concentration

  Nitrates: enhance hypotensive effect

  Sex Hormones: *oestrogens and combined oral contraceptives* antagonise hypotensive effect

  Sympathomimetics: *see* Sympathomimetics (main list)

  Ulcer-healing Drugs: *carbenoxolone* antagonises hypotensive effect

Methylphenobarbitone see Barbiturates
Methylprednisolone see Corticosteroids
Metipranolol see Beta-blockers
Metirosine
Antipsychotics: increased risk of extrapyramidal effects
Dopaminergics: antagonism
Metoclopramide
Analgesics: increased absorption of *aspirin and paracetamol* (enhanced effect); *opioid analgesics* antagonise effect on gastro-intestinal activity

Metoclopramide (*continued*)
Antimuscarinics: antagonism of effect on gastro-intestinal activity
Antipsychotics: increased risk of extrapyramidal effects
Dopaminergics: antagonism of hypoprolactinaemic effect of *bromocriptine*; increased plasma concentration of *levodopa*
Lithium: increased risk of extrapyramidal effects and possibility of neurotoxicity
Tetrabenazine: increased risk of extrapyramidal effects
Metolazone see Diuretics (thiazide-related)
Metoprolol see Beta-blockers
Metronidazole
Alcohol: disulfiram-like reaction
- Anticoagulants: effect of *nicoumalone and warfarin* enhanced
- Antiepileptics: *metronidazole* inhibits metabolism of *phenytoin* (increased plasma-phenytoin concentration); *phenobarbitone* accelerates metabolism of *metronidazole* (reduced plasma-metronidazole concentration)

  Disulfiram: psychotic reactions reported
  Lithium: increased toxicity reported
  Ulcer-healing Drugs: *cimetidine* inhibits metabolism (increased plasma-metronidazole concentration)
Mexiletine
Analgesics: *opioid analgesics* delay absorption
- *other* Anti-arrhythmics: increased myocardial depression with any combination of *anti-arrhythmics*

  Antibacterials: *rifampicin* accelerates metabolism (reduced plasma-mexiletine concentration)
  Anti-epileptics: *phenytoin* accelerates metabolism (reduced plasma-mexiletine concentration)
  Antimuscarinics: *atropine* delays absorption
  Diuretics: action of *mexiletine* antagonised by hypokalaemia due to *acetazolamide, loop diuretics, and thiazides;* interaction with *acetazolamide* no longer considered significant
  Theophylline: plasma-theophylline concentration increased
Mianserin
Alcohol: enhanced effect
Antiepileptics: antagonism (convulsive threshold lowered); reduced antidepressant effect (reduced plasma-mianserin concentration)
Anxiolytics and Hypnotics: enhanced effect
Miconazole
- Anticoagulants: effect of *nicoumalone and warfarin* enhanced
- Antidiabetics: effect of *sulphonylureas* enhanced
- Antiepileptics: effect of *phenytoin* enhanced

  other Antifungals: *amphotericin* antagonises effect
Mifepristone
Analgesics: manufacturer recommends avoid *aspirin* and *NSAIDs* until 8–12 days after *mifepristone* administration
Minocycline see Tetracyclines
Minoxidil see Hydralazine for general hypotensive interactions
Monoamine-oxidase Inhibitors see MAOIs
Monosulfiram
Alcohol: disulfiram-like reaction
Morphine see Opioid Analgesics
Muscle Relaxants
Alcohol: enhanced sedative effect with *baclofen*
- Anti-arrhythmics: *procainamide* and *quinidine* enhance muscle relaxant effect

Muscle Relaxants (*continued*)
- Antibacterials: effect of *non-depolarising muscle relaxants such as tubocurarine* enhanced by *aminoglycosides, azlocillin, clindamycin* and *polymyxins*

  Antihypertensives: enhanced hypotensive effect with *baclofen*

  Anxiolytics and Hypnotics: enhanced sedative effect with *baclofen*

  Beta-blockers: *propranolol* enhances muscle relaxant effect

  Calcium-channel Blockers: *nifedipine* and *verapamil* enhance effect of *non-depolarising muscle relaxants such as tubocurarine*; hypotension, myocardial depression, and hyperkalaemia reported with intravenous *dantrolene* and *verapamil*

  Cardiac Glycosides: arrhythmias if *suxamethonium* given with *digoxin*

  Cholinergics: *demecarium* and *ecothiopate* eye-drops, and *neostigmine*, and *pyridostigmine* enhance effect of *suxamethonium* but antagonise effect of *non-depolarising muscle relaxants such as tubocurarine*

  Cytotoxics: *cyclophosphamide* and *thiotepa* enhance effect of *suxamethonium*

  Lithium: *lithium* enhances muscle relaxant effect

  Magnesium Salts: *parenteral magnesium* enhances effect of *non-depolarising muscle relaxants such as tubocurarine*

Nabilone
  Alcohol: sedative effect of *nabilone* enhanced

  Anxiolytics and Hypnotics: enhanced sedative effect

Nabumetone *see* NSAIDs
Nadolol *see* Beta-blockers
Nalbuphine *see* Opioid Analgesics
Nalidixic Acid *see* 4-Quinolones
Nandrolone *see* Anabolic Steroids
Naproxen *see* NSAIDs
Nefopam
- Antidepressants: manufacturer recommends avoid *MAOIs*

  Antimuscarinics: increased side-effects

Neomycin *see* Aminoglycosides
Neostigmine *see* Cholinergics
Netilmicin *see* Aminoglycosides
Nicardipine *see* Calcium-channel Blockers
Nicoumalone *see* Warfarin
Nifedipine *see* Calcium-channel Blockers
Nimodipine *see* Calcium-channel Blockers
Nimorazole alcohol interaction *as for* Metronidazole
Nitrates *see* Glyceryl Trinitrate
Nitrazepam *see* Benzodiazepines and other Anxiolytics and Hypnotics
Nitrofurantoin
  Uricosurics: *probenecid* reduces excretion of *nitrofurantoin* (risk of toxicity)

Nitroprusside *as for* Hydralazine
Nizatidine *see* Histamine H2-antagonists
Noradrenaline *see* Sympathomimetics
Norfloxacin *see* 4-Quinolones
Nortriptyline *see* Antidepressants, Tricyclic
NSAIDs (*see also* Aspirin)
  Anion-exchange Resins: *cholestyramine* reduces absorption of *phenylbutazone*

  Antacids and Adsorbents: *antacids* reduce absorption of *diflunisal*
- Antibacterials: *NSAIDs* increase risk of convulsions with *4-quinolones*

  Anticoagulants: *see* Warfarin
- Antidiabetics: effect of *sulphonylureas* enhanced by *azapropazone* and *phenylbutazone*

NSAIDs (*continued*)
- Antiepileptics: effect of *phenytoin* enhanced by *azapropazone* and *phenylbutazone*

  Antihypertensives: antagonism of hypotensive effect; increased risk of renal failure with *ACE inhibitors* and increased risk of hyperkalaemia on administration of *ACE inhibitors* with *indomethacin* and possibly other *NSAIDs*

  Cardiac Glycosides: *NSAIDs* may exacerbate heart failure, reduce GFR, and increase plasma-cardiac glycoside concentration
- Cyclosporin: increased risk of nephrotoxicity
- Cytotoxics: excretion of *methotrexate* reduced by aspirin, azapropazone, diclofenac, indomethacin, ketoprofen, naproxen, phenylbutazone and probably other *NSAIDs* (increased risk of toxicity)

  Diuretics: risk of nephrotoxicity of *NSAIDs* increased; *NSAIDs* notably *indomethacin* antagonise diuretic effect; *indomethacin* and possibly other *NSAIDs* increase risk of hyperkalaemia with *potassium-sparing diuretics*; occasional reports of decreased renal function when *indomethacin* given with *triamterene*
- Lithium: excretion of *lithium* reduced by *diclofenac, ibuprofen, indomethacin, mefenamic acid, naproxen, phenylbutazone, piroxicam,* and probably other *NSAIDs* (possibility of toxicity)

  Mifepristone: manufacturer recommends avoid *aspirin* and *NSAIDs* until 8–12 days after *mifepristone* administration

  Thyroxine: false low total plasma-thyroxine concentration with *phenylbutazone*

  Uricosurics: *probenecid* delays excretion of *indomethacin, ketoprofen,* and *naproxen* (raised plasma concentrations)

Octreotide
  Antidiabetics: reduces *insulin and antidiabetic drug* requirements in diabetes mellitus

  Cyclosporin: absorption of *cyclosporin* reduced (reduced plasma concentration)

Oestrogens *see* Contraceptives, Oral
Ofloxacin *see* 4-Quinolones
Omeprazole
- Anticoagulants: effects of *warfarin* enhanced
- Antiepileptics: effects of *phenytoin* enhanced

  Anxiolytics and Hypnotics: metabolism of *diazepam* inhibited (increased effect possible)

Opioid Analgesics
  Anti-arrhythmics: delayed absorption of *mexiletine*

  Antibacterials: *rifampicin* accelerates metabolism of *methadone* (reduced effect); *erythromycin* increases plasma concentration of *alfentanil*
- Anticoagulants: *dextropropoxyphene* may enhance effect of *nicoumalone* and *warfarin*

  Antidepressants: CNS excitation or depression (hypertension or hypotension) if *pethidine* and possibly other opioid analgesics given to patients receiving *MAOIs*
- Antiepileptics: *dextropropoxyphene* enhances effect of *carbamazepine*

  Anxiolytics and Hypnotics: enhanced sedative effect

  Cisapride: possible antagonism of gastro-intestinal effect

  Domperidone and Metoclopramide: antagonism of gastro-intestinal effects

  Dopaminergics: hyperpyrexia and CNS toxicity reported with *selegiline*

  Ulcer-healing Drugs: *cimetidine* inhibits metabolism of opioid analgesics notably *pethidine* (increased plasma concentration)

Orciprenaline *see* Sympathomimetics
Orphenadrine *see* Antimuscarinics
Oxatomide *see* Antihistamines
Oxazepam *see* Benzodiazepines and other Anxiolytics and Hypnotics
Oxprenolol *see* Beta-blockers
Oxybutynin *see* Antimuscarinics
Oxymetazoline *see* Sympathomimetics
Oxymetholone *see* Anabolic Steroids
Oxypertine *see* Phenothiazines and other Antipsychotics
Oxytetracycline *see* Tetracyclines
Pamidronate Sodium *see* Bisphosphonates
Pancuronium *see* Muscle Relaxants (non-depolarising)
Papaveretum *see* Opioid Analgesics
Paracetamol
  Anion-exchange Resins: *cholestyramine* reduces absorption of *paracetamol*
  Anticoagulants: prolonged regular use of *paracetamol* possibly enhances *warfarin*
  Antivirals: regular use of *paracetamol* possibly reduces metabolism of *zidovudine* (increased risk of neutropenia)
  Domperidone and Metoclopramide: *metoclopramide* accelerates absorption of *paracetamol* (enhanced effect)
Paroxetine *see* Antidepressants, Serotonin-uptake Inhibitor
Pemoline *see* Sympathomimetics
Penbutolol *see* Beta-blockers
Penicillamine
  Antacids and Adsorbents: *antacids* reduce absorption
  Iron: reduced absorption of *penicillamine*
  Zinc: reduced absorption of *penicillamine*
Penicillins
  Antacids: reduced absorption of *pivampicillin*
  Anticoagulants: *see* Phenindione and Warfarin
  Guar Gum: reduced absorption of *phenoxymethylpenicillin*
  Muscle Relaxants: effects of *non-depolarising muscle relaxants* such as *tubocurarine* enhanced by *azlocillin*
  Probenecid: reduced excretion of *penicillins*
  Sex Hormones: *see* Contraceptives, Oral
Pentaerythritol Tetranitrate *see* Glyceryl Trinitrate
Pentazocine *see* Opioid Analgesics
Pergolide
  Antipsychotics: antagonism of effect
Pericyazine *see* Phenothiazines and other Antipsychotics
Perindopril *see* ACE Inhibitors
Perphenazine *see* Phenothiazines and other Antipsychotics
Pethidine *see* Opioid Analgesics
Phenazocine *see* Opioid Analgesics
Phenelzine *see* MAOIs
Phenindamine *see* Antihistamines
Phenindione
• Anabolic Steroids: anticoagulant effect enhanced by *oxymetholone, stanozolol* and others
• Analgesics: anticoagulant effect enhanced by *aspirin*
  Anion-exchange Resins: anticoagulant effect enhanced or reduced by *cholestyramine*
  Antibacterials: although studies have failed to demonstrate interaction common experience in anticoagulant clinics is that prothrombin time can be prolonged by course of *oral broad-spectrum antibiotic such as ampicillin* (may also apply to antibiotics given for local action on gut such as *neomycin*)

Phenindione (*continued*)
• Antiplatelet Drugs: anticoagulant effect enhanced by *aspirin and dipyridamole*
• Clofibrate Group: enhanced anticoagulant effect
• Sex Hormones: anticoagulant effect antagonised by *oral contraceptives*
• Thyroxine: enhanced anticoagulant effect
• Vitamins: anticoagulant effect antagonised by vitamin K (present in some enteral feeds)
Pheniramine *see* Antihistamines
Phenobarbitone *see* Barbiturates
Phenoperidine *see* Opioid Analgesics
Phenothiazines and other Antipsychotics
  Alcohol: enhanced sedative effect
• Anaesthetics: enhanced hypotensive effect
  Antacids: reduced absorption of *phenothiazines*
  Anti-arrhythmics: increased risk of ventricular arrhythmias with drugs which prolong QT interval
  Antibacterials: *rifampicin* accelerates metabolism of *haloperidol* (reduced plasma-haloperidol concentration)
• Antidepressants: increased plasma concentrations and increased antimuscarinic effects notably on administration of *tricyclics* with *phenothiazines*; *fluoxetine* increases plasma concentration of *haloperidol*; *oxypertine* causes CNS excitation and hypertension with *MAOIs*
• Antiepileptics: antagonism (convulsive threshold lowered); *carbamazepine* accelerates metabolism of *haloperidol* (reduced plasma concentration); *phenytoin* accelerates metabolism of *clozapine*
  Antihypertensives: enhanced hypotensive effect; higher doses of *chlorpromazine* antagonise hypotensive effect of *adrenergic neurone blockers*; severe postural hypotension on administration of *ACE inhibitors* with *chlorpromazine and possibly other antipsychotics*; increased risk of extrapyramidal effects on administration of *methyldopa* and *metirosine*
  Antimuscarinics: antimuscarinic side-effects of *phenothiazines* increased (but reduced plasma concentrations)
  Anxiolytics and Hypnotics: enhanced sedative effect
  Beta-blockers: *propranolol* increases plasma concentration of *chlorpromazine*
  Calcium-channel Blockers: enhanced hypotensive effect
  Desferrioxamine: manufacturer advises avoid *prochlorperazine*
  Diuretics: hypokalaemia increases risk of ventricular arrhythmias with *pimozide*
  Domperidone and Metoclopramide: increased risk of extrapyramidal effects with *metoclopramide*
  Dopaminergics: antagonism of hypoprolactinaemic and antiparkinsonian effects of *bromocriptine*; antagonism of effect of *levodopa, lysuride,* and *pergolide*
  Lithium: increased risk of extrapyramidal effects and possibility of neurotoxicity with *clozapine, haloperidol and phenothiazines*
  Tetrabenazine: increased risk of extrapyramidal effects
  Ulcer-healing Drugs: *cimetidine* may enhance effects of *chlorpromazine, clozapine,* and possibly *other antipsychotics*
Phenoxymethylpenicillin *see* Penicillins
Phentermine *see* Sympathomimetics
Phenylbutazone *see* NSAIDs
Phenylephrine *see* Sympathomimetics
Phenylpropanolamine *see* Sympathomimetics

Phenytoin

- Analgesics: plasma-phenytoin concentration increased by *aspirin, azapropazone,* and *phenylbutazone*

  Antacids: reduced *phenytoin* absorption
- Anti-arrhythmics: *amiodarone* increases plasma-phenytoin concentration; *phenytoin* reduces plasma concentrations of *disopyramide, mexiletine,* and *quinidine*
- Antibacterials: plasma-phenytoin concentration increased by *chloramphenicol, cycloserine, isoniazid,* and *metronidazole*; plasma-phenytoin concentration and antifolate effect increased by *co-trimoxazole* and *trimethoprim*; plasma phenytoin concentration reduced by *rifampicin*; plasma concentration of *doxycycline* reduced by *phenytoin*
- Anticoagulants: metabolism of *nicoumalone* and *warfarin* accelerated (possibility of reduced anticoagulant effect, but enhancement also reported)
- Antidepressants: antagonism of anticonvulsant effect (convulsive threshold lowered); *viloxazine* increases plasma-phenytoin concentration; *phenytoin* reduces plasma concentrations of *mianserin, paroxetine,* and *tricyclics*

  Antidiabetics: plasma-phenytoin concentration transiently increased by *tolbutamide* (possibility of toxicity)
- other Antiepileptics: concomitant administration of two or more antiepileptics may enhance toxicity without a corresponding increase in antiepileptic effect; moreover interactions between individual antiepileptics can complicate monitoring of treatment; interactions include enhanced effects, increased sedation, and reductions in plasma concentrations
- Antifungals: plasma-phenytoin concentration increased by *fluconazole, ketoconazole,* and *miconazole*; plasma concentration of *ketoconazole* and possibly others reduced

  Antimalarials: increased risk of antifolate effect with *pyrimethamine* (includes Fansidar® and Maloprim®)

  Antiplatelet Drugs: plasma-phenytoin concentration increased by *aspirin*
- Antipsychotics: antagonism of anticonvulsant effect (convulsive threshold lowered); *phenytoin* accelerates metabolism of *clozapine*

  Calcium-channel Blockers: *diltiazem* increases plasma concentration of *phenytoin*; effect of *felodipine, isradipine* and probably *nicardipine, nifedipine,* and *verapamil* reduced

  Cardiac Glycosides: metabolism of *digitoxin* only accelerated (reduced effect)
- Corticosteroids: metabolism of *corticosteroids* accelerated (reduced effect)
- Cyclosporin: metabolism of *cyclosporin* accelerated (reduced plasma concentration)

  Cytotoxics: reduced absorption of *phenytoin*; increased anti-folate effect with *methotrexate*
- Disulfiram: plasma-phenytoin concentration increased

  Diuretics: increased risk of osteomalacia with *carbonic anhydrase inhibitors*

  Food: some *enteral foods* may interfere with absorption of *phenytoin*

  Lithium: neurotoxicity may occur without increased plasma-lithium concentration
- Sex Hormones: metabolism of *gestrinone, tibolone,* and *oral contraceptives* accelerated (reduced contraceptive effect, important: see p. 291)

  Theophylline: metabolism of *theophylline* accelerated (reduced plasma-theophylline concentration)

Phenytoin (continued)

Thyroxine: metabolism of *thyroxine* accelerated (may increase thyroxine requirements in hypothyroidism)

- Ulcer-healing Drugs: *cimetidine* inhibits metabolism (increased plasma-phenytoin concentration); *sucralfate* reduces absorption; *omeprazole* enhances effect of *phenytoin*
- Uricosurics: plasma-phenytoin concentration increased by *sulphinpyrazone*

  Vaccines: effect enhanced by *influenza vaccine*

  Vitamins: plasma-phenytoin concentration occasionally reduced by *folic acid*; *vitamin D* requirements possibly increased

Physostigmine see Cholinergics

Phytomenadione see Vitamins (Vitamin K)

Pimozide see Phenothiazines and other Antipsychotics (CSM: see also p. 151)

Pindolol see Beta-blockers

Pipenzolate see Antimuscarinics

Piperazine

other Anthelmintics: antagonism of *pyrantel*

Pipothiazine see Phenothiazines and other Antipsychotics

Pirbuterol see Sympathomimetics, Beta$_2$

Piretanide see Diuretics (loop)

Piroxicam see NSAIDs

Pivampicillin see Penicillins

Pizotifen

Antihypertensives: hypotensive effect of *adrenergic neurone blockers* antagonised

Poldine see Antimuscarinics

Polymyxins (see also Aminoglycosides)

Muscle Relaxants: enhanced muscle relaxant effect

Polythiazide see Diuretics (thiazides)

Potassium Salts (includes Salt Substitutes)

- Antihypertensives: hyperkalaemia with *ACE inhibitors*
- Cyclosporin: increased risk of hyperkalaemia
- Diuretics: hyperkalaemia with *potassium-sparing diuretics*

Pravastatin

Clofibrate Group: increased risk of myopathy

Cyclosporin: increased risk of myopathy

Prazosin see Alpha-blockers (post-synaptic)

Prednisolone see Corticosteroids

Prednisone see Corticosteroids

Primaquine

other Antimalarials: *mepacrine* increases plasma concentration of *primaquine* (risk of toxicity)

Primidone see Barbiturates and Primidone

Probenecid

Analgesics: *aspirin* antagonises effect; excretion of *indomethacin, ketoprofen,* and *naproxen* delayed (increased plasma concentrations)

Antibacterials: reduced excretion of *cephalosporins, cinoxacin, dapsone, nalidixic acid, nitrofurantoin,* and *penicillins* (increased plasma-concentrations); antagonism by *pyrazinamide*

Antihypertensives: reduced excretion of *captopril*

Antivirals: reduced excretion of *acyclovir* and *zidovudine* (increased plasma concentrations and risk of toxicity)

- Cytotoxics: reduced excretion of *methotrexate* (increased risk of toxicity)

Procainamide

- other Anti-arrhythmics: *amiodarone* increases procainamide-plasma concentrations; increased myocardial depression with any anti-arrhythmic

Antibacterials: *trimethoprim* increases plasma concentration of *procainamide*

Procainamide (*continued*)
Cholinergics: antagonism of effect of *neostigmine* and *pyridostigmine*
- Muscle Relaxants: muscle relaxant effect enhanced
- Ulcer-healing Drugs: *cimetidine* inhibits excretion (increased plasma-procainamide concentration)

Procarbazine
Alcohol: disulfiram-like reaction

Prochlorperazine see Phenothiazines and other Antipsychotics

Procyclidine see Antimuscarinics

Progestogens (*see also* Contraceptives, Oral)
- Cyclosporin: increased plasma-cyclosporin concentration (inhibition of metabolism)

Proguanil
- Anticoagulants: effect of warfarin possibly enhanced

Promazine see Phenothiazines and other Antipsychotics

Promethazine see Antihistamines

Propafenone
other Anti-arrhythmics: *quinidine* increases plasma concentration of *propafenone*; increased myocardial depression with any *anti-arrhythmic*
Antibacterials: *rifampicin* reduces plasma concentration of *propafenone*
- Anticoagulants: increased plasma concentration of *warfarin* and *nicoumalone* (enhanced effect)
- Cardiac Glycosides: increased plasma concentrations of *digoxin* (halve maintenance dose of digoxin)
Cholinergics: possible antagonism of effect of *neostigmine* and *pyridostigmine*
- Ulcer-healing Drugs: *cimetidine* increases plasma-propafenone concentration

Propantheline see Antimuscarinics

Propranolol see Beta-Blockers

Protriptyline see Antidepressants, Tricyclic

Pyrantel
other Anthelmintics: antagonism of *piperazine*

Pyrazinamide
Uricosurics: antagonism of *probenecid* and *sulphinpyrazone*

Pyridostigmine see Cholinergics

Pyridoxine see Vitamins

Pyrimethamine
Antibacterials: increased antifolate effect with *cotrimoxazole* and *trimethoprim*
Antiepileptics: increased antifolate effect with *phenytoin*
Cytotoxics: increased antifolate effect with *methotrexate*

Quinalbarbitone see Barbiturates and Primidone

Quinapril see ACE Inhibitors

Quinidine
Antacids: reduced excretion in alkaline urine (plasma-quinidine concentration occasionally increased)
- *other* Anti-arrhythmics: *amiodarone* increases plasma-quinidine concentrations (and increases risk of ventricular arrhythmias); plasma concentration of *propafenone* increased; increased myocardial depression with *any anti-arrhythmic*
Antibacterials: *rifampicin* accelerates metabolism (reduced plasma-quinidine concentration)
Anticoagulants: effect of *nicoumalone and warfarin* may be enhanced
Antiepileptics: *phenobarbitone, phenytoin,* and *primidone* accelerate metabolism (reduced plasma-quinidine concentration)
Barbiturates: *see under* Antiepileptics, above

Quinidine (*continued*)
- Calcium-channel Blockers: *verapamil* increases plasma-quinidine concentration (possibility of extreme hypotension)
- Cardiac Glycosides: plasma concentration of *digoxin* increased (halve digoxin maintenance dose)
Cholinergics: antagonism of effect of *neostigmine* and *pyridostigmine*
- Diuretics: *acetazolamide* reduces excretion (plasma-quinidine concentration occasionally increased); quinidine toxicity increased if hypokalaemia occurs with *acetazolamide, loop diuretics, and thiazides*
- Muscle Relaxants: muscle relaxant effect enhanced
- Ulcer-healing Drugs: *cimetidine* inhibits metabolism (increased plasma-quinidine concentration)

Quinine
other Antimalarials: see Mefloquine
- Cardiac Glycosides: plasma concentration of *digoxin* increased (halve digoxin maintenance dose); includes use of quinine for cramps
Ulcer-healing Drugs: *cimetidine* inhibits metabolism (increased plasma-quinine concentration)

4-Quinolones
- Analgesics: increased risk of convulsions with *NSAIDs*
Antacids and Adsorbents: *antacids* reduce absorption of *ciprofloxacin, norfloxacin* and *ofloxacin*
- Anticoagulants: anticoagulant effect of *nicoumalone* and *warfarin* enhanced by *ciprofloxacin, enoxacin, nalidixic acid,* and *norfloxacin*
Cyclosporin: increased risk of nephrotoxicity
Iron: absorption of *ciprofloxacin, norfloxacin,* and *ofloxacin* reduced by *oral iron*
- Theophylline: *ciprofloxacin, enoxacin,* and *norfloxacin* increase plasma-theophylline concentration
Ulcer-healing Drugs: *sucralfate* reduces absorption of *ciprofloxacin, norfloxacin,* and *ofloxacin*
Uricosurics: *probenecid* reduces excretion of *cinoxacin* and *nalidixic acid* (increased side-effects)
Zinc Salts: *zinc* reduces absorption of *ciprofloxacin*

Rabies Vaccine see p. 452

Ramipril see ACE Inhibitors

Ranitidine see Histamine H2-antagonists

Remoxipride
Domperidone and Metoclopramide: increased risk of extrapyramidal effects with *metoclopramide*
Dopaminergics: antagonism of hypoprolactinaemic and antiparkinsonian effects of *bromocriptine*; antagonism of effect of *levodopa, lysuride* and *pergolide*
Tetrabenazine: increased risk of extrapyramidal effects

Reproterol see Sympathomimetics, Beta₂

Rifampicin
Analgesics: metabolism of *methadone* accelerated (reduced effect)
Antacids: reduced absorption of *rifampicin*
Anti-arrhythmics: metabolism accelerated—reduced plasma concentrations of *disopyramide, mexiletine, propafenone,* and *quinidine*
other Antibacterials: metabolism of *chloramphenicol* accelerated (reduced plasma concentration); plasma concentration of *dapsone* reduced
- Anticoagulants: metabolism of *nicoumalone* and *warfarin* accelerated (reduced anticoagulant effect)
- Antidiabetics: metabolism of *chlorpropamide, tolbutamide* and possibly other *sulphonylureas* accelerated (reduced effect)

Rifampicin (*continued*)
- Antiepileptics: metabolism of *phenytoin* accelerated (reduced plasma concentration)
  Antifungals: metabolism of *fluconazole, itraconazole and ketoconazole* accelerated (reduced plasma concentrations); plasma concentration of *terbinafine* reduced
  Antipsychotics: metabolism of *haloperidol* accelerated (reduced plasma concentration)
  Anxiolytics and Hypnotics: metabolism of *diazepam* accelerated (reduced plasma concentration)
  Beta-blockers: metabolism of *bisoprolol* and *propranolol* accelerated (reduced plasma concentration)
  Calcium-channel Blockers: metabolism of *verapamil and possibly isradipine* and *nifedipine* accelerated (reduced plasma concentration)
  Cardiac glycosides: metabolism of *digitoxin* only accelerated (reduced effect)
- Corticosteroids: metabolism of *corticosteroids* accelerated (reduced effect)
- Cyclosporin: metabolism accelerated (reduced plasma-cyclosporin concentration)
- Sex Hormones: metabolism accelerated (contraceptive effect of *both combined and progestogen-only oral contraceptives* reduced, important: see p. 291)
  Theophylline: metabolism accelerated (reduced plasma-theophylline concentration)
  Thyroxine: metabolism of *thyroxine* accelerated (may increase requirements in hypothyroidism)
  Ulcer-healing Drugs: metabolism of *cimetidine* accelerated (reduced plasma concentration)

Rimiterol *see* Sympathomimetics, Beta$_2$
Ritodrine *see* Sympathomimetics, Beta$_2$
Rowachol®
  Anticoagulants: effect of *nicoumalone and warfarin* may be reduced
Salbutamol *see* Sympathomimetics, Beta$_2$
Salmeterol *see* Sympathomimetics, Beta$_2$
Salt Substitutes *see* Potassium salts
Selegiline
  Analgesics: hyperpyrexia and CNS toxicity with *pethidine*
Sertraline *see* Antidepressants, Serotonin-uptake Inhibitor
Simvastatin
- Anticoagulants: effect of *nicoumalone and warfarin* may be enhanced
  Cyclosporin: increased risk of myopathy
  other Lipid-lowering Drugs: increased risk of myopathy with *clofibrate group*
Sodium Bicarbonate *see* Antacids and Adsorbents
Sodium Clodronate *see* Bisphosphonates
Sodium Valproate *see* Valproate
Sotalol *see* Beta-blockers
Spectinomycin
  Lithium: increased toxicity reported
Spironolactone *see* Diuretics (potassium-sparing)
Stanozolol *see* Anabolic Steroids
Streptomycin *see* Aminoglycosides
Sucralfate
  Antibacterials: reduced absorption of *ciprofloxacin, norfloxacin, ofloxacin,* and *tetracycline*
- Anticoagulants: absorption of *warfarin* possibly reduced
- Antiepileptics: reduced absorption of *phenytoin*
  Cardiac Glycosides: absorption of *cardiac glycosides* possibly reduced
Sulfadoxine *see* Co-trimoxazole and Sulphonamides
Sulfametopyrazine *see* Co-trimoxazole and Sulphonamides

Sulindac *see* NSAIDs
Sulphadiazine *see* Co-trimoxazole and Sulphonamides
Sulphadimidine *see* Co-trimoxazole and Sulphonamides
Sulphinpyrazone
  Analgesics: *aspirin* antagonises uricosuric effect
  Antibacterials: *pyrazinamide* antagonises effect
- Anticoagulants: anticoagulant effect of *nicoumalone and warfarin* enhanced
- Antidiabetics: effect of *sulphonylureas* enhanced
- Antiepileptics: plasma concentration of *phenytoin* increased
  Theophylline: plasma-theophylline concentration reduced
Sulphonamides *see* Co-trimoxazole and Sulphonamides
Sulphonylureas *see* Antidiabetics
Sulpiride *see* Phenothiazines and other Antipsychotics
Sumatriptan
- Antidepressants: risk of CNS toxicity with *MAOIs* and *serotonin-uptake inhibitors*
- Ergotamine: increased risk of vasospasm
- Lithium: risk of CNS toxicity
Suxamethonium *see* Muscle Relaxants
Sympathomimetics (*see below* for Beta$_2$-Sympathomimetics)
- Anaesthetics: risk of arrhythmias if *adrenaline and isoprenaline* given with *volatile anaesthetics*
- Antidepressants: with *tricyclics* administration of *adrenaline and noradrenaline* may cause hypertension and arrhythmias (but local anaesthetics with adrenaline appear to be safe); with *MAOIs* administration of inotropics such as *dopamine* and *dopexamine* may cause hypertensive crisis; also with *MAOIs* administration of *dexamphetamine and other amphetamines, dexfenfluramine, diethylpropion, ephedrine, fenfluramine, isometheptene, mazindol, pemoline, phentermine, phenylephrine, phenylpropanolamine,* and *pseudoephedrine* may cause hypertensive crisis (these drugs are contained in anorectics or cold and cough remedies)
  Antihypertensives: sympathomimetics in *anorectics and cold and cough remedies* (*see* above) antagonise hypotensive effect of *adrenergic neurone blockers;* hypotensive effect of some other antihypertensives may be enhanced by *dexfenfluramine and fenfluramine*
- Beta-blockers: severe hypertension with *adrenaline and noradrenaline* (especially with non-selective beta-blockers); severe hypertension also possible with sympathomimetics in *anorectics and cold and cough remedies, see* above
  Respiratory Stimulants: risk of hypertension with *doxapram*
  other Sympathomimetics: *dopexamine* possibly potentiates effect of *adrenaline* and *noradrenaline*
Sympathomimetics, Beta$_2$
  Corticosteroids: increased risk of hypokalaemia if high doses of *corticosteroids* given with high doses of *fenoterol, pirbuterol, reproterol, rimiterol, ritodrine, salbutamol, salmeterol, terbutaline* and *tulobuterol*
  Theophylline: increased risk of hypokalaemia if given with high doses of *fenoterol, pirbuterol, reproterol, rimiterol, ritodrine, salbutamol, salmeterol, terbutaline,* and *tulobuterol*
Tamoxifen
- Anticoagulants: anticoagulant effect of *nicoumalone and warfarin* enhanced

Temazepam see Benzodiazepines and other Anxiolytics and Hypnotics
Tenoxicam see NSAIDs
Terazosin see Alpha-blockers (post-synaptic)
Terbinafine
  Antibacterials: plasma concentration reduced by *rifampicin*
  Ulcer-healing Drugs: plasma concentration increased by *cimetidine*
Terbutaline see Sympathomimetics, Beta$_2$
Terfenadine see Antihistamines
Tetrabenazine (general extrapyramidal interactions *as for* phenothiazines)
  • Antidepressants: CNS excitation and hypertension with *MAOIs*
Tetracyclines
  Antacids: reduced absorption
  Anticoagulants: *see* Phenindione and Warfarin
  Antiepileptics: *carbamazepine, phenobarbitone, phenytoin, and primidone* increase metabolism of *doxycycline* (reduced plasma concentration)
  Antihypertensives: *quinapril* reduces absorption (tablets contain magnesium carbonate excipient)
  Barbiturates: *see under* Antiepileptics, above
  Calcium Salts: reduced absorption of *tetracyclines*
  Dairy products: reduced absorption (except *doxycycline* and *minocycline*)
  Iron: absorption of *oral iron* reduced by *tetracyclines* and *vice versa*
  Sex Hormones: *see* Contraceptives, Oral (main list)
  Ulcer-healing Drugs: *bismuth chelate* and *sucralfate* reduce absorption
  Zinc Salts: reduced absorption (and *vice versa*)
Theophylline
  Anaesthetics: increased risk of arrhythmias with *halothane*
  Anthelmintics: *thiabendazole* may increase plasma-theophylline concentration
  Anti-arrhythmics: antagonism of anti-arrhythmic effect of *adenosine*; plasma-theophylline concentration increased by *mexiletine*
  • Antibacterials: plasma-theophylline concentration increased by *ciprofloxacin, enoxacin, erythromycin,* and *norfloxacin* and possibly increased by *isoniazid*; plasma-theophylline concentration reduced by *rifampicin*
  Antidepressants: plasma-theophylline concentration increased by *viloxazine*
  Antiepileptics: plasma-theophylline concentration reduced by *carbamazepine, phenobarbitone, phenytoin, and primidone*
  Antifungals: plasma-theophylline concentration possibly increased by *fluconazole*
  Barbiturates: *see under* Antiepileptics, above
  Beta-blockers: should be avoided on pharmacological grounds (bronchospasm)
  • Calcium-channel Blockers: plasma-theophylline concentration increased by *diltiazem* and *verapamil*
  Disulfiram: increases plasma-theophylline concentration
  Hormone Antagonists: plasma-theophylline concentration reduced by *aminoglutethimide*
  Interferons: plasma-theophylline concentration increased
  Lithium: *lithium* excretion accelerated (reduced plasma-lithium concentration)
  Respiratory Stimulants: increased CNS stimulation
  Sex Hormones: plasma-theophylline concentration increased by *combined oral contraceptives*

Theophylline (continued)
  Sympathomimetics: increased risk of hypokalaemia if *theophylline* given with high doses of *fenoterol, pirbuterol, reproterol, rimiterol, ritodrine, salbutamol, salmeterol, terbutaline,* and *tulobuterol*
  • Ulcer-healing Drugs: plasma-theophylline concentration increased by *cimetidine*
  Uricosurics: plasma-theophylline concentration reduced by *sulphinpyrazone*
  Vaccines: plasma-theophylline concentration occasionally increased by *influenza vaccine*
Thiabendazole
  Theophylline: plasma concentration may be increased
Thiazides see Diuretics
Thiethylperazine see Phenothiazines and other Antipsychotics
Thiopentone see Barbiturates and Primidone
Thioridazine see Phenothiazines and other Antipsychotics
Thiotepa
  Muscle Relaxants: effect of *suxamethonium* enhanced
Thyroxine
  Analgesics: false low total plasma-thyroxine concentration with *phenylbutazone*
  Anion-exchange Resins: absorption of *thyroxine* reduced by *cholestyramine*
  Antibacterials: *rifampicin* accelerates metabolism of thyroxine (may increase requirements in hypothyroidism)
  • Anticoagulants: effect of *nicoumalone, phenindione,* and *warfarin* enhanced
  Antiepileptics: *carbamazepine, phenobarbitone, phenytoin, and primidone* accelerate metabolism of *thyroxine* (may increase requirements in hypothyroidism)
  Barbiturates: *see under* Antiepileptics, above
  Beta-blockers: metabolism of propranolol accelerated (reduced effect)
Tiaprofenic Acid see NSAIDs
Tibolone
  Antibacterials: *rifampicin* accelerates metabolism (reduced plasma concentration)
  Antiepileptics: *carbamazepine, phenobarbitone, phenytoin, and primidone* accelerate metabolism (reduced plasma concentration)
Timolol see Beta-blockers
Tinidazole alcohol interaction *as for* Metronidazole
Tobramycin see Aminoglycosides
Tocainide
  other Anti-arrhythmics: increased myocardial depression with any anti-arrhythmic
  Beta-blockers: increased risk of bradycardia and myocardial depression
  Diuretics: effect of *tocainide* antagonised by hypokalaemia with *acetazolamide*, loop diuretics, and thiazides
Tolazamide see Antidiabetics (sulphonylurea)
Tolbutamide see Antidiabetics (sulphonylurea)
Tolmetin see NSAIDs
Tranylcypromine see MAOIs
Trazodone
  Alcohol: enhanced sedative effect
  • other Antidepressants: interaction with *MAOIs* possible (avoid for at least 2 weeks after stopping MAOI)
  Antiepileptics: antagonism of anticonvulsant effect
  Anxiolytics and Hypnotics: enhanced sedative effect

Triamcinolone see Corticosteroids
Triamterene see Diuretics (potassium-sparing)
Triclofos see Chloral
Trientine
  Iron: absorption of *oral iron* reduced
Trifluoperazine see Phenothiazines and other Antipsychotics
Trifluperidol see Phenothiazines and other Antipsychotics
Trilostane
  Diuretics: increased risk of hyperkalaemia with *potassium-sparing diuretics*
Trimeprazine see Antihistamines
Trimethoprim
  Anti-arrhythmics: plasma concentration of *procainamide* increased
  Anticoagulants: effect of *nicoumalone* and *warfarin* possibly enhanced
  Antidiabetics: effect of *sulphonylureas* enhanced
  Antiepileptics: antifolate effect of *phenytoin* increased
  Antimalarials: increased risk of antifolate effect with *pyrimethamine* (ingredient of *Fansidar*® and *Maloprim*®)
  Cytotoxics: antifolate effect of *methotrexate* increased
Trimipramine see Antidepressants, Tricyclic
Triprolidine see Antihistamines
Tropicamide see Antimuscarinics
Tryptophan
• *other* Antidepressants: CNS excitation and confusion with *MAOIs* (reduce tryptophan dose); agitation and nausea with *fluoxetine, fluvoxamine, paroxetine, and sertraline*
Tubocurarine see Muscle Relaxants (non-depolarising)
Tulobuterol see Sympathomimetics, Beta$_2$
Typhoid Vaccine see p. 453
Ulcer-healing Drugs see individual drugs
Uricosurics see individual drugs
Vaccines see Influenza Vaccine (p. 488), Rabies Vaccine (p. 452), Typhoid Vaccine (p. 453)
Valproate
  Analgesics: *aspirin* enhances effect
• Antidepressants: antagonism of anticonvulsant effect (convulsive threshold lowered)
• *other* Antiepileptics: concomitant administration of two or more antiepileptics may enhance toxicity without a corresponding increase in antiepileptic effect; moreover, interactions between individual antiepileptics can complicate monitoring of treatment; interactions include enhanced effects, increased sedation, and reductions in plasma concentrations
• Antipsychotics: antagonism of anticonvulsant effect (convulsive threshold lowered)
Vancomycin
  Anion-exchange Resins: antagonism of *oral vancomycin* by *cholestyramine*
  other Antibacterials: increased risk of ototoxicity and nephrotoxicity with *aminoglycosides and capreomycin*
  Diuretics: increased risk of ototoxicity with *loop diuretics*
Vecuronium see Muscle Relaxants (non-depolarising)
Verapamil see Calcium-channel blockers
Vigabatrin
  other Antiepileptics: *vigabatrin* lowers plasma concentration of *phenytoin*

Viloxazine
• Antiepileptics: increased plasma concentrations of *carbamazepine* and *phenytoin*
  Theophylline: increased plasma-theophylline concentration
Vitamins
• Anticoagulants: anticoagulant effect of *nicoumalone, phenindione, and warfarin* antagonised by *vitamin K* (present in some enteral feeds)
  Antiepileptics: *folic acid* occasionally reduces plasma-phenytoin concentration; *vitamin D* requirements possibly increased by *carbamazepine, phenobarbitone, phenytoin,* and *primidone*
  Dopaminergics: effect of *levodopa* antagonised by *pyridoxine* (unless a dopa decarboxylase inhibitor also given)
Warfarin
• Alcohol: enhanced anticoagulant effect
  Allopurinol: anticoagulant effect possibly enhanced
• Anabolic Steroids: *oxymetholone, stanozolol and others* enhance anticoagulant effect
• Analgesics: *aspirin* increases risk of bleeding due to antiplatelet effect; anticoagulant effect seriously enhanced by *azapropazone* (see also p. 330) and *phenylbutazone*, and possibly enhanced by *diflunisal, flurbiprofen, mefenamic acid, piroxicam, sulindac,* and possibly *other NSAIDs*; anticoagulant effect possibly also enhanced by *dextropropoxyphene* and by prolonged regular use of *paracetamol*
• Anion-exchange Resins: *cholestyramine* may enhance or reduce anticoagulant effect
• Anti-arrhythmics: *amiodarone and propafenone* enhance anticoagulant effect; *quinidine* may enhance anticoagulant effect
• Antibacterials: anticoagulant effect reduced by *rifampicin*; anticoagulant effect enhanced by *aztreonam, cephamandole, chloramphenicol, ciprofloxacin, co-trimoxazole, erythromycin, metronidazole,* and *sulphonamides*; anticoagulant effect possibly also enhanced by *azithromycin, enoxacin, nalidixic acid, neomycin, norfloxacin, tetracyclines,* and *trimethoprim*; although studies have failed to demonstrate interaction, common experience in anticoagulant clinics is that prothrombin time can be prolonged by few seconds following course of oral broad-spectrum antibiotic, such as ampicillin (may also apply to antibiotics given for local action on gut such as neomycin)
• Antidepressants: *fluvoxamine and paroxetine* may enhance anticoagulant effect
• Antiepileptics: reduced anticoagulant effect with *carbamazepine, phenobarbitone, and primidone*; both reduced and enhanced effects reported with *phenytoin*
• Antifungals: anticoagulant effect reduced by *griseofulvin*; anticoagulant effect enhanced by *fluconazole, itraconazole, ketoconazole, and miconazole*
• Antimalarials: anticoagulant effect possibly enhanced by *proguanil*
• Antiplatelet Drugs: *aspirin and dipyridamole* increase risk of bleeding due to antiplatelet effect
  Anxiolytics and Hypnotics: *chloral* may transiently enhance anticoagulant effect
• Barbiturates: anticoagulant effect reduced
• Clofibrate Group: enhanced anticoagulant effect
• Cytotoxics: anticoagulant effect possibly enhanced by *ifosfamide*

Warfarin (*continued*)
- Disulfiram: enhanced anticoagulant effect
- Hormone Antagonists: *aminoglutethimide* reduces anticoagulant effect; *danazol, flutamide,* and *tamoxifen* enhance anticoagulant effect
  Rowachol®: may reduce anticoagulant effect
- Sex Hormones: *oral contraceptives* reduce anticoagulant effect
- Simvastatin: may enhance anticoagulant effect
- Thyroxine: enhanced anticoagulant effect
- Ulcer-healing Drugs: *sucralfate* possibly reduces anticoagulant effect (reduced absorption); *cimetidine* and *omeprazole* enhance anticoagulant effect
- Uricosurics: *sulphinpyrazone* enhances anticoagulant effect
  Vaccines: influenza vaccine occasionally enhances anticoagulant effect
- Vitamins: *vitamin K* reduces anticoagulant effect; major changes in diet (especially involving vegetables) may affect control; vitamin K also present in some enteral feeds

Xamoterol
Beta-blockers: antagonism of effect of *xamoterol* and reduction in beta-blockade

Xipamide *see* Diuretics (thiazide-related)
Xylometazoline *see* Sympathomimetics
Zidovudine
  Note. Increased risk of toxicity with other nephrotoxic and myelosuppressive drugs
  Analgesics: regular use of *paracetamol* possibly reduces metabolism of *zidovudine* (increased risk of neutropenia
  other Antivirals: extreme lethargy reported on administration of *intravenous acyclovir*; profound myelosuppression with *ganciclovir*
  Uricosurics: *probenecid* increases plasma-zidovudine concentration and risk of toxicity

Zinc
  Antibacterials: reduced absorption of *ciprofloxacin*; *tetracyclines* reduce absorption of *zinc* (and *vice versa*)
  Iron: reduced absorption of *oral iron* (and *vice versa*)
  Penicillamine: reduced absorption of *penicillamine*

Zopiclone (general sedative interactions *as for* Benzodiazepines and other Anxiolytics and Hypnotics)
Zuclopenthixol *see* Phenothiazines and other Antipsychotics

Appendix 2: Liver Disease

Liver disease may alter the response to drugs in several ways as indicated below, and drug prescribing should be kept to a minimum in all patients with severe liver disease. The main problems occur in patients with jaundice, ascites, or evidence of encephalopathy.

IMPAIRED DRUG METABOLISM. Metabolism by the liver is the main route of elimination for many drugs, but the hepatic reserve appears to be large and liver disease has to be severe before important changes in drug metabolism occur. Routine liver-function tests are a poor guide to the capacity of the liver to metabolise drugs, and in the individual patient it is not possible to predict the extent to which the metabolism of a particular drug may be impaired.

A few drugs, e.g. rifampicin and fusidic acid, are excreted in the bile unchanged and may accumulate in patients with intrahepatic or extrahepatic obstructive jaundice.

HYPOPROTEINAEMIA. The hypoalbuminaemia in severe liver disease is associated with reduced protein binding and increased toxicity of some highly protein-bound drugs such as phenytoin and prednisolone.

REDUCED CLOTTING. Reduced hepatic synthesis of blood-clotting factors, indicated by a prolonged prothrombin time, increases the sensitivity to oral anticoagulants such as warfarin and phenindione.

HEPATIC ENCEPHALOPATHY. In severe liver disease many drugs can further impair cerebral function and may precipitate hepatic encephalopathy. These include all sedative drugs, opioid analgesics, those diuretics that produce hypokalaemia, and drugs that cause constipation.

FLUID OVERLOAD. Oedema and ascites in chronic liver disease may be exacerbated by drugs that give rise to fluid retention, e.g. NSAIDs, corticosteroids, and carbenoxolone.

HEPATOTOXIC DRUGS. Hepatotoxicity is either dose-related or unpredictable (idiosyncratic). Drugs causing dose-related toxicity may do so at lower doses than in patients with normal liver function, and some drugs producing reactions of the idiosyncratic kind do so more frequently in patients with liver disease. These drugs should be avoided.

Table of drugs to be avoided or used with caution in liver disease

The list of drugs given below is not comprehensive and is based on current information concerning the use of these drugs in therapeutic dosage. Products introduced or amended since publication of BNF No. 23 (March 1992) are underlined.

Drugs	Comment
Acemetacin *see* NSAIDs	
Acrivastine *see* Antihistamines	
Alfentanil *see* Opioid Analgesics	
Alprazolam *see* Anxiolytics and Hypnotics	
Aminophylline *see* Theophylline	
Amitriptyline *see* Antidepressants, Tricyclic	
Amlodipine	Reduce dose
Amoxapine *see* Antidepressants, Tricyclic	
Anabolic Steroids	Preferably avoid—dose-related toxicity
Analgesics *see* NSAIDs and Opioid Analgesics	
Androgens	Preferably avoid—dose-related toxicity with some, and produce fluid retention
Antacids	In patients with fluid retention, avoid those containing large amounts of sodium, e.g. magnesium trisilicate mixture, Gaviscon®. Avoid those causing constipation—can precipitate coma
Anticoagulants, Oral	Avoid, especially if prothrombin time is already prolonged
Antidepressants, MAOI *see* MAOIs	
Antidepressants, Serotonin-uptake Inhibitor	Reduce dose in severe liver disease
Antidepressants, Tricyclic (and related)	Tricyclics preferable to MAOIs but sedative effects increased; iprindole may cause idiosyncratic hepatotoxicity; lofepramine contra-indicated
Antihistamines	Avoid—may precipitate coma; terfenadine see also p. 127
Antipsychotics	All can precipitate coma; phenothiazines are hepatotoxic
Anxiolytics and Hypnotics	All can precipitate coma; small dose of oxazepam or temazepam probably safest; reduce oral dose of chlormethiazole
Aspirin	Avoid—increased risk of gastro-intestinal bleeding
Astemizole *see* Antihistamines	
Auranofin *see* Gold	
Aurothiomalate *see* Gold	
Azapropazone *see* NSAIDs	
Azatadine *see* Antihistamines	
Azathioprine	May need dose reduction
Bendrofluazide *see* Thiazides	
Benorylate [aspirin-paracetamol ester] *see* Aspirin	
Benperidol *see* Antipsychotics	
Benzodiazepines *see* Anxiolytics and Hypnotics	
Beta-blockers *see* individual drugs	
Bezafibrate	Avoid in severe liver disease
Bromazepam *see* Anxiolytics and Hypnotics	

Appendix 2: Liver disease

Table of drugs to be avoided or used with caution in liver disease (*continued*)

Drugs	Comment
Brompheniramine *see* Antihistamines	
Bumetanide *see* Loop Diuretics	
Bupivacaine *see* Lignocaine	
Buprenorphine *see* Opioid Analgesics	
Butriptyline *see* Antidepressants	
Carbenoxolone	Produces sodium and water retention and hypokalaemia
Cetirizine *see* Antihistamines	
Chenodeoxycholic Acid	Avoid in chronic liver disease; patients with non-functioning gall-bladder do not respond
Chloral Hydrate *see* Anxiolytics and Hypnotics	
Chloramphenicol	Avoid—increased risk of bone-marrow depression
Chlordiazepoxide *see* Anxiolytics and Hypnotics	
Chlormethiazole	Reduce oral dose; *see* Anxiolytics and Hypnotics
Chlormezanone *see* Anxiolytics and Hypnotics	
Chlorothiazide *see* Thiazides	
Chlorpheniramine *see* Antihistamines	
Chlorpromazine *see* Antipsychotics	
Chlorpropamide *see* Sulphonylureas	
Chlorthalidone *see* Thiazides	
Cholestyramine	Interferes with absorption of fat-soluble vitamins and may aggravate malabsorption in primary biliary cirrhosis
Choline Magnesium Trisalicylate *see* Aspirin	
Choline Theophyllinate *see* Theophylline	
Cimetidine	Increased risk of confusion; reduce dose
Cinnarizine *see* Antihistamines	
Cisapride	Halve dose initially
Clemastine *see* Antihistamines	
Clindamycin	Reduce dose
Clobazam *see* Anxiolytics and Hypnotics	
Clofibrate	Avoid in severe liver disease
Clomiphene	Avoid in severe liver disease
Clomipramine *see* Antidepressants, Tricyclic	
Clopamide *see* Thiazides	
Clorazepate *see* Anxiolytics and Hypnotics	
Clozapine *see* Antipsychotics	
Codeine *see* Opioid Analgesics	
Contraceptives, Oral	Avoid in active liver disease and in patients with a history of pruritus or cholestasis during pregnancy
Cyclizine *see* Antihistamines	
Cyclofenil	Avoid in severe liver disease
Cyclopenthiazide *see* Thiazides	
Cyproheptadine *see* Antihistamines	
Cyproterone Acetate	Avoid—dose-related toxicity
Dantrolene	Avoid—may cause severe liver damage
Dehydrocholic Acid	Avoid in intra-hepatic cholestasis or complete biliary obstruction
Desipramine *see* Antidepressants, Tricyclic	
Dextromethorphan *see* Opioid Analgesics	
Dextromoramide *see* Opioid Analgesics	
Dextropropoxyphene *see* Opioid Analgesics	
Diamorphine *see* Opioid Analgesics	
Diazepam *see* Anxiolytics and Hypnotics	
Diclofenac *see* NSAIDs	
Diflunisal *see* NSAIDs	
Dihydrocodeine *see* Opioid Analgesics	
Diltiazem	Reduce dose
Dimenhydrinate *see* Antihistamines	
Dimethindene *see* Antihistamines	
Diphenoxylate *see* Opioid Analgesics	
Diphenylpyraline *see* Antihistamines	
Dipipanone *see* Opioid Analgesics	
Dothiepin *see* Antidepressants, Tricyclic	
Doxepin *see* Antidepressants, Tricyclic	
Doxorubicin	Reduce dose according to bilirubin concentration
Droperidol *see* Antipsychotics	
Epirubicin	Reduce dose according to bilirubin concentration
Ergotamine	Avoid in severe liver disease—risk of toxicity increased
Erythromycin	May cause idiosyncratic hepatotoxicity
Ethacrynic Acid *see* Loop Diuretics	
Etodolac *see* NSAIDs	
Etretinate	Avoid—further impairment of liver function may occur
Felodipine	Reduce dose
Fenbufen *see* NSAIDs	
Fenofibrate *see* Clofibrate	
Fenoprofen *see* NSAIDs	
Fentanyl *see* Opioid Analgesics	
Flecainide	Avoid (or reduce dose) in severe liver disease
Flunitrazepam *see* Anxiolytics and Hypnotics	
Fluoxetine *see* Antidepressants, Serotonin-uptake Inhibitor	
Flupenthixol *see* Antipsychotics	
Fluphenazine *see* Antipsychotics	
Flurazepam *see* Anxiolytics and Hypnotics	
Flurbiprofen *see* NSAIDs	
Fluspirilene *see* Antipsychotics	
Fluvoxamine *see* Antidepressants, Serotonin-uptake Inhibitor	
Frusemide *see* Loop Diuretics	
Fusidic Acid	Impaired biliary excretion; may be increased risk of hepatotoxicity; avoid or reduce dose
Gemfibrozil	Avoid in severe liver disease
Glibenclamide *see* Sulphonylureas	
Gliclazide *see* Sulphonylureas	
Glipizide *see* Sulphonylureas	
Gliquidone *see* Sulphonylureas	
Gold (auranofin, aurothiomalate)	Avoid in severe liver disease—hepatotoxicity may occur
Haloperidol *see* Antipsychotics	
Hydrochlorothiazide *see* Thiazides	
Hydroflumethiazide *see* Thiazides	
Hydroxyzine *see* Antihistamines	
Hypnotics *see* Anxiolytics and Hypnotics	
Ibuprofen *see* NSAIDs	
Idarubicin	Reduce dose according to bilirubin concentration
Imipramine *see* Antidepressants, Tricyclic	
Indapamide *see* Thiazides	
Indomethacin *see* NSAIDs	
Iprindole *see* Antidepressants, Tricyclic (and related)	
Isocarboxazid *see* MAOIs	
Isoniazid	Avoid—idiosyncratic hepatotoxicity more common
Isotretinoin	Avoid—*see* Etretinate

Appendix 2: Liver disease 501

Table of drugs to be avoided or used with caution in liver disease (*continued*)

Drugs	Comment
Isradipine	Reduce dose
Itraconazole	Avoid—toxicity with related drugs
Ketoconazole	Induces hepatitis-like reaction; may accumulate in severe liver disease; contra-indicated unless no alternative
Ketoprofen *see* NSAIDs	
Ketorolac *see* NSAIDs	
Ketotifen *see* Antihistamines	
Labetalol	Avoid—severe hepatocellular injury reported
Lignocaine	Avoid (or reduce dose) in severe liver disease
Lofepramine *see* Antidepressants, Tricyclic	
Loop Diuretics	Hypokalaemia may precipitate coma; potassium-sparing diuretic should be used to prevent this; increased risk of hypomagnesaemia in alcoholic cirrhosis
Loprazolam *see* Anxiolytics and Hypnotics	
Lorazepam *see* Anxiolytics and Hypnotics	
Lormetazepam *see* Anxiolytics and Hypnotics	
Loxapine *see* Antipsychotics	
Magnesium Salts	Avoid in hepatic coma if risk of renal failure
MAOIs	May cause idiosyncratic hepatotoxicity
Maprotiline *see* Antidepressants, Tricyclic (and related)	
Mebhydrolin *see* Antihistamines	
Medazepam *see* Anxiolytics and Hypnotics	
Mefenamic Acid *see* NSAIDs	
Mefruside *see* Thiazides	
Meprobamate *see* Anxiolytics and Hypnotics	
Meptazinol *see* Opioid Analgesics	
Mequitazine *see* Antihistamines	
Metformin	Avoid—increased risk of lactic acidosis
Methadone *see* Opioid Analgesics	
Methohexitone	Avoid or reduce dose
Methotrexate	Dose-related toxicity—avoid in non-malignant conditions (e.g. psoriasis)
Methotrimeprazine *see* Antipsychotics	
Methoxsalen	Avoid or reduce dose
Methyclothiazide *see* Thiazides	
Methyldopa	Avoid—increased risk of hepatotoxicity
Metoclopramide	Reduce dose in severe liver disease
Metolazone *see* Thiazides	
Metoprolol	Reduce oral dose
Metronidazole	Reduce dose in severe liver disease
Mexiletine	Avoid (or reduce dose) in severe liver disease
Mianserin *see* Antidepressants, Tricyclic (and related)	
Monoamine-oxidase Inhibitors *see* MAOIs	
Morphine *see* Opioid Analgesics	
Nabumetone *see* NSAIDs	
Nalbuphine *see* Opioid Analgesics	
Nalidixic Acid	Partially conjugated in liver
Nandrolone *see* Anabolic Steroids	
Naproxen *see* NSAIDs	
Narcotic Analgesics *see* Opioid Analgesics	
Nicardipine	Reduce dose
Nifedipine	Reduce dose
Niridazole	Increased CNS toxicity in patients with cirrhosis or portal-systemic shunts
Nitrazepam *see* Anxiolytics and Hypnotics	
Nitroprusside	Avoid in severe liver disease
Nortriptyline *see* Antidepressants, Tricyclic	
NSAIDs	Increased risk of gastro-intestinal bleeding and can cause fluid retention
Oestrogens	Avoid; *see also* Contraceptives, oral
Omeprazole	In severe liver disease not more than 20 mg daily should be needed
Ondansetron	Reduce dose; not more than 8 mg daily in severe liver disease
Opioid Analgesics	Avoid—may precipitate coma
Oral Contraceptives *see* Contraceptives, Oral	
Oxatomide *see* Antihistamines	
Oxazepam *see* Anxiolytics and Hypnotics	
Oxprenolol	Reduce oral dose
Oxymetholone *see* Anabolic Steroids	
Oxypertine *see* Antipsychotics	
Papaveretum *see* Opioid Analgesics	
Paracetamol	Dose-related toxicity—avoid large doses
Paroxetine *see* Antidepressants, Serotonin-uptake Inhibitor	
Pentazocine *see* Opioid Analgesics	
Pericyazine *see* Antipsychotics	
Perphenazine *see* Antipsychotics	
Pethidine *see* Opioid Analgesics	
Phenazocine *see* Opioid Analgesics	
Phenelzine *see* MAOIs	
Phenindamine *see* Antihistamines	
Pheniramine *see* Antihistamines	
Phenobarbitone	May precipitate coma
Phenoperidine *see* Opioid Analgesics	
Phenothiazines *see* Antipsychotics	
Phenylbutazone *see* NSAIDs	
Phenytoin	Reduce dose to avoid toxicity
Pholcodine *see* Opioid Analgesics	
Pimozide *see* Antipsychotics	
Pipothiazine *see* Antipsychotics	
Piretanide *see* Loop Diuretics	
Piroxicam *see* NSAIDs	
Plicamycin	Avoid if possible (increased risk of toxicity)
Polythiazide *see* Thiazides	
Prednisolone	Side-effects more common
Prednisone	Prednisolone is preferable (prednisone needs conversion to prednisolone by liver before active)
Primidone	May precipitate coma
Procainamide	Avoid or reduce dose
Prochlorperazine *see* Antipsychotics	
Progestogens	Avoid; *see also* Contraceptives, Oral
Promazine *see* Antipsychotics	
Promethazine *see* Antihistamines	
Propafenone	Reduce dose
Propranolol	Reduce oral dose

Table of drugs to be avoided or used with caution in liver disease (continued)

Drugs	Comment
Protriptyline *see* Antidepressants, Tricyclic	
Pyrazinamide	Avoid—idiosyncratic hepatotoxicity more common
Ranitidine	Increased risk of confusion; reduce dose
Rifampicin	Impaired elimination; may be increased risk of hepatotoxicity; avoid or do not exceed 8 mg/kg daily
Salsalate *see* Aspirin	
Sertraline *see* Antidepressants, Serotonin-uptake Inhibitor	
Simvastatin	Avoid—hepatotoxic
Sodium Aurothiomalate *see* Gold	
Sodium Fusidate *see* Fusidic Acid	
Sodium Nitroprusside *see* Nitroprusside	
Sodium Valproate *see* Valproate	
Stanozolol *see* Anabolic Steroids	
Sulindac *see* NSAIDs	
Sulphonylureas	Increased risk of hypoglycaemia in severe liver disease; avoid or use small dose; can produce jaundice
Suxamethonium	Prolonged apnoea may occur in severe liver disease due to reduced hepatic synthesis of pseudocholinesterase
Temazepam *see* Anxiolytics and Hypnotics	
Tenoxicam *see* NSAIDs	
Terbinafine	Reduce dose
Terfenadine *see* Antihistamines	
Testosterone *see* Androgens	
Tetracyclines	Avoid—dose-related toxicity by i/v route
Theophylline	Reduce dose

Drugs	Comment
Thiazides	Hypokalaemia may precipitate coma (potassium-sparing diuretic can prevent); increased risk of hypomagnesaemia in alcoholic cirrhosis
Thiethylperazine *see* Antipsychotics	
Thiopentone	Reduce dose for induction in severe liver disease
Thioridazine *see* Antipsychotics	
Tiaprofenic acid *see* NSAIDs	
Tibolone	Avoid in severe liver disease
Tocainide	Avoid (or reduce dose) in severe liver disease
Tolazamide *see* Sulphonylureas	
Tolbutamide *see* Sulphonylureas	
Tolmetin *see* NSAIDs	
Tranylcypromine *see* MAOIs	
Trazodone *see* Antidepressants, Tricyclic (and related)	
Triclofos *see* Anxiolytics and Hypnotics	
Trifluoperazine *see* Antipsychotics	
Trifluperidol *see* Antipsychotics	
Trimeprazine *see* Antihistamines	
Trimipramine *see* Antidepressants, Tricyclic	
Triprolidine *see* Antihistamines	
Valproate	Avoid if possible—hepatotoxicity and liver failure may occasionally occur (usually in first 6 months)
Verapamil	Reduce oral dose
Zidovudine	Accumulation may occur
Zopiclone	Reduce dose
Zuclopenthixol *see* Antipsychotics	

Appendix 3: Renal Impairment

The use of drugs in patients with reduced renal function can give rise to problems for several reasons:

- failure to excrete a drug or its metabolites may produce toxicity;
- sensitivity to some drugs is increased even if elimination is unimpaired;
- many side-effects are tolerated poorly by patients in renal failure;
- some drugs cease to be effective when renal function is reduced.

Many of these problems can be avoided by reducing the dose or by using alternative drugs.

Principles of dose adjustment in renal impairment

The level of renal function below which the dose of a drug must be reduced depends on whether the drug is eliminated entirely by renal excretion or is partly metabolised, and on how toxic it is.

For many drugs with only minor or no dose-related side-effects very precise modification of the dose regimen is unnecessary and a simple scheme for dose reduction is sufficient.

For more toxic drugs with a small safety margin dose regimens based on glomerular filtration rate should be used. For those where both efficacy and toxicity are closely related to plasma concentrations recommended regimens should be seen only as a guide to initial treatment; subsequent treatment must be adjusted according to clinical response and plasma concentration.

The total daily maintenance dose of a drug can be reduced either by reducing the size of the individual doses or by increasing the interval between doses. For some drugs, if the size of the maintenance dose is reduced it will be important to give a loading dose if an immediate effect is required. This is because when a patient is given a regular dose of any drug it takes more than five times the half-life to achieve steady-state plasma concentrations. As the plasma half-life of drugs excreted by the kidney is prolonged in renal failure it may take many days for the reduced dosage to achieve a therapeutic plasma concentration. The loading dose should usually be the same size as the initial dose for a patient with normal renal function.

Nephrotoxic drugs should, if possible, be avoided in patients with renal disease because the consequences of nephrotoxicity are likely to be more serious when the renal reserve is already reduced.

Use of dosage table

Dose recommendations are based on the severity of renal impairment. This is expressed in terms of glomerular filtration rate (GFR), usually measured by the **creatinine clearance**. The serum-creatinine concentration can be used instead as a measure of renal function but is only a rough guide unless corrected for age, weight, and sex. Nomograms are available for making the correction and should be used where accuracy is important.

Renal impairment is arbitrarily divided into 3 grades:

Grade	GFR	Serum creatinine (approx.)
Mild	20–50 mL/min	150–300 μmol/litre
Moderate	10–20 mL/min	300–700 μmol/litre
Severe	< 10 mL/min	> 700 μmol/litre

Note. Conversion factors are:
Litres/24 hours = mL/minute × 1.44
mL/minute = Litres/24 hours × 0.69

Renal function declines with age; many elderly patients have a glomerular filtration rate below 50 mL/minute which, because of reduced muscle mass, may not be indicated by a raised serum creatinine. It is wise to assume at least mild impairment of renal function when prescribing for the elderly.

The following table may be used as a guide to drugs which are known to require a reduction in dose in renal impairment, and to those which are potentially harmful or are ineffective. Drug prescribing should be kept to the minimum in all patients with severe renal disease.

If renal impairment is considered likely on clinical grounds renal function should be checked before prescribing **any** drug which requires dose modification even when renal impairment is mild.

Table of drugs to be avoided or used with caution in renal impairment

Products introduced or amended since publication of BNF No. 23 (March 1992) are underlined.

Drug and Degree of impairment	Comment	Drug and Degree of impairment	Comment
Acebutolol *see* Beta-blockers		Acipimox	
Acemetacin *see* NSAIDs		Mild	Reduce dose
Acetazolamide		Acrivastine	
Mild	Avoid; metabolic acidosis	Moderate	Avoid; excreted by kidney

Appendix 3: Renal impairment

Table of drugs to be avoided or used with caution in renal impairment (*continued*)

Drug and Degree of impairment	Comment	Drug and Degree of impairment	Comment
Acyclovir		**Bacampicillin**	
Mild	Reduce dose; possible transient increase in plasma urea	Severe	Reduce dose; rashes more common
Alcuronium *see* Tubocurarine		**Baclofen**	
Alfentanil *see* Opioid Analgesics		Mild	Use smaller doses; excreted by kidney
Allopurinol		Bendrofluazide *see* Thiazides	
Moderate	Max. 200 mg daily; increased toxicity; rashes	Benorylate [aspirin-paracetamol ester] *see* Aspirin	
Severe	Max. 100 mg daily	Benperidol *see* Antipsychotics	
Alprazolam *see* Anxiolytics and Hypnotics		Benzodiazepines *see* Anxiolytics and Hypnotics	
Alteplase		**Benzylpenicillin**	
Moderate	Risk of hyperkalaemia	Severe	Max. 6 g daily; neurotoxicity—high doses may cause convulsions
Aluminium Salts			
Severe	Aluminium is absorbed and may accumulate	**Beta-blockers**	
Amantadine		Moderate	Start with small dose of acebutolol (active metabolite accumulates); reduce dose of atenolol, nadolol, pindolol, sotalol (all excreted unchanged)
Mild to moderate	Reduce dose; excreted by kidney		
Severe	Avoid		
Amikacin *see* Aminoglycosides			
Amiloride *see* Potassium-sparing Diuretics		Severe	Start with small dose; higher plasma concentrations after oral administration; may reduce renal blood flow and adversely affect renal function in severe impairment
Aminoglycosides			
Mild	Reduce dose; monitor plasma concentrations; ototoxic; nephrotoxic		
Amiodarone			
Moderate	Accumulation of iodine may increase risk of thyroid dysfunction	Betaxolol *see* Beta-blockers	
		Bethanidine	
		Moderate	Avoid; increased postural hypotension; decrease in renal blood flow
Amoxycillin			
Severe	Reduce dose; rashes more common	**Bezafibrate**	
Amphotericin		Mild to moderate	Reduce dose; further deterioration in renal function
Mild	Use only if no alternative; nephrotoxic	Severe	Avoid
Ampicillin		Bicarbonate *see* Sodium Bicarbonate	
Severe	Reduce dose; rashes more common	Bisoprolol *see* Beta-blockers	
		Bleomycin	
Amylobarbitone		Moderate	Reduce dose
Severe	Reduce dose; active metabolite accumulates	Bromazepam *see* Anxiolytics and Hypnotics	
Analgesics *see* Opioid Analgesics and NSAIDs		**Bumetanide**	
Antipsychotics		Moderate	May need high doses
Severe	Start with small doses; increased cerebral sensitivity; *see also* Sulpiride	Buprenorphine *see* Opioid Analgesics	
		Capreomycin	
Anxiolytics and Hypnotics		Mild	Reduce dose; nephrotoxic; ototoxic
Severe	Start with small doses; increased cerebral sensitivity	**Captopril**	
Aspirin		Mild	Reduce dose and monitor response; avoid if possible; excreted by kidney; hyperkalaemia and other side-effects more common (but specialised role in some forms of renal disease)
Severe	Avoid; fluid retention; deterioration in renal function; increased risk of gastro-intestinal bleeding		
Atenolol *see* Beta-blockers			
Auranofin *see* Gold			
Aurothiomalate *see* Gold		**Carbenicillin**	
Azapropazone *see* NSAIDs (excreted by kidney)		Moderate	Reduce dose; neurotoxic; may produce bleeding diathesis; 1 g contains 5.4 mmol sodium
Azathioprine			
Severe	Reduce dose		
Azlocillin			
Moderate	Reduce dose	**Carbenoxolone**	
Aztreonam		Moderate	Avoid; fluid retention
Moderate	Reduce dose	Carboplatin *see* Cisplatin	
		Carteolol *see* Beta-blockers	

Appendix 3: Renal impairment

Table of drugs to be avoided or used with caution in renal impairment (*continued*)

Drug and Degree of impairment	Comment
Cefadroxil	
Moderate	Reduce dose
Cefixime	
Moderate	Reduce dose
Cefodizime	
Moderate	Reduce dose
Cefotaxime	
Severe	Use half dose
Cefoxitin	
Mild	Reduce dose
Cefsulodin	
Moderate	Reduce dose
Ceftazidime	
Mild	Reduce dose
Ceftizoxime	
Mild	Reduce dose
Cefuroxime	
Mild	Reduce parenteral dose
Celiprolol *see* Beta-blockers	
Cephalexin	
Severe	Max. 500 mg daily
Cephamandole	
Mild	Reduce dose
Cephazolin	
Mild	Reduce dose
Cephradine	
Mild	Reduce dose
Cetirizine	
Moderate	Use half dose
Chloral Hydrate *see* Anxiolytics and Hypnotics	
Chloramphenicol	
Severe	Avoid unless no alternative; dose-related depression of haematopoiesis
Chlordiazepoxide *see* Anxiolytics and Hypnotics	
Chlormethiazole *see* Anxiolytics and Hypnotics	
Chlormezanone *see* Anxiolytics and Hypnotics	
Chloroquine	
Mild to moderate	Reduce dose; only on prolonged use
Severe	Avoid
Chlorothiazide *see* Thiazides	
Chlorpromazine *see* Antipsychotics	
Chlorpropamide	
Mild	Avoid; tolbutamide and gliquidone suitable alternatives
Chlorthalidone *see* Thiazides	
Choline Magnesium Trisalicylate *see* Aspirin	
Cilazapril	
Mild	Reduce dose and monitor response; avoid if possible; *see also* Captopril
Cimetidine	
Moderate	400–600 mg daily; occasional risk of confusion
Severe	400 mg daily
Cinoxacin	
Moderate	Avoid; nausea, rashes
Ciprofloxacin	
Moderate	Use half dose
Cisapride	
Moderate	Start with half dose
Cisplatin	
Mild	Avoid if possible; nephrotoxic

Drug and Degree of impairmant	Comment
Clarithromycin	
Moderate	Reduce dose
Clavulanic acid [ingredient] *see* Co-amoxiclav, Timentin®	
Clobazam *see* Anxiolytics and Hypnotics	
Clodronate sodium	
Moderate	Avoid
Clofibrate	
Mild to moderate	Reduce dose; further deterioration in renal function; myopathy
Severe	Avoid
Clopamide *see* Thiazides	
Clorazepate *see* Anxiolytics and Hypnotics	
Clozapine *see* Antipsychotics	
Co-amoxiclav	
Moderate	Reduce dose
Codeine	
Moderate	Avoid; increased and prolonged effect; *see also* Opioid Analgesics
Colchicine	
Severe	Avoid or reduce dose if no alternative
Colistin	
Mild	Reduce dose; nephrotoxic; neurotoxic
Colven®	
Severe	Avoid; high sodium content
Co-trimoxazole	
Moderate	Reduce dose; rashes and blood disorders; may cause further deterioration in renal function
Cyclopenthiazide *see* Thiazides	
Cyclophosphamide	
Moderate	Reduce dose
Cycloserine	
Mild to moderate	Reduce dose
Severe	Avoid
Cyclosporin *see* section 8.2.2	
Debrisoquine	
Moderate	Avoid; increased postural hypotension; decrease in renal blood flow
De-Nol®, De-Noltab®	
Severe	Avoid
Dextromethorphan *see* Opioid Analgesics	
Dextromoramide *see* Opioid Analgesics	
Dextropropoxyphene	
Severe	Avoid; increased CNS toxicity
Diamorphine *see* Opioid Analgesics	
Diazepam *see* Anxiolytics and Hypnotics	
Diazoxide	
Severe	75–150 mg i/v; increased sensitivity to hypotensive effect
Dicapen®	
Severe	Reduce dose
Diclofenac *see* NSAIDs	
Diflunisal *see* NSAIDs (excreted by kidney)	
Digitoxin	
Severe	Max. 100 micrograms daily; *see also* Digoxin

Appendix 3: Renal impairment

Table of drugs to be avoided or used with caution in renal impairment (*continued*)

Drug and Degree of impairment	Comment	Drug and Degree of impairment	Comment
Digoxin		**Fluoxetine**	
Mild	250 micrograms daily; toxicity increased by electrolyte disturbances	Moderate	Start with smaller dose
		Severe	Avoid
Moderate	125–250 micrograms daily	**Flupenthixol** *see* Antipsychotics	
Severe	Up to 125 micrograms daily	**Fluphenazine** *see* Antipsychotics	
Dihydrocodeine		**Flurazepam** *see* Anxiolytics and Hypnotics	
Moderate	Avoid; increased and prolonged effect; *see also* Opioid Analgesics	**Flurbiprofen** *see* NSAIDs	
		Fluspirilene *see* Antipsychotics	
Diphenoxylate *see* Opioid Analgesics		**Fluvoxamine**	
Dipipanone *see* Opioid Analgesics		Moderate	Start with smaller dose
Disopyramide		**Foscarnet**	
Mild	100 mg every 8 hours *or* 150 mg every 12 hours	Mild	Reduce dose; consult data sheet
Moderate	100 mg every 12 hours	**Fosinopril**	
Severe	150 mg every 24 hours	Mild	Start with 10 mg daily; *see also* Captopril
Domperidone		**Frusemide**	
Severe	Reduce dose by 30–50%	Moderate	May need high doses; deafness may follow rapid i/v injection
Droperidol *see* Antipsychotics			
Enalapril			
Mild	Reduce dose and monitor response; avoid if possible; *see also* Captopril	***Fybogel*®**	
		Severe	Avoid; contains 7 mmol potassium per sachet
Enoxacin		**Gallamine**	
Moderate	Max. 400 mg daily	Moderate	Avoid; prolonged paralysis
Ephedrine		**Ganciclovir**	
Severe	Avoid; increased CNS toxicity	Mild	Reduce dose; consult data sheet
Ergotamine		***Gaviscon*®**	
Moderate	Avoid; nausea and vomiting; risk of renal vasoconstriction	Severe	Avoid; high sodium content
		Gemfibrozil	
Erythromycin		Severe	Start with 900 mg daily
Severe	Max. 1.5 g daily (ototoxicity)	**Gentamicin** *see* Aminoglycosides	
Ethacrynic Acid		**Glibenclamide**	
Severe	Avoid; ototoxic	Severe	Avoid; increased risk of prolonged hypoglycaemia
Ethambutol			
Mild	Reduce dose; optic nerve damage	**Gliclazide**	
		Severe	Start with small dose; increased risk of hypoglycaemia
Etidronate Disodium			
Mild	Max. 5 mg/kg daily; excreted by kidney	**Glipizide**	
Moderate	Avoid	Severe	Start with small dose; increased risk of hypoglycaemia
Etodolac *see* NSAIDs			
Etoposide		**Gliquidone**	
Mild	Reduce dose	Severe	May need dose reduction; increased risk of hypoglycaemia
Etretinate			
Mild	Avoid; increased risk of toxicity	**Gold** (auranofin, aurothiomalate)	
		Mild	Avoid; nephrotoxic
Famotidine		**Guanethidine**	
Severe	Reduce dose	Moderate	Avoid; increased postural hypotension and decrease in renal blood flow
Fenbufen *see* NSAIDs			
Fenofibrate			
Mild	200 mg daily	**Haloperidol** *see* Antipsychotics	
Moderate	100 mg daily	**Hexamine**	
Fenoprofen *see* NSAIDs		Mild	Avoid; ineffective
Fentanyl *see* Opioid Analgesics		**Hydralazine**	
Flecainide		Moderate	Start with small dose; increased hypotensive effect
Mild	Reduce dose		
Fluconazole		**Hydrochlorothiazide** *see* Thiazides	
Mild	Reduce dose for multiple dose therapy	**Hydroflumethiazide** *see* Thiazides	
		Hydroxychloroquine	
Flucytosine		Mild to moderate	Reduce dose; only on prolonged use
Mild	Reduce dose	Severe	Avoid
Flunitrazepam *see* Anxiolytics and Hypnotics			

Appendix 3: Renal impairment

Table of drugs to be avoided or used with caution in renal impairment (*continued*)

Drug and Degree of impairment	Comment
Hypnotics *see* Anxiolytics and Hypnotics	
Ibuprofen *see* NSAIDs	
Idarubicin	
Mild	Reduce dose
Ifosfamide	
Moderate	Reduce dose
Indapamide *see* Thiazides	
Indomethacin *see* NSAIDs	
Inosine Pranobex	
Mild	Avoid; metabolised to uric acid
Insulin	
Severe	May need dose reduction; insulin requirements fall; compensatory response to hypoglycaemia is impaired
Isoniazid	
Severe	Max. 200 mg daily; peripheral neuropathy
Isotretinoin	
Mild	Avoid; increased risk of toxicity
Kanamycin *see* Aminoglycosides	
Ketoprofen *see* NSAIDs	
Ketorolac *see* NSAIDs	
Lisinopril	
Mild	Reduce dose and monitor response; *see also* Captopril
Lithium	
Mild	Avoid if possible or reduce dose and monitor plasma concentration carefully
Moderate	Avoid
Loprazolam *see* Anxiolytics and Hypnotics	
Lorazepam *see* Anxiolytics and Hypnotics	
Lormetazepam *see* Anxiolytics and Hypnotics	
Loxapine *see* Antipsychotics	
Magnesium Salts	
Moderate	Avoid or reduce dose; increased risk of toxicity; magnesium carbonate mixture and magnesium trisilicate mixture also have high sodium content
Medazepam *see* Anxiolytics and Hypnotics	
Mefenamic Acid *see* NSAIDs	
Mefruside *see* Thiazides	
<u>Mefloquine</u>	
Mild	Avoid prophylactic use
Melphalan	
Moderate	Reduce dose
Meprobamate *see* Anxiolytics and Hypnotics	
Meptazinol *see* Opioid Analgesics	
Mercaptopurine	
Moderate	Reduce dose
Mesalazine	
Mild	Avoid; nephrotoxic
Metformin	
Mild	Avoid; increased risk of lactic acidosis
Methadone *see* Opioid Analgesics	
Methocarbamol	
Mild	Avoid; increased plasma urea and acidosis due to solvent in injection
Methotrexate	
Mild	Reduce dose; accumulates; nephrotoxic
Moderate	Avoid
Methotrimeprazine *see* Antipsychotics	
Methyclothiazide *see* Thiazides	
Methyldopa	
Moderate	Start with small dose; increased sensitivity to hypotensive and sedative effect
Metoclopramide	
Severe	Avoid or use small dose; increased risk of extrapyramidal reactions
Metolazone *see* Thiazides	
Metoprolol *see* Beta-blockers	
Milrinone	
Mild	Reduce dose and monitor response
Morphine	
Moderate	Avoid; increased and prolonged effect; *see also* Opioid Analgesics
Nabumetone *see* NSAIDs	
Nadolol *see* Beta-blockers	
Nalbuphine *see* Opioid Analgesics	
Nalidixic Acid	
Moderate	Avoid; increased risk of nausea, vomiting, rashes, photosensitivity; ineffective because of inadequate urine concentration
Naproxen *see* NSAIDs	
Narcotic Analgesics *see* Opioid Analgesics	
Neomycin	
Mild	Avoid; ototoxic; nephrotoxic
Netilmicin *see* Aminoglycosides	
Nicardipine	
Moderate	Start with small dose
Nifedipine	
Moderate	Start with small dose; reversible deterioration in renal function has been reported
Nitrazepam *see* Anxiolytics and Hypnotics	
Nitrofurantoin	
Mild	Avoid; peripheral neuropathy; ineffective because of inadequate urine concentrations
Nitroprusside	
Moderate	Avoid prolonged use
Nizatidine	
Mild	150 mg daily
Moderate	150 mg on alternate days
Norfloxacin	
Moderate	Use half dose
Severe	Avoid
NSAIDs	
Mild	Avoid if possible; deterioration in renal function (**important**: see section 10.1.1); sodium and water retention

Appendix 3: Renal impairment

Table of drugs to be avoided or used with caution in renal impairment (*continued*)

Drug and Degree of impairment	Comment
Ofloxacin	
Mild	Use half dose
Moderate	100 mg every 48 hours
Opioid Analgesics	
Moderate	Use small doses—avoid codeine, dihydrocodeine, morphine; increased cerebral sensitivity; *see also* individual entries
Severe	Avoid dextropropoxyphene, pethidine
Oxazepam *see* Anxiolytics and Hypnotics	
Oxprenolol *see* Beta-blockers	
Oxypertine *see* Antipsychotics	
Pamidronate Disodium	
Severe	Divide daily dose
Pancuronium *see* Tubucurarine	
Papaveretum *see* Opioid Analgesics	
Paroxetine	
Moderate	Start with smaller dose
Penbutolol *see* Beta-blockers	
Penicillamine	
Mild	Avoid if possible or reduce dose; nephrotoxic
Pentamidine	
Mild	Reduce dose; consult data sheet
Pentazocine *see* Opioid Analgesics	
Pericyazine *see* Antipsychotics	
Perindopril	
Mild	Reduce dose and monitor response; *see also* Captopril
Perphenazine *see* Antipsychotics	
Pethidine	
Severe	Avoid; increased CNS toxicity; *see also* Opioid Analgesics
Phenazocine *see* Opioid Analgesics	
Phenobarbitone	
Severe	Avoid large doses
Phenoperidine *see* Opioid Analgesics	
Phenothiazines *see* Antipsychotics	
Phenylbutazone *see* NSAIDs	
Pholcodine *see* Opioid Analgesics	
Pimozide *see* Antipsychotics	
Pindolol *see* Beta-blockers	
Piperacillin	
Moderate	Reduce dose
Piperazine	
Severe	Reduce dose; neurotoxic
Pipothiazine *see* Antipsychotics	
Piroxicam *see* NSAIDs	
Pivampicillin	
Severe	Reduce dose; rashes more common
Plicamycin	
Moderate	Avoid if possible
Polythiazide *see* Thiazides	
Potassium Salts	
Moderate	Avoid routine use; high risk of hyperkalaemia

Drug and Degree of impairment	Comment
Potassium-sparing Diuretics	
Mild	Monitor plasma K^+; high risk of hyperkalaemia in renal impairment; amiloride excreted by kidney unchanged
Moderate	Avoid
Povidone-iodine	
Severe	Avoid regular application to inflamed or broken mucosa
Prazosin	
Severe	Start with small dose; increased sensitivity to hypotensive effect and possible CNS toxicity
Primaxin®	
Mild	Reduce dose
Primidone	
Severe	Avoid large doses
Probenecid	
Moderate	Avoid; ineffective and toxicity increased
Procainamide	
Mild	Avoid or reduce dose
Procarbazine	
Moderate	Reduce dose
Prochlorperazine *see* Antipsychotics	
Proguanil	
Severe	Avoid or reduce dose; increased risk of haematological toxicity
Promazine *see* Antipsychotics	
Propranolol *see* Beta-blockers	
Propylthiouracil	
Mild	Reduce dose
Pseudoephedrine	
Severe	Avoid; increased CNS toxicity
Quinapril	
Mild	Start with 2.5 mg daily; *see also* Captopril
Ramipril	
Mild	Start with 1.25 mg daily; *see also* Captopril
Ranitidine	
Severe	Use half normal dose; occasional risk of confusion
Regulan®	
Severe	Avoid; contains 6.4 mmol potassium per sachet
Remoxipride *see* Antipsychotics	
Salicylates *see* Aspirin	
Salsalate *see* Aspirin	
Salt Substitutes	
Moderate	Avoid routine use; high risk of hyperkalaemia
Sertraline	Manufacturer recommends avoid
Sodium Aurothiomalate *see* Gold	
Sodium Bicarbonate	
Severe	Avoid; specialised role in some forms of renal disease
Sodium Nitroprusside *see* Nitroprusside	
Sodium Salts	
Severe	Avoid

Appendix 3: Renal impairment

Table of drugs to be avoided or used with caution in renal impairment (*continued*)

Drug and Degree of impairment	Comment	Drug and Degree of impairmant	Comment
Solpadeine®		Thiethylperazine *see* Antipsychotics	
Severe	Avoid; high sodium content	Thioguanine	
Sotalol *see* Beta-blockers		Moderate	Reduce dose
Spironolactone *see* Potassium-sparing Diuretics		Thioridazine *see* Antipsychotics	
Streptomycin *see* Aminoglycosides		Tiaprofenic Acid *see* NSAIDs	
Sucralfate		Ticarcillin	
Severe	Avoid; aluminium is absorbed and may accumulate	Moderate	Reduce dose; 1 g contains 5.3 mmol sodium
		Timentin®	
Sulbactam		Moderate	Reduce dose
Moderate	Reduce dose	Timolol *see* Beta-blockers	
Sulfametopyrazine *see* Sulphonamides		Tobramycin *see* Aminoglycosides	
Sulindac *see* NSAIDs (excreted by kidney)		Tocainide	
Sulphadiazine		Mild	Reduce dose
Severe	Avoid; high risk of crystalluria	Tolazamide	
Sulphadimidine *see* Sulphonamides		Severe	May need dose reduction; increased risk of hypoglycaemia
Sulphasalazine			
Severe	Ensure high fluid intake; rashes and blood disorders; crystalluria a risk	Tolbutamide	
		Severe	May need dose reduction; increased risk of hypoglycaemia
Sulphinpyrazone			
Moderate	Avoid; ineffective as uricosuric	Tolmetin *see* NSAIDs (excreted by kidney)	
		Triamterene *see* Potassium-sparing Diuretics	
Sulphonamides		Triclofos *see* Anxiolytics and Hypnotics	
Moderate	Ensure high fluid intake; rashes and blood disorders; crystalluria a risk	Trifluoperazine *see* Antipsychotics	
		Trifluperidol *see* Antipsychotics	
		Trimethoprim	
Sulphonylureas *see under* individual drugs		Moderate	Reduce dose
Sulpiride		Tubocurarine	
Moderate	Avoid if possible, or reduce dose	Moderate	Reduce dose; prolonged paralysis with large or repeated doses
Teicoplanin			
Mild	Reduce dose after 4 days	Tulobuterol	
Temazepam *see* Anxiolytics and Hypnotics		Mild	May need dose reduction; excreted by kidney
Temocillin			
Moderate	Reduce dose	Vancomycin	
Tenoxicam *see* NSAIDs		Mild	Avoid parenteral use if possible; ototoxic; nephrotoxic
Terbinafine			
Mild	Use half normal dose		
Tetracyclines (except doxycycline and minocycline)		Vecuronium *see* Tubocurarine	
Mild	Avoid—use doxycycline or minocycline if necessary; anti-anabolic effect, increased plasma urea, further deterioration in renal function	Vigabatrin	
		Mild	Reduce dose; excreted by kidney
		Xamoterol	
		Moderate	Reduce dose; excreted by kidney
Thiazides and Related Diuretics (except metolazone)		Xipamide *see* Thiazides	
		Zidovudine	
Moderate	Avoid; ineffective (metolazone remains effective but risk of excessive diuresis)	Mild	Excreted by kidney; increased risk of toxicity
		Zuclopenthixol *see* Antipsychotics	

Appendix 4: Pregnancy

Drugs can have harmful effects on the fetus at any time during pregnancy. Experience with many drugs in pregnancy is limited.

During the *first trimester* they may produce congenital malformations (teratogenesis), and the period of greatest risk is from the third to the eleventh week of pregnancy.

During the *second* and *third trimesters* drugs may affect the growth and functional development of the fetus or have toxic effects on fetal tissues; and drugs given shortly before term or during labour may have adverse effects on labour or on the neonate after delivery.

The following table lists drugs which may have harmful effects in pregnancy and indicates the trimester of risk.

The table is based on human data but information on *animal* studies has been included for some newer drugs when its omission might be misleading.

> Drugs should be prescribed in pregnancy only if the expected benefit to the mother is thought to be greater than the risk to the fetus, and all drugs should be avoided if possible during the first trimester. Drugs which have been extensively used in pregnancy and appear to be usually safe should be prescribed in preference to new or untried drugs; and the smallest effective dose should be used.
>
> Few drugs have been shown conclusively to be teratogenic in man but no drug is safe beyond all doubt in early pregnancy. Screening procedures are available where there is a known risk of certain defects.
>
> It should be noted that the BNF provides independent advice and may not always agree with the data sheets.
>
> Absence of a drug from the list does not imply safety.

Table of drugs to be avoided or used with caution in pregnancy
Products introduced or amended since publication of BNF No. 23 (March 1992) are <u>underlined</u>.

Drug (Trimester of risk)	Comments
ACE Inhibitors (2, 3)	Avoid; may adversely affect fetal and neonatal blood pressure control and renal function; also possible skull defects and oligohydramnios; toxicity in *animal* studies
Acebutolol *see* Beta-blockers	
Acemetacin *see* NSAIDs	
Acetazolamide *see* Diuretics	
Acetohexamide *see* Sulphonylureas	
Acrivastine *see* Antihistamines	
Alclometasone *see* Corticosteroids	
Alcohol (1, 2)	Regular daily drinking is teratogenic ('fetal alcohol syndrome') and may cause growth retardation; occasional single drinks are probably safe
(3)	Withdrawal syndrome may occur in babies of alcoholic mothers
Alfentanil *see* Opioid Analgesics	
Allyloestrenol *see* Progestogens	
Alprazolam *see* Anxiolytics and Hypnotics	
Alteplase *see* Streptokinase	
Amikacin *see* Aminoglycosides	
Amiloride *see* Diuretics	
Aminoglutethimide	Avoid; toxicity in *animal* studies and may affect fetal sexual development
Aminoglycosides (2, 3)	Auditory or vestibular nerve damage; risk greatest with streptomycin; probably very small with gentamicin and tobramycin
Aminophylline *see* Theophylline	

Drug (Trimester of risk)	Comments
Amiodarone (2, 3)	Possible risk of neonatal goitre; use only if no alternative
Amitriptyline *see* Antidepressants, Tricyclic	
Amlodipine *see* Calcium-channel Blockers	
Amoxapine *see* Antidepressants, Tricyclic	
Amylobarbitone *see* Barbiturates	
Anabolic Steroids (1, 2, 3)	Masculinisation of female fetus
Anaesthetics, General (3)	Depress neonatal respiration
Anaesthetics, Local (3)	With large doses, neonatal respiratory depression, hypotonia, and bradycardia after paracervical or epidural block
Analgesics *see* Opioid Analgesics and NSAIDs	
Androgens (1, 2, 3)	Masculinisation of female fetus
Anistreplase *see* Streptokinase	
Anticoagulants	
Heparin (1, 2, 3)	Osteoporosis has been reported after prolonged use
Oral Anticoagulants (1, 2, 3)	Congenital malformations; fetal and neonatal haemorrhage See also section 2.8
Antidepressants	
Fluoxetine, Fluvoxamine, MAOIs, Paroxetine, Sertraline (1, 2, 3)	No evidence of harm but manufacturers advise avoid unless compelling reasons
Tricyclic (and related) (3)	Tachycardia, irritability, muscle spasms, and convulsions in neonate reported occasionally

Appendix 4: Pregnancy

Table of drugs to be avoided or used with caution in pregnancy (*continued*)

Drug (Trimester of risk)	Comments	Drug (Trimester of risk)	Comments
Antiepileptics	Benefit of treatment outweighs risk to fetus; risk of teratogenicity greater if more than one drug used; **important:** see also carbamazepine, ethosuximide, phenobarbitone, phenytoin, valproate, and section 4.8	Benzodiazepines *see* Anxiolytics and Hypnotics	
		Beta-blockers (3)	May cause intra-uterine growth retardation, neonatal hypoglycaemia, and bradycardia; risk greater in severe hypertension
		Betamethasone *see* Corticosteroids	
		Betaxolol *see* Beta-blockers	
		Bethanidine *see* Guanethidine	
Antihistamines	No evidence of teratogenicity; some packs of antihistamines sold to the public carry warning to avoid in pregnancy; manufacturer of astemizole advises toxicity at high doses in *animal* studies	Bezafibrate *see* Clofibrate	
		Bisoprolol *see* Beta-blockers	
		Bisphosphonates	Manufacturers advise avoid (on theoretical grounds)
		Bromazepam *see* Anxiolytics and Hypnotics	
		Brompheniramine *see* Antihistamines	
		Budesonide *see* Corticosteroids	
		Bumetanide *see* Diuretics	
Antimalarials (1, 3)	Benefit of prophylaxis and treatment in malaria outweighs risk; **important:** *see also* individual drugs	Bupivacaine *see* Anaesthetics, Local	
		Buprenorphine *see* Opioid Analgesics	
		Butriptyline *see* Antidepressants, Tricyclic	
Antipsychotics (3)	Extrapyramidal effects in neonate occasionally reported	Calcium-channel Blockers	May inhibit labour and manufacturers advise that diltiazem and some dihydropyridines are teratogenic in *animals*
Anxiolytics and Hypnotics (3)	Depress neonatal respiration. Benzodiazepines cause neonatal drowsiness, hypotonia, and withdrawal symptoms; avoid large doses and regular use; short-acting benzodiazepines preferable to long-acting		
		Capreomycin	Manufacturer advises teratogenic in *animal* studies
		Captopril *see* ACE Inhibitors	
		Carbamazepine (1)	May be small risk of teratogenesis including increased risk of neural tube defects (screening advised); *see also* Antiepileptics
Aspirin (3)	Impaired platelet function and risk of haemorrhage; delayed onset and increased duration of labour with increased blood loss; avoid analgesic doses if possible in last week (low doses probably not harmful); with high doses, closure of fetal ductus arteriosus *in utero* and possibly persistent pulmonary hypertension of newborn; kernicterus in jaundiced neonates	Carbenoxolone (3)	Avoid; causes sodium retention with oedema
		Carbimazole (2, 3)	Neonatal goitre and hypothyroidism. Has been associated with aplasia cutis of the neonate
		Celiprolol *see* Beta-blockers	
		Cetirizine *see* Antihistamines	
		Chenodeoxycholic Acid (1, 2, 3)	Theoretical risk of effects on fetal metabolism
		Chloral hydrate *see* Anxiolytics and Hypnotics	
		Chloramphenicol (3)	Neonatal 'grey syndrome'
Astemizole *see* Antihistamines		Chlordiazepoxide *see* Anxiolytics and Hypnotics	
Atenolol *see* Beta-blockers		Chlormethiazole *see* Anxiolytics and Hypnotics	
Auranofin *see* Gold		Chlormezanone *see* Anxiolytics and Hypnotics	
Aurothiomalate *see* Gold		Chloroquine *see* Antimalarials	
Azapropazone *see* NSAIDs		Chlorothiazide *see* Diuretics	
Azatadine *see* Antihistamines		Chlorpheniramine *see* Antihistamines	
Azathioprine (1)	Spontaneous abortion may be more common (see section 8.1)	Chlorpromazine *see* Antipsychotics	
		Chlorpropamide *see* Sulphonylureas	
Azelastine *see* Antihistamines		Chlorprothixene *see* Antipsychotics	
Aztreonam	Manufacturer advises avoid (but no evidence of teratogenicity)	Chlortetracycline *see* Tetracyclines	
		Chlorthalidone *see* Diuretics	
		Choline magnesium trisalicylate *see* Aspirin	
Barbiturates (3)	Withdrawal effects in neonate; *see also* Phenobarbitone	Cilazapril *see* ACE Inhibitors	
		Cinnarizine *see* Antihistamines	
		Ciprofloxacin *see* 4-Quinolones	
Beclomethasone *see* Corticosteroids		Cisapride	Manufacturer advises avoid
Bendrofluazide *see* Diuretics		Clemastine *see* Antihistamines	
Benorylate [aspirin-paracetamol ester] *see* Aspirin		Clobazam *see* Anxiolytics and Hypnotics	
Benperidol *see* Antipsychotics		Clobetasol *see* Corticosteroids	
Benserazide [ingredient] *see* Madopar®		Clobetasone *see* Corticosteroids	

Table of drugs to be avoided or used with caution in pregnancy (continued)

Drug (Trimester of risk)	Comments
Clodronate sodium *see* Bisphosphonates	
Clofibrate (1, 2, 3)	Avoid—theoretical possibility of interference with embryonic growth and development due to anticholesterol effect
Clomiphene	Possible effects on fetal development
Clomipramine *see* Antidepressants, Tricyclic	
Clomocycline *see* Tetracyclines	
Clonazepam *see* Antiepileptics	
Clorazepate *see* Anxiolytics and Hypnotics	
Clozapine	Manufacturer advises avoid
Codeine *see* Opioid Analgesics	
Contraceptives, Oral	Epidemiological evidence suggests no harmful effects on fetus
Corticosteroids (2, 3)	Benefit of treatment, e.g. in asthma, outweighs risk; high doses (>10 mg prednisolone daily) may produce fetal and neonatal adrenal suppression; corticosteroid cover required by mother during labour
Co-trimoxazole (1)	Possible teratogenic risk (trimethoprim a folate antagonist)
(3)	Neonatal haemolysis and methaemoglobinaemia; fear of increased risk of kernicterus in neonates appears to be unfounded
Cyclizine *see* Antihistamines	
Cyclopenthiazide *see* Diuretics	
Cyclopropane *see* Anaesthetics, General	
Cyclosporin	May cause fetal growth retardation; *see also* section 8.1
Cyproheptadine *see* Antihistamines	
Cyproterone [ingredient] *see* Dianette®	
Cytotoxic drugs (1)	Most are teratogenic; *see* section 8.1
Danazol (1, 2, 3)	Has weak androgenic effects and virilisation of female fetus reported
Dapsone (3)	Neonatal haemolysis and methaemoglobinaemia; folate supplements should be given to mother
Debrisoquine *see* Guanethidine	
Demeclocycline *see* Tetracyclines	
Desferrioxamine	Manufacturer advises toxicity in *animal* studies
Desipramine *see* Antidepressants, Tricyclic	
Desonide *see* Corticosteroids	
Desoxymethasone *see* Corticosteroids	
Dexamethasone *see* Corticosteroids	
Dextromethorphan *see* Opioid Analgesics	
Dextromoramide *see* Opioid Analgesics	
Dextropropoxyphene *see* Opioid Analgesics	
Diamorphine *see* Opioid Analgesics	
Dianette® (1, 2, 3)	Feminisation of male fetus (due to cyproterone)
Diazepam *see* Anxiolytics and Hypnotics	
Diazoxide (2, 3)	Prolonged use may produce alopecia and impaired glucose tolerance in neonate; inhibits uterine activity during labour
Diclofenac *see* NSAIDs	
Diethylpropion	Avoid—congenital malformations reported to CSM
Diflucortolone *see* Corticosteroids	
Diflunisal *see* NSAIDs	
Dihydrocodeine *see* Opioid Analgesics	
Dihydroergotamine *see* Ergotamine	
Diltiazem *see* Calcium-channel Blockers	
Dimenhydrinate *see* Antihistamines	
Dimethindene *see* Antihistamines	
Diphenhydramine *see* Antihistamines	
Diphenoxylate *see* Opioid Analgesics	
Diphenylpyraline *see* Antihistamines	
Dipipanone *see* Opioid Analgesics	
Disodium Etidronate *see* Bisphosphonates	
Disodium Pamidronate *see* Bisphosphonates	
Disopyramide (3)	May induce labour
Distigmine	Manufacturer advises avoid (may stimulate uterine contractions)
Disulfiram (1)	High concentrations of acetaldehyde which occur in presence of alcohol may be teratogenic
Diuretics (3)	Not used to treat hypertension in pregnancy; thiazides may cause neonatal thrombocytopenia
Dothiepin *see* Antidepressants, Tricyclic	
Doxepin *see* Antidepressants, Tricyclic	
Doxycycline *see* Tetracyclines	
Droperidol *see* Antipsychotics	
Dydrogesterone *see* Progestogens	
Enalapril *see* ACE Inhibitors	
Enflurane *see* Anaesthetics, General	
Enoxacin *see* 4-Quinolones	
Ergotamine (1, 2, 3)	Oxytocic effects on the pregnant uterus
Ethacrynic acid *see* Diuretics	
Ether *see* Anaesthetics, General	
Ethinyloestradiol *see* Contraceptives, Oral	
Ethionamide (1)	May be teratogenic
Ethosuximide (1)	May possibly be teratogenic; *see* Antiepileptics
Etidronate Disodium *see* Bisphosphonates	
Etodolac *see* NSAIDs	
Etomidate *see* Anaesthetics, General	
Etretinate (1, 2, 3)	Teratogenic; effective contraception must be used for at least 1 month before treatment, during treatment, and for at least two years after stopping

Appendix 4: Pregnancy 513

Table of drugs to be avoided or used with caution in pregnancy (*continued*)

Drug (Trimester of risk)	Comments
Fansidar[®]	
(1)	Possible teratogenic risk (pyrimethamine a folate antagonist)
(3)	Neonatal haemolysis and methaemoglobinaemia; fear of increased risk of kernicterus in neonates appears to be unfounded *see also* Antimalarials
Felodipine *see* Calcium-channel Blockers	
Fenbufen *see* NSAIDs	
Fenofibrate (1, 2, 3)	Manufacturer advises toxicity in *animal* studies; *see also* Clofibrate
Fenoprofen *see* NSAIDs	
Fentanyl *see* Opioid Analgesics	
Flecainide	Manufacturer advises toxicity in *animal* studies
Fluclorolone *see* Corticosteroids	
Fluconazole	Manufacturer advises toxicity at high doses in *animal* studies
Flucytosine (1)	Possible teratogenic risk
Flunitrazepam *see* Anxiolytics and Hypnotics	
Fluocinolone *see* Corticosteroids	
Fluocinonide *see* Corticosteroids	
Fluocortolone *see* Corticosteroids	
Fluoxetine *see* Antidepressants	
Flupenthixol *see* Antipsychotics	
Fluphenazine *see* Antipsychotics	
Flurandrenolone *see* Corticosteroids	
Flurazepam *see* Anxiolytics and Hypnotics	
Flurbiprofen *see* NSAIDs	
Fluspirilene *see* Antipsychotics	
Fluvoxamine *see* Antidepressants	
Foscarnet	Manufacturer advises avoid
Fosinopril *see* ACE Inhibitors	
Frusemide *see* Diuretics	
Ganciclovir	Avoid—teratogenic risk
Gemfibrozil *see* Clofibrate	
Gentamicin *see* Aminoglycosides	
Gestrinone (1, 2, 3)	Avoid
Glibenclamide *see* Sulphonylureas	
Gliclazide *see* Sulphonylureas	
Glipizide *see* Sulphonylureas	
Gliquidone *see* Sulphonylureas	
Gold	
Auranofin	Manufacturer advises teratogenicity in *animal* studies; effective contraception should be used during and for at least 6 months after treatment
Aurothiomalate (1, 2, 3)	No good evidence of harm but avoid if possible
Griseofulvin	CRM advises avoid (fetotoxicity and teratogenicity in *animals*)
Growth Hormone	Avoid on theoretical grounds
Guanethidine (3)	Postural hypotension and reduced uteroplacental perfusion; should not be used to treat hypertension in pregnancy

Drug (Trimester of risk)	Comments
Halcinonide *see* Corticosteroids	
Halofantrine (1)	Manufacturer advises teratogenicity in *animal* studies
Haloperidol *see* Antipsychotics	
Halothane *see* Anaesthetics, General	
Heparin *see* Anticoagulants	
Hydralazine (1)	Manufacturer advises toxicity in *animal* studies
Hydrochlorothiazide *see* Diuretics	
Hydrocortisone *see* Corticosteroids	
Hydroflumethiazide *see* Diuretics	
Hydroxychloroquine	Avoid for rheumatic disease (but for malaria *see* Antimalarials)
Hydroxyprogesterone *see* Progestogens	
Hydroxyzine *see* Antihistamines	
Hypnotics *see* Anxiolytics and Hypnotics	
Ibuprofen *see* NSAIDs	
Idoxuridine	Manufacturers advise toxicity in *animal* studies
Imipramine *see* Antidepressants, Tricyclic	
Immunosuppressants *see* section 8.1	
Indapamide *see* Diuretics	
Indomethacin *see* NSAIDs	
Interferons	Manufacturers recommend avoid unless compelling reasons; not for chronic active hepatitis during pregnancy
Iodine and Iodides (2, 3)	Neonatal goitre and hypothyroidism
Radioactive iodine (1, 2, 3)	Permanent hypothyroidism—avoid
Iprindole *see* Antidepressants, Tricyclic (and related)	
Isoflurane *see* Anaesthetics, General	
Isotretinoin (1, 2, 3)	Teratogenic; effective contraception must be used for at least 1 month before treatment, during treatment and for at least 1 month after stopping
Isradipine *see* Calcium-channel Blockers	
Itraconazole	Manufacturer advises toxicity in *animal* studies
Kanamycin *see* Aminoglycosides	
Ketamine *see* Anaesthetics, General	
Ketoconazole	Manufacturer advises teratogenicity in *animal* studies; packs carry a warning to avoid in pregnancy
Ketoprofen *see* NSAIDs	
Ketorolac *see* NSAIDs	
Ketotifen *see* Antihistamines	
Labetalol *see* Beta-blockers	
Lamotrigine *see* Antiepileptics	
Levodopa	Manufacturers advise toxicity in *animal* studies
Lignocaine *see* Anaesthetics, Local	
Lindane	Manufacturer advises toxicity in *animal* studies
Lisinopril *see* ACE Inhibitors	

Appendix 4: Pregnancy

Table of drugs to be avoided or used with caution in pregnancy (*continued*)

Drug (Trimester of risk)	Comments
Lithium (1, 2, 3)	Dose requirements increased; congenital malformations; neonatal goitre reported; lithium toxicity (hypotonia and cyanosis) in neonate if maternal therapy poorly controlled
Lofepramine *see* Antidepressants, Tricyclic	
Loprazolam *see* Anxiolytics and Hypnotics	
Loratadine *see* Antihistamines	
Lorazepam *see* Anxiolytics and Hypnotics	
Lormetazepam *see* Anxiolytics and Hypnotics	
Lymecycline *see* Tetracyclines	
Madopar® *see* Levodopa	
Maloprim®	
(1)	Possible teratogenic risk (pyrimethamine a folate antagonist)
(3)	Neonatal haemolysis and methaemoglobinaemia (due to dapsone); folate supplements should be given to mother *see also* Antimalarials
Maprotiline *see* Antidepressants, Tricyclic (and related)	
Mebendazole	Manufacturer advises toxicity in *animal* studies
Mebhydrolin *see* Antihistamines	
Medazepam *see* Anxiolytics and Hypnotics	
Mefenamic Acid *see* NSAIDs	
Mefloquine (1)	Manufacturer advises teratogenicity in *animal* studies; avoid for prophylaxis, *see* p. 244
Mefruside *see* Diuretics	
Meprobamate *see* Anxiolytics and Hypnotics	
Meptazinol *see* Opioid Analgesics	
Mesterolone *see* Androgens	
Mestranol *see* Contraceptives, Oral	
Metaraminol (1, 2, 3)	Avoid—may reduce placental perfusion
Metformin (1, 2, 3)	Avoid
Methadone *see* Opioid Analgesics	
Methohexitone *see* Anaesthetics, General	
Methotrimeprazine *see* Antipsychotics	
Methyclothiazide *see* Diuretics	
Methylphenobarbitone *see* Antiepileptics	
Methylprednisolone *see* Corticosteroids	
Metolazone *see* Diuretics	
Metoprolol *see* Beta-blockers	
Metronidazole	Manufacturer advises avoidance of high-dose regimens
Metyrapone	Avoid (may impair biosynthesis of fetal-placental steroids)
Mianserin *see* Antidepressants, Tricyclic (and related)	
Mifepristone	Manufacturer advises that if treatment fails, essential that pregnancy be terminated by another method
Minocycline *see* Tetracyclines	
Minoxidil (3)	Neonatal hirsutism reported
Misoprostol (1, 2, 3)	Avoid; increases uterine tone
Morphine *see* Opioid Analgesics	
Nabumetone *see* NSAIDs	
Nadolol *see* Beta-blockers	
Nafarelin	Avoid
Nalbuphine *see* Opioid Analgesics	
Nalidixic acid *see* 4-Quinolones	
Nandrolone *see* Anabolic Steroids	
Naproxen *see* NSAIDs	
Narcotic Analgesics *see* Opioid Analgesics	
Neomycin *see* Aminoglycosides	
Neostigmine (3)	Neonatal myasthenia with large doses
Netilmicin *see* Aminoglycosides	
Nicardipine *see* Calcium-channel Blockers	
Nicoumalone *see* Anticoagulants	
Nifedipine *see* Calcium-channel Blockers	
Nimodipine *see* Calcium-channel Blockers	
Nitrazepam *see* Anxiolytics and Hypnotics	
Nitrofurantoin (3)	May produce neonatal haemolysis if used at term
Nitrous oxide *see* Anaesthetics, General	
Noradrenaline (1, 2, 3)	Avoid—may reduce placental perfusion
Norfloxacin *see* 4-Quinolones	
Nortriptyline *see* Antidepressants, Tricyclic	
NSAIDs (3)	With regular use closure of fetal ductus arteriosus *in utero* and possibly persistent pulmonary hypertension of the newborn. Delayed onset and increased duration of labour
Octreotide (1, 2, 3)	Avoid; possible effect on fetal growth
Oestrogens *see* Contraceptives, Oral	
Ofloxacin *see* 4-Quinolones	
Omeprazole	Manufacturer advises toxicity in *animal* studies
Opioid Analgesics	
(1)	Avoid papaveretum (contains noscapine which may be teratogenic)
(3)	Depress neonatal respiration; withdrawal effects in neonates of dependent mothers; gastric stasis and risk of inhalation pneumonia in mother during labour
Oxatomide *see* Antihistamines	
Oxazepam *see* Anxiolytics and Hypnotics	
Oxprenolol *see* Beta-blockers	
Oxypertine *see* Antipsychotics	
Oxytetracycline *see* Tetracyclines	
Pamidronate Disodium *see* Bisphosphonates	
Papaveretum *see* Opioid Analgesics	
Paroxetine *see* Antidepressants	
Penbutolol *see* Beta-blockers	
Penicillamine (1, 2, 3)	Fetal abnormalities reported rarely; avoid if possible
Pentazocine *see* Opioid Analgesics	
Pericyazine *see* Antipsychotics	
Perindopril *see* ACE Inhibitors	

Table of drugs to be avoided or used with caution in pregnancy (*continued*)

Drug (Trimester of risk)	Comments
Perphenazine *see* Antipsychotics	
Pethidine *see* Opioid Analgesics	
Phenindamine *see* Antihistamines	
Phenindione *see* Anticoagulants	
Pheniramine *see* Antihistamines	
Phenobarbitone (1, 3)	Congenital malformations. Neonatal bleeding tendency—prophylactic vitamin K$_1$ should be given; *see also* Antiepileptics
Phenoperidine *see* Opioid Analgesics	
Phenothiazines *see* Antipsychotics	
Phenytoin (1, 3)	Congenital malformations. Folate supplements should be given to mother (reduced absorption). Neonatal bleeding tendency—prophylactic vitamin K$_1$ should be given. Caution in interpreting plasma concentrations—bound may be reduced but free (i.e. effective) unchanged; *see also* Antiepileptics
Pholcodine *see* Opioid Analgesics	
Pimozide *see* Antipsychotics	
Pindolol *see* Beta-blockers	
Piperazine	No clinical evidence of harm but packs sold to the general public carry a warning to avoid in pregnancy except on medical advice
Pipothiazine *see* Antipsychotics	
Piroxicam *see* NSAIDs	
Podophyllum resin (1, 2, 3)	Avoid—neonatal death and teratogenesis have been reported
Polythiazide *see* Diuretics	
Povidone-iodine (2, 3)	Sufficient iodine may be absorbed to affect the fetal thyroid
Pravastatin *see* Clofibrate	
Prednisolone *see* Corticosteroids	
Prednisone *see* Corticosteroids	
Prilocaine (3)	Neonatal methaemoglobinaemia; *see also* Anaesthetics, Local
Primaquine (3)	Neonatal haemolysis and methaemoglobinaemia; *see also* Antimalarials
Primidone *see* Antiepileptics	
Probucol *see* Clofibrate	
Procaine (3)	Neonatal methaemoglobinaemia; *see also* Anaesthetics, Local
Prochlorperazine *see* Antipsychotics	
Progestogens (1)	High doses may possibly be teratogenic
Proguanil	Folate supplements should be given to mother; *see also* Antimalarials
Promazine *see* Antipsychotics	
Promethazine *see* Antihistamines	
Propofol *see* Anaesthetics, General	
Propranolol *see* Beta-blockers	
Propylthiouracil (2, 3)	Neonatal goitre and hypothyroidism
Prothionamide (1)	May be teratogenic
Protriptyline *see* Antidepressants, Tricyclic	
Pyridostigmine (3)	Neonatal myasthenia with large doses
Pyrimethamine (1)	Possible teratogenic risk (folate antagonist); folate supplements should be given to mother; *see also* Antimalarials
Quinapril *see* ACE Inhibitors	
Quinine (1)	High doses are teratogenic; but in malaria benefit of treatment outweighs risk
4-Quinolones (1, 2, 3)	Arthropathy in *animal* studies
Ramipril *see* ACE inhibitors	
Remoxipride *see* Antipsychotics	
Rifampicin (1)	Manufacturers advise very high doses teratogenic in *animal* studies
(3)	Risk of neonatal bleeding may be increased
Salbutamol (3)	Large parenteral doses given at term for asthma could delay onset of labour
Salicylates *see* Aspirin	
Salsalate *see* Aspirin	
Sertraline *see* Antidepressants	
Simvastatin	Manufacturer advises toxicity in *animal* studies
Sodium Aurothiomalate *see* Gold	
Sodium Clodronate *see* Bisphosphonates	
Sodium Valproate *see* Valproate	
Sotalol *see* Beta-blockers	
Spironolactone	Manufacturers advise toxicity in *animal* studies
Stanozolol *see* Anabolic Steroids	
Stilboestrol (1)	High doses associated with vaginal carcinoma, urogenital abnormalities, and reduced fertility in female offspring
Streptokinase (1, 2, 3)	Possibility of premature separation of placenta in first 18 weeks; theoretical possibility of fetal haemorrhage throughout pregnancy; avoid postpartum use—maternal haemorrhage
Streptomycin *see* Aminoglycosides	
Sulfadoxine *see* Sulphonamides	
Sulfametopyrazine *see* Sulphonamides	
Sulindac *see* NSAIDs	
Sulphadiazine *see* Sulphonamides	
Sulphadimidine *see* Sulphonamides	
Sulphasalazine (3)	Theoretical risk of neonatal haemolysis; folate supplements should be given to mother

Appendix 4: Pregnancy

Table of drugs to be avoided or used with caution in pregnancy (*continued*)

Drug (Trimester of risk)	Comments
Sulphonamides (3)	Neonatal haemolysis and methaemoglobinaemia; fear of increased risk of kernicterus in neonates appears to be unfounded
Sulphonylureas (3)	Neonatal hypoglycaemia; insulin is normally substituted in all diabetics; if oral drugs are used therapy should be stopped at least 2 days before delivery
Sulpiride *see* Antipsychotics	
Tamoxifen	Possible effects on fetal development
Temazepam *see* Anxiolytics and Hypnotics	
Tenoxicam *see* NSAIDS	
Terbutaline (3)	Large parenteral doses given at term for asthma could delay onset of labour
Terfenadine *see* Antihistamines	
Testosterone *see* Androgens	
Tetracyclines (2, 3)	Dental discoloration; maternal hepatotoxicity with large parenteral doses
Theophylline (3)	Neonatal irritability and apnoea have been reported
Thiabendazole (1)	Teratogenic in *animal* studies
Thiazides (3)	May cause neonatal thrombocytopenia; *see also* Diuretics
Thiethylperazine *see* Antipsychotics	
Thiopentone *see* Anaesthetics, General	
Thioridazine *see* Antipsychotics	
Tiaprofenic acid *see* NSAIDs	
Timolol *see* Beta-blockers	
Tinidazole	Manufacturer advises avoid in first trimester
Tobramycin *see* Aminoglycosides	
Tocainide	Manufacturer advises toxicity in *animal* studies
Tolbutamide *see* Sulphonylureas	
Tolmetin *see* NSAIDs	

Drug (Trimester of risk)	Comments
Trazodone *see* Antidepressants, Tricyclic (and related)	
Triamcinolone *see* Corticosteroids	
Triamterene *see* Diuretics	
Tribavirin	Manufacturer advises avoid
Triclofos *see* Anxiolytics and Hypnotics	
Trifluoperazine *see* Antipsychotics	
Trifluperidol *see* Antipsychotics	
Trilostane (1, 2, 3)	Interferes with placental sex hormone production
Trimeprazine *see* Antihistamines	
Trimetaphan (3)	Avoid. Risk of paralytic ileus in newborn
Trimethoprim (1)	Possible teratogenic risk (folate antagonist)
Trimipramine *see* Antidepressants, Tricyclic	
Triprolidine *see* Antihistamines	
Urokinase (1, 2, 3)	Possibility of premature separation of placenta in first 18 weeks; theoretical possibility of fetal haemorrhage throughout pregnancy; avoid postpartum use—maternal haemorrhage
Vaccines (live) (1)	Theoretical risk of congenital malformations; see section 14.1
Valproate (1, 3)	Increased risk of neural tube defects (screening advised); neonatal bleeding and hepatotoxicity also reported; *see also* Antiepileptics
Verapamil *see* Calcium-channel Blockers	
Vigabatrin	Manufacturer advises toxicity in *animal* studies; *see also* Antiepileptics
Viloxazine *see* Antidepressants, Tricyclic (and related)	
Vitamin A (1)	Excessive doses may be teratogenic; *see also* p. 350
Warfarin *see* Anticoagulants	
Xamoterol	Manufacturer advises toxicity in *animal* studies
Xipamide *see* Diuretics	
Zuclopenthixol *see* Antipsychotics	

Appendix 5: Breast-feeding

Administration of some drugs to nursing mothers may cause toxicity in the infant (e.g. ergotamine), whereas administration of others (e.g. digoxin), has little effect on the neonate. Some drugs inhibit lactation (e.g. bromocriptine).

Toxicity to the infant can occur if the drug enters the milk in pharmacologically significant quantities. Milk concentrations of some drugs (e.g. iodides), may exceed those in the maternal plasma so that therapeutic doses in the mother may cause toxicity to the infant. Some drugs inhibit the infant's sucking reflex (e.g. phenobarbitone). Drugs in breast milk may, at least theoretically, cause hypersensitivity in the infant even when concentrations are too low for a pharmacological effect.

The following table lists drugs:

which should be used with caution or which are contra-indicated in breast-feeding for the reasons given above;

which, on present evidence, may be given to the mother during breast-feeding, because they are excreted in milk in amounts which are too small to be harmful to the infant;

which are not known to be harmful to the infant although they are present in milk in significant amounts.

For many drugs there is insufficient evidence available to provide guidance and it is advisable only to administer essential drugs to a mother during breast-feeding. Because of the inadequacy of currently available information on drugs in breast milk the following table should be used only as a guide; absence from the table does not imply safety.

Table of drugs excreted in breast milk
Products introduced or amended since publication of BNF No. 23 (March 1992) are underlined.

Drug	Comments
Acebutolol *see* Beta-blockers	
Acetazolamide	Amount too small to be harmful
Acetohexamide *see* Sulphonylureas	
Acrivastine *see* Antihistamines	
Alcohol	Large amounts may affect infant and reduce milk consumption
Alfacalcidol *see* Vitamin D	
Alprazolam *see* Benzodiazepines	
Aminophylline *see* Theophylline	
Amiodarone	Avoid; present in milk in significant amounts; theoretical risk from release of iodine; *see also* Iodine
Amitriptyline *see* Antidepressants, Tricyclic	
Amoxapine *see* Antidepressants, Tricyclic	
Amphetamines	Significant amount in milk. Avoid
Amylobarbitone *see* Barbiturates	
Androgens	Avoid; may cause masculinisation in the female infant or precocious development in the male infant; high doses suppress lactation
Anthraquinones	Avoid; large doses may cause increased gastric motility and diarrhoea (particularly cascara and danthron)
Anticoagulants, Oral	Risk of haemorrhage; increased by vitamin-K deficiency; warfarin appears safe but phenindione should be avoided
Antidepressants, Tricyclic (and related)	Amount of tricyclic antidepressants (including related drugs such as mianserin and trazodone) too small to be harmful; accumulation of doxepin metabolite may cause sedation and respiratory depression
Antihistamines	Significant amount of some but not known to be harmful; drowsiness in infant reported with clemastine
Antipsychotics	Although amount excreted in milk probably too small to be harmful, *animal studies indicate possible adverse effects* of these drugs on developing nervous system therefore avoid unless absolutely necessary; drowsiness in infant reported with chlorpromazine; significant amount of sulpiride excreted in milk (best avoided)
Aspirin	Avoid—possible risk of Reye's syndrome; regular use of high doses could impair platelet function and produce hypoprothrombinaemia in infant if neonatal vitamin K stores low
Astemizole *see* Antihistamines	
Atenolol *see* Beta-blockers	
Atropine	May possibly have antimuscarinic effects in infants
Auranofin *see* Gold	
Aurothiomalate *see* Gold	
Azatadine *see* Antihistamines	
Baclofen	Amount too small to be harmful
Barbiturates	Avoid if possible (*see also* phenobarbitone); large doses may produce drowsiness
Bendrofluazide *see* Thiazides	
Benperidol *see* Antipsychotics	
Benzodiazepines	Avoid repeated doses; lethargy and weight loss may occur in infant

Appendix 5: Breast-feeding

Table of drugs excreted in breast milk (*continued*)

Drug	Comments
Beta-blockers and Labetalol	Monitor infant; possible toxicity due to beta-blockade but amount of most beta-blockers excreted in milk too small to affect infant; acebutolol, atenolol, nadolol, and sotalol are present in greater amounts than other beta-blockers
Betamethasone *see* Corticosteroids	
Betaxolol *see* Beta-blockers	
Bisoprolol *see* Beta-blockers	
Bromazepam *see* Benzodiazepines	
Bromide salts	Avoid; sedation and rash in infant
Bromocriptine	Suppresses lactation
Brompheniramine *see* Antihistamines	
Buprenorphine	Amount too small to be harmful
Butobarbitone *see* Barbiturates	
Butriptyline *see* Antidepressants, Tricyclic	
Caffeine	Regular intake of large amounts can affect infant
Calciferol *see* Vitamin D	
Calcitonin	Avoid; inhibits lactation in *animals*
Calcitriol *see* Vitamin D	
Captopril	Amount too small to be harmful
Carbamazepine	Amount too small to be harmful
Carbimazole	Amounts in milk may be sufficient to affect neonatal thyroid function (but *see also* section 6.2.2)
Carisoprodol	Concentrated in milk; no adverse effects reported but best avoided
Cascara *see* Anthraquinones	
Celiprolol *see* Beta-blockers	
Cetirizine *see* Antihistamines	
Chloral Hydrate	Sedation in infant
Chloramphenicol	Use another antibiotic; may cause bone-marrow toxicity in infant; concentration in milk usually insufficient to cause 'grey syndrome'
Chlordiazepoxide *see* Benzodiazepines	
Chlormethiazole	Amount too small to be harmful
Chloroquine	Amount too small to be harmful
Chlorothiazide *see* Thiazides	
Chlorpheniramine *see* Antihistamines	
Chlorpromazine	Drowsiness in infant reported; *see* Antipsychotics
Chlorpropamide *see* Sulphonylureas	
Chlortetracycline *see* Tetracyclines	
Chlorthalidone *see* Thiazides	
Cholecalciferol *see* Vitamin D	
Cimetidine	Significant amount but not known to be harmful
Ciprofloxacin	High concentrations in breast milk
Cisapride	Amount too small to be harmful

Drug	Comments
Clavulanic acid (in co-amoxiclav, Timentin®)	Amount too small to be harmful
Clemastine *see* Antihistamines	
Clobazam *see* Benzodiazepines	
Clomipramine *see* Antidepressants, Tricyclic	
Clomocycline *see* Tetracyclines	
Clorazepate *see* Benzodiazepines	
Clozapine *see* Antipsychotics	
Codeine	Amount too small to be harmful
Colchicine	Caution because of its cytotoxicity
Contraceptives, Oral	Oestrogen/progestogen contraceptives usually have little effect on milk flow; in some women, usually when lactation not well established, suppression may occur; one report of neonatal folate deficiency; progestogen-only contraceptives do not appear to adversely affect established milk flow
Corticosteroids	Continuous therapy with high doses (>10 mg prednisolone daily) could possibly affect infant's adrenal function—monitor carefully
Cortisone Acetate *see* Corticosteroids	
Co-trimoxazole	Small risk of kernicterus in jaundiced infants and of haemolysis in G6PD-deficient infants (due to sulphamethoxazole)
Cough mixtures containing iodides	Use alternative cough mixtures; *see* Iodine
Cyclopenthiazide *see* Thiazides	
Cycloserine	Amount too small to be harmful
Cyclosporin	Caution—excreted in milk
Cyproheptadine *see* Antihistamines	
Cyproterone Acetate	Caution; possibility of anti-androgen effects in neonate
Cytotoxics	Discontinue breast-feeding
Danazol	No data available but avoid because of possible androgenic effects in infant
Danthron *see* Anthraquinones	
Dapsone	Haemolytic anaemia; although significant amount in milk risk to infant very small
Demeclocycline *see* Tetracyclines	
Desipramine *see* Antidepressants, Tricyclic	
Dexamethasone *see* Corticosteroids	
Dexamphetamine *see* Amphetamines	
Dextropropoxyphene	Amount too small to be harmful

Table of drugs excreted in breast milk (*continued*)

Drug	Comments
Diamorphine	Therapeutic doses unlikely to affect infant; withdrawal symptoms in infants of dependent mothers; breast-feeding no longer considered best method of treating dependence in offspring of dependent mothers and should be stopped
Diazepam *see* Benzodiazepines	
Diclofenac	Amount too small to be harmful
Digoxin	Amount too small to be harmful
Dihydrotachysterol *see* Vitamin D	
Diltiazem	Significant amount but not known to be harmful
Dimethindene *see* Antihistamines	
Diphenylpyraline *see* Antihistamines	
Disopyramide	Amount too small to be harmful
Domperidone	Amount probably too small to be harmful
Dothiepin *see* Antidepressants, Tricyclic	
Doxepin *see* Antidepressants, Tricyclic	
Doxycycline *see* Tetracyclines	
Droperidol *see* Antipsychotics	
Enalapril	Amount too small to be harmful
Enoxacin	High concentrations in breast milk in *animals*
Ephedrine	Irritability and disturbed sleep reported
Ergocalciferol *see* Vitamin D	
Ergotamine	Avoid where possible; ergotism may occur in infant; repeated doses may inhibit lactation
Erythromycin	Only small amounts in milk
Ethambutol	Amount too small to be harmful
Ethamsylate	Significant amount but not known to be harmful
Ethosuximide	Significant amount; hyperexcitability and poor suckling reported
Etretinate	Avoid
Famotidine	Amount too small to be harmful
Fansidar®	Small risk of kernicterus in jaundiced infants and of haemolysis in G6PD-deficient infants (due to sulfadoxine)
Fenbufen	Amount too small to be harmful
Fenoprofen	Amount too small to be harmful
Flunitrazepam *see* Benzodiazepines	
Fluoxetine	Only small amounts in milk but could accumulate in infant
Flupenthixol *see* Antipsychotics	
Fluphenazine *see* Antipsychotics	
Flurazepam *see* Benzodiazepines	
Flurbiprofen	Amount too small to be harmful
Fluvoxamine	Amount too small to be harmful
Frusemide	Amount too small to be harmful
Ganciclovir	Avoid
Glibenclamide *see* Sulphonylureas	
Gliclazide *see* Sulphonylureas	
Glipizide *see* Sulphonylureas	
Gliquidone *see* Sulphonylureas	
Glymidine *see* Sulphonylureas	
Gold (auranofin, aurothiomalate)	Caution—excreted in milk; theoretical possibility of rashes and idiosyncratic reactions
Halofantrine	Avoid
Haloperidol *see* Antipsychotics	
Heparin	Amount too small to be harmful
Hydrochlorothiazide *see* Thiazides	
Hydrocortisone *see* Corticosteroids	
Hydroflumethiazide *see* Thiazides	
Hydroxychloroquine	Amount too small to be harmful
Hydroxyzine *see* Antihistamines	
Hyoscine	Amount too small to be harmful
Ibuprofen	Amount too small to be harmful
Idoxuridine	May possibly make milk taste unpleasant
Imipramine *see* Antidepressants, Tricyclic	
Indapamide *see* Thiazides	
Indomethacin	Amount probably too small to be harmful but convulsions reported in one infant
Insulin	Amount too small to be harmful
Iodine	Stop breast-feeding; danger of neonatal hypothyroidism or goitre; appears to be concentrated in milk
Radioactive iodine	Breast-feeding contra-indicated after therapeutic doses. With diagnostic doses withhold breast-feeding for at least 24 hours
Iprindole *see* Antidepressants, Tricyclic (and related)	
Isoniazid	Monitor infant for possible toxicity; theoretical risk of convulsions and neuropathy; prophylactic pyridoxine advisable in mother and infant
Isotretinoin	Avoid
Ketoprofen	Amount too small to be harmful
Ketotifen *see* Antihistamines	
Labetalol *see* Beta-blockers	
Liothyronine	May interfere with neonatal screening for hypothyroidism

Table of drugs excreted in breast milk (continued)

Drug	Comments
Lithium salts	Monitor infant for possible intoxication; low incidence of adverse effects but increased by continuous ingestion; good control of maternal plasma concentrations minimises the risk
Lofepramine *see* Antidepressants, Tricyclic	
Loprazolam *see* Benzodiazepines	
Lorazepam *see* Benzodiazepines	
Lormetazepam *see* Benzodiazepines	
Lymecycline *see* Tetracyclines	
Lysuride	May suppress lactation
Maloprim®	Haemolytic anaemia (due to dapsone); risk to infant very small
Maprotiline *see* Antidepressants, Tricyclic (and related)	
Mebeverine	Amount too small to be harmful
Mebhydrolin *see* Antihistamines	
Medazepam *see* Benzodiazepines	
Mefenamic Acid	Amount too small to be harmful
Mefloquine	Avoid
Mefruside *see* Thiazides	
Meprobamate	Avoid; concentration in milk may exceed maternal plasma concentrations fourfold and may cause drowsiness in infant
Mequitazine *see* Antihistamines	
Mesalazine	Diarrhoea reported
Methadone	Withdrawal symptoms in infant; breast-feeding permissible during maintenance but dose should be as low as possible and baby monitored to avoid sedation
Methotrimeprazine *see* Antipsychotics	
Methyclothiazide *see* Thiazides	
Methyldopa	Amount too small to be harmful
Methylprednisolone *see* Corticosteroids	
Metoclopramide	Amount probably too small to be harmful
Metolazone *see* Thiazides	
Metoprolol *see* Beta-blockers	
Metronidazole	Significant amount in milk; avoid for 24 hours after large single doses; may give a bitter taste to the milk
Mexiletine	Amount too small to be harmful
Mianserin *see* Antidepressants, Tricyclic (and related)	
Minocycline *see* Tetracyclines	
Minoxidil	Significant amount but not known to be harmful
Morphine	Therapeutic doses unlikely to affect infant; withdrawal symptoms in infants of dependent mothers; breast-feeding not best method of treating dependence in offspring and should be stopped
Nadolol *see* Beta-blockers	
Nalidixic Acid	Risk to infant very small but one case of haemolytic anaemia reported
Naproxen	Amount too small to be harmful
Nefopam	Amount too small to be harmful
Nicoumalone *see* Anticoagulants, Oral	
Nifedipine	Amount too small to be harmful but manufacturer advises avoid
Nitrazepam *see* Benzodiazepines	
Nitrofurantoin	Only small amounts in milk but could be enough to produce haemolysis in G6PD-deficient infants
Nizatidine	Amount too small to be harmful
Nortriptyline *see* Antidepressants, Tricyclic	
NSAIDs *see* individual entries	
Octreotide	Avoid
Oestrogens	High doses suppress lactation but *see also* Contraceptives, Oral
Opioid Analgesics *see* individual entries	
Oxatomide *see* Antihistamines	
Oxazepam *see* Benzodiazepines	
Oxprenolol *see* Beta-blockers	
Oxypertine *see* Antipsychotics	
Oxytetracycline *see* Tetracyclines	
Paracetamol	Amount too small to be harmful
Penbutolol *see* Beta-blockers	
Pergolide	May suppress lactation
Pericyazine *see* Antipsychotics	
Perphenazine *see* Antipsychotics	
Phenindamine *see* Antihistamines	
Phenindione *see* Anticoagulants, Oral	
Pheniramine *see* Antihistamines	
Phenobarbitone	Avoid when possible; drowsiness may occur but risk probably small; one report of methaemoglobinaemia with phenobarbitone and phenytoin
Phenolphthalein	Avoid; increased gastric motility, diarrhoea, and possibly rash
Phenytoin	Amount too small to be harmful
Pimozide *see* Antipsychotics	
Pindolol *see* Beta-blockers	
Pirenzepine	Amount too small to be harmful
Piroxicam	Amount too small to be harmful
Polythiazide *see* Thiazides	
Povidone-iodine	Avoid; iodine absorbed from vaginal preparations is concentrated in milk
Prednisolone *see* Corticosteroids	
Prednisone *see* Corticosteroids	
Primidone *see* Phenobarbitone	
Prochlorperazine *see* Antipsychotics	
Progestogens	High doses suppress lactation but *see also* Contraceptives, Oral

Table of drugs excreted in breast milk (*continued*)

Drug	Comments
Promazine *see* Antipsychotics	
Promethazine *see* Antihistamines	
Propranolol *see* Beta-blockers	
Propylthiouracil	Monitor infant's thyroid status but amounts in milk probably too small to affect infant; high doses might affect neonatal thyroid function
Protriptyline *see* Antidepressants, Tricyclic	
Pseudoephedrine	Amount too small to be harmful
Pyrazinamide	Amount too small to be harmful
Pyridostigmine	Amount too small to be harmful
Pyrimethamine	Significant amount but not known to be harmful
Quinalbarbitone *see* Barbiturates	
Quinidine	Significant amount but not known to be harmful
Ranitidine	Significant amount but not known to be harmful
Rifampicin	Amount too small to be harmful
Senna *see* Anthraquinones	
Sodium Valproate *see* Valproate	
Sotalol *see* Beta-blockers	
Sulfametopyrazine *see* Sulphonamides	
Sulphadiazine *see* Sulphonamides	
Sulphadimidine *see* Sulphonamides	
Sulphasalazine	Small amounts in milk but bloody diarrhoea has been reported; theoretical risk of neonatal haemolysis especially in G6PD-deficient infants
Sulphonamides	Small risk of kernicterus in jaundiced infants particularly with long-acting sulphonamides, and of haemolysis in G6PD-deficient infants
Sulphonylureas	Caution; theoretical possibility of hypoglycaemia in infant
Sulpiride	Best avoided; significant amounts in milk; *see also* Antipsychotics
Temazepam *see* Benzodiazepines	
Terbutaline	Amount too small to be harmful
Terfenadine *see* Antihistamines	
Tetracyclines	Some authorities recommend avoidance but absorption and therefore discoloration of teeth in infant probably prevented by chelation with calcium in milk
Theophylline	Irritability in infant reported; modified-release preparations probably safe
Thiamine	Severely thiamine-deficient mothers should avoid breast-feeding as toxic methylglyoxal excreted in milk
Thiazides	Amount too small to be harmful; large doses may suppress lactation
Thiethylperazine *see* Antipsychotics	
Thioridazine *see* Antipsychotics	
Thyroxine	May interfere with neonatal screening for hypothyroidism
Tiaprofenic acid	Amount too small to be harmful
Timolol *see* Beta-blockers	
Tolazamide *see* Sulphonylureas	
Tolbutamide *see* Sulphonylureas	
Tolmetin	Amount too small to be harmful
Trazodone	Amount too small to be harmful
Triamcinolone *see* Corticosteroids	
Trifluoperazine *see* Antipsychotics	
Trifluperidol *see* Antipsychotics	
Trimeprazine *see* Antihistamines	
Trimipramine *see* Antidepressants, Tricyclic	
Triprolidine *see* Antihistamines	
Valproate	Amount too small to be harmful
Verapamil	Amount too small to be harmful
Viloxazine *see* Antidepressants, Tricyclic (and related)	
Vitamin A	Theoretical risk of toxicity in infants of mothers taking large doses
Vitamin D (and related compounds)	Caution with high doses; may cause hypercalcaemia in infant
Warfarin *see* Anticoagulants, Oral	
Xipamide *see* Thiazides	
Zopiclone	Amount too small to be harmful
Zuclopenthixol *see* Antipsychotics	

Appendix 6: Intravenous Additives

INTRAVENOUS ADDITIVE POLICIES. A local policy on the addition of drugs to intravenous fluids should be drawn up by a multi-disciplinary team in each Health Authority and issued as a document to the members of staff concerned.

Centralised additive services are provided in a number of hospital pharmacy departments and should be used in preference to making additions on wards.

The information that follows should be read in conjunction with local policy documents.

Guidelines

1. Drugs should only be added to infusion containers when constant plasma concentrations are needed or when the administration of a more concentrated solution would be harmful.
2. In general, only one drug should be added to any infusion container and the components should be compatible. Ready-prepared solutions should be used whenever possible. Drugs should not normally be added to blood products, mannitol, or sodium bicarbonate. Only specially formulated additives should be used with fat emulsions or amino-acid solutions (see section 9.3).
3. Solutions should be thoroughly mixed by shaking and checked for absence of particulate matter before use.
4. Strict asepsis should be maintained throughout and in general the giving set should not be used for more than 24 hours.
5. The infusion container should be labelled with the patient's name, the name and quantity of additives, and the date and time of addition (and the new expiry date or time). Such additional labelling should not interfere with information on the manufacturer's label that is still valid. When possible, containers should be retained for a period after use in case they are needed for investigation.
6. It is good practice to examine intravenous infusions from time to time while they are running. If cloudiness, crystallisation, change of colour, or any other sign of interaction or contamination is observed the infusion should be discontinued.

Problems

MICROBIAL CONTAMINATION. The accidental entry and subsequent growth of micro-organisms converts the infusion fluid pathway into a potential vehicle for infection with micro-organisms, particularly species of Candida, Enterobacter, and Klebsiella. Ready-prepared infusions containing the additional drugs, or infusions prepared by an additive service (when available) should therefore be used in preference to making extemporaneous additions to infusion containers on wards etc. However, when this is necessary strict aseptic procedure should be followed.

INCOMPATIBILITY. Physical and chemical incompatibilities may occur with loss of potency, increase in toxicity, or other adverse effect. The solutions may become opalescent or precipitation may occur, but in many instances there is no visual indication of incompatibility. Interaction may take place at any point in the infusion fluid pathway, and the potential for incompatibility is increased when more than one substance is added to the infusion fluid.

Common incompatibilities. Precipitation reactions are numerous and varied and may occur as a result of pH, concentration changes, 'salting-out' effects, complexation or other chemical changes. Precipitation or other particle formation must be avoided since, apart from loss of control of dosage on administration, it may initiate or exacerbate adverse effects. This is particularly important in the case of drugs which have been implicated in either thrombophlebitis (e.g. diazepam) or in skin sloughing or necrosis caused by extravasation (e.g. sodium bicarbonate and certain cytotoxic drugs). It is also especially important to effect solution of colloidal drugs and to prevent their subsequent precipitation in order to avoid a pyrogenic reaction (e.g. amphotericin).

It is considered undesirable to mix beta-lactam antibiotics, such as semi-synthetic penicillins and cephalosporins, with proteinaceous materials on the grounds that immunogenic and allergenic conjugates could be formed.

A number of preparations undergo significant loss of potency when added singly or in combination to large volume infusions. Examples include ampicillin in infusions that contain glucose or lactates, mustine hydrochloride in isotonic saline and gentamicin/carbenicillin combinations. The breakdown products of dacarbazine have been implicated in adverse effects.

Blood. Because of the large number of incompatibilities, drugs should not normally be added to blood and blood products for infusion purposes. Examples of incompatibility with blood include hypertonic mannitol solutions (irreversible crenation of red cells), dextrans (rouleaux formation and interference with cross-matching), glucose (clumping of red cells), and oxytocin (inactivated).

If the giving set is not changed after the administration of blood, but used for other infusion fluids, a fibrin clot may form which, apart from blocking the set, increases the likelihood of microbial growth.

Intravenous fat emulsions may break down with coalescence of fat globules and separation of phases when additions such as antibiotics or electrolytes are made, thus increasing the possibility of embolism. Only specially formulated products such as Vitlipid N® (see section 9.3) may be added to appropriate intravenous fat emulsions.

Other infusions that frequently give rise to incompatibility include amino acids, mannitol, and sodium bicarbonate.

Bactericides such as chlorocresol 0.1% or

phenylmercuric nitrate 0.001% are present in some injection solutions. The total volume of such solutions added to a container for infusion on one occasion should not exceed 15 mL.

Method

Ready-prepared infusions should be used whenever available. **Potassium chloride** is usually available in concentrations of 20, 27, and 40 mmol/litre in sodium chloride intravenous infusion (0.9%), glucose intravenous infusion (5%) or sodium chloride and glucose intravenous infusion. **Lignocaine hydrochloride** is usually available in concentrations of 0.1 or 0.2% in glucose intravenous infusion (5%).

When addition is required to be made extemporaneously, any product reconstitution instructions such as those relating to concentration, vehicle, mixing, and handling precautions should be strictly followed using an aseptic technique throughout. Once the product has been reconstituted, addition to the infusion fluid should be made immediately in order to minimise microbial contamination and, with certain products, to prevent degradation or other formulation change which may occur; e.g. reconstituted ampicillin injection degrades rapidly on standing, and also may form polymers which could cause sensitivity reactions.

It is also important in certain instances that an infusion fluid of specific pH be used. **Amphotericin** injection requires dilution in glucose injection of pH greater than 4.2 and **frusemide** injection should be added to infusions of pH greater than 5.5.

When drug additions are made it is important to mix thoroughly; additions should not be made to an infusion container that has been connected to a giving set, as mixing is hampered. If the solutions are not thoroughly mixed a concentrated layer of the additive may form owing to differences in density. **Potassium chloride** is particularly prone to this 'layering' effect when added without adequate mixing to infusions packed in non-rigid infusion containers; if such a mixture is administered it may have a serious effect on the heart.

A time limit between addition and completion of administration must be imposed for certain admixtures to guarantee satisfactory drug potency and compatibility. For admixtures in which degradation occurs without the formation of toxic substances, an acceptable limit is the time taken for 10% decomposition of the drug. When toxic substances are produced stricter limits may be imposed. Because of the risk of microbial contamination a maximum time limit of 12 hours should be imposed for additions made elsewhere than in hospital pharmacies offering central additive service.

Certain injections must be protected from light during continuous infusion to minimise oxidation, e.g. amphotericin, dacarbazine, and sodium nitroprusside.

Dilution with a small volume of an appropriate vehicle and administration using a motorised infusion pump is advocated for preparations such as heparin where strict control over administration is required. In this case the appropriate dose may be dissolved in a convenient volume (e.g. 24 to 48 mL) of sodium chloride intravenous infusion (0.9%).

Use of table

The table lists preparations given by three methods:
  continuous infusion,
  intermittent infusion, and
  addition *via* the drip tubing.

Drugs for **continuous infusion** must be diluted in a large volume infusion. Penicillins and cephalosporins are not usually given by continuous infusion because of stability problems and because adequate plasma and tissue concentrations are best obtained by intermittent infusion. Where it is necessary to administer them by continuous infusion, detailed literature should be consulted.

Drugs that are both compatible and clinically suitable may be given by **intermittent infusion** in a relatively small volume of infusion over a short period of time, e.g. 100 mL in 30 minutes. The method is used if the product is incompatible or unstable over the period necessary for continuous infusion; the limited stability of ampicillin or amoxycillin in large volume glucose or lactate infusions may be overcome in this way.

Intermittent infusion is also used if adequate plasma and tissue concentrations are not produced by continuous infusion as in the case of drugs such as carbenicillin, dacarbazine, gentamicin, and ticarcillin.

An in-line burette may be used for intermittent infusion techniques in order to achieve strict control over the time and rate of administration, especially for infants and children and in intensive care units. Intermittent infusion may also make use of the 'piggy-back' technique provided that no additions are made to the primary infusion. In this method the drug is added to a small secondary container connected to a Y-type injection site on the primary infusion giving set; the secondary solution is usually infused within 30 minutes.

Addition *via* the drip tubing is indicated for a number of cytotoxic drugs in order to minimise extravasation. The preparation is added aseptically *via* the rubber septum of the injection site of a fast-running infusion. In general, drug preparations intended for a bolus effect should be given directly into a separate vein where possible. Failing this, administration may be made *via* the drip tubing provided that the preparation is compatible with the infusion fluid when given in this manner.

Appendix 6: Intravenous additives

Table of drugs given by intravenous infusion

Covers addition to glucose 5 and 10%, Sodium chloride 0.9%, Compound sodium chloride (Ringer's solution), and Compound sodium lactate (Hartmann's solution). Compatibility with glucose 5% and with sodium chloride 0.9% indicates compatibility with any strength of sodium chloride and glucose infusion. Infusion of a large volume of hypotonic solution should be avoided therefore care should be taken if water for injections is used. The information in the Table relates to the proprietary preparations indicated; for other preparations suitability should be checked with the manufacturer

Drug	Infusion method
Acetylcysteine *Parvolex*®	Continuous *in* Glucose 5%
See Emergency Treatment of Poisoning	
Aclarubicin hydrochloride *Aclacin*®	Intermittent *in* Glucose 5% *or* Sodium chloride 0.9%
Dissolve initially in 10 mL water for injections or sodium chloride 0.9% then dilute with 200–500 mL infusion fluid to a concentration of 200–500 micrograms/mL; give over 30–60 minutes and protect from light during administration; pH of glucose infusion should be between 5 and 6	
Acyclovir sodium *Zovirax IV*®	Intermittent *in* Sodium chloride 0.9% *or* Sodium chloride and glucose *or* Compound sodium lactate
Initially reconstitute to 25 mg/mL in water for injections or sodium chloride 0.9% then dilute to not more than 5 mg/mL with the infusion fluid; minimum volume 50 mL; to be given over 1 hour; alternatively, may be administered in a concentration of 25 mg/mL using a suitable infusion pump and given over 1 hour	
Aldesleukin *Proleukin*®	Continuous *in* Glucose 5%
Reconstitute each vial with 1.2 mL water for injections (do not shake or allow to foam); dilute in up to 500 mL glucose 5% containing albumin 0.1% (albumin added and thoroughly mixed in glucose 5% solution before adding aldesleukin); polypropylene, PVC, polyolefine, or glass containers with polyethylene or PVC giving sets may be used; do not use in-line filter	
Alfentanil hydrochloride *Rapifen*® preparations	Continuous *or* intermittent *in* Glucose 5% *or* Sodium chloride 0.9% *or* Compound sodium lactate
Alprostadil *Prostin VR*®	Continuous *in* Glucose 5% *or* Sodium chloride 0.9%
Amikacin sulphate *Amikin*®	Intermittent *in* Glucose 5% *or* Sodium chloride 0.9% *or* Compound sodium lactate
To be given over 30 minutes	
Aminophylline	Continuous *in* Glucose 5% *or* Sodium chloride 0.9% *or* Compound sodium lactate

Drug	Infusion method
Amiodarone hydrochloride *Cordarone X*®	Continuous *or* intermittent *in* Glucose 5%
Suggested initial infusion volume 250 mL given over 20–120 minutes; for repeat infusions up to 1.2 g in a maximum volume of 500 mL; incompatible with sodium chloride infusion	
Amoxycillin sodium *Amoxil*®	[1]Intermittent *in* Glucose 5% *or* Sodium chloride 0.9%
Reconstituted solutions diluted and given without delay; suggested volume 100 mL given over 30–60 minutes	
	via drip tubing *in* Glucose 5% *or* Sodium chloride 0.9% *or* Ringer's solution *or* Compound sodium lactate
Amphotericin (liposomal) *AmBisome*®	Intermittent *in* Glucose 5%
Reconstitute each vial with 12 mL water for injections (both vial and water for injections should be cooled to 2–8°C before reconstitution) and shake vigorously; incubate reconstituted vial at 65°C for 10 minutes and allow to cool to room temperature; withdraw requisite dose from vial and introduce into infusion fluid through the 5 micron filter provided to produce a final concentration of 500 micrograms/mL; infuse over 30–60 minutes; incompatible with sodium chloride solutions, flush existing intravenous line with glucose 5% or use separate line	
Amphotericin sodium deoxycholate complex *Fungizone*®	Continuous *in* Glucose 5%
Dissolve thoroughly at reconstitution stage; preparation must be diluted in a large volume infusion; pH of the glucose must not be below 4.2 (check each container); protect from light; suggested infusion time 6 hours	
Ampicillin sodium *Penbritin*®	[1]Intermittent *in* Glucose 5% *or* Sodium chloride 0.9%
Reconstituted solutions diluted and given without delay; suggested volume 100 mL given over 30–60 minutes	
	via drip tubing *in* Glucose 5% *or* Sodium chloride 0.9% *or* Ringer's solution *or* Compound sodium lactate

1. Continuous infusion not usually recommended

Appendix 6: Intravenous additives

Drug	Infusion method
Ampicillin/cloxacillin (sodium salts) *Ampiclox®*	Intermittent *in* Glucose 5% *or* Sodium chloride 0.9% Reconstituted solutions diluted and given without delay; suggested volume 100 mL given over 30–60 minutes
	via drip tubing *in* Glucose 5% *or* Sodium chloride 0.9% *or* Ringer's solution *or* Compound sodium lactate
Ampicillin/sulbactam (sodium salts) *Dicapen®*	[1]Intermittent *in* Glucose 5% *or* Sodium chloride 0.9% *or* Water for injections Reconstituted solutions diluted and given without delay; give over 15–30 minutes
Amsacrine *Amsidine®*	Intermittent *in* Glucose 5% Reconstitute with diluent provided and dilute to suggested volume 500 mL; give over 60–90 minutes; use glass syringes; incompatible with sodium chloride infusion
Ancrod *Arvin®*	Continuous *in* Sodium chloride 0.9% Suggested volume 50–500 mL given over 4–12 hours
Atenolol *Tenormin®*	Intermittent *in* Glucose 5% *or* Sodium chloride 0.9% Suggested infusion time 20 minutes
Atracurium besylate *Tracrium®*	Continuous *in* Glucose 5% *or* Sodium chloride 0.9% *or* Compound sodium lactate Stability varies with diluent
Azathioprine *Imuran®*	*via* drip tubing *in* Glucose 5% *or* Sodium chloride 0.9% Reconstituted solutions should be administered without delay
Azlocillin sodium *Securopen®* (5 g)	Intermittent *in* Glucose 5 and 10% *or* Sodium chloride 0.9% *or* Ringer's solution Intermittent infusion suggested for doses over 2 g; to be given over 20–30 minutes
Aztreonam *Azactam®*	Intermittent *in* Glucose 5% *or* Sodium chloride 0.9% *or* Ringer's solution *or* Compound sodium lactate Dissolve initially in water for injections (1 g per 3 mL) then dilute to a concentration of less than 20 mg/mL; to be given over 20–60 minutes
Benzylpenicillin sodium *Crystapen®*	[1]Intermittent *in* Glucose 5% *or* Sodium chloride 0.9% Suggested volume 100 mL given over 30–60 minutes
Betamethasone sodium phosphate *Betnesol®*	Continuous *or* intermittent *or* *via* drip tubing *in* Glucose 5% *or* Sodium chloride 0.9%
Bleomycin sulphate	Intermittent *in* Sodium chloride 0.9% To be given slowly; suggested volume 200 mL
Bumetanide *Burinex®*	Intermittent *in* Glucose 5% *or* Sodium chloride 0.9% Suggested volume 500 mL given over 30–60 minutes
Calcium gluconate	Continuous *in* Glucose 5% *or* Sodium chloride 0.9% Avoid bicarbonates, phosphates, or sulphates
Carbenicillin sodium *Pyopen®*	Intermittent *in* Glucose 5% *or* Water for injections Suggested volume 100 mL given over 30–40 minutes
Carboplatin *Paraplatin®*	Continuous *in* Glucose 5% *or* Sodium chloride 0.9% Final concentration as low as 500 micrograms/mL; give over 15–60 minutes
Carmustine *BiCNU®*	Intermittent *in* Glucose 5% *or* Sodium chloride 0.9% Reconstitute with diluent provided; give over 1–2 hours
Cefodizime sodium *Timecef®*	Intermittent *in* Glucose 5% *or* Sodium chloride 0.9% *or* Ringer's solution *or* Compound sodium lactate *or* Water for injections Dissolve in 40 mL infusion fluid and give over up to 30 minutes
Cefotaxime sodium *Claforan®*	Intermittent *in* Glucose 5% *or* Sodium chloride 0.9% *or* Compound sodium lactate *or* Water for injections Suggested volume 40–100 mL given over 20–60 minutes
Cefoxitin sodium *Mefoxin®*	[1]Intermittent *or* *via* drip tubing *in* Glucose 5 and 10% *or* Sodium chloride 0.9%
Cefsulodin sodium *Monaspor®*	[1]Intermittent *or* *via* drip tubing *in* Glucose 5% *or* Sodium chloride 0.9%
Ceftazidime pentahydrate *Fortum®*	Intermittent *or* *via* drip tubing *in* Glucose 5 and 10% *or* Sodium chloride 0.9% *or* Compound sodium lactate *or* Water for injections

1. Continuous infusion not usually recommended

Appendix 6: Intravenous additives

Drug	Infusion method
Ceftizoxime sodium Cefizox®	Continuous *or* intermittent *or via* drip tubing *in* Glucose 5 and 10% *or* Sodium chloride 0.9% *or* Ringer's solution *or* Compound sodium lactate

Suggested volume 50–100 mL

Cefuroxime sodium Zinacef®	Intermittent *or via* drip tubing *in* Glucose 5% *or* Sodium chloride 0.9% *or* Compound sodium lactate

Suggested volume 50–100 mL given over 30 minutes

Cephamandole nafate Kefadol®	[1]Intermittent *or via* drip tubing *in* Glucose 5 and 10% *or* Sodium chloride 0.9% *or* Water for injections
Cephazolin sodium Kefzol®	[1]Intermittent *or via* drip tubing *in* Glucose 5 and 10% *or* Sodium chloride 0.9% *or* Compound sodium lactate *or* Water for injections
Cephradine Velosef®	Continuous *or* intermittent *in* Glucose 5 and 10% *or* Sodium chloride 0.9% *or* Ringer's solution *or* Compound sodium lactate *or* Water for injections

Reconstituted solutions diluted and given without delay; max. 8 hours between addition and completion of administration

Chloramphenicol sodium succinate Kemicetine®	Intermittent *or via* drip tubing *in* Glucose 5% *or* Sodium chloride 0.9%
Chloroquine sulphate Nivaquine® See also section 5.4.1	Continuous *in* Sodium chloride 0.9%
Cimetidine Tagamet®	Continuous *or* intermittent *in* Glucose 5% *or* Sodium chloride 0.9%

For intermittent infusion suggested volume 100 mL given over 30–60 minutes

Cisplatin	Continuous *in* Sodium chloride 0.9% *or* Sodium chloride and glucose

Suggested volume 1 litre given over 6–8 hours

Drug	Infusion method
Clindamycin phosphate Dalacin C®	Continuous *or* intermittent *in* Glucose 5% *or* Sodium chloride 0.9%

Dilute to a concentration of 300 mg in 50 mL; give each 300 mg over at least 10 minutes (1.2 g over at least 45 minutes)

Clomipramine Anafranil®	Intermittent *in* Glucose 5% *or* Sodium chloride 0.9%

Suggested volume 125–500 mL given over 45–120 minutes

Clonazepam Rivotril®	Intermittent *in* Glucose 5 and 10% *or* Sodium chloride 0.9%

Suggested volume 250 mL

Cloxacillin sodium Orbenin®	[1]Intermittent *in* Glucose 5% *or* Sodium chloride 0.9%

Suggested volume 100 mL given over 30–60 minutes

	via drip tubing *in* Glucose 5% *or* Sodium chloride 0.9% *or* Ringer's solution *or* Compound sodium lactate
Co-amoxiclav Augmentin®	Intermittent *in* Sodium chloride 0.9% *or* Water for injections; see also package leaflet

Suggested volume 50–100 mL given over 30–40 minutes and completed within 2 hours of reconstitution

	via drip tubing *in* Glucose 5% *or* Sodium chloride 0.9%
Co-fluampicil (sodium salts) Magnapen®	Intermittent *in* Glucose 5% *or* Sodium chloride 0.9%

Reconstituted solutions diluted and given without delay; suggested volume 100 mL given over 30–60 minutes

	via drip tubing *in* Glucose 5% *or* Sodium chloride 0.9% *or* Ringer's solution *or* Compound sodium lactate
Colistin sulphomethate sodium Colomycin®	Continuous *or* intermittent *in* Glucose 5% *or* Sodium chloride 0.9% *or* Ringer's solution

Max. 6 hours between addition and completion of administration

Co-trimoxazole Septrin® for infusion	Continuous *in* Glucose 5 and 10% *or* Sodium chloride 0.9% *or* Ringer's solution

Dilute contents of 1 ampoule (5 mL) to 125 mL, 2 ampoules (10 mL) to 250 mL or 3 ampoules (15 mL) to 500 mL; if fluid restriction necessary, 1 ampoule may be diluted with 75 mL glucose 5%

---

1. Continuous infusion not usually recommended

Appendix 6: Intravenous additives 527

Drug	Infusion method
Cyclophosphamide Endoxana®	Intermittent *or* *via* drip tubing *in* Glucose 5% *or* Sodium chloride 0.9% *or* Water for injections

For intermittent infusion suggested volume 50–100 mL given over 5–15 minutes; max. 30 minutes between addition and completion of administration

	via drip tubing *in* Glucose 5%
Cyclosporin Sandimmun®	Continuous *in* Glucose 5% *or* Sodium chloride 0.9%

Dilute to a concentration of 50 mg in 20–100 mL; give over 2–6 hours

Cytarabine Alexan®, Cytosar®	Continuous *or* intermittent *or* *via* drip tubing *in* Glucose 5% *or* Sodium chloride 0.9%

Reconstitute *Cytosar®* with the diluent provided; check container for haze or precipitate during administration

Dacarbazine DTIC-Dome®	Intermittent *in* Glucose 5% *or* Sodium chloride 0.9%

Suggested volume 125–250 mL given over 15–30 minutes; protect infusion from light

Dactinomycin Cosmegen Lyovac®	*via* drip tubing *in* Glucose 5% *or* Sodium chloride 0.9%

Reconstitute with water for injections

Desferrioxamine **mesylate** Desferal®	Continuous *or* intermittent *in* Glucose 5% *or* Sodium chloride 0.9%

Dexamethasone **sodium phosphate** Decadron®, Dexamethasone (Organon)	Continuous *or* intermittent *or* *via* drip tubing *in* Glucose 5% *or* Sodium chloride 0.9%

Dexamethasone (Organon) can also be infused in Glucose 10% *or* Ringer's solution *or* Compound sodium lactate

Diazepam (solution) Valium®	Continuous *in* Glucose 5% *or* Sodium chloride 0.9%

Dilute to a concentration of not more than 40 mg in 500 mL; max. 6 hours between addition and completion of administration; adsorbed to some extent by the plastics of the infusion set

Diazepam (emulsion) Diazemuls®	Continuous *in* Glucose 5 and 10%

May be diluted to a max. concentration of 200 mg in 500 mL; max. 6 hours between addition and completion of administration; adsorbed to some extent by the plastics of the infusion set

	via drip tubing *in* Glucose 5 and 10% *or* Sodium chloride 0.9%

Adsorbed to some extent by the plastics of the infusion set

Drug	Infusion method
Digoxin Lanoxin®	Continuous *in* Glucose 5% *or* Sodium chloride 0.9%

To be given slowly; see also section 2.1.1

Digoxin-specific **antibody fragments** Digibind®	Intermittent *in* Sodium chloride 0.9%

Dissolve initially in water for injections (4 mL/vial) then dilute with the sodium chloride 0.9% and give through a 0.22 micron sterile, disposable filter over 20 minutes

Dinoprostone Prostin E2®	Continuous *or* intermittent *in* Glucose 5% *or* Sodium chloride 0.9%

Disodium etidronate Didronel IV®	Continuous *in* Sodium chloride 0.9%

Dilute in large-volume infusion, suggested minimum volume 250 mL; minimum period of infusion 2 hours

Disodium **pamidronate** Aredia®	Continuous *in* Sodium chloride 0.9%

Dilute to a concentration of 15 mg in 125 mL and give each 15 mg over at least 1 hour; not to be given with infusion fluids containing calcium

Disopyramide **phosphate** Rythmodan®	Continuous *or* intermittent *in* Glucose 5% *or* Sodium chloride 0.9% *or* Ringer's solution *or* Compound sodium lactate

Max. rate by continuous infusion 20–30 mg/hour (or 400 micrograms/kg/hour)

Dobutamine **hydrochloride** Dobutrex® Solution	Continuous *in* Glucose 5% *or* Sodium chloride 0.9%

Dilute to a concentration of 0.5–1 mg/mL; give higher concentration (max. 5 mg/mL) with infusion pump; incompatible with bicarbonate

Dopamine **hydrochloride** Intropin®	Continuous *in* Glucose 5% *or* Sodium chloride 0.9% *or* Compound sodium lactate

Dilute to a concentration of 1.6 mg/mL; incompatible with bicarbonate

Dopexamine **hydrochloride** Dopacard®	Continuous *in* Glucose 5% *or* Sodium chloride 0.9%

Dilute to a concentration of 400 or 800 micrograms/mL; give *via* infusion pump or other device which provides accurate control of rate; contact with metal should be minimised; incompatible with bicarbonate

1. Continuous infusion not usually recommended

Appendix 6: Intravenous additives

Drug	Infusion method
Doxorubicin hydrochloride *Doxorubicin Rapid Dissolution*, *Doxorubicin Solution* (both Farmitalia Carlo Erba) Reconstitute *Doxorubicin Rapid Dissolution* with water for injections or sodium chloride 0.9% (10 mg in 5 mL, 50 mg in 25 mL); give over 2–3 minutes	*via* drip tubing *in* Glucose 5% *or* Sodium chloride 0.9%
Electrolytes *Addiphos*® Suggested volume 500 mL	Continuous *in* Glucose 5 and 10%
Enoximone *Perfan*® Dilute to a concentration of 2.5 mg/mL; incompatible with glucose solutions; use only plastic containers or syringes	Continuous *or* intermittent *in* Sodium chloride 0.9% *or* Water for injections
Epirubicin hydrochloride *Pharmorubicin*® Rapid Dissolution *Pharmorubicin*® Solution Reconstitute *Pharmorubicin*® Rapid Dissolution with sodium chloride 0.9% or with water for injections (10 mg in 5 mL, 20 mg in 10 mL, 50 mg in 25 mL); give over 3–5 minutes	*via* drip tubing *in* Sodium chloride 0.9%
Epoprostenol *Flolan*® Reconstitute with the diluent provided (pH 10.5) to make a concentrate; use this concentrate within 12 hours and store at 2°–8°C; dilute with not more than 6 times the volume of sodium chloride 0.9% before use	Intermittent *in* Sodium chloride 0.9%
Erythromycin lactobionate *Erythrocin*® Dissolve initially in water for injections (1 g in 20 mL) then dilute to a concentration of 1 mg/mL for continuous infusion and 1–5 mg/mL for intermittent infusion	Continuous *or* intermittent *in* Glucose 5% (neutralised with sodium bicarbonate) *or* Sodium chloride 0.9% *or* Compound sodium lactate
Ethacrynic acid (sodium salt) *Edecrin*® pH of glucose infusion should be adjusted to above 5	*via* drip tubing *in* Glucose 5% *or* Sodium chloride 0.9%
Ethanol Dilute to a concentration of 5–10%	Continuous *in* Glucose 5% *or* Sodium chloride 0.9% *or* Ringer's solution *or* Compound sodium lactate
Etoposide *Vepesid*® Dilute to a concentration of not more than 250 micrograms/mL and give over not less than 30 minutes and not more than 6 hours; check container for haze or precipitate during administration; may dissolve certain types of filter	Intermittent *in* Sodium chloride 0.9%
Filgrastim *Neupogen*® For a filgrastim concentration of less than 1 500 000 units/mL (15 micrograms/mL) albumin solution (human serum albumin) is added to produce a final albumin concentration of 2 mg/mL; should not be diluted to a filgrastim concentration of less than 200 000 units/mL (2 micrograms/mL) and should not be diluted with sodium chloride solution	Intermittent *in* Glucose 5%
Flecainide acetate *Tambocor*® Minimum volume in infusion fluids containing chlorides 500 mL	Continuous *or* intermittent *in* Glucose 5% *or* Sodium chloride 0.9% *or* Compound sodium lactate
Flucloxacillin sodium *Floxapen*® Suggested volume 100 mL given over 30–60 minutes	[1]Intermittent *in* Glucose 5% *or* Sodium chloride 0.9% *via* drip tubing *in* Glucose 5% *or* Sodium chloride 0.9% *or* Ringer's solution *or* Compound sodium lactate
Flumazenil *Anexate*®	Continuous *in* Glucose 5% *or* Sodium chloride 0.9%
Fluorouracil sodium For continuous infusion suggested volume 500 mL given over 4 hours	Continuous *or via* drip tubing *in* Glucose 5%
Folinic acid (calcium salt) *Calcium Leucovorin*®, *Refolinon*® *Calcium Leucovorin*® can also be infused in Glucose 5 and 10% *or* Compound sodium lactate	Continuous *in* Sodium chloride 0.9%
Foscarnet trisodium *Foscavir*® Dilute to a concentration of 12 mg/mL or less for infusion into peripheral vein (undiluted solution *via* central venous line only)	Continuous *in* Glucose 5%
Frusemide (sodium salt) *Lasix*® Infusion pH must be above 5.5; glucose solutions are unsuitable	Continuous *in* Sodium chloride 0.9% *or* Ringer's solution
Fusidic acid (diethanolamine salt) *Fucidin*® Reconstitute with the buffer solution provided and dilute to a max. concentration of diethanolamine fusidate 1.16 mg/mL (= sodium fusidate 1 mg/mL); to be given over not less than 6 hours; incompatible if glucose solution too acidic	Continuous *in* Glucose 5% (but see below) *or* Sodium chloride 0.9%

1. Continuous infusion not usually recommended

Appendix 6: Intravenous additives

Drug	Infusion method
Ganciclovir (sodium salt) *Cymevene®*	Intermittent *in* Glucose 5% *or* Sodium chloride 0.9% *or* Ringer's solution *or* Compound sodium lactate

Reconstitute initially in water for injections (500 mg/10 mL) then dilute to not more than 10 mg/mL with infusion fluid (usually 100 mL); infuse over 1 hour

Drug	Infusion method
Gentamicin sulphate *Cidomycin®*	Intermittent *or via* drip tubing *in* Glucose 5% *or* Sodium chloride 0.9%

Suggested volume for intermittent infusion 50–100 mL given over 20 minutes

Drug	Infusion method
Glyceryl trinitrate *Nitrocine®*, *Nitronal®*, *Tridil®*	Continuous *in* Glucose 5% *or* Sodium chloride 0.9%

For *Tridil®* dilute to a concentration of not more than 400 micrograms/mL; for *Nitrocine®* suggested infusion concentration 100 micrograms/mL; incompatible with polyvinyl chloride infusion containers such as Viaflex® or Steriflex®; use glass or polyethylene containers or give *via* a syringe pump

Drug	Infusion method
Granisetron hydrochloride *Kytril®*	Intermittent *in* Glucose 5% *or* Sodium chloride 0.9% *or* Compound sodium lactate

Dilute 3 mL in 20–50 mL infusion fluid and give over 5 minutes

Drug	Infusion method
HA-1A *Centoxin®*	Single infusion *in* Sodium chloride 0.9%

Inject solution (20 mL) through a 0.2 or 0.22 micron sterile, low protein binding filter into 50 mL infusion fluid; give over 15–30 minutes

Drug	Infusion method
Heparin sodium	Continuous *in* Glucose 5% *or* Sodium chloride 0.9%

Administration with a motorised pump may be advisable

Drug	Infusion method
Hydralazine hydrochloride *Apresoline®*	Continuous *in* Sodium chloride 0.9% *or* Ringer's solution

Suggested infusion volume 500 mL

Drug	Infusion method
Hydrocortisone sodium phosphate *Efcortesol®*	Continuous *or* intermittent *or via* drip tubing *in* Glucose 5% *or* Sodium chloride 0.9%

Drug	Infusion method
Hydrocortisone sodium succinate *Efcortelan Soluble®*, *Solu-Cortef®*	Continuous *or* intermittent *or via* drip tubing *in* Glucose 5% *or* Sodium chloride 0.9%

Drug	Infusion method
Idarubicin hydrochloride *Zavedos®*	*via* drip tubing *in* Sodium chloride 0.9%

Reconstitute with water for injections; give over 5–10 minutes

Drug	Infusion method
Ifosfamide *Mitoxana®*	Continuous *or* intermittent *or via* drip tubing *in* Glucose 5% *or* Sodium chloride 0.9%

For continuous infusion, suggested volume 3 litres given over 24 hours; for intermittent infusion, give over 30–120 minutes

Drug	Infusion method
Imipenem/cilastatin (sodium salt) *Primaxin®*	[1]Intermittent *in* Glucose 5% *or* Sodium chloride 0.9% *or* Water for injections

Dilute to a concentration of 5 mg (as imipenem)/mL; infuse 250–500 mg (as imipenem) over 20–30 minutes, 1 g over 40–60 minutes

Drug	Infusion method
Insulin (soluble)	Continuous *in* Sodium chloride 0.9% *or* Compound sodium lactate

Adsorbed to some extent by plastics of infusion set; see also section 6.1.3; ensure insulin is not injected into 'dead space' of injection port of the infusion bag

Drug	Infusion method
Iron dextran *Imferon®*	Intermittent *in* Glucose 5% *or* Sodium chloride 0.9%

Suggested volume 500 mL.

Drug	Infusion method
Isoprenaline hydrochloride *Saventrine IV®*	Continuous *in* Glucose 5% *or* Sodium chloride and glucose

Dilute in a large-volume infusion; suggested minimum volume 500 mL; pH of the infusion must be below 5.

Drug	Infusion method
Isosorbide dinitrate *Cedocard IV®*, *Isoket 0.05%®*, *Isoket 0.1%®*	Continuous *in* Glucose 5% *or* Sodium chloride 0.9%

Adsorbed to some extent by polyvinyl chloride infusion containers; preferably use glass or polyethylene containers or give *via* a syringe pump; *Isoket 0.05%®* can alternatively be administered undiluted using a syringe pump with a glass or rigid plastic syringe

Drug	Infusion method
Isoxsuprine hydrochloride *Duvadilan®*	Continuous *in* Glucose 5% *or* Sodium chloride 0.9%

Suggested infusion concentration 0.02%

Drug	Infusion method
Kanamycin sulphate *Kannasyn®*	Intermittent *in* Glucose 5% *or* Sodium chloride 0.9%

Dilute to 2.5 mg/mL and give at a rate of 3–4 mL/minute

Drug	Infusion method
Ketamine hydrochloride *Ketalar®*	Continuous *in* Glucose 5% *or* Sodium chloride 0.9%

Dilute to 1 mg/mL; microdrip infusion for maintenance of anaesthesia

Drug	Infusion method
Labetalol hydrochloride *Trandate®*	Intermittent *in* Glucose 5% *or* Sodium chloride and glucose

Dilute to a concentration of 1 mg/mL; suggested volume 200 mL; adjust rate with in-line burette

---

1. Continuous infusion not usually recommended

Drug	Infusion method
Lignocaine hydrochloride Xylocard 20%®	Continuous *in* Glucose 5% *or* Sodium chloride 0.9% *or* Ringer's solution
Suggested infusion concentration 0.2%; use ready-prepared solution when available	
Mecillinam Selexidin®	Intermittent *in* Glucose 5% *or* Sodium chloride 0.9%
Reconstituted solutions diluted and given without delay; suggested infusion time 15–30 minutes	
Melphalan Alkeran®	Continuous *or* *via* drip tubing *in* Sodium chloride 0.9%
Reconstitute with the solvent and diluent provided then dilute with infusion fluid; max. 2 hours between addition and completion of administration	
Mesna Uromitexan®	Continuous *or* *via* drip tubing *in* Glucose 5% *or* Sodium chloride 0.9%
Max. 24 hours between addition and completion of administration	
Metaraminol tartrate Aramine®	Continuous *or* *via* drip tubing *in* Glucose 5% *or* Sodium chloride 0.9% *or* Ringer's solution *or* Compound sodium lactate
Suggested infusion volume 500 mL	
Methicillin sodium Celbenin®	[1]Intermittent *in* Glucose 5% *or* Sodium chloride 0.9%
Suggested volume 100 mL given over 30–60 minutes	
	via drip tubing *in* Glucose 5% *or* Sodium chloride 0.9% *or* Ringer's solution *or* Compound sodium lactate
Methocarbamol Robaxin®	Intermittent *in* Glucose 5% *or* Sodium chloride 0.9%
Dilute to a concentration of not less than 1 g in 250 mL	
Methotrexate sodium Methotrexate (Lederle)	Continuous *or* *via* drip tubing *in* Glucose 5% *or* Sodium chloride 0.9% *or* Compound sodium lactate *or* Ringer's solution
Dilute in a large-volume infusion; max. 24 hours between addition and completion of administration	
Methyldopate hydrochloride Aldomet®	Intermittent *in* Glucose 5%
Suggested volume 100 mL given over 30–60 minutes	

Drug	Infusion method
Methylprednisolone sodium succinate Solu-Medrone®	Continuous *or* intermittent *or* *via* drip tubing *in* Glucose 5% *or* Sodium chloride 0.9%
Metoclopramide hydrochloride Maxolon High Dose®	Continuous *or* intermittent *in* Glucose 5% *or* Sodium chloride 0.9% *or* Compound sodium lactate
Loading dose, dilute with 50–100 mL and give over 15–30 minutes; maintenance dose, dilute with 500 mL and give over 8–12 hours; for intermittent infusion dilute with at least 50 mL and give over at least 15 minutes	
Mexiletine hydrochloride Mexitil®	Continuous *in* Glucose 5% *or* Sodium chloride 0.9%
Mezlocillin sodium Baypen® (5 g)	Intermittent *in* Glucose 5 and 10% *or* Sodium chloride 0.9% *or* Ringer's solution *or* Water for injections
Suggested volume 50 mL given over 15–20 minutes	
Miconazole Daktarin®	Continuous *or* intermittent *in* Glucose 5% *or* Sodium chloride 0.9%
Minimum period of infusion 30 minutes; for intermittent infusion suggested volume 200–500 mL	
Milrinone Primacor®	Continuous *in* Glucose 5% *or* Sodium chloride 0.9%
Dilute to a suggested concentration of 200 micrograms/mL	
Mitozantrone hydrochloride Novantrone®	*via* drip tubing *in* Glucose 5% *or* Sodium chloride 0.9%
Suggested volume at least 50 mL given over at least 3–5 minutes	
Mustine hydrochloride (Boots)	*via* drip tubing *in* Glucose 5% *or* Sodium chloride 0.9%
Naftidrofuryl oxalate Praxilene Forte®	Intermittent *in* Glucose 5 and 10% *or* Sodium chloride 0.9%
Suggested volume 250–500 mL given over 90–120 minutes	
Naloxone Min-I-Jet® Naloxone Hydrochloride, Narcan®	Continuous *in* Glucose 5% *or* Sodium chloride 0.9%
Dilute to a concentration of 4 micrograms/mL	
Netilmicin sulphate Netillin®	Intermittent *or* *via* drip tubing *in* Glucose 5 and 10% *or* Sodium chloride 0.9%
For intermittent infusion suggested volume 50–200 mL given over 90–120 minutes	

1. Continuous infusion not usually recommended

Drug	Infusion method
Nimodipine Nimotop®	*via* drip tubing *in* Glucose 5% *or* Sodium chloride 0.9% *or* Ringer's solution

Not to be added to infusion container; administer *via* an infusion pump through a Y-piece into a central catheter; incompatible with polyvinyl chloride giving sets or containers

Noradrenaline solution strong sterile Levophed®	Continuous *in* Glucose 5% *or* Sodium chloride and glucose

Dilute in a large-volume infusion; pH of the infusion solution must be below 6

Ondansetron hydrochloride Zofran®	Continuous *or* intermittent *in* Glucose 5% *or* Sodium chloride 0.9% *or* Ringer's solution
Oxytocin Syntocinon®	Continuous *in* Glucose 5% *or* Sodium chloride 0.9% *or* Ringer's solution

Dilute in a large-volume infusion

Pentamidine isethionate Pentacarinat®	Intermittent *in* Glucose 5% *or* Sodium chloride 0.9%

Dissolve initially in water for injections (300 mg in 3–5 mL) then dilute in 50–250 mL; give over at least 60 minutes

Phenoxybenzamine hydrochloride Dibenyline®	Intermittent *in* Sodium chloride 0.9%

Dilute in 200–500 mL infusion; give over at least 2 hours; max. 4 hours between dilution and completion of administration

Phentolamine mesylate Rogitine®	Intermittent *in* Glucose 5% *or* Sodium chloride 0.9%
Phenylephrine hydrochloride	Intermittent *in* Glucose 5% *or* Sodium chloride 0.9%
Piperacillin sodium Pipril®	Intermittent *in* Glucose 5% *or* Sodium chloride 0.9% *or* Compound sodium lactate *or* Water for injections

Minimum volume 50 mL given over 20–40 minutes

Plicamycin Mithracin®	Continuous *in* Glucose 5% *or* Sodium chloride 0.9%

Reconstitute 2.5 mg with 4.9 mL water for injections then dilute appropriate dose to suggested volume 1000 mL given over 4–6 hours

Polymyxin B sulphate Aerosporin®	Continuous *or* intermittent *in* Glucose 5%

Suggested volume of intermittent infusion, 200–500 mL given over 60–120 minutes

Drug	Infusion method
Potassium canrenoate Spiroctan-M®	Intermittent *in* Glucose 5% *or* Sodium chloride 0.9%

Suggested volume 250 mL

Potassium chloride	Continuous *in* Glucose 5% *or* Sodium chloride 0.9%

Dilute in a large-volume infusion; mix thoroughly to avoid 'layering', especially in non-rigid infusion containers; use ready-prepared solutions when possible

Procainamide hydrochloride Pronestyl®	Continuous *or* intermittent *in* Glucose 5%

For maintenance, dilute to a concentration of *either* 2 mg/mL and give at a rate of 1–3 mL/minute *or* 4 mg/mL and give at a rate of 0.5–1.5 mL/minute

Propofol Diprivan®	*via* drip tubing *in* Glucose 5% *or* Sodium chloride 0.9%

Not to be mixed with other therapeutic agents or infusion fluids; to be administered *via* a Y-piece close to injection site

Continuous *in* Glucose 5%

Dilute to a concentration not exceeding 2 mg/mL; administer using suitable device to control infusion rate; use glass or PVC containers (if PVC bag used it should be full—withdraw volume of infusion fluid equal to that of propofol to be added); propofol may alternatively be infused undiluted using a suitable infusion pump

Quinine dihydrochloride	Continuous *in* Sodium chloride 0.9%

To be given over 4 hours; see also section 5.4.1

Ranitidine hydrochloride Zantac®	Intermittent *in* Glucose 5% *or* Sodium chloride 0.9% *or* Compound sodium lactate
Rifampicin Rifadin®, Rimactane®	Intermittent *in* Glucose 5 and 10% *or* Sodium chloride 0.9% *or* Ringer's solution

Reconstitute with solvent provided then dilute with 250 mL (Rimactane®) or 500 mL (Rifadin®) infusion fluid; give over 2–3 hours

Ritodrine hydrochloride Yutopar®	Continuous *in* Glucose 5% *or* Sodium chloride 0.9%

Dilute in a large-volume infusion

Salbutamol sulphate Ventolin® For Intravenous Infusion	Continuous *in* Glucose 5% *or* Sodium chloride 0.9%

Suggested volume 500 mL as a solution containing 10 micrograms/mL

Salcatonin Miacalcic®	Continuous *in* Sodium chloride 0.9%

Diluted solution given without delay; dilute in 500 mL and give over at least 6 hours; glass or hard plastic containers should not be used; approx. 20% loss of potency on dilution (take into account when calculating dose)

1. Continuous infusion not usually recommended

Appendix 6: Intravenous additives

Drug	Infusion method
Sodium calciumedetate Ledclair®	Continuous *in* Glucose 5% *or* Sodium chloride 0.9%
Dilute to a concentration of not more than 3%; suggested volume 250–500 mL given over at least 1 hour	
Sodium clodronate Bonefos® Concentrate, Loron®	Continuous *in* Sodium chloride 0.9%
Dilute 300 mg in 500 mL infusion fluid and give over at least 2 hours; Bonefos® Concentrate can also be infused in Glucose 5%	
Sodium nitroprusside Nipride®	Continuous *in* Glucose 5% *or* Sodium chloride 0.9% *or* Ringer's solution *or* Compound sodium lactate
Reconstitute with solvent provided then dilute immediately with 250–1000 mL infusion fluid; preferably infuse *via* infusion device to allow precise control; protect infusion from light	
Sodium valproate Epilim®	Continuous *or* intermittent *in* Glucose 5% *or* Sodium chloride 0.9%
Reconstitute with solvent provided then dilute with infusion fluid	
Streptokinase Kabikinase®, Streptase®	Continuous *in* Sodium chloride 0.9%
Kabikinase® can also be infused in Glucose 5%	
Sulphadiazine sodium	Continuous *in* Sodium chloride 0.9%
Suggested volume 500 mL; ampoule solution has a pH of over 10	
Suxamethonium chloride Anectine®, Scoline®	Continuous *in* Glucose 5% *or* Sodium chloride 0.9%
Teicoplanin Targocid®	[1]Intermittent *in* Glucose 5% *or* Sodium chloride 0.9% *or* Compound sodium lactate
Reconstitute initially with water for injections provided; infuse over 30 minutes	
Temocillin sodium Temopen®	Intermittent *in* Glucose 5% *or* Sodium chloride 0.9% *or* Ringer's solution *or* Compound sodium lactate
Dissolve initially in water for injections (500 mg in 10 mL; 1–2 g in 20 mL) then dilute with infusion fluid and give over 30–40 minutes	
Terbutaline sulphate Bricanyl®	Continuous *in* Glucose 5% *or* Sodium chloride 0.9%
Suggested volume 500 mL; to be given over 8–10 hours	
Tetracosactrin Synacthen®	Continuous *in* Glucose 5% *or* Sodium chloride 0.9%
Suggested volume 500 mL given over 6 hours	
Tetracycline hydrochloride Achromycin Intravenous®	Continuous *in* Glucose 5% *or* Sodium chloride 0.9% *or* Compound sodium lactate
Reconstitute initially with water for injections (250 mg in 5 mL, 500 mg in 10 mL) then dilute to at least 100 mL (max. 1 litre) and give at a rate not exceeding 100 mL in 5 minutes preferably through a 0.22 micron filter	
Theophylline (solubilised with lysine) Labophylline®	Continuous *in* Glucose 5% *or* Sodium chloride 0.9%
Ticarcillin sodium Ticar®	Intermittent *in* Glucose 5% *or* Water for injections
Suggested volume 100–150 mL given over 30–40 minutes	
Ticarcillin sodium/ clavulanic acid Timentin®	Intermittent *in* Glucose 5% *or* Water for injections
Suggested volume glucose 5%, 50–150 mL (depending on dose) or water for injections, 25–100 mL; given over 30–40 minutes	
Tobramycin sulphate Nebcin®	Intermittent *or via* drip tubing *in* Glucose 5% *or* Sodium chloride 0.9%
For adult intermittent infusion suggested volume 50–100 mL (children proportionately smaller volume) given over 20–60 minutes	
Tocainide hydrochloride Tonocard®	Intermittent *in* Glucose 5% *or* Sodium chloride 0.9%
Suggested volume 50–100 mL given over 15–30 minutes	
Treosulfan Treosulfan (Leo)	Intermittent *in* Water for injections
Infusion suggested for doses above 5 g; dilute to a concentration of 5 g in 100 mL	
Trimetaphan camsylate Arfonad®	Intermittent *in* Glucose 5% *or* Sodium chloride 0.9%
Suggested infusion concentration 0.05–0.1%; suggested volume 100–500 mL	
Trimethoprim lactate Monotrim® Syraprim®	*via* drip tubing *in* Glucose 5%
Monotrim® can also be infused *via* drip tubing in Sodium chloride 0.9% *or* Compound sodium lactate; Syraprim® can also be given by intermittent infusion in Glucose 5%	
Trisodium edetate Limclair®	Continuous *in* Glucose 5% *or* Sodium chloride 0.9%
Suggested volume 500 mL given over 2–3 hours	
Urokinase Urokinase (Leo)	Continuous *in* Sodium chloride 0.9%

1. Continuous infusion not usually recommended

Appendix 6: Intravenous additives

Drug	Infusion method
Vancomycin hydrochloride *Vancocin*®	[1]Intermittent *in* Glucose 5% *or* Sodium chloride 0.9%

Reconstitute 500 mg with 10 mL water for injections and dilute to 100–200 mL with infusion fluid; give over at least 60 minutes (rate not to exceed 10 mg/minute for doses over 500 mg); use continuous infusion only if intermittent not feasible

Vasopressin, synthetic *Pitressin*®	Intermittent *in* Glucose 5%

Suggested concentration 20 units/100 mL given over 15 minutes

Vecuronium bromide *Norcuron*®	Continuous *in* Glucose 5% *or* Sodium chloride 0.9% *or* Ringer's solution

Reconstitute with the solvent provided

Vinblastine sulphate *Velbe*®	*via* drip tubing *in* Sodium chloride 0.9% *or* Water for injections

Reconstitute with the diluent provided

Vincristine sulphate *Oncovin*®	*via* drip tubing *in* Sodium chloride 0.9% *or* Water for injections

Reconstitute with the diluent provided

Drug	Infusion method
Vindesine sulphate *Eldisine*®	*via* drip tubing *in* Glucose 5% *or* Sodium chloride 0.9%

Reconstitute with the diluent provided

Vitamins B & C *Parentrovite IVHP*®	Intermittent *or via* drip tubing *in* Glucose 5% *or* Sodium chloride 0.9%

Ampoule contents should be mixed, diluted, and administered without delay; give over 10 minutes (see CSM advice, section 9.6.2)

Vitamins, multiple

Multibionta®	Intermittent *in* Glucose 5% *or* Sodium chloride 0.9%

Dilute 10 mL in not less than 250 mL of infusion fluid (adults); see also section 9.3

Solivito N®	Intermittent *in* Glucose 5 and 10%

Suggested volume 500–1000 mL given over 2–3 hours; see also section 9.3

Zidovudine *Retrovir*®	Intermittent *in* Glucose 5%

Dilute to a concentration of 2 mg/mL or 4 mg/mL and give over 1 hour

---

1. Continuous infusion not usually recommended

Appendix 7: Borderline Substances

In certain conditions some foods (and toilet preparations) have characteristics of drugs and the Advisory Committee on Borderline Substances advises as to the circumstances in which such substances may be regarded as drugs. Prescriptions issued in accordance with the Committee's advice and endorsed 'ACBS' will normally not be investigated.

> General Practitioners are reminded that the ACBS recommends products on the basis that they may be regarded as drugs for the treatment of specified conditions. Doctors should satisfy themselves that the products can safely be prescribed, that patients are adequately monitored and that, where necessary, expert hospital supervision is available.

FOODS WHICH MAY BE PRESCRIBED ON FP10

Note. This is a list of food products which the ACBS has approved. The clinical condition for which the product has approval follows each entry.

Aglutella® (Ultrapharm)
Rice, low protein. Net price 500 g = £3.95

AL 110® (Nestle)
Powder, protein 14 g, fat 25 g, carbohydrate 55.3 g, energy 2100 kJ (502 kcal)/100 g with vitamins and minerals. Net price 400 g = £7.27. For proven lactose intolerance in pre-school children, galactosaemia, and galactokinase deficiency

Albumaid® (Scientific Hospital Supplies)
RVHB, powder, amino acid mixture, methionine-free. Net price 200 g = £31.05. For homocystinuria
RVHB complete, powder, amino acid mixture, methionine-free, with vitamins, minerals, and trace elements. Net price 200 g = £31.05. For homocystinuria
XP, powder, amino acids 40%, carbohydrate 50%, fat nil, phenylalanine not more than 10 mg per 100 g, with vitamins, minerals, and trace elements. Net price 200 g = £15.81. For phenylketonuria
XP Concentrate, powder, amino acids 85%, carbohydrate and fat nil, phenylalanine not more than 25 mg per 100 g, with vitamins, minerals, and trace elements. Net price 200 g = £30.20. For phenylketonuria

Alcoholic Beverages see under Rectified Spirit

Alembicol D® (Alembic Products)
Fractionated coconut oil. Net price 4 kg = £66.64. For steatorrhoea associated with cystic fibrosis of the pancreas, intestinal lymphangiectasia, surgery of the intestine, chronic liver disease, liver cirrhosis, other proven malabsorption syndromes; and in a ketogenic diet in the management of epilepsy

Alfare® (Nestle)
Powder, protein 16.5 g, fat 24 g, carbohydrate 51.7 g, energy 2010 kJ (480 kcal)/100 g with vitamins and minerals. Net price 400 g = £5.49. For disaccharide and whole protein intolerance, or where amino acids or peptides are indicated in conjunction with medium chain triglycerides

Aminogran® (UCB Pharma)
Food Supplement, powder, containing all essential amino acids except phenylalanine, for use with mineral mixture (see below). Net price 500 g = £43.87. For phenylketonuria
Mineral Mixture, powder, containing all appropriate minerals for use with the above food supplement and other synthetic diets. Net price 250 g = £7.43. For phenylketonuria and as a mineral supplement in synthetic diets

Analog® (Scientific Hospital Supplies)
MSUD, powder, essential and non-essential amino acids 15.5% except isoleucine, leucine and valine, with carbohydrate, fat, vitamins, minerals, and trace elements. Net price 400 g = £17.99. For maple syrup urine disease
RVHB, powder, essential and non-essential amino acids 15.5% except methionine, with carbohydrate, fat, vitamins, minerals, and trace elements. Net price 400 g = £17.99. For hypermethioninaemia; homocystinuria
XLys, powder, essential and non-essential amino acids 15.5% except lysine, with carbohydrate, fat, vitamins, minerals, and trace elements. Net price 400 g = £17.99. For hyperlysinaemia
XMet, Thre, Val, Isoleu, powder, essential and non-essential amino acids 15.5% except methionine, threonine, valine and low isoleucine, with carbohydrate, fat, vitamins, minerals, and trace elements. Net price 400 g = £17.99. For methylmalonic or propionic acidaemia
XP, powder, essential and non-essential amino acids 15.5% except phenylalanine, with carbohydrate, fat, vitamins, minerals, and trace elements. Net price 400 g = £15.00. For phenylketonuria
XPhen, Tyr, powder, essential and non-essential amino acids 15.5% except phenylalanine and tyrosine, with carbohydrate, fat, vitamins, minerals and trace elements. Net price 400 g = £17.99. For tyrosinaemia

Aproten® (Ultrapharm)
Various products, gluten-free, low protein, low Na^+ and K^+. Net prices: anellini 500 g = £3.95; biscuits 180 g (36) = £2.80; bread mix 250 g = £2.00; cake mix 300 g = £2.10; crispbread 240 g = £3.95; ditalini 500 g = £3.95; flour 300 g = £1.84; rigatini 500 g = £3.95; spaghetti 500 g = £3.95; tagliatelle 250 g = £2.10. For phenylketonuria; similar amino acid abnormalities; renal failure; liver failure and liver cirrhosis; gluten-sensitive enteropathies including steatorrhoea due to gluten sensitivity, coeliac disease, and dermatitis herpetiformis

Arnott® (Ultrapharm)
Rice Cookies, gluten-free. Net price 200 g = £1.32. For gluten-sensitive enteropathies including steatorrhoea due to gluten sensitivity, coeliac disease, and dermatitis herpetiformis

Bi-Aglut® (Ultrapharm)
Biscuits, gluten-free. Net price 180 g (36) = £2.60
Cracker toast, gluten-, lactose-, and milk-protein-free. Net price 240 g (40) = £3.45. For gluten-sensitive enteropathies including steatorrhoea due to gluten sensitivity, coeliac disease, dermatitis herpetiformis

Calogen® (Scientific Hospital Supplies)
Emulsion, arachis oil 50% in water. Net price 250 mL = £2.69; 1 litre = £9.72. For renal failure and other conditions requiring a high-fluid, low-fluid, low-electrolyte diet, disorders of amino acid metabolism or carbohydrate absorption; in a ketogenic diet in the management of epilepsy

Caloreen® (Roussel)
Powder, water-soluble dextrins, with less than 1.8 mmol of Na^+ and 0.3 mmol of K^+/100 g. Net price 250 g = £1.38; 5 kg = £22.54. For renal failure; liver cirrhosis; disaccharide intolerance (without isomaltose intolerance), disorders of amino acid metabolism (and other similar disorders) and/or whole protein intolerance); malabsorption states and other conditions (including proven hypoglycaemia) requiring a high energy, low fluid intake, whether or not sodium and/or potassium restriction is essential

Carobel, Instant® (Cow & Gate)
Powder, carob seed flour. Net price 45 g = £1.98. For thickening feeds in the treatment of vomiting

Casilan® (Crookes)
Powder, whole protein, containing all essential amino

acids, 90% with less than 0.1% Na⁺. Net price 250 g = £4.20. For biochemically proven hypoproteinaemia

Clinifeed® (Roussel)

Clinifeed 400, protein 15 g, carbohydrate 55 g, fat 13.4 g, energy 1674 kJ (400 kcal)/375 mL, with vitamins and minerals, vanilla flavour. Fructose-free. Net price 375-mL can = £1.10

Clinifeed Protein Rich, protein 30 g, carbohydrate 70 g, fat 11 g, energy 2092 kJ (500 kcal)/375 mL, with vitamins and minerals, vanilla flavour. Fructose- and lactose-free. Net price 375-mL can = £1.23

Both for use as necessary nutritional supplements prescribed on medical grounds for: short bowel syndrome, intractable malabsorption, pre-operative preparation of patients who are undernourished, treatment for those with proven inflammatory bowel disease, treatment following total gastrectomy, dysphagia, bowel fistulas, disease-related malnutrition, continuous ambulatory peritoneal dialysis (CAPD), and haemodialysis. Not to be prescribed for any child under one year

Clinifeed Favour, protein 14.1 g, carbohydrate 49.9 g, fat 14.6 g, energy 1575 kJ (375 kcal)/375 mL, with vitamins and minerals, neutral flavour. Lactose-, fructose-, and sucrose-free. Net price 375-mL can = 88p

Clinifeed Iso, protein 10.5 g, carbohydrate 49.2 g, fat 15.4 g, energy 1575 kJ (375 kcal)/375 mL, with vitamins and minerals, vanilla flavour. Fructose- and sucrose-free, and low sodium. Net price 375-mL can = £1.24

Both for use as the sole source of nutrition or as necessary nutritional supplements prescribed on medical grounds for: short bowel syndrome, intractable malabsorption, pre-operative preparation of patients who are undernourished, treatment for those with proven inflammatory bowel disease, treatment following total gastrectomy, dysphagia, bowel fistulas, disease-related malnutrition. Not to be prescribed for any child under one year, unsuitable as a sole source of nutrition for young children up to 5 years of age

Clinutren® (Clintec Nutrition)

Clinutren 1.0, liquid, protein 10 g, carbohydrate 31.8 g, fat 9.5 g, energy 1045 kJ (250 kcal)/250 mL with vitamins, minerals, and trace elements. Cholesterol-, gluten-, and lactose-free. Strawberry, vanilla, chocolate, and neutral flavours. Net price 250-mL can = 81p. For use as the sole source of nutrition or as a necessary nutritional supplement prescribed on medical grounds for: short bowel syndrome, intractable malabsorption, pre-operative preparation of patients who are undernourished, treatment for those with proven inflammatory bowel disease, treatment following total gastrectomy, dysphagia, bowel fistulas, disease-related malnutrition. Not to be prescribed for any child under one year, unsuitable as a sole source of nutrition for young children up to 5 years of age

Clinutren 1.5, liquid, protein 15 g, carbohydrate 42.5 g, fat 16.9 g, energy 1570 kJ (375 kcal)/250 mL with vitamins, minerals, and trace elements. Cholesterol-, gluten-, and lactose-free. Strawberry, vanilla, and chocolate flavours. Net price 250-mL can = £1.08. As a necessary nutritional supplement prescribed on medical grounds for: short bowel syndrome, intractable malabsorption, pre-operative preparation of patients who are undernourished, treatment for those with proven inflammatory bowel disease, treatment following total gastrectomy, dysphagia, bowel fistulas, disease-related malnutrition. Not to be prescribed for any child under one year

Comminuted Chicken Meat (Cow & Gate)

Suspension (aqueous). Net price 128 g = £1.02. For carbohydrate intolerance in association with possible or proven intolerance of milk; glucose and galactose intolerance

Corn flour and corn starch. For hypoglycaemia associated with glycogen-storage disease

Corn oil (maize oil). Net price 100 mL = 37p. For familial hypercholesterolaemia

Appendix 7: Borderline substances 535

Dialamine® (Scientific Hospital Supplies)

Powder, essential amino acids 30%, with carbohydrate 62%, energy 1500 kJ (360 kcal)/100 g, with ascorbic acid, minerals, and trace elements. Flavour: orange. Net price 200 g = £14.41. For oral feeding where essential amino acid supplements are required; e.g. chronic renal failure, hypoproteinaemia, wound fistula leakage with excessive protein loss, conditions requiring a controlled nitrogen intake, and haemodialysis

dp® (Nutricia)

Cookies, low-protein, butterscotch- or chocolate flavoured chip cookies. Net price 170 g = £4.90. For phenylketonuria; similar amino acid abnormalities; renal failure; liver failure and liver cirrhosis

Duocal® (Scientific Hospital Supplies)

Liquid, emulsion providing carbohydrate 23.4 g, fat 7.1 g, energy 628 kJ/100 mL. Low-electrolyte, gluten-, lactose-, and protein-free. Net price 250 mL = £1.51; 1 litre = £5.36

Super Soluble Powder, carbohydrate 72.7 g, fat 22.3 g, energy 1988 kJ/100 g. Low electrolyte, gluten-, protein-, and lactose-free. Net price 400 g = £9.78.

Both for renal failure; liver cirrhosis; disaccharide intolerance (without isomaltose intolerance), disorders of amino acid metabolism (and other similar disorders), and/or whole protein intolerance; malabsorption states and other conditions requiring a high energy, low fluid intake, whether or not sodium and/or potassium restriction is essential

Elemental 028® (Scientific Hospital Supplies)

Powder, amino acids 12%, carbohydrate 70.5–72%, fat 6.64%, energy 1544–1568 kJ (364–370 kcal)/100 g with vitamins and minerals. For preparation with water before use. Net price 100-g box (orange flavoured or plain) = £3.61. For use as the sole source of nutrition or as a necessary nutritional supplement prescribed on medical grounds for: short-bowel syndrome, intractable malabsorption, treatment for proven inflammatory bowel disease, bowel fistulas. Not to be prescribed for any child under one year, unsuitable as a sole source of nutrition for young children up to 5 years of age

Ener-G® (General Designs)

Gluten-free. Rice bread (sliced), brown, net price 200 g = £1.73; 400 g = £3.45, white, 200 g = £1.73. Tapioca bread (sliced), 200 g = £1.73. Rice pasta (shells, small shells, lasagna, and vermicelli), 454 g = £3.00; spaghetti, 447 g = £3.00; tagliatelle, 300 g = £3.00; cannelloni, 285 g = £3.00. For gluten-sensitive enteropathies including steatorrhoea due to gluten sensitivity, coeliac disease, and dermatitis herpetiformis

Enrich® (Abbott)

Liquid with dietary fibre, providing protein 9.4 g, carbohydrate 38.3 g (including 5 g as dietary fibre), fat 8.8 g, energy 1090 kJ (260 kcal)/250 mL with vitamins and minerals. Lactose- and gluten-free. Vanilla and chocolate flavours. Net price 250-mL can = £1.66. For use as the sole source of nutrition or as a necessary nutritional supplement prescribed on medical grounds for: short-bowel syndrome, intractable malabsorption, pre-operative preparation of patients who are undernourished, treatment for proven inflammatory bowel disease, treatment following total gastrectomy, dysphagia, disease-related malnutrition. Not to be prescribed for any child under one year, unsuitable as a sole source of nutrition for young children up to 5 years of age

Ensure® (Abbott)

Liquid, protein 3.7%, fat 3.7%, carbohydrate 14.5%, with minerals and vitamins, lactose- and gluten-free, energy 1050 kJ (253 kcal)/250 mL. Vanilla flavour. Net price 237-mL bottle = £1.51; 250-mL can = £1.40; 946-mL can = £5.60. Chocolate, blackcurrant, coffee, eggnog, and nut flavours. Net price 237-mL can = £1.40. Chicken, mushroom, and asparagus flavours. Net price 250-mL can = £1.40.

Powder, same composition as Ensure liquid when reconstituted. Net price 400 g = £5.93

Both for use as the sole source of nutrition or as a

necessary nutritional supplement prescribed on medical grounds for: short bowel syndrome, intractable malabsorption, pre-operative preparation of patients who are undernourished, treatment for proven inflammatory bowel disease, treatment following total gastrectomy, dysphagia, bowel fistulas, disease-related malnutrition. Neither to be prescribed for any child under one year, unsuitable as a sole source of nutrition for young children up to 5 years of age

Ensure Plus® (Abbott)
Liquid, protein 6.3%, fat 5%, carbohydrate 20%, with vitamins and minerals, lactose- and gluten-free, energy 1570 kJ (375 kcal)/250 mL. Vanilla flavour. Net price 250-mL can = £1.75; 500-mL bottle = £3.50. Caramel, chocolate, strawberry, and vanilla flavours. Net price 200-mL Tetrapak = £1.44. As a necessary nutritional supplement prescribed on medical grounds for: short bowel syndrome, intractable malabsorption, pre-operative preparation of patients who are undernourished, treatment for those with proven inflammatory bowel disease, treatment following total gastrectomy, dysphagia, bowel fistulas, disease-related malnutrition, continuous ambulatory peritoneal dialysis (CAPD), and haemodialysis. Not to be prescribed for any child under one year

Farley's Gluten-free biscuits (Farley)
Biscuits. Net price 200 g = £1.14. For gluten-sensitive enteropathies including steatorrhoea due to gluten sensitivity, coeliac disease and dermatitis herpetiformis

Flexical® (Bristol-Myers)
Powder, protein 9.9%, carbohydrate 67%, fat 15% with vitamins and minerals. Gluten- and lactose-free. Net price 454 g = £9.36. For use as the sole source of nutrition or as a necessary nutritional supplement prescribed on medical grounds for: short-bowel syndrome, intractable malabsorption, treatment for those with proven inflammatory bowel disease, bowel fistulas. Not to be prescribed for any child under one year, unsuitable as a sole source of nutrition for young children up to 5 years of age

Forceval Protein® (Unigreg)
Powder, calcium caseinate 60%, carbohydrate 30%, with vitamins and minerals, providing not less than 55% protein, not more than 1% of fat, not more than 0.12% of Na$^+$. Lactose- and gluten-free. Vanilla, strawberry, and neutral flavours. Net price 300 g = £12.00; 8 × 15-g sachets = £5.12. For biochemically proven hypoproteinaemia

Formula MCT(1) see under MCT(1)
Formula S® see **Nutrilon Soya®**
Fortical® (Cow & Gate)
Liquid, glucose polymers providing carbohydrate 61.5 g/100 mL. Low-electrolyte, protein-free. Flavours: apple, apricot, black currant, lemon, orange, and neutral. Net price 200 mL = £1.00. For renal failure; liver cirrhosis, disaccharide intolerance (without maltose intolerance), disorders of amino acid metabolism, and/or whole protein intolerance, malabsorption states, or other conditions including proven hypoglycaemia requiring a high-energy, low-fluid, low-electrolyte diet

Fortimel® (Cow & Gate)
Liquid, protein 19.4 g, carbohydrate 20.8 g, fat 4.2 g, energy 840 kJ (200 kcal)/200 mL with vitamins and minerals. Vanilla, strawberry, chocolate, coffee, apricot, and forest fruits flavours. Net price 200-mL carton = 79p. As a necessary nutritional supplement prescribed on medical grounds for the treatment of: short bowel syndrome, intractable malabsorption, pre-operative preparation of patients who are undernourished, treatment for those with proven inflammatory bowel disease, treatment following total gastrectomy, dysphagia, bowel fistulas, disease-related malnutrition. Not to be prescribed for any child under one year

Fortipudding® (Cow & Gate)
Semi-solid, protein 15.3 g, carbohydrate 24 g, fat 4.5 g, energy 825 kJ (196 kcal)/150 g with vitamins and minerals. Vanilla, chocolate, and coffee flavours. Net price

150-g tub = 87p. As a necessary nutritional supplement prescribed on medical grounds for: short bowel syndrome, intractable malabsorption, pre-operative preparation of patients who are undernourished, treatment for those with proven inflammatory bowel disease, treatment following total gastrectomy, dysphagia, bowel fistulas, disease-related malnutrition or growth failure, continuous ambulatory peritoneal dialysis (CAPD) and haemodialysis. Not to be prescribed for any child under one year

Fortisip® (Cow & Gate)
Liquid, protein 10 g, carbohydrate 35.8 g, fat 13 g, energy 1260 kJ (300 kcal)/200 mL, with vitamins and minerals. Gluten-free and low lactose. Vanilla, banana, orange, strawberry, tropical fruits, mushroom, and neutral flavours. Net price 200 mL = £1.19. As a necessary nutritional supplement prescribed on medical grounds for: short-bowel syndrome, intractable malabsorption, pre-operative preparation of patients who are undernourished, treatment for proven inflammatory bowel disease, treatment following total gastrectomy, dysphagia, bowel fistulas, disease-related malnutrition. Not to be prescribed for any child under one year

Fortison® see **Nutrison®**
Fresenius OPD® (Fresenius)
Liquid, protein 22.5 g, carbohydrate 75 g, fat 13 g, energy 2460 kJ (500 kcal) /500 mL, with vitamins, minerals, and trace elements. Gluten-free, and low lactose. Net price 500-mL bottle = £3.50. As a necessary nutritional supplement prescribed on medical grounds for the treatment of: short bowel syndrome, intractable malabsorption, pre-operative preparation of patients who are undernourished, treatment for those with proven inflammatory bowel disease, treatment following total gastrectomy, dysphagia, bowel fistulas, disease-related malnutrition. Not to be prescribed for any child under one year; unsuitable as a sole source of nutrition for young children up to 5 years of age

Fresubin® (Fresenius)
Liquid, protein 7.6 g, carbohydrate 27.6 g, fat 6.8 g, energy 840 kJ (200 kcal)/200 mL with vitamins and minerals. Gluten-free, low lactose and cholesterol. Net price 200-mL carton (nut, peach, black currant, chocolate, mocha, and vanilla flavours) = 99p; 500-mL bottle (nut, peach, and vanilla flavours) = £2.25. For use as the sole source of nutrition or as a necessary nutritional supplement prescribed on medical grounds for: short-bowel syndrome, intractable malabsorption, pre-operative preparation of patients who are undernourished, treatment for proven inflammatory bowel disease, treatment following total gastrectomy, dysphagia, bowel fistulas, disease-related malnutrition, and Refsum's disease. Not to be prescribed for any child under one year, unsuitable as a sole source of nutrition for young children up to 5 years of age

High Energy Liquid, protein 13.2 g, carbohydrate 44.4 g, fat 13.7 g, energy 1491 kJ (355 kcal)/236 mL with vitamins and minerals. Gluten-free, cholesterol-free and low lactose. Vanilla, chocolate and strawberry flavours. Net price 236-mL Tetrabrik = £1.40. For indications, see under Fresubin liquid (except Refsum's disease). Not to be prescribed for any child under 2 years, unsuitable as a sole source of nutrition for young children up to 5 years of age

Fresubin Plus F® (Fresenius)
Liquid foods with dietary fibre in 2 formulations. For use as the sole source of nutrition or as a necessary nutritional supplement prescribed on medical grounds for: short-bowel syndrome, intractable malabsorption, pre-operative preparation of patients who are undernourished, treatment for proven inflammatory bowel disease, treatment following total gastrectomy, dysphagia, disease-related malnutrition. Not to be prescribed for any child under 2 years, unsuitable as a sole source of nutrition for young children up to 5 years of age

Muesli-flavour, milk protein, cereals, coconut, sunflower oil, vitamins and minerals providing protein 19 g, fat 17 g, carbohydrate 69 g, fibre 5 g, energy 2100 kJ (500 kcal)/500 mL. Low sodium, lactose, and cholesterol. Net price 200-mL carton = £1.15; 500-mL bottle = £2.65

Vegetable soup-flavour, milk protein, beef fat and protein, sunflower oil, maize starch, vitamins and minerals providing protein 19 g, fat 17 g, carbohydrate 69 g, fibre 3 g, energy 2100 kJ (500 kcal)/500 mL. Gluten-free, low sodium, lactose, and cholesterol. Net price 200-mL bottle = £1.30

Fresubin 750® (Fresenius)
Liquid, protein 37.5 g, carbohydrate 85 g, fat 30 g, energy 3150 kJ (750 kcal)/500 mL with vitamins, minerals, and trace elements. Gluten-free and low lactose. Vanilla flavour. Net price 500-mL bottle = £2.40. As a necessary nutritional supplement prescribed on medical grounds for the treatment of: short bowel syndrome, intractable malabsorption, pre-operative preparation of patients who are undernourished, treatment for those with proven inflammatory bowel disease, treatment following total gastrectomy, dysphagia, bowel fistulas, disease-related malnutrition, continuous ambulatory peritoneal dialysis (CAPD), and haemodialysis. Not to be prescribed for any child under one year. A maximum of 500 mL per day to be taken by dialysis patients

Fructose (laevulose). For proven glucose/galactose intolerance

Galactomin® (Cow & Gate)
Formula 17 (new formula), powder, protein 14.5 g, fat 25.9 g, carbohydrate 56.9 g, mineral salts 3.4 g/100 g. Used as a 13.1% solution with additional vitamins in place of milk. Net price 400 g = £8.35. For proven lactose intolerance in preschool children, galactosaemia and galactokinase deficiency

Formula 19 (new formula), powder, protein 14.6 g, fat 30.8 g, carbohydrate 49.7 g (fructose as carbohydrate source), mineral salts 2.1 g/100 g, with vitamins. Used as a 12.9% solution in place of milk. Net price 400 g = £18.35. For glucose plus galactose intolerance

Generaid® (Scientific Hospital Supplies)
Powder, whey protein and additional branched-chain amino acids (protein equivalent 81%). Net price 200 g = £16.85. For patients with chronic liver disease and/or porto-hepatic encephalopathy

GF Dietary® (Nutricia)
Biscuits, gluten-free. Net price 150 g = £1.01. For gluten-sensitive enteropathies including steatorrhoea due to gluten sensitivity, coeliac disease, and dermatitis herpetiformis

Glucose (dextrose monohydrate). Net price 100 g = 14p. For glycogen storage disease and sucrose/isomaltose intolerance

Glutafin® (Nutricia)
Gluten-free. Bread (whole or sliced), net price 400-g loaf = £2.14. Fibre bread (whole or sliced), 400-g loaf = £2.14. Mix, 500 g = £4.48. Baking mix, 500 g = £4.48. Fibre mix, 500 g = £4.48. Biscuits, savoury or tea, 125 g = £1.37. Biscuits, digestive or sweet, 150 g = £1.37. Biscuits, 200 g = £3.06. Crackers, 200 g = £2.23. High fibre crackers, 200 g = £1.87. Pasta (macaroni, pasta spirals, or spaghetti shortcut), 250 g = £2.44. For gluten-sensitive enteropathies including steatorrhoea due to gluten sensitivity, coeliac disease, and dermatitis herpetiformis

Gluten-free biscuits and **crackers**, see under Farley and GF

Hepatic-Aid II® (Kendall)
Powder, amino acids 4.4%, carbohydrate 16.8%, fat 3.6% when reconstituted. Low sodium and electrolytes; mineral and vitamin supplementation is required. Flavours: chocolate, chocolate mint, custard, and eggnog. Net price per packet = £7.95. For patients with chronic liver disease and/or porto-hepatic encephalopathy

Hycal® (SmithKline Beecham Brands)
Liquid, protein-free, low-electrolyte, glucose syrup solids 49.5%. Flavours, blackcurrant, lemon, orange, and raspberry. Net price 171 mL = 69p. For renal failure; liver cirrhosis or other conditions requiring a high-energy, low-fluid, low-electrolyte diet

Instant Carobel see **Carobel, Instant**

Isomil® (Abbott)
Powder, protein 1.8%, carbohydrate 6.9%, fat 4.69% with vitamins and minerals when reconstituted. Lactose-free. Net price 400 g = £3.20. For proven lactose intolerance in preschool children, galactokinase deficiency, galactosaemia, and proven whole cow's milk sensitivity

Jevity® (Abbott)
Liquid, protein 4.2%, fat 3.5%, carbohydrate 13.4%, dietary fibre 1.36%, with vitamins and minerals. Gluten-, lactose, and sucrose-free. Net price 500-mL bottle = £3.50. For use as the sole source of nutrition or as a necessary nutritional supplement prescribed on medical grounds for: short bowel syndrome, intractable malabsorption, pre-operative preparation of patients who are undernourished, treatment for those with proven inflammatory bowel disease, treatment following total gastrectomy, dysphagia, disease-related malnutrition. Not to be prescribed for any child under 2 years, unsuitable as a sole source of nutrition for young children up to 5 years of age

Juvela® (Scientific Hospital Supplies)
Gluten-free. Corn mix, fibre mix, and flour mix, net price 500 g = £4.48. Bread (whole or sliced), 400-g loaf = £2.14. Fibre bread (sliced and unsliced), 400-g loaf = £2.14. For gluten-sensitive enteropathies including steatorrhoea due to gluten sensitivity, coeliac disease, and dermatitis herpetiformis

Low Protein. Mix, net price 500 g = £4.08. Bread, (whole or sliced) 400-g loaf = £2.14. Biscuits, chocolate chip, orange, and cinnamon flavour, 150 g = £4.48. For phenylketonuria and similar amino-acid abnormalities; renal failure; liver failure and liver cirrhosis; gluten-sensitive enteropathies, see above

Kindergen® **P R O D** (Scientific Hospital Supplies)
Powder, protein 7.6 g, carbohydrate 60.6 g, fat 26.1 g, energy 2060 kJ (492 kcal)/100 g with vitamins and minerals. Net price 400 g = £10.30. For complete nutritional support or supplementary feeding for infants and children with chronic renal failure who are receiving peritoneal rapid overnight dialysis

Liga® (Jacobs Bakery)
Rusks, egg- and gluten-free. Net price 24 = 75p. For gluten-sensitive enteropathies including steatorrhoea due to gluten sensitivity, coeliac disease, and dermatitis herpetiformis

Liquigen® (Scientific Hospital Supplies)
Emulsion, medium chain triglycerides 52%. Net price 250 mL = £4.17; 1 litre = £15.45. For steatorrhoea associated with cystic fibrosis of the pancreas; intestinal lymphangiectasia, surgery of the intestine; chronic liver disease and liver cirrhosis; other proven malabsorption syndromes; ketogenic diet in the management of epilepsy; type I hyperlipoproteinaemia

Liquisorb® (Merck)
Liquid, protein 20 g, carbohydrate 59 g, fat 20 g, energy 2095 kJ (500 kcal)/500 mL with vitamins and minerals. Gluten-free, low lactose. Banana, vanilla, chocolate, strawberry, and neutral flavours. Net price 500-mL bottle = £1.90. Strawberry and vanilla flavours only. Net price 200-mL Tetrapak = 78p. For use as the sole source of nutrition or as a necessary nutritional supplement prescribed on medical grounds for: short bowel syndrome, intractable malabsorption, pre-operative preparation of patients who are undernourished, treatment for proven inflammatory bowel disease, treatment following total gastrectomy, dysphagia, bowel fistulas, disease-related malnutrition. Not to be prescribed for any child under one year, unsuitable as a sole source of nutrition for young children up to 5 years of age

High energy liquid, protein 30 g, carbohydrate 87.5 g, fat 30 g, energy 3150 kJ (750 kcal)/500 mL, with vitamins, minerals and trace elements. Gluten-free and low lactose. Net price 500-mL bottle = £2.60. As a necessary nutritional supplement prescribed on medical grounds for the treatment of: short bowel syndrome, intractable malabsorption, pre-operative preparation of patients who are undernourished, treatment for those with proven inflammatory bowel disease, treatment following total gastrectomy, dysphagia, bowel fistulas, disease-related malnutrition. Not to be prescribed for any child under one year. A maximum of 500 mL per day to be taken by dialysis patients

Liquisorbon MCT® (Merck)
Liquid, protein 25 g, carbohydrate 61.5 g, fat 16.5 g, energy 2095 kJ (500 kcal)/500 mL with vitamins and minerals. Gluten- and fructose-free, low lactose. Strawberry, vanilla, and neutral flavours. Net price 500 mL = £2.65. As a necessary nutritional supplement prescribed on medical grounds for the treatment of: short bowel syndrome, intractable malabsorption, pre-operative preparation of patients who are undernourished, treatment for those with proven inflammatory bowel disease, treatment following total gastrectomy, dysphagia, bowel fistulas, disease-related malnutrition. Not to be prescribed for any child under one year

Locasol New Formula® (Cow & Gate)
Powder, protein 14.6 g, carbohydrate 56.5 g, fat 26.1 g, mineral salts 1.9 g, not more than 55 mg of $Ca^{2+}/100$ g and vitamins. Used as a 13.1% solution in place of milk. Net price 400 g = £9.29. For calcium intolerance

Lofenalac® (Bristol-Myers)
Powder, protein 15%, carbohydrate 60%, fat 18%, phenylalanine not more than 0.1% with vitamins and minerals. Gluten-, sucrose-, and lactose-free. Net price 450 g = £8.00. For phenylketonuria

Loprofin® (Nutricia)
Low protein. Sweet biscuits, 150 g = £1.37; *chocolate cream-filled biscuits*, 125 g = £1.37; *crackers*, 150 g = £1.87; *cookies* (chocolate chip or cinnamon), 100 g = £4.48; *wafers* (orange, vanilla, or chocolate), 100 g = £1.34. For phenylketonuria and similar amino acid abnormalities; renal failure; liver failure and liver cirrhosis
Low protein/gluten-free. Bread (sliced or whole), net price 400-g loaf = £2.14. *Mix*, 500 g = £4.48. *Pasta* (macaroni, pasta spirals or spaghetti short-cut), 250 g = £2.44. For phenylketonuria and similar amino-acid abnormalities; renal failure; liver failure and liver cirrhosis; gluten-sensitive enteropathies including steatorrhoea due to gluten sensitivity, coeliac disease, and dermatitis herpetiformis
PKU Drink, protein 1 g (phenylalanine 30 mg), lactose 9.4 g, fat 4 g, energy 300 kJ (72 kcal)/200 mL. Net price 200-mL bottle = 44p. For phenylketonuria

Lorenzo's Oil (Scientific Hospital Supplies)
Liquid, glycerol trioleate oil 4 parts, glycerol trierucate oil 1 part. Net price 710 mL = £55.91. For biochemically proven and/or clinically manifest adrenoleukodystrophy

Low Protein Drink (Milupa)
Powder, protein 0.4%, carbohydrate 5.1%, fat 2% when reconstituted. Net price 400 g = £5.75. For inherited disorders of amino acid metabolism in childhood
Note. Termed Milupa lpd by manufacturer

Maxamaid® (Scientific Hospital Supplies)
MSUD, powder, essential and non-essential amino acids 30% except isoleucine, leucine, and valine, with carbohydrate, fat less than 0.5%, vitamins, minerals, and trace elements. Net price 575 g = £44.74. For maple syrup urine disease
RVHB, powder, essential and non-essential amino acids 30% except methionine, with carbohydrate, fat less than 0.5%, vitamins, minerals, and trace elements. Net price 575 g = £44.74. For hypermethioninaemia, homocystinuria
XLys, powder, essential and non-essential amino acids 30% except lysine, with carbohydrate, fat less than 0.5%, vitamins, minerals, and trace elements. Net price 575 g = £44.74. For hyperlysinaemia
XLys, Try, powder, essential and non-essential amino acids 30% except lysine and tryptophan, with carbohydrate, fat less than 0.5%, vitamins, minerals, and trace elements. Net price 575 g = £44.74. For glutaric aciduria
XMet, Thre, Val, Isoleu, powder, essential and non-essential amino acids 30% except methionine, threonine, valine and low isoleucine, with carbohydrate, fat less than 0.5%, vitamins, minerals, and trace elements. Net price 575 g = £44.74. For methylmalonic or propionic acidaemia
XP, essential and non-essential amino acids 30% except phenylalanine, with carbohydrate, vitamins, minerals, and trace elements; Net price 25-g bar = 79p; powder (orange-flavoured or unflavoured), 575 g = £34.78. For phenylketonuria. Not to be prescribed for children under 2 years of age
XP Concentrate, powder, essential and non-essential amino acids 65% except phenylalanine, with carbohydrate, fat less than 0.5%, vitamins, minerals, and trace elements. Unflavoured. Net price 200 g = £33.79. For phenylketonuria. Not to be prescribed for children under 2 years of age
XPhen, Tyr, powder, essential and non-essential amino acids 30% except phenylalanine and tyrosine, with carbohydrate, fat less than 0.5%, vitamins, minerals, and trace elements. Net price 575 g = £44.74. For tyrosinaemia

Maxamum® (Scientific Hospital Supplies)
MSUD, powder, essential and non-essential amino acids 47% except isoleucine, leucine, and valine, with carbohydrate, fat less than 0.5%, vitamins, minerals, and trace elements. Orange-flavoured. Net price 200 g = £24.95. For maple syrup urine disease. Not recommended for children under 8 years.
RVHB, powder, essential and non-essential amino acids 47% except methionine, with carbohydrate, fat less than 0.5%, vitamins, minerals, and trace elements. Unflavoured. Net price 200 g = £24.95. For hypermethioninaemia, homocystinuria. Not recommended for children under 8 years
XMet, Thre, Val, Isoleu, powder, essential and non-essential amino acids 47% except methionine, threonine, valine, and low isoleucine, with carbohydrate, fat less than 0.5%, vitamins, minerals, and trace elements. Unflavoured. Net price 200 g = £24.95. For methylmalonic or propionic acidaemia. Not recommended for children under 8 years
XP, powder, essential and non-essential amino acids 47% except phenylalanine, with carbohydrates, vitamins, minerals, and trace elements. Orange-flavoured or unflavoured. Net price 575 g = £55.72. For phenylketonuria. Not to be prescribed for children under 8 years

Maxijul® (Scientific Hospital Supplies)
Liquid, carbohydrate 50%, with potassium 0.004%, sodium 0.023%. Gluten-, lactose-, and fructose-free. Flavours: black currant, lemon and lime, orange, and natural. Net price 200 mL = 69p
Super Soluble Powder, glucose polymer, potassium 0.004%, sodium 0.046%. Gluten-, lactose-, and fructose-free. Net price 4 × 140-g sachet pack = £2.44, 200 g = £1.39, 2.5 kg = £11.50.
Both for renal failure; liver cirrhosis; disaccharide intolerance (without isomaltose intolerance); disorders of amino acid metabolism (and other similar disorders) and/or whole protein intolerance; malabsorption states and other conditions, including proven hypoglycaemia, requiring a high-energy, low-fluid intake

Maxijul LE® (Scientific Hospital Supplies)
Powder, modification of Maxijul with lower concentrations of sodium and potassium. Net price 100 g = £1.02, 2 kg = £13.50. For indications, see under Maxijul where sodium and/or potassium restriction is also essential

Maxipro HBV® Super Soluble (Scientific Hospital Supplies)
Powder, whey protein and additional amino acids (protein equivalent 80%). Net price 200 g = £4.92; 1 kg = £19.67. For biochemically proven hypoproteinaemia. Not to be prescribed for any child under one year; unsuitable as a sole source of nutrition

Maxisorb® (Scientific Hospital Supplies)
Powder, protein 12 g, carbohydrate 9 g, fat 6 g, energy 565 kJ (135 kcal)/30 g with minerals. Vanilla, strawberry and chocolate flavours. Net price 5 × 30-g sachets = £1.96. As a necessary nutritional supplement prescribed on medical grounds for: short bowel syndrome, intractable malabsorption, pre-operative preparation of patients who are undernourished, treatment for those with proven inflammatory bowel disease, treatment following total gastrectomy, dysphagia, bowel fistulas, disease-related malnutrition, continuous ambulatory peritoneal dialysis (CAPD) and haemodialysis. Not to be prescribed for any child under one year

MCT Oil
Triglycerides from medium chain fatty acids. For steatorrhoea associated with cystic fibrosis of the pancreas; intestinal lymphangiectasia; surgery of the intestine; chronic liver disease and liver cirrhosis; other proven malabsorption syndromes; in a ketogenic diet in the management of epilepsy; in type I hyperlipoproteinaemia
Available from Bristol-Myers (net price 950 mL = £7.80); Cow & Gate (net price 1 litre = £13.06); Scientific Hospital Supplies (net price 250 mL = £3.21)

MCT (1)® (Cow & Gate)
Powder, protein 25.6%, carbohydrate 40.6%, medium chain triglycerides 28%, when used as a 12.5% solution. Low in lactose and sucrose-free. Net price 400 g = £6.82. For steatorrhoea associated with cystic fibrosis of the pancreas; intestinal lymphangiectasia; chronic liver disease; surgery of the intestine in infants

MCT Pepdite® (Scientific Hospital Supplies)
Powder, essential and non-essential amino acids, peptides, medium chain triglycerides, monoglyceride of sunflower oil, with carbohydrate, fat, vitamins, minerals, and trace elements.
MCT Pepdite 0–2. Net price 400 g = £10.82
MCT Pepdite 2+. Net price 400 g = £10.82
Both for disorders in which a high intake of medium chain triglyceride is beneficial

Metabolic Mineral Mixture® (Scientific Hospital Supplies)
Powder, essential mineral salts. Net price 100 g = £5.33. For mineral supplementation in synthetic diets

Milupa® Low Protein Drink see under **Low Protein Drink**

Milupa® PKU2 and PKU3 see under **PKU2 and PKU3**

Minafen® (Cow & Gate)
Powder, equivalent of 12.5% protein, carbohydrate 48%, fat 31%, not more than 0.02% of phenylalanine. For use as 13.1% solution with additional vitamins. Net price 400 g = £12.00. For phenylketonuria

MSUD Aid® (Scientific Hospital Supplies)
Powder, containing full range of amino acids except isoleucine, leucine, and valine, with vitamins, minerals, and trace elements. Net price 200 g = £32.38. For maple syrup urine disease

Neocate® (Scientific Hospital Supplies)
Powder, essential and non-essential amino acids, maltodextrin, fat, vitamins, minerals, and trace elements. Net price 400 g = £15.09. For proven whole protein intolerance, short bowel syndrome, intractable malabsorption, proven inflammatory bowel disease, and bowel fistulas

Nestargel® (Nestlé)
Powder, carob seed flour 96.5%, calcium lactate 3.5%. Net price 125 g = £3.46. For infants and children with galactokinase deficiency, galactosaemia, proven lactose and/or sucrose intolerance in pre-school children, proven sensitivity to whole protein

Nutramigen® (Bristol-Myers)
Powder, protein 13%, carbohydrate 62%, fat 18% with vitamins and minerals. Gluten-, sucrose-, and lactose-free. Net price 425 g = £7.00. For disaccharide and/or whole protein intolerance where additional medium chain triglyceride is not indicated

Nutrilon Soya® (Cow & Gate) [formerly Formula S®]
Powder, carbohydrate 7.1%, fat 3.6%, and protein 1.8% with vitamins and minerals when used as a 12.7% solution. Net price 450 g = £2.96. For proven lactose and associated sucrose intolerance in pre-school children, galactokinase deficiency, galactosaemia, and proven whole cow's milk sensitivity

Nutrison® (Cow & Gate) [formerly Fortison®]
Energy-plus, liquid, protein 30 g, carbohydrate 92 g, fat 29 g, energy 3200 kJ (755 kcal)/500 mL. Net price 500 mL = £2.46. 1 litre (Steriflo®) = £5.15. As a necessary nutritional supplement prescribed on medical grounds for: short bowel syndrome, intractable malabsorption, pre-operative preparation of patients who are undernourished, treatment for those with proven inflammatory bowel disease, treatment following total gastrectomy, dysphagia, bowel fistulas, disease-related malnutrition. Not to be prescribed for any child under one year
Fibre, liquid, protein 20 g, carbohydrate 61.5 g, fat 19.5 g, fibre 7.5 g, energy 2125 kJ (505 kcal)/500 mL. Net price 500-mL bottle = £2.18; 1 litre (Steriflo®) = £4.56. For use as the sole source of nutrition or as a necessary nutritional supplement prescribed on medical grounds for: short bowel syndrome, intractable malabsorption, pre-operative preparation of patients who are undernourished, treatment for those with proven inflammatory bowel disease, treatment following total gastrectomy, dysphagia, disease-related malnutrition. Not to be prescribed for any child under two years, unsuitable as a sole source of nutrition for young children up to 5 years of age
Paediatric, liquid, protein 5.4 g, carbohydrate 24.4 g, fat 9 g, energy 850 kJ (202 kcal)/200 mL. Net price 200-mL bottle = £1.58. For use as the sole source of nutrition or as a necessary nutritional supplement prescribed on medical grounds for: short bowel syndrome, intractable malabsorption, pre-operative preparation of patients who are undernourished, dysphagia, bowel fistulas, disease-related malnutrition or growth failure. Not to be prescribed for any child under one year
Soya, liquid, protein 20 g, carbohydrate 61.5 g, fat 19.5 g, energy 2125 kJ (505 kcal)/500 mL, with vitamins and minerals. Gluten-free. Net price 500 mL = £2.55; 1 litre (Steriflo®) = £5.34. For milk intolerance and lactose intolerance. Not to be prescribed for any child under one year, unsuitable as a sole source of nutrition for young children up to 5 years of age
Standard, liquid, protein 20 g, carbohydrate 61.5 g, fat 19.5 g, energy 2125 kJ (505 kcal)/500 mL, with vitamins and minerals. Net price 500 mL = £2.10; 1 litre (Steriflo®) = £4.39. For use as the sole source of nutrition or as a necessary nutritional supplement prescribed on medical grounds for: short bowel syndrome, intractable malabsorption, pre-operative preparation of patients who are undernourished, treatment for those with proven inflammatory bowel disease, treatment following total gastrectomy, dysphagia, bowel fistulas, disease-related malnutrition. Not to be prescribed for any child under one year, unsuitable as a sole source of nutrition for young children up to 5 years of age

Osmolite® (Abbott)
Liquid, protein 10.5 g, carbohydrate 33.4 g, fat 8.7 g, energy 1050 kJ (250 kcal)/250 mL with vitamins and minerals. Gluten- and lactose-free. Net price 250-mL can = £1.49; 500-mL bottle = £2.98. For use as the sole source of nutrition or as a necessary nutritional supplement prescribed on medical grounds for: short-bowel

syndrome, intractable malabsorption, pre-operative preparation of patients who are undernourished, treatment for proven inflammatory bowel disease, treatment following total gastrectomy, dysphagia, bowel fistulas, disease-related malnutrition. Not to be prescribed for any child under one year, unsuitable as a sole source of nutrition for young children up to 5 years of age

OsterSoy® (Farley)
Powder, providing protein 2%, carbohydrate 7%, fat 3.8% with vitamins and minerals when reconstituted. Gluten-, sucrose-, and lactose-free. Net price 450 g = £2.89. For proven lactose and sucrose intolerance in preschool children, galactokinase deficiency, galactosaemia, and proven whole cow's milk protein sensitivity

Paediasure® (Abbott)
Liquid, protein 3%, fat 5%, carbohydrate 11%, with minerals and vitamins, gluten-free, energy 995 kJ (238 kcal)/237 mL. Vanilla flavour. Net price 237-mL can = £2.03. For use as the sole source of nutrition or as a necessary nutritional supplement prescribed on medical grounds for: short-bowel syndrome, intractable malabsorption, pre-operative preparation of patients who are undernourished, dysphagia, bowel fistulas; and disease-related malnutrition or growth failure. Not to be prescribed for any child under one year

Paediatric Seravit® (Scientific Hospital Supplies)
Powder, vitamins, minerals, low sodium and potassium, and trace elements. Net price 100 g = £5.08
For vitamin and mineral supplementation in restrictive therapeutic diets in infants and children

Pastariso® (General Designs)
Gluten-free. Brown rice pasta (spaghetti, elbow macaroni, fusilli, mini elbows, spirals, and twists), net price 284 g = £1.87; fettucini, 227 g = £1.87. For gluten-sensitive enteropathies including steatorrhoea due to gluten sensitivity, coeliac disease and dermatitis herpetiformis

Pepdite® (Scientific Hospital Supplies)
Powder, essential and non-essential amino acids, peptides, with carbohydrate, fat, vitamins, minerals, and trace elements.
Pepdite 0–2. Providing 1925 kJ (460 kcal)/100 g. Net price 400 g = £9.84
Pepdite 2+. Providing 1787 kJ (425 kcal)/100 g. Net price 400 g = £9.84
Both for disaccharide and/or whole protein intolerance, or where amino acids or peptides are indicated in conjunction with medium chain triglycerides

Peptamen® (Clintec Nutrition)
Liquid, protein 4%, carbohydrate 12.7%, fat 3.9%, energy 420 kJ (100 kcal)/100 mL, with vitamins and minerals. Lactose- and gluten-free. Unflavoured. Net price 500 mL = £5.75. Orange and strawberry flavours. Net price 250-mL can = £2.95. For use as the sole source of nutrition or as a necessary nutritional supplement prescribed on medical grounds for: short bowel syndrome, intractable malabsorption, treatment for proven inflammatory bowel disease, bowel fistulas. Not to be prescribed for any child under one year, unsuitable as a sole source of nutrition for young children up to 5 years of age

Pepti-2000 LF® (Cow & Gate)
Liquid, protein 20 g, fat 5 g, carbohydrate 94 g, energy 2100 kJ (500 kcal)/500 mL with vitamins and minerals. Gluten-free. Net price 500 mL = £2.70.
Powder, same composition as Pepti-2000 LF liquid when reconstituted. Net price 126-g sachet = £3.70.
For use as the sole source of nutrition or as a necessary nutritional supplement prescribed on medical grounds for: short bowel syndrome, intractable malabsorption, treatment for those with proven inflammatory bowel disease, bowel fistulas. Not to be prescribed for any child under one year, unsuitable as a sole source of nutrition for young children up to 5 years of age

Pepti-Junior® (Cow & Gate)
Powder, protein 15.3 g, fat 28.3 g, carbohydrate 55.1 g, energy 2140 kJ (507 kcal)/100 g with vitamins and minerals. Used as a 13.1% solution in place of milk. Net price 400 g = £7.18. For disaccharide and/or whole protein intolerance or where amino acids and peptides are indicated in conjunction with medium chain triglycerides

Peptisorb® (Merck)
Liquid, amino acids and peptides 3.75%, carbohydrate 18.75%, fat 1.11%, with vitamins and minerals, low lactose, and fructose- and gluten-free, energy 2100 kJ (500 kcal)/500 mL. Net price 500 mL = £4.60. For use as the sole source of nutrition or as a necessary nutritional supplement prescribed on medical grounds for: short bowel syndrome, intractable malabsorption, treatment for those with proven inflammatory bowel disease, bowel fistulas. Not to be prescribed for any child under one year; unsuitable as a sole source of nutrition for young children up to 5 years of age

Peptisorbon® (Merck)
Powder, amino acids and peptides 18%, carbohydrate 70%, fat 5.3%, with vitamins and minerals, low lactose, and fructose- and gluten-free, energy 1393 kJ (333 kcal)/sachet. Net price 83.3-g sachet = £2.07. As a necessary nutritional supplement prescribed on medical grounds for the treatment of: short bowel syndrome, intractable malabsorption, pre-operative preparation of patients who are undernourished, treatment for those with proven inflammatory bowel disease, treatment following total gastrectomy, dysphagia, bowel fistulas, disease-related malnutrition. Not to be prescribed for any child under one year

PK Aid 3® (Scientific Hospital Supplies)
Powder, containing essential and non-essential amino acids except phenylalanine. Net price 500 g = £79.00. For phenylketonuria

PKU 2® (Milupa)
Granules, containing essential and non-essential amino acids except phenylalanine; with vitamins, minerals, trace elements, 7.1% sucrose. Flavour: vanilla. Net price 500 g = £38.16. For phenylketonuria

PKU 3® (Milupa)
Granules, containing essential and non-essential amino acids except phenylalanine, vitamins, minerals, and trace elements, with 3.4% sucrose. Flavour vanilla. Net price 500 g = £38.16. For phenylketonuria, not recommended for child under 8 years

Polial® (Ultrapharm)
Biscuits. Gluten- and lactose-free. Net price 200-g pack = £2.85. For gluten-sensitive enteropathies including steatorrhea due to gluten sensitivity, coeliac disease, and dermatitis herpetiformis

Polycal® (Cow & Gate)
Powder, glucose, maltose, and polysaccharides, providing 1610kJ (380kcal)/100 g. Net price 400 g = £2.60; 900 g = £4.62
For renal failure; liver cirrhosis; disaccharide intolerance (without isomaltose intolerance); disorders of amino acid metabolism (and other similar disorders) and/or whole protein intolerance; malabsorption states and other conditions, including proven hypoglycaemia requiring a high-energy, low-fluid intake, whether or not sodium and/or potassium restriction is essential

Polycose® (Abbott)
Powder, glucose polymers, providing carbohydrate 94 g, energy 1600 kJ (380 kcal)/100 g. Net price 350-g can = £2.99. For renal failure; liver cirrhosis; disaccharide intolerance (without isomaltose intolerance); disorders of amino acid metabolism (and other similar disorders) and/or whole protein intolerance; malabsorption states and other conditions, including proven hypoglycaemia requiring a high-energy, low-fluid intake, whether or not sodium and/or potassium restriction is essential

Appendix 7: Borderline substances 541

Portagen® (Bristol-Myers)
Powder, protein 16.5%, carbohydrate 54%, fat 22% with vitamins and minerals. Gluten- and lactose-free. Net price 454 g = £6.23. For disorders in which a high intake of medium chain triglycerides is beneficial

Pregestimil® (Bristol-Myers)
Powder, protein 12.8%, carbohydrate 61.6%, fat 18.3% with vitamins and minerals. Gluten-, sucrose-, and lactose-free. Net price 450 g = £8.01. For disaccharide and/or whole protein intolerance or where amino acids or peptides are indicated in conjunction with medium chain triglycerides

Prejomin® (Milupa)
Granules, protein 13.3 g, carbohydrate 57 g, fat 24.2 g, energy 2090 kJ (499 kcal)/100 g, with vitamins and minerals. Gluten-free. For preparation with water before use. Net price 400 g = £7.50. For disaccharide and/or whole protein intolerance where additional medium chain triglyceride is indicated

ProMod® (Abbott)
Powder, protein 75.8%, carbohydrate 10.2%, fat 9.1%. Gluten-free. Net price 275-g can = £7.99. For biochemically proven hypoproteinaemia

Prosobee® (Bristol-Myers)
Liquid concentrate, protein 4.1%, carbohydrate 13.7%, fat 7.2% with vitamins and minerals. Gluten-, sucrose-, and lactose-free. Net price 385 mL = £1.39
Powder, protein 15.6%, carbohydrate 51.4%, fat 27.9% with vitamins and minerals. Gluten-, sucrose-, and lactose-free. Net price 400 g = £3.56. For proven lactose and associated sucrose intolerance in pre-school children, galactokinase deficiency, galactosaemia, and proven whole cow's milk sensitivity

Protein Forte® (Fresenius)
Liquid, protein 20 g, carbohydrate 19 g, fat 5.2 g, energy 840 kJ (200 kcal)/200 mL, with vitamins, minerals, and trace elements. Gluten-free. Vanilla, strawberry, and chocolate flavours. Net price 200-mL tetrabrik = 95p. As a necessary nutritional supplement prescribed on medical grounds for: short bowel syndrome, intractable malabsorption, pre-operative preparation of patients who are undernourished, treatment for those with proven inflammatory bowel disease, treatment following total gastrectomy, dysphagia, bowel fistulas, disease-related malnutrition, continuous ambulatory peritoneal dialysis (CAPD) and haemodialysis. Not to be prescribed for any child under one year

Protifar® (Cow & Gate)
Powder, protein 88.5%. Low lactose, gluten- and sucrose-free. Net price 225 g = £5.20. For biochemically proven hypoproteinaemia

Provide® (Fresenius)
Liquid, protein 9 g, carbohydrate 28 g, fat less than 1 g, energy 630 kJ (250 kcal)/250 mL with vitamins and minerals. Gluten- and lactose-free. Apple, lemon and lime, and tropical fruit flavour. Net price 250-mL tetrabrik = £1.15. As a necessary nutritional supplement prescribed on medical grounds for: short bowel syndrome, intractable malabsorption, pre-operative preparation of patients who are undernourished, treatment for those with proven inflammatory bowel disease, treatment following total gastrectomy, dysphagia, bowel fistulas, disease-related malnutrition. Not to be prescribed for any child under one year

Reabilan® (Roussel)
Liquid, protein 11.8 g, carbohydrate 49.3 g, fat 14.6 g, energy 1575 kJ (375 kcal)/375 mL with vitamins and minerals. Gluten- and lactose-free. Net price 375 mL = £3.08. For use as the sole source of nutrition or as a necessary nutritional supplement prescribed on medical grounds for: short bowel syndrome, intractable malabsorption, treatment for those with inflammatory bowel disease, bowel fistulas. Not to be prescribed for any child under 1 year, unsuitable as a sole source of nutrition for young children up to 5 years of age

Rectified Spirit. Where the therapeutic qualities of alcohol are required rectified spirit (suitably flavoured and diluted) should be prescribed

Rite-Diet® (Nutricia)
Gluten-free. Flour mix. Net price 500 g = £2.90. Bread mix. 500 g (brown) = £2.90; white, 500 g = £2.90. Bread (white). 400 g = £2.14. High-fibre bread (with soya bran). 400 g = £2.14. For gluten-sensitive enteropathies including steatorrhoea due to gluten sensitivity, coeliac disease, and dermatitis herpetiformis
Low protein/gluten-free. Baking mix. Net price 500 g = £2.90. Flour mix. 400 g = £2.90. Bread; 227 g = £1.45. Bread with soya bran; 280 g = £1.45. Bread (with or without salt). 227 g = £1.45. White bread (with added fibre). 400 g = £2.14. For phenylketonuria and similar amino-acid abnormalities; renal failure; liver failure and liver cirrhosis; gluten-sensitive enteropathies including steatorrhoea due to gluten sensitivity, coeliac disease, and dermatitis herpetiformis
Low sodium. Bread containing protein 8.5%, carbohydrate 53.8%, fat 5.5%, Na$^+$ 0.01%, K$^+$ 0.055%. Net price 227 g = £1.32. For conditions in which a low-sodium diet is indicated

Schar® (Ultrapharm)
Gluten-free, Bread. Net price 250 g = £1.41. Bread rolls, 200 g = £1.41. Bread mix, 500 g = £3.95. Cake mix, 500 g = £3.95. Crackers, 200 g = £2.15. Crispbread, 250 g = £2.82. Pasta (fusilli, penne, rigatoni, tagliatelle), 250 g = £1.90; spaghetti, 500 g = £3.41. Pizza bases, 250 g = £4.12. Savoy biscuits, 200 g = £2.15. For gluten-sensitive enteropathies including steatorrhoea due to gluten sensitivity, coeliac disease, and dermatitis herpetiformis

SHS Modjul® Flavour System (Scientific Hospital Supplies)
Powder, blackcurrant, orange, pineapple, and savoury tomato flavours. Net price 100 g = £4.87
For use with any unflavoured products based on peptides or amino acids

Sunflower oil. Net price 100 mL = 31p. For familial hypercholesterolaemia (non-drug for multiple sclerosis)

Sunnyvale® (Everfresh)
Mixed grain bread, gluten-free. Net price 400 g = £1.12. For gluten-sensitive enteropathies including steatorrhoea due to gluten sensitivity, coeliac disease and dermatitis herpetiformis

Super Soluble Maxijul®, see under Maxijul®

Supplimen® (Clintec)
Product discontinued

Triosorbon® (Merck)
Powder, protein 19%, carbohydrate 56%, fat 19%, with vitamins and minerals. Gluten-free. Net price 85-g sachet = £1.66. For use as the sole source of nutrition or as a necessary nutritional supplement prescribed on medical grounds for: short-bowel syndrome, intractable malabsorption, pre-operative preparation of patients who are undernourished, treatment for proven inflammatory bowel disease, treatment following total gastrectomy, dysphagia, bowel fistulas, disease-related malnutrition. Not to be prescribed for any child under one year, unsuitable as a sole source of nutrition for young children up to 5 years of age

Tritamyl® (Procea)
Flour, self-raising (starch-based), gluten- and lactose-free. Net price 2 kg = £5.86. For gluten-sensitive enteropathies including steatorrhoea due to gluten sensitivity, coeliac disease, and dermatitis herpetiformis

Trufree® (Cantassium)
Gluten-free, wheat-free flours. For gluten-sensitive enteropathies including steatorrhoea due to gluten-sensitivity, coeliac disease, and dermatitis herpetiformis
No. 1 (formerly bread mix 420 g). Net price 1 kg = £3.71
No. 2 with rice bran (formerly bread with rice bran 410 g). Net price 1 kg = £4.46
No. 3 for Cantabread® (formerly Cantabread mix). Net price 1 kg = £4.84
No. 4 white. Net price 1 kg = £3.71
No. 5 brown. Net price 1 kg = £3.71
No. 6 plain (formerly Trufree plain flour). Net price 1 kg = £3.53
No. 7 self-raising (formerly Trufree self-raising flour). Net price 1 kg = £3.71
Ultra® (Ultrapharm)
Gluten-free. High-fibre bread. Net price 500 g = £3.26. Crackerbread, 100 g = £1.72. For gluten-sensitive enteropathies including steatorrhea due to gluten sensitivity, coeliac disease and dermatitis herpetiformis
Low protein/gluten-free. Brown bread (canned). Net price 500 g = £3.80. White bread (canned), 350 g = £2.75. For phenylketonuria (not canned brown bread) and similar amino-acid abnormalities; renal failure, liver failure, and liver cirrhosis; gluten-sensitive enteropathies including steatorrhoea due to gluten sensitivity, coeliac disease, and dermatitis herpetiformis
Wysoy® (Wyeth)
Powder, carbohydrate 6.9%, fat 3.6%, and protein 2.1% with vitamins and minerals when reconstituted. Net price 430 g = £3.10; 860 g = £5.93. For proven lactose and associated sucrose intolerance in pre-school children, galactokinase deficiency, galactosaemia and proven whole cows milk sensitivity

CONDITIONS FOR WHICH FOODS MAY BE PRESCRIBED ON FP10

Note. This is a list of clinical conditions for which the ACBS has approved food products. It is essential to check the list of products (above) for availability.

Adrenoleukodystrophy: Lorenzo's Oil.
Amino acid metabolic disorders and similar protein disorders: low protein drink (Milupa); see also phenylketonuria; histidinaemia; homocystinuria; maple syrup urine disease; synthetic diets; low-protein products.
Anorexia nervosa: see malnutrition (disease-related)
Bowel fistulas: Clinifeed 400[1], Favour, Iso and Protein Rich[1]; Clinutren 1.0 and 1.5[1]; Elemental 028; Enrich; Ensure; Ensure Plus[1]; Ensure Powder; Flexical; Fortimel[1]; Fortipudding[1]; Fortisip[1]; Fresenius OPD[1]; Fresubin Liquid, High Energy, Sip Feeds Plus F and 750[1]; Jevity; Liquisorb High Energy[1]; Liquisorb feed and drink; Liquisorbon MCT[1]; Maxisorb[1]; Nutrison Energy Plus[1], Fibre, Paediatric and Standard; Osmolite; Paediasure; Peptamen; Pepti-2000 LF; Peptisorb; Peptisorbon; Protein Forte[1]; Provide[1]; Reabilan; Supplimen[1]; Triosorbon.
Calcium intolerance: Locasol New Formula.
Carbohydrate malabsorption: Calogen. See also synthetic diets; malabsorption states.
Disaccharide intolerance (without isomaltose intolerance): Alfare; Caloreen; Duocal, Super Soluble and Duocal Liquid; Maxijul LE, Liquid, Super Soluble; Pepti-Junior; Polycal; Polycose powder. See also lactose intolerance; lactose with sucrose intolerance.

---

1. As a supplement only
2. Defined as a condition of intolerance to an intake of the relevant disaccharide confirmed by demonstrated clinical benefit of effectiveness of disaccharide free diet, and presence of reducing substances or excessive acid in stools, low concentration of corresponding disaccharidase enzyme on intestinal biopsy, or breath tests, or lactose tolerance tests.

Glucose and galactose intolerance: Comminuted chicken meat (Cow & Gate); Fructose Galactomin Formula 19 (fructose formula).
Isomaltose intolerance: Glucose (dextrose).
Lactose intolerance[2]: AL110; Comminuted chicken meat (Cow & Gate); Galactomin Formula 17 (new formula); Isomil powder; Nutramigen; Nutrilon Soya; Nutrison Soya; Ostersoy; Pepdite; Portagen; Pregestimil; Prejomin; Prosobee; Wysoy.
Lactose with sucrose intolerance[2]: Comminuted Chicken Meat (Cow & Gate); Galactomin Formula 17 (new formula); Nutramigen; Nutrilon Soya; Ostersoy; Pepti-Junior; Pregestimil; Prejomin; Prosobee; Wysoy.
Sucrose intolerance[2]: Glucose (dextrose) and see also synthetic diets; malabsorption states; lactose with sucrose intolerance.
Cirrhosis of the liver and chronic liver disease: see liver disease.
Coeliac disease: see gluten-sensitive enteropathies.
Continuous Ambulatory Peritoneal Dialysis (CAPD): see dialysis.
Cystic fibrosis: see malabsorption states.
Dermatitis Herpetiformis: see gluten sensitive enteropathies.
Dialysis: nutritional supplements for haemodialysis or continuous ambulatory peritoneal dialysis (CAPD) patients: Clinifeed 400 and Protein Rich; Ensure Plus; Fortipudding; Fresubin 750; Kindergen PROD; Maxisorb; Protein Forte.
Disaccharide intolerance: see carbohydrate malabsorption.
Dysphagia (associated with: intrinsic disease of the oesophagus, e.g. oesophagitis; neuromuscular disorders, e.g. multiple sclerosis and motor neurone disease; major surgery and/or radiotherapy for cancer of the upper digestive tract; protracted severe inflammatory disease of the upper digestive tract, e.g. Stevens-Johnson syndrome and epidermolysis bullosa): Clinifeed 400[1], Favour, Iso and Protein Rich[1]; Clinutren 1.0 and 1.5[1]; Enrich; Ensure; Ensure Plus[1]; Ensure Powder; Fortimel[1], Fortipudding[1]; Fortisip[1]; Fresenius OPD[1]; Fresubin Liquid, High Energy, Sip Feeds, Plus F and 750[1]; Jevity; Liquisorb High Energy[1]; Liquisorb feed and drink; Liquisorbon MCT[1]; Maxisorb[1]; Nutrison Energy Plus[1], Fibre, Paediatric and Standard; Osmolite; Paediasure; Peptisorbon; Protein Forte[1]; Provide[1]; Supplimen[1]; Triosorbon.
Epilepsy (ketogenic diet in): Alembicol D; Calogen; Liquigen; Medium-Chain Triglyceride Oil (MCT).
Flavouring for use with any unflavoured product based on peptides or amino acids: SHS Flavour Modjul
Galactokinase deficiency and galactosaemia: AL 110; Galactomin Formula 17 (new formula); Isomil powder; Nutrilon Soya; Ostersoy; Prosobee Liquid and Powder; Wysoy.
Gastrectomy (total): Clinifeed 400[1], Favour, Iso and Protein Rich[1], Clinutren 1.0 and 1.5[1]; Enrich; Ensure; Ensure Plus[1]; Ensure Powder; Fortimel[1]; Fortipudding[1]; Fortisip[1]; Fresenius OPD[1]; Fresubin Liquid, High Energy, Sip Feeds, Plus F and 750[1]; Jevity; Liquisorb High Energy[1]; Liquisorb Feed and Drink; Liquisorbon MCT[1]; Maxisorb[1]; Nutrison Energy Plus[1]; Fibre and Standard; Osmolite; Peptisorbon; Protein Forte[1]; Provide[1]; Supplimen[1]; Triosorbon.
Glucose/galactose intolerance: Comminuted Chicken Meat (Cow & Gate); Galactomin Formula 19 (fructose formula); also see carbohydrate malabsorption.
Glutaric aciduria: Maxamaid XLys, Try
Gluten-sensitive enteropathies: Aproten products (anellini, biscuits, breadmix, cake mix, crispbread, ditalini, flour, rigatini, spaghetti, tagliatelle); Arnott gluten-free rice cookies; Bi-Aglut biscuits, flour, and gluten-free toast; Ener-G brown and white rice bread, gluten-free tapioca bread, gluten-free rice pasta (cannelloni, lasagna, shells, small shells, spaghetti, tagliatelli, ver-

Appendix 7: Borderline substances

micelli); Glutafin bread, fibre bread, mix, fibre mix, biscuits (digestive, savoury, sweet (without chocolate or sultanas), tea), crackers, high fibre crackers and pasta (spirals, macaroni, spaghetti short-cut); Gluten-free biscuits (Farley); Gluten-free biscuits (Nutricia); Juvela gluten-free corn mix, gluten-free loaf and high-fibre loaf (sliced and unsliced), gluten-free mix and fibre mix; Juvela low-protein loaf (sliced and unsliced) and low-protein mix; Liga gluten-free rusks (Jacobs); Loprofin bread, mix, pasta (macaroni, pasta spirals, spaghetti short-cut); Pastariso gluten-free brown rice, pasta (elbow macaroni, fettucini, fusilli, mini elbows, spaghetti, spirals, twists); Polial gluten-free biscuits; Rite-Diet gluten-free high-fibre bread (with added soya-bran); Rite-Diet gluten-free white bread 400 g; Rite-Diet gluten-free white bread mix; Rite-Diet gluten-free brown bread mix; Rite-Diet gluten-free bread with soya bran (dispensed in tin); Rite-Diet gluten-free high-fibre crackers; Rite-Diet baking mix; Rite-Diet low-protein flour mix; Rite-Diet gluten-free flour mix; Rite-Diet gluten-free low-protein bread (dispensed in tin, with or without salt); Rite-Diet low-protein white bread (with added fibre); Schar gluten-free bread, bread mix, bread rolls, crackers, crispbread, pasta (fusilli, penne, rigatoni, spaghetti, tagliatelli), pizza base, savoy biscuits; Schar gluten-free low-protein cake mix; Sunnyvale gluten-free bread; Tritamyl gluten-free flour; Tritamyl PK flour; Trufree special dietary flours No. 1, No. 2 with rice bran, No. 3 for Cantabread, No. 4 white, No. 5 brown, No. 6 plain, No. 7 self-raising; Ultra gluten-free High-Fibre bread; Ultra gluten-free crackerbread, Ultra gluten-free, low-protein bread rolls; Ultra low-protein, gluten-free canned bread (brown and white); Ultra white gluten-free, low-protein bread (sliced and unsliced).

Glycogen storage disease: Caloreen; Corn Flour or Corn Starch; Glucose (dextrose); Maxijul LE, Liquid, and Super Soluble; Polycal; Polycose.

Growth Failure (secondary to disease related anorexia): Fortipudding; Nutrison Paediatric; Paediasure.

Haemodialysis: see dialysis.

Histidinaemia: HF(2), and see also low-protein products; synthetic diets.

Homocystinuria: Albumaid RVHB X Methionine; Albumaid RVHB Complete X Methionine, Analog RVHB; Maxamaid RVHB; Maxamum RVHB, and see also low-protein products; synthetic diets.

Hypercholesterolaemia (familial): Corn oil; Sunflower oil.

Hyperlipoproteinaemia type 1: Liquigen; Medium Chain Triglyceride Oil.

Hyperlysinaemia: Analog XLys; Maxamaid XLys

Hypermethioninaemia: Analog RVHB; Maxamaid RVHB; Maxamum RVHB.

Hypoglycaemia: Caloreen; Corn Flour or Corn Starch; Maxijul LE, Liquid, and Super Soluble; Polycal; Polycose, and see also glycogen storage disease.

Hypoproteinaemia: Casilan; Dialamine; Forceval Protein; Maxipro HBV Super Soluble; ProMod; Protifar.

Inflammatory Bowel Disease: Clinifeed 400[1], Favour, Iso and Protein Rich[1]; Clinutren 1.0 and 1.5[1]; Elemental 028; Enrich; Ensure; Ensure Plus[1]; Ensure Powder; Flexical; Fortimel[1]; Fortipudding[1]; Fortisip[1]; Fresenius OPD[1]; Fresubin Liquid, High energy, Sip Feeds, Plus F and 750[1]; Jevity; Liquisorb High Energy[1]; Liquisorb Feed and Drink; Liquisorbon MCT[1]; Maxisorb[1]; Nutrison Energy Plus[1], Fibre and Standard; Osmolite; Peptamen; Pepti-2000 LF; Peptisorb; Peptisorbon; Protein Forte[1]; Provide[1]; Reabilan; Supplimen[1]; Triosorbon.

Intestinal lymphangiectasia: see malabsorption states.
Intestinal surgery: see malabsorption states.
Isomaltose intolerance: see carbohydrate malabsorption.
Lactose intolerance: see carbohydrate malabsorption.
Liver disease (i.e. chronic liver disease, cirrhosis): Aglutella low-protein rice; Alembicol D; Aproten products (anellini, biscuits, bread mix, cake mix, crispbread, ditalini, flour, rigatini, spaghetti, tagliatelle); Caloreen; dp Low-Protein butterscotch-flavoured or chocolate-flavoured chip cookies; Duocal, Super Soluble, and Duocal Liquid; Fortical; Generaid; Hepatic Aid; Hycal; Juvela gluten-free low-protein (chocolate chip, orange, and cinnamon flavour) cookies; Juvela low-protein loaf (sliced and unsliced) and low-protein flour mix; Liquigen; Loprofin gluten-free low-protein bread, mix, pasta (macaroni, spaghetti short-cut, pasta spirals); Loprofin low-protein sweet biscuits, chocolate cream-filled biscuits, crackers, cookies (chocolate chip, cinnamon), wafers (orange, chocolate, vanilla); Maxijul LE, Liquid, and Super Soluble; MCT (1) Powder; Medium Chain Triglyceride Oil; Polycal; Polycose; Portagen; Rite-Diet gluten-free low-protein bread (dispensed in tin with or without salt); Rite-Diet low-protein white bread (with added fibre); Rite-Diet low-protein baking mix; Rite-Diet low-protein flour mix; Ultra gluten-free, low-protein bread rolls; Ultra low-protein, gluten-free canned bread (brown and white); Ultra white gluten-free, low protein bread (sliced and unsliced).

Low-protein products: Aglutella low-protein rice; Aproten products (anellini, biscuits, bread mix, cake mix, crispbread, ditalini, flour, rigatini, spaghetti, tagliatelle); dp Low-Protein butterscotch-flavoured or chocolate-flavoured chip cookies*; Juvela gluten-free low-protein (chocolate chip, orange, and cinnamon flavour) cookies*; Juvela low-protein loaf (sliced and unsliced); Juvela low-protein mix; Loprofin gluten-free low-protein bread, mix, pasta (macaroni, spaghetti short-cut, pasta spirals); Loprofin low-protein sweet biscuits, chocolate cream-filled biscuits, crackers, cookies (chocolate chip, cinnamon), wafers (orange, chocolate, vanilla); Rite-Diet gluten-free low-protein bread (dispensed in tin, with or without salt); Rite-Diet low-protein white bread (with added fibre); Rite-Diet low-protein flour mix; Ultra gluten-free, low-protein bread rolls; Ultra low-protein, gluten-free canned brown bread (except for phenylketonuria); Ultra low-protein, gluten-free canned white bread; Ultra white gluten-free, low-protein bread (sliced and unsliced).

*Not prescribable on ACBS for coeliac disease, dermatitis herpetiformis, steatorrhoea due to gluten sensitivity

Malabsorption states: (see also gluten-sensitive enteropathies; liver disease; carbohydrate malabsorption; intestinal lymphangiectasia; milk intolerance and synthetic diets).

(a) Protein sources: Albumaid Complete; Comminuted Chicken Meat (Cow & Gate); Duocal, Super Soluble, and Duocal Liquid; Forceval Protein; Maxipro HBV; MCT Pepdite; Neocate; Pepdite.

(b) Fat: Alembicol D; Calogen; Liquigen; Medium Chain Triglyceride Oil; MCT Pepdite.

(c) Carbohydrate: Caloreen; Fortical; Hycal; Maxijul LE, Liquid, and Super Soluble; Polycal; Polycose.

(d) Complete Feeds. For use as the sole source of nutrition or as a necessary nutritional supplement prescribed on medical grounds: Clinifeed Favour and Iso; Clinutren 1.0; Elemental 028; Enrich; Ensure; Ensure Powder; Flexical; Fresubin Liquid, High Energy, Sip Feeds, and Plus F; Jevity; Liquisorb feed and drink, MCT (1) Powder (with appropriate vitamin and mineral supplements); MCT Pepdite; Nutrison Fibre, Paediatric and Standard; Osmolite; Paediasure; Pepdite; Peptamen; Pepti-2000 LF; Pepti-Junior; Peptisorb; Portagen; Pregestimil; Reabilan; Triosorbon.

(e) Nutritional supplements. Necessary nutritional supplements prescribed on medical grounds: Clinifeed 400 and Protein Rich; Clinutren 1.5; Ensure Plus; Fortimel; Fortipudding; Fortisip; Fresenius OPD; Fresubin 750; Liquisorb High Energy; Liquisorbon MCT; Maxisorb; Nutrison Energy Plus; Peptisorbon; Protein Forte; Provide; Supplimen.

- (f) Minerals: Aminogran Mineral Mixture; Metabolic Mineral Mixture.
- (g) Vitamins: As appropriate, and see synthetic diets.
- (h) Vitamins and Minerals: Paediatric Seravit

Malnutrition (disease-related): Clinifeed 400[1], Favour, Iso and Protein Rich; Clinutren 1.0 and 1.5[1]; Enrich; Ensure; Ensure Plus; Ensure Powder; Fortimel[1]; Fortipudding[1]; Fortisip[1]; Fresenus OPD[1]; Fresubin Liquid, High Energy, Sip Feeds, Plus F and 750[1]; Jevity; Liquisorb High Energy[1]; Liquisorb Feed and Drink; Liquisorbon MCT[1]; Maxisorb[1]; Nutrison Energy Plus[1], Fibre, Paediatric and Standard; Osmolite; Paediasure; Peptisorbon; Protein Forte[1]; Provide[1]; Supplimen[1]; Triosorbon.

Maple syrup urine disease: Analog MSUD; Maxamaid MSUD; Maxamum MSUD; MSUD Aid, and see also low-protein products; synthetic diets.

Methylmalonic or propionic acidaemia: Analog XMet, Thre, Val, Isoleu; Maxamaid XMet, Thre, Val, Isoleu; Maxamum XMet, Thre, Val, Isoleu.

Milk protein sensitivity: Comminuted Chicken Meat (Cow & Gate); Isomil powder; Nutramigen; Nutrilon Soya; Nutrison Soya; Ostersoy; Pregestimil; Prosobee Liquid and powder; Wysoy, and see also synthetic diets.

Neoplasia-related (associated) cachexia (anorexia): see **Malnutrition (disease-related)**

Nutritional support for adults (for precise conditions for which these products have ACBS approval, see products above):

- A. (a) Nutritionally complete feeds. For use as the sole source of nutrition or as a necessary nutritional supplement prescribed on medical grounds for:
  - (i) Gluten-Free: Clinifeed Iso; Fresubin Liquid, Sip Feeds, High Energy, and Plus F (vegetable soup flavour only); Liquisorb feed and drink; Nutrison Fibre and Standard; Triosorbon.
  - (ii) Lactose-free: Clinifeed Favour; Clinutren 1.0.
  - (iii) Lactose- and Gluten-Free: Enrich; Ensure, Ensure Powder; Osmolite.
  - (iv) Containing fibre: Enrich; Fresubin Plus F; Jevity; Nutrison Fibre.
  - (v) Elemental Feeds: Elemental 028; Flexical; Peptamen; Pepti-2000 LF; Peptisorb; Reabilan.
- B. **Nutritional source supplements;** see synthetic diets; malabsorption states.
  - (a) General supplements. Necessary nutritional supplements prescribed on medical grounds: Clinifeed 400 and Protein Rich; Clinutren 1.5; Ensure Plus; Fortimel; Fortipudding; Fortisip; Fresenius OPD; Fresubin 750; Liquisorb High Energy; Liquisorbon MCT; Maxisorb; Nutrison Energy Plus; Peptisorbon; Protein Forte; Provide; Supplimen.
  - (b) Carbohydrates; lactose-free and gluten-free: Caloreen*; Super-Soluble Duocal, and Duocal Liquid*; Fortical*; Hycal*; Maxijul LE*, Liquid, and Super Soluble*; Polycal; Polycose.
    *Have low electrolyte content.
  - (c) Fat: Alembicol D; Calogen; MCT Oil; Liquigen.
  - (d) Nitrogen: Albumaid Complete (hydrolysed protein based); Casilan (whole protein based, low-sodium); Forceval Protein (whole protein based, low-sodium); Maxipro HBV (whole protein based, low-sodium); Pro-Mod (whey protein based, low-sodium).
  - (e) Minerals: Aminogran Mineral Mixture; Metabolic Mineral Mixture.

Phenylketonuria: Aglutelle low-protein rice; Albumaid XP and XP Concentrate; Aminogran Food Supplement and Mineral Mixture; Analog XP; Aproten products (annellini, biscuits, bread mix, cake mix, crispbread, ditalini, flour, rigatini, spaghetti, tagliatelle); Calogen; Caloreen; dp Low-Protein butterscotch-flavoured or chocolate-flavoured chip cookies; Juvela low-protein loaf (sliced and unsliced); Juvela gluten-free low-protein (chocolate chip, orange, and cinnamon flavour) cookies; Juvela low-protein mix; Lofenalac; Loprofin gluten-free, low-protein bread, mix and pasta (macaroni, spaghetti short-cut, pasta spirals); Loprofin low-protein sweet biscuits, chocolate cream-filled biscuits, crackers, cookies (chocolate chip, cinnamon), wafers (orange, chocolate, vanilla); Loprofin PKU drink; Maxamaid XP; Maxamaid XP bar; Maxamaid XP Concentrate; Metabolic Mineral Mixture; Milupa PKU2 and PKU3; Minafen; PK Aid 3; Polycal; Polycose liquid and powder; Rite-Diet gluten-free low-protein bread (dispensed in tin, with or without salt); Rite-Diet low-protein white bread (with added fibre); Rite-Diet low-protein baking mix; Rite-Diet low-protein flour mix; Ultra gluten-free, low-protein bread rolls; Ultra low-protein, gluten-free canned white bread; Ultra white gluten-free, low protein bread (sliced and unsliced) and see low-protein products and synthetic diets.

Propionic acidaemia: Analog X Met, Thre, Val, Isoleu; Maxamaid X Met, Thre, Val, Isoleu.

Renal dialysis: see dialysis.

Protein intolerance: see milk protein sensitivity, whole protein sensitivity, low-protein products, synthetic diets, and amino acid metabolic disorders.

Refsum's Disease: Fresubin Liquid and Sip Feeds.

Renal failure: Aglutella low-protein rice; Aproten products (annellini, biscuits, bread mix, cake mix, crispbread, ditalini, flour, rigatini, spaghetti, tagliatelle); Calogen; Caloreen; Dialamine; dp Low-Protein butterscotch-flavoured or chocolate-flavoured chip cookies; Super-Soluble Duocal and Duocal Liquid; Fortical; Hycal; Juvela gluten-free low-protein (chocolate chip, orange, and cinnamon flavour) cookies; Juvela low-protein loaf (sliced and unsliced) and low-protein flour mix; Loprofin gluten-free, low-protein bread, mix and pasta (macaroni, spaghetti short-cut, pasta spirals); Loprofin low-protein sweet biscuits, chocolate cream-filled biscuits, crackers, cookies (chocolate chip, cinnamon), wafers (orange, chocolate, vanilla); Maxijul LE, Liquid, and Super Soluble; Polycal; Polycose liquid and powder; Rite-Diet gluten-free low-protein bread (dispensed in tin, with or without salt); Rite-Diet low-protein white bread (with added fibre); Rite-Diet low-protein flour mix; Rite-Diet low-protein baking mix; Rite-Diet low-sodium bread; Ultra gluten-free, low-protein bread rolls; Ultra low-protein, gluten-free canned bread (brown and white); Ultra white gluten-free, low-protein bread (sliced and unsliced).

Short bowel syndrome: see malabsorption states.

Sicca Syndrome: Glandosane; Luborant; Saliva Orthana; Salivace.

Sodium dietary reduction: Rite-Diet low-sodium bread.

Sucrose intolerance: see carbohydrate malabsorption.

Synthetic diets:
- (a) Fat: Alembicol D; Calogen; Liquigen; Medium Chain Triglyceride Oil.
- (b) Carbohydrate: Caloreen; Fortical; Hycal; Maxijul LE, Liquid (and orange), Super Soluble; Polycal; Polycose powder.
- (c) Minerals: Aminogran Mineral Mixture; Metabolic Mineral Mixture.
- (d) Protein sources: see malabsorption states, complete feeds.
- (e) Vitamins: as appropriate and see malabsorption states, nutritional support for adults.
- (f) Vitamins and Minerals: Paediatric Seravit.

Tyrosinaemia: Analog XPhen, Tyr; Maxamaid XPhen, Tyr.

Vomiting in infancy: Instant Carobel, Nestargel.

Whole protein sensitivity[2]**:** Alfare; MCT Pepdite; Neocate; Nutramigen; Pepdite; Pepti-Junior; Pregestimil; Prejomin.

Xerostomia: Glandosane; Luborant; Saliva Orthana; Salivace.

---

1. As a supplement only
2. Defined as: intolerance to whole protein, proven by at least two withdrawal and challenge tests, as suggested by an accurate dietary history.

CONDITIONS FOR WHICH TOILET PREPARATIONS MAY BE PRESCRIBED ON FP10

Note. This is a list of clinical conditions for which the ACBS has approved toilet preparations. For details of the preparations see Chapter 13.

Acne: Ionax scrub.
Birthmarks: see disfiguring skin lesions.
Dermatitis (includes contact, atopic and infective dermatoses, eczema and pruritic dermatoses): Aveeno Bath Oil; Aveeno Cream; Aveeno sachets (regular and oilated); Bath E45; Betadine Skin Cleanser and Foam; Genisol; Polytar Emollient, Liquid, and Plus; Ster-Zac Bath Concentrate; T/Gel shampoo; Vaseline Dermacare Cream and Lotion; Wash E45.
Dermatitis herpetiformis: see gluten-sensitive enteropathies.
Disfiguring skin lesions (birthmarks, mutilating lesions and scars): Boots Covering Cream; Covermark products; Dermablend Cover Creme, Leg Cover, and Setting Powder; Dermacolor Camouflage cream and fixing powder; Keromask masking cream and finishing powder; Veil Cover cream and Finishing Powder. (Cleansing Creams, Cleansing Milks, and Cleansing Lotions are excluded.)
Disinfectants (antiseptics): drugs only when ordered in such quantities and with such directions as are appropriate for the treatment of patients. Not to be regarded as drugs if ordered for general hygienic purposes.
Eczema: see dermatitis.
Photodermatoses (skin protection in): Almay Total Sunblock Cream and Lip protector; Coppertone Supershade, and Sunstick 15 and Ultrashade 23; Piz Buin Sunblock Lotion 24; RoC Opaque Total Sunblock Cream SPF 15 A & B (Colourless and tinted); RoC Sunscreen Stick; Spectraban 15; Spectraban Ultra; Sun E45 Cream 25; Sun E45 Lotion 15; Uvistat Sun Cream 15 and 30; Uvistat Lipscreen 15; Uvistat Sun Block Cream 20.
Pruritus: see dermatitis.
Psoriasis: see scaling of the scalp.
Scabies: Tetmosol.
Scaling of the scalp (psoriasis, dandruff, eczema): Alphosyl; Betadine shampoo; Capitol; Ceanel Concentrate; Gelcotar; Genisol; Ionil T; Polytar Emollient, Liquid, and Plus; T/Gel shampoo.

Appendix 8: Cautionary and Advisory Labels for Dispensed Medicines

Numbers following the preparation entries in the BNF correspond to the code numbers of the cautionary labels that pharmacists are recommended to add when dispensing. It is also expected that pharmacists will counsel patients when necessary.

Counselling needs to be related to the age, experience, background, and understanding of the individual patient. The pharmacist should ensure that the patient understands how to take or use the medicine and how to follow the correct dosage schedule. Any effects of the medicine on driving or work, any foods or medicines to be avoided, and what to do if a dose is missed should also be explained. Other matters, such as the possibility of staining of the clothes or skin by a medicine should also be mentioned.

For some preparations there is a special need for counselling, such as an unusual method or time of administration or a potential interaction with a common food or domestic remedy, and this is indicated where necessary.

ORIGINAL PACKS. Many preparations are now dispensed in unbroken original packs that bear complete instructions for the patient or provide a leaflet addressed to the patient. These labels or leaflets should not normally be obscured or removed. Where it is known that such instructions are provided with an original pack intended for the patient no label has been listed under the preparation. Label 10 may be used where appropriate. Leaflets are available from various sources advising on the administration of preparations such as eye-drops, eye ointments, inhalers, and suppositories.

SCOPE OF LABELS. In general no label recommendations have been made for injections on the assumption that they will be administered by a health professional or a well-instructed patient. The labelling is not exhaustive and pharmacists are recommended to use their professional discretion in labelling new preparations and those for which no labels are shown.

Individual labelling advice is not given on the administration of the large variety of antacids. In the absence of instructions from the prescriber, and if on enquiry the patient has had no verbal instructions, the directions given under 'Dose' should be used on the label.

It is recognised that there may be occasions when pharmacists will use their knowledge and professional discretion and decide to omit one or more of the recommended labels for a particular patient. In this case counselling is of the utmost importance. There may also be an occasion when a prescriber does not wish additional cautionary labels to be used, in which case the prescription should be endorsed 'NCL' (no cautionary labels). The exact wording that is required instead should then be specified on the prescription.

Pharmacists have traditionally labelled medicines with various wordings in addition to those directions specified on the prescription. Such labels include 'Shake the bottle', 'For external use only', and 'Store in a cool place', as well as 'Discard .... days after opening' and 'Do not use after ....', which apply particularly to antibiotic mixtures, diluted liquid and topical preparations, and to eye-drops. Although not listed in the BNF these labels should continue to be used when appropriate; indeed, 'For external use only' is a legal requirement on external liquid preparations, while 'Keep out of the reach of children' is a legal requirement on all dispensed medicines.

It is the usual practice for patients to take standard tablets with water or other liquid and for this reason no separate label has been recommended.

The label or labels for each preparation are recommended after careful consideration of the information available. However, it is recognised that in some cases this information may be either incomplete or open to a different interpretation. The Executive Editor will therefore be grateful to receive any constructive comments on the labelling suggested for any preparation.

Recommended label wordings

Wordings which can be given as separate warnings are labels 1–19 and labels 29–33. Wordings which can be incorporated in an appropriate position in the directions for dosage or administration are labels 21–28. A label has been omitted for number 20.

If separate labels are used it is recommended that the wordings be used without modification. If changes are made to suit computer requirements, care should be taken to retain the sense of the original.

(1) Warning. May cause drowsiness

To be used on *preparations for children* containing antihistamines, or other preparations given to children where the warnings of label 2 on driving or alcohol would not be appropriate.

(2) Warning. May cause drowsiness. If affected do not drive or operate machinery. Avoid alcoholic drink

To be used on *preparations for adults that can cause drowsiness*, thereby affecting the ability to drive and operate hazardous machinery; label 1 is more appropriate for children. *It is an offence to drive while under the influence of drink or drugs.*

Some of these preparations only cause drowsiness in the first few days of treatment and some only cause drowsiness in higher doses.

In such cases the patient should be told that the advice applies until the effects have worn off. However many of these preparations can produce a slowing of reaction time and a loss of mental concentration that can have the same effects as drowsiness.

Avoidance of alcoholic drink is recommended because the effects of CNS depressants are enhanced by alcohol. Strict prohibition however could lead to some patients not taking the medicine. Pharmacists should therefore explain the risk and encourage compliance, particularly in patients who may think they already tolerate the effects of alcohol (see also label 3). Queries from patients with epilepsy regarding fitness to drive should be referred back to the patient's doctor.

Side-effects unrelated to drowsiness that may affect a patient's ability to drive or operate machinery safely include *blurred vision, dizziness, or nausea*. In general, no label has been recommended to cover these cases, but the patient should be suitably counselled.

(3) Warning. May cause drowsiness. If affected do not drive or operate machinery

To be used on *preparations containing monoamine-oxidase inhibitors*; the warning to avoid alcohol and dealcoholised (low alcohol) drink is covered by the MAOI treatment card.

(4) Warning. Avoid alcoholic drink

To be used on *preparations where a reaction such as flushing may occur if alcohol is taken* (e.g. metronidazole and chlorpropamide). Alcohol may also enhance the hypoglycaemia produced by some oral antidiabetic drugs but routine application of a warning label is not considered necessary.

(5) Do not take indigestion remedies at the same time of day as this medicine

To be used with label 25 on *preparations coated to resist gastric acid* (e.g. enteric-coated tablets). This is to avoid the possibility of premature dissolution of the coating in the presence of an alkaline pH.

Label 5 also applies to drugs such as ciprofloxacin and ketoconazole *where the absorption is significantly affected by antacids*; the usual period of avoidance recommended is 2 to 4 hours.

(6) Do not take iron preparations or indigestion remedies at the same time of day as this medicine

To be used on *preparations containing doxycycline, minocycline, and penicillamine*. These drugs chelate iron and calcium ions and are less well absorbed when given with iron or calcium-containing antacids. If necessary these incompatible preparations may be given about two hours apart.

(7) Do not take milk, iron preparations or indigestion remedies at the same time of day as this medicine

To be used on *preparations containing tetracyclines that chelate iron, calcium, and magnesium* and are thus less available for absorption; if it is necessary to give milk, iron or antacids, the usual period of avoidance is about 2 hours. Doxycycline and minocycline are less liable to form chelates and therefore only require label 6 (see above).

(8) Do not stop taking this medicine except on your doctor's advice

To be used on *preparations that contain a drug which is required to be taken over long periods without the patient necessarily perceiving any benefit* (e.g. antituberculous drugs).

Also to be used on *preparations that contain a drug whose withdrawal is likely to be a particular hazard* (e.g. clonidine for hypertension). Label 10 (see below) is more appropriate for corticosteroids.

(9) Take at regular intervals. Complete the prescribed course unless otherwise directed

To be used on *preparations where a course of treatment should be completed* to reduce the incidence of relapse, the development of resistance, or failure of treatment.

The preparations are antimicrobial drugs given by mouth. Very occasionally, some may have severe side-effects (e.g. diarrhoea in patients receiving clindamycin) and in such cases the patient may need to be advised of reasons for stopping treatment quickly and returning to the doctor.

(10) Warning. Follow the printed instructions you have been given with this medicine

To be used particularly on *preparations containing anticoagulants, lithium, monoamine-oxidase inhibitors, and oral corticosteroids*. The appropriate treatment card should be given to the patient and any necessary explanations given.

This label may also be used on other preparations to remind the patient of the instructions that have been given.

(11) Avoid exposure of skin to direct sunlight or sun lamps

To be used *on preparations that may cause phototoxic or photoallergic reactions* if the patient is exposed to ultraviolet radiation. Many drugs other than those listed (e.g. phenothiazines and sulphonamides) may on rare occasions cause reactions in susceptible patients. Exposure to high intensity ultraviolet radiation from sunray lamps and sunbeds is particularly likely to cause reactions.

(12) Do not take anything containing aspirin while taking this medicine

To be used *on preparations containing probenecid and sulphinpyrazone* whose activity is reduced by aspirin.

Label 12 should not be used for anticoagulants since label 10 is more appropriate.

(13) Dissolve or mix with water before taking

To be used on *preparations that are intended to be dissolved in water* (e.g. soluble tablets) or *mixed with water* (e.g. powders, granules) before use. In a few cases other liquids such as fruit juice or milk may be used.

(14) This medicine may colour the urine

To be used on *preparations that may cause the patient's urine to turn an unusual colour*. These include phenolphthalein (alkaline urine pink), triamterene (blue under some lights), levodopa (dark reddish), and rifampicin (red).

(15) Caution flammable: keep away from fire or flames

To be used on *preparations containing sufficient flammable solvent to render them flammable if exposed to a naked flame.*

(16) Allow to dissolve under the tongue. Do not transfer from this container. Keep tightly closed. Discard eight weeks after opening

To be used on *glyceryl trinitrate tablets* to remind the patient not to transfer the tablets to plastic or less suitable containers.

(17) Do not take more than . . . . in 24 hours

To be used on *preparations for the treatment of acute migraine* except those containing ergotamine, for which label 18 is used. The dose form should be specified, e.g. tablets or capsules.

It may also be used on preparations for which no dose has been specified by the prescriber.

(18) Do not take more than . . . in 24 hours or . . . in any one week

To be used on preparations containing ergotamine. The dose form should be specified, e.g. tablets or suppositories.

(19) Warning. Causes drowsiness which may continue the next day. If affected do not drive or operate machinery. Avoid alcoholic drink

To be used on *preparations containing hypnotics prescribed to be taken at night*. On the rare occasions (e.g. nitrazepam in epilepsy) when hypnotics are prescribed for daytime administration this label would clearly not be appropriate. Also to be used as *an alternative to the label 2 wording* (the choice being at the discretion of the pharmacist) *for anxiolytics prescribed to be taken at night*.

It is hoped that this wording will convey adequately the problem of residual morning sedation after taking 'sleeping tablets'.

(21) . . . with or after food

To be used on *preparations that are liable to cause gastric irritation*, or *those that are better absorbed with food*.

Patients should be advised that a *small amount of food is sufficient*.

(22) . . . half to one hour before food

To be used on some preparations (e.g. propantheline) *whose absorption is thereby improved*. Most oral antibiotics require label 23 instead (see below),

(23) . . . an hour before food or on an empty stomach

To be used on *oral antibiotics whose absorption may be reduced by the presence of food and acid in the stomach.*

(24) . . . sucked or chewed

To be used on *preparations that should be sucked or chewed.*

The pharmacist should use discretion as to which of these words is appropriate.

(25) . . . swallowed whole, not chewed

To be used on *preparations that are enteric coated or designed for modified-release.*

Also to be used on *preparations that taste very unpleasant or may damage the mouth* if not swallowed whole.

(26) . . . dissolved under the tongue

To be used on *preparations designed for sublingual use*. Patients should be advised to hold under the tongue and avoid swallowing until dissolved. The buccal mucosa between the gum and cheek is occasionally specified by the prescriber.

(27) . . . with plenty of water

To be used on *preparations that should be well diluted* (e.g. chloral hydrate), *where a high fluid intake is required* (e.g. sulphonamides), or *where water is required to aid the action* (e.g. methylcellulose). The patient should be advised that 'plenty' means at least 150 mL (about a tumblerful). In most cases fruit juice, tea, or coffee may be used.

(28) To be spread thinly . . .

To be used on *external corticosteroid preparations*.

(29) Do not take more than 2 at any one time. Do not take more than 8 in 24 hours

To be used on containers of dispensed *solid dose preparations containing paracetamol for adults when the instruction on the label indicates that the dose can be taken on an 'as required' basis*. The dose form should be specified, e.g. tablets or capsules.

This label has been introduced because of the serious consequences of overdosage with paracetamol.

(30) Contains paracetamol

To be used on containers of dispensed *preparations containing paracetamol when the name on the label does not include the word 'paracetamol'.*

(31) Contains aspirin and paracetamol

To be used on containers of dispensed *preparations containing aspirin and paracetamol* (e.g. benorylate), *when the name on the label does not include the words 'aspirin' and 'paracetamol'.*

(32) Contains aspirin

To be used on containers of dispensed *preparations containing aspirin when the name on the label does not include the word 'aspirin'.*

(33) Contains an aspirin-like medicine

To be used on containers of dispensed *preparations containing a salicylate derivative.*

Appendix 8: Cautionary and advisory labels 549

Products and their labels

Products introduced or amended since publication of BNF No. 23 (March 1992) are <u>underlined</u>.
Proprietary names are in italics.
C = counselling advised; see BNF = consult product entry in BNF.

Acebutolol, 8
Acemetacin, 21, C, driving
Acetazolamide, 3
Acetazolamide m/r, 3, 25
Acetylcysteine gran, 13
Achromycin, 7, 9, 23, C, posture
Acipimox, 21
Acrivastine, C, driving, alcohol, see BNF
<u>Acrosoxacin</u>, 2, 23
Actifed, 2
Actifed Compound, 2
Actifed Expectorant, 2
Actinac, 28
Actonorm pdr, 13
Acupan, 2, 14 (urine pink)
Acyclovir susp and tabs, 9
Adalat caps, 21, C, see BNF
Adalat LA, 25
<u>*Adalat Retard*</u>, 21, 25
Adcortyl external preps, 28
Adcortyl with Graneodin, 28
Adizem preps, 25
AeroBec, 8, C, dose
AeroBec Forte, 8, 10 steroid card, C, dose
Agarol, 14
Akineton, 2
Alcopar, 13
Aldomet, 3, 8
<u>*Algipan spray*</u>, 15
Algitec, C, chew thoroughly
Alimix, C, administration
Allegron, 2
Allopurinol, 8, 21, 27
Alophen, e/c (alkaline urine pink)
<u>*Alphodith*</u>, 10 patient information leaflet, 28
Alphosyl HC, 28
Aloxiprin, 12, 21
Alphaderm, 28
Alprazolam, 2
Alrheumat, 21
Alvedon, 30
Alvercol, 25, 27, C, administration, see BNF
Amantadine, C, driving
Ambaxin, 9
Aminophylline m/r, see preps
Amiodarone, 11
Amitriptyline, 2
Amitriptyline m/r, 2, 25
Amorolfine, 10 patient information leaflet
Amoxapine, 2
Amoxil, 9
Amoxil dispersible tabs and sachets, 9, 13
Amoxil Fiztab, 9, 10 patient information leaflet
Amoxil paed susp, 9, C, use of pipette
Amoxycillin, 9
Amoxycillin chewable tabs, 9, 10 patient information leaflet
Amoxycillin dispersible tabs and sachets, 9, 13
Amphotericin loz, 9, 24, C, after food
Amphotericin mixt (g.i.), 9, C, use of pipette
Amphotericin mixt (mouth), 9, C, use of pipette, hold in mouth, after food
Amphotericin tabs, 9
Ampicillin, 9, 23
Ampiclox Neonatal, 9, C, use of pipette
Amylobarbitone, 19
Amytal, 19
Anafranil, 2
Anafranil m/r, 2, 25
Androcur, 2, 21
Angettes-75, 32

Anhydrol Forte, 15
Anquil, 2
Antabuse, 2, C, alcohol reaction, see BNF
Antacids, see BNF dosage statements
Antepsin, 5, C, administration, see BNF
Anthranol preps, 28
Anticoagulants, oral, 10 anticoagulant card
Antihistamines (see individual preparations)
Antipressan, 8
Anturan, 21
Apisate, 25, C, driving
APP pdr, 13
Apsin VK, 9, 23
Arelix, 21
Arpimycin, 9
Arpicolin, C, driving
Artane, C, before or after food, driving, see BNF
Arythmol, 21, 25
Asacol, 5, 25
Ascorbic acid, effervescent, 13
Ascorbic acid tabs (500 mg), 24
Asendis, 2
Aspav, 2, 13, 21, 32
Aspellin, 15
Aspirin and papaveretum dispersible tabs, 2, 13, 21, also 32 (if 'aspirin' not on label)
Aspirin dispersible tabs, 13, 21, also 32 (if 'aspirin' not on label)
Aspirin effervescent, 13, also 32 (if 'aspirin' not on label)
Aspirin e/c, 5, 25, also 32 (if 'aspirin' not on label)
Aspirin m/r, 25, also 32 (if 'aspirin' not on label)
Aspirin tabs, 21, also 32 (if 'aspirin' not on label)
Aspirin, paracetamol and codeine tabs, 21, 29, also 31 (if 'aspirin' and 'paracetamol' not on label)
Astemizole, C, driving, alcohol, see BNF
Atarax, 2
Atenolol, 8
Ativan, 2 or 19
Atromid-S, 21
Augmentin, 9
Augmentin dispersible tabs, 9, 13
Auranofin, 21
Aureocort, 28
Aureomycin, 7, 9, 23
Aventyl, 2
Avloclor, 5
Avomine, 2
Azapropazone, 21, C, see BNF
Azatadine, 2
<u>Azithromycin</u>, 5, 9, 23

Bacampicillin, 9
Baclofen, 2, 8
Bactrim, 9
Bactrim dispersible tabs, 9, 13
Baratol, 2
Baxan, 9
Becloforte preps, 8, 10 steroid card, C, dose
Beclomethasone external preps, 28
Beclomethasone inhalations, 8, 10 steroid card (high-dose preparations only), C, dose
Becodisks, 8, C, dose
Becotide preps, 8, C, dose
Bedranol S.R., 8, 25
Bendogen, 21
Benemid, 12, 21, 27
Benoral susp and tabs, 21, 31

Benoral gran, 13, 21, 31
Benorylate, 21, 31
Benorylate gran, 13, 21, 31
Benperidol, 2
Benylin adult preps, 2
Benylin paediatric preps, 1
Benzathine penicillin, 9
Benzhexol, C, before or after food, driving, see BNF
Benzoin tincture, cpd, 15
Benztropine, 2
Bephenium, 13
Berkolol, 8
Beta-Adalat, 8, 25
Beta-Cardone, 8
Betahistine, 21
Betaloc, 8
Betaloc-SA, 8, 25
Betamethasone inj, 10 steroid card
Betamethasone tab, 10 steroid card, 21
Betamethasone external preps, 28
Betamethasone scalp application, 15, 28
Betaxolol tabs, 8
Bethanechol, 22
Bethanidine, 21
Betim, 8
Betnelan, 10 steroid card, 21
Betnesol injection, 10 steroid card
Betnesol tabs, 10 steroid card, 13, 21
Betnovate external preps, 28
Betnovate scalp application, 15, 28
Betnovate-RD, 28
Bezafibrate, 21
Bezalip, 21
Bezalip-Mono, 21, 25
Biogastrone, 21
Biophylline syr, 21
Biophylline tabs, 25
Biorphen, C, driving
Biperiden, 2
Bisacodyl tabs, 5, 25
Bisoprolol, 8
Blocadren, 8
Bolvidon, 2, 25
Bonefos, C, food and calcium, see BNF
Bradilan, 5, 25
Bricanyl SA, 25
Britiazim, 25
Brocadopa, 14 (urine reddish), 21
Broflex, C, before or after food, driving, see BNF
Bromazepam, 2
Bromocriptine, 21, C, hypotensive reactions
Brompheniramine, 2
Brufen, 21
Brufen gran, 13, 21
Brufen Retard, 25, 27
Buccastem, 2, C, administration, see BNF
Budesonide external preps, 28
Budesonide inhalations, 8, 10 steroid card (high-dose preparations only), C, dose
Buprenorphine, 2, 26
Burinex K, 25, 27, C, posture, see BNF
<u>*Buserelin nasal spray*</u>, C, nasal decongestants, see BNF
Buspar, C, driving
Buspirone, C, driving
Butacote, 5, 21, 25
Butobarbitone, 19
Butriptyline, 2

Cacit, 13
Cafadol, 29, 30
Cafergot, 18, C, dosage
Calcichew, 24
<u>*Calcichew D3*</u>, 24

550 Appendix 8: Cautionary and advisory labels

Calcidrink, 13
Calcisorb, 13, 21, C, may be sprinkled on food
Calcium-500, 25
Calcium carbonate tabs, chewable, 24
Calcium carbonate tabs and gran effervescent, 13
Calcium gluconate tabs, 24
Calcium Resonium, 13
Calcium and ergocalciferol tabs, C, administration, see BNF
Calmurid HC, 28
Calpol susp, 30
Calpol Extra, 29, 30
Camcolit 250 tabs, 10 lithium card, C, fluid and salt intake
Camcolit 400 tabs, 10 lithium card, 25, C, fluid and salt intake
Canesten HC, 28
Canesten spray, 15
Caprin, 5, 25, 32
Carbachol, 22
Carbamazepine chewable, 3, 21, 24
Carbamazepine liq and tabs, 3
Carbamazepine m/r, 3, 25
Carbenoxolone sodium, see preps
Carbo-Cort, 28
Cardinol, 8
Carisoma, 2
Carisoprodol, 2
Carteolol tabs, 8
Cartrol, 8
Carylderm lotion, 15
Catapres, 3, 8
Catapres Perlongets, 3, 8, 25
Caved-S, 24
Cedocard Retard, 25
Cefaclor, 9
Cefadroxil, 9
Cefixime, 9
Cefuroxime susp, 9, 21
Cefuroxime sachets, 9, 13, 21
Cefuroxime tab, 9, 21, 25
Celance, C, hypotensive reactions, see BNF
Celectol, 8, 22
Celevac (constip. or diarrhoea), C, administration, see BNF
Celevac tabs (anorectic), C, administration, see BNF
Celiprolol, 8, 22
Centyl K, 25, 27, C, posture, see BNF
Cephalexin, 9
Cephradine, 9
Ceporex caps, mixts, and tabs, 9
Ceporex paed drops, 9, C, use of pipette
Cesamet, 2
Cetirizine, C, driving, alcohol, see BNF
Chloral hydrate, 19, 27
Chloral paed elixir, 1, 27
Chloral mixt, 19, 27
Chlordiazepoxide, 2
Chlormethiazole, 19
Chlormezanone, 2 or 19
Chloroquine, 5
Chlorpheniramine, 2
Chlorpromazine mixts and supps, 2
Chlorpromazine tabs, 2
Chlorpropamide, 4
Chlortetracycline, 7, 9, 23
Cholestyramine, 13, C, avoid other drugs at same time
Choline magnesium trisalicylate, 21, 33
Choline theophyllinate m/r, 25
Cimetidine chewable tabs, C, administration
Cimetidine effervescent tabs, 13
Cinnarizine, 2
Cinobac, 9
Cinoxacin, 9
Ciprofloxacin, 5, 9, 25, C, driving
Ciproxin tabs, 5, 9, 25, C, driving
Cisapride, C, administration
Citramag, 10 patient information leaflet, 13, C, administration
Citrical, 13
Clarithromycin, 9
Clarityn, C, driving, alcohol, see BNF

Clemastine, 2
Clindamycin, 9, 27, C, diarrhoea
Clinoril, 21
Clobazam, 2 or 19
Clobetasol external preps, 28
Clobetasol scalp application, 15, 28
Clofazimine, 8, 14 (urine red), 21
Clofibrate, 21
Clomipramine, 2
Clomipramine m/r, 2, 25
Clonazepam, 2
Clonidine see Catapres
Clonidine m/r, 3, 8, 25
Clopixol, 2
Clorazepate, 2 or 19
Clotrimazole spray, 15
Cloxacillin, 9, 23
Clozapine, 2, 10 patient information leaflet
Clozaril, 2, 10 patient information leaflet
Coal tar paint, 15
Co-amoxiclav, 9
Co-amoxiclav dispersible tabs, 9, 13
Cobadex, 28
Co-beneldopa, 14 (urine reddish), 21
Co-beneldopa dispersible tabs, 14 (urine reddish), 21, C, administration, see BNF
Co-beneldopa m/r, 5, 14 (urine reddish), 25
Co-Betaloc, 8
Co-Betaloc SA, 8, 25
Co-careldopa, 14 (urine reddish), 21
Co-careldopa m/r, 14 (urine reddish), 25
Co-codamol caps and tabs, 29, 30
Co-codamol dispersible tabs, 13, 29, 30
Co-codaprin dispersible tabs, 13, 21, 32
Co-codaprin tabs, 21, 32
Codafen Continus, 2, 21, 25
Codalax, 14 (urine red)
Co-danthramer, 14 (urine red)
Co-danthrusate, 14 (urine red)
Codeine phosphate syr and tabs, 2
Co-dergocrine, 22
Co-dydramol, 21, 29, 30
Co-fluampicil, 9, 23
Cogentin, 2
Colestid, 13, C, avoid other drugs at same time
Colestipol, 13, C, avoid other drugs at same time
Collodion, flexible, 15
Colofac, 22
Colpermin, 5, 22, 25
Colven sachets, 13, 22, C, administration, see BNF
Complement Continus, 25
Comprecin, 9
Concordin, 2, 11
Condyline, 15
Co-prenozide, 8, 25
Co-proxamol, 2, 10 patient information leaflet, 29, 30
Coracten, 2
Cordarone X, 11
Cordgard, 8
Corgaretic, 8
Corticosteroid external preps, 28
Corticosteroid tabs, 10 steroid card, 21
Corticosteroid injections (systemic), 10 steroid card
Cortisone tab, 10 steroid card, 21
Cortistab, 10 steroid card, 21
Cortisyl, 10 steroid card, 21
Cosalgesic, 2, 10 patient information leaflet, 29, 30
Co-tenidone, 8
Co-trimoxazole mixts and tabs, 9
Co-trimoxazole dispersible tabs, 9, 13
Coversyl, 22
Creon preps, C, see BNF
Cuplex, 15
Cyclizine, 2
Cyclophosphamide, 27
Cycloserine caps, 2, 8

Cyclosporin solution, C, administration
Cyproheptadine, 2
Cyprostat, 3, 21
Cyproterone, see preps
Cystrin, 3

Daktacort, 28
Daktarin oral gel, 9, C, hold in mouth, after food
Daktarin tabs, 9, 21
Dalacin C, 9, 27, C, diarrhoea
Dalmane, 19
Daneral SA, 2, 25
Dantrium, 2
Dantrolene, 2
Dapsone, 8
Davenol, 2
Decadron inj, 10 steroid card
Decadron tabs, 10 steroid card, 21
Decortisyl, 10 steroid card, 21
Deltacortril e/c, 5, 10 steroid card, 25
Deltastab inj, 10 steroid card
Deltastab tabs, 10 steroid card, 21
Demeclocycline, 7, 9, 11, 23
Demser, 2
De-Nol, C, administration, see BNF
De-Noltab, C, administration, see BNF
Depixol, 2
Depo-Medrone (systemic), 10 steroid card
Deponit, 10 patient information leaflet, C, administration, see BNF
Derbac C preps, 10 patient information leaflet
Dermovate cream and oint, 28
Dermovate scalp application, 15, 28
Dermovate-NN, 28
Deseril, 2, 21
Desipramine, 2
Desoxymethasone external preps, 28
Destolit, 21
Deteclo, 7, 9, 11, 23, C, posture
Dexamethasone inj, 10 steroid card
Dexamethasone tabs, 10 steroid card, 21
Dexamphetamine, C, driving
Dexedrine, C, driving
Dextromoramide, 2
Dextropropoxyphene, 2
DHC Continus, 2, 25
Diabinese, 4
Diamorphine preps, 2
Diamox tabs, 3
Diamox SR, 3, 25
Diazepam, 2 or 19
Diclofenac dispersible tabs, 13, 21
Diclofenac e/c, 5, 25
Diclofenac m/r, 21, 25
Diconal, 2
Didronel, C, food and calcium, see BNF
Didronel PMO, 10 patient information leaflet, C, food and calcium
Diethylpropion m/r, 25, C, driving
Diflucan 50 and 200 mg, 9
Diflucan susp, 9
Diflucortolone external preps, 28
Diflunisal, 21, 25, C, avoid aluminium hydroxide
Digoxin elixir, C, use of pipette
Dihydrocodeine, 2, 21
Dihydrocodeine m/r, 2, 25
Diloxanide, 9
Diltiazem, 25
Dimenhydrinate, 2
Dimethicone, see paediatric prep
Dimethindene m/r, 2, 25
Dimotane, 2
Dimotane Expectorant, 2
Dimotane LA, 2, 25
Dimotane Plus, 2
Dimotane Plus LA, 2, 25
Dimotane Plus, Paediatric, 1
Dimotane with Codeine, 2
Dimotane with Codeine Paediatric, 1
Dimotapp elixir, 2
Dimotapp paed elixir, 1
Dimotapp LA, 2, 25, C, gluten

Appendix 8: Cautionary and advisory labels 551

Dindevan, 10 anticoagulant card, 14 (urine pink)
Diocalm Junior, 13
Dioderm, 28
Dioralyte, 13
Dipentum, 21
Diphenhydramine, 2
Diphenylpyraline m/r, 2, 25
Diprosalic, 28
Diprosone, 28
Dipyridamole, 22
Dirythmin SA, 25
Disalcid, 21, 33
Disipal, C, driving
Disodium etidronate, C, food and calcium, see BNF
Disopyramide m/r, 25
Disprol, 30
Distaclor, 9
Distalgesic, 2, 10 patient information leaflet, 29, 30
Distamine, 6, 22
Distigmine, 22
Disulfiram, 2, C, alcohol reaction, see BNF
Dithranol preps, 28
Dithrocream preps, 28
Dithrolan, 28
Ditropan, 3
Diumide-K Continus, 25, 27, C, posture, see BNF
Dolmatil, 2
Dolobid, 21, 25, C, avoid aluminium hydroxide
Doloxene, 2
Doloxene Compound, 2, 21, 32
Doralese, 2
Dormonoct, 19
Dothiepin, 2
Doxepin, 2
Doxycycline caps and tabs, 6, 9, 27, C, posture, see BNF
Dozic, 2
Dramamine, 2
Driclor, 15
Droleptan, 2
Droperidol, 2
Dulcolax tabs, 5, 25
Duofilm, 15
Duromine, 25, C, driving
Dyazide, 14 (urine blue in some lights), 21
Dyspamet tabs, C, administration
Dytac, 14 (urine blue in some lights), 21
Dytide, 14 (urine blue in some lights), 21

Econacort, 28
Ecostatin spray, 15
Edecrin, 21
Efcortelan external preps, 28
Efcortelan soluble, 10 steroid card
Efcortesol, 10 steroid card
Effercitrate, 13
Elantan preps, 25
Electrolade, 13
Electrolyte pdr (see individual preparations)
Emcor preps, 8
Emeside, 2
Emflex, 21, C, driving
En-De-Kay mouthwash, C, food and drink, see BNF
Endoxana, 27
Enoxacin, 9
Entamizole, 4, 9, 21, 25
Epanutin caps, 27, C, administration, see BNF
Epanutin Infatabs, 24
Epanutin susp, C, administration, see BNF
Epifoam, 28
Epilim e/c tabs, 5, 25
Epogam, C, administration, see BNF
Equagesic, 2, 21, 32
Equanil, 2
Eradacin, 2, 23
Ergotamine, 18, C, dosage
Erycen tabs, 5, 9, 25

Erymax, 5, 9, 25
Erythrocin, 9
Erythromid, 5, 9, 25
Erythromid DS, 5, 9, 25
Erythromycin estolate, 9
Erythromycin ethyl succinate, 9
Erythromycin ethyl succinate gran, 9, 13
Erythromycin stearate tabs, 9
Erythromycin tabs, 5, 9, 25
Erythroped, 9
Erythroped sachets, 9, 13
Erythroped A tabs, 9
Erythroped A sachets, 9, 13
Eskornade Spansule, 2, 25
Eskornade syrup, 2
Estracombi, 10 patient information leaflet, C, administration, see BNF
Estracyt, 21, C, dairy products, see BNF
Estraderm TTS, 10 patient information leaflet, C, administration, see BNF
Estrapak-50, 10 patient information leaflet, C, administration, see BNF
Estramustine, 21, C, dairy products, see BNF
Ethacrynic acid, 21
Ethambutol, 8
Ethosuximide, 2
Etidronate, C, food and calcium, see BNF
Etodolac, 21
Etretinate, 10 patient information card, 17
Eumovate external preps, 28
Eurax-Hydrocortisone, 28
Evadyne, 2
Exolan, 28
Expulin, 2
Expulin (paed), 1
Expurhin, 1

Fabahistin, 2
Fabrol, 13
Farlutal 500 mg tabs, 27
Fasigyn, 4, 9, 21, 25
Faverin, 2, 5, 25, C, driving, see BNF
Fefol, 25
Fefol-Vit, 25
Fefol Z, 25
Felbinac foam, 15
Feldene caps, 21
Feldene dispersible tabs, 13, 21
Felodipine m/r, 25
Fenbid, 25
Fenbufen, 21
Fenbufen effervescent tabs, 13, 21
Fenfluramine m/r, 2, 25
Fenofibrate, 21
Fenoprofen, 21
Fenopron, 21
Fenostil Retard, 2, 25
Fentazin, 2
Feospan, 25
Feospan Z, 25
Ferrocap, 25
Ferrocap-F 350, 25
Ferrocontin Continus, 25
Ferrocontin Folic Continus, 25
Ferrograd, 25
Ferrograd Z, 25
Ferrograd Folic, 25
Ferrous salts m/r see preps
Ferrous sulphate paed mixt, 27
Fesovit, 25
Fesovit Z, 25
Flagyl S, 4, 9, 23
Flagyl supps, 4, 9
Flagyl tabs, 4, 9, 21, 25, 27
Flemoxin Solutab, 9, 13
Flexin Continus preps, 21, 25, C, driving
Florinef, 10 steroid card
Floxapen, 9, 23
Fluanxol, C, administration
Fluclorolone external preps, 28
Flucloxacillin, 9, 23
Fluconazole 50 and 200 mg, 9
Fluconazole susp, 9

Fludrocortisone, 10 steroid card
Flunitrazepam, 19
Fluocinolone external preps, 28
Fluocinonide external preps, 28
Fluocinonide scalp lotion, 15, 28
Fluocortolone external preps, 28
Fluorigard mouthwash, C, food and drink, see BNF
Fluorouracil caps, 21
Fluoxetine, C, driving, see BNF
Flupenthixol, see preps
Fluphenazine, 2
Flurandrenolone external preps, 28
Flurazepam, 19
Flurbiprofen, 21
Flurbiprofen m/r, 21, 25
Fluvoxamine, 2, 5, 25, C, driving, see BNF
Fortagesic, 2, 21, 29, 30
Fortral caps and tabs, 2, 21
Fortral supps, 2
Franol, 21
Franol Plus, 21
Frisium, 2 or 19
Froben, 21
Froben SR, 21, 25
Frusene, 14 (urine blue in some lights), 21
Fucibet, 28
Fucidin susp, 9, 21
Fucidin tabs, 9
Fucidin H, 28
Fulcin, 9, 21, C, driving
Full Marks lotion, 15
Fungilin loz, 9, 24, C, after food
Fungilin susp (g.i.), 9, C, use of pipette
Fungilin susp (mouth), 9, C, use of pipette, hold in mouth, after food
Fungilin tabs, 9
Furadantin, 9, 14 (urine yellow or brown), 21
Furamide, 9
Fybogel, 13, C, administration, see BNF
Fybranta, 24, 27, C, administration, see BNF

Galake, 21, 29, 30
Gamanil, 2
Gamolenic acid in evening primrose oil, C, administration, see BNF
Gastrobid Continus, 25
Gastromax, 22, 25
Gastrozepin, 22
Genticin HC, 28
Gluco-lyte, 13
Glucophage, 21
Glyceryl trinitrate patch, see preps
Glyceryl trinitrate m/r, 25
Glyceryl trinitrate tabs, 16
Glytrin Spray, 10 patient information leaflet
Gregoderm, 28
Griseofulvin, 9, 21, C, driving
Grisovin, 9, 21, C, driving
GTN 300 mcg, 16
Guanor Expectorant, 2
Guar gum, see preps
Guarem, 13, C, food, administration, see BNF
Guarina, 13, C, food

Haelan, 28
Haelan-C, 28
Halciderm Topical, 28
Halcinonide external preps, 28
Haldol, 2
Half-Inderal LA, 8, 25
Haloperidol, 2
Haymine, 2, 25
Heminevrin, 19
Hexamine, 9
Hiprex, 9
Hismanal, C, driving, alcohol, see BNF
Histalix, 2
Histryl, 2, 25
Histryl (paed), 1, 25
Hollister skin gel, 15
Hydergine, 22

Hydrocal, 28
Hydrocortisone inj, 10 steroid card
Hydrocortisone external preps, 28
Hydrocortisone tabs, 10 steroid card, 21
Hydrocortisone butyrate external preps, 28
Hydrocortisone butyrate scalp lotion, 15, 28
Hydrocortistab inj, 10 steroid card
Hydrocortistab external preps, 28
Hydrocortistab tabs, 10 steroid card, 21
Hydrocortisyl, 28
Hydrocortone, 10 steroid card, 21
Hydromet, 3, 8
Hydroxychloroquine, 5
Hydroxyzine, 2
Hygroton-K, 25, 27, C, posture, see BNF
Hyoscine, 2
Hypovase, 3, C, dose, see BNF
Hytrin, 3, C, dose, see BNF

Ibuprofen, 2
Ibuprofen gran, 13, 21
Ibuprofen m/r, 25, 27
Ilosone, 25
Imdur, 25
Imigran, 3, 10 patient information leaflet
Imipramine, 2
Imperacin, 7, 9, 23
Imunovir, 9
Inderal, 8
Inderal-LA, 8, 25
Inderetic, 8
Inderex, 8, 25
Indocid caps and susp, 21, C, driving
Indocid-R, 21, 25, C, driving
Indolar SR, 21, 25, C, driving
Indomethacin caps and mixt, 21, C, driving
Indomethacin m/r, see preps
Indomethacin supps, C, driving
Indomod, 25, C, driving
Indoramin, 2
Industrial methylated spirit, 15
Infacol, C, use of dropper
Inosine pranobex, 9
Insulin, C, see BNF
Intal Spincaps and inhalers, 8
Integrin, 2
Iodine Solution, Aqueous, 27
Ionamin, 25, C, driving
Ipral, 9
Iprindole, 2
Ismo Retard, 25
Ismo tabs, 25
Isocarboxazid, 3, 10 MAOI card
Isogel, 13, C, administration, see BNF
Isoket Retard, 25
Isoniazid elixir and tabs, 8, 22
Isoprenaline sulphate tabs, 26
Isordil (sublingual), 26
Isordil Tembids, 25
Isosorbide dinitrate m/r, 25
Isosorbide mononitrate, 25
Isosorbide mononitrate m/r, 25
Isotrate, 25
Isotretinoin, 10 patient information card, 21
Ispaghula, 13, C, administration, see BNF
Itraconazole, 5, 9, 21, 25

Junifen, 21

Kalspare, 14 (urine blue in some lights), 21
Kalten, 8
Kay-Cee-L, 21
Keflex, 9
Kelfizine W tabs, 9,13
Kemadrin, C, driving
Kenalog (systemic), 10 steroid card
Kerlone, 8
Kest, 14 (alkaline urine pink)
Ketoconazole tabs and susp, 5, 9, 21
Ketoprofen caps, 21
Ketotifen, 2, 8, 21

Kiditard, 25
Kinidin Durules, 25
Klaricid, 9
Klean-Prep, C, administration, see BNF
Kloref, 13, 21
Kloref-S, 13, 21
Konakion tabs, 24

Labetalol, 8, 21
Laboprin DL, 13, 21, 33
Labrocol, 8, 21
Lactitol, C, administration, see BNF
Lamisil, 9
Lanoxin-PG elixir, C, use of pipette
Largactil, 2
Lariam, 21, 25, 27
Larodopa, 14 (urine reddish), 21
Lasikal, 25, 27, C, posture, see BNF
Lasipressin, 8
Lasix + K, 25, 27, C, posture, see BNF
Lasma, 25
Ledercort external preps, 28
Ledercort tabs, 10 steroid card, 21
Lederfen, 21
Lederfen F, 13
Lederkyn, 9, 27
Ledermycin, 7, 9, 11, 23
Lentizol, 2, 25
Leo K, 25, 27, C, posture, see BNF
Levodopa, 14 (urine reddish), 21
Levodopa m/r, 5, 14 (urine reddish), 25
Lexotan, 2
Li-Liquid, 10 lithium card, C, fluid and salt intake
Limbitrol, 2
Lingraine, 18, 26, C, dosage
Lioresal, 2, 8
Lipantil, 21
Liquid paraffin/phenolphthalein mixt, 14 (alkaline urine pink)
Liskonum, 10 lithium card, 25, C, fluid and salt intake
Litarex, 10 lithium card, 25, C, fluid and salt intake
Lithium carbonate, 10 lithium card, C, fluid and salt intake
Lithium carbonate m/r, 10 lithium card, 25, C, fluid and salt intake
Lithium citrate liq, 10 lithium card, C, fluid and salt intake
Lithium citrate m/r, 10 lithium card, 25, C, fluid and salt intake
Lobak, 2, 29, 30
Loceryl, 10 patient information leaflet
Locoid cream and oint, 28
Locoid scalp lotion, 15, 28
Locoid C, 28
Lodine, 21
Lofepramine, 2
Loprazolam, 19
Lopresor, 8
Lopresor SR, 8, 25
Lopresoretic, 8
Loratadine, C, driving, alcohol, see BNF
Lorazepam, 2 or 19
Lormetazepam, 19
Loron caps, 10 patient information leaflet, C, food and calcium, see BNF
Losec, 25
Lotriderm, 28
Loxapac, 2
Loxapine, 2
Ludiomil, 2
Lurselle, 21
Lustral, 21
Lyclear Dermal cream, 10 patient information leaflet
Lymecycline, 6, 9
Lysuride, 21, C, hypotensive reactions

Macrodantin, 9, 14 (urine yellow or brown), 21
Madopar, 14 (urine reddish), 21

Madopar dispersible tabs, 14 (urine reddish), 21, C, administration, see BNF
Madopar CR, 5, 14 (urine reddish), 25
Magnapen, 9, 23
Magnesium citrate effervescent pdr, 10 patient information leaflet, 13, C, administration
Magnesium sulphate, 13
Magnesium trisilicate oral pdr, cpd, 13
Manevac, 25, 27
Maprotiline, 2
Marevan, 10 anticoagulant card
Marplan, 3, 10 MAOI card
Maxepa, 21
Maxolon paed liquid, C, use of pipette
Maxolon SR, 25
Mazindol, C, driving
Mebeverine, 22
Mebhydrolin, 2
Medazepam, 2
Medihaler-ergotamine, 18, C, dosage
Medised susp, 1, 30
Medrone tabs, 10 steroid card, 21
Mefenamic acid caps, paed susp, and tabs, 21
Mefenamic acid dispersible tabs, 13, 21
Mefloquine, 21, 25, 27
Melleril, 2
Menthol and benzoin inhalation, 15
Mepacrine, 4, 9, 14, 21
Meprobamate, 2
Meptazinol, 2
Meptid, 2
Mequitazine, 2
Mesalazine e/c, 5, 25
Mesalazine m/r, 25
Metamucil, 13, C, administration, see BNF
Metformin, 21
Methadone, 2
Methixene, 2
Methocarbamol, 2
Methotrimeprazine, 2
Methylcellulose (constip. or diarrhoea), C, administration, see BNF
Methylcellulose tabs (anorectic), C, administration, see BNF
Methylcysteine, 5, 22, 25
Methyldopa, 3, 8
Methylphenobarbitone, 2
Methylprednisolone external preps, 28
Methylprednisolone inj, 10 steroid card
Methylprednisolone tabs, 10 steroid card, 21
Methysergide, 2, 21
Metirosine, 2
Metoclopramide paed liquid, C, use of pipette
Metoclopramide m/r, see preps
Metopirone, 21
Metoprolol, 8
Metoprolol m/r, see preps
Metosyn cream and oint, 28
Metosyn scalp lotion, 15, 28
Metrogel, 10 patient information leaflet
Metrolyl supps, 4, 9
Metronidazole gel, see preps
Metronidazole mixt, 4, 9, 23
Metronidazole supps, 4, 9
Metronidazole tabs, 4, 9, 21, 25, 27
Metyrapone, 21
Mexiletine m/r, 25
Mexitil PL Perlongets, 25
Mianserin, 2, 25
Miconazole oral gel, 9, C, hold in mouth, after food
Miconazole tabs, 9, 21
Mictral, 9, 11, 23
Midrid, 17, 30
Mifegyne, 10 patient information leaflet
Mifepristone, 10 patient information leaflet

Migraleve, 2, 17, 30
Migravess, 13, 17, 32 (should **not** have label 30)
Migravess Forte, 13, 17, 32 (should **not** have label 30)
Migril, 2, 18, C, dosage
Mildison, 28
Minocin, 6, 9
Minocin MR, 6, 25
Minocycline, 6, 9
Minocycline m/r, 6, 25
Mintec, 5, 22, 25
Mintezol, 3, 21, 24
Miraxid tabs, 9, 21, 27, C, posture, see BNF
Miraxid paed sachets, 9, 13, 21
Mobiflex, 21
Moditen, 2
Modrasone, 28
Moducren, 8
Mogadon, 19
Molipaxin, 2, 21
Molipaxin CR, 2, 21, 25
Monit preps, 25
Mono-Cedocard, 25
Monocor, 8
Monosulfiram, 4, 15
Monotrim, 9
Morphine preps, 2
Morphine m/r, 2, 25
Motipress, 2
Motival, 2
MST Continus, 2, 25
Muripsin, 21
Myambutol, 8
Mycardol, 22
Mynah, 8, 23
Myotonine Chloride, 22
Mysoline, 2
Mysteclin, 7, 9, 23, C, posture

Nabilone, 2
Nabumetone, 21, 25
Nabumetone susp, 21
Nadolol, 8
Nafarelin spray, 10 patient information leaflet, C, nasal decongestants, see BNF
Naftidrofuryl, 25, 27
Nalcrom, 22, C, administration, see BNF
Nalidixic acid, 9, 11
Napratec, 21
Naprosyn EC, 5, 21
Naprosyn granules, 13, 21
Naprosyn tabs and susp, 21
Naproxen e/c, 5, 25
Naproxen granules, 13, 21
Naproxen tabs and susp, 21
Nardil, 3, 10 MAOI card
Narphen, 2
Natulan, 4
Naxogin, 4, 21
Nedocromil sodium inhalation, 8
Nefopam, 2, 14 (urine pink)
Negram, 9, 11
Neo-Medrone, 28
Neo-NaClex-K, 25, 27, C, posture, BNF
Nepenthe, 2
Nerisone, 28
Nerisone Forte, 28
Neulactil, 2
Nicofuranose, 5, 25
Nicotinic acid tabs, 21
Nicoumalone, 10 anticoagulant card
Nidazol, 4, 9, 21, 25, 27
Nifedipine caps, 21, C, see BNF
Nifedipine m/r, see preps
Nifensar XL, 21, 25
Niferex elixir, C, infants, use of dropper
Nilstim, C, administration
Nimorazole, 4, 21
Nitoman, 2
Nitrazepam, 19
Nitro-Dur, 10 patient information leaflet, C, see BNF
Nitrocontin Continus, 25
Nitrofurantoin tabs, 9, 14 (urine yellow or brown), 21

Nivaquine, 5
Nizoral, 5, 9, 21
Nobrium, 2
Noctec, 19, 27
Nordox, 6, 9, 27, C, posture, see BNF
Norfloxacin, 5, 9
Normacol preps, 25, 27, C, administration, see BNF
Normax, 14 (urine red)
Normison, 19
Nortriptyline, 2
Norval, 2, 25
Nozinan, 2
Nuelin, 21
Nuelin SA preps, 25
Nu-K, 25, 27, C, see BNF
Nu-Seals Aspirin, 5, 25, 32
Nutrizym GR, C, administration, see BNF
Nycopren, 5, 25
Nystadermal, 28
Nystaform-HC, 28
Nystan pastilles, 9, 24, C, after food
Nystan susp (g.i.), 9, C, use of pipette
Nystan susp (mouth), 9, C, use of pipette, hold in mouth, after food
Nystan tabs, 9
Nystatin mixt (g.i.), 9, C, use of pipette
Nystatin mixt (mouth), 9, C, use of pipette, hold in mouth, after food
Nystatin pastilles, 9, 24, C, after food
Nystatin tabs, 9
Nystatin-Dome (g.i.), 9, C, use of 1-mL spoon
Nystatin-Dome (mouth), 9, C, use of 1-mL spoon, hold in mouth, after food

Ocusert Pilo, C, method of use
Oestriol, 25
Ofloxacin, 5, 9, 11, C, driving
Olbetam, 21
Olsalazine, 21
Omeprazole, 25
Opilon, 21
Opium tincture, 2
Optimine, 2
Oramorph, 2
Orap, 2
Orbenin, 9, 23
Orphenadrine, C, driving
Orudis caps, 21
Oruvail, 21, 25
Ovestin, 25
Oxatomide, 2
Oxazepam, 2
Oxerutins, 21
Oxpentifylline m/r, 21, 25
Oxprenolol, 8
Oxprenolol m/r, 8, 25
Oxybutynin, 3
Oxypertine, 2
Oxytetracycline, 7, 9, 23

Palaprin Forte, 21, 33
Paludrine, 21
Pameton, 29, 30
Panadol tabs, 29, 30
Panadol Soluble, 13, 29, 30
Panadol susp, 30
Pancrease caps, C, administration, see BNF
Pancreatin, see BNF
Pancrex gran, 25, C, dose, see BNF
Pancrex V Forte tabs, 5, 25, C, dose, see BNF
Pancrex V caps, 125 caps and pdr, C, administration, see BNF
Pancrex V tabs, 5, 25, C, dose, see BNF
Paracetamol liq and supps, 30 (if 'paracetamol' not on label)
Paracetamol tabs, 29, also 30 if 'paracetamol' not on label
Paracetamol tabs, soluble, 13, 29, also 30 if 'paracetamol' not on label
Paramax sachets, 13, 17, 30
Paramax tabs, 17, 30
Parlodel, 21, C, hypotensive reactions

Parnate, 3, 10 MAOI card
Paroven, 21
Paroxetine, 21, 25, C, driving, see BNF
Parstelin, 3, 10 MAOI card
Paxofen, 21
Pecram, 25
Penbritin caps and syrup, 9, 23
Penbritin paed syrup, 9, 23, C, use of pipette
Pendramine, 6, 22
Penicillamine, 6, 22
Penidural paed drops, 9, C, use of pipette
Penidural susp, 9
Pentaerythritol tetranitrate, 22
Pentaerythritol tetranitrate m/r, 22, 25
Pentasa tabs, 25
Pentazocine caps and tabs, 2, 21
Pentazocine supps, 2
Pentobarbitone, 19
Peppermint oil caps, 5, 22, 25
Percutol, C, administration, see BNF
Pergolide, C, hypotensive reactions, see BNF
Periactin, 2
Pericyazine, 2
Perindopril, 22
Permethrin dermal cream, 10 patient information leaflet
Perphenazine, 2
Persantin, 22
Pertofran, 2
Pethidine, 2
Pevaryl TC, 28
Phasal, 10 lithium card, 25, C, fluid and salt intake
Phenazocine, 2
Phenelzine, 3, 10 MAOI card
Phenergan, 2
Phenethicillin, 9, 23
Phenindamine, 2
Phenindione, 10 anticoagulant card, 14 (urine pink)
Pheniramine m/r, 2, 25
Phenobarbitone elixir and tabs, 2
Phenolphthalein, 14 (alkaline urine pink)
Phenothrin lotion, 15
Phenoxymethylpenicillin, 9, 23
Phensedyl, 2
Phentermine m/r, 25, C, driving
Phenylbutazone, e/c, 5, 21, 25
Phenytoin caps and tabs, 27, C, administration, see BNF
Phenytoin chewable tabs, 24
Phenytoin susp, C, administration, see BNF
Phosphate-Sandoz, 13
Phyllocontin Continus, 25
Physeptone, 2
Phytomenadione, 24
Picolax, 10 patient information leaflet, 13, C, see BNF
Pimozide, 2
Pindolol, 8
Piperazine powder, 13
Pirenzepine, 22
Piretanide, 21
Piriton, 2
Piroxicam caps, 21
Piroxicam dispersible tabs, 13, 21
Pivampicillin sachets, 5, 9, 13, 21
Pivampicillin susp and tabs, 5, 9, 21
Pivmecillinam susp, 9, 21
Pivmecillinam tabs, 9, 21, 27, C, posture, see BNF
Pizotifen, 2
Plaquenil, 5
Platet, 13, 32
Plendil, 25
Podophyllin paint cpd, 15, C, application, see BNF
Polynoxylin loz, 9, 24, C, after food
Ponderax Pacaps, 2, 25
Pondocillin sachets, 5, 9, 13, 21
Pondocillin susp and tabs, 5, 9, 21
Pondocillin Plus, 9, 21, 27, C, posture, see BNF
Ponstan, 21
Ponstan Dispersible, 13, 21

Appendix 8: Cautionary and advisory labels

Potaba caps and tabs, 21
Potaba Envules, 13, 21
Potassium chloride m/r, see preps
Potassium citrate mixt, 27
Potassium effervescent tabs, 13, 21
Praxilene, 25, 27
Prazosin, 3, C, dose, see BNF
Precortisyl, 10 steroid card, 21
Precortisyl Forte, 10 steroid card, 21
Prednesol, 10 steroid card, 13, 21
Prednisolone inj, 10 steroid card
Prednisolone tabs, 10 steroid card, 21
Prednisolone e/c, 5, 10 steroid card, 25
Prednisone, 10 steroid card, 21
Preferid, 28
Prefil, 22, 27, C, administration
Prepulsid, C, administration
Prestim, 8
Prestim Forte, 8
Priadel liq, 10 lithium card, C, fluid and salt intake, see BNF
Priadel tabs, 10 lithium card, 25, C, fluid and salt intake, see BNF
Primalan, 2
Primidone, 2
Prioderm lotion, 15
Pripsen, 13
Pro-Actidil, 2, 25
Pro-Banthine, 23
Probenecid, 12, 21, 27
Probucol, 21
Procainamide Durules, 25
Procarbazine, 4
Prochlorperazine, 2
Prochlorperazine m/r, 2, 25
Prochlorperazine buccal tabs, 2, C, administration, see BNF
Prochlorperazine sachets, 2, 13
Proctofibe, C, administration, see BNF
Procyclidine, C, driving
Progesic, 21
Proguanil, 21
Promazine, 2
Promethazine, 2
Prominal, 2
Prondol, 2
Propaderm, 28
Propafenone, 21, 25
Propain, 2, 29, 30
Propantheline, 23
Propranolol, 8
Propranolol m/r, 8, 25
Prothiaden, 8
Prothionamide, 8, 21
Protriptyline, 2, 11
Pro-Vent, 25
Prozac, C, driving, see BNF
Psoradrate, 28
Psorin, 28
Pulmicort, 8, 10 steroid card, C, dose
Pulmicort LS, 8, C, dose
Pulmicort Respules, 8, 10 steroid card, C, dose
Pyrazinamide, 8
Pyrogastrone liquid, 21
Pyrogastrone tabs, 21, 24

Questran preps, 13, C, avoid other drugs at same time
Quinalbarbitone, 19
Quinidine m/r, 25
Quinocort, 28
Quinoderm with Hydrocortisone, 28

Ranitidine dispersible and effervescent tabs, 13
Rapolyte, 13
Redoxon effervescent, 13
Redoxon (500 mg), 24
Regulan, 13, C, administration, see BNF
Rehidrat, 13
Relifex, 21, 25
Relifex susp, 21
Remedeine preps, 2, 21, 29, 30
Remoxipride m/r, 3, 25
Resonium A, 13
Restandol, 21, 25

Retrovir syrup, C, use of oral syringe
Revanil, 21, C, hypotensive reactions
Rheumacin SR, 21, 25, C, driving
Rheumox, 21, C, see BNF
Rhumalgan, 5, 25
Ridaura, 21
Rifadin, 8, 14 (urine orange-red), 22, C, soft lenses
Rifampicin caps and mixt, 8, 14 (urine orange-red), 22, C, soft lenses
Rifater, 8, 14 (urine orange-red), 22, C, soft lenses
Rifinah, 8, 14 (urine orange-red), 22, C, soft lenses
Rimactane, 8, 14 (urine orange-red), 22, C, soft lenses
Rimactazid, 8, 14 (urine orange-red), 22, C, soft lenses
Rivotril, 2
Roaccutane, 10 patient information card, 21
Robaxin, 2
Robaxisal Forte, 2, 21, 32
Rohypnol, 19
Ronicol Timespan, 25
Rowachol, 22
Rowatinex caps, 25
Roxiam, 3, 25
Rythmodan Retard, 25

Sabidal SR, 25
Sabril, 3
Safapryn, 5, 25
Safapryn-Co, 5, 25
Salactol, 15
Salatac, 15
Salazopyrin, 14 (urine orange-yellow), C, soft lenses
Salazopyrin EN-tabs, 5, 14 (urine orange-yellow) 25, C, soft lenses
Salbutamol m/r, see preps
Salicylic acid collodion, 15
Salicylic acid lotion, 15
Salofalk, 5, 25
Salsalate, 21, 33
Salts latex adhesive soln, 15
Salts 'SPR' plaster remover, 15
Sandimmun solution, C, administration
Sando-K, 13, 21
Sandocal, 13
Sanomigran, 2
Scopoderm TTS, 2, C, administration, see BNF
Secadrex, 8
Seconal, 19
Sectral, 8
Securon SR, 25
Selexid susp, 9, 13, 21
Selexid tabs, 9, 21, 27, C, posture, see BNF
Semprex, C, driving, alcohol, see BNF
Sential, 28
Septrin susp and tabs, 9
Septrin dispersible tabs, 9, 13
Serc, 21
Serenace, 2
Seroxat, 21, 25, C, driving, see BNF
Sertraline, 21
Sevredol, 2
Sinemet CR, 14 (urine reddish), 25
Sinemet preps, 14 (urine reddish), 21
Sinequan, 2
Sinthrome, 10 anticoagulant card
Sintisone, 10 steroid card, 21
Slo-Indo, 21, 25, C, driving
Slo-Phyllin, 25 or C, administration, see BNF
Sloprolol, 8, 25
Slow Sodium, 25
Slow-Fe, 25
Slow-Fe Folic, 25
Slow-K, 25, 27, C, posture, see BNF
Slow-Pren, 8, 25
Slow-Trasicor, 8, 25
Sodium Amytal, 19
Sodium bicarbonate pdr, 13
Sodium cellulose phosphate, 13, 21, C, may be sprinkled on food
Sodium chloride m/r, 25

Sodium chloride tabs, 13
Sodium chloride and glucose oral pdr, cpd, 13
Sodium chloride solution-tabs, 13
Sodium clodronate, C, food and calcium, see BNF
Sodium cromoglycate (oral), 22, C, administration, see BNF
Sodium cromoglycate inhalations, 8
Sodium fusidate susp, 9, 21
Sodium fusidate tabs, 9
Sodium picosulphate pdr, 10 patient information leaflet, 13, C, see BNF
Sodium valproate e/c, 5, 25
Solpadeine caps, 29, 30
Solpadeine effervescent tabs, 13, 29, 30
Solpadol, 2, 13, 29, 30
Solu-Cortef, 10 steroid card
Solu-Medrone, 10 steroid card
Solvazinc, 13, 21
Somnite, 19
Soneryl, 19
Soni-Slo, 25
Sorbichew, 24
Sorbid-SA, 25
Sotacor, 8
Sotalol, 8
Sotazide, 8
Sparine, 2
Sporanox, 5, 9, 21, 25
SRM-Rhotard, 2, 25
Stelazine syrup and tabs, 2
Stelazine Spansule, 2, 25
Stemetil, 2
Stemetil Eff, 2, 13
Sterculia, C, administration, see BNF
Stiedex, 28
Stugeron, 2
Stugeron Forte, 2
Sucralfate, 5, C, administration, see BNF
Sudafed linct, 2
Sudafed Plus, 2
Sudafed SA, 25
Suleo-C lotion, 15
Suleo-M, 15
Sulfametopyrazine, 9, 13
Sulindac, 21
Sulphadiazine, 9, 27
Sulphadimidine, 9, 27
Sulphasalazine e/c, 5, 14 (urine orange-yellow), 25, C, soft lenses
Sulphasalazine, 14 (urine orange-yellow), C, soft lenses
Sulphinpyrazone, 12, 21
Sulpiride, 2
Sulpitil, 2
Sultamicillin, 9
Sumatriptan, 3, 10 patient information leaflet
Suprax, 9
Suprecur, C, nasal decongestants, see BNF
Suprefact nasal spray, C, nasal decongestants, see BNF
Surgam tabs, 21
Surgam SA caps, 21, 25
Surgical spirit, 15
Surmontil, 2
Suscard Buccal, C, administration, see BNF
Sustac, 25
Sustamycin, 7, 9, 23, 25
Symmetrel, C, driving
Synalar external preps, 28
Synarel, 10 patient information leaflet, C, nasal decongestants, see BNF
Syndol, 2, 29, 30
Synflex, 21

Tagamet effervescent tabs, 13
Tarcortin, 28
Tarivid, 5, 9, 11, C, driving
Tavegil, 2
Tegretol Chewtabs, 3, 21, 24
Tegretol liq and tabs, 3
Tegretol Retard, 3, 25

Appendix 8: Cautionary and advisory labels 555

Temazepam, 19
Temgesic, 2, 26
Tenif, 8, 25
Tenoret 50, 8
Tenoretic, 8
Tenormin, 8
Tenoxicam, 21
Tenuate Dospan, 25, C, driving
Terazosin, 3, C, dose, see BNF
Terbinafine, 9
Terbutaline m/r, 25
Terfenadine, C, driving, alcohol, see BNF
Teronac, C, driving
Terra-Cortril oint and spray, 28
Terra-Cortril Nystatin, 28
Terramycin, 7, 9, 23
Testosterone undecanoate caps, 21, 25
Tetmosol, 4, 15
Tetrabenazine, 2
Tetrabid, 7, 9, 23, 25
Tetrachel, 7, 9, 23, C, posture
Tetracycline, 7, 9, 23, C, posture
Tetracycline mouthbath, see BNF
Tetralysal preps, 6, 9
Theo-Dur, 25
Theophylline, 21
Theophylline m/r, see preps
Thephorin, 2
Thiabendazole, 3, 21, 24
Thiethylperazine tabs, 2
Thioridazine, 2
Thymoxamine, 21
Tiaprofenic acid tabs, 21
Tiaprofenic acid m/r, 21, 25
Tigason, 10 patient information card, 21
Tilade, 8
Tildiem preps, 25
Timodine, 28
Timolol, 8
Tinidazole tabs, 4, 9, 21, 25
Tinset, 2, 21
Tixylix, 1 or 2
Tofranil, 2
Tolectin, 21
Tolerzide, 8
Tolmetin, 21
Topilar, 28
Torecan tabs, 2
Trancopal, 2 or 19
Trandate, 8, 21
Transiderm-Nitro, 10 patient information leaflet, C, administration, see BNF
Tranxene, 2 or 19
Tranylcypromine, 3, 10 MAOI card
Trasicor, 8

Trasidrex, 8, 25
Traxam foam, 15
Trazodone, 2, 21
Trazodone m/r, 2, 21, 25
Tremonil, 2
Trental m/r, 21, 25
Treosulfan, 25
Tri-Adcortyl external preps, 28
Triamcinolone inj, 10 steroid card
Triamcinolone external preps, 28
Triamcinolone tabs, 10 steroid card, 21
Triamco, 14 (urine blue in some lights), 21
Triamterene, 14 (urine blue in some lights), 21
Tri-Cicatrin, 28
Triclofos sodium, 19
Trientine, 6, 22
Trifluoperazine, 2
Trifluperidol, 2
Trifyba, C, administration, see BNF
Trilisate, 21, 33
Triludan, C, driving, alcohol, see BNF
Trimeprazine, 2
Trimethoprim mixt and tabs, 9
Trimipramine, 2
Trimopan, 9
Trimovate, 28
Triominic, 2
Triperidol, 2
Tripotassium dicitratobismuthate, C, administration, see BNF
Triprolidine m/r, 2, 25
Triptafen preps, 2
Tropium, 2
Tryptizol caps, 2, 25
Tryptizol mixt and tabs, 2
Tuinal, 19
Tylex, 2, 29, 30
Typhoid vaccine, oral, 23, 25, C, administration, see BNF

Ubretid, 22
Ucerax, 2
Ultradil Plain, 28
Ultralanum Plain, 28
Unasyn tabs, 9
Uniflu with Gregovite C, 2
Uniphyllin Continus, 25
Univer, 25
Uriben, 9, 11
Ursodeoxycholic acid, 21
Ursofalk, 21
Utinor, 5, 9

Valium, 2 or 19
Vallergan, 2
Valoid, 2

Veganin, 21, 29, 31
Velosef, 9
Ventide, 8, C, dose
Ventolin CR, 25, 27
Verapamil m/r, 25
Vertigon, 2, 25
Vibramycin caps, 6, 9, 27, C, posture, see BNF
Vibramycin-D, 6, 9, 13
Vigabatrin, 3
Viloxazine, 2
Vioform-Hydrocortisone, 28
Visclair, 5, 22, 25
Viskaldix, 8
Visken, 8
Vita-E Gelucaps, 24
Vivalan, 2
Vivotif, 23, 25, C, administration, see BNF
Volmax, 25
Voltarol dispersible tabs, 13, 21
Voltarol tabs, 5, 25
Voltarol 75 mg SR and *Retard,* 21, 25

Warfarin, 10 anticoagulant card
Warfarin WBP, 10 anticoagulant card
Warticon, 15
Welldorm, 19, 27

Xanax, 2

Z Span, 25
Zaditen, 2, 8, 21
Zadstat supps, 4, 9
Zantac dispersible and effervescent tabs, 13
Zarontin, 2
Zidovudine syrup, C, use of oral syringe
Zimovane, 19
Zinamide, 8
Zincomed, 21
Zinc sulphate, 21
Zinnat sachets, 9, 13, 21
Zinnat susp, 9, 21
Zinnat tabs, 9, 21, 25
Zirtek, C, driving, alcohol, see BNF
Zithromax, 5, 9, 23
Zopiclone, 19
Zovirax susp and tabs, 9
Zuclopenthixol, 2
Zyloric, 8, 21, 27

Dental Practitioners' Formulary

List of Dental Preparations

The following list has been approved by the appropriate Secretaries of State, and the preparations therein may be prescribed by dental practitioners on form FP14 (GP14 in Scotland).

Sugar-free versions, where available, are preferred.

Acyclovir Cream, DPF
Acyclovir Oral Suspension, DPF
Acyclovir Tablets 200 mg, DPF
Amoxycillin Capsules, BP
Amoxycillin Injection, DPF
Amoxycillin Oral Powder, DPF
Amoxycillin Oral Suspension, BP
Amoxycillin Tablets, Dispersible, DPF
Amphotericin Lozenges, BP
Amphotericin Oral Suspension, DPF
Amphotericin Tablets, DPF
Ampicillin Capsules, BP
Ampicillin Oral Suspension, BP
Artificial Saliva, DPF
Ascorbic Acid Tablets, BP
Aspirin Tablets, Dispersible, BP[1]
Benzydamine Mouthwash, DPF
Benzydamine Oral Spray, DPF
Benzylpenicillin Injection, BP
Carbamazepine Tablets, BP
Carmellose Gelatin Paste, DPF
Cephalexin Capsules, BP
Cephalexin Oral Suspension, DPF
Cephalexin Tablets, BP
Cephradine Capsules, BP
Cephradine Injection, DPF
Cephradine Oral Solution, DPF
Chlorhexidine Gluconate gels containing at least 1 per cent
Chlorhexidine Mouthwash, DPF[2]
Chlorpheniramine Tablets, BP
Choline Salicylate Dental Gel, BP
Clindamycin Capsules, BP
Clindamycin Injection, DPF
Clindamycin Oral Suspension, Paediatric, DPF
Co-trimoxazole Oral Suspension, BP
Co-trimoxazole Oral Suspension, Paediatric, BP
Co-trimoxazole Tablets, BP
Co-trimoxazole Tablets, Dispersible, BP
Co-trimoxazole Tablets, Paediatric, BP
Diazepam Oral Solution, BP
Diazepam Tablets, BP
Diflunisal Tablets, BP
Dihydrocodeine Tablets, BP
Doxycycline Capsules 100 mg, BP
Ephedrine Nasal Drops, BP
Erythromycin Ethyl Succinate Oral Suspension, DPF
Erythromycin Ethyl Succinate Oral Suspension, Paediatric, DPF
Erythromycin Ethyl Succinate Tablets, DPF
Erythromycin Lactobionate Intravenous Infusion, BP
Erythromycin Stearate Tablets, BP
Erythromycin Tablets, BP
Hydrocortisone Cream, BP
Hydrocortisone Lozenges, BPC
Hydrocortisone and Miconazole Cream, DPF
Hydrocortisone and Miconazole Ointment, DPF
Hydrogen Peroxide Mouthwash, DPF
Ibuprofen Oral Suspension, DPF
Ibuprofen Tablets, BP
Idoxuridine 5% in Dimethyl Sulphoxide, DPF
Lignocaine 5% Ointment, DPF
Menthol and Eucalyptus Inhalation, BP 1980[3]
Metronidazole Oral Suspension, DPF
Metronidazole Tablets, BP
Miconazole Oral Gel, DPF
Mouthwash Solution-tablets, DPF
Nitrazepam Tablets, BP
Nystatin Ointment, BP
Nystatin Oral Suspension, BP
Nystatin Pastilles, DPF
Nystatin Tablets, BP
Oxytetracycline Capsules, BP
Oxytetracycline Tablets, BP
Paracetamol Oral Suspension, Paediatric, BP[4]
Paracetamol Tablets, BP
Paracetamol Tablets, Dispersible, DPF
Penicillin Triple Injection, BPC
Pethidine Tablets, BP
Phenoxymethylpenicillin Capsules, BP [not currently available]
Phenoxymethylpenicillin Oral Solution, BP
Phenoxymethylpenicillin Tablets, BP
Povidone-iodine Mouthwash, DPF
Promethazine Hydrochloride Tablets, BP
Promethazine Oral Solution, BP
Sodium Chloride Mouthwash, Compound, BP
Sodium Fluoride Oral Drops, DPF[5]
Sodium Fluoride Tablets, DPF[5]
Sodium Fusidate Ointment, BP
 (former title Fusidic Acid Ointment, DPF)
Sodium Perborate Mouthwash, DPF
Temazepam Capsules, DPF
Temazepam Oral Solution, BP
Temazepam Tablets, DPF
Tetracycline Capsules, BP
Tetracycline Tablets, BP
Thymol Glycerin, Compound, BP
Triamcinolone Dental Paste, BP
Vitamin B Tablets, Compound, Strong, BPC
Zinc Sulphate Mouthwash, DPF
 [not currently available]

---

1. Addendum 1989 to BP 1988 has directed that when soluble aspirin tablets are prescribed, dispersible aspirin tablets should be dispensed.
2. This includes spray presentation
3. This preparation does not appear in BP 1988
4. BP 1988 directs that when Paediatric Paracetamol Oral Suspension or Paediatric Paracetamol Mixture is prescribed and no strength stated Paracetamol Oral Suspension 120 mg/5 mL should be dispensed
5. With effect from 1 January, 1993

Dental Practitioner's Formulary

Details of DPF preparations

Preparations on the List of Dental Preparations which are not included in the BP or BPC are described as follows in the DPF.

Although brand names have sometimes been included for identification purposes preparations on the list should be prescribed by non-proprietary name.

PoM Acyclovir Cream, (proprietary product: *Zovirax Cream*), acyclovir 5%

PoM Acyclovir Oral Suspension, (proprietary product: *Zovirax Suspension*), acyclovir 200 mg/5 mL

PoM Acyclovir Tablets 200 mg, (proprietary product: *Zovirax Tablets*), acyclovir 200 mg

PoM Amoxycillin Injection, sterile powder for reconstitution

PoM Amoxycillin Oral Powder (proprietary products: *Amoxil Sachets SF*), amoxycillin 750 mg and 3 g (as trihydrate)

PoM Amoxycillin Tablets Dispersible, (proprietary products: *Amoxil Dispersible Tablets*, amoxycillin 500 mg (as trihydrate); *Flemoxin Solutab*, amoxycillin 375 mg and 750 mg (as trihydrate))

PoM Amphotericin Oral Suspension (proprietary product: *Fungilin Suspension*), amphotericin 100 mg/mL

PoM Amphotericin Tablets (proprietary product: *Fungilin Tablets*), amphotericin 100 mg

Artificial Saliva, consists of sorbitol 1.8 g, carmellose sodium (sodium carboxymethylcellulose) 390 mg, dibasic potassium phosphate 48.23 mg, potassium chloride 37.5 mg, monobasic potassium phosphate 21.97 mg, calcium chloride 9.972 mg, magnesium chloride 3.528 mg, sodium fluoride 258 micrograms/60 mL, with preservatives and colouring agents (proprietary product: *Luborant*)

Benzydamine Mouthwash (proprietary product: *Difflam Oral Rinse*), benzydamine hydrochloride 0.15%

Benzydamine Oral Spray, (proprietary product: *Difflam Spray*), benzydamine hydrochloride 0.15%

Carmellose Gelatin Paste (proprietary product: *Orabase Paste*), gelatin, pectin, carmellose sodium, 16.58% of each in a suitable basis

PoM Cephalexin Oral Suspension, cephalexin 125 mg, 250 mg, or 500 mg/5 mL (may be powder for reconstitution or ready prepared)

PoM Cephradine Injection (proprietary product: *Velosef Injection*), sterile powder for reconstitution

PoM Cephradine Oral Solution (proprietary product: *Velosef Syrup*), cephradine 250 mg/5 mL when reconstituted with water

Chlorhexidine Gel (proprietary product: *Corsodyl Dental Gel*), chlorhexidine gluconate 1%

Chlorhexidine Mouthwash (proprietary products: *Corsodyl Mouthwash, Corsodyl Spray*), chlorhexidine gluconate 0.2%

PoM Clindamycin Injection (proprietary product: *Dalacin C Phosphate Sterile Solution*), clindamycin 150 mg (as phosphate)/mL

PoM Clindamycin Oral Suspension, Paediatric (proprietary product: *Dalacin C Paediatric Suspension*), clindamycin 75 mg (as hydrochloride palmitate)/5 mL when reconstituted with purified water (freshly boiled and cooled)

PoM Erythromycin Ethyl Succinate Oral Suspension (proprietary product: *Erythroped, Erythroped SF, Erythroped Suspension Forte*), erythromycin 250 mg and 500 mg (as ethyl succinate)/5 mL when reconstituted with water

PoM Erythromycin Ethyl Succinate Oral Suspension, Paediatric (proprietary products: *Erythroped PI, Erythroped PI SF*), erythromycin 125 mg (as ethyl succinate)/5 mL when reconstituted with water

PoM Erythromycin Ethyl Succinate Tablets (proprietary product: *Erythroped A*), erythromycin ethyl succinate 500 mg

PoM Hydrocortisone and Miconazole Cream (proprietary product: *Daktacort Cream*), hydrocortisone 1%, miconazole nitrate 2%

PoM Hydrocortisone and Miconazole Ointment (proprietary product: *Daktacort Ointment*), hydrocortisone 1%, miconazole nitrate 2%

Hydrogen Peroxide Mouthwash consists of hydrogen peroxide solution (6%), BP

PoM Ibuprofen Oral Suspension (proprietary product: *Junifen*), ibuprofen 100 mg/5 mL

PoM Idoxuridine 5% in Dimethyl Sulphoxide, idoxuridine 5% in dimethyl sulphoxide

Lignocaine 5% Ointment, lignocaine 5% in a suitable basis

PoM Metronidazole Oral Suspension (proprietary product: *Flagyl S*), metronidazole 200 mg (as benzoate)/5 mL

Miconazole Oral Gel (proprietary product: *Daktarin Oral Gel*), miconazole 25 mg/mL

Mouthwash Solution-tablets, DPF, consist of tablets which may contain antimicrobial, colouring and flavouring agents in a suitable soluble effervescent basis to make a mouthwash suitable for dental purposes

PoM Nystatin Pastilles (proprietary product: *Nystan Pastilles*), nystatin 100 000 units

Paracetamol Tablets, Dispersible (proprietary product: *Panadol Soluble*), paracetamol 500 mg in an effervescent basis

Povidone-iodine Mouthwash (proprietary product: *Betadine Mouthwash*), povidone-iodine 1%

Sodium Fluoride Oral Drops, see section 9.5.3

Sodium Fluoride Tablets, see section 9.5.3

Sodium Perborate Mouthwash, (proprietary product: *Bocasan Mouthwash*), sodium perborate 68.6%

PoM Temazepam Capsules, DPF, temazepam 10, 15, 20 and 30 mg

Note. Temazepam Capsules DPF are soft gelatin capsules

PoM Temazepam Tablets, temazepam 10 and 20 mg

Zinc Sulphate Mouthwash, consists of zinc sulphate lotion, BP. Directions for use: dilute 1 part with 4 parts of warm water

Note. Not currently available

Index of Manufacturers

Abbott
Abbott Laboratories Ltd,
Abbott House, Moorbridge Rd,
Maidenhead, Berks SL6 8JG.
(0628) 773355

A&H
Allen & Hanburys Ltd,
Stockley Park West, Uxbridge,
Middx UB11 1BT.
081-990 9888

Alcon
Alcon Laboratories (UK) Ltd,
Imperial Way, Watford, Herts
WD2 4YR.
(0923) 246133

Alembic Products
Alembic Products Ltd,
Unit 4, Brymau 2 Estate,
River Lane, Saltney,
Chester, Cheshire CH4 8RQ.
(0244) 680147

Allergan
Allergan Ltd,
Coronation Rd, High Wycombe,
Bucks HP12 3SH.
(0494) 444722

Alpha
Alpha Therapeutic UK Ltd,
Howlett Way, Fison Way
Industrial Estate, Thetford,
Norfolk IP24 1HZ.
(0842) 764260

APS
Approved Prescription Services
Ltd,
Water St, Towngate, Wyke,
Bradford, West Yorks
BD12 9AF.
(0274) 606974

Armour
Armour Pharmaceutical Co. Ltd,
St. Leonards House,
St. Leonards Rd, Eastbourne,
East Sussex BN21 3YG.
(0323) 410200

Arun
Arun Products Ltd,
Contact De Witt

Ashbourne
Ashbourne Pharmaceuticals Ltd,
Ferro Fields,
Scaldwell Rd, Brixworth,
Northampton NN6 9EN.
(0604) 882190

ASTA Medica
ASTA Medica Ltd,
168 Cowley Rd, Cambridge
CB4 4DL
(0223) 423434

Astra
Astra Pharmaceuticals Ltd,
Home Park Estate,
Kings Langley,
Herts WD4 8DH.
(0923) 266191

Astra Meditec
Astra Meditec Ltd,
PO Box 13, Stroud, Glos
GL5 3DL.
(0453) 833377

Bailey, Robert
Robert Bailey & Son plc,
Dysart St, Great Moor,
Stockport, Cheshire
SK2 7PF.
061-483 1133

Baker Norton
Division of Norton Healthcare
Contact Norton

Bard
C.R. Bard International Ltd,
Forest House, Brighton Rd,
Crawley, West Sussex
RH11 9BP.
(0293) 27888

Baxter
Baxter Healthcare Ltd,
Caxton Way, Thetford, Norfolk
IP24 3SE.
(0842) 754581

Bayer
Bayer UK Ltd,
Pharmaceutical Business Group,
Bayer House, Strawberry Hill,
Newbury, Berks RG13 1JA.
(0635) 39000

Bayer Diagnostics
Bayer Diagnostics UK Ltd,
Ames Division, Evans House,
Hamilton Close, Basingstoke,
Hants RG21 2YE.
(0256) 29181

Baypharm
Contact Bayer.

Becton Dickinson
Becton Dickinson UK Ltd,
Between Towns Rd,
Cowley, Oxford,
Oxon OX4 3LY.
(0865) 777722

Beecham
Beecham Research,
Contact SmithKline Beecham

Beecham Products
see SmithKline Beecham Brands

Beiersdorf
Beiersdorf UK Ltd,
Yeomans Drive, Blakelands,
Milton Keynes,
Bucks MK14 5LS.
(0908) 211444

Bell and Croyden
John Bell and Croyden,
54 Wigmore St, London
W1H 0AU.
071-935 5555

Bencard
Contact SmithKline Beecham

Bengué
Bengué & Co. Ltd.
Contact Syntex

Berk
Berk Pharmaceuticals Ltd,
Water St, Towngate, Wyke,
Bradford, West Yorks
BD12 9AF.
(0274) 690696

Beta
Beta Medical Products Ltd,
Valley Lodge, Bakewell Rd,
Matlock, Derbyshire
DE4 3BN
(0629) 582198

BHR
BHR Pharmaceuticals Ltd,
41 Centenary Business Centre,
Hammond Close,
Attleborough Fields, Nuneaton,
Warwickshire CV11 6RY.
(0203) 353742

Bio Diagnostics
Bio Diagnostics Ltd,
Upton Industrial Estate,
Rectory Rd, Upton-upon-Severn,
Worcs WR8 0XL.
(0684) 592262

Bioglan
Bioglan Laboratories Ltd,
1 The Cam Centre
Wilbury Way, Hitchin,
Herts SG4 0TW.
(0462) 438444

Bio-Medical
Bio-Medical Services,
BMS Laboratories Ltd,
River View Rd, Beverley,
North Humberside HU17 0LD.
(0482) 860228

Biorex
Biorex Laboratories Ltd,
2 Crossfield Chambers, Gladbeck
Way, Enfield, Middx EN2 7HT.
081-366 9301

Biotest
Biotest (UK) Ltd,
Unit 21A Monkspath Business
Park, Highlands Rd, Shirley,
Solihull, West Midlands
B90 4NZ.
021-733 3393

Blake
Thomas Blake & Co,
The Byre House, Fearby,
Nr. Masham, North Yorkshire
HG4 4NF.
(0765) 689042

BM Diagnostics
Boehringer Mannheim
(Diagnostics & Biochemicals)
Ltd,
Bell Lane, Lewes,
East Sussex BN7 1LG.
(0273) 480444

Index of manufacturers

Body's Care
Body's Care Centre Ltd,
631 London Rd,
Westcliffe-on-Sea, Essex
SS0 9PE.
(0702) 337339

Boehringer Ingelheim
Boehringer Ingelheim Ltd,
Ellesfield Ave, Bracknell, Berks
RG12 4YS.
(0344) 424600

Boehringer Mannheim
Boehringer Mannheim UK
(Pharmaceuticals) Ltd,
Simpson Parkway, Kirkton
Campus, Livingston, West
Lothian EH54 7BH.
(0506) 412512

Boots
The Boots Co. plc,
1 Thane Rd West, Nottingham
NG2 3AA.
(0602) 506255

BPL
Bio Products Laboratory,
Dagger Lane, Elstree, Herts
WD6 3BX.
081-905 1818

Braun
B. Braun (Medical) Ltd,
Braun House, 13–14 Farmbrough
Close, Aylesbury Vale Industrial
Park, Aylesbury, Bucks
HP20 1DQ.
(0296) 393900

Brevit
Brevit Hospital Products,
Unit 6, Carter Hire Complex,
Wilson Way, Redruth, Cornwall
TR15 3QT.
(0209) 219097

Bristol-Myers
Bristol-Myers Squibb
Pharmaceuticals Ltd,
141–149 Staines Rd, Hounslow,
Middx TW3 3JA.
081-572 7422

Britannia
Britannia Pharmaceuticals Ltd,
Forum House, 41–75 Brighton
Rd, Redhill, Surrey RH1 6YS.
(0737) 773741

BritCair
BritCair Ltd,
Division of CV Laboratories Ltd,
Gordon House, Gordon Rd,
Aldershot, Hants GU11 1LD.
(0252) 333314

Brocades
Brocades (Great Britain) Ltd,
Brocades House, Pyrford Rd,
West Byfleet, Surrey KT14 6RA.
(0932) 345535

David Bull
David Bull Laboratories,
Spartan Close, Tachbrook Park,
Warwick CV34 6RS.
(0926) 451515

Bullen
C.S. Bullen Ltd,
3–7 Moss St, Liverpool L6 1EY.
051-207 6995

Bullen & Smears
Bullen & Smears Ltd,
99 Kempston St, Liverpool
L3 8HE.
051-207 1239

Burgess
Edwin Burgess Ltd,
Contact Leo.

Cabot
see Solco Basle

Cambmac
Cambmac Instruments Ltd,
Pembroke Ave, Waterbeach,
Cambridge CB5 9PY.
(0223) 441144

Cambridge
Cambridge Laboratories,
Richmond House,
Old Brewery Court,
Sandyford Rd,
Newcastle upon Tyne NE2 1XG.
091-261 5950

Camp
Camp Ltd,
Northgate House,
Staple Gardens, Winchester,
Hants SO23 8ST.
(0962) 55248

Cantassium
The Cantassium Company,
Larkhall Laboratories,
225 Putney Bridge Rd,
London SW15 2PY.
081-874 1130

Centocor
Centocor BV,
Einsteinweg 101,
2333 CB Leiden,
The Netherlands.
0800-898461

Chancellor
Chancellor Group Ltd,
see Consolidated

Charwell
Charwell Pharmaceuticals Ltd,
Charwell House, Wilsom Rd,
Alton, Hants GU34 2TJ.
(0420) 84801

Ciba
CIBA Laboratories,
Wimblehurst Rd, Horsham, West
Sussex RH12 4AB.
(0403) 272827

Cilag
Cilag Ltd,
PO Box 79, Saunderton, High
Wycombe, Bucks HP14 4HJ.
(0494) 563541

Clement Clarke
Clement Clarke International
Ltd,
Airmed House, Edinburgh Way,
Harlow, Essex CM20 2ED.
(0279) 414969

CliniFlex
CliniFlex Ltd,
Contact CliniMed.

CliniMed
CliniMed Ltd,
Cavell House, Knaves Beech
Way, Loudwater, High
Wycombe, Bucks HP10 9QY.
(0628) 850100

Clintec
Clintec Nutrition Ltd,
Shaftesbury Court,
18 Chalvey Park, Slough,
Berks SL1 2HT.
(0753) 550800

Coloplast
Coloplast Ltd,
Peterborough Business Park,
Peterborough PE2 0FX.
(0733) 239898

Concept
Concept Pharmaceuticals Ltd
see Fabre

Consolidated
Consolidated Chemicals Ltd,
Abbey Rd,
The Industrial Estate,
Wrexham, Clywd LL13 9PW.
(0978) 661351

ConvaTec
ConvaTec Ltd,
Harrington House, Milton Rd,
Ickenham, Uxbridge, Middx
UB10 8PU.
(0895) 678888

Cow & Gate
Cow & Gate Ltd,
Newmarket Ave, Whitehorse
Business Park,
Trowbridge, Wilts BA14 0XQ.
(0225) 768381

Cox
A. H. Cox & Co Ltd,
Whiddon Valley, Barnstaple,
Devon EX32 8NS.
(0271) 75001

CP
CP Pharmaceuticals Ltd,
Ash Rd North, Wrexham
Industrial Estate, Wrexham,
Clwyd LL13 9UF.
(0978) 661261

Crookes
Crookes Healthcare Ltd,
PO Box 94, 1 Thane Rd West,
Nottingham NG2 3AA.
(0602) 507431

Cupal
Cupal Ltd,
Pharmaceutical Laboratories,
King St, Blackburn, Lancs
BB2 2DX.
(0254) 580321

Cusi
Cusi (UK) Ltd,
8A Liphook Rd, Haslemere,
Surrey GU27 1NL.
(0428) 61078

Cussons
Cussons (UK) Ltd,
Kersal Vale, Manchester
M7 0GL.
061-792 6111

Index of manufacturers

Cutter
Contact Bayer.

Cuxson
Cuxson, Gerrard & Co. (IMS) Ltd,
Oldbury, Warley,
West Midlands B69 3BB.
021-552 1355

Cyanamid
Contact Lederle.

Daniels
Richard Daniel & Son Ltd,
Mansfield Rd, Derby DE1 3RE.
(0332) 40671

Davis & Geck
Contact Lederle.

DDC
DDC (London) Ltd,
158 Notting Hill Gate,
London W11 3GQ.
071-229 4224

DDD
DDD Ltd,
94 Rickmansworth Rd,
Watford, Herts WD1 7JJ.
(0923) 229251

DDSA
DDSA Pharmaceuticals Ltd,
310 Old Brompton Rd, London
SW5 9JQ.
071-373 7884

De Vilbiss
De Vilbiss Health Care UK Ltd,
Airlinks, Spitfire Way, Heston,
Middx TW5 9NR.
Dial 100 and ask for 'Freephone
Oxygen Concentrator'

De Witt
E. C. De Witt & Co Ltd,
62–64 East Barnet Rd, New
Barnet, Herts EN4 8RQ.
081-441 9310

Delandale
Delandale Laboratories Ltd,
Delandale House, 37 Old Dover
Rd, Canterbury, Kent CT1 3JF.
(0227) 766353

Dental Health
Dental Health Products Ltd,
Broughton House, 33 Earl St,
Maidstone, Kent ME14 1PF.
(0622) 762269

DePuy
DePuy Healthcare,
47 Great George St,
Leeds LS1 3BB.
(0532) 430028

Dermal
Dermal Laboratories Ltd,
Tatmore Place, Gosmore,
Hitchin, Herts SG4 7QR.
(0462) 458866

Dermalex
Contact Sanofi.

DF
Duncan, Flockhart & Co Ltd,
Division of Glaxo Laboratories
Ltd
Contact Glaxo

Dispersa
Dispersa (United Kingdom) Ltd,
Flanders Rd, Hedge End,
Southampton SO3 3LG.
(0489) 785399

Dista
Dista Products Ltd,
Contact Lilly.

Dow Corning
Dow Corning Ltd,
Kings Court, 185 Kings Rd,
Reading, Berks RG1 4EX.
(0734) 596888

Downs
Contact Simcare

Drew
John Drew (London) Ltd,
433 Uxbridge Rd, Ealing,
London W5 3NT.
081-992 0381

Du Pont
Du Pont Pharmaceuticals Ltd,
Avenue One, Letchworth
Garden City, Herts
SG4 2HU.
(0462) 488200

Dumex
Dumex Ltd,
Longwick Rd, Princes
Risborough, Aylesbury,
Bucks HP17 9UZ.
(0844) 274414

Duphar
Duphar Laboratories Ltd,
Gaters Hill, West End,
Southampton SO3 3JD.
(0703) 472281

Dylade
Contact Fresenius Ltd.

Eastern
Eastern Pharmaceuticals Ltd,
Coomb House, 7 St Johns Rd,
Isleworth, Middx TW7 6NA.
081-569 8174

Elida Gibbs
Elida Gibbs Ltd,
Coal Rd, Seacroft, Leeds
LS14 2AR.
(0532) 737473

Ellis
Ellis, Son & Paramore Ltd,
Spring Street Works,
Sheffield S3 8PB.
(0742) 738921

EMS
EMS Medical Ltd,
Unit 3, Stroud Industrial Estate,
Oldends Lane, Stonehouse, Glos
GL10 2DG.
(0453) 791791

EuroCetus
EuroCetus UK Ltd,
Salamander Quay West,
Park Lane, Harefield,
Middx UB9 6NY.
(0895) 824087

Evans
Evans Medical Ltd,
Langhurst, Horsham,
Sussex RH12 4QD.
(0403) 41400

Everfresh
Everfresh Natural Foods,
Gatehouse Close, Aylesbury,
Bucks HP19 3DE.
(0296) 25333

Fabre
Pierre Fabre Ltd,
Shelley Court, Shelley Close,
Headington, Oxon OX3 8HB.
(0865) 742525

Farillon
Farillon Ltd,
Ashton Rd, Harold Hill,
Romford, Essex
RM3 8UE.
(04023) 71136

Farley
Farley Health Products Ltd,
Torr Lane, Plymouth PL3 5UA.
(0752) 24151

Farmitalia Carlo Erba
Farmitalia Carlo Erba Ltd,
Italia House, 23 Grosvenor Rd,
St. Albans, Herts AL1 3AW.
(0727) 40041

Ferraris
Ferraris Development &
Engineering Co Ltd,
26 Lea Valley Trading Estate,
Angel Rd, Edmonton,
London N18 3JD.
081-807 3636

Ferring
Ferring Pharmaceuticals Ltd,
11 Mount Rd, Feltham, Middx
TW13 6AR.
081-898 8396

Fisons
Fisons plc,
Pharmaceutical Division,
Coleorton Hall,
Coleorton, Leics LE6 4GP.
(0509) 634000

Fournier
Fournier Pharmaceuticals Ltd,
19–20 Progress Business Centre,
Whittle Parkway,
Slough SL1 6DQ.
(0628) 660552

Fox
C. H. Fox Ltd,
22 Tavistock St, London
WC2E 7PY
071-240 3111

FP
Family Planning Sales Ltd,
28 Kelburne Rd, Cowley, Oxford
OX4 3SZ.
(0865) 772486

Fresenius
Fresenius Ltd,
6–8 Christleton Court, Stuart Rd,
Manor Park, Runcorn, Cheshire
WA7 1ST.
(0928) 580058

Fry
Fry Surgical International Ltd,
Unit 17, Goldsworth Park
Trading Estate, Woking, Surrey
GU21 3BA.
(0483) 721404

Index of manufacturers

Galderma
Galderma (UK) Ltd,
Contact Alcon.
(0923) 210180

Galen
Galen Ltd,
Seagoe Industrial Estate,
Craigavon, Northern Ireland
BT63 5UA.
(0762) 334974

Garnier
Laboratoires Garnier,
Golden Ltd,
PO Box 5, Pontyclun, Glam
CF7 8XW.
(0443) 237456

Geigy
Geigy Pharmaceuticals.
see Ciba

Geistlich
Geistlich Sons Ltd,
Newton Bank, Long Lane,
Chester CH2 3QZ.
(0244) 347534

General Designs
General Designs Ltd,
PO Box 38E, Worcester Park,
Surrey KT4 7LX.
081-337 9366

Generics
Generics (UK) Ltd,
12 Station Close, Potters Bar,
Herts EN6 1TL.
(0707) 44556

GF Supplies
see Nutricia

Glaxo
Glaxo Laboratories Ltd,
Stockley Park West,
Uxbridge, Middx UB11 1BT.
081-990 9444

Glenwood
Glenwood Laboratories Ltd,
Jenkins Dale, Chatham,
Kent ME4 5RD.
(0634) 830535

Gold Cross
Gold Cross Pharmaceuticals.
Contact Searle.

Goldshield
Goldshield Pharmaceuticals Ltd,
Bensham House, Bensham Lane,
Thornton Heath, Surrey
CR7 7EQ.
081-684 3664

Graseby Medical
Graseby Medical Ltd,
Colonial Way, Watford, Herts
WD2 4LG.
(0923) 246434

Henleys
Henleys Medical Supplies Ltd,
Brownfields, Welwyn Garden
City, Herts AL7 1AN.
(0707) 333164

Hillcross
Hillcross Pharmaceuticals,
Primrose Mill, Harrison St,
Briercliffe, Burnley BB10 2HP.
(0282) 830042

Hoechst
Hoechst UK Ltd,
Pharmaceutical Division, Hoechst
House, Salisbury Rd, Hounslow,
Middx TW4 6JH.
081-570 7712

Hollister
Hollister Ltd,
Rectory Court, 42 Broad St,
Wokingham, Berks RG11 1AB.
(0734) 775545

Hospital Management & Supplies
Hospital Management and
Supplies Ltd,
Selinas Lane, Dagenham, Essex
RM8 1QD.
081-593 7511

Hough
Hough, Hoseason & Co. Ltd,
22 Chapel St, Levenshulme,
Manchester M19 3PT.
061-224 3271

Hypoguard
Hypoguard Ltd,
Dock Lane, Melton,
Woodbridge, Suffolk IP12 1PE.
(03943) 7333

ICI
ICI Pharmaceuticals,
Kings Court, Water Lane,
Wilmslow, Cheshire SK9 5AZ.
(0625) 535999

Immuno
Immuno Ltd,
Arctic House, Rye Lane, Dunton
Green, Nr Sevenoaks, Kent
TN14 5HB.
(0732) 458101

IMS
International Medication Systems
(UK) Ltd,
11 Royal Oak Way South,
Daventry, Northants NN11 5PJ.
(0327) 703231

Incare
Incare Medical Products,
Contact Hollister

Innovex
Innovex Medical
Contact Nova

Intercare
Intercare Products Ltd,
7 The Business Centre,
Molly Millars Lane, Wokingham,
Berks RG11 2QZ.
(0734) 790345

Invicta
Contact Pfizer.

Iolab
Iolab,
Enterprise House, Station Rd,
Loudwater, High Wycombe,
Bucks HP10 9UG.
(0494) 461096

J&J
Johnson & Johnson Patient Care
Ltd,
Coronation Rd, Ascot,
Berks SL5 9EY.
(0990) 872626

Jackson
Ernest Jackson & Co. Ltd,
Crediton, Devon EX17 3AP.
(03632) 2251

Jacobs
The Jacobs Bakery Ltd,
Suttons Business Park,
Earley, Reading, Berks
RG6 1AZ.
(0734) 492000

Janssen
Janssen Pharmaceutical Ltd,
Grove, Wantage, Oxon
OX12 0DQ.
(0235) 772966

JLB
JLB Textiles Ltd,
Unit 2B, St Columb Industrial
Estate, St Columb Major,
Cornwall TR9 6SF.
(0637) 880065

K & K-Greeff
K & K-Greeff Ltd,
Suffolk House, George St,
Croydon CR9 3QL.
081-686 0544

K/L
K/L Pharmaceuticals Ltd,
25 Macadam Place, South
Newmoor Industrial Estate,
Irvine KA11 4HP.
(0294) 215951

Kabi Pharmacia
Kabi Pharmacia Ltd,
Davy Ave, Knowlhill,
Milton Keynes MK5 8PH.
(0908) 661101

Kendall
The Kendall Company (UK) Ltd,
Pool, Redruth,
Cornwall TR15 3QN.
(0209) 215151

Kendall-Lastonet
Contact Kendall.

Kerfoot
Thomas Kerfoot & Co. Ltd,
Vale of Bardsley, Ashton-under-
Lyne, Lancs OL7 9RR.
061-330 4531

Knoll
Knoll Ltd,
Fleming House, 71 King St,
Maidenhead, Berks SL6 1DU.
(0628) 776360

LAB
Laboratories for Applied Biology
Ltd,
91 Amhurst Park, London
N16 5DR.
081-800 2252

Laerdal
Laerdal Medical Ltd,
Laerdal House, Goodmead Rd,
Orpington, Kent BR6 0HX.
(0689) 76634

Index of manufacturers

Lagap
Lagap Pharmaceuticals Ltd,
37 Woolmer Way, Bordon,
Hants GU35 9QE.
(0420) 478301

Lamberts
Lamberts (Dalston) Ltd,
Dalston House, Hastings St,
Luton, Beds LU1 5BW.
(0582) 400711

Lederle
Lederle Laboratories,
Cyanamid House, Fareham Rd,
Gosport, Hants PO13 0AS.
(0329) 224000

Leo
Leo Laboratories Ltd,
Longwick Rd, Princes
Risborough, Aylesbury, Bucks
HP17 9RR.
(08444) 7333

Lilly
Eli Lilly & Co Ltd,
Dextra Court, Chapel Hill,
Basingstoke, Hants RG21 2SY.
(0256) 473241

Lipha
Lipha Pharmaceuticals Ltd,
Harrier House, High St,
West Drayton, Middx
UB7 7QG.
(0895) 449331

Lorex
Lorex Pharmaceuticals Ltd,
see Searle.
(0494) 526188

Loveridge
J. M. Loveridge plc,
Southbrook Rd, Southampton
SO9 3LT.
(0703) 228411

Loxley
Loxley Medical,
Unit 5D, Carnaby Industrial
Estate, Bridlington, North
Humberside YO15 3QY.
(0262) 603979

LRC
LRC Products Ltd,
North Circular Rd, Chingford,
London E4 8QA.
081-527 2377

Lundbeck
Lundbeck Ltd,
Sunningdale House,
Caldecott Lake Business Park,
Caldecott, Milton Keynes
MK7 8BR.
(0908) 649966

3M
3M Health Care Ltd,
3M House, Morley St,
Loughborough, Leics LE11 1EP.
(0509) 611611

Macfarlan Smith
Macfarlan Smith Ltd,
Wheatfield Rd, Edinburgh
EH11 2QA.
031-337 2434

Martindale
Martindale Pharmaceuticals Ltd,
Bampton Rd, Harold Hill,
Romford, Essex RM3 8UG.
(0708) 386660

Mediplus
Mediplus Ltd,
Unit C2, Thames Industrial
Estate, Fieldhouse Lane,
Marlow, Bucks SL7 1TB.
(0628) 483581

MediSense
MediSense Britain Ltd,
PO Box 2159, Coleshill,
Birmingham B46 1HZ.
(0675) 467044

Medo
Medo Pharmaceuticals Ltd.
Contact Schwarz.

Mepra-pharm
Mepra-pharm,
Brent House, Kenton Rd,
Harrow, Middx HA3 8DA.
081-907 4332

Merck
E. Merck Pharmaceuticals,
Winchester Rd, Four Marks,
Alton, Hants GU34 5HB.
(0420) 64011

Merieux
Merieux UK,
Clivemont House, Clivemont Rd,
Maidenhead, Berks SL6 7BU.
(0628) 785291

Merrell
Marion Merrell Dow Ltd,
Lakeside House, Stockley Park,
Uxbridge, Middx UB11 1BE.
081-848 3456

Milupa
Milupa Ltd, Milupa House,
Uxbridge Rd, Hillingdon,
Middx UB10 0NE.
081-573 9966

MMG
MMG (Europe) Ltd,
157 Redland Rd,
Bristol BS6 6YE.
(0272) 736883

Molnlycke
Molnlycke Ltd,
Southfields Rd,
Dunstable, Beds LU6 3EJ.
(0582) 600211

Monmouth
Monmouth Pharmaceuticals,
3/4 Huxley Rd,
The Surrey Research Park,
Guildford, Surrey GU2 5RE.
(0483) 65299

Morson
Thomas Morson Pharmaceuticals,
Contact MSD

MSD
Merck Sharp & Dohme Ltd,
Hertford Rd, Hoddesdon, Herts
EN11 9BU.
(0992) 467272

Napp
Napp Laboratories Ltd,
Cambridge Science Park, Milton
Rd, Cambridge CB4 4GW.
(0223) 424444

Nationwide Ostomy
Nationwide Ostomy Supplies
Ltd,
North West House, 62 Oakhill
Trading Estate, Walkden,
Manchester M28 5PT.
(0204) 709255

Nestlé
Nestlé Co. Ltd,
St. George's House, Croydon
CR9 1NR.
081-686 3333

Network Management
Network Management Ltd,
Christy Estate, North Lane,
Aldershot, Hants GU12 4QP.
(0252) 29911

Neutrogena
Neutrogena (UK) Ltd,
2 Mansfield Rd, South Croydon,
Surrey CR2 6HN.
081-680 5504

Nicholas
Nicholas Laboratories Ltd.
Contact Roche.

Nordic
Nordic Pharmaceuticals Ltd,
Contact Ferring.
081-898 8665

Norgine
Norgine Ltd,
116 London Rd, Headington,
Oxford OX3 9BA.
(0865) 750717

Norma
Norma Chemicals Ltd,
Contact Wallace Mfg.

North West
North West Medical Supplies
Ltd,
Green Arms Rd, Bolton
BL7 0ND.
(0204) 852383

North West Ostomy
see Nationwide Ostomy

Norton
H. N. Norton & Co. Ltd,
Gemini House, Flex Meadow,
Harlow, Essex CM19 5TJ.
(0279) 426666

Norwich Eaton
Norwich Eaton Ltd,
New Sandgate House, City Rd,
Newcastle upon Tyne
NE99 1YD.
091-222 1882

Novex
Novex Pharma Ltd,
Innovex House,
Reading Rd,
Henley-on-Thames RG9 1EL.
(0491) 578171

Index of manufacturers

Novo Nordisk
Novo Nordisk Pharmaceutical Ltd,
Novo Nordisk House, Broadfield Park, Brighton Rd, Pease Pottage, Crawley, West Sussex RH11 9RT.
(0293) 613555

Nutricia
Nutricia Dietary Products Ltd, 494–496 Honeypot Lane, Stanmore, Middx HA7 1JH.
081-951 5155

Nycomed
Nycomed (UK) Ltd, Nycomed House, 2111 Coventry Rd, Sheldon, Birmingham B26 3EA.
021-742 2444

Omnicare
The Omnicare Group Ltd, Unit 7E, Blacknest Works, Blacknest, Nr. Alton, Hants GU34 4PX.
Dial 100 and ask for 'Freephone Omnicare Oxygen'

Oral B Labs
Oral B Laboratories Ltd, Gatehouse Rd, Aylesbury, Bucks HP19 3ED.
(0296) 32601

Organon
Organon Laboratories Ltd, Cambridge Science Park, Milton Rd, Cambridge, CB4 4FL.
(0223) 423445

Organon-Teknika
Organon-Teknika Ltd,
see Organon
(0223) 423650

Ortho
Ortho Pharmaceutical Ltd
Contact Cilag

Owen Mumford
Owen Mumford Ltd, Brook Hill, Woodstock, Oxford OX7 1TU.
(0993) 812021

Oxford Nutrition
Oxford Nutrition Ltd, PO Box 31, Oxford OX4 3UH.
(0865) 716323

Oxygen Therapy Co Ltd
The Oxygen Therapy Co Ltd, Dumballs Rd, Cardiff CF1 6JE.
(0800) 373580

Paines & Byrne
Paines & Byrne Ltd, Pabyrn Laboratories, 177 Bilton Rd, Perivale, Greenford, Middx UB6 7HG.
081-997 1143

Panpharma
Panpharma Ltd, Hayes Gate House, 27 Uxbridge Rd, Hayes, Middx UB4 0JN.
081-561 8774

Payne
S G & P Payne, Percy House, Brook St, Hyde, Cheshire SK14 2NS.
061-367 8561

P-D
Parke-Davis Medical, Lambert Court, Chestnut Ave, Eastleigh, Hants SO5 3ZQ.
(0703) 620500

Penn
Penn Pharmaceuticals Ltd, Tafarnaubach Industrial Estate, Tredegar, Gwent, NP2 3AA.
(0495) 711711

Pennine
Pennine Healthcare, Pontefract St, Ascot Drive Industrial Estate, Derby DE2 8JD.
(0332) 384489

Perstorp
Perstorp Pharma Ltd, Wound-Care Division, Studio 1, Intec 2, Wade Rd, Basingstoke, Hants RG24 0NE.
(0256) 477868

Pfizer
Pfizer Ltd, Sandwich, Kent CT13 9NJ.
(0304) 616161

Pharma-Plast
Pharma-Plast Ltd, Thornhill Rd, North Moons Moat, Redditch, Worcs B98 9NL.
(0527) 64222

Pharmax
Pharmax Ltd, Bourne Rd, Bexley, Kent DA5 1NX.
(0322) 550550

Philip Harris
Philip Harris Medical Ltd, Hazelwell Lane, Birmingham B30 2PS.
021-433 3030

Phillips Yeast
Phillips Yeast Products Ltd, Park Royal Rd, London NW10 7JX.
081-965 7533

Pickles
J. Pickles & Sons, Beech House, 62 High St, Knaresborough, N. Yorks HG5 0EA.
(0423) 867314

Portex
Portex Ltd, Hythe, Kent CT21 6JL.
(0303) 260551

Porton
Porton Products Ltd, 1 Bath Rd, Maidenhead, Berks SL6 4UH.
(0628) 771417

Procea
Procea, Alexandra Road, Dublin 1.
(0001) 741741

Procter & Gamble
Procter & Gamble Ltd, Rusham Park, Whitehall Lane, Egham, Surrey TW20 9NW.
(0784) 434422

Quinoderm Ltd
Quinoderm Ltd, Manchester Rd, Oldham, Lancs OL8 4PB.
061-624 9307

Rand Rocket
Rand Rocket Ltd, ABCare House, Hownsgill Industrial Park, Consett, County Durham DH8 7NU.
(0207) 591099

R&C
Reckitt & Colman, Pharmaceutical Division, Dansom Lane, Hull HU8 7DS.
(0482) 26151

Regent
Regent Laboratories Ltd, Cunard Rd, London NW10 6PN.
081-965 3637

Renacare
Contact Martindale
(0708) 384455

Rendell
W. J. Rendell Ltd, Ickleford Manor, Hitchin, Herts SG5 3XE.
(0462) 32596

Rhône-Poulenc Rorer
Rhône-Poulenc Rorer Ltd, 52 St Leonards Rd, Eastbourne, East Sussex BN21 3YG.
(0323) 21422

Richborough
Contact Pfizer.

Rima
Rima Pharmaceuticals Ltd, 214–216 St James's Rd, Croydon, Surrey CR0 2BW.
081-683 1266

RMT
RMT Products Ltd, 57A Soulbury Rd, Leighton Buzzard, Beds LU7 7RW.
(0525) 374523

Robinsons
Robinson Healthcare
Hipper House, Chesterfield, Derbyshire S40 1YF.
(0246) 220022

RoC
Laboratoires RoC UK Ltd, Silver City House, 62 Brompton Rd, London SW3 1BW.
071-823 9223

Roche
Roche Products Ltd, PO Box 8, Welwyn Garden City, Herts AL7 3AY.
(0707) 328128

Index of manufacturers

Rona
Contact Lipha.

Roterpharma
Roterpharma Ltd,
Littleton House, Littleton Rd,
Ashford, Middx TW15 1UU.
(0784) 248279

Roussel
Roussel Laboratories Ltd,
Broadwater Park, North Orbital
Rd, Uxbridge, Middx UB9 5HP.
(0895) 834343

RP Drugs
RP Drugs Ltd,
RPD House, Yorkdale Industrial
Park, Braithwaite St, Leeds
LS11 9XE.
(0532) 441400

Rüsch
Rüsch UK Ltd,
PO Box 138,
Cressex Industrial Estate,
High Wycombe, Bucks
HP12 3NB.
(0494) 532761

Rybar
Rybar Laboratories Ltd,
30 Sycamore Rd, Amersham,
Bucks HP6 5DR.
(0494) 722741

Sallis
E. Sallis Ltd,
Vernon Works, Waterford St,
Old Basford, Nottingham
NG6 0DH.
(0602) 787841

Salts
Salt & Son Ltd,
Saltair House, Lord St,
Heartlands, Birmingham
B7 4DS.
021-359 5123

Sandoz
Sandoz Pharmaceuticals,
Frimley Business Park, Frimley,
Camberley, Surrey GU16 5SG.
(0276) 692255

Sanofi Winthrop
Sanofi Winthrop Ltd,
Onslow St, Guildford, Surrey
GU1 4YS.
(0483) 505515

Sara Lee
Sara Lee Household & Personal
Care (UK) Ltd,
225 Bath Rd, Slough SL1 4AU.
(0753) 523971

Schering Health Care
Schering Health Care Ltd,
The Brow, Burgess Hill, West
Sussex RH15 9NE.
(0444) 232323

Schering-Plough
Schering-Plough Ltd,
Mildenhall, Bury St. Edmunds,
Suffolk IP28 7AX.
(0638) 716321

Scholl
Scholl Consumer Products Ltd,
475 Capability Green, Luton,
Beds LU1 3LU.
(0582) 482929

Schwarz
Schwarz Pharma Ltd,
Schwarz House, East St,
Chesham, Bucks HP5 1DG.
(0494) 772071

Scientific Hospital Supplies
Scientific Hospital Supplies
Group UK Ltd,
100 Wavertree Boulevard,
Wavertree Technology Park,
Liverpool L7 9PT.
051-228 1992

Scotia
Scotia Pharmaceuticals Ltd,
Units 26–29,
Surrey Technical Centre,
The Research Park,
40 Occam Rd, Guildford,
Surrey GU2 5YH.
(0483) 304408

Searle
Searle Pharmaceuticals,
PO Box 53, Lane End Rd, High
Wycombe, Bucks HP12 4HL.
(0494) 521124

Serono
Serono Laboratories (UK) Ltd,
99 Bridge Rd. East, Welwyn
Garden City, Herts AL7 1BG.
(0707) 331972

Servier
Servier Laboratories Ltd,
Fulmer Hall, Windmill Rd,
Fulmer, Slough SL3 6HH.
(0753) 662744

Seton
Seton Healthcare,
Seton Healthcare Group plc,
Tubiton House, Medlock St,
Oldham, Lancs OL1 3HS.
061-652 2222

Seton-Prebbles
As Seton

Seven Seas
Seven Seas Ltd,
Hedon Rd, Marfleet, Hull
HU9 5NJ.
(0482) 75234

Seward
Seward Medical,
131 Great Suffolk St, London
SE1 1PP.
071-357 6527

Shannon
T.J. Shannon Ltd,
59 Bradford St, Bolton
BL2 1HT.
(0204) 21789

Shaw
A.H. Shaw and Partners Ltd,
Manor Rd, Ossett, West
Yorkshire WF5 0LF.
(0924) 273474

Sherwood
Sherwood Medical Industries
Ltd,
County Oak Way, Crawley,
West Sussex RH11 7YQ.
(0293) 534501

Shire
Shire Pharmaceuticals Ltd,
1 Viscount Court, South Way,
Andover, Hants SP10 5NW.
(0264) 333455

Simcare
Simcare,
Peter Rd, Lancing,
West Sussex BN15 8TJ.
(0903) 761122

Simpla
Simpla Plastics Ltd,
Cardiff Business Park, Cardiff
CF4 5WF.
(0222) 747000

Sinclair
Sinclair Pharmaceuticals Ltd,
Borough Rd, Godalming, Surrey
GU7 2AB.
(0483) 426644

S&N
Smith & Nephew Medical Ltd,
PO Box 81, 101 Hessle Rd, Hull
HU3 2BN.
(0482) 25181

S&N Pharm.
Smith & Nephew
Pharmaceuticals Ltd,
Bampton Rd, Harold Hill,
Romford, Essex RM3 8SL.
(04023) 49333

SK&F
Smith Kline & French
Laboratories,
Contact SmithKline Beecham

SmithKline Beecham
SmithKline Beecham
Pharmaceuticals,
SmithKline Beecham plc,
Mundells, Welwyn Garden City,
Herts AL7 1EY.
(0707) 325111

SmithKline Beecham Brands
SmithKline Beecham Consumer
Brands,
St Georges Ave, Weybridge,
Surrey KT13 0DE.
(0932) 822000

SNBTS
Scottish National Blood
Transfusion Service,
Protein Fractionation Centre,
21 Ellen's Glen Rd,
Edinburgh EH17 7QT.
031-664 2317

Spodefell
Spodefell Ltd,
5 Inverness Mews, London
W2 3QJ.
071-229 9125

Squibb
E.R. Squibb & Sons Ltd,
see Bristol-Myers.

Index of manufacturers

Squibb Surgicare
As Squibb

Stafford-Miller
Stafford-Miller Ltd,
Broadwater Rd, Welwyn Garden City, Herts AL7 3SP.
(0707) 331001

STD Pharmaceutical
STD Pharmaceutical Products,
Fields Yard, Plough Lane,
Hereford HR4 0EL.
(0432) 53684

Steeper
Steeper (Orthopaedic) Ltd,
59 North Worple Way, Mortlake, London SW14 8PS.
081-878 8633

Steriseal
Steriseal Ltd,
Thornhill Rd, Redditch,
Worcs B98 9NL.
(0527) 64222

Sterling Health
Sterling-Winthrop Group Ltd,
Contact Sanofi Winthrop.

Sterwin
Contact Sanofi Winthrop.

Stiefel
Stiefel Laboratories (UK) Ltd,
Holtspur Lane, Wooburn Green,
High Wycombe,
Bucks HP10 0AU
(0628) 524966

Storz
Storz Ophthalmics
Contact Lederle

Stuart
Contact ICI.

Syntex
Syntex Pharmaceuticals Ltd,
Syntex House, St. Ives Rd,
Maidenhead, Berks SL6 1RD.
(0628) 33191

Texlastic
Texlastic Ltd,
Unit 3, 28 Charter St, Leicester LE1 3UD.
(0533) 626682

Thackraycare
see DePuy

Thames
see Consolidated.

Thornton & Ross
Thornton & Ross Ltd,
Linthwaite Laboratories,
Huddersfield HD7 5QH.
(0484) 842217

Tillomed
Tillomed Laboratories Ltd,
Unit 2, Campus 5,
Letchworth Business Park,
Letchworth Garden City,
Herts SG6 2JF.
(0462) 480344

Tillotts
Contact Farmitalia Carlo Erba

Torbet
Torbet Laboratories Ltd,
Broughton House, 33 Earl St,
Maidstone, Kent ME14 1PF.
(0622) 762269

Tosara
Tosara Products Ltd,
Baldoyle Industrial Estate,
Grange Rd, Dublin 13.
(0001) 392212

Typharm
Typharm Ltd,
14 Parkstone Rd, Poole,
Dorset BH15 2PG.
(04254) 79711

UCB Pharma
UCB Pharma Ltd,
Star House, 69 Clarendon Rd,
Watford,
Herts WD1 1DJ.
(0923) 248011

Ultra
Ultra Laboratories Ltd,
Trinity Trading Estate,
Tribune Drive, Sittingbourne,
Kent ME10 2PG.
(0795) 70953

Ultrapharm
Ultrapharm Ltd,
PO Box 18, Henley-on-Thames,
Oxon RG9 2AW.
(0491) 578016

Unigreg
Unigreg Ltd,
Enterprise House, 181 Garth Rd,
Morden, Surrey SM4 4LL.
081-330 1421

Universal
Universal Hospital Supplies,
313 Chase Rd, London N14 6JA.
081-882 6444

Upjohn
Upjohn Ltd,
Fleming Way, Crawley, West Sussex RH10 2NJ.
(0293) 531133

Vernon-Carus
Vernon-Carus Ltd,
Hoddlesden Mills,
Hoddlesden, Darwen,
Lancs BB3 3NW.
(0254) 701383

Vestar
Vestar Ltd, 51 Cambridge Place,
Hills Rd, Cambridge CB2 1NS.
(0223) 461380

Vestric
Vestric Ltd,
West Lane, Runcorn, Cheshire WA7 2PE.
(0928) 717070

Vitabiotics
Vitabiotics Ltd,
Vitabiotics House, 3 Bashley Rd,
London NW10 6SU.
081-963 0999

Vitalograph
Vitalograph Ltd,
Maids Moreton House,
Buckingham MK18 1SW.
(0280) 822811

Vygon
Vygon (UK) Ltd,
Bridge Rd, Cirencester,
Glos GL7 1PT.
(0285) 67051

Wallace Mfg
Wallace Manufacturing Chemists,
15 Cochrane Mews,
London NW8 6NY.
071-722 9166

Ward
Ward Surgical Appliance Co Ltd,
57A Brightwell Ave,
Westcliffe-on-Sea, Essex
SS0 9EB.
(0702) 354064

WBP
WB Pharmaceuticals Ltd,
Contact Boehringer Ingelheim

Welfare Foods
see Nutricia.

Welland
Welland Medical Ltd,
15 Pelham Court, Broadfield,
Crawley, West Sussex
RH11 9AZ.
(0293) 615455

Wellcome
The Wellcome Foundation Ltd,
Wellcome Medical Division,
Crewe Hall, Crewe, Cheshire
CW1 1UB.
(0270) 583151

Whitehall
Whitehall Laboratories,
11 Chenies St,
London WC1E 7ET.
071-636 8080

Willis
S. R. Willis & Sons Ltd,
176 Albion Rd, London
N16 9JR.
071-254 7373

Windsor
Contact Boehringer Ingelheim.

W-L
Warner Lambert UK Ltd,
Contact P-D.

Wyeth
Wyeth Laboratories,
Huntercombe Lane South,
Taplow, Maidenhead, Berks
SL6 0PH.
(0628) 604377

Zeal
G.H. Zeal Ltd,
8 Lombard Rd, Merton,
London SW19 3UU.
081-542 2283

Zyma
Zyma Healthcare
Mill Rd, Holmwood
Dorking, Surrey RH5 4NU.
(0306) 742800

Index

Where an entry is followed by more than one page reference, the principal reference is printed in **bold** type. Proprietary (trade) names are printed in *italic* type.

100 plus, 309
AAA, 396
Abbreviations, *inside front cover*, 2
    latin, *inside back cover*, 4
    of units, 4
Abdominal surgery, antibacterial prophylaxis, 203
Abidec, capsules, xiii
Abidec drops, 354
Abortion,
    habitual, 271
    haemorrhage, 284
    induction, 284
Abrasive agents, acne, 415
Absence seizures, 186
    atypical, 186
Absorbent cotton, 438
    hospital quality, 438
Absorbent cotton gauze, 438
Absorbent cotton ribbon gauze, 438
    viscose and, 438
Absorbent dressing, perforated film, 438
Absorbent lint, 438
Absorbent muslin, 438
Absorbent pads, 438
ABVD therapy, 318
AC Vax, 449
Acanthamoeba keratitis, 377
Acaricides, 428
ACBS, 534–45
    alcoholic beverages, 541
    disinfectants, 545
    foods, 534–42
    toilet preparations, 545
Accupro, 89
Accuseal adaptor, 306
Accuseal drainage bag, 305
Accuseal extension tube, 306
Accuseal leg bag, 304
ACE inhibitors, 87
    pregnancy, 510
    renal failure, 87
    see also individual drugs
Acebutolol, 77
Acemetacin, 360
Acepril, 87
Acetazolamide, 384
    breast-feeding, 517
    diuretic, 69
    epilepsy, 185, 186, **189**
    glaucoma, 382, **384**
    preparations, 384
    renal failure, 503

Acetest, 259
Acetic acid [ingredient], 290
Acetomenaphthone [ingredient], 354
Acetoxyl preparations, 417
Acetylcholine chloride, 386
Acetylcysteine, 133
    cystic fibrosis, 134
    eye, 385
    granules, 134
    infusion table, 524
    poisoning, 18
Acezide, 87
Achlorhydria, 59
Achromycin, 216
    ear, 390
    eye, 378
    Topical, 425
Acid aspiration, 31
Acidification of urine, 299
Acidosis, metabolic, 337
Aci-Jel, 290
Acipimox, 110
    renal failure, 503
Acitretin, xii
Acknowledgements, x
Aclacin, 314
Aclarubicin, 314
    infusion table, 524
Acne, 215, **415**
    ACBS, 545
Acnegel, 417
Acnidazil, 417
Acrivastine, 126, **127**
    renal failure, 503
Acrolein, 312
Acromegaly, 281
Acrosoxacin, 231, **232**
    see also 4-Quinolones
ACTH *see* Corticotrophin
Actifed, 137
    Compound Linctus, 136
    Expectorant, 136
Actilyse, 107
Actinac, 417
Actinomycin D *see* Dactinomycin
Actinomycosis, 203
Actisorb Plus, 439
Actonorm gel, 26
Actonorm powder, 28
Actraphane 30/70, Human, 254
Actrapid, Human, 252
Actrapid, Human Penfill, 252
Actron, 176
Acupan, 176

Acyclovir, 238
    herpes simplex, 238
        buccal, 396
        eye, 379
        genital, 238, 290, 427
        labialis, 427
    herpes zoster, 238
    infusion table, 524
    preparations, 238
        cream, 427
        eye ointment, 379
    renal failure, 504
Adalat preparations, 95
Adcortyl, 411
    in *Orabase*, 395
    Intra-articular/Intradermal, 366
    with *Graneodin* cream, 411
Addamel, 344
Addicts, notification of, 9
Addiphos, 344
    infusion table, 528
Addison's disease, 262
Additives,
    details provided, 2
    skin preparations and, 399
Additrace, 344
Adenocor, 71
Adenosine, 70
Adexolin, 350
ADH, 278
Adhesive, surgical tissue, 430
Adhesive dressings, 437
Adhesive films, 439
Adhesive remover, 54
Adhesive (Simcare), 50, 53
Adifax, 167
Adizem preparations, 94
Adrenal function test, 275
Adrenal hyperplasia, 264
Adrenal insufficiency, 262
Adrenal suppression, 263
    metyrapone, 283
    topical corticosteroids, 404
Adrenalectomy, 262
Adrenaline, 131
    anaphylaxis, 130
    cardiac arrest, 98
    eye, 383
    local anaesthesia, 473
Adrenergic neurone blocking drugs, 84
Adrenoceptor stimulants, 113
Adrenoleukodystrophy,
    ACBS, 542
Adriamycin, 315

Index 567

ADROIT, 10
Adsorbents, poisoning, 17
Adverse reactions, reporting, 10
Advisory and cautionary labels *see* Cautionary and advisory labels
Advisory Committee on Borderline Substances *see* ACBS
AeroBec preparations, 123–4
Aerolin preparations, 116
Aerosporin, 224
Afrazine nasal spray, 393
Agammaglobulinaemia, congenital, 455
Agarol, 43
Agiolax, 42
Aglutella, 534
AIDS, 239
  vaccines and, 442
Airstrip, 437
Akineton, 196
AL-110, 534
Albendazole, 249
Albucid, 378
Albumaid preparations, 534
Albumin solution, 340
Albuminar preparations, 340
Albustix, 259
Albutein preparations, 340
Albym Test, 260
Alclometasone dipropionate, 407
Alcobon, 236
Alcoderm, 400
Alcohol,
  ACBS, 541
  breast-feeding, 517
  dependence, 197
  hypnotic, 141
  infusion table, 528
  nutrition, 342
  poisoning by, 17
  pregnancy, 510
  skin, 431
  withdrawal, 141
Alcoholism, 197
  vitamin B, 350
Alcopar, 249
Alcuronium, 469
Aldactide preparations, 68
Aldactone, 67
Aldesleukin, 321
  infusion table, 524
Aldomet, 84
Aldosterone antagonists, 67
Alembicol D, 534
Alexa, 302
Alexan preparations, 316
Alfacalcidol, 352
Alfare, 534
Alfentanil, 466
  infusion table, 524
Algesal, 375
Algicon, 26
Alginates, 26
  dressings, 440
Algipan, 375

Algitec preparations, 32
Alimix, 30
Alka-Donna preparations, xiii
Alkalinisation of urine, 298
Alka-Seltzer, 176
Alkeran, 313
Alkylating drugs, 312–13
Allantoin [ingredient], 413, 417, 422, 430
Allbee with C, 354
Allegron, 160
Aller-eze, 128
Allergen extract vaccines, 130
Allergic disorders, 126–31, 264
  conjunctivitis, 380
  rhinitis, 391
Allergic emergencies, 130
Allergy, diagnosis of, 130
Alleyvn, 440
All-Flex diaphragm, 296
Alloferin, 469
Allopurinol, 370
  preparations, 370
  renal failure, 504
Allyloestrenol, 271, **272**
Almay sun preparations, 420
Almevax, 452
Almodan, 206
Almond oil, 390
Alnide, 381
Alomide, 380
Alopecia, cytotoxic drugs, 311
Alophen, 43
Aloxiprin, 173
Alpha Keri Bath Oil, 402
Alpha tocopheryl acetate, 353
Alpha-adrenoceptor blocking drugs, 85
Alphaderm, 405
Alphavase, 86
Alphodith, 414
Alphosyl, 413
Alphosyl HC, 414
Alphosyl shampoo, 422
Alprazolam, 142, **143**
Alprostadil, 286
  infusion table, 524
Alrheumat, 362
Altacite Plus preparations, 26
Altacite preparations, 25
Alteplase, 106, **107**
  renal failure, 504
Alu-Cap,
  antacid, 24
  hyperphosphataemia, 348
Aludrox, 24
Aludrox SA, xiii
Aluhyde, 28
Aluminium acetate,
  ear-drops, 388
  lotion, 433
Aluminium chloride, 434
Aluminium hydroxide, 24
  antacid, 24
  diarrhoea, 38
  hyperphosphataemia, 348
  renal failure, 504

Aluminium hydroxide–magnesium carbonate co-dried gel, 24
Aluminium hydroxychloride, 434
Alupent preparations, 118
Alvedon, 174
Alvercol, 29
Alverine, 29
Amantadine, 194
  parkinsonism, 193, **194**
  preparations, 194
  renal failure, 504
  viral infections, 238
Ambaxin, 208
Ambilhar, 249
AmBisome, 235
Amenorrhoea, primary, 268
Amethocaine, 475
  eye, 385
Amfipen, 207
Amikacin, 218, **219**
  infusion table, 524
Amikin, 219
Amilco, 68
Amilmaxco, 68
Amiloride, 66, **67**
  preparations, 67
    compound, 68
  see also Diuretics, potassium-sparing
Amilospare, 67
Amino acids, intravenous nutrition, 342
  branched chain, 343
Aminobenzoic acid, 350, 420
Aminoglutethimide, 323
  pregnancy, 510
Aminoglycosides, 217–9
  ear, 388, 390
  pregnancy, 510
  renal failure, 504
Aminogran, 534
Aminophylline, 119, **121**
  infusion table, 524
  preparations, 121
  see also Theophylline
Aminoplasmal preparations, 343
Aminoplex preparations, 343
Aminosalicylic acid, 37
Amiodarone, 71
  breast-feeding, 517
  infusion table, 524
  pregnancy, 510
  renal failure, 504
Amitriptyline, 158
  preparations, 159
Amix, 206
Amlodipine, 94
  liver disease, 499
  see also Calcium-channel blockers
Ammonia, poisoning by, 21
Ammonia and ipecacuanha mixture, 136
Ammonium chloride mixture, morphine and, 136

568 Index

Amnivent, 121
Amoebiasis, 245
Amoebic abscess, 245
Amoebic dysentery, 245
Amoebicides, 245
Amoram, 206
Amorolfine, 425
Amoxapine, 158, **159**
Amoxil preparations, 206–7
Amoxycillin, **206**, 233
   infusion table, 524
   preparations, 206
   renal failure, 504
Amphetamines, 165
   abuse, 7
   breast-feeding, 517
   poisoning by, 20
Amphotericin, 234, **235**
   bladder infections, 299
   infusion table, 524
   mouth, 395
   preparations, 235
      lozenges, 396
      oral suspension, 396
   renal failure, 504
Amphotericin (liposomal), 234, 235
   infusion table, 524
Ampicillin, **206**, 233
   flucloxacillin with, 206, **208**
   infusion table, 524
   preparations, 206
   renal failure, 504
   sulbactam with, 206
Ampicillin/cloxacillin, infusion table, 525
Ampicillin/sulbactam, infusion table, 525
Ampiclox, 207
   infusion table, 525
Amrit, 206
Amsacrine, 318
   infusion table, 525
Amsidine, 318
Amylobarbitone, 145
   renal failure, 504
Amytal, 145
Anabolic steroids, 274
   anaemias, 331
   liver disease, 499
   pregnancy, 510
Anacal, 46
Anadin preparations, 176
   Anadin Ibuprofen, 359
Anaemias, 326–34
   aplastic, 331
   chronic renal failure, 332
   haemolytic, 331
   hypoplastic, 331
   iron-deficiency, 326–30
   megaloblastic, 330
   pernicious, 330
   sideroblastic, 331
Anaesthesia,
   analgesics, 466–9
   antimuscarinics, 462
   corticosteroids, 263, 459
   driving, 458

Anaesthesia (*continued*)—
   general, 458–62
      inhalational, 461
      intravenous, 459–61
   local, 472–5
      eye, 385
      mouth, 394–7
      rectal, 45
      skin, 403
   muscle relaxants, 469–71
   pregnancy, 510
Anaesthetics *see* Anaesthesia
Anaflex, 430
Anafranil preparations, 159
Analeptics, 131
Analgesics, 172–84
   compound, 173
   non-opioid, 173–6
   NSAIDs, 173
      anaesthesia, 466
      liver disease, 501
      poisoning by, 18
      pregnancy, 514
      renal failure, 507
      rheumatic diseases, 357–64
      topical, 374
   opioid, 177
      anaesthesia, 466
      choice, 177
      cough suppressants, 134–5
      dependence on, 7
      diarrhoea, 36
      liver disease, 501
      oral solutions, 178
      poisoning by, 18
      pregnancy, 514
      renal failure, 508
Analog preparations, 534
Anaphylaxis, 126, **130**
Anapolon-50, 332
Ancrod, 103
   infusion table, 525
Ancrod antivenom, 104
Ancylostomiasis, 248
Andrews Answer, 176
Androcur, 274
Androgens, 273
   breast-feeding, 517
   liver disease, 499
   malignant disease, 322
   pregnancy, 510
Anectine, 471
Anethaine, 404
Anexate, 472
Angettes-75, 106
Angilol, 77
Angina,
   beta-blockers, 76
   calcium-channel blockers, 93
   nitrates, 90
Angioedema, **131**, 264
   hereditary, 107, 131, 275, 282
Angiopine, 95

Angiotensin-converting enzyme inhibitors *see* ACE inhibitors
Angiozem, 94
Anhydrol Forte, 434
Anistreplase, 106, **107**
Ankylosing spondylitis, 359, 363, 365
Anodesyn, 46
Anorectics, 166–7
Anorexia, neoplasia-related, ACBS, 544
Anorexia nervosa, ACBS, 542
Anquil, 148
Antabuse, 198
Antacids, 24–7
   alginates and, 26–7
   aluminium, 24
   bismuth, 27
   calcium, 27
   dimethicone and, 26
   liver disease, 499
   magnesium, 24
Antazoline, 380
Antepar tablets, xiii
Antepsin, 34
Anthelmintics, 247–9
Anthisan cream, 404
Anthranol , 414
Anthraquinones, 41
   breast-feeding, 517
Anthrax, 203
   vaccine, 444
Anti-androgens, 274
Anti-arrhythmic drugs, 69–75
Antibacterials, 199–234
   acne, 416
   choice, 199
   diarrhoea, 35
   ear, 388–90
   eye, 377–8
   prophylaxis, 202–3
   skin, 423
   summary of therapy, 200
   vaginal, 289
Antibiotic policies, 199
Antibiotic sensitivity, 199
Antibiotics *see* Antibacterials
Anticholinergic drugs *see* Antimuscarinics
Anticholinergic syndrome, 462
Anticholinesterases, 371
   anaesthesia, 471
Anticoagulant treatment booklets, 105
Anticoagulants, 102
   oral, 104
      breast-feeding, 517
      liver disease, 499
      reversal, 104
      surgery, 459
   parenteral, 102
   pregnancy, 510
Anticonvulsants *see* Anti-epileptics
Anti-D (Rh $_0$) immunoglobulin, 456

Antidepressants, 157–65
  choice, 158
  compound, 163
  liver disease, 499
  poisoning by, 19
  pregnancy, 510
  see also Monoamine-oxidase inhibitors
  serotonin-uptake inhibitor, 164
  surgery, 459
  tricyclic, 157–61
    breast-feeding, 517
    diabetic neuropathy, 258
    enuresis, 298
    MAOIs with, 162
    migraine, 184
  withdrawal, 157–8
Antidiabetic drugs, 250–9
  oral, 255–7
Antidiarrhoeal drugs see Diarrhoea
Antidiuretic hormone, 278
  antagonist, 279
  inappropriate secretion, 279
Anti-emetics, 167–72
  cytotoxic therapy and, 311
  migraine, 182
Antiepileptics, 185–92
  pregnancy, 511
  surgery, 459
Antifibrinolytic drugs, 107
Antifungal drugs, 234–7
  anogenital, 288–9
  skin, 425
Antigiardial drugs, 246
Antihaemophilic fraction, human, 108
Antihistamines, 126–8
  allergic emergencies, 130
  allergy, 126
  breast-feeding, 517
  cough preparations, 136
  eye, 380
  liver disease, 499
  nasal allergy, 391
  nasal decongestants, 137
  nausea and vertigo, 167–8
  pregnancy, 511
  skin, 403
Antihypertensives, 81–9
  ACE inhibitors, 87
  adrenergic neurone blockers, 84
  alpha-blockers, 85
  beta-blockers, 76
  calcium-channel blockers, 93
  centrally acting, 84
  ganglion blockers, 89
  vasodilator, 83
Anti-inflammatory analgesics see Analgesics, NSAIDs
Antileprotic drugs, 229
Antilymphocyte immunoglobulin, 319

Antimalarials, 240–5
  pregnancy, 511
Antimanic drugs, 155
Antimetabolites, 315
Antimigraine drugs, 182
Antimotility drugs, 36
Antimuscarinics,
  antipsychotics and, 146
  bronchodilator, 118
  eye, 381
  gastro-intestinal, 28–9
  gustatory sweating, 259
  parkinsonism, 195
  premedication, 462
  quaternary ammonium, 28–9
  urinary tract, 297
Antineoplastic drugs, 310–25
  see also Cytotoxic drugs
Anti-oestrogens, 275, 322
Antiperspirants, 434
Antiplatelet drugs, 105
Antipressan, 78
Antiprotozoal drugs, 240–7
Antipruritics, topical, 403
Antipsychotics, 145–55
  breast-feeding, 517
  depot injections, 153
  equivalent doses,
    depot, 153
    oral, 147
  liver disease, 499
  mania, 155
  pregnancy, 511
  renal failure, 504
  withdrawal, 147
Antipyretics, 173
Antirabies immunoglobulin, 455
Antiseptics, 431
  ACBS, 545
  lozenges, 396
  sprays, oropharynx, 396
  vaginal preparations, 290
Antiserum, 444
Antispasmodics, 27–31
Antitetanus immunoglobulin, 455–6
Antithyroid drugs, 260–2
Antituberculous drugs, 226–9
Antitussives, 134–7
Antivaricella-zoster immunoglobulin, 455, 456
Antivenoms, 22
Antiviral drugs, 237–40
  eye, 379
  skin, 427
Antoin, xiii
Anturan, 371
Anugesic-HC, 46
Anusol, 46
Anusol-HC, 46
Anxiety, 142
  antipsychotics, 146
Anxiolytics, 138, 142–5
  anaesthesia, 463
  benzodiazepines, 142–4
  liver disease, 499

Anxiolytics (*continued*)—
  poisoning by, 19
  pregnancy, 511
  renal failure, 504
  withdrawal, 138
APD, 280
Aphthous ulcers, 394
Apisate, 167
APP preparations, 31
Appetite stimulants, 355
Appetite suppressants, 166–7
Appliances,
  colostomy, 48–58
  ileostomy, 50–8
  incontinence, 302–9
    accessories, 305–6
    adhesives, 303
    belts, 302
    drainable dribbling, 302
    fixing strips, 303
    leg bags, 304–5
    night drainage bags, 305
    sheaths, 302–3
    suspensory systems, 305
    tubing, 305–6
  urinal systems, 306–9
  urinary disorders, 300–9
  urostomy, 300–2
Applications, definition, 399
Apresoline, 83
Aprinox, 64
Aproten preparations, 534
Aprotinin, 107, **108**
  injection, 108
APSAC, 107
Apsifen, 359
Apsin, 204
Apsolol, 77
Apsolox, 80
Aqua, 305
Aquadrate, 402
Aquadry adhesive, 304
Aquadry, drainage bag, 304
Aquadry leg bag, 304
Aquadry, leg strap, 304
Aquadry pouch, 302
Aquadry sheaths, 303
Aquadry urinal, 307
Aqueous cream, 400
Arachis oil,
  cradle cap, 422
  enema, 43
Aradolene, xiii
Aramine, 101
Aredia, 280
Arelix, 66
Arfonad, 89
Argipressin (*Pitressin*), 278
Argyle catheters, 309
Argyle drainage bag, 305
Argyle leg bag, 304
Argyle strap, 306
Argyle tube, 306
Arilvax, 454

Index

Arnott, 534
Arpicolin, 196
Arpimycin, 220
Arret, 37
Arrhythmias, 69
   poisoning and, 16
   supraventricular, 61, 69
   ventricular, 70
Artane, 196
Arterial occlusion, 104
Arteritis, temporal, 365
Arthritis, 357
   juvenile, 357, 367
   psoriatic, 366
   rheumatoid, 357–69
   septic, 201
Arthrofen, 359
Arthrosin, 363
Artificial saliva, 398
Artracin, 362
Arvin, 104
Arvin Antidote, 104
Arythmol, 75
5-ASA, 37
Asacol, 38
Ascabiol, 428
Ascaricides, 248
Ascaris, 248
Ascorbic acid, 352
   acidification of urine, 299
   iron excretion, 333
   preparations, 352
Asendis, 159
Aserbine, 434
Asilone, 26
Askit, 176
Asparaginase, 318
Aspav, 174
Aspellin, 375
Aspirin, 173
   analgesia, 173
   antiplatelet, 105, **106**
   breast-feeding, 517
   liver disease, 499
   migraine, 182
   myocardial infarction, 106
   poisoning by, 17
   pregnancy, 511
   preparations, 173
      antiplatelet, 106
      compound, 173–4, 176
   renal failure, 504
   Reye's syndrome and, 173
   rheumatic disease, 357, **358**
Aspirin–paracetamol ester *see* Benorylate
Aspro preparations, 176
Astemizole, 126, **127**
   pregnancy, 511
Asthma, 113
   emergency treatment, 114
   nocturnal, 114, 119
   pregnancy, 114
   prophylaxis, 122, 125
Astringents,
   ear, 388
   skin, 431
AT-10, 353

Atarax, 129
Atenix, 78
AtenixCo, 78
Atenolol, 78
   infusion table, 525
   preparations, 78
Atensine, 143
Athlete's foot, 425
Ativan injection, **144**, 465
Ativan tablets, 144
Atmocol, 54
Atonic seizures, 186
Atracurium, 469
   infusion table, 525
Atrial fibrillation, 61, 69, 104
Atrial flutter, 69
Atromid-S, 110
Atropine sulphate,
   anticholinesterases and, 471
   antispasmodic, 28
   bradycardia, 70, 462
   breast-feeding, 517
   eye, 381
   organophosphorus poisoning, 22
   premedication, 462
   preparations, 463
      eye, 381
Atrovent preparations, 119
Audax, 390
Audicort, 389
Audinorm, 391
Augmentin, 208
   infusion table, 526
Auranofin, 367
   see also Gold
Aureocort, 411
Aureomycin, 216
   eye, 377
   skin, 424
Aurothiomalate, 367
   see also Gold
Autoclix, 255
Autopen, 254
Aveeno bath preparations, 402
Aveeno cream, 400
Aventyl, 160
Avloclor, 243
Avomine, 172
Axid, 33
Azactam, 215
Azamune, 319
Azapropazone, 358, **360**
   gout, 369
   renal failure, 504
Azatadine, 127
Azathioprine, 319
   infusion table, 525
   liver disease, 499
   myasthenia gravis, 372
   pregnancy, 511
   preparations, 319
   renal failure, 504
   rheumatic disease, 369
   ulcerative colitis, 37
Azelastine, 391

Azidothymidine, 239
Azithromycin, 220, **221**
Azlocillin, 209
   infusion table, 525
   renal failure, 504
AZT, 239
Aztreonam, 214, **215**
   infusion table, 525
   pregnancy, 511
   renal failure, 504

Bacampicillin, 206, **208**
   renal failure, 504
Bacillus Calmette-Guerin vaccine, 444
   isoniazid-resistant, 445
   percutaneous, 445
Back pain, 357
Baclofen, 373
   breast-feeding, 517
   preparations, 373
   renal failure, 504
Baclospas, 373
Bacterial vaginosis, 230
Bactericides, in infusions, 522
Bacteroides fragilis infections, 209, 211, 221, 230
Bactigras, 439
Bactrim preparations, 225
   paediatric tablets, xiii
Bactroban, 423
   nasal, 394
BAL, 21
Balanced Salt Solution, 386
Baldness, male-pattern, 423
Balmandol, 402
Balmosa, 375
Balneum preparations, 402
   with Tar, 413
Baltar, 422
Bandages, 435–7
   medicated, 436
Banimax, 176
Baratol, 85
Barbiturates, 145
   breast-feeding, 517
   poisoning by, 19
   pregnancy, 511
   regulations, 7
Bard Absorption Dressing, 439
Barquinol HC, xiii
Barrier preparations, 402
Bath additives,
   coal tar, 413
   emollient, 402
Baxan, 212
Baycaron, 65
Bayolin, 375
Baypen, xiii
BC-500, 354
BC 500 with Iron, xiii
BCG vaccine, 444
B-D Microfine, 255
B-D Pen, 254
B-D Safe-clip, 255
Becloforte preparations, 124

Index 571

Beclomethasone dipropionate,
    asthma, 122, **123**
    nasal allergy, 391
    skin, 407
Becodisks, 124
Beconase preparations, 391
Becosym, 351
Becotide preparations, 124
Bedranol SR, 77
Bedsores, 402
Bee sting allergy preparations, 130
Beechams cough and cold preparations, 176
Behavioural disturbances, 146
Belladonna, 28
Bellocarb, 28
Benadon, 351
Bendogen, 85
Bendrofluazide, 63
    preparations, 64
Benemid, 371
Benerva, 350
Benerva Compound, 351
Benethamine penicillin, 203, **204**
Bengue's Balsam, 375
Bengue's Balsam SG, 375
Benoral, 358
Benorylate,
    analgesia, 173, **175**
    preparations, 358
    rheumatic disease, 358
Benoxinate *see* Oxybuprocaine
Benoxyl preparations, 417
Benperidol, 147, **148**
Benserazide, 192
    levodopa with, 192
Bentonite, 21
Benylin cold preparations, 176
Benylin cough preparations, 136
Benzagel preparations, 417
Benzalkonium chloride, 432
Benzalkonium chloride-bromine adduct, 419
Benzalkonium lozenges, 396
Benzathine penicillin, 204
Benzhexol, 195, **196**, 197
Benzocaine, 475
    [ingredient], 375
    lozenges, compound, 395
    mouth, 395, 396
Benzodiazepines, 138
    anaesthesia, 463
    antagonist, 471
    anxiolytics, 142–4
    breast-feeding, 517
    epilepsy, 189
    hypnotics, 139
    muscle spasm, 373
    poisoning by, 19
    pregnancy, 511
    withdrawal, 138
Benzoic acid ointment, compound, 425
Benzoin tincture, compound, 134

Benzoyl peroxide,
    acne, 417
    ringworm, 425
Benzthiazide, 64
Benztropine, 195, **196**
Benzydamine, 394
    cream, 375
Benzyl benzoate, 428
Benzylpenicillin, 203
    eye-drops, 386
    infusion table, 525
    injection, 204
    renal failure, 504
Beogex, 45
Bephenium, 248
Bergamot oil, 420
Berkamil, 67
Berkaprine, 319
Berkatens, 96
Berkmycen, 217
Berkolol, 77
Berkozide, 64
Berotec preparations, 117
Beta, 50, 53
Beta-Adalat, 78
Beta-adrenoceptor blocking drugs, 75–81
    anaesthesia, 458
    angina, 76
    anxiety, 144
    arrhythmias, 71, **76**
    breast-feeding, 518
    diuretics with, 76
    eye, 382, **383–4**
    hypertension, 76
    migraine, 184
    myocardial infarction, 76
    pregnancy, 511
    renal failure, 504
    thyrotoxicosis, 76, 261
    verapamil and, 70
Beta-adrenoceptor stimulants,
    asthma, 113–18
    premature labour, 287
Beta-blockers *see* Beta-adrenoceptor blocking drugs
Beta-Cardone, 81
Betadur CR, 77
Betagan, 384
Betahistine, 168
Beta-lactamases, 203
Betaloc preparations, 79
Betamethasone, 263, 264, **266**
Betamethasone dipropionate, 408
Betamethasone sodium phosphate,
    infusion table, 525
    preparations, 266
        ear, 388
        eye, 379
        nose, 391

Betamethasone valerate,
    haemorrhoids [ingredient], 46
    skin, 407–8
Beta-Prograne, 77
Betaxolol, 78
    eye, 383, **384**
Bethanechol,
    laxative, 41
    urinary retention, 296, **297**
Bethanidine, 85
    renal failure, 504
Betim, 81
Betnelan, 266
Betnesol, 266
    ear, 388
    eye, 379
    nose, 391
Betnesol-N, 389
    ear, 389
    eye, 379
    nose, 393
Betnovate preparations
    rectal, 46
    skin, 407–8
Betoptic, 384
Bezafibrate, 109, **110**
    liver disease, 499
    renal failure, 504
Bezalip preparations, 110
Bi-Aglut, 534
Bicarbonate
    intravenous, 339
    oral, 337
    see also Sodium bicarbonate
Bicillin, 204
BiCNU, 312
Biguanides, 257
Bilarcil, 249
Bilharziasis, 249
Biliary-tract infection, 200
Biltricide, 249
BiNovum, 293
Biocath, 309
Bioclusive, 439
Biofilm, 440
Biogastrone, 35
Biophylline preparations, 120
Bioplex, 395
Biopore, 48
Bioral Gel, 395
Biorphen, 196
Biotin, 350
Biotrol, 48, 51
Biperiden, 196
Biphosphonates *see* Bisphosphonates
Bipolar depression *see* Manic depression
Birkbeck, 52
Birthmarks, ACBS, 545
Bisacodyl, 41
    preparations, 41
Bismuth chelate, 33, **34**

Bismuth subgallate suppositories, compound, 46
Bisoprolol, 78
Bisphosphonates, 280
    hypercalcaemia, 346
    pregnancy, 511
Bitters, 355
BJ6 eye-drops, 385
Bladder,
    blood clot dissolution, 299
    irrigations, 299
        cytotoxic, 299
Blemix, 217
Blenderm, 437
Bleomycin, 314
    infusion table, 525
    renal failure, 504
Blepharitis, 386
Blocadren, 81
Blood,
    drugs affecting, 326–34
    incompatibilities, 522
Blood clot dissolution, bladder, 299
Blue line webbing, 436
BM-Test 1-44, 259
Bocasan, 397
Body-surface, dosage and, 11
Body-weight, dosage and, 11
Bolus injections, 523
Bolvidon, 161
Bone metabolism, drugs affecting, 279
Bone tumours, analgesia, 173
Bonefos, 281
Bone-marrow suppression, cytotoxic drugs, 311
Bonjela, 395
Boots Covering Cream, 421
Borderline substances *see* ACBS
Botulinum A toxin–haemagglutinin complex, 197
Botulinum antitoxin, 445
Botulism antitoxin, 445
Bowel cleansing solutions, 45
Bowel fistulas, ACBS, 542
Bowel sterilisation, 218
Bradilan, 111
Bradosol, 396
Bradosol Plus, 396
Bradycardia, 70
    anaesthesia, 462
Bran, 40
Brand names, symbol, 2
Brasivol, 416
Breast cancer, 314, 315, 317, 319–24
Breast disease, benign, 281
Breast pain, 281, **283**, 415
Breast-feeding, prescribing during, 517–21
Brelomax, 118
Bretylate, 74
Bretylium, 73, **74**
Brevibloc, xii
Brevinor, 292
Bricanyl preparations, 116

Brietal Sodium, 460
Britiazim, 94
Brocadopa, 193
Broflex, 196
Brolene, 378
Bromazepam, 142, **143**
Bromides, breast-feeding, 518
Bromocriptine, 281
    acromegaly, 281
    breast disease, benign, 281
    breast-feeding, 518
    galactorrhoea, 281
    hypogonadism, 281
    lactation suppression, 281
    neuroleptic malignant syndrome, 146
    parkinsonism, 193, **194**
    preparations, 194, 281
    prolactinoma, 281
Brompheniramine, 127
Bronchial carcinoma, 317
Bronchiectasis, 133, 134
Bronchilator, xiii
Bronchitis, 113, 118, 133, 134, 200
Bronchodil inhaler, 117
Bronchodilators, 113–22
    adrenoceptor stimulant, 113
    antimuscarinic, 118
    compound, 121
    surgery, 459
    sympathomimetic, 113
    theophylline, 119
Bronchospasm, 113
Brucellosis, 215, 229
Brufen preparations, 360
Brugia malayi, 249
Brulidine, 430
BSA, 11
Bubble U, 303
Buccastem, 172
Buclizine [ingredient], 182
Budesonide,
    asthma, 122, **124**
    nasal allergy, 392
    skin, 408
Bufexamac, 414
Bumetanide, 65, **66**
    infusion table, 525
    renal failure, 504
Buminate preparations, 340
Bupivacaine, 474
Buprenorphine, 177, **179**
    anaesthesia, 467
    breast-feeding, 518
Burinex, 66
Burinex A, 68
Burinex K, 69
Burns,
    infected, 423
    plasma and plasma substitutes, 340
Buscopan, 29
Buserelin, 323
    endometriosis, 282
    prostate cancer, 323
Buspar, 144

Buspirone, 144
Busulphan, 312
Butacote, 363
Butobarbitone, 145
Butriptyline, 158, **159**
Butyrophenones, 146

Cachexia, neoplasia-related, ACBS, 544
Cacit, 346
Cadexomer iodine, 440
Cafadol, 176
Cafergot, 183
Caffeine, 165, 173
    breast-feeding, 518
Calaband, 436
Calabren, 256
Caladryl preparations, 404
Calamine, 403
    preparations, 403
    coal tar and, 413
Calcichew, 346
Calcichew D3, 352
Calcidrink, 346
Calciferol, 352
    preparations, 352–3
Calcilat, 95
Calcimax, 354
Calciparine, 103
Calcipotriol, 412, **414**
Calcisorb, 347
Calcitare, 279
Calcitonin, **279**, 347
    breast-feeding, 518
Calcitonin (pork), 279
Calcitriol, 352
Calcium-500, 346
Calcium alginate dressings, 440
Calcium and ergocalciferol tablets, 352
Calcium and vitamin D tablets, 352
Calcium balance, maintenance, 279
Calcium carbonate, 346, **348**
    antacid, 27
    supplements, 346
Calcium chloride injection, 346
Calcium folinate, 317
Calcium gluconate, 346
    infusion table, 525
    injection, 346
    tablets, 346
Calcium intolerance, ACBS, 542
Calcium lactate tablets, 346
Calcium leucovorin, 317
Calcium Resonium, 336
Calcium salts, 346
Calcium supplements, 346
Calcium-channel blockers, 93
    angina, 93
    hypertension, 93
    migraine, 184
    pregnancy, 511
Calcium-Sandoz, 346
Calgel, 397

Calluses, 418
Callusolve, 419
Calmurid, 402
   solution, 422
Calmurid HC, 405
Calogen, 534
Caloreen, 534
Calpol preparations, 174, 176
   Extra, 176
Calsynar, 280
CAM, 118
Camcolit preparations, 156
Camouflaging preparations, 421
Camphor [ingredient], 375
Campylobacter enteritis, 35, 200, 220
Campylobacter pylori, 33
Candidiasis, 234–7
   intestinal, 234–7
   oropharyngeal, 234–7, **395**
   perianal, 45
   skin, 425
   systemic, 234–7
   vaginal, 234–6, **288**
   vulval, 288
Canesten,
   anogenital, 289
   ear, 389
   skin, 426
Canesten-HC, 406
Cannabis, regulations, 7
Canrenoate, 67
   infusion table, 531
   see also Aldosterone antagonists
Cantabread, 542
Cantil, 29
Capasal, 422
Capastat, 227
Capitol, 422
Caplenal, 370
Capoten, 87
Capozide, 87
Capreomycin, 227
   pregnancy, 511
   renal failure, 504
Caprin, 173
Caps, contraceptive, 296
Capsicin [ingredient], 375
Capsicum [ingredient], 375
Captopril, 87
   breast-feeding, 518
   pregnancy, 511
   renal failure, 504
   see also ACE inhibitors
Carace, 88
Carace Plus, 88
Carbachol,
   glaucoma, 382
   preparations, 297
      eye-drops, 382
   urinary retention, 296
Carbalax, 45
Carbamazepine,
   breast-feeding, 518
   diabetes insipidus, 278
   diabetic neuropathy, 258

Carbamazepine (*continued*)—
   epilepsy, 185, **186**
   manic depression, 157
   poisoning, elimination, 17
   pregnancy, 511
   preparations, 186
   trigeminal neuralgia, 182
Carbaryl, 428
Carbellon, 26
Carbenicillin, 209, **210**
   infusion table, 525
   renal failure, 504
Carbenoxolone, 35
   liver disease, 500
   mouth, 394
   pregnancy, 511
   preparations, 35
      mouth, 395
   renal failure, 504
Carbidopa, 192
   levodopa with, 192
Carbimazole, 261
   breast-feeding, 518
   pregnancy, 511
Carbocisteine, 134
   preparations, 134
Carbo-Cort, 414
Carbo-Dome, 412, **413**
Carbohydrate malabsorption, ACBS, 542
Carbomix, 17
Carbon monoxide poisoning, 21
Carbonet, 439
Carbonic anhydrase inhibitors, 69
   glaucoma, 384
Carboplatin, 318
   infusion table, 525
Carboprost, 284
Carbosorb, 439
Cardene, 95
Cardiac arrest, **98**, 340
   resuscitation, 99
Cardiac glycosides, 61
   arrhythmias, 70
Cardiac *see also* Heart
Cardiacap, xiii
Cardinol, 77
Cardinol, 85
Careline drainage bag, 305
Careline leg bag, 304
Carisoma, 374
Carisoprodol, 374
   breast-feeding, 518
Carmellose, 394
   gelatin preparations, 395
Carmustine, 312
   infusion table, 525
Carobel, Instant, 534
Carpal tunnel syndrome, 365
Carshalton, 54, 302
Carteolol,
   cardiovascular, 78
   eye, 383, **384**
Cartrol, 78
Carylderm, 429
Cascara, 41
Casilan, 534

Castor oil, 41
Catapres preparations, 84
Catarrh, vernal, 380
Catarrh-Ex, 176
Catheter maintenance, 300
Catheters, urethral, 309
Cautionary and advisory labels, 546–55
   counselling, 546
   key, *inside back cover*
   leaflets, 546
   list of products, 549–55
   'NCL', 546
   original packs, 546
   scope, 546
Caved-S, 35
Cavendish, 53
CCNU, 312, **313**
Ceanel Concentrate, 422
Cedilanid, xiii
Cedocard , 92
Cedocard IV, 92
Cedocard Retard, 92
Cef . . . *see also* Ceph . . .
Cefaclor, 211
Cefadroxil, 211, **212**
   renal failure, 505
Cefixime, 211, **212**
   renal failure, 505
Cefizox, 213
Cefodizime, 211, **212**
   infusion table, 525
   renal failure, 505
Cefotaxime, 211, **212**
   infusion table, 525
   renal failure, 505
Cefoxitin, 211, **212**
   infusion table, 525
   renal failure, 505
Cefsulodin, 211, **212**
   infusion table, 525
   renal failure, 505
Ceftazidime, 211, **213**
   infusion table, 525
   renal failure, 505
Ceftizoxime, 211, **213**
   infusion table, 526
   renal failure, 505
Cefuroxime, 211, **213**
   infusion table, 526
   renal failure, 505
Cefuroxime axetil, 211, **213**
Celance, 195
Celbenin, 205
Celectol, 79
Celevac tablets, 41, 166
Celiprolol, 76, 79
Cellosene, 438
Cellulitis, 201
Cellulose wadding, 438
Cellulose wadding tissue, gauze and, 438
Centoxin, 456
Central nervous stimulants, 165
Centyl, 64
Centyl K, 69
Ceph . . . *see also* Cef . . .

574 Index

Cephalexin, 211, **213**
   preparations, 214
   renal failure, 505
Cephalosporins, 211–14
   third generation, 211
Cephamandole, 211, **214**
   infusion table, 526
   renal failure, 505
Cephamycins, 211
Cephazolin, 211, **214**
   infusion table, 526
   renal failure, 505
Cephradine, 211, **214**
   infusion table, 526
   renal failure, 505
Ceporex, 214
Cerebrovase, 106
Cerumol, 391
Cervagem, 285
Cesamet, 171
Cetavlex, 430
Cetirizine, 126, **127**
   renal failure, 505
Cetrimide, 430, **432**
   cream, 430
Cetylpyridinium, 397
C-Film, 295
Charcoal,
   activated, 17
   dressings, 439
   haemoperfusion, 17
Chemotrim, 225
Chendol, 58
Chenodeoxycholic acid, 58
   liver disease, 500
   pregnancy, 511
Chenofalk, 59
Chicken meat, comminuted, 535
Chickenpox, 238
Chilblains, 441
Children,
   medicine storage, 3
   prescribing for, 11
Children's Vitamin Drops, 350
Child-resistant containers, 3
Chiron adhesives, 54
Chiron barrier cream, 57
Chiron pouches, 50, 53
   urostomy, 302
Chironair, 54
Chironseal, 50
Chlamydia, 215
Chloractil, 148
Chloral betaine, 141
Chloral hydrate, 140
   breast-feeding, 518
   preparations, 140
Chlorambucil, 312
   rheumatoid arthritis, 369
Chloramphenicol, 222
   breast-feeding, 518
   ear, 388, **389**
   eye, 377
   infusion table, 526
   liver disease, 500
   pregnancy, 511

Chloramphenicol (continued)—
   preparations, 222
   ear, 389
   eye, **377**, 380
   renal failure, 505
Chlorasept, 431
Chloraseptic mouthwash, 397
Chlorasol, 433
Chlordiazepoxide, 142, **143**
Chlorhexidine, 430, **431**
   bladder infections, 299
   dressing, gauze, 439
   mouth, 394, 396, **397**
   nose, 393
   skin disinfection, 431
     cream, 430
     dusting powder, 431
Chlorinated lime and boric acid solution, 432
Chlorinated soda solution, surgical, 433
Chlorine poisoning, 21
Chlormethiazole, 141
   anaesthesia, 464
   breast-feeding, 518
   liver disease, 500
   status epilepticus, 190, **191**
Chlormezanone, 144
   muscle spasm, 374
Chloromycetin, 222
   eye, 377
   Hydrocortisone, 380
Chloroquine,
   breast-feeding, 518
   infusion table, 526
   malaria, 241–3
   preparations, 243
   renal failure, 505
   rheumatic disease, 366, **368**
Chlorothiazide, 64
Chlorpheniramine, 126, **128**
   preparations, 128
Chlorpromazine, 147
   anaesthesia, 464
   breast-feeding, 518
   hiccup, 147
   nausea, 168
   preparations, 148
   psychoses, 147
   terminal care, 13
Chlorpropamide, 255, **256**
   diabetes insipidus, 278
   preparations, 256
   renal failure, 505
Chlortetracycline, 216
   eye, 377
   skin, 423, **424**
Chlorthalidone, 63, **64**
   diabetes insipidus, 278
Cholecalciferol, 352
Choledyl, 121
Cholera vaccine, 446
   travel, 457
Cholestyramine, 109
   diarrhoea, 38, **39**
   hypercholesterolaemia, 109

Cholestyramine (continued)—
   liver disease, 500
   pruritus, 109
Choline, 350
Choline magnesium trisalicylate, 358
Choline salicylate, 390
   dental gel, 394, **395**
Choline theophyllinate, 119, **121**
Cholinergic crises, 371
Cholinesterase inhibitors, 371, 471
Cho/Vac, 436
Choreas, 197
Choriocarcinoma, 315
Chorionic gonadotrophin, 276
Chymotrypsin, eye, 386
Cicatrin preparations, 423
Cidomycin, 219
   ear, 389
   eye, 377
Cidomycin Topical, 424
Cigarette smoking, 198
Cilastatin, 215
   imipenem with, 215
Cilazapril, 88
   renal failure, 505
   see also ACE inhibitors
Cilest, 292
Cimetidine, 31
   breast-feeding, 518
   infusion table, 526
   liver disease, 500
   preparations, 32
   renal failure, 505
Cinazière, 169
Cinnarizine, 169
   nausea and vertigo, 168
   vascular disease, 97
Cinobac, 232
Cinoxacin, 231, **232**
   renal failure, 505
   see also 4-Quinolones
Ciprofloxacin, 231, **232**, 233
   breast-feeding, 518
   Campylobacter infections, 35
   renal failure, 505
   see also 4-Quinolones
Ciproxin, 232
Cirrhosis, ACBS, 542
Cisapride, 30
   breast-feeding, 518
   liver disease, 500
   pregnancy, 511
   renal failure, 505
Cisplatin, 318
   infusion table, 526
   renal failure, 505
Citanest preparations, 475
Citramag, 44
Citrical, 346
Claforan, 212
Clairvan, 132

Index 575

Clarithromycin, 220, **221**
   renal failure, 505
Clarityn, 127
Classic, 48, 51, 301
Classification changes, xi
Clavulanic acid, 206
   amoxycillin with, 206, **208**
   breast-feeding, 518
   ticarcillin with, 209, **210**
Cleansers, skin, 431
Clemastine, 128
   breast-feeding, 517
Clexane, 103
Clickcount, 255
Climaval, 269
Clindamycin, 221
   infusion table, 526
   liver disease, 500
   preparations, 221–2
      acne, 416
Clinicide, 429
Clinifeed preparations, 535
CliniFlex dressings, 439
CliniShield barrier wipes, 57
Clinistix, 259
Clinitar, 413
   shampoo, 422
Clinitest, 259
Clinoril, 364
Clinutren preparations, 535
Clioquinol,
   diarrhoea, 36
   ear, 388, **389**
   skin [ingredient], 407
Clobazam, 142, **143**
   capsules, 143
   epilepsy, 185
Clobetasol propionate, 408–9
Clobetasone butyrate,
   eye, 379
   skin, 409
Clodronate sodium, 280, **281**
   infusion table, 532
   renal failure, 505
Clofazimine, 229, **230**
Clofibrate, 109, **110**
   liver disease, 500
   pregnancy, 512
   renal failure, 505
Clomid, 275
Clomiphene, 275
   liver disease, 500
   pregnancy, 512
Clomipramine, 158, **159**
   infusion table, 526
Clonazepam, 185, 186, **189**
   infusion table, 526
   myoclonus, 373
   status epilepticus, 190
Clonidine, 84
   hypertension, 84
   menopausal flushing, 184
   migraine, 184
   Tourette syndrome, 197
Clopamide, 64
Clopixol, 153, 155
Clopixol Acuphase, 153
Clopixol Conc, 155

Clorazepate, 142, **144**
Clorhexitulle, 439
Clostet, 453
Clotrimazole,
   anogenital, 289
   ear, 389
   skin, 425, **426**
   vaginal, 289
Cloxacillin, 204, 205
   infusion table, 526
Clozapine, 147, **148**
   pregnancy, 512
Clozaril, 149
CMV, 239
Coal tar, 412, **413**
   preparations, 413–14
   scalp, 421
Co-amilofruse preparations, 68
Co-amilozide preparations, 68
Co-amoxiclav, 206, **208**, 233
   breast-feeding, 518
   infusion table, 526
   renal failure, 505
Cobadex, 405
Cobalin-H, 331
Coban, 436
Co-beneldopa, 192, **193**
Co-Betaloc preparations, 80
Cocaine, 166
   eye-drops, 385
      homatropine and, 385
   local anaesthesia, 475
   poisoning by, 20
   prescribing for addicts, 9
Co-careldopa, 192, **194**
Co-codamol preparations, 174
Co-codaprin preparations, 173
Cocois, 413
Codafen Continus, 360
Codalax preparations, 42
Coda-Med, 176
Codanin, 176
Co-danthramer preparations, 42
Co-danthrusate preparations, 42
Codeine, 179
   breast-feeding, 518
   cough suppressant, 134
   diarrhoea, 36
      diabetic, 258
   pain, 177, **179**
   preparations, 36, **179**
      compound, 173–6
      linctuses, 134–5
   renal failure, 505
Co-dergocrine mesylate, 97
Codis, 176
Co-dydramol tablets, 175
Coeliac disease, ACBS, 542
Co-fluampicil, 206, **208**
   infusion table, 526
Co-flumactone preparations, 68
Cogentin, 196
Cohepress, 436
Cohesive extensible bandages, 436

Cohesive strips, 304
Cohflex, 49, 52
Cojene, 176
Colchicine, 369, **370**
   breast-feeding, 518
   renal failure, 505
   tablets, 370
Coldrex preparations, 176
Colds, 352
Colestid, 109
Colestipol, 109
Colfosceril palmitate, 132
Colgen, xiii
Colifoam, 39
Colistin, 224
   eye-drops, 386
   infusion table, 526
   renal failure, 505
   skin, 424
Colitis,
   pseudomembranous, 38
   ulcerative, 37–9
Collodion,
   definition, 399
   flexible, 430
   salicylic acid, 419
Colloid dressings, 439
Colodress, 48
Colofac, 29
Colomycin, 224, 424
Colostomy Plus, 54
Colostomy products, 48–58
Colpermin, 30
Coltapaste, 437
Colven, 30
   renal failure, 505
Coma,
   hyperglycaemic, 257
   hyperosmolar nonketotic, 257
   hypoglycaemic, 258
   hypothyroid, 260
   insulin, 258
   ketoacidotic, 257
Co-magaldrox, xi
Combantrin, 248
Comfeel dressings, 440
Comfeel preparations, 57
Comfort, 48, 305
Comixco, 225
Comox, 225
Complement Continus, 351
Comprecin, 232
Concavit, 354
Concordin, 161
Condyline, 419
Condylomata acuminata, 419
Conjugated oestrogens, 270
   vaginal, 288
Conjunctivitis, 201, 377
   allergic, 380
Conn's syndrome, 66
Conotrane, 403
Conova-30, 292
Conseal, 48
Contact lenses, 387
Containers, child-resistant, 3
Contents, vi

Contraceptives, 290–6
  devices, 295–6
  oral, 290–4
    breast-feeding, 518
    combined, 290–3
    emergency, 293
    interactions, 291
    liver disease, 500
    missed pill, 291
    phased, 293
    pregnancy, 512
    progestogen-only, 294
    surgery, **291**, 459
  parenteral, 294–5
  spermicidal, 295
Contrapain Femafen, 359
Contrast media, adverse reaction reporting, 10
Controlled drugs, 7–9
  see also preparations identified by **CD** throughout BNF
  travel abroad, 8
Conveen, 303
Conveen drainage bag, 305
Conveen leg bag, 304
Conveen sheath, 303
Conversions, approximate, 6
Convulsions
  febrile, 192
  poisoning and, 16
  see also Epilepsy
Coparvax, 320
Co-phenotrope, 36
Copholco, 136
Coppertone preparations, 420
Co-prenozide, 80
Co-proxamol tablets, 175
  poisoning, 18
Coracten, 95
Cordarone X, 72
Cordilox, 96
Corgard, 80
Corgaretic preparations, 80
Corlan, 395
Corn oil, 535
Corn starch, 535
Corneal ulcer, 379
Cornflour, 535
Coro-Nitro Spray, 90
Corsodyl preparations, 397
Corticosteroids, 262–7
  adrenal suppression, 263
  adrenalectomy, 262
  allergic emergencies, 131
  allergy, 264
    nasal, 391
  anaesthesia, 263, 459
  aphthous ulcers, 394
  asthma, 122
    emergency, 114
  blood disorders, 331
  breast-feeding, 518
  cancer, 319
  cautions, 263
  children, 265
  Crohn's disease, 37
  ear, 388–90

Corticosteroids (*continued*)—
  epilepsy, 186
  equivalent doses, 262
  eye, 377, **379**
  haemorrhoids, 46
  hypercalcaemia, 347
  hypophysectomy, 262
  immunosuppression, 319
  myasthenia gravis, 371, 372
  pregnancy, 512
  proctitis, 39
  replacement therapy, 262
  rheumatic disease, 364–6
  side-effects, 263
  skin,
    acne, 416
    eczema, 404–11
    psoriasis, 412
  ulcerative colitis, 37, **39**
Corticotrophin, 275
Cortisol, 262
Cortisone acetate, 266
  preparations, 266
  replacement therapy, 262
Cortistab, 266
Cortisyl, 266
Corwin, 100
Corynebacterium parvum
  vaccine, 320
Cosalgesic, 175
Cosmegen Lyovac, 314
Cosuric, 370
Cotazym, xiii
Co-tenidone, 78
Cotfil, 438
Co-triamterzide, xi
Co-trimoxazole, 224
  breast-feeding, 518
  infusion table, 526
  pregnancy, 512
  renal failure, 505
Cotton, absorbent, 438
Cotton and rubber elastic bandage, 436
  heavy, 436
Cotton conforming bandage, 435
Cotton crepe bandage, 436
Cotton gauze, absorbent, 438
Cotton ribbon gauze, absorbent, 438
  viscose and, 438
Cotton stockinette, 435
Cotton stretch bandage, 436
Cotton suspensory bandage, 436
Cough preparations,
  compound, 136
  breast-feeding, 518
Cough suppressants, 134
Coughcaps, 135
Coumarins, 104
Counter-irritants, 375
Covering creams *see* Camouflaging preparations
Covermark preparations, 421
Coversyl, 89

Crab lice, 428
Cradle cap, 422
Cramps, nocturnal, 373
Creams, definition, 399
Creams, suitable quantities, 399
Creatinine clearance, dosage and, 503
Cremalgin, 375
Creon preparations, 59–60
Crepe bandage, 436
  cotton, 436
Cretinism *see* Hypothyroidism, neonatal
Crinx, 435
Crisantaspase, 318
Crohn's disease, 37
Cromogen, 125
Cromoglycate *see* Sodium cromoglycate
Crotamiton, 403
  scabies, 428
Cryotherapy, 420
Cryptococcosis, 235–7
Crystal violet, 434
  paint, 434
Crystapen, 204
Cullen's (Mrs.), 176
Cupanol, 174, 176
Cuplex, 419
Cuprofen, 359
Cushing's syndrome, 283
  corticosteroid-induced, 263
CX Antiseptic Dusting Powder, 431
Cyanides, poisoning by, 20
Cyanocobalamin, 331
  preparations, 331
Cyclandelate, 98
Cyclimorph preparations, 179
Cyclizine, 168, **169**
Cyclobral, 98
Cyclocaps (salbutamol), 116
Cyclofenil, 275
  liver disease, 500
Cyclogest, 271
Cyclohaler, 122
Cyclopenthiazide, 64
Cyclopentolate, 381
Cyclophosphamide, 312
  infusion table, 527
  renal failure, 505
  rheumatic disease, 369
Cycloplegics, 381
Cyclo-Progynova, 269
Cycloserine, 227, **228**
  breast-feeding, 518
  capsules, 228
  renal failure, 505
Cyclospasmol, xiii
Cyclosporin, 319, **320**
  breast-feeding, 518
  infusion table, 527
  pregnancy, 512
Cyklokapron, 108
Cymevene, 240
Cyproheptadine, 128
  migraine, 184

Index 577

Cyprostat, 324
Cyproterone acetate, 274
  acne, 416, **418**
  breast-feeding, 518
  liver disease, 500
  male hypersexuality, 274
  malignant disease, 323, **324**
Cystic fibrosis, 59
  ACBS, 542
  acetylcysteine, 134
Cystinuria, 355
Cystitis, 298
  haemorrhagic, 313
  interstitial, 299
Cystrin, 298
Cytacon, 331
Cytamen, 331
Cytarabine, 315
  infusion table, 527
  preparations, 316
Cytomegalovirus infections, 239
Cytosar, 316
Cytotec, 34
Cytotoxic drugs, 310–25
  alopecia, 311
  bladder instillation, 299
  bone-marrow suppression, 311
  breast-feeding, 518
  CRM handling guidelines, 310
  dosage, 310
  extravasation, 310
  hypercalcaemia, 310
  hyperuricaemia, 310
  immunosuppressants, 319
  nausea and vomiting, 311
  pregnancy, 311, 512
  regimens, 310

Dacarbazine, 318
  infusion table, 527
Dactinomycin, 314
  infusion table, 527
Dakin's solution, 433
Daktacort, 406
Daktarin, 236
  skin, 426
Daktarin Oral Gel, 396
Dalacin C, 221–2
Dalacin T preparations, 416
Dalivit, 354
Dalmane, 140
Dalteparin, 103
Danazol, 282
  breast-feeding, 518
  pregnancy, 512
Dandruff, 421
  ACBS, 545
Daneral-SA, 129
Danol, 282
Dansac, 48, 51
Danthron, 41
Dantrium, 373
Dantrium Intravenous, 472
Dantrolene, 373
  liver disease, 500
  malignant hyperthermia, 472
  neuroleptic malignant syndrome, 146
Daonil, 256
Dapsone, 230
  breast-feeding, 518
  dermatitis herpetiformis, 230
  leprosy, 229
  malaria, 244
  poisoning, elimination, 17
  pregnancy, 512
  pyrimethamine with, see Maloprim
  tablets, 230
Daranide, 384
Daraprim, 244
Darier's disease, 413
Davenol, 136
Day Nurse, 176
DDAVP, 279
De Witt's analgesic pills, 176
Debrisan, 440
Debrisoquine, 85
  renal failure, 505
Decadron preparations, 266, 365
Deca-Durabolin, 275
Deca-Durabolin-100, 331
Declinax, 85
Decortisyl, 267
Defective medicines, 10
Dehydrocholic acid, 58, **59**
  liver disease, 500
Delfen foam, 295
Deltacortril Enteric, 265
Deltastab, 265, 366
Demecarium bromide, 382
Demeclocycline, 216
  hyponatraemia, 279
Dementia, 97
Demix, 217
Demser, 89
Demulcent cough preparations, 135
Dendritic ulcer, 379
De-Nol, 34
  renal failure, 505
De-Noltab, 34
  renal failure, 505
Dental caries prophylaxis, 348
Dental infections, 201
Dental Practitioners' Formulary, 556–7
Dental preparations, approved list, 556–7
Dental prophylaxis, 202
Dependence see Drug dependence
Depixol, 149, 154
Depixol Conc, 154
Depixol Low Volume, 154
Depo-Medrone, 267, 366
  with Lidocaine, 366
Deponit, 91
Depo-Provera,
  contraception, 294
  gynaecology, 272
  malignant disease, 322
Depostat, 322
Depression, 155
  antipsychotics, 146
  manic, 155
Dequacaine, 397
Dequadin, 396
Dequalinium, 396
Derbac-C, 428
Derbac-M, 429
Dermablend preparations, 421
Dermacare, Vaseline, 401
Dermacolor preparations, 421
Derma-gard, 57
Dermalex, 430
Dermatitis, ACBS, 545
Dermatitis herpetiformis, 230
  ACBS, 545
Dermatological preparations see Skin preparations
Dermatophyte infections, 234–7
Dermiflex, 440
Dermovate, 408
Dermovate-NN, 409
Deseril, 184
Desferal, 19
Desferrioxamine, 19
  eye, 386
  infusion table, 527
  iron overload, 333
  poisoning, 19
  pregnancy, 512
Desipramine, 158, **159**
Desloughing agents, 434
Desmopressin, 278
  nocturnal enuresis, 298
Desmospray, 279
Desogestrel [ingredient], 292
Desoxymethasone, 409
Destolit, 59
Detelco, 216
Dexamethasone, 263, 264, **266**
  eye, 379
  rheumatic disease, 365
  suppression test, 264
Dexamethasone sodium phosphate, 266
  infusion table, 527
Dexamphetamine, 165
Dexa-Rhinaspray, 393
Dexedrine, 165
Dexfenfluramine, 166
Dextran intravenous infusions, 341
Dextranomer, 440
Dextraven-110, 342
Dextrolyte, 336
Dextromethorphan, 135
Dextromoramide, 177, **179**

Dextropropoxyphene, 177, **180**
 breast-feeding, 518
 poisoning by, 18
 preparations, 180
  compound, 175
 renal failure, 505
Dextrose monohydrate, 339, 537
Dextrostix, 259
DF-118, 180
DHC Continus, 180
Diabetamide, 256
Diabetes insipidus, 278
 diagnosis, 278
Diabetes mellitus, 250–9
 diagnosis, 260
 monitoring
  meters, 259
  test strips, 259
Diabetic ketoacidosis, **257**, 338, 339
Diabetic neuropathy, 258
Diabinese, 256
Diabur Test 5000, 259
Dialamine, 535
Dialysis, ACBS, 542
Diamicron, 256
Diamorphine, 177, **180**
 breast-feeding, 519
 cough, 135
 pain, 177
  chronic, 12, 177
 preparations, 180
  linctus, 135
 prescribing for addicts, 9
Diamox preparations, 384
 Sustets, xiii
Dianette, 416, **418**
 pregnancy, 512
Diaphine, 180
Diaphragms, contraceptive, 296
Diarphen, 36
Diarrest, 36
Diarrhoea, 35, **336**
Diastix, 259
Diazemuls, 143, 190
 anaesthesia, 465
Diazepam, 142
 anaesthesia, 463, **464**
 anxiety, 142
 febrile convulsions, 192
 hypnotic, 139
 infusion table, 527
 muscle spasm, 373
 preparations, 143
 status epilepticus, 190
Diazoxide, 83
 hypertension, 83
 hypoglycaemia, 258
 pregnancy, 512
 preparations,
  injection, 83
  oral, 258
 renal failure, 505
Dibenyline, 86

Dicapen, 208
 infusion table, 525
 renal failure, 505
Dichloralphenazone, 141
Dichlorphenamide, 384
 diuretic, 69
 glaucoma, 384
Diclofenac, 358, **360**
 breast-feeding, 519
 gout, 369
 preparations, 360
  topical, 375
 ureteric colic, 298, **360**
Diclozip, 360
Dicobalt edetate, 20
Diconal, 180
 prescribing for addicts, 9
Dicyclomine, 28
Dicynene, 108
Didronel preparations, 280
Dienoestrol cream, 288
Diethylcarbamazine, 249
Diethylpropion, 166, **167**
 pregnancy, 512
Difflam cream, 375
Difflam oral rinse, 394
Difflam spray, 394
Diflucan, 236
Diflucortolone valerate, 409
Diflunisal, 175
 pain, 175
 preparations, 361
 renal failure, 505
 rheumatic disease, 358, **361**
Digibind, 62
Digitoxin, 61, **62**
 poisoning, elimination, 17
 preparations, 62
 renal failure, 505
Digoxin, 61
 breast-feeding, 519
 infusion table, 527
 poisoning, 17, **61**
 preparations, 62
 renal failure, 506
Digoxin-specific antibody fragments, 61, **62**
 infusion table, 527
Dihydergot, 183
Dihydrocodeine, 177, **180**
 preparations, 180
  compound, 175
 renal failure, 506
Dihydroergotamine, 182, **183**
Dihydropyridine calcium-channel blockers, 93
Dihydrotachysterol, 352, **353**
Dihydroxycholecalciferol, 352
Dijex, 24
Diloxanide furoate, 245
Diltiazem, 94
 breast-feeding, 519
 liver disease, 500
 preparations, 94
 see also Calcium-channel blockers
Dimenhydrinate, 168, **169**
Dimercaprol, 21

Dimethicone [antacid], 26
Dimethindene, 128
Dimethyl sulphoxide, 427
 interstitial cystitis, 299
Dimetriose, 282
Dimotane, 128
Dimotane Co preparations, 136
Dimotane Expectorant, 136
Dimotane LA, 128
Dimotane Plus preparations, 137
Dimotapp preparations, 137
Dimyril, 135
Dindevan, 105
Dinoprost, 285
Dinoprostone, 284–5
 infusion table, 527
Diocalm Junior, 336
Diocalm Ultra, 37
Dioctyl, 42
 ear, 391
Dioctyl sodium sulphosuccinate *see* Docusate sodium
Dioderm, 405
Dioralyte, 337
Diovol, 26
Dipentum, 39
Diphenhydramine, 128
Diphenoxylate, 36
 see also Analgesics, opioid
Diphenylbutylpiperidines, 146
Diphenylpyraline, 128
Diphosphonates *see* Bisphosphonates
Diphtheria, 203, 446
 antitoxin, 446, **447**
 prophylaxis, 202
 vaccination, 443
Diphtheria vaccine, 446
 for adults, 447
 tetanus, pertussis and, 446
 tetanus and, 446
Dipipanone, 177, **180**
 prescribing for addicts, 9
Dipivefrine, 383
Dipotassium clorazepate *see* Clorazepate
Dip/Ser, 447
Dip/Vac/Ads, 446
Dip/Vac/Ads for Adults, 447
Diprivan, 461
Diprobase, 401
Diprosalic, 408
Diprosone, 408
Dipyridamole, 105, **106**
 preparations, 106
Dirythmin SA, 72
Disaccharide intolerance, ACBS, 542
Disalcid, 358
Discontinued preparations, xiii
Disfiguring skin lesions, ACBS, 545
Disinfectants, 431–4
 ACBS, 545
Disipal, 196
Disodium cromoglycate *see* Sodium cromoglycate

Index 579

Disodium etidronate, 280
   infusion table, 527
   renal failure, 506
Disodium pamidronate, 280
   infusion table, 527
   renal failure, 508
Disopyramide, 71, **72**
   breast-feeding, 519
   infusion table, 527
   pregnancy, 512
   preparations, 72
   renal failure, 506
Disprin preparations, 176
Disprol preparations, 174, 176
Distaclor, 212
Distalgesic, 175
Distamine, 368
Distaquaine V-K tablets, 204
Distigmine, 372
   laxative, 41
   myasthenia gravis, 371
   pregnancy, 512
   urinary retention, 296, **297**
Disulfiram, 197
   pregnancy, 512
Dithranol, 412, **414**
   preparations, 414
Dithranol triacetate, 414
Dithrocream, 412, **414**
Dithrolan, 414
Ditropan, 298
Diumide-K Continus, 69
Diuresis, forced, 17
Diuretics, 63–9
   beta-blockers with, 76
   carbonic anhydrase inhibitors, 69
   loop, 65
      hypercalcaemia, 346
      liver disease, 501
   mercurial, 69
   osmotic, 69
   potassium and, 69, 335
   potassium-sparing, 66
      renal failure, 508
      with other diuretics, 68
   pregnancy, 512
   see also Thiazides
Diurexan, 65
Diverticular disease, 28, 38
Dixarit, 184
Doan's backache pills, 176
Dobutamine, 98
   infusion table, 527
Dobutrex solution, 98
Docusate sodium, 42
   ear, 391
   laxative, 41, **42**
Do-Do tablets, 122
Dolmatil, 152
Dolobid, 361
Doloxene, 180
Doloxene Compound, 174
Domette bandage, 435
Domical, 159

Domiphen [ingredient], 396
Domperidone, 169
   breast-feeding, 519
   gastro-intestinal, 30
   nausea, 168
   renal failure, 506
Donald Rose, 53
Dopacard, 100
Dopa-decarboxylase inhibitors, 192
Dopamet, 84
Dopamine, 98
   infusion table, 527
   preparations, 100
Dopaminergic drugs,
   endocrine, 281
   parkinsonism, 192
Dopexamine, 98, **100**
   infusion table, 527
Dopram, 132, 471
Dor, 54
Doralese, 86
Dormonoct, 140
Dose changes, xi
Doses, 2
   children, 11
   elderly, 14
   liver disease, 499–502
   renal impairment, 503–9
Dothapax, 160
Dothiepin, 158, **160**
Double Check, 295
Dovonex, 414
Dow Corning preparations, 54, 304
   Silastic catheter, 309
Doxapram, 131
   anaesthesia, 471
Doxazosin, 85
Doxepin, 158, **160**
Doxorubicin, 314
   bladder, 299
   infusion table, 528
   liver disease, 500
   preparations, 315
Doxycycline, 215, **216**
   preparations, 217
Doxylamine [ingredient], 176
Doxylar, 217
Dozic, 150
dp Cookies, 535
Dracontiasis, 249
Dramamine, 169
Drapolene, 430
Dressing pack, sterile, 438
   non-woven pads with, 438
Dressing packs, multiple, 435
Dressings, 435–41
Dribblet, 302
Driclor, 435
Dristan, 176
Drogenil, 324
Droleptan, 149, 465
Droperidol, 149
   anaesthesia, 465
Drug allergy, 126
Drug dependence, 7–9
   management, 197

Drug information services, xiv
Drug interactions, 476–98
   MAOIs, 162, 489
Dry mouth, 398
Dryaid, 303, 304
Dryptal, 66
DTIC-Dome, 318
DT/Vac/Ads, 446
DT/Vac/FT, 446
DTPer/Vac, 446
DTPer/Vac/Ads, 446
Dual block, 470
   diagnosis, 470
Dubam, 375
Ductus arteriosus,
   closure, 286
   patency, 286
Dulcolax, 41
Dumas Vault Cap, 296
Dumping syndrome, 257
Duocal, 535
Duofilm, 419
Duovent, 122
Duphalac, 44
Duphaston, 272
Durabolin, 275
Duracreme, 295
Duracel, 295
Durex diaphragms, 296
Duromine, 167
Dusting powders, 403
   definition, 399
Duvadilan, 287
Dyazide, 68
Dydrogesterone, 271, **272**
Dynese, 25
Dysentery, amoebic, 245
Dysentery, bacillary *see* Shigellosis
Dysman preparations, 363
Dysmenorrhoea, 173, 271
Dyspamet, 32
Dyspepsia, 24–31
Dysphagia, ACBS, 542
Dysport, 197
Dystonias, 195
   drug-induced, 195
Dytac, 67
Dytide, 68

E45 bath, 402
E45 cream, 401
E45 wash, 401
Eakin, 49, 52
Ear, 388–91
   infections, 388
   wax, removal, 390
Easifix, 435
Easychange, 49, 54
Ebufac, 359
EC-1 pouch, 50, 53
Eclampsia, 82
Econacort, 406
Econazole,
   anogenital, 289
   skin, 425, **426**
   vaginal, 289

Ecostatin,
 anogenital, 289
 skin, 426
Ecothiopate iodide, 382
Ectopic beats, 69
Eczederm, 403
Eczema, 411–12
 ACBS, 545
 ear, 388
Edecrin, 66
Edrophonium, 372
 anaesthesia, 471
 myasthenia gravis, 371, **372**
Eesiban, 436
Efalith, 422
Efamast, 415
Efcortelan cream, 405
Efcortelan ointment, 405
Efcortelan Soluble, 267
Efcortesol, 267
Effercitrate, 298
Effico, 355
Efudix, 316
Elantan preparations, 93
Elastic adhesive bandage, 436
 half-spread, 436
 ventilated, 436
Elastic adhesive dressing, 437
Elastic adhesive plaster, 437
Elastic web bandage, 436
 without foot loop, 436
Elasticated net surgical tubular stockinette, 435
Elasticated surgical tubular stockinette, 435
 foam padded, 435
Elasticated tubular bandage, 435
Elasticated viscose stockinette, 435
Elastoplast, 437
Elastoplast bandage, 436
Elastoweb, 436
Elavil, 159
Eldepryl, 195
Elderly,
 diuretics and, 63
 hypertension in, 82
 prescribing for, 14
Eldisine, 317
Electroconvulsive therapy, 157
Electrolade, 337
Electrolyte and water replacement,
 intravenous, 338–42
 oral, 334–8
Electrolyte infusions, usual strengths, 334
Electrolytes, infusion table, 528
Elemental-028, 535
Elkamol, 176
Elohes-6%, 342
Eltroxin, 260
Eludril aerosol spray, 397
Eludril mouthwash, 397
Elyzol, xiii
Emblon, 324
Emcor, 78

Emergency supply, 6
Emeside, 187
Emesis,
 drug-induced, 168
 in poisoning, 16
Emflex, 360
Eminase, 107
Emla, 474
Emmolate, 402
Emollients, 400–2
 eczema, 411
Emphysema, 113
Emulsiderm, 402
Emulsifying ointment, 400
Enalapril, 88
 breast-feeding, 519
 pregnancy, 512
 renal failure, 506
 see also ACE inhibitors
Enbucrilate, 430
Encephalopathy, hepatic, 44, 499
En-De-Kay preparations, 349
Endobulin, 455
Endocarditis, 200, 221
 prophylaxis, 202
Endometrial cancer, 321–2
Endometriosis, 271, 282
Endoxana, 313
Enduron, 65
Ener-G, 535
Energy, intravenous nutrition, 342
Enflurane, 461, **462**
Engerix B, 448
Enoxacin, 231, **232**
 breast-feeding, 519
 renal failure, 506
 see also 4-Quinolones
Enoxaparin, 103
Enoximone, 62
 infusion table, 528
Enrich, 535
Ensure preparations, 535–6
Entamizole, 245
Entamoeba histolytica, 245
Enteric infections, 200, 220
Enterobiasis, 247
Entonox, 462
Enuresis, nocturnal, 298
Enzyme induction, 476
Enzymes,
 eye, 386
 fibrinolytic, 106
 ulcers, 434
EP, 176
Epanutin preparations, 188
 Ready Mixed Parenteral, 192
Ephedrine, 118
 anaesthesia, 101
 breast-feeding, 519
 bronchospasm, 118
 diabetic neuropathy, 259
 nocturnal enuresis, 298
 preparations, 118
  injection, 101
  nasal drops, 393
 renal failure, 506

Ephynal, 353
Epifoam, 406
Epifrin, 383
Epiglottitis, 200, 222
Epilepsy, 185–92
 driving, 185
 ketogenic diet, ACBS, 542
 pregnancy, 185
 status, 190
Epilim, 189
Epirubicin, 314, **315**
 infusion table, 528
 liver disease, 500
Epoetin, 332
Epogam preparations, 415
Epoprostenol, 104
 infusion table, 528
Eppy, 383
Eprex, 332
Epsom salts, 44
Equagesic, 174
Equanil, 145
Eradacin, 232
Ergocalciferol, 352
Ergometrine, 284, **285**
 preparations, 285
 tablets, xiii
Ergotamine, 182, **183**
 breast-feeding, 519
 liver disease, 500
 pregnancy, 512
 renal failure, 506
Ervevax, 452
Erwinase, 318
Erycen, 220
Erymax, 220
Erysipelas, 201
Erythrocin, 220
Erythromid preparations, 220–1
Erythromycin, **220**, 233
 acne, 416
 breast-feeding, 519
 Campylobacter infections, 35
 ear, 390
 infusion table, 528
 liver disease, 500
 preparations, 220
  topical, 416–17
 renal failure, 506
Erythroped preparations, 220–1
Erythropoietin, 332
Eschmann Folatex, 309
Eschmann Folatex S, 309
Eserine, 382
Esidrex, 64
Eskamel, 417
Eskornade, 137
Esmolol, xii
Estracombi, 270
Estracyt, 313
Estraderm TTS, 269
Estradurin, 321
Estragest TTS, 270
Estramustine, 312, **313**
Estrapak, 270
Estropipate, 271

Ete, 439
Ethacrynic acid, 65, **66**
　　infusion table, 528
　　renal failure, 506
Ethambutol, 226, 227, **228**
　　breast-feeding, 519
　　renal failure, 506
Ethamivan, 132
Ethamsylate, 108
　　breast-feeding, 519
Ethanol, 342
　　infusion table, 528
　　see also Alcohol
Ethanolamine oleate, 112
Ethinyloestradiol, 268
　　acne, 416
　　contraception, 292–3
　　malignant disease, 321
　　tablets, 269
Ethionamide, 229
　　pregnancy, 512
Ethoheptazine [ingredient], 174
Ethosuximide, 186
　　breast-feeding, 519
　　pregnancy, 512
Ethynodiol diacetate [ingredient], 292
Etidronate disodium, 280
　　infusion table, 527
　　renal failure, 506
Etodolac, 359, **361**
Etomidate, 459, **460**
Etoposide, 317
　　infusion table, 528
　　renal failure, 506
Etretinate, 412, **415**
　　breast-feeding, 519
　　liver disease, 500
　　pregnancy, 512
　　renal failure, 506
Eudemine injection, 83
Eudemine [oral], 258
Euglucon, 256
Eugynon-30, 292
Eumovate, 409
　　eye, 379
Eumovate-N, 379
Eurax, 403
Eurax-Hydrocortisone, 406
Eusol, 432
Evadyne, 159
Evening primrose oil, gamolenic acid in, 415
ExacTech,
　　meter, 259
　　test strips, 259
Exelderm, 427
Exfoliative dermatitis, 264
Exirel, 117
Exolan, 414
Exosurf Neonatal, 132
Expectorants, 135
Expelix, 248
Expulin, 136
Expurhin, 137
Extension plaster, 436
Exterol, 391

Extrapyramidal symptoms,
　　antipsychotics and, 146
　　treatment, 195
Eye, 376–87
　　preparations,
　　　　antibacterial, 377–8
　　　　antifungal, 378
　　　　anti-infective, 376–9
　　　　anti-inflammatory, 379–81
　　　　antiviral, 379
　　　　corticosteroid, 379–80
　　　　cycloplegics, 381
　　　　effects on contact lenses, 387
　　　　glaucoma, 382
　　　　microbial contamination, 376
　　　　miotics, 382
　　　　mydriatics, 381
Eye lotions, 376
Eye ointments, 376
Eye-drops, 376

Fabahistin, 129
Fabrol, 134
Factor VIII fraction, 108
Factor VIII inhibitor bypassing fraction, 108
Factor IX fraction, 108
Faecal softeners, 43
Famotidine, 31, **32**
　　breast-feeding, 519
　　renal failure, 506
Fanalgic, 176
Fansidar, 241, **244**
　　breast-feeding, 519
　　pregnancy, 513
Farlutal, 322
Fasigyn, 231
Fat emulsions, intravenous, 342, 522
Faverin, 164
Febrile convulsions, 192
Fectrim preparations, 225
Fefol, 328
Fefol Z, 329
Fefol-Vit, 329
Feiba Immuno, 108
Felbinac *(Traxam)*, 375
Feldene preparations, 364
　　gel, 375
Felodipine, 94
　　liver disease, 500
Felypressin, 475
Femeron, 289
Femigraine, 176
Feminax, 176
Femodene, 292
Femodene ED, 292
Femulen, 294
Fenbid, 360
Fenbufen, 358, **361**
　　breast-feeding, 519
Fenfluramine, 166, **167**
Fennings preparations, 176

Fenofibrate, 109, **110**
　　pregnancy, 513
　　renal failure, 506
Fenoprofen,
　　analgesia, 175
　　breast-feeding, 519
　　rheumatic disease, 358, **361**
Fenopron preparations, 361
Fenostil Retard, 128
Fenoterol, 113, **117**
Fentanyl, 466, **467**
　　preparations, 467
Fentazin, 151
Feospan, 327
Ferfolic SV, 328
Fergon, 327
Ferric salts, 326
Ferrocap, 327
Ferrocap-F-350, 328
Ferrocontin Continus, 327
Ferrocontin Folic Continus, 328
Ferrograd, 327
Ferrograd C, 329
Ferrograd Folic, 328
Ferromyn, 328
Ferrous fumarate, 327
Ferrous gluconate, 327
Ferrous glycine sulphate, 327
Ferrous salts, 326
Ferrous succinate, 327
Ferrous sulphate, 326, **327**
　　preparations, 327
　　　　compound tablets, 329
Fersaday, 327
Fersamal, 327
Fertility,
　　female, 275, 277
　　male, 276
Fertility thermometer, 296
Fertiral, 277
Fesovit preparations, 329
Fibracol, 440
Fibrinolytic drugs, 106
Fibrosing alveolitis, 132
Filaricides, 249
Filgrastim, 334
　　infusion table, 528
Finasteride, xii
First Choice, 301
Fish oils, hyperlipidaemia, 111
Fissure, anal, 46
Fits *see* Epilepsy
Flagyl preparations, 231
Flamazine, 424
Flavouring, ACBS, 542
Flavoxate, 297
Flaxedil, 470
Flecainide, 71, **72**
　　infusion table, 528
　　liver disease, 500
　　pregnancy, 513
　　renal failure, 506
Flemoxin Solutab, 207
Fletchers' enemas, 43–4
　　Enemette, 42
Flexible collodion, 430

582 Index

Flexical, 536
Flexin Continus preparations, 362
Flexipore-6000, 439
Flexoplast, 436, 437
Flixonase, 392
Flolan, 104
Florinef, 262
Floxapen, 205
Flu-Amp, 209
Fluanxol, 164
Fluclomix, 205
Fluclorolone acetonide, 409
Flucloxacillin, 204, **205**
　ampicillin with, 206, **208**
　ear, 388
　infusion table, 528
　preparations, 205
Fluconazole, 235
　pregnancy, 513
　renal failure, 506
Flucytosine, 235, **236**
　pregnancy, 513
　renal failure, 506
Fludrocortisone, 262
　diabetic neuropathy, 259
Fluid and electrolyte replacement, 334–42
Fluid overload, liver disease, 499
Flumazenil, 19, 471
　infusion table, 528
Flunisolide, 392
Flunitrazepam, 139, **140**
Fluocinolone acetonide, 409
Fluocinonide, 410
Fluocortolone, 410
Fluor-a-day, 348
Fluorescein, 386
Fluoride, 348
　preparations, 349
Fluorigard preparations, 349
Fluorometholone, 380
Fluorouracil, 315, **316**
　infusion table, 528
　preparations, 316
Fluothane, 462
Fluoxetine, 164
　breast-feeding, 519
　renal failure, 506
Flupenthixol, 163
　depot injections, 154
　depression, 157, **164**
　psychoses, 147, **149**, 154
　tablets,
　　depression, 164
　　psychoses, 149
Flupenthixol decanoate, 154
Fluphenazine, 147, **149**, **154**
　depot injections, 154
　tablets, 149
Fluphenazine decanoate, 154
Flurandrenolone, 410
Flurazepam, 139, **140**
Flurbiprofen, 361
　breast-feeding, 519
　diabetic neuropathy, 259

Flurbiprofen (*continued*)—
　eye, 386
　rheumatic disease, 358, **361**
Flurex preparations, 176
Fluspirilene, 154
Flutamide, 323, **324**
Fluticasone, 392
Fluvirin, 448
Fluvoxamine, 164
　breast-feeding, 519
　renal failure, 506
Fluzone, 448
FML, 380
FML-Neo, 380
Foam dressings, 440
Folate deficiency, 330
Folate rescue, 316
Folex-350, 328
Foley catheter, 309
Folic acid, 330, **331**
　preparations, 331
　iron and, 328
Folicin, 329
Folinic acid, 316
　infusion table, 528
Folinic acid rescue, 316
Follicle-stimulating hormone, 276
Fomac, 29
Foods for special diets, 345
　ACBS, 534–42
　vitamin supplements, 354
Forced diuresis, alkaline, 17
Forceval, 354
Forceval Protein, 536
Forest Breeze, 54
Formaldehyde, 419
　preparations, 419
Formula S, 539
Formulary, Dental, 556–7
Fortagesic, 175
Fortical, 536
Fortimel, 536
Fortipudding, 536
Fortisip, 536
Fortison, 539
Fortral, 181
Fortum, 213
Foscarnet, 239, **240**
　infusion table, 528
　pregnancy, 513
　renal failure, 506
Foscavir, 240
Fosfestrol, 321
Fosinopril, 88
　pregnancy, 513
　renal failure, 506
　see also ACE inhibitors
Fragmin, 103
Framycetin,
　ear [ingredient], 390
　eye, 377
　skin, 423
　　dressing, 439
Franol preparations, 122
Franolyn Expect, 122
FreAmine-III preparations, 343
Fresenius OPD, 536

Fresh frozen plasma, 109
'Freshly prepared', 2
Fresubin preparations, 536–7
Frisium, 143
Froben preparations, 361
Fructose, 342, 537
Frumax, 66
Frumil preparations, 68
Frusemide, 65
　breast-feeding, 519
　infusion table, 528
　preparations, 66
　renal failure, 506
Frusene, 68
FSH, 276
Fucibet, 408
Fucidin, 222
　skin, 424
Fucidin H, 406
Fucidin Intertulle, 439
Fucithalmic, 377
Fulcin, 236
Full Marks preparations, 430
Fuller's earth, 21
Fungal infections, 234–9
　anogenital, 288
　eye, 378
　oral, 395
　skin, 425
Fungilin, 235
　mouth, 396
Fungizone, 235
Furadantin, 234
Furamide, 245
Fusafungine [ingredient], 396
Fusidic acid, 222
　eye, 377
　infusion table, 528
　liver disease, 500
　preparations, 222
　　eye, 377
　　skin, 424, 439
　skin, 424
Fybogel, 40
　renal failure, 506
Fybranta, 40
Fynnon, 176

Galactokinase deficiency, 542
Galactomin, 537
Galactorrhoea, 281
Galactosaemia, ACBS, 542
Galactose intolerance, ACBS, 542
Galake, 175
Galcodine, 134–5
Galenamet, 32
Galenamox, 206
Galenphol, 135
Galfer, 327
Galfer FA, 328
Galfloxin, 205
Gallamine, 469, **470**
　renal failure, 506
Gallstones, 58
Galpseud, 137
Gamanil, 160

Gamimune-N, 455
Gamma benzene hexachloride *see* Lindane
Gamma globulin, 454
Gammabulin, 455
Gamolenic acid, 415
   breast pain, 283, 415
   eczema, 412, **415**
Ganciclovir, 239
   breast-feeding, 519
   infusion table, 529
   pregnancy, 513
   renal failure, 506
Ganda, 383
Ganglion-blocking drugs, 89
Garamycin,
   ear, 389
   eye, 377
Gardenal Sodium, 187
Gardnerella vaginalis, 230
Gargles, 397
Gas cylinders, 458
Gas-gangrene, 203
   prophylaxis, 202
Gastrectomy,
   ACBS, 542
   iron therapy, 326
   vitamin B_{12}, 330
Gastric emptying, poisoning and, 16
Gastrils, 24
Gastrobid Continus, 170
Gastrocote, 26
Gastro-enteritis, 35, 200
Gastroflux, 170
Gastro-intestinal system, 24–59
   electrolytes, 334
Gastromax, 171
Gastron, 26
Gastrozepin, 33
Gauze, cotton ribbon, absorbent, 438
   viscose and, 438
Gauze and cellulose wadding tissue, 438
Gauze and cotton tissue, 438
Gauze swabs, 438
   filmated, 438
Gaviscon, 26
   infant, 26
   liver disease, 499
   renal failure, 506
G-CSF, 334
Geangin, 96
Gee's linctus, 136
Gel dressings, 439
Gelatin infusion, 341, **342**
Gelcosal, 413
Gelcotar gel, 413
Gelcotar liquid, 422
Geliperm, 440
Gelofusine, 342
Gelusil, 24
Gemeprost, 284, **285**
Gemfibrozil, 109, **110**
   liver disease, 500
   renal failure, 506
Generaid, 537

General anaesthesia *see* Anaesthesia, general
Generic prescribing, 2
Genisol, 422
Genotropin preparations, 277
Gentamicin, 218
   ear, 389
   eye, 377
   infusion table, 529
   injections, 218–9
   skin, 424
Gentian mixture, acid, 355
Gentian mixture, alkaline, 355
Gentian violet *see* Crystal violet
Genticin, 219
   ear, 389
   eye, 377
   skin, 425
Genticin HC, 406
Gentisone HC, 389, 406
Gentran preparations, 341
German measles *see* Rubella
Gestanin, 272
Gestodene [ingredient], 292
Gestone, 272
Gestrinone, 282
   pregnancy, 513
Gestronol, 322
Giardia lamblia, 246
Giardiasis, 246
Gilles de la Tourette syndrome *see* Tourette syndrome
Givitol, 329
Glandosane, 398
Glaucoma, 382–4
   steroid, 379
Glibenclamide, 255, **256**
   preparations, 256
   renal failure, 506
Glibenese, 256
Gliclazide, 255, **256**
   renal failure, 506
Glipizide, 256
   renal failure, 506
Gliquidone, 256
   renal failure, 506
Glomerular filtration rate, dosage and, 503
Glucagon, 258
   injection, 258
Glucocorticoids,
   equivalent doses, 262
   replacement therapy, 262
Glucolet, 255
Gluco-lyte, 337
Glucometer, 259
Glucophage, 257
Glucoplex preparations, 343
Glucose, 339
   hypoglycaemia, 258
   infusion, 339
      potassium chloride and, 339
      sodium chloride and, 338
   intravenous nutrition, 342
   oral rehydration, 336
   special diets, 537

Glucose (*continued*)—
   tests, 259–60
      tolerance, 260
Glucose intolerance, ACBS, 542
Glucose 6-phosphate dehydrogenase deficiency, 333
   see also G6PD
Glucostix, 259
Glue ear, 390
Glurenorm, 256
Glutafin, 537
Glutamic acid hydrochloride, 59
Glutaraldehyde, 419
Glutaric aciduria, ACBS, 542
Glutarol, 419
Gluten, presence of, 2
Gluten enteropathy, ACBS, 542
Gluten-free biscuits, 536, 537
Gluten-free products, ACBS, 542–3
Glycavent, 125
Glycerin suppositories, 42
Glycerin thymol compound mouthwash, 394, 397, **398**
Glycerol,
   glaucoma, 384
   suppositories, 41, **42**
Glyceryl trinitrate, 90
   infusion table, 529
   preparations, 90–1
Glycine irrigation solution, 299–300
Glycogen storage disease, ACBS, 543
Glycopeptide antibiotics, 223
Glycopyrronium, 462, **463**
Glykola, xiii
Glypressin, 279
Glytrin Spray, 91
Goitre, 260
Gold, 366, **367**
   breast-feeding, 519
   liver disease, 500
   pregnancy, 513
   renal failure, 506
Golfer's elbow, 365
Golytely, xiii
Gonadorelin, 277
Gonadotraphon LH, 276
Gonadotrophin, chorionic, 276
Gonadotrophin-releasing hormone, 277
   malignant disease, 323
Gonadotrophins, 276
Gonorrhoea, 201, 203, 222
Goserelin, 323, **324**
   endometriosis, 282
   malignant disease, 324
Gout, 369–71
G6PD deficiency, 333
   drugs to be avoided in, 333
Gramicidin [ingredient], 378, 390
Gramoxone, poisoning by, 21
Grand mal, 185

584 Index

Graneodin, 424
Granisetron, 168, **169**
    infusion table, 529
Granuflex, 440
Granulocyte colony stimulating factor, 334
Gregoderm, 406
Griseofulvin, 235, **236**
    pregnancy, 513
    preparations, 236
Grisovin, 236
Growth failure, ACBS, 543
Growth hormone, 276, **277**
    pregnancy, 513
GTN 300 mcg, 91
Guanethidine, 84
    eye, 383
    hypertension, 85
    pregnancy, 513
    renal failure, 506
Guanor Expectorant, 136
Guar gum, 257
Guardian, 49, 52, 301
Guarem, 257
Guarina, 257
Guinea worm infections, 249
Gynatren, xiii
Gyno-Daktarin preparations, 289
Gynol-II, 295
Gyno-Pevaryl preparations, 289

HA-1A, 456
    infusion table, 529
Haelan, 410
Haelan-C, 410–11
Haemaccel, 342
Haemodialysis, 17
    ACBS, 543
Haemolytic anaemia, 331
    G6PD deficiency, 333
Haemolytic disease of newborn, prevention, 456
Haemoperfusion, 17
Haemophilia, 108
    mild to moderate, 278
Haemophilus influenzae type b (Hib), 447
    prophylaxis, 202
    vaccination, 443
    vaccine, 447
Haemorrhage, 108
    abortion, 284
    gastro-intestinal, 31
    postpartum, 284
Haemorrhoids, 45–7
Haemostatics, 107
Hainsworth, 50, 53
Halciderm Topical, 411
Halcinonide, 411
Halcion, xiii
Haldol, 150
Haldol Decanoate, 154
Haleraid, 122
Half Securon SR, xii
Halfan, 243

Half-Inderal LA, 77
Halibut-liver oil capsules, 350
Halofantrine, 241, **243**
    breast-feeding, 519
    pregnancy, 513
Haloperidol, 149, 154
    hiccup, 147
    movement disorders, 197
    preparations, 149–50
        depot, 154
    psychoses, 147, **149**, **154**
    terminal care, 13
Haloperidol decanoate, 154
Halothane, 461, **462**
Halycitrol, 350
Hamamelis, 45
    suppositories, zinc oxide and, 46
Hamarin, 370
Hansen's disease, 229
Harmogen, 271
Hartmann's solution *see* Sodium lactate intravenous infusion, compound
Havrix, 447
Hay fever, 126, 391
Haymine, 137
HBIG, 455
HCG, 276
Head lice, 428
Headache, 173
    migraine, 182
Heaf test, 445
Healonid, 386
Heart failure,
    ACE inhibitors, 87
    cardiac glycosides, 61
    diuretics, 63
    vasodilators, 90
Heart *see also* Cardiac
Hedex preparations, 176
Height–weight charts, 11
Helicobacter pylori, 31, 32
Helminth infections, 247–9
Hemabate, 284
Heminevrin, 141
    infusion, 191, 464
Hepanutrin, 343
Heparin, 102
    breast-feeding, 519
    infusion table, 529
    low molecular weight, 102, 103
    pregnancy, 510
Heparin preparations, 102–3
    flushes, 103
Heparinoid [ingredient], 46, 375, 441
Hepatic encephalopathy, 44, 218, 499
Hepatic-Aid II, 537
Hepatic *see also* Liver
Hepatitis,
    chronic active, 264, 355
    infectious, 454

Hepatitis A, 447
    international travel, 457
    normal immunoglobulin, 454
    vaccination, 443
    vaccine, 447
Hepatitis B, 447, 455
    high-risk groups, 448
    specific immunoglobulin, 455–6
    vaccination, 443
    vaccine, 447
Hepatolenticular degeneration *see* Wilson's disease
Hepatotoxicity, 499
Hep-Flush, 103
HeplexAmine, 343
Heplok, 103
Hepsal, 103
Hereditary angioedema *see* Angioedema, hereditary
Heritage Cohesive/Sheath, 303
Heritage extension tube, 306
Heritage leg bag, 304
Heritage sheath collar pack, 304
Heroin *see* Diamorphine
Herpes infections, 238
    eye, 379
    genital, 290
    immunoglobulin, 455, 456
    mouth, 396
    skin, 427
Herpid, 427
Hespan, 342
Hetastarch, 341, **342**
Hetrazan, 249
Hewletts cream, 401
Hexachlorophane, 431, **433**
Hexamine, 233, **234**
    renal failure, 506
Hexetidine, 397
Hexopal, 97
HGH, 277
Hib, 447
Hibidil, xiii
Hibiscrub, 431
Hibisol, 431
Hibitane preparations, 431–2
Hiccup, 147, 197
Hioxyl, 434
Hiprex, 234
Hirsutism, 274, 416
Hirudoid, 441
Hismanal, 127
Histalix, 136
Histamine H$_1$-antagonists, 126
Histamine H$_2$-antagonists, 31
Histidinaemia, ACBS, 543
Histoacryl, 430
Histofreezer, 420
Histryl, 128
HIV infections, 239
HNIG, 454
Hodgkin's disease, 312, 318–19
HolliGard, 49
Homatropine, 381
    eye-drops, 381
        cocaine and, 385

Index 585

Homocystinuria, ACBS, 543
Honvan, 321
Hookworm infections, 248
Hormone antagonists,
 hypersexuality, 274
 malignant disease, 322
Hormone replacement,
 androgens, 273
 oestrogens, 267
  vaginal, 288
 progestogens, 268
Hormonin, 269
Hosiery, elastic, 441
HRF, 277
HRT, 267
HTIG, 455
Human Actraphane 30/70, 254
Human Actrapid, 252
Human Actrapid Penfill, 252
Human antihaemophilic
 fraction, 108
Human Factor IX fraction, 108
Human Initard 50/50, 254
Human Insulatard, 253
Human Mixtard 30/70, 254
Human Monotard, 252
Human Protaphane, 253
Human Protaphane Penfill, 253
Human Ultratard, 253
Human Velosulin, 252
Humatrope, 277
Humegon, 276
Humiderm, 401
Humotet, 456
Humulin I, 253
Humulin Lente, 252
Humulin M preparations, 254
Humulin S, 252
Humulin Zn, 253
Huntington's chorea, 197
Hyalase, 374
Hyaluronidase, 374
 [ingredient], 441
Hyate C, 108
Hycal, 537
Hydergine, 97
Hydralazine, 83
 infusion table, 529
 pregnancy, 513
 renal failure, 506
Hydrea, 318
Hydrenox, 64
Hydrocal, 406
Hydrochlorothiazide, 64
Hydrocolloid dressings, 440
Hydrocortisone, 264, **266**
 colitis, 39
 haemorrhoids, 46
 preparations, 266
  eye, 380
  mouth, 395
  rectal, 39
  rectal (compound), 46–7
  skin, 405–7
  skin, miconazole and, 406
 proctitis, 39

Hydrocortisone (*continued*)—
 replacement therapy, 262
 skin, 405
Hydrocortisone acetate,
 eye, 380
 rheumatic disease, 365
Hydrocortisone butyrate, 407
Hydrocortisone sodium phosphate, 267
 infusion table, 529
Hydrocortisone sodium succinate, 267
 infusion table, 529
Hydrocortistab, 266, 366
 skin, 405
Hydrocortisyl cream, 405
Hydrocortisyl ointment, 405
Hydrocortone, 266
Hydroflumethiazide, 64
Hydrogel dressings, 439
Hydrogen peroxide, 434
 mouthwash, 397
 solutions, 434
Hydromet, 84
Hydromol, 401
Hydromol Emollient, 402
HydroSaluric, 64
Hydrotalcite, 24, **25**
 preparations, 25
Hydrous ointment, 400
Hydroxocobalamin, 330
 injection, 331
Hydroxyapatite (*Ossopan*), 346
Hydroxychloroquine, 366, **368**
 breast-feeding, 519
 pregnancy, 513
 renal failure, 506
Hydroxycholecalciferol, 352
Hydroxyethylcellulose, 385
Hydroxyprogesterone, 271, **272**
Hydroxyquinoline [ingredient], 406
Hydroxyurea, 318
Hydroxyzine, 129
Hygroton, 64
Hygroton-K, 69
Hyoscine butylbromide, 28
Hyoscine hydrobromide,
 breast-feeding, 519
 eye, 381
 nausea and vertigo, 167, **170**
 premedication, 462, **463**
Hypal-2, 437
Hyperactive children, 165
Hyperaldosteronism, 283
Hypercal, xiii
Hypercalcaemia, 279, 310, 314, **346**
Hypercholesterolaemia, 109
 ACBS, 543
Hyperdrol, xiii
Hyperglycaemia, 250–7
 coma, 257
Hyperhidrosis, 434
Hyperkalaemia, 336, 339, 346

Hyperkeratosis, 412
Hyperlipidaemia, 109
Hyperlipoproteinaemia,
 ACBS, 543
Hyperlysinaemia, ACBS, 543
Hypermethioninaemia, ACBS, 543
Hyperphosphataemia, 348
Hypersensitivity *see* Allergy
Hypersexuality, 274
Hypertane-50, 68
Hypertension, 63, 76, **81**, 87, 93
 crisis, 82
 elderly, 82
 malignant, 82
 pregnancy, 82
 pulmonary, 133
 systolic, 82
Hyperthyroidism *see* Thyrotoxicosis
Hyperuricaemia, 310, 370
Hypnomidate, 460
Hypnotics, 139–42
 liver disease, 499
 poisoning by, 19
 pregnancy, 511
 renal failure, 504
 withdrawal, 138
Hypnovel, 465
Hypocalcaemia, 346
Hypochlorhydria, 59
Hypochlorite, 433
Hypocount meters, 259
Hypodermic equipment,
 insulin, 254
Hypodermoclysis, 374
Hypogammaglobulinaemia, 455
Hypoglycaemia, 251, 258
 ACBS, 543
 acute, 258
 chronic, 258
Hypogonadism, 267, 273
Hypoguard test strips, 259
Hypokalaemia, 339
 diuretics and, 63
Hypomagnesaemia, 347
Hypoparathyroidism, 346, 352
Hypophysectomy, 262
Hypopituitarism, 262, 273, 276
Hypoproteinaemia
 ACBS, 543
 liver disease, 499
Hyposensitisation, 130
Hypotears, 386
Hypotension
 controlled, 458
 poisoning and, 16
 sympathomimetics, 101
Hypothalamic hormones, 277
Hypothermia,
 antipsychotics and, 146
 poisoning and, 16
Hypothyroidism, 260
 neonatal, 260
Hypovase, 86
Hypovolaemia, 340–2
Hypoxaemia, 132

586 Index

Hypromellose, 385
  eye-drops, 385
Hypurin Isophane, 253
Hypurin Lente, 252
Hypurin Neutral, 252
Hypurin Protamine Zinc, 253
Hysterectomy, antibacterial prophylaxis, 203
Hytrin, 86

Ibrufhalal, 359
Ibugel, 375
Ibular, 359
Ibuleve, 375
Ibuprofen, 359
  analgesia, 175
  breast-feeding, 519
  fever in children, 175
  preparations, 359–60
    Junifen, 175
    topical, 375
  rheumatic disease, 358, **359**
Ichthammol, 412, **414**
  preparations, 414
Ichthopaste, 437
Ichthyosis, 400
Icthaband, 437
Idarubicin, 314, **315**
  infusion table, 529
  liver disease, 500
  renal failure, 507
Idoxene, 379
Idoxuridine, 238
  breast-feeding, 519
  eye, 379
  mouth, 396
  pregnancy, 513
  skin, 427
Iduridin, 428
Ifosfamide, 312, **313**
  infusion table, 529
  renal failure, 507
Ileo-B, 51
Ileodress, 51
Ileostomy products, 50–8
Ilosone, 221
Ilube, 385
Imbrilon preparations, 362
Imdur, 93
Imferon, 330
Imidazole antifungal drugs, 234
Imigran preparations, 183
Imipenem, 214, **215**
Imipenem/cilastatin, infusion table, 529
Imipramine, 158, **160**
Immravax, 449
Immunisation, 442
  international travel, 457
  programmes, 443
Immunity,
  active, 442
  passive, 444
Immunodeficiency, 455
  syndrome, acquired, 239

Immunoglobulins, 444, **454–6**
  anti-D (Rh$_0$), 456
  antilymphocyte, 319
  hepatitis B, 455–6
  normal, 454–5
  rabies, 455–6
  tetanus, 455–6
  varicella-zoster, 455–6
Immunoprin, 319
Immunostimulants, 320
Immunosuppressants,
  malignant disease, 319
  myasthenia gravis, 372
  rheumatic disease, 366, **369**
Imodium, 37
Imperacin, 217
Impetigo, 201, 423
  scalp, 422
Impotence, 273, **300**
Imunovir, 238
Imuran, 319
Inadine, 439
Incontiaid leg bag, 304
Incontiaid sheath, 303
Incontiaid sheath holder, 304
Incontinence, urinary, 297
Indapamide, 63, **64**
Indaxa, 64
Inderal preparations, 77
Inderetic, 77
Inderex, 77
Indian hemp *see* Cannabis
Indocid preparations, 362
  PDA, 286
Indolar SR, 362
Indomax preparations, 362
Indomethacin, 361
  breast-feeding, 519
  ductus closure, 286
  gout, 369
  preparations, 362
    injection, 286
  rheumatic disease, 359, **361**
Indomod, 362
Indoramin, 85
  urinary tract, **86**, 297
Infacol, 27
Infant Gaviscon see Gaviscon
Infections,
  amoebic, 245
  antisera, 444
  bladder, 234
    mycotic, 299
  ear, 388
  eye, 376–9
  fungal, 234–7
  helminth, 247–9
  immunoglobulins, 444
  nail, fungal, 235–7
  oropharyngeal, 395
  protozoal, 240–7
  skin, 423
  trichomonal, 245
  vaccines, 442
  vaginal, 288
  viral, 237–40
  vulval, 288

Infertility,
  female, 275, 277
  male, 276
Inflammatory bowel disease, ACBS, 543
Inflammatory diseases,
  corticosteroids, 264
    local injections, 365
  rheumatic, 357–69
Influenza,
  prophylaxis, 238
  vaccination, 443
Influenza vaccines, 448
  split virion, 448
  surface antigen, 448
Influvac Sub-unit, 448
Information services,
  drugs, xiv
  poisons, 15
Inhalations, 134
  aromatic, 134
  steam, 133, 392
Inhaler devices, 122
Initard 50/50, 254
Initard 50/50, Human, 254
Innovace, 88
Innozide, 88
Inosine pranobex, 238
  renal failure, 507
Inositol, 350
Inositol nicotinate, 97
Inotropic drugs, positive, 61, 98
Inoven, 359
Insect stings, 22, 126
Insecticides, poisoning by, 22
Insomnia, 139
Instillagel, 474
Insulatard, 253
Insulatard, Human, 253
Insulin, 250–4
  biphasic, 252, **253**
    isophane, 252, **253**
  breast-feeding, 519
  human, 251
  infusion table, 529
  isophane, 252, **253**
    biphasic, 252, **253**
    NPH, 253
    protamine, 253
  neutral, 251
  protamine zinc, 252, 253
  renal failure, 507
  soluble, 251
  subcutaneous infusion, 250
  zinc suspension, 252
    amorphous, 252
    crystalline, 253
    mixed, 252
Insulin injection equipment, 254
Intal preparations, 125–6
Integrin, 150
Interactions, 476–98
  MAOIs, 162, 489
Interferons, 320
  pregnancy, 513

Index 587

International travel, immunisation for, 457
Intersurgical 005 mask, 133
Intersurgical 010 mask, 133
Intralgin, 375
Intralipid preparations, 343
Intrasite, 440
Intra-uterine devices, 295
Intraval Sodium, 460
Intravenous infusions, 338–45
   addition to, 522–33
Intravenous nutrition, 342–5
Intron A, 320
Intropin, 100
Iodides, pregnancy, 513
Iodine, 261
   breast-feeding, 519
   pregnancy, 513
   preparations,
      oral solution, 261
      skin, 433
   radioactive, 261
      breast-feeding, 519
      pregnancy, 513
Iodoflex paste, 440
Iodosorb preparations, 440
Ionamin, 167
Ionax Scrub, 416
Ionil T, 422
Ipecacuanha,
   and morphine mixture, 136
   emetic mixture, paediatric, 17
Ipral, 226
Ipratropium, 119
   asthma, 118
   rhinorrhoea, 392, **393**
Iprindole, 158, **161**
Iridocyclitis, 381
Iron,
   deficiency, 326
   overload, 333
   poisoning by, 19
   preparations, 327–30
      compound, 329
      folic acid and, 328
      infusion table, 529
      iron dextran, 329, **330**
      iron sorbitol, 329, **330**
      modified-release, 326
   therapy,
      oral, 326–9
      parenteral, 329
Irritable bowel syndrome, 28, 37
Ischaemic attacks, 104
Ischaemic disease of limbs, 341
Isib, 92
Island dressings, 437
Ismelin, 85
   eye-drops, 383
Ismo preparations, 93
Isoaminile citrate, 135
Isoaminile linctus, 135
Isocarboxazid, 162, **163**
Isoconazole, 289
Isoflurane, 461, **462**
Isogel, 40

Isoket injection, 92
Isoket Retard, 92
Isomaltose intolerance, ACBS, 543
Isometheptene mucate, 183
Isomide preparations, 72
Isomil, 537
Isoniazid, 226, 227, **228**
   breast-feeding, 519
   liver disease, 500
   preparations, 228
   renal failure, 507
Isoprenaline, 100
   bronchospasm, 118
   infusion table, 529
   inotropic, 98
Isopto,
   Alkaline, 385
   Atropine, 381
   Carbachol, 382
   Carpine, 383
   Frin, 385
   Plain, 385
Isordil, 92
Isordil Tembids, 92
Isosorbide dinitrate, 90, **92**
   infusion table, 529
   preparations, 92
Isosorbide mononitrate, 90, **92**
   preparations, 92
Isotrate, 93
Isotretinoin, 416, **418**
   breast-feeding, 519
   liver disease, 500
   pregnancy, 513
   renal failure, 507
   topical, xii
Isotrex, xii
Isoxsuprine, 287
   infusion table, 529
Ispaghula, 40
   constipation, 40
   diarrhoea, 36
Isradipine, 94, **95**
   liver disease, 501
   see also Calcium-channel blockers
Istin, 94
Itraconazole, 235, **236**
   liver disease, 501
   pregnancy, 513
IUDs, 295
Ivermectin, 249
IZS, 252
   amorph, 252
   cryst, 253

Jacques, 309
Jectofer, 330
Jelonet, 439
Jevity, 537
Jexin, 470
Joint diseases, 357–71
   corticosteroid injections, 365
Joy-rides, 170
Junifen, 175

Junior Lemsip, 176
Juvela preparations, 537

Kabiglobulin, 455
Kabikinase, 107
Kala-azar, 246
Kalspare preparations, 68
Kalten, 78
Kaltocarb, 440
Kaltoclude, 440
Kaltostat preparations, 440
Kamillosan, 401
Kanamycin, 218, **219**
   infusion table, 529
Kannasyn, 219
Kaodene, 36
Kaolin, 36
   preparations, 36
      morphine and, 37
Kaolin poultices, 375
Kaopectate, 36
Karaya gum preparations, 57
Karvol, 134
Kawasaki syndrome, 455
Kay-Cee-L, 335
Kefadol, 214
Keflex, 214
Kefzol, 214
Kelfizine W, 225
Kelocyanor, 20
Kemadrin, 196
Kemicetine, 222
Kenalog, Intra-articular/Intramuscular, 267, 366
   Intramuscular only, 267
Keratolytics,
   acne, 415
   eczema, 411
   warts and calluses, 418
Keratosis follicularis, 413
Keri lotion, 401
Kerlone, 78
Keromask preparations, 421
Kest, 43
Ketalar, 460
Ketamine, 460
   infusion table, 529
Ketoconazole, 235, **237**
   anogenital, 289
   liver disease, 501
   pregnancy, 513
   scalp, 422, **426**
   skin, 426
Ketoprofen, 358, **362**, 369
   breast-feeding, 519
   preparations, 362
   topical, 375
Ketorolac, 466
Ketostix, 259
Ketotifen, 125
Ketovite, 354
Ketur Test, 259
K-Flex, 48, 51
Kiditard, 73
Kidney *see* Renal

Kindergen PROD, 537
Kinidin Durules, 73
Kipper bag, 304–5, 307
Klaricid, 220
Klean-Prep, 45
Kling, 435
KLN, 36
Kloref preparations, 335
Knitted viscose dressing, primary, 438
Koenig Rutzen, 52, 301
Kolanticon, 28
Kombo, 49, 52
Konakion, 354
Korsakoff's psychosis, 350
Kwells, 170
Kytril, 169

Labelling, cautionary and advisory *see* Cautionary and advisory labels
Labetalol, 76, **79**
 breast-feeding, 518
 infusion table, 529
 liver disease, 501
 preparations, 79
Labiton, 355
Labophylline, 120
Laboprin DL, 176
Labosept, 396
Labour,
 analgesia, 177
 induction, 284
 premature, 287
Labrocol, 79
Labyrinthine disorders, 167–8
Lachesine eye-drops, xiii
Lachrymation, excessive, 386
Lacri-Lube, 385
Lactation, suppression, 268, **281**
Lacticare, 401
Lactitol, 44
Lactose intolerance, ACBS, 542
Lactose with sucrose intolerance, ACBS, 542
Lactulose, 44
 preparations, 44
Ladropen, 205
Laevulose *see* Fructose
Lamictal, 190
Lamisil, 237
 cream, xiii
Lamotrigine, 185, **189**
Lamprene, 230
Lanolin *see* Wool fat, hydrous
Lanoxin preparations, 62
Lanvis, 316
Laractone, 67
Laraflex, 363
Laratrim, 225
Largactil, **148**, 464
Lariam, 244
Larodopa, 193
Lasikal, 69
Lasilactone, 68
Lasipressin, 80

Lasix, 66
Lasix+K, 69
Lasma, 120
Lasonil, 441
Lasoride, 68
Lassar's paste, 415
Lastogrip, 435
Laxatives, 40–5
 bulk-forming, 40
 faecal softeners, 43
 osmotic, 44
 stimulant, 41
Laxoberal, 43
Ledclair, 21
Ledercort, 267, 411
 ointment, xiii
Lederfen preparations, 361
Ledermycin, 216
Lederspan, 366
Left ventricular failure, 120
Legionnaires' disease, 220
Leishmaniacides, 246
Leishmaniasis, 246
Lem-Plus preparations, 176
Lemsip preparations, 176
Lenbul, 50, 300
Lenium, 422
Lentard MC, 252
Lentizol, 159
Leo K, 335
Lepra reactions, 230
Leprosy, 229–30
Leptospirosis, 203, 215
Leucovorin, 316
Leukaemia,
 acute, 314, 317
  lymphoblastic, 315, 318, 319
 chronic lymphocytic, 312
 chronic myeloid, 312, 318, 320
 CNS, prophylaxis, 315
 hairy cell, 320
 lymphoid, 331
Leukeran, 312
Leukopor, 437
Leukosilk, 437
Leuprorelin, 324
 endometriosis, 283
 prostate cancer, 323
Levamisole, 248
Levobunolol, 383, **384**
Levodopa, 192, **193**
 benserazide with, 192
 carbidopa with, 192
 pregnancy, 513
Levonorgestrel [ingredient], 292
Levophed, 101
Lexotan, 143
Lexpec, 331
Lexpec with Iron, 328
Lexpec with Iron-M, 328
LH, 276
LH–RH, 277
Libanil, 256
Librium, 143
Librofem, 359

Lice, 428
Lidifen, 359
Lidocaine *see* Lignocaine
Lidocaton, 474
Liga, 537
Light White, 52, 301
Lignocaine, 473
 arrhythmias, 73, **74**
 diabetic neuropathy, 258
 eye, 385
 infusion table, 530
 liver disease, 501
 local anaesthesia, 474
  urethral pain, 298
 preparations,
  infusions, 74
  injections, 74
  local, 474
Lignostab, 474
Li-Liquid, 156
Limbitrol, 163
Limclair, 347
Limited list *see* preparations identified by NHS throughout BNF
Limone, 54
Lincocin, xiii
Lindane, 428, **429**
 pregnancy, 513
Lingraine, 183
Liniments, 375
Lint, absorbent, 438
Lioresal, 373
Liothyronine, 260
 breast-feeding, 519
Lipantil, 110
Lipid-lowering drugs, 109
Lipobase, 401
Lipofundin preparations, 343
Lipostat, 111
Liquid paraffin, 43
 emulsion, 43
  magnesium hydroxide and, 44
 eye, 385
Liquifilm Tears, 386
Liquigen, 537
Liquisorb, 537
Liquisorbon MCT, 538
Liquorice, deglycyrrhizinised, 35
Lisinopril, 88
 pregnancy, 513
 renal failure, 507
 see also ACE inhibitors
Liskonum, 156
Litarex, 156
Lithium, 155
 breast-feeding, 520
 mania, 155
 poisoning by, 19
 pregnancy, 514
 recurrent depression, 155
 renal failure, 507
 scalp, 422
 surgery, 459
Lithium carbonate, 156
Lithium citrate, 156

Index 589

Lithium succinate, 422
Lithofalk, 59
Little Ones, 51
Liver disease,
    ACBS, 543
    prescribing in, 499–502
Livial, 271
Loa loa, 249
Lobak, 175
Locabiotal, 393, 396
Local anaesthetics *see* Anaesthesia, local
Locasol New Formula, 538
Loceryl, 425
Locoid, 407
Locoid C, 407
Locorten-Vioform, 389
Lodine, 361
Lodoxamide, 380
Loestrin-20, 292
Loestrin-30, 292
Lofenalac, 538
Lofepramine, 158, **160**
Lofric, 309
Logynon, 293
Logynon ED, 293
Lomodex preparations, 341
Lomotil, 36
Lomustine, 312, **313**
Loniten, 83
Loop diuretics *see* Diuretics, loop
Loperamide, 36
    diarrhoea, 36
    preparations, 37
LOP-F7, 50
Lopid preparations, 110
Loprazolam, 139, **140**
Lopresor preparations, 79–80
Lopresoretic, 80
Lo-profile, 301
Loprofin, 538
LOP-U, 300
Loratadine, 126, **127**
Lorazepam, 142, **144**
    anaesthesia, 464, **465**
    preparations, 144
    status epilepticus, 190, **191**
Lorenzo's Oil, 538
Lormetazepam, 139, **140**
Loron, 281
Losec, 35
Lotions,
    definition, 399
    eye, 376
    suitable quantities, 399
Lotriderm, 408
Low protein drink, 538
Low sodium content (antacids), 24
Low-protein products, ACBS, 543
Loxapac, 150
Loxapine, 147, **150**
LSD *see* Lysergide
Luborant, 398
Ludiomil, 161

Lugol's solution, 261
Lupus erythematosus,
    discoid, 367
    systemic, 264, 365, 367, 369
Lurselle, 111
Lustral, 165
Luteinising hormone, 276
Lyclear, 430
Lyme disease, 215
    children, 203
Lymecycline, 217
Lymphangiectasia, intestinal, ACBS, 543
Lymphogranuloma venereum, 215
Lymphoma, 312–15, 317, 319
Lyofoam, 440
Lyofoam C, 439
Lypressin, 278, **279**
Lysergic acid diethylamide *see* Lysergide
Lysergide, regulations, 7
Lysuride, 193, **195**
    breast-feeding, 520

Maalox, 25
Maalox Plus, 27
Maalox TC, 25
Macpak, 305
Macrodantin, 234
Macrodex, 341
Macrodom, 303
Macrodom Plus, 303
Macrofix, 435
Macrolides, 220
Madopar preparations, 193
    pregnancy, 514
Magaldrate, 24, **25**
    preparations, 25
Magnapen, 209
    infusion table, 526
Magnesia, cream of, 44
Magnesium carbonate, 24, **25**
    preparations, 25
    renal failure, 507
Magnesium chloride, 347
Magnesium citrate, 44
Magnesium hydroxide, 44
    preparations, 44
        liquid paraffin, 44
Magnesium salts, 44, 347
    renal failure, 507
Magnesium sulphate, 44
    enema, 44
    liver disease, 501
    nutrition, 347
    paste, 430
Magnesium trisilicate, 24, **25**
    liver disease, 499
    preparations, 25
    renal failure, 507
Maize oil, 535
Malabsorption syndromes, 37
    ACBS, 543
    electrolytes, 334–8
    magnesium, 347
    vitamin K, 353

Malaria, 240–45
    prophylaxis, 242–3
    treatment, 241
Malathion, 428, **429**
Malignant disease, 310–25
    bladder, 299
    hormone antagonists, 322
    pain, 177
        bone, 173
    sex hormones, 321–2
Malignant effusions, 312, 314, 320
Malignant hyperthermia, 472
    antagonists, 472
Malix, 256
Malnutrition, disease-related, ACBS, 544
Maloprim, 242, 243, **245**
    breast-feeding, 520
    pregnancy, 514
Mammary dysplasia, 282
Manevac, 42
Mania, 146, 155
Manic depression, 155
Mannitol, 69
    glaucoma, 384
    preparations, 69
Mantoux test, 445
Manufacturers, index of, 558
Manusept, 433
MAOIs *see* Monoamine-oxidase inhibitors
Maple syrup urine disease, ACBS, 544
Maprotiline, 158, **161**
Marcain preparations, 474–5
Marevan, 105
Marplan, 163
Marvelon, 292
Marzine RF, 169
Masse Breast Cream, 401
Mastalgia, 281, **283**, 415
Maxamaid preparations, 538
Maxamum preparations, 538
Maxepa, 111
Maxidex, 379
Maxijul preparations, 538
Maxipro HBV Super Soluble, 539
Maxisorb, 539
Maxitrol, 380
Maxivent, 116
Maxolon preparations, 170
Maxtrex, 316
Mazindol, 166, **167**
MC Mask, 133
mc pouches, 48, 51
MCR-50, 93
MCT Oil, 539
MCT Pepdite, 539
MCT(1) Powder, 539
Measles,
    immunoglobulin, 455
    vaccination, 443
    vaccine, 448
        MMR, 449
        mumps, rubella and, 449

Mebendazole, **247**, 248
   pregnancy, 514
Mebeverine, 29
   breast-feeding, 520
Mebhydrolin, 129
Mecillinam, 210
   infusion table, 530
Mectizan, 249
Medazepam, 142, **144**
Medicated bandages, 436
Medicoal, 17
Medihaler-epi, 131
Medihaler-Ergotamine, 183
Medihaler-Iso preparations, 118
Medilave gel, 397
Medimates, 303
Medised, 176
Medrone, 267
Medroxyprogesterone, 272, 321, 322
   contraception, 294
   malignant disease, 321
   menstrual disorders, 271, **272**
Mefenamic acid,
   analgesia, 175
   breast-feeding, 520
   menorrhagia, 175
   preparations, 363
   rheumatic disease, 359, **362**
Mefloquine, 241, **243**
   breast-feeding, 520
   pregnancy, 514
   renal failure, 507
Mefoxin, 212
Mefruside, 64
Megace, 322
Megestrol, 321, **322**
Melanoma, 318
Melleril, 152
Melolin, 438
Melolite, 439
Melphalan, 312, **313**
   infusion table, 530
   renal failure, 507
Menadiol sodium phosphate, 353, **354**
Mendelson's syndrome, 31
Mengivac (A + C), 450
Meniere's disease, 167–8
Meningeal carcinoma, 315
Meningitis,
   cryptococcal, 236
   haemophilus, 200, 222
   listerial, 200
   meningococcal, 200
      prophylaxis, 202, 215
      vaccine, 449
   pneumococcal, 200
Meningococcal vaccine, 449
Menopausal symptoms, 184, **268**
Menophase, Syntex, 269
Menorrhagia, 107, 175, 271, 282
Menotrophin, 276
Menstrual disorders, 271
Menthol [ingredient], 375

Menthol inhalation,
   benzoin and, 134
   eucalyptus and, 134
Menzol, 273
Mepacrine, 246
   rheumatic disease, 369
Mepenzolate, 28, **29**
Mepranix, 79
Meprobamate, 144, **145**
   breast-feeding, 520
   muscle spasm, 374
Meptazinol, 180
   anaesthesia, 466, **467**
   analgesia, 177, **180**
Meptid, 181, 467
Mequitazine, 129
Merbentyl preparations, 28
Mercaptopurine, 315, **316**
   renal failure, 507
Mercilon, 292
Mercuric oxide eye ointment, 377
Meredith, 304
Merieux Inactivated Rabies Vaccine, 452
Merocaine, 397
Merocet solution, 397
Merocets, 396
Mersalyl, 69
Mesalazine, 37, **38**
   breast-feeding, 520
   renal failure, 507
Mesna, 312, **313**
   infusion table, 530
Mesorb, 439
Mesterolone, 274
Mestinon, 372
Mestranol, 269
Metabolic Mineral Mixture, 539
Metalpha, 84
Metamucil, 40
Metanium, 403
Metaraminol, 101
   infusion table, 530
   pregnancy, 514
Metatone, 355
Metenix-5, 65
Meterfolic, 328
Metformin, 257
   liver disease, 501
   pregnancy, 514
   preparations, 257
   renal failure, 507
Methadone, 177, **181**, 198
   breast-feeding, 520
   cough, 135
   preparations, 181
      linctus, 135
      mixture (1 mg/mL), 198
Methaemoglobinaemia, 475
Methenamine *see* Hexamine
Methicillin, 205
   infusion table, 530
Methionine, 18
   tablets, 18
Methixene, 196

Methocarbamol, 374
   infusion table, 530
   renal failure, 507
Methohexitone, 459, **460**
   liver disease, 501
Methotrexate, 315, **316**
   infusion table, 530
   liver disease, 501
   preparations, 316
   psoriasis, 412
   renal failure, 507
   rheumatic disease, 369
Methotrimeprazine, 150
   psychoses, 150
   terminal care, 13, **150**
Methoxamine, 101
Methoxsalen, 412
   liver disease, 501
Methyclothiazide, 65
Methyl salicylate [ingredient], 427
Methylated spirit, industrial, 431
Methylcellulose, 40, **41**
   constipation, 40
   diarrhoea, 36
   obesity, 166
   preparations, 41
Methylcysteine, 134
Methyldopa, 84
   breast-feeding, 520
   infusion table, 530
   liver disease, 501
   preparations, 84
   renal failure, 507
Methyldopate hydrochloride, 84
Methylene blue, 475
Methylmalonic, propionic acidaemia, ACBS, 544
Methylphenobarbitone, 187
Methylprednisolone, 267
Methylprednisolone acetate, 267
   rheumatic disease, 366
   skin, 411
Methylprednisolone sodium succinate, 267
   infusion table, 530
Methysergide, 184
Metipranolol, 383, **384**
Metirosine, 89
Metoclopramide, 170
   breast-feeding, 520
   gastro-intestinal, 30
   infusion table, 530
   liver disease, 501
   migraine, 182
   nausea, 168, **170**
   preparations, 170
   renal failure, 507
Metolazone, 63, **65**
   renal failure, 509
Metopirone, 283
Metoprolol, 79
   liver disease, 501
   migraine, 184
   preparations, 79

Index 591

Metosyn, 410
Metramid, 170
Metriphonate, 249
Metrodin, 276
Metrogel, 425
Metrolyl, 231
Metronidazole, 230
    amoebiasis, 245
    breast-feeding, 520
    Crohn's disease, 37
    giardiasis, 246
    guinea worm, 249
    liver disease, 501
    pregnancy, 514
    preparations, 231
        tumours, 425
    protozoal infections, 245
    skin, 425
    trichomoniasis, 245
    ulcerative gingivitis, 395
Metrotop, 425
Metyrapone, 283
    pregnancy, 514
Mexiletine, 73, **74**
    breast-feeding, 520
    diabetic neuropathy, 258
    infusion table, 530
    liver disease, 501
Mexitil preparations, 74
MFV-Ject, 448
Miacalcic, 280
Mianserin, 158, **161**
    preparations, 161
Micolette, 45
Miconazole, 235, **237**
    infusion table, 530
    oral gel, 396
    skin, 425, **426**
        hydrocortisone and, 406
    vaginal, 289
Micralax, 45
Micral-Test, 260
Microgynon-30, 292
Micronor, 294
Micropore, 437
Microval, 294
Mictral, 233
Midamor, 67
Midazolam, 464, **465**
Midrid, 176, 183
Mifegyne, 287
Mifepristone, 286
    pregnancy, 514
Migrafen, 359
Migraine, 182–4
Migraleve, 176, 182
Migravess, 182
Migril, 183
Mildison, 405
Milk, drugs in, 517–21
Milk intolerance, ACBS, 544
Milk-alkali syndrome, 27
Milrinone, 62
    infusion table, 530
    renal failure, 507
Milupa Low Protein Drink, 539

Milupa lpd, 539
Milupa PKU preparations, 539
Minafen, 539
Mineralocorticoids, 262
    replacement therapy, 262
Minihep preparations, 103
Min-I-Jet,
    Adrenaline, 98, 131
    Atropine sulphate, 463
    Bretylium, 74
    Calcium Chloride, 346
    Frusemide, 66
    Glucose, 339
    Isoprenaline, 100
    Lignocaine, 74
        Adrenaline with, 473
    Mannitol, 69
    Naloxone, 19
    Sodium bicarbonate, 340
Minims,
    Amethocaine, 385
    Artificial Tears, 385
    Atropine Sulphate, 381
    Benoxinate (Oxybuprocaine), 385
    Chloramphenicol, 377
    Cyclopentolate, 381
    Fluorescein Sodium, 386
    Gentamicin, 378
    Homatropine, 381
    Lignocaine and Fluorescein, 385
    Metipranolol, 384
    Neomycin Sulphate, 378
    Phenylephrine, 382
    Pilocarpine Nitrate, 383
    Prednisolone, 380
    Rose Bengal, 386
    Sodium Chloride, 386
    Sulphacetamide, 378
    Tropicamide, 382
Mini-Wright, 122
Minocin preparations, 217
Minocycline, 215, **217**
Minodiab, 256
Minoxidil, 83
    breast-feeding, 520
    hypertension, 83
    pregnancy, 514
    scalp, 423
Mintec, 30
Mintezol, 249
Minulet, 284
Miochol, 386
Miotics, 382
Miradol, 176
Miraxid, 209
Misoprostol, 34
    naproxen with, 363
    pregnancy, 514
'Missed pill', 294
Misuse of drugs, 7
    Act, 8
    Regulations 1985, 8
Mitcham, 302
Mithracin, 315
Mithramycin *see* Plicamycin

Mitobronitol, 312
Mitomycin, 314, **315**
    bladder, 299
Mitomycin C Kyowa, 315
Mitoxana, 313
Mitozantrone, 314, **315**
    infusion table, 530
Mixtard 30/70 preparations, 254
MMR vaccine, 449
MMR-II, 449
Mobiflex, 364
Mobilan, 362
Modecate preparations, 154
Moditen, 149
Modrasone, 407
Modrenal, 283
Moducren, 81
Moduret-25, 68
Moduretic, 68
Mogadon, 139
Molcer, 391
Molipaxin, 161
Monaspor, 212
Monit preparations, 93
Monoamine-oxidase inhibitors, 162
    liver disease, 501
    surgery, 459
    treatment card, 162
Monoamine-oxidase-B inhibitors, 193
Mono-Cedocard preparations, 93
Monoclate-P, 108
Monocor, 78
Monolet lancets, 255
Monoparin preparations, 102–3
Monosulfiram, 428, **429**
Monotard, Human, 252
Monotrim, 226
Monovent syrup, 116
Monphytol, 427
MOPP therapy, 319
Morhulin, 401
Morphine, 178
    anaesthesia, 467
    breast-feeding, 520
    cough, 135
    pain, 177
        chronic, 12, 177
    preparations, 178–9
        anaesthesia, 467
        kaolin and, 37
    renal failure, 507
Morsep, 401
Motilium, 169
Motion sickness, 168
Motipress, 163
Motival, 163
Motrin, 359
Mountain sickness, 69
Mouth ulceration, 394
Mouthwash solution-tablets, 398
Mouthwashes, 397
Movelat, 375
Movement disorders, 197

MS-36, 255
MST Continus, 178
    terminal care, 12
MSUD Aid, 539
Mucaine, 27
Mucodyne, 134
Mucogel, 25
Mucolytics, 133
Mu-Cron, 176
Multibionta, 345
    infusion table, 533
Multiload IUDs, 296
Multiparin, 103
Multivitamin preparations, 354
Mumps vaccination, 443
Mumps vaccine, 450
Mumpsvax, 450
Mupirocin, 423
    ointment, 423
    nasal, 394
Muripsin, 59
Muscle relaxants,
    anaesthesia, 469–71
    skeletal, 372–3
Muscle spasm, 372
Musculoskeletal disorders, rheumatic, 357–69
Muslin, absorbent, 438
Mustine, 312, **313**
    infusion table, 530
    injection, 313
Myambutol, 228
Myasthenia gravis, 371
    diagnosis, 371
Mycardol, 93
Mycifradin, 219
Mycoplasma infections, 215
Mycota, 427
Mydriacyl, 382
Mydriatics, 381
Mydrilate, 381
Myelobromol, 312
Myeloma, 312
Myelomatosis, 331
Myleran, 312
Mynah preparations, 228
    Mynah-200, xiii
Myocardial infarction,
    arrhythmias, 70
    beta-blockers, 76
    thrombolytics, 106
Myoclonic seizures, 186
Myocrisin, 367
Myometrial relaxants, 287
Myotonine, 297
Mysoline, 187
Mysteclin, 216
Myxoedema, 260

N-A Dressing, 438
Nabilone, 168, **171**
Nabumetone, 359, **363**
Nacton, 29
Nadolol, 80
    migraine, 184
    thyrotoxicosis, 261
Nafarelin, 282, **283**
    pregnancy, 514

Naftidrofuryl oxalate, 98
    infusion table, 530
Nail infections (fungal), 235–7, 425
Nalbuphine, 181
    anaesthesia, 467
    analgesia, 177, **181**
Nalcrom, 40
Nalidixic acid, 231, **232**, 233
    breast-feeding, 520
    liver disease, 501
    renal failure, 507
    see also 4-Quinolones
Nalorex, 198
Naloxone,
    anaesthesia, 471
    infusion table, 530
    poisoning, 18
    preparations, 19
    neonatal, 472
Naltrexone, 198
'Named patient', 4
Nandrolone decanoate, 275
    aplastic anaemia, 331
Nandrolone phenylpropionate, 275
Naphazoline [ingredient], 380
Napkin rash, 403
Napratec, 363
Naprosyn preparations, 363
Naproxen, 363
    breast-feeding, 520
    gout, 369
    pain, 176
    preparations, 363
        misoprostol with, 363
    rheumatic disease, 358, **363**
Narcan, 19
Narcan Neonatal, 472
Narcolepsy, 165
Narcotic analgesics *see* Analgesics, opioid
Narcotic antagonists *see* Opioid antagonists
Nardil, 163
Narphen, 182
Nasal allergy, 391
Nasal congestion, 391–3
Nasal decongestants,
    systemic, 126, **136**
    topical, 392
Naseptin, 394
Natrilix, 64
Natuderm, 401
Natulan, 319
Nausea, 168
    cytotoxic drugs, 311
    pregnancy, 168
Navidrex, 64
Navispare, 68
Naxogin-500, xiii
'NCL' prescriptions, 546
Nebacumab, xi
Nebcin, 219
Nebuhaler, 122
Necatoriasis, 248
Nedocromil, 125

Needles, insulin, 255
    clipping device, 255
Nefopam, 173, **176**
    breast-feeding, 520
Negram, 233
Nelaton catheter, 309
Neocate, 539
Neocon-1/35, 292
Neo-Cortef, 389
    ear, 389
    eye, 380
Neo-Cytamen, 331
Neogest, 294
Neo-Lidocaton, 474
Neo-Medrone, 411
Neo-Mercazole, 261
Neomycin, 218, **219**
    ear, 388, **389**
    eye, 377, **378**
    preparations, 219
        ear, 389
        eye, 378
        skin, 423
    renal failure, 507
    skin, 423
Neo-NaClex, 64
Neo-NaClex-K, 69
Neosporin, 378
Neostigmine, 371, 372
    anaesthesia, 471
    laxative, 41
    myasthenia gravis, 371, **372**
    pregnancy, 514
Neotigason, xii
Nepenthe oral solution, 179
Nephramine, 343
Nephril, 65
Nephrotic syndrome, 264
Nericur, 417
Nerisone preparations, 409
Nestargel, 539
Netelast, 435
Netillin, 219
Netilmicin, 218, **219**
    infusion table, 530
Neulactil, 151
Neupogen, 334
Neuralgia, trigeminal, 182
Neuroleptanalgesia, 467
Neuroleptic malignant syndrome, 146
Neuroleptics *see* Antipsychotics
Neuromuscular blocking drugs, 469
Neuromuscular disorders, 371
Neuropathy, compression, 365
Neutropenias, 331, 334
New preparations, xii–xiii
Nicardipine, 93, **95**
    liver disease, 501
    renal failure, 507
    see also Calcium-channel blockers
Niclosamide, 248
Nicofuranose, 110, **111**
Nicorette preparations, 198
Nicotinamide, 350, **351**
    tablets, 351

Index 593

Nicotinates [ingredient], 375
Nicotine products, xii, 198
Nicotinell TTS, xii
Nicotinic acid, 110, **111**
    tablets, 111
    vascular disease, 97
Nicotinyl alcohol, 97
Nicoumalone, 105
Nifedipine, 93, **95**
    breast-feeding, 520
    liver disease, 501
    preparations, 95
    renal failure, 507
    see also Calcium-channel blockers
Nifensar XL, 96
Niferex preparations, 328
Night Nurse, 176
Nikethamide, 132
Nilodor, 54
Nilstim, 166
Nimodipine, 94, **96**
    infusion table, 531
Nimorazole, 246
    trichomoniasis, 245
    ulcerative gingivitis, 395
Nimotop, 96
Nipride, 84
Niridazole, 249
    liver disease, 501
Nitoman, 197
Nitrates,
    angina, 90
    heart failure, 90
Nitrazepam, 139
    preparations, 139
Nitrocine, 91
Nitrocontin Continus, 91
Nitro-Dur, 91
Nitrofurantoin, 233, **234**
    breast-feeding, 520
    pregnancy, 514
    renal failure, 507
Nitrolingual Spray, 91
Nitronal, 91
Nitroprusside, 83
    infusion table, 532
    liver disease, 501
    preparations, 84
    renal failure, 507
Nitrous oxide, 462
Nitrous oxide–oxygen, 462
Nivaquine, 243
Nivemycin, 219
Nizatidine, 31, **32**
    breast-feeding, 520
    renal failure, 507
Nizoral, 237, 289
    topical, 426
Nobrium, 144
Noctec, 140
Nocturnal enuresis, 298
Noltam, 324
Nolvadex preparations, 324
Nonoxinol [ingredient], 295
Non-woven swabs, 438
    filmated, 438

Noradrenaline, 101
    infusion table, 531
    pregnancy, 514
Noratex, xiii
Norcuron, 470
Norditropin preparations, 277
Nordox, 217
Norethisterone, 273
    contraception, 292–5
    malignant disease, 322
    menstrual disorders, 271
Norethisterone acetate, 292
    malignant disease, 322
Norethisterone enanthate, 294
Norflex, 374
Norfloxacin, 231, **232**
    eye, 377, **378**
    renal failure, 507
    see also 4-Quinolones
Norgalax Micro-enema, 42
Norgestimate [ingredient], 292
Norgeston, 294
Norgestrel *see* Levonorgestrel
Noriday, 294
Norimin, 292
Norinyl-1, 293
Noristerat, 295
Normacol Antispasmodic, 29
Normacol preparations, 41
Normal immunoglobulin *see* Immunoglobulins, normal
'Normal saline', 338
Normasol, 431
    eye, 386
Normax, 42
Normetic, xiii
Noroxin, 378
Nortriptyline, 158, **160**
Norval, 161
Nose *see* Nasal
Novagard, 296
Novantrone, 315
Novaprin, 359
Novaruca, 419
Nova-T, 296
NovoPen-II, 254
Nozinan, 150
'NP' labelling, 3
NSAIDs (Non-steroidal anti-inflammatory drugs) *see* Analgesics
Nubain, 181, 468
Nuelin preparations, 120
Nu-K, 335
Nulacin, 27
Nurofen, 359
Nurse Sykes Powders, 176
Nu-Seals Aspirin, 173, 176
Nutracel preparations, 343
Nutramigen, 539
Nutraplus, 402
Nutrilon Soya, 539
Nutrison, 539
Nutrition, 342–5
    ACBS, 534
    enteral, 345
    intravenous, 342–5
    supplements, 344–5

Nutrition (*continued*)—
    oral, 345
    total parenteral, 342–5
Nutritional supplements, ACBS, 544
Nutrizym GR, 60
Nuvelle, 270
Nycopren, 363
Nylon and viscose stretch bandage, 435
Nystadermal, 411
Nystaform, 426
Nystaform-HC, 406
Nystan, 237
    anogenital, 289
    mouth, 396
    skin, 426
Nystatin, 234, **237**
    anogenital, 289
        perianal, 45
        vaginal, 289
        vulval, 289
    mouth, 396
    skin, 425, **426**
Nystatin-Dome, 237
    mouth, 396

Obesity, 166–7
Obstructive airways disease, 113, 131, 133
Octovit, 329
Octoxinol [ingredient], 295
Octreotide, 325
    breast-feeding, 520
    pregnancy, 514
Ocufen, 386
Ocusert Pilo preparations, 383
Ocuserts, 376
Oedema, 63
    cerebral, 69, 264
Oesophageal varices, 278
Oesophagitis, 24, 31
Oestradiol, 269
    preparations, 269–70
        implants, 269
        vaginal, 288
Oestradiol valerate, 269
Oestrifen, 324
Oestriol, 270
    preparations, 270
        vaginal, 288
Oestrogens, 267–71
    breast-feeding, 520
    conjugated, 270
    HRT, 267–71
    liver disease, 501
    malignant disease, 321
    oral contraceptives, 290
    surgery, 459
    vaginal, 288
Ofloxacin, 231, **233**
    renal failure, 508
    see also 4-Quinolones
Oilatum,
    cream, 401
    Emollient, 402
    shower emollient, 401

Ointments,
    definition, 400
    eye, 376
    suitable quantities, 399
Olbetam, 110
Oligospermia, 276
Olive oil, 390
    cradle cap, 422
Olsalazine, 37, **39**
Omega-3 marine triglycerides, 111
Omeprazole, 34
    liver disease, 501
    pregnancy, 514
Omiderm, 439
Omni, 50, 53
Omnopon, 468
Onchocerciasis, 249
Oncovin, 317
Ondansetron, 168, **171**
    infusion table, 531
    liver disease, 501
One-alpha, 353
Onychomycosis see Nail infections
Open-wove bandage, 435
Operidine, 469
Ophthaine, 385
Ophthalmic preparations see Eye preparations
Opiate squill linctus, 136
Opilon, 97
Opioid analgesics see Analgesics, opioid
Opioid antagonists, 471
    poisoning, 18
OPR-F, 51
OPR-U, 300
Opsite, 439
Opticrom, 381
Optimine, 127
OPV, 451
Orabase, 395
Orabet, 257
Orahesive, 395
Oral contraceptives see Contraceptives, oral
Oral hypoglycaemic drugs see Antidiabetic drugs, oral
Oral rehydration, 336
    preparations, 336
    WHO formula, 337
Oral rehydration salts, 336
Oral syringes, 2
Oral-B Fluoride, 348
Oralcer, 396
Oraldene, 397
Oramorph, 178
    Unit Dose Vials, xiii
Orap, 151
Orbenin, 205
Orciprenaline, 118
Organophosphorus insecticides, poisoning by, 22
Orimeten, 323
Oropharynx, 394–8
    anti-infective drugs, 395–6

Orovite preparations, 354
    syrup, xiii
Orphenadrine citrate, 374
Orphenadrine hydrochloride, 195, **196**
ORS, 336
ORT, 336
Ortho diaphragm, 296
Ortho Dienoestrol, 288
Ortho Gyne T, 296
Ortho Gyne T Slimline, 296
Ortho-Creme, 295
Orthoforms, 295
Ortho-Gynest, 288
Ortho-Gynol, 295
Ortho-Novin 1/50, 293
Ortho-White diaphragm, 296
Orudis, 362
Oruvail, 362
Oruvail gel, 375
Osmolite, 539
Ossopan, 346
Osteoarthritis, 357
Osteoarthrosis, 357
Osteomyelitis, 201, 221, 222
Osteoporosis,
    anabolic steroids, 274
    calcium, 346
    disodium etidronate, 280
    HRT, 268
OsterSoy, 540
Ostobon, 54
Ostopore, 49, 52
Otitis externa, 201, 388
Otitis media, 201, 390
Otomize, 389
Otosporin, 390
Otrivine, 393
Otrivine-Antistin, 380
Ouabain, 70
Ovarian cancer, 312, 318
Ovestin cream, 288
Ovestin tablets, 270
Ovran, 292
Ovran-30, 292
Ovranette, 292
Ovysmen, 292
Oxamniquine, 249
Oxatomide, 129
Oxazepam, 142, **144**
Oxerutins, 97
Oxethazaine [ingredient], 27
Oxitropium, 119
Oxivent, 119
Oxpentifylline, 97
Oxprenolol, 80
    liver disease, 501
    preparations, 80
Oxybenzone, 421
Oxybuprocaine, 385
Oxybutynin, 297–8
Oxycodone suppositories, 177
Oxygen, 132
    concentrators, 133
    cylinders, 132
Oxymetazoline, 393
Oxymetholone, 331
Oxymycin, 217

Oxypertine, 147, **150**
    preparations, 150
Oxyphenbutazone eye ointment, 380, **381**
Oxyphenisatin, 41, **42**
Oxyprenix SR, 80
Oxytetracycline, 217
Oxytetramix, 217
Oxytocin, 284, **286**
    infusion table, 531

Pacifene, 359
PACT, 1
Padimate O, 420
Paediasure, 540
Paediatric doses, 11
Paediatric Seravit, 540
Paget's disease of bone, 279, 280
Pain, 173–84
    bone, 173, 280
    dressings, 462
    intra-operative, 466
    musculoskeletal, 173, 374
    obstetric, 462
    postoperative, 466
    rheumatic, 357–64
    terminal care, 177
    urethral, 298
    visceral, 177
Palaprin Forte, 173, 176
Paldesic, 174, 176
Palex, 49
Palfium, 180
Paludrine, 244
Pamergan P100, 181, 468
Pameton, 176
Pamidronate disodium, 280
    infusion table, 527
    renal failure, 508
Panadeine, 174, 176
Panadol preparations, 174, 176
Panaleve preparations, 176
Pancrease, 60
Pancreatin, 59
    preparations, 59
Pancreatitis, chronic, 59
Pancrex, 60
Pancrex V, 60
Pancuronium, 469, **470**
Panerel, 176
Panic attacks, 142, 157
Panmycin, xiii
Panoxyl preparations, 417
Panthenol, 350
Pantothenic acid, 350
Papaveretum,
    anaesthesia, 468
    pregnancy, 514
    preparations, 468
    with aspirin (Aspav), 174
Papaverine (impotence), 300
Paracetamol, 173, **174**
    breast-feeding, 520
    dextropropoxyphene and, 175
    febrile convulsions, 192

Index

Paracetamol (*continued*)—
  liver disease, 501
  migraine, 182
  poisoning by, 18
  post-immunisation pyrexia, 444
  preparations, 174
    compound, 174–6
Paracets, 176
Paracodol, 174, 176
Paraffin
  white soft, 400
  yellow soft, 400
    eye, 386
Paraffin gauze dressing, 439
Parake, 174
Paraldehyde, 190, **191**
  injection, 191
Paramax, 182
Paramin, 176
Paramol, 175, 176
Paraplatin, 318
Paraproteinaemias, 331
Paraquat, poisoning by, 21
Parasiticidal preparations, 428
Parasympathomimetics,
  anaesthesia, 470
  laxative, 41
  myasthenia gravis, 371
  urinary retention, 296
Paratulle, 439
Parenteral nutrition, 342–5
  infusion fluids, 343–4
Parentrovite, 351
  infusion table, 533
Parfenac, 414
Parkinsonism, 192–6
  drug-induced, 146, 195
  idiopathic, 192
  post-encephalitic, 192
Parlodel, 194, 281
Parmid, 170
Parnate, 163
Paroven, 97
Paroxetine, 164
  renal failure, 508
Parstelin, 163
Partial seizures, 185
Partobulin, 456
Parvolex, 18
Pastariso, 540
Pastes, definition, 400
Patents, 3
Pavacol-D, 135
Pavulon, 470
pc pouches, 48, 51
Peak flow meters, 122
PEC high compression bandage, 436
Pecram, 121
Ped-El, 345
Pediculosis, 428
Pelvic inflammatory disease, 201
Pemoline, 165
Pemphigus, 264
Penbritin, 207
Penbutolol, 80

Pendramine, 368
Penicillamine, 355, **368**
  chronic hepatitis, 355
  cystinuria, 355
  poisoning, 21
  pregnancy, 514
  preparations, 368
  renal failure, 508
  rheumatic disease, 366, **367–8**
  Wilson's disease, 355
Penicillin G *see* Benzylpenicillin
Penicillin triple injection, [= *Triplopen*], 204
Penicillin V *see* Phenoxymethylpenicillin
Penicillin VK *see* Phenoxymethylpenicillin
Penicillinases, 203
Penicillins, 203–11
  antipseudomonal, 209
  broad-spectrum, 206
  penicillinase-resistant, 204
  penicillinase-sensitive, 203
Penidural, 204
Peniflow, 303
Penject, 254
PenMix preparations, 254
Pentacarinat, 247
Pentaerythritol tetranitrate, 93
Pentamidine isethionate, 246, **247**
  infusion table, 531
  leishmaniasis, 247
  renal failure, 508
Pentasa, 39
Pentazocine, 177, **181**
  preparations, 181
Pentostam, 246
Peoplecare,
  belts, 302
  drip urinal, 302
  urinal systems, 307
Pepcid, 32
Pepdite, 540
Peppermint oil, 29, **30**
Peptamen, 540
Pepti-2000 LF, 540
Pepti-Junior, 540
Peptimax, 32
Peptisorb, 540
Peptisorbon, 540
Percutol, 91
Perfan, 62
Perfect, 48
Perforated film absorbent dressing, 438
Perfron, 439
Pergolide, 193, **195**
  breast-feeding, 520
Pergonal, 276
Periactin, 128
Pericyazine, 150
Perifusin, 343
Perindopril, 88
  pregnancy, 514
  renal failure, 508
  see also ACE inhibitors

Peritonitis, 200
Permethrin, 428, **429**
Permitabs, 434
Per/Vac, 450
Perphenazine, 151
  nausea, 168, **171**
  psychoses, 151
Persantin, 106
Pertofran, 159
Pertussis, 220
  vaccination, 443
  vaccine, 450
    diphtheria, tetanus, and, 446
Pethidine, 181
  anaesthesia, 468
  analgesia, 177, **181**
  preparations, 181, 468
  renal failure, 508
Petit mal, 186
Petrolagar, 43
Petroleum jelly, 400
Petroleum products, poisoning by, 17
Pevaryl, 426
  anogenital, 289
Pevaryl TC, 411
Peyronie's disease, 352
Phaeochromocytoma, 76, 85, 89
Pharmalgen, 130
Pharmorubicin preparations, 315
Pharyngitis *see* Throat infections
Pharynx *see* Oropharynx
Phasal, 156
Phenazocine, 177, **181**
Phenelzine, 162
Phenergan, 129
Phenindamine, 129
Phenindione, 104, **105**
Pheniramine, 129
Phenobarbitone, 187
  breast-feeding, 520
  epilepsy, 186, **187**
    status, 190
  liver disease, 501
  poisoning, elimination, 17
  pregnancy, 515
  preparations, 187
  renal failure, 508
Phenol, 397
  haemorrhoids, 47
  injection, oily, 47
Phenolphthalein, 43
  breast-feeding, 520
  [ingredient], 43
Phenoperidine, 468
Phenothiazines, 146
  classification, 146
  diabetic neuropathy, 258
  nausea, 168
  poisoning by, 20
  psychoses, 146–54
Phenothrin, 428, **430**
Phenoxybenzamine, 85, **86**
  infusion table, 531

Phenoxymethylpenicillin, 203, **204**
  preparations, 204
Phensedyl, 136
Phensic preparations, 176
Phentermine, 166, **167**
Phentolamine, 85, **86**
  impotence, 300
  infusion table, 531
Phenylbutazone, 359, **363**
Phenylephrine,
  eye-drops, 382
  hypotension, 101
  infusion table, 531
  injection 1%, 102
  nose, 393
Phenylketonuria, ACBS, 544
Phenylpropanolamine, nasal decongestants, 137
Phenytoin, 186
  arrhythmias, 73, 74
  breast-feeding, 520
  epilepsy, 185, **187**
    status, 190, **191**
  liver disease, 501
  poisoning, elimination, 17
  pregnancy, 515
  preparations, 188, 192
  trigeminal neuralgia, 182
pHiso-med, 432
Phobia, 162
Phoenix, 50
Pholcodine, 135
  preparations, 135
Pholcomed preparations, 135
PhorPain, 359
Phosgene, poisoning by, 21
Phosphate supplements, 347–8
Phosphate-binding agents, 348
Phosphates,
  enema, 44, 45
  hypercalcaemia, 347
  intravenous, 347
Phosphate-Sandoz, 348
Phosphodiesterase inhibitors, 62
Pholine iodide, 382
Phosphorus, 347–8
Photodermatoses, 420
  ACBS, 545
Phyllocontin Continus, 121
Physeptone, 181
Physiological saline, 338
Physostigmine, 382
  eye-drops, 382
    pilocarpine and, 382
Phytex, 427
Phytocil cream, 427
Phytocil powder, 427
Phytomenadione, 353, **354**
Picolax, 43
Piggy-back technique, 523
Pilocarpine, 382
  eye-drops, 382
    physostigmine and, 382
Pimozide, 147, **151**
  Tourette syndrome, 197

Pindolol, 80
Pinworm infections, 247
Pipenzolate, 28, **29**
Piperacillin, 209, **210**
  infusion table, 531
  renal failure, 508
Piperazine, 247, **248**
  pregnancy, 515
  preparations, 248
  renal failure, 508
Piperazine oestrone sulphate, 271
Piportil Depot, 155
Pipothiazine palmitate, 155
Pipril, 210
Piptal, 29
Piptalin, 29
Pirbuterol, 117
Pirenzepine, 33
  breast-feeding, 520
Piretanide, 65, **66**
Piriton, 128
Piroxicam, 364
  breast-feeding, 520
  gout, 369
  preparations, 364
  topical, 375
  rheumatic disease, 359, **364**
Pirozip, 364
Pitressin, 278
Pituitary function test, 283
Pituitary hormones, 275
  anterior, 275–7
  posterior, 278–9
Pityriasis capitis, 421
Pityriasis versicolor, 235
Pivampicillin, 206, **209**
  renal failure, 508
Pivmecillinam, 210
Piz Buin preparations, 420
Pizotifen, 184
PK Aid 3, 540
PKU preparations, 540
Plaque, 397
Plaquenil, 369
Plasma, 340
  fresh frozen, 109
Plasma and plasma substitutes, 340–2
Plasma concentrations, 6
  electrolytes, 334
Plasma protein solution, 341
Plasma-Lyte preparations, 343
Plasmapheresis, myasthenia gravis, 371
Plasmatein, 341
Plasters, 437
Plastic wound dressings, 437
Platet, 106
Plendil, 94
Plesmet, 327
Pleural effusions, 216
Plicamycin, 314, **315**
  hypercalcaemia, 346
  infusion table, 531
  liver disease, 501
  renal failure, 508
Pluserix MMR, 449

Pneumococcal infection,
  prophylaxis, 202
  vaccination, 443
  vaccine, 450
Pneumococcal vaccine, 450
Pneumocystis pneumonia, 225, 246
Pneumonia, 132, 200
Pneumovax II, 451
Podophyllin, 418, **419**
  pregnancy, 515
  preparations, 419–20
Podophyllotoxin, 419
Podophyllum resin *see* Podophyllin
Poisoning, 15–22
  active elimination, 17
  adsorbents, 17
  hospital admission, 16
  information services, 15
Poisons information services, 15
Poldine, 28, **29**
Polial, 540
Poliomyelitis,
  vaccination, 443
  vaccines, 451
  travel, 457
Pollen allergy preparations, 130
Pollon-eze, 127
Pol/Vac (Inact), 451
Pol/Vac (Oral), 451
Polyamide, elastane, and cotton compression bandage, 436
Polyamide and cellulose contour bandage, 435
Polyarteritis nodosa, 264, 365
Polybactrin, 424
  Soluble GU, xiii
Polycal, 540
Polycose, 540
Polycrol preparations, xiii
Polyene antifungal drugs, 234
Polyestradiol, 321
Polyfax, 424
  eye, 378
Polygeline, 342
Polymyalgia rheumatica, 365
Polymyositis, 365, 369
Polymyxin B, 224
  ear, 390
  eye, 378
  infusion table, 531
  skin, 424
Polymyxins, 223–4
  ear, 388, 390
Polysaccharide-iron complex, 328
Polystyrene sulphonate resins, 336
Polytar,
  Emollient, 413
  Liquid, 422
  Plus, 422
Polythiazide, 65
Polytrim, 378

Index 597

Polyurethane foam dressing, 440
Polyvinyl alcohol, 386
Ponderax, 167
Pondocillin, 209
Pondocillin Plus, 209
Ponstan preparations, 363
Poroplast, 436
Porous flexible adhesive bandage, 436
Porphyrias, acute, 355
  drugs to be avoided in, 356
Portabag, 305
Portabelt, 305
Portagen, 541
Portal hypertension, 77
Portasheath, 303
Posalfilin, 419
Posey, 302, 303
Potaba, 352
Potable water, 338
Potassium aminobenzoate, 352
Potassium bicarbonate, 337, **338**
  tablets, effervescent, 338
Potassium canrenoate see Canrenoate
Potassium chloride, 335, 339
  infusion,
    glucose and, 339
    sodium chloride and, 339
    sodium chloride, glucose and, 339
  infusion table, 531
  solution, strong, 339
  tablets, 335
Potassium citrate, 298
  preparations, 298
  renal failure, 508
Potassium permanganate, 434
  solution, 431, **434**
Potassium supplements, 335
  diuretic with, 69
  renal failure, 508
Potassium tablets, 335
  effervescent, 338
Povidone-iodine,
  breast-feeding, 520
  mouthwash, 398
  oropharynx, 394, **398**
  pregnancy, 515
  renal failure, 508
  skin, 433
    dressing, 439
  vaginal, 290
Powerin, 176
PPF, 341
Pragmatar, 413
Pralidoxime mesylate, 22
Pramoxine [ingredient], 406
Pravastatin, 111
Praxilene, 98
Praziquantel, 248, 249
Prazosin, 86
  cardiovascular, 85
  renal failure, 508
  urinary tract, **86**, 297

Precortisyl preparations, 265
Pred Forte, 380
Predenema, 39
Predfoam, 39
Prednesol, 266
Prednisolone, 263, **265**
  asthma, 123
  Crohn's disease, 39
  haemorrhoids, 47
  lepra reactions, 230
  liver disease, 501
  myasthenia gravis, 372
  pregnancy, 512
  preparations, 265
    injection, 366
    rectal, 39
    rectal (compound), 47
    tablets, 265
  proctitis, 39
  rheumatic disease, 365
  ulcerative colitis, 39
Prednisolone acetate
  eye, 380
  rheumatic disease, 366
Prednisolone sodium phosphate, 266
  ear, 389
  eye, 380
Prednisolone steaglate, 266
Prednisone, 263, **267**
  liver disease, 501
  tablets, 267
Predsol,
  ear, 389
  eye, 380
  rectal, 39
Predsol-N, 389
  ear, 389
  eye, 380
Preface, x
Preferid, 408
Prefil, 166
Pregaday, 328
Pregestimil, 541
Pregnancy,
  anticoagulants, 105
  asthma and, 114
  epilepsy and, 185
  hypertension in, 82
  iron, 326
    folic acid and, 328
  prescribing in, 510–16
  termination, 284
Pregnavite Forte F, 329
Pregnyl, 276
Prejomin, 541
Premarin cream, 288
Premarin tablets, 270
Premedication, 462
  children, 463
Premenstrual syndrome, 271, 350
Premium, 49, 52
Prempak-C, 270
Prentif Cavity Rim Cervical Cap, 296
Prepadine, 160
Prepidil, 285

Prepulsid, 30
Prescal, 95
Prescribing, 1–5
  ACBS, 534
  addicts, 9
  analyses and cost, 1
  breast-feeding, 517–21
  children, 11
  computer-generated, 5
  controlled drugs, 7
  elderly, 14
  generic, 2
  instalments, 7
  liver disease, 499–502
  'named patient', 4
  non-proprietary, 2
  pregnancy, 510–16
  renal impairment, 503–9
  sport, inside front cover, 23
  terminal care, 12
Prescription forms,
  FP14, 556
  FP10HP(ad), 7
  FP10(MDA), 7
  GP14, 556
  HBP(A), 7
  security, 3
Prescription-only medicines see preparations identified by PoM throughout BNF
Pressure sores, 402
Prestim preparations, 81
Priadel, 156
Prices, 1
Prilocaine, 475
  pregnancy, 515
Primacor, 62
Primalan, 129
Primaquine, 241, **244**
  pregnancy, 515
  tablets, 244
Primaxin, 215
  infusion table, 529
  renal failure, 508
Primene, 343
Primidone, 187
  liver disease, 501
  renal failure, 508
  tremor, 197
Primolut Depot, 272
Primolut N, 273
Primoteston Depot, 273
Primperan, 170
Prioderm, 429
Pripsen, 248
Pro-Actidil, 130
Pro-Banthine, 29
Probenecid, 370, **371**
  antibiotics and, 202
  renal failure, 508
Probucol, 111
Procainamide, 71, **73**
  Durules, 73
  infusion table, 531
  liver disease, 501
  renal failure, 508

Procaine, 475
  injection, 475
  pregnancy, 515
Procaine penicillin, 203, **204**
Procarbazine, 319
  renal failure, 508
Prochlorperazine, 168
  nausea and vertigo, 168, **171**
  preparations, 172
  psychoses, 151
Proctitis, 37, 39
Proctofibe, 40
Proctofoam HC, 46
Proctosedyl, 46
Procyclidine, 195, **196**
  preparations, 196
Profasi, 276
Profilate-SD, 108
Proflavine cream, 430
Proflex, 359, 375
Progesic, 175
Progesterone, 271
  preparations, 272
Progestogens, 271–3
  breast-feeding, 520
  liver disease, 501
  malignant disease, 321
  oral contraceptives, 294
    oestrogens and, 290
  pregnancy, 515
Progress, 306
Proguanil, 242, **244**
  pregnancy, 515
  renal failure, 508
Progynova, 269
Prolactinoma, 281
Proleukin, 321
Prolintane, 166
Proluton Depot, 272
Promazine, 147, **151**
  preparations, 152
Promethazine, 129
  allergic disorders, 126, **129**
  anaesthesia, 465
  hypnotic, 141, **142**
  nausea and vertigo, 168, **172**
Promethazine hydrochloride preparations, 129
Promethazine theoclate preparations, 172
Prominal, 187
ProMod, 541
Prondol, 161
Pronestyl, 73
Propaderm, 407
Propaderm-A, xiii
Propafenone, 73, **74**
  liver disease, 501
Propain, 176
Propamidine isethionate, 377, **378**
Propanix, 77
Propantheline, 29
  gastro-intestinal, 28, **29**
  urinary tract, 297, **298**

Prophylaxis, antibacterial, 202
Propine, 383
Propofol, 460, **461**
  infusion table, 531
Propranolol, 77
  cardiovascular, 77
  liver disease, 501
  migraine, 184
  preparations, 77
  see also Beta-adrenoceptor blocking drugs
  thyrotoxicosis, 261
  tremor, 197
Proprietary names, symbol, 2
Propylthiouracil, 261, **262**
  breast-feeding, 521
  pregnancy, 515
  renal failure, 508
  tablets, 262
Prosaid, 363
Proscar, xii
Prosobee, 541
Prostacyclin *see* Epoprostenol
Prostaglandins, 284–6
  anticoagulant, 104
  gastro-intestinal, 34
Prostap SR, 324
Prostate cancer, 312, 321–4
Prostatic hypertrophy, benign, 85, **297**
Prostatitis, 201, 233
Prostigmin, 372
  anaesthesia, 471
Prostin E2, 285
Prostin F2 alpha, 285
Prostin VR, 286
Prosulf, 105
Protamine sulphate, 102, **105**
  injection, 105
Protaphane, Human, 253
Protaphane, Human Penfill, 253
Protein, intravenous nutrition, 342
Protein Forte, 541
Protein intolerance, ACBS, 544
Protein sensitivity, ACBS, 544
Prothiaden, 160
Prothionamide, 227
  leprosy, 229
  pregnancy, 515
Protifar, 541
Protirelin, 278
Protozoal infections, 240–7
Protriptyline, 158, **160**
Pro-Vent, 120
Provera, 272
  malignant disease, 322
Provide, 541
Pro-Viron, 274
Proxymetacaine, 385
Prozac, 164
Prozière, 172
Pruritus, 126
  ACBS, 545
Pruritus ani, 45

Pseudoephedrine,
  breast-feeding, 521
  cough preparations, 136
  nasal decongestants, 137
  renal failure, 508
Pseudomembranous colitis, 38, 223, 230
Pseudomonas aeruginosa infections, 209, 217, 223
  eye, 377
Psittacosis, 215
Psoradrate, 412, **414**
Psoralens, 412
Psoriasis, 412
  Ingram's method, 412
  PUVA, 412
Psoriatic arthropathy, 369
Psoriderm preparations, 413–14
  scalp, 422
PsoriGel, 413
Psorin, 414
Psychoses, 145–55
Puberty, delayed, 273, 276
Pubic lice, 428
Pulmadil preparations, 117
Pulmicort preparations, 124–5
Pulmonary embolism, 106, 132
Pump-Hep, 103
Pur-In Isophane, 253
Pur-In Mix preparations, 254
Pur-In Neutral, 252
Pur-In Pen, 254
Puri-Nethol, 316
Purpura, thrombocytopenic, 333
PUVA, 412
Pyelonephritis, 201, 233
Pyodermas, scalp, 422
Pyopen, 210
Pyralvex, 395
Pyrantel, 247, **248**
Pyrazinamide, 226, 227, **228**
  breast-feeding, 521
  liver disease, 502
Pyrexia, 173
  post-immunisation, 444
Pyridostigmine, 371, **372**
  breast-feeding, 521
  laxative, 41
  pregnancy, 515
Pyridoxine, 350, **351**
  anaemias, 331
Pyrimethamine, 244
  breast-feeding, 521
  dapsone with, 244
  malaria, 244
  pregnancy, 515
  sulfadoxine with, 244
  toxoplasmosis, 246
Pyrithione zinc shampoos, 421
Pyrogastrone, 35

Q-fever, 215
Quaternary ammonium compounds, 28
Quellada, 429
Questran preparations, 109
Quinaband, 437

Index 599

Quinalbarbitone, 145
Quinapril, 89
    pregnancy, 515
    renal failure, 508
    see also ACE inhibitors
Quinidine, 71, **73**
    breast-feeding, 521
    preparations, 73
Quinine, 244
    infusion table, 531
    malaria, 241
    nocturnal cramps, 373
    poisoning, elimination, 17
    pregnancy, 515
    preparations, 245
Quinocort, 406
Quinoderm, 417
    with Hydrocortisone, 417
4-Quinolones, 231–3
    pregnancy, 515
Quinoped, 425

R.B.C., 404
Rabies immunoglobulin, 455–6
Rabies vaccine, 451
Rabro, xiii
Radiation sickness, 168
Ramipril, 89
    pregnancy, 515
    renal failure, 508
    see also ACE inhibitors
Ranitidine, 31, **33**
    breast-feeding, 521
    infusion table, 531
    liver disease, 502
    renal failure, 508
Rapifen, 467
Rapitard MC, 253
Rashes, allergic, 126
Rastinon, 256
Rauwolfia alkaloids, 84
Raymed, 51, 301
Raynaud's syndrome, 86, 95, **97**
Razoxane, 319
Razoxin, 319
Reabilan, 541
'Recently prepared', 3
Recormon, 332
Recormon S, xiii
Red eye, 377, 379
Red line webbing, 436
Redeptin, 154
Redifit, 50, 53
Rediflow, 302
Rediform, 435
Rediseal, 50
Redoxon, 352
Reflolux meter, 259
Refolinon, 317
Refsum's disease, ACBS, 544
Regaine, 423
Regal, 438
Regard, 303, 305
Regard drainage bag, 305
Regulan, 41
    renal failure, 508
Rehibin, 275

Rehidrat, 337
Rehydration,
    oral, 336
    parenteral, 338
Relaxit, 45
Relcofen, 359
Release-II, 439
Relefact LH–RH, 277
Relefact LH–RH/TRH, 277
Reliacath, 309
Reliaseal, 54
Reliasheath, 302
Relifex, 363
Remedeine, 175
Remnos, 139
Remoxipride, 147, **152**
Renal colic *see* Ureteric colic
Renal excretion, interactions affecting, 476
Renal impairment,
    ACBS, 544
    prescribing in, 503–9
Reproterol, 117
Resiston One, 392
Resolve, 176
Resonium A, 336
Resorcinol,
    rectal, 45
    skin, 417
Respiratory depression,
    poisoning, 16
    postoperative, 471
Respiratory distress syndrome, 132
Respiratory failure, 131
Respiratory stimulants, 131
Respiratory syncytial virus infections, 240
Restandol, 273
Resuscitation,
    cardiopulmonary, 99
Retin-A, 415, **418**
Retinoids,
    acne, 415–16
    psoriasis, 413
Retinol, 350
Retrovir, 239
Revanil, 195
Reye's syndrome, aspirin and, 173
Rezolve, 54
Rheomacrodex, 341
Rhesus incompatibility, 456
Rheuflex, 363
Rheumacin SR, 362
Rheumatic diseases, 357–69
    rubefacients, 374
Rheumatic fever, 264
    prophylaxis, 202
Rheumatism, palindromic, 367
Rheumatoid arthritis, 357–69
Rheumox, 360
Rhinitis,
    allergic, 126, 391
    medicamentosa, 391
    vasomotor, 126, 391, 392
Rhinocort preparations, 392
Rhinolast, 391

Rhumalgan, 360
Ribavirin *see* Tribavirin
Ribbed cotton and viscose surgical tubular stockinette, 435
Riboflavine, 350, **351**
Rickets, hypophosphataemic, 347
Rickettsia, 215
Ridaura, 367
Rifadin, 228
Rifampicin, 226, 227, **228**
    breast-feeding, 521
    infusion table, 531
    leprosy, 229
    liver disease, 502
    pregnancy, 515
    preparations, 229
Rifater, 229
Rifinah preparations, 229
Rikospray Silicone, xiii
Rimacid, 362
Rimacillin, 207
Rimactane, 229
Rimactazid preparations, 229
Rimadol, 176
Rimafen, 359
Rimapam, 143
Rimapurinol, 370
Rimifon, 228
Rimiterol, 113, **117**
Rimoxallin, 206
Rimso-50, 299
Rinatec, 393
Ringer-Lactate solution, 338
Ringer's solution, 338
Ringworm infection *see* Dermatophyte infection
Riplex Jacques, 309
Rite-Diet preparations, 541
Ritodrine, 287
    infusion table, 531
Rivotril, 189, 191
Roaccutane, 418
Ro-A-Vit, 350
Robaxin preparations, 374
Robaxisal Forte, 174
Robinul injection, 463
Robinul-Neostigmine, 471
RoC sun preparations, 421
Rocaltrol, 353
Roccal preparations, 432
Roferon-A, 320
Rogitine, 86
Rohypnol, 140
Rommix, 220
Rondo, 122
Ronicol, 97
Rose bengal, 386
Rosoxacin *see* Acrosoxacin
Rotahaler, 122
Roter, 27
Rotersept, 432
Roundworm infections, 248
Rowachol, 59
Rowatinex, 299
Roxiam, 152
Rubavax, 452
Rubefacients, 374

600 Index

Rubella,
  normal immunoglobulin, 455
  vaccination, 443
  vaccine, 452
Rub/Vac (Live), 452
Rusyde, 66
Rutosides, 97
Rynacrom preparations, 392
Rythmodan preparations, 72

Sabidal SR-270, 121
Sabril, 190
Saizen, 277
Salactol, 419
Salatac, 419
Salazopyrin, 38
  rheumatic disease, 369
Salbulin preparations, 116
Salbutamol, 115
  asthma, 113–16
  infusion table, 531
  pregnancy, 515
  premature labour, 287
  preparations, 115–16
    Cyclocaps, 116
Salbuvent preparations, 115–16
Salcatonin, 279
  infusion table, 531
Salger, 52
Salicylates,
  aphthous ulcers, 395
  poisoning by, 17
  rheumatic disease, 357, **358**
  topical, 375
Salicylic acid,
  fungal skin infections, 426
  hyperkeratoses, 412, 418
  preparations, 415
    acne, 418
    coal tar and, 413
    warts and calluses, 418
Saline, physiological, 338, 431
Saline purgatives, 44
Saliva, artificial, 398
Saliva Orthana, 398
Salmeterol, 113, **117**
Salmonellosis, 35, 200, 210
Salofalk, 39
Salonair, 375
Salpingitis, 215
Salsalate, 358
Salt substitutes, 335
  renal failure, 508
Saltair preparations, 54, 57
Saluric, 64
Salzone, 174, 176
Sandimmun, 320
Sandocal preparations, 346
Sandoglobulin, 455
Sando-K, 335
Sandostatin, 325
Sanomigran, 184
Sassco, 50, 53
Saventrine preparations, 100
Savloclens, xiii
Savlodil, xiii

Savlon Dry, 433
Savlon Hospital Concentrate, 432
Scabies, 428
  ACBS, 545
Scalp preparations, ACBS, 545
Scanpor, 437
Schacht, 48, 51
Schar, 541
Schering PC4, 293
Scheriproct, 47
Scherisorb, 440
Schick test, 447
Schistosoma, 249
Schistosomicides, 249
Schizophrenia, 146
Scleritis, 379
Scleroderma, 352
Sclerosants, 112
Scoline, 471
Scopoderm TTS, 170
Scopolamine see Hyoscine
Scottish Prescribing Analysis, 1
Scurvy, 352
Seborrhoeic dermatitis, scalp, 422
Secaderm, 441
Secadrex, 77
Seconal Sodium, 145
Sectral, 77
Secure, 436
Securon preparations, 96
Securopen, 209
Sedation, anaesthesia, 463–9
Sedatives, 138
  see also Anxiolytics
Seldane, 127
Select-A-Jet Dopamine, 100
Select-A-Jet Lignocaine, 74
Selegiline, 193, **195**
Selenium sulphide, 422
Selexid, 211
Selexidin, 210
Selsun, 422
Semi-Daonil, 256
Semipermeable adhesive film, 439
Semitard MC, 252
Semprex, 127
Senna, 41, **42**
  preparations, 42
Senokot, 42
Sential, 406
Sential E, 402
Septic shock, 264
Septicaemia, initial therapy, 201
Septrin preparations, 225
  paediatric dispersible tablets, xiii
Serc, 168
Serenace, 150
Serevent, 118
Serophene, 275
Serotonin-uptake inhibitor antidepressants see Antidepressants, serotonin-uptake inhibitor

Serotulle, 439
Seroxat, 165
Sertraline, 164, **165**
  renal failure, 508
Seton Urisac, 304
Setopress, 436
Sevredol suppositories, 179
Sevredol tablets, 178
Sex hormones, 267–74
  androgens, 273
    antagonists, 274
  malignant disease, 321–2
  oestrogens, 267–71
    antagonists, 275, 322
  progestogens, 271–3
Sexual deviation, 147, 274
SH-420, 322
Shampoos, 421
  ACBS, 545
Shigellosis, 35, 200
Shingles, 238
Shock, 98, 101, 264, 341
  anaphylactic, **130**, 264
  cardiogenic, 98
  septic, 264
Short bowel syndrome, ACBS, 544
SHS Modjul Flavour, 541
Sicca syndrome, ACBS, 544
Silastic, 309, 441
Silgrip, 306
Silicone foam cavity wound dressing, 441
Silver sulphadiazine, 423, **424**
Simeco, 27
Simpla urine bags, 305
Simpla gel, 57
Simplaseel, 50, 53
Simple eye ointment, 386
Simple linctus, 136
  paediatric, 136
Simplene, 383
Simplicity, 49, 52, 302
Simvastatin, 111, **112**
  liver disease, 502
  pregnancy, 515
Sinemet preparations, 194
Sine-Off, 176
Sinequan, 160
Sinthrome, 105
Sintisone, xiii
Sinusitis, 201
Sinutab, 176
Siopel, 403
Skin preparations,
  additives, 399
  anaesthetic, 403
  antibacterial, 423
  antipruritic, 403
  antiviral, 427
  barrier, 402–3
  cleansing, 431–3
  corticosteroids, 405–11
  emollient, 400–2
  stoma, 57–8
  ulcers, 434
Slimline, 48
Slinky, 435

Slo-Indo, 362
Slo-Phyllin, 120
Sloprolol, 77
Slow Sodium, 336
Slow-Fe, 327
Slow-Fe Folic, 328
Slow-K, 335
Slow-Trasicor, 80
8SM, 108
Smallpox vaccine, 452
Smoking, cigarette, 198
Snake bites, 22
Snake-bite antivenom, 22
Sno Phenicol, 377
Sno Pilo, 383
Sno Tears, 386
Soap,
 soft, 432
  enema, 41
 spirit, 432
 substitutes, 432
Soda mint tablets, 27
Sodium acid phosphate, 348
Sodium Amytal, 145
Sodium aurothiomalate, 367
 see also Gold
Sodium bicarbonate, 27, 337, 339, 340
 antacid preparations, 27
 capsules, 337
 ear drops, 391
 intravenous infusion, 340
 renal failure, 508
 urine alkalinisation, 298, **299**
Sodium calciumedetate, 21
 infusion table, 532
Sodium carboxymethyl cellulose *see* Carmellose sodium
Sodium cellulose phosphate, 347
Sodium chloride, 336, 338
 bladder irrigation, 299
 eye, 376, 386
 infusion, 338
  glucose and, 338
  hypercalcaemia, 346
  potassium chloride and, 339
  potassium chloride, glucose and, 339
 mouthwash, compound, 397, **398**
 nose, 392
 oropharynx, 398
 solution,
  eye, 386
  skin cleansing, 431
 tablets, 336
Sodium citrate,
 bladder irrigation, 299
 rectal, 45
 renal failure, 508

Sodium clodronate, 280, **281**
 infusion table, 532
 renal failure, 505
Sodium cromoglycate, 125
 asthma, 125
 eye, 380
 food allergy, 39
 nose, 391, **392**
Sodium fluoride, 348–9
Sodium fusidate, 222, 424
 dressing, 439
 ointment (*Fucidin*), 424
 see also Fusidic acid
Sodium hyaluronate, 386
Sodium ironedetate, 328
Sodium lactate, 340
 intravenous infusion, 340
  compound, 338
Sodium nitrite, 20
Sodium nitroprusside *see* Nitroprusside
Sodium perborate, 397
 mouthwash, 397
Sodium picosulphate, 43
 preparations, 43
Sodium restriction, ACBS, 544
Sodium stibogluconate, 246
Sodium tetradecyl sulphate, 112
Sodium thiosulphate, 20
Sodium valproate *see* Valproate
Sofradex, 390
 ear, 390
 eye, 380
Soframycin, 423
 ear, 390
 eye, 377
Sofra-Tulle, 439
Soft Simplastic, 309
Solarcaine, 404
Solivito-N, 345
 infusion table, 533
Solo, 49, 53
Solpadeine, 176
 renal failure, 509
Solpadol, 174
Solu-Cortef, 267
Solu-Medrone, 267
Solvazinc, 349
Solvents, ear wax removal, 390
Somatotrophin, 277
Somatropin, 277
Sominex, 129
Somnite, 139
Soneryl, 145
Soni-Slo, 92
Sorbichew, 92
Sorbid SA, 92
Sorbitol, 342
Sorbitrate, 92
Sorbsan preparations, 440
Sotacor, 81
Sotalol, 81
 thyrotoxicosis, 261
Sotazide, 81
Soyacal preparations, 344
SP Cold Relief capsules, 176
SPA, 1

Sparine, 152
Spasmonal, 29
Spasticity, 372
Spectinomycin, 223
Spectraban, 421
Spectralgen preparations, 130
Spermicides, 295
Spinhaler insufflator, 125
Spiramycin, toxoplasmosis, 246
Spirit
 industrial methylated, 431
 surgical, 431
Spiroctan, 67
Spiroctan-M, 67
Spirolone, 67
Spironolactone, 66, **67**
 pregnancy, 515
 preparations, 67
  compound, 68
 see also Aldosterone antagonists
Spirospare, 67
Splenectomy, pneumococcal vaccine and, 450
Sporanox, 236
Sport, prescribing and, *inside front cover*, 23
Sprilon, 403
Sputum liquefaction, 133
Spyroflex, 439
Spyrosorb, 439
SR-F, 51
SRM-Rhotard, 178
 terminal care, 12
SR-U, 300
Stabillin V-K, 204
Stafoxil, 205
Stanozolol, 275
Staril, 88
Status epilepticus, 190
Staycept, 295
Stayform, 435
STD, 112
Steam inhalation, 133, 392
Stelazine, 153
Stemetil, 172
Sterac, 431
Sterculia, 41
 constipation, 40, **41**
 diarrhoea, 36
 obesity, 166
Sterexidine, 432
Steri-Neb Cromogen, 125
Steri-Neb Salamol, 116
Steroid cards, 265
Steroids, anabolic, 274
Ster-Zac preparations, 433
Stesolid, **143**, 190
Stiedex, 409
Stiemycin, 416
Stilboestrol, 321, 323
 pregnancy, 515
 vaginal, 288
Still's disease *see* Arthritis, juvenile

Index

Stimulants
  central nervous, 165
  respiratory, 131
Stings, 22
Stockinette, cotton, 435
Stockinette, elasticated viscose, 435
Stockinette, surgical tubular
  cotton, 435
  elastic net, 435
  elasticated, 435
    foam padded, 435
  ribbed cotton and viscose, 435
Stokes-Adams attacks, 98
Stoma, drugs and, 47
Stoma products, 48–58
  adhesives, 54
  belts, 55
  caps and dressings, 58
  closed pouches, 49–50
  closures, 54
  covers, 55
  filters and bridges, 56
  flanges, 56
  irrigation appliances, 57
  plates and shields, 57
  skin, 57
  tubing, 58
Stoma Urine, 301
Stomahesive, 57
Stomaseal, 54
Stomatitis, 395
Stomobar, 57
Stomogel, 54
Stomosol, 57
Streptase, 107
Streptokinase, 106, **107**
  infusion table, 532
  pregnancy, 515
Streptokinase-streptodornase, 434
Streptomycin, 226, 227, **229**
  injection, 229
Stretch bandage, cotton, 436
Stromba, 275
Strongyloidiasis, 249
Stugeron, 169
Stugeron Forte, 97
Sublimaze, 467
Sucralfate, 33, **34**
  renal failure, 509
Sucrose intolerance, ACBS, 542
Sudafed preparations, 136–7
Sudafed-Co, 176
Sudocrem, 401
'Sugar-free', definition, 2
Sugar-free liquid medicines *see* preparations identified by 'sugar-free' throughout BNF
Sulbactam, 206
  ampicillin with, 206, **207**
  renal failure, 509
Sulconazole, 425, **427**
Suleo-C, 429
Suleo-M, 429
Sulfa . . . *see also* Sulpha . . .

Sulfadoxine, malaria, 244
  pyrimethamine with, *see Fansidar*
Sulfametopyrazine, 224, **225**
Sulindac, 359, **364**
  gout, 369
  preparations, 364
  renal failure, 509
Sulpha . . . *see also* Sulfa . . .
Sulphacetamide, 377, **378**
Sulphadiazine, 225
  infusion table, 532
  preparations, 225
  renal failure, 509
  toxoplasmosis, 246
Sulphadiazine, silver, 424
Sulphadimethoxine, trachoma, 378
Sulphadimidine, 225
  tablets, 225
Sulphamethoxazole, trimethoprim with, *see* Co-trimoxazole
Sulphasalazine, 37, **38**
  breast-feeding, 521
  Crohn's disease, 37
  pregnancy, 515
  preparations, 38
  renal failure, 509
  rheumatic disease, 366, **369**
  ulcerative colitis, 37
Sulphinpyrazone, 370, **371**
  renal failure, 509
Sulphonamides, 224–6
  breast-feeding, 521
  pregnancy, 516
  renal failure, 509
  vaginal, 290
Sulphonylureas, 255–6
  breast-feeding, 521
  liver disease, 502
  pregnancy, 516
Sulphur, 417
  preparations, 417–18
Sulphur dioxide, poisoning, 21
Sulpiride, 147, **152**
  breast-feeding, 521
  renal failure, 509
  Tourette syndrome, 197
Sulpitil, 152
Sultamicillin, 208
Sultrin, 290
Sumatriptan, 182, **183**
Sun E45 preparations, 421
Sun protection factor, 420
Sunflower oil, 541
Sunnyvale, 541
Sunscreens, 420
  ACBS, 545
Supasac, 49
Supplementary vitamin tablets for infants, 354
Supplimen, 541
Suprax, 212
Suprecur, 282
Suprefact, 323
Suramin, 249
Surbex T, 354

Surgam preparations, 364
Surgery,
  long-term medication and, 459
  tetanus vaccine, 453
Surgical adhesive tapes, 437
Surgical spirit, 431
Surgical tissue adhesive, 430
Surgicare System-2, 48, 51
  urostomy, 301
Surgipad, 438
Surmontil, 161
Suscard Buccal, 91
Suspensory bandage, cotton, 436
Sustac, 91
Sustamycin, 216
Sustanon preparations, 274
Suxamethonium, 470
  infusion table, 532
  liver disease, 502
Swabs, 438
Sween, 54
Symbols, *inside front cover*
Symmetrel, 194
Sympathomimetics, 98
  asthma, 113
  decongestants, 392
  inotropic, 98
  premature labour, 287
  urinary tract, 298
  vasoconstrictor, 101
Symphony, 50
Synacthen, 276
Synacthen Depot, 276
Synalar preparations, 410
Synarel, 283
Syndol, 176
Synflex, 176
Synkavit tablets, 354
Synogist, xiii
Synphase, 293
Syntaris, 392
Syntex Menophase, 269
Synthamin preparations, 344
Synthamix preparations, 344
Synthetic diets, ACBS, 544
Syntocinon, 286
Syntometrine, 284, **286**
Syntopressin, 279
Syphilis, 201, 203
Syraprim, xiii
Syringe driver, terminal care, 12
Syringes,
  insulin, 255
  oral, 2
Sytron, 328

Tachycardias *see* Arrhythmias
Taenia solium, 248
Taenicides, 248
Tagamet, 32
Talc dusting powder, 403
Talpen, xiii
Tambocor, 73

Tamofen, 324
Tamoxifen, 275, 322, **324**
    pregnancy, 516
    preparations, 324
Tampovagan Stilboestrol and Lactic Acid, 288
Tancolin, 136
Tanderil eye ointment, 381
    chloramphenicol and, xiii
Tapes, surgical adhesive, 437
Tapeworm infections, 248
Tar *see* Coal tar
Tarband, 437
Tarcortin, 414
Tardive dyskinesia, 146
Targocid, 223
Tarivid, 233
Tartrazine, presence of, 2
Tavegil, 128
Tear deficiency, 385
Tears, artificial, 385
Tears, excessive, 386
Tears Naturale, 385
Teejel, 395
Teflox, xiii
Tegaderm, 439
Tegasorb, 440
Tegretol preparations, 186
Teicoplanin, 223
    infusion table, 532
    renal failure, 509
Telangiectasia, hereditary haemorrhagic, 268
Telfa, 438
Temafloxacin, 231
Temazepam, 139, **140**
    anaesthesia, 464, **465**
    preparations, 140
        hard gelatin capsules, xiii
        Planpak, xiii
Temgesic, 179
Temocillin, 205
    infusion table, 532
    renal failure, 509
Temopen, 206
Tendinitis, 365
Tenif, 78
Tennis elbow, 365
Tenoret-50, 78
Tenoretic, 78
Tenormin preparations, 78
Tenoxicam, 359, **364**
Tensilon, 372, 471
Tensium, 143
Tensogrip, 435
Tensopress, 436
Tenuate Dospan, 167
Teoptic, 384
Teratogenesis, 510
Teratoma of testis, 317, 318
Terazosin, 85, **86**
Terbinafine, 235, **237**
    liver disease, 502
    renal failure, 509
    topical, xiii

Terbutaline, 116
    asthma, 113–16
    breast-feeding, 521
    infusion table, 532
    pregnancy, 516
    premature labour, 287
Tercoda, xiii
Terfenadine, 126, **127**
Terlipressin, 279
Terminal care,
    analgesic solution, 178
    prescribing in, 12
Teronac, 167
Terpenes, gall bladder, 58
Terpoin, 136
Terra-Cortril, 406
    ear, 390
    Nystatin, 406
Terramycin, 217
Tertroxin, 260
Testosterone esters, 273
Testosterone implants, 274
Tetanus, 203
    muscle spasm, 373–4
    toxoids, 453
    vaccination, 443
    vaccine, 453
        adsorbed, 453
        diphtheria, pertussis and, 446
        diphtheria and, 446
Tetanus immunoglobulin, 455–6
Tetany, hypocalcaemic, 346
Tetavax, 453
Tetmosol, 429
Tet/Vac/Ads, 453
Tet/Vac/FT, 453
Tetrabenazine, 197
Tetrabid-Organon, 216
Tetrachel, 216
Tetracosactrin, 263, 275, **276**
    infusion table, 532
Tetracycline, 216
    acne, 416
    aphthous ulcers, 394, **395**
    breast-feeding, 521
    diabetic diarrhoea, 258
    infusion table, 532
    liver disease, 502
    malaria, 241
    pregnancy, 516
    preparations, 216
        ear, 390
        eye, 378
        mouth, 395
        skin, 425
        skin, acne, 417
    renal failure, 509
Tetracyclines, 215–17
    see also Tetracycline
Tetralysal-300, 217
Texagrip, 435
Texas Catheter, 303
Textube, 435
T-Gel, 422
Thalamonal, 467
Thalassaemia, 333

Theo-Dur, 120
Theophylline, 119, **120**
    breast-feeding, 521
    infusion table, 532
    liver disease, 502
    poisoning, elimination, 17
    poisoning by, 20
    pregnancy, 516
    preparations, 120–1
Thephorin, 129
Thermometer, fertility, 296
Thiabendazole, 249
    pregnancy, 516
Thiamine, 350
    breast-feeding, 521
    preparations, 350–1
Thiazides, 63
    breast-feeding, 521
    diabetes insipidus, 278
    liver disease, 502
    pregnancy, 516
    renal failure, 509
    see also Diuretics
Thiethylperazine, 168, **172**
Thioguanine, 316
    renal failure, 509
Thiopentone, 459, **460**
    liver disease, 502
    preparations, 460
Thioridazine, 147, **152**
    preparations, 152
Thiotepa, 299, 312, **313**
    injection, 313
Thioxanthenes, 147
Thovaline, xiii
Threadworm infections, 247
Throat infections, 201
Thrombocytopenias, 331
Thrombocytopenic purpura, 333, 455
Thrombo-embolism, 104
    peripheral, 341
    pulmonary, 106, 132
Thrombolytics, 106
Thrombosis,
    antiplatelet drugs, 105
    deep-vein, 102, 104
    prophylaxis, 102
    venous, 106
Thrush *see* Candidiasis
Thymol, 398
    glycerin, compound, 394, 398
Thymoxamine, 97
Thyroid antagonists, 260–2
Thyroid carcinoma, 260
Thyroid function test, 277
Thyroid hormones, 260
Thyroid storm, 261
Thyroidectomy, 260
Thyrotoxic crisis, 261
Thyrotoxicosis, 261
    beta-blockers, 76, 261
Thyrotrophin-releasing hormone, 277
Thyroxine, 260
    breast-feeding, 521

604 Index

Tiaprofenic acid, 358, **364**
   breast-feeding, 521
   preparations, 364
Tibolone, 271
   liver disease, 502
Ticar, 210
Ticarcillin, 209, **210**
   infusion table, 532
   renal failure, 509
Ticarcillin/clavulanic acid,
   infusion table, 532
Tics, 197
Tielle, 440
Tigason, 415
Tilade Mint, 126
Tildiem preparations, 94
Timecef, 212
Timentin, 210
   breast-feeding, 518
   infusion table, 532
   renal failure, 509
Timodine, 407
Timolol, 81
   cardiovascular, 81
   eye, 383, **384**
   migraine, 184
Timoped, xiii
Timoptol, 384
   preservative-free, xiii
Tinaderm-M, 426
Tinea infections, 235, 425
Tinidazole, 230, **231**
   amoebiasis, 245
   giardiasis, 246
   pregnancy, 516
   protozoal infections, 245
Tinset, 129
Tioconazole, 427
Tisept, 432
Titanium dioxide, 420
   bandage, 436
Titralac, 348
Tixylix, 136
Tobralex, 378
Tobramycin, 218, **219**
   eye, 377, **378**
   infusion table, 532
Tocainide, 73, **75**
   infusion table, 532
   liver disease, 502
   pregnancy, 516
   renal failure, 509
Tocopherols, 353
Tofranil, 160
Toilet preparations, ACBS, 545
Tolanase, 256
Tolazamide, 256
   renal failure, 509
Tolbutamide, 255, **256**
   preparations, 256
   renal failure, 509
Tolectin, 364
Tolerzide, 81
Tolmetin, 359, **364**
   breast-feeding, 521
   renal failure, 509
Tolu linctus, compound, paediatric, 136
Tonic seizures, 186

Tonic-clonic seizures, 185
Tonics, 355
Tonocard, 75
   injection, xiii
Tonsillitis *see* Throat infections
Topal, 27
Topicycline, 417
Topilar, 409
Topper-8, 438
Toptabs, 176
Toradol, 466
Torecan preparations, 172
   suppositories, xiii
Torsion dystonias, 197
Torulopsosis, 235
Tosmilen, 382
Total parenteral, nutrition, 342–5
Totamol, 78
Tourette syndrome, 197
Toxoplasma choroidoretinitis, 246
Toxoplasmosis, 246
TPN, 342
Trachoma, 215, 378
Tracrium, 469
Trade marks, symbol, 2
Tramazoline [ingredient], 393
Tramil, 176
Trancopal, 145
Trandate, 79
Tranexamic acid, 107, **108**
Tranquillisers, 138–57
Transacryl, 54
Transfusion reactions, 331
Transiderm-Nitro, 91
Transite Film Dressing, 439
Translet appliance, 49
Translet, skin, 57
Translet solutions, 54
Transplant rejection, 319
Transvasin, 375
Tranxene, 144
Tranylcypromine, 162, **163**
Trasicor, 80
Trasidrex, 80
Trasylol, 108
Travasept-100, 432
Travel, vaccination for, 457
Travel sickness, 168
Travellers' diarrhoea, 35, 457
Travogyn, 289
   cream, xiii
Traxam, 375
Trazodone, 158, **161**
   breast-feeding, 521
Treatment cards,
   anticoagulant, 105
   MAOI, 162
   steroid, 265
Tremonil, 196
Tremors, 197
Trental, 97
Treosulfan, 312, **313**
   infusion table, 532
   preparations, 313
Tretinoin, 415, **418**
TRH, 277

TRH-Roche, 278
Tri-Adcortyl, 411
Tri-Adcortyl Otic, 390
Triadene, 293
Triamaxco, 68
Triamcinolone, 267
Triamcinolone acetonide, 267
   dental paste, 395
   rheumatic disease, 366
   skin, 411
Triamcinolone hexacetonide,
   rheumatic disease, 366
Triamco, 68
Triamterene, 66, **67**
   preparations, 67
     compound, 68
   see also Diuretics, potassium-sparing
Triangular calico bandage, 435
Triazolam, xiii
Triazole antifungal drugs, 235
Tribaviran, 240
   pregnancy, 516
Tribiotic, 424
Trichomonacides, 245
Trichomonal infections, 245
Tri-Cicatrin, 407
Triclofos, 140, **141**
   elixir, 141
Triclosan, 433
Tricotex, 438
Tricyclic antidepressants *see* Antidepressants, tricyclic
Trident, 304
Tridil, 91
Trientine, 355
   capsules, 355
Trifluoperazine, 152
   nausea, 168, **172**
   preparations, 153
   psychoses, 147, **152**
Trifluperidol, 153
Tri-form, 305
Trifyba, 40
Trigeminal neuralgia, 182
Tri-iodothyronine, 260
Trilisate, 358
Trilostane, 283
   pregnancy, 516
Triludan, 127
Trimeprazine, 130
   allergic disorders, 126, **130**
   anaesthesia, 466
Trimetaphan camsylate, 89
   infusion table, 532
   pregnancy, 516
Trimethoprim, 224, **225**, 233
   ear, 390
   infusion table, 532
   pregnancy, 516
   preparations, 226
     co-trimoxazole, 225
   renal failure, 509
   sulphamethoxazole with, *see* Co-trimoxazole
Tri-Minulet, 293
Trimipramine, 158, **161**
Trimogal, 226

Trimopan, 226
Trimovate, 409
  ointment, xiii
Trinordiol, 293
TriNovum and *ED*, 293
Triogesic, 137, 176
Triominic, 137
Triosorbon, 541
Triperidol, 153
Triple penicillin injection, 204
Triple vaccine, **446**, 453
Triplopen, 204
Tripotassium
  dicitratobismuthate, 33
Triprolidine, 130
Triptafen preparations, 163
Trisequens preparations, 270
Trisodium edetate, 347
  eye, **347**, 386
  infusion table, 532
Tritace, 89
Tritamyl, 541
Trivax and *AD*, 446
Trobicin, 223
Tropical diseases, advice, 240
Tropicamide, 381, **382**
Tropium, 143
Trosyl, 427
Trufree, 542
Trypanocides, 246
Trypanosomiasis, 246
Tryptizol, 159
Tryptophan, 164
Tubarine, 470
Tubegauz, 435
Tuberculin PPD, 445
Tuberculosis,
  diagnosis, 445
  prophylaxis, 202
  treatment, 226–9
  vaccination, 443, 444
  travel, 457
Tubifast, 435
Tubigrip, 435
Tubipad, 435
Tubocurarine, 469, **470**
  renal failure, 509
Tub/Vac/BCG, Dried, 445
Tub/Vac/BCG (Perc), 445
Tubular gauze bandage, 435
Tuinal, 145
Tulle dressings, 439
Tulobuterol, 118
  renal failure, 509
Turbohaler,
  Bricanyl, 116
  Pulmicort, 125
Turner syndrome, 276
Two's Company, 295
Tylex, 174
Typhim Vi, 454
Typhoid fever, 200
Typhoid vaccine, 453
  oral, 453
  polysaccharide, 453
  travel, 457
  whole cell, 453
Typhoid/Vac, 453

Tyrosinaemia, ACBS, 544
Tyrothricin [ingredient], 397
Tyrozets, 397

Ubretid, 297
Ucerax, 129
Ukidan, 107
Ulcerative colitis, 37–9
Ulcerative gingivitis, 395
Ulcer-healing drugs, 31–5
Ulcers,
  aphthous, 394
  duodenal, 31
  gastric, 31
  Hunner's, 299
  mouth, 394
  skin, 434
Ultra preparations, 542
Ultrabase, 401
Ultradil Plain, 410
Ultralanum Plain, 410
Ultraproct, 47
Ultrasil, 309
Ultratard, Human, 253
Ultraviolet radiation, 420
Unasyn, 208
Undecenoates, 425, **427**
Unguentum Merck, 401
Unicap M, 329
Unicap T, 329
Unicorn, 305
Uniflu with Gregovite C, 137, 176
Unigest, 27
Unihep, 103
Unilet lancets, 255
Uniparin preparations, 103
Uniphyllin Continus, 121
Uniroid, 47
Unisept, 432
Unisomnia, 139
United, 53
United skin barrier paste, 57
Units, 6
Unitulle, 439
Univer, 96
Urea, skin, 400
Ureteric colic, 298
Urethral catheters, 309
Urethritis, non-gonococcal, 201, 215
Uriben, 233
Uricosuric drugs, 370
Uridom, 303
UriDrain, 303
Uridrop, 303
Urifix, 303, 304
Uriflex preparations, 300
Urihesive, 304
Uriliner, 303
Urinary,
  frequency, 297
  incontinence, 297
  infections, 201, 233
  pH adjustment, 299
  retention, 296
Urine tests, 259
Uriplan bag strap, 306

Uriplan catheter, 309
Uriplan drainage bag, 305
Uriplan leg bag, 304
Uriplan McGuire, 306
Uriplan sheath, 302
Urisac, 305
Urisac tapes, 306
Uriseal, 303
Urispas, 297
Uristrip, 303, 304
URO-2002, 301
Uro sheath, 302
Uro-Flo drainage bag, 305
Uro-Flo leg bag, 304
Uro-Flo Mk 2, 303
Uro-Flo sheath, 303
Uro-Flo strap, 306
Urofollitrophin, 276
Urokinase, 106, **107**
  infusion table, 532
  pregnancy, 516
Uromitexan, 313
Urosheath adaptor, 305
Uro-Tainer preparations, 300
Ursodeoxycholic acid, 58, **59**
Ursofalk, 59
Urticaria, 126
Uterine bleeding, 284
Uterine relaxants, 287
Uterine stimulants, 284–6
Utinor, 233
Utovlan, 273
Uveitis, 379
Uvistat preparations, 421

Vaccination,
  programmes, 443
  travel, 457
Vaccines, 442–54
  allergen extract, 130
  contra-indications, 442
  post-immunisation
    pyrexia, 444
  pregnancy, 442, 516
  side-effects, 442
  storage and use, 444
Vagifem, 288
Vaginitis,
  candidal, 288
  menopausal, 268, 288
  non-specific *see* Vaginosis, bacterial
Vaginosis, bacterial, 230
Vaginyl, 231
Valenac, 360
Valium, **143**, 190, 465
Vallergan, 130
Valoid, 169
Valproate, 185, **188**
  breast-feeding, 521
  infusion table, 532
  liver disease, 502
  pregnancy, 516
  preparations, 189
Valrox, 363
Vamin preparations, 344
Vaminolact, 344
Vancocin, 223

Index

Vancomycin, 223
　infusion table, 533
　renal failure, 509
Vansil, 248
Vapour-permeable adhesive film, 439
Varicella, 238
Varicella-zoster immunoglobulin, 455–6
Variclene, 434
Varicose veins, 112, 441
Varidase Topical, 434
Var/Vac, 452
Vasaten, 78
Vascace, 88
Vascardin, 92
Vaseline Dermacare, 401
Vasetic, 68
Vasocon A, 380
Vasoconstrictors, 101
　local anaesthesia, 473
Vasodilators, 90–8
　antihypertensive, 83
　cerebral, 97
　peripheral, 97
Vasogen, 403
Vasopressin, 278
　infusion table, 533
Vasoxine, 101
Vasyrol, 106
V-Cil-K, xiii
VEC high compression bandage, 436
Vecuronium, 469, **470**
　infusion table, 533
Veganin, 176
Veil preparations, 421
Velbe, 317
Velosef, 214
Velosulin, 252
Velosulin, Human, 252
Velosulin Cartridge, xiii
Venoglobulin, 455
Venticaire mask, 133
Ventide, 124
Ventilatory failure, 131
Ventimask, 133
Ventodisks, 116
Ventolin preparations, 115–16
Vepesid, 317
Veracur, 419
Verapamil, 96
　angina, 93
　arrhythmias, 70
　beta-blockers and, 70
　breast-feeding, 521
　hypertension, 93
　liver disease, 502
　preparations, 96
　see also Calcium-channel blockers
Veripaque, 42
Vermox, 247
Verrucas, 418
Verrugon, 419
Vertigo, 168
Vertigon, 172
Verucasep, 419
Vesagex, 430
Vestibular disorders, 167–8
Vibramycin preparations, 217
Vibrocil, 393
Vick cold preparations, 176
Vicks Ultra Chloraseptic, 397
Videne dusting powder, 433
Vidopen, 207
Vigabatrin, 185, 189, **190**
　pregnancy, 516
　renal failure, 509
Vigam, 455
Vigilon, 440
Vigranon B, 351
Villescon, 166
Viloxazine, 158, **162**
Vimule Cap, 296
Vinblastine, 317
　infusion table, 533
Vinca alkaloids, 317
Vincent's infection, 395
Vincristine, 317
　infusion table, 533
Vindesine, 317
　infusion table, 533
Vioform-Hydrocortisone, 407
Viral infections, 237–40
Virazid, 240
Virormone, 274
Virudox, 428
Virudox, 428
Visclair, 134
Viscopaste PB7, 436
Viscose, elastane, and cotton compression bandage, 436
Viskaldix, 81
Visken, 81
Vista-Methasone,
　ear, 389
　eye, 379
　nose, 391
Vista-Methasone N, 389
　ear, 389
　eye, 379
　nose, 393
Vita-E, 353, 402
Vitalograph Pulmo-Aide, 122
Vitamin A, 350
　breast-feeding, 521
　pregnancy, 516
　preparations, 350
　　vitamin D and, 350
Vitamin B group, 350
　preparations, 350–1
　　B and C injection, 351, 533
Vitamin B_{12}, 330
Vitamin C, 352
　see also Ascorbic acid
Vitamin D, 352
　breast-feeding, 521
　preparations, 352–3
Vitamin deficiency, 349
Vitamin E, 353
　preparations, 353
Vitamin K, 353
　preparations, 354
Vitamin tablets for infants, supplementary, 354
Vitamins, 349–54
　multivitamin preparations, 354
　　infusion table, 533
　parenteral, 344–5
Vitamins capsules, 354
Vitlipid-N, 345
Vitrimix KV, 344
Vivalan, 162
Vivotif, 454
Volital, 165
Volmax, 115
Volraman, 360
Voltarol preparations, 360–1
　Emulgel, 375
Volumatic, 122
Volume expansion, 340–2
Vomiting, 167–8
　cytotoxic drugs, 311
　in infancy, ACBS, 544
　pregnancy, 168
Vulvitis, candidal, 288

Warfarin, 104, **105**
　tablets, 105
Warticon, 420
Warts, 418
Wasp sting allergy, preparations, 130
Water, 338
　for injections, 340
　potable, 338
Waxsol, 391
Webbing, blue line, 436
Webbing, red line, 436
Welldorm, 141
Wellferon, 320
Wernicke's encephalopathy, 350
Whitfield's ointment, 425
Whooping cough see Pertussis
Wilson's disease, 355
Withdrawal,
　alcohol, 141
　anxiolytics, 138
　hypnotics, 138
Withdrawn drugs, prescribing of, 4
Wolff-Parkinson-White syndrome, 70–1
Worm infestation, 247–9
Wound dressings, 438
　pads, 438
Wound management products, 435–41
Wright pocket peak flow meter, 122
Wuchereria bancrofti, 249
Wysoy, 542

Xamoterol, 98, **100**
　pregnancy, 516
　renal failure, 509
Xanax, 143
Xanthine bronchodilators see Theophylline

Index 607

Xanthine-oxidase inhibitor, 370
Xanthomax, 370
Xerostomia, ACBS, 544
Xipamide, 63, **65**
Xtend, 304
Xuret, 65
Xylocaine, 474
Xylocard, 74
Xylometazoline,
  eye, 380
  nasal preparations, 393
Xyloproct, 47
Xylotox, 474

8Y, 108
Yaws, 203
Yeasts, 234–7
Yellow cards, *inside back cover*, 10
Yellow fever vaccine, 454
  travel, 457
Yel/Vac, 454
Yomesan, 248
Yutopar, 287

Z Span, 349
Zaditen, 126
Zadstat, 231
Zagreb antivenom, 22
Zantac, 33
Zarontin, 187
Zavedos, 315
ZeaSORB, 403
Zenalb, 340

Zentel, 249
Zestoretic, 88
Zestril, 88
Zidovudine, 239
  infusion table, 533
  liver disease, 502
  renal failure, 509
ZIG, 455
Zimovane, 142
Zinacef, 213
Zinamide, 228
Zinc cream, 400
  ichthammol and, 414
Zinc deficiency, 349
Zinc dusting-powder, starch, talc and, 403
Zinc eye preparations, 386
Zinc ointment, 400
  castor oil and, 400
Zinc oral preparations, 349
Zinc oxide plaster, 437
Zinc oxide suppositories, hamamelis and, 46
Zinc paste,
  coal tar and, 413
  salicylic acid and, 415
Zinc paste bandage, 436
  calamine, clioquinol and, 436
  calamine and, 436
  coal tar and, 437
  ichthammol and, 437
Zinc sulphate preparations,
  capsules, 349
  eye-drops, 386

Zinc sulphate preparations (*continued*)—
  lotion, xiii
  mouthwash, xiii
  tablets, 349
Zinc tape, adhesive, 437
Zincaband, 436
Zincomed, 349
Zineryt, 417
Zirtek, 127
Zinnat, 213
Zithromax, 221
Zocor, 112
Zofran, 171
Zoladex, 324
Zollinger-Ellison syndrome, 31
Zonulysin, 386
Zopiclone, 141, **142**
  breast-feeding, 521
  liver disease, 502
Zopla, 54
Zoster *see* Herpes infections
Zovirax preparations, 238
  cream, 427
  eye ointment, 379
Zuclopenthixol, 147, **153**, 154, **155**
  depot injections, 155
  tablets, 153
Zuclopenthixol acetate, 153
Zuclopenthixol decanoate, 155
Zuclopenthixol dihydrochloride, 153
Zumenon, xiii
Zyloric, 370
Zymafluor, 349

IN CONFIDENCE — COMMITTEE ON SAFETY OF MEDICINES (For advice on reporting reactions see *Adverse Reactions to Drugs* section of BNF)

REPORT ON SUSPECTED ADVERSE DRUG REACTIONS

PATIENT'S DETAILS SURNAME _____ OTHER NAMES _____

DATE OF BIRTH (OR AGE) _____ SEX: M ☐ F ☐ WEIGHT (kg) [___]

Hospital if relevant _____ Hospital Number _____ Consultant in charge/GP Principal _____

SUSPECTED DRUG (Give brand name of drug and batch number if known) _____ ROUTE _____ DAILY DOSE _____

DATE STARTED _____ DATE STOPPED _____ THERAPEUTIC INDICATION _____

SUSPECTED REACTIONS

_____

_____

_____

DATE REACTION STARTED _____ DATE REACTION ENDED _____

OUTCOME (e.g. fatal, recovered, continuing) _____

SEND TO CSM, FREEPOST, London SW8 5BR
OR if you are in one of the following NHS regions:
TO CSM Mersey, FREEPOST, Liverpool L3 3AB
OR CSM West Midlands, FREEPOST, Birmingham B15 1BR
OR CSM Northern, FREEPOST 1085, Newcastle upon Tyne NE1 1BR
OR CSM Wales, FREEPOST, Cardiff CF4 1ZZ

REPORTING DOCTOR

Name _____

Address _____

_____

_____

Telephone _____ Specialty _____

Signature _____ Date _____

If you would like information about other reports associated with the suspected drug, tick here ☐

PTO

OTHER DRUGS TAKEN IN THE LAST 3 MONTHS INCLUDING SELF-MEDICATION **Give brand name if known** Write **none** if no other drug has been taken	ROUTE	DAILY DOSE	DATE DRUG STARTED	DATE DRUG STOPPED	THERAPEUTIC INDICATION

Additional information including medical history, investigations, known allergies, suspected drug interactions relevant to the reaction and LMP for drugs taken during pregnancy.

_____

_____

_____

IN CONFIDENCE — COMMITTEE ON SAFETY OF MEDICINES (For advice on reporting reactions see *Adverse Reactions to Drugs* section of BNF)

REPORT ON SUSPECTED ADVERSE DRUG REACTIONS

PATIENT'S DETAILS SURNAME _____ OTHER NAMES _____

DATE OF BIRTH (OR AGE) _____ SEX: M ☐ F ☐ WEIGHT (kg) _____

Hospital if relevant _____ Hospital Number _____ Consultant in charge/GP Principal _____

SUSPECTED DRUG (Give brand name of drug and batch number if known) _____

DATE STARTED _____ DATE STOPPED _____ ROUTE _____ DAILY DOSE _____

THERAPEUTIC INDICATION _____

SUSPECTED REACTIONS

_____
_____
_____

DATE REACTION STARTED _____ DATE REACTION ENDED _____

OUTCOME (e.g. fatal, recovered, continuing) _____

SEND TO CSM, FREEPOST, London SW8 5BR
OR if you are in one of the following NHS regions:
TO CSM Mersey, FREEPOST, Liverpool L3 3AB
OR CSM West Midlands, FREEPOST, Birmingham B15 1BR
OR CSM Northern, FREEPOST 1085, Newcastle upon Tyne NE1 1BR
OR CSM Wales, FREEPOST, Cardiff CF4 1ZZ

REPORTING DOCTOR

Name _____
Address _____
_____
_____

Telephone _____ Specialty _____
Signature _____ Date _____

If you would like information about other reports associated with the suspected drug, tick here ☐

PTO

OTHER DRUGS TAKEN IN THE LAST 3 MONTHS INCLUDING SELF-MEDICATION **Give brand name if known** Write **none** if no other drug has been taken	ROUTE	DAILY DOSE	DATE DRUG STARTED	DATE DRUG STOPPED	THERAPEUTIC INDICATION

Additional information including medical history, investigations, known allergies, suspected drug interactions relevant to the reaction and LMP for drugs taken during pregnancy.

IN CONFIDENCE — COMMITTEE ON SAFETY OF MEDICINES

REPORT ON SUSPECTED ADVERSE DRUG REACTIONS

(For advice on reporting reactions see *Adverse Reactions to Drugs* section of BNF)

PATIENT'S DETAILS SURNAME _____ OTHER NAMES _____
DATE OF BIRTH (OR AGE) _____ SEX: M ☐ F ☐ WEIGHT (kg) ☐
Hospital if relevant _____ Hospital Number _____ Consultant in charge/GP Principal _____

SUSPECTED DRUG (Give brand name of drug and batch number if known) _____ ROUTE _____ DAILY DOSE _____
DATE STARTED _____ DATE STOPPED _____ THERAPEUTIC INDICATION _____

SUSPECTED REACTIONS

_____
_____
_____

DATE REACTION STARTED _____ DATE REACTION ENDED _____

OUTCOME (e.g. fatal, recovered, continuing) _____

SEND TO CSM, FREEPOST, London SW8 5BR
OR if you are in one of the following NHS regions:
TO CSM Mersey, FREEPOST, Liverpool L3 3AB
OR CSM West Midlands, FREEPOST, Birmingham B15 1BR
OR CSM Northern, FREEPOST 1085, Newcastle upon Tyne NE1 1BR
OR CSM Wales, FREEPOST, Cardiff CF4 1ZZ

REPORTING DOCTOR

Name _____
Address _____
_____
_____

Telephone _____ Specialty _____
Signature _____ Date _____

If you would like information about other reports associated with the suspected drug, tick here ☐

PTO

OTHER DRUGS TAKEN IN THE LAST 3 MONTHS INCLUDING SELF-MEDICATION **Give brand name if known** Write **none** if no other drug has been taken	ROUTE	DAILY DOSE	DATE DRUG STARTED	DATE DRUG STOPPED	THERAPEUTIC INDICATION

Additional information including medical history, investigations, known allergies, suspected drug interactions relevant to the reaction and LMP for drugs taken during pregnancy.

_____

_____

_____

IN CONFIDENCE — COMMITTEE ON SAFETY OF MEDICINES (For advice on reporting reactions see
REPORT ON SUSPECTED ADVERSE DRUG REACTIONS *Adverse Reactions to Drugs* section of BNF)

PATIENT'S DETAILS SURNAME _____ OTHER NAMES _____
DATE OF BIRTH (OR AGE) _____ SEX: M ☐ F ☐ WEIGHT (kg) [ ]
Hospital if relevant _____ Hospital Number _____ Consultant in charge/GP Principal _____

SUSPECTED DRUG (Give brand name of drug and batch number if known) _____ ROUTE _____ DAILY DOSE _____
DATE STARTED _____ DATE STOPPED _____ THERAPEUTIC INDICATION _____

SUSPECTED REACTIONS
_____
_____
_____

DATE REACTION STARTED _____ DATE REACTION ENDED _____

OUTCOME (e.g. fatal, recovered, continuing) _____

SEND TO CSM, FREEPOST, London SW8 5BR
OR if you are in one of the following NHS regions:
TO CSM Mersey, FREEPOST, Liverpool L3 3AB
OR CSM West Midlands, FREEPOST, Birmingham B15 1BR
OR CSM Northern, FREEPOST 1085, Newcastle upon Tyne NE1 1BR
OR CSM Wales, FREEPOST, Cardiff CF4 1ZZ

REPORTING DOCTOR
Name _____
Address _____
_____
_____

Telephone _____ Specialty _____
Signature _____ Date _____

If you would like information about other reports associated with the suspected drug, tick here ☐

PTO

OTHER DRUGS TAKEN IN THE LAST 3 MONTHS INCLUDING SELF-MEDICATION **Give brand name if known** Write **none** if no other drug has been taken	ROUTE	DAILY DOSE	DATE DRUG STARTED	DATE DRUG STOPPED	THERAPEUTIC INDICATION

Additional information including medical history, investigations, known allergies, suspected drug interactions relevant to the reaction and LMP for drugs taken during pregnancy.

_____

_____

_____